# MEDICAL

EIGHTEENTH
EDITION

# MICROBIOLOGY

## A GUIDE TO MICROBIAL INFECTIONS:
### PATHOGENESIS, IMMUNITY, LABORATORY DIAGNOSIS AND CONTROL

EDITED BY

**David Greenwood** BSc PhD DSc FRCPath

Emeritus Professor of Antimicrobial Science, University of Nottingham Medical School,
Nottingham, UK

**Mike Barer** BSc MBBS MSc PhD FRCPath

Professor of Clinical Microbiology, Department of Infection, Immunity and Inflammation,
University of Leicester Medical School, Leicester, UK

**Richard Slack** MA MB BChir FRCPath FRSPH DRCOG

Formerly Senior Lecturer, Division of Microbiology, University of Nottingham Medical School,
Nottingham, UK; Honorary Consultant in Communicable Disease Control and Regional
Microbiologist, Health Protection Agency, East Midlands, UK

**Will Irving** MA, MB BChir, MRCP, PhD, FRCPath

Professor and Honorary Consultant in Virology, University of Nottingham and Nottingham
University Hospitals NHS Trust, Department of Microbiology, Queen's Medical Centre,
Nottingham, UK

CHURCHILL
LIVINGSTONE

ELSEVIER

EDINBURGH   LONDON   NEW YORK   OXFORD   PHILADELPHIA   ST LOUIS   SYDNEY   TORONTO   2012

## CHURCHILL
## LIVINGSTONE
### ELSEVIER

© 2012 Elsevier Ltd. All rights reserved, except Chapter 21
© Crown Copyright 2012/DSTL.

| | |
|---|---|
| First edition 1925 | Eleventh edition 1965 |
| Second edition 1928 | Twelfth edition (Vol. 1) 1973 |
| Third edition 1931 | Twelfth edition (Vol. 2) 1975 |
| Fourth edition 1934 | Thirteenth edition (Vol. 1) 1978 |
| Fifth edition 1938 | Thirteenth edition (Vol. 2) 1980 |
| Sixth edition 1942 | Fourteenth edition 1992 |
| Seventh edition 1945 | Fifteenth edition 1997 |
| Eighth edition 1948 | Sixteenth edition 2002 |
| Ninth edition 1953 | Seventeenth edition 2007 |
| Tenth edition 1960 | Eighteenth edition 2012 |

ISBN: 9780702040894
International ISBN: 9780702040900

**British Library Cataloguing in Publication Data**
A catalogue record for this book is available from the British Library

**Library of Congress Cataloging in Publication Data**
A catalog record for this book is available from the Library of Congress

**ELSEVIER** your source for books, journals and multimedia in the health sciences
www.elsevierhealth.com

Working together to grow
libraries in developing countries
www.elsevier.com | www.bookaid.org | www.sabre.org
ELSEVIER    BOOK AID International    Sabre Foundation

The publisher's policy is to use paper manufactured from sustainable forests

Printed in China

# MEDICAL
EIGHTEENTH
EDITION
# MICROBIOLOGY

*Commissioning Editor:* Jeremy Bowes/Timothy Horne
*Development Editor:* Carole McMurray
*Project Manager:* Andrew Riley
*Designer:* Stewart Larking
*Illustration Manager:* Jennifer Rose
*Illustrator:* Antbits

This classic introductory text has served medical students, trainees in the clinical practice of infection and non-clinical scientists throughout the world for nearly 90 years. The overall aims of the book have been set out in earlier editions and we reproduce the preface to the previous edition so that the reader may understand its origins and general philosophy. The global scope is particularly important; infection is international and capable of rapid dissemination. For this reason we have once again been at pains to ensure that all aspects of microbial disease are fully covered, not just those organisms and conditions that that tend to take centre stage in countries with advanced health care provision. We are aware of and value the cosmopolitan nature of our readership and hope that this revision will continue to serve those who wish to learn about microbes and infection wherever they may be.

While much medical teaching takes an integrative approach deploying a multi-disciplinary analysis of every presenting complaint, this text remains rooted in the discipline of microbiology and is steeped in the view that an understanding of the biology of micro-organisms that associate with human beings provides an essential building block for both practice and research. A well trained practitioner in infection should first understand the organisms, then the pathological processes with which they are associated and finally the means by which the resulting diseases may be diagnosed, treated and ultimately prevented. Most other texts start either with the clinical syndromes and work back to the organisms; or with the therapeutic agents used in infection, identifying the organisms against which they are effective and the clinical situations for which they are appropriate. Specialists in infection need to be adept in all three approaches but we take the view that the first, organism-centred approach is the best place for medical students and trainees to start.

In an era when we may know the genome sequence of a newly isolated organism within days of its isolation and when intricate molecular details of the mechanisms underlying the pathogenesis of many infections are understood, the knowledge that may be considered essential to our understanding of infection is constantly shifting. The present revision takes into account those developments that impact on the clinical practice of infection and those that we hope will inspire the reader to achieve new insights.

Finally, we must once again earnestly thank our international team of contributors – some veterans of several previous editions, others new to the task and bringing welcome new insights – who, for little reward, find time in their very busy lives to share their expertise with our readership. We are also grateful to the expert team at Elsevier, who have seen the book through to publication with courtesy and skill.

D.G.
M.R.B
R.C.B.S.
W.I
Nottingham, Leicester
March, 2012

**From the Preface to the 17th edition:** It is now more than 80 years since the first appearance of this textbook's illustrious forerunner – Mackie and McCartney's *Introduction to Practical Bacteriology as Applied to Medicine and Public Health*. When that classic text first appeared in 1925, the requirements of medical students, then thought to include a need to be fully conversant with laboratory methods, could be encompassed in a small-format handbook of less than 300 pages. At that time, virology scarcely existed, immunology was in its infancy, parasitology was regarded as a subject of study necessary only for prospective colonial doctors, effective treatment of microbial disease was almost non-existent and molecular biology was unknown. Medical students are, thankfully, no longer expected to be familiar with what goes on in microbiology laboratories, except insofar as they need to be able to use laboratory services and interpret the results emanating from them in an intelligent fashion, but this has been replaced by an unmanageable corpus of clinical knowledge that encompasses not only the burgeoning subjects of bacteriology, virology, mycology and parasitology, but also the related disciplines of immunology, antimicrobial chemotherapy and epidemiology. Such has been the explosion in knowledge that one can only sympathize with today's student doctors in their struggle to master the basic facets of medical microbiology that will impinge daily on their professional lives.

Of course, all the information one could ever need is now available at the click of a mouse via the internet – that vast, unregulated agglomeration of the good the bad and the ugly – yet textbooks remain stubbornly popular with students, at least for core subjects. This should not be surprising, as a good textbook offers a uniquely user-friendly source of knowledge, assembled by experts familiar with the needs of students and presented in an accessible format, clearly written and logically arranged. Such, at any rate, have been the defining features of previous manifestations of this textbook, a tradition that we believe this new edition fully upholds.

As before, the 17th edition of *Medical Microbiology* strives to bridge the gap between texts that deal with microbiology in a traditional organism-based way and the more modern approaches that take microbial diseases as the starting point or attempt to view the subject from an immunological or epidemiological perspective. Thus, a thorough overview of microbial biology is followed by a consideration of the principles of the body's immunological response to various types of micro-organism, before moving on to consider bacteria, viruses, fungi and parasites individually. The content of these 'systematic' chapters is heavily biased towards understanding the associated diseases, their pathogenesis, clinical features, epidemiology and control. A final section integrates what has gone before in terms of the day-to-day practicalities of the diagnosis of infection, its treatment and avoidance.

In our experience, students of medicine and allied health-care sciences are among the most motivated of all students: it is rare to find one who does not harbour a genuine desire to become a safe and knowledgeable doctor or health-care professional. For our part we sincerely hope that we have provided a text that will help them to fulfil these ambitions in the context of the intrinsically fascinating subject of medical microbiology. For the first time, we have included 'key point' boxes in each chapter to highlight issues that are of particular relevance to the topic. These are intended to provide students with signposts to a wider understanding of key issues and are certainly not meant to represent 'all the student needs to remember' on a particular theme. To use them in such a way would impoverish the student's understanding of the subject and negate the whole purpose of the text. Make no mistake: a thorough knowledge of infection in all its guises is as necessary to the practice of medicine today as it ever was.

In addition to the specific suggestions provided at the end of individual chapters, the following internet sites, most of which offer diverse links to sources of further information, are recommended as the starting point for searches of information on microbial topics.

American Society for Microbiology:
www.asm.org

Centers for Disease Control and Prevention:
www.cdc.gov

CDC National Center for Infectious Diseases:
www.cdc.gov/ncidod/index.htm

Health Protection Agency (formerly Public Health Laboratory Service):
www.hpa.org.uk

Medscape:
www.medscape.com/InfectiousDiseases

Oregon Health Sciences University:
www.ohsuhealth.com

PubMed (National Library of Medicine):
www.ncbi.nlm.nih.gov/PubMed/

Society for General Microbiology:
www.sgm.ac.uk

University of Leicester: http://www.le.ac.uk/bs/medbiobrochure/welcome.htm

World Health Organization:
www.who.int/en/

**D. A. A. Ala'Aldeen**
Molecular Bacteriology and Immunology Group
Division of Microbiology and Infectious Diseases
University Hospital
Queen's Medical Centre
Nottingham NG7 2UH
UK

**R. P. Allaker**
Institute of Dentistry
Queen Mary, University of London
4 Newark Street
London E1 2AT
UK

**H. S. Atkins**
Department of Biomedical Sciences
Defence Science and Technology Laboratory
Porton Down
Salisbury SP4 0JQ
UK

**A. C. Banyard**
Wildlife Zoonoses and Vector-borne Diseases
Research Group
Animal Health and Veterinary Laboratories Agency
(AHVLA, Weybridge)
New Haw
Addlestone
Surrey KT15 3NB
UK

**M. R. Barer**
Department of Infection, Immunity and
Inflammation
University of Leicester
Medical Sciences Building
University Road
Leicester LE1 9HN
UK

**A. D. T. Barrett**
Department of Pathology
University of Texas Medical Branch
301 University Boulevard
Galveston
Texas 77555-0609
USA

**S. M. Burns**
Department of Laboratory Medicine
Royal Infirmary of Edinburgh
51 Little France Crescent
Edinburgh EH16 4SA
UK

**H. Chart**
Laboratory of Gastrointestinal Pathogens
Health Protection Agency
61 Colindale Avenue
London NW9 5EQ
UK

**A. Cockayne**
Centre for Biomolecular Sciences
University of Nottingham
University Park
Nottingham NG7 2RD
UK

**M. J. Corbel**
24 The Approach
Two Mile Ash
Milton Keynes MK8 8PA
UK

**H. A. Cubie**
Scottish HPV Reference Laboratory
Royal Infirmary of Edinburgh
51 Little France Crescent
Edinburgh
EH16 4SA
UK

**W. D. Cubitt**
Mallard House
26 Riverside Gardens
Peterborough, PE36GE
UK

**N. A. Cunliffe**
Department of Clinical Infection, Microbiology &
Immunology
Institute of Infection & Global Health
University of Liverpool
Apex Building,
8 West Derby Street,
Liverpool L69 7BE
UK

**K. S. Cuschieri**
Scottish HPV Reference Laboratory
Royal Infirmary of Edinburgh
51 Little France Crescent
Edinburgh
EH16 4SA
UK

**G. F. S. Edwards**
Scottish Legionella Haemophilus Meningococcus
and Pneumococcus Reference Laboratory
Stobhill Hospital
NHS Greater Glasgow and Clyde
133 Balornock Road
Glasgow G21 3UW
UK

**D. Falzarano**
National Institute of Allergy and Infectious Diseases
2A122 903 S 4th Street
Hamilton, MT, USA

**H. Feldmann**
National Institute of Allergy and Infectious Diseases
2A122 903 S 4th Street
Hamilton, MT, USA

**A. R. Fooks**
Wildlife Zoonoses and Vector-borne Diseases
Research Group
Animal Health and Veterinary Laboratories Agency
(AHVLA, Weybridge)
New Haw
Addlestone
Surrey KT15 3NB
UK

**D. Goldberg**
NHS National Services Scotland
Health Protection Scotland
Meridian Court
5 Cadogan Street
Glasgow G2 6QE
UK

**J. R. W. Govan**
Cystic Fibrosis Group
Centre for Infectious Diseases
University of Edinburgh Medical School
The Chancellor's Building
49 Little France Crescent
Edinburgh EH16 4SB
UK

**J. M. Grange**
Advanced Therapies Centre B2
London Clinic Cancer Centre
22 Devonshire Place
London W1G 6JA
UK

**D. Greenwood**
11 Perry Road
Sherwood
Nottingham NG5 3AD
UK

**D. M. Healy**
Wildlife Zoonoses and Vector-borne Diseases
Research Group
Animal Health and Veterinary Laboratories Agency
(AHVLA, Weybridge)
New Haw
Addlestone
Surrey KT15 3NB
UK

**L. Hesketh**
Lancashire Teaching Hospitals
NHS Foundation Trust
Preston
Lancashire PR1 8UY
UK

**J. Hood**
Department of Clinical Microbiology
Glasgow Royal Infirmary
Glasgow G4 0SF
UK

**H. Humphreys**
Department of Clinical Microbiology
Royal College of Surgeons in Ireland
Education and Research Centre
Beaumont Hospital
Smurfit Building
Dublin 9
Ireland

**J. W. Ironside**
National CJD Research & Surveillance Unit
University of Edinburgh
Western General Hospital
Edinburgh
EH4 2XU
UK

**W. L. Irving**
Department of Microbiology
Queen's Medical Centre
Nottingham NG7 2UH
UK

**I. Johannessen**
Department of Laboratory Medicine
Royal Infirmary of Edinburgh
51 Little France Crescent
Edinburgh EH16 4SA
UK

**J. M. Ketley**
Department of Genetics
University of Leicester
Adrian Building
University Road
Leicester LE1 7RH
UK

**M. Kilian**
Institute of Medical Microbiology & Immunology
University of Aarhus
The Bartholin Building
DK-8000 Aarhus C
Denmark

**D. Mabey**
London School of Hygiene and Tropical Medicine
Keppel Street
London WC1E 7HT
UK

**C. R. Madeley**
Burnfoot
Stocksfield
Northumberland NE43 7TN
UK

**J. McLauchlin**
Food Water and Environmental Microbiology
Centre for Infections
Health Protection Agency
61 Colindale Avenue
London NW9 5EQ
UK

**P. J. Molyneaux**
Department of Medical Microbiology
Aberdeen Royal Infirmary
Foresterhill
Aberdeen AB25 2ZN
UK

**O. Nakagomi**
Department of Molecular Microbiology and
Immunology
Nagasaki University
Nagasaki 852-8523
Japan

**M. Norval**
Biomedical Sciences
University of Edinburgh Medical School
Teviot Place
Edinburgh EH8 9AG
UK

**M. M. Ogilvie**
62/3 Blacket Place
Edinburgh EH9 1RJ
UK

**N. Oldfield**
Molecular Bacteriology & Immunology Group
Centre for Biomolecular Sciences
University of Nottingham
Nottingham NG7 2RD
UK

**R. W. Peeling**
London School of Hygiene and Tropical Medicine
Keppel Street
London WC1E 7HT
UK

**J. S. M. Peiris**
School of Public Health
Li Ka Shing Faculty of Medicine
The University of Hong Kong
Sassoon Rd
Pokfulam
Hong Kong
China

**T. H. Pennington**
Emeritus Professor of Bacteriology
University of Aberdeen
Medical School Building
Foresterhill
Aberdeen AB25 2ZD
UK

**M. Picardeau**
Unité de Biologie des Spirochètes
Institut Pasteur
28 Rue de Docteur Roux
75724 Paris Cedex 15
France

**T. L. Pitt**
Centre for Infections
Health Protection Agency
61 Colindale Avenue
London NW9 5EQ
UK

**N. W. Preston**
448 Manchester Road
Stockport SK4 5DL
UK

**D. Reid**
29 Arkleston Road
Paisley PA1 3TE
UK

**P. Riegel**
Laboratory of Bacteriology
University Hospitals of Strasbourg
3 Rue Koeberle
F-67000 Strasbourg
France

**T. V. Riley**
The University of Western Australia and
Division of Microbiology & Infectious Diseases
Path West Laboratory Medicine
Queen Elizabeth II Medical Centre
Nedlands 6009
Western Australia

**R. C. Russell**
Department of Medical Entomology
University of Sydney and Westmead Hospital
NSW 2006
Australia

**D. Safronetz**
National Institute of Allergy and Infectious
Diseases
2A122 903 S 4th Street
Hamilton, MT, USA

**Peter Simmonds**
Laboratory for Clinical and Molecular Virology
University of Edinburgh
Summerhall
Edinburgh EH9 1QH
UK

**M. P. E. Slack**
Haemophilus Reference Unit
Respiratory & Systemic Infection Laboratory
Microbiology Services Division
Health Protection Agency
61 Colindale Avenue
London
NW9 5EQ
UK

**R. C. B. Slack**
Lane House
Marsh Road
Llanrhidian
Swansea SA3 1ER
UK

**J. Stewart**
Biomedical Teaching Organisation
School of Biomedical Sciences
The University of Edinburgh Medical School
Teviot Place
Edinburgh EH8 9AG
UK

**Y. A. Taha**
Division of Microbiology and Infectious Diseases
Nottingham University Hospitals NHS Trust
Queen's Medical Centre
Nottingham NG7 2UH
UK

**D. Taylor-Robinson**
6 Vache Mews
Vache Lane
Chalfont St Giles
Buckinghamshire HP8 4UT
UK

**J. E. Thwaite**
Department of Biomedical Sciences
Defence Science and Technology Laboratory
Porton Down
Salisbury SP4 0JQ
UK

**C. Y. W. Tong**
Department of Infectious Diseases
Guy's and St. Thomas' NHS Trust and King's
College London School of Medicine St. Thomas'
Hospital
Westminster Bridge Road
London SE1 7EH
UK

**K. J. Towner**
Department of Clinical Microbiology
University Hospital
Queen's Medical Centre
Nottingham NG7 2UH
UK

**A. H. M. Van Vliet**
Institute of Food Research
Foodborne Bacterial Pathogens Programme
Colney Lane
Norwich NR4 7UA
UK

**D. H. Walker**
Department of Pathology
University of Texas Medical Branch at Galveston
Galveston
Texas 77555-0609
USA

**D. W. Warnock**
Division of Bacterial and Mycotic Diseases
National Center for Infectious Diseases
Centers for Disease Control and Prevention
1600 Clifton Road NE, Mailstop G-11
Atlanta
Georgia 30333
USA

**S. C. Weaver**
Institute for Human Infections and Immunity and
Department of Pathology
University of Texas Medical Branch at Galveston
301 University Boulevard
Galveston
Texas 77555-0610
USA

**K. G. Wooldridge**
Molecular Bacteriology & Immunology Group
Centre for Biomolecular Sciences
University of Nottingham
Nottingham NG7 2RD
UK

**X.-J. Yu**
Department of Pathology
University of Texas Medical Branch at Galveston
301 University Boulevard
Galveston
Texas 77555-0609
USA

**M. Zambon**
Microbiology Services Division
Colindale Helath Protection Agency
61 Colindale Avenue
London NW9 5EQ
UK

# CONTENTS

# PART 1
## MICROBIAL BIOLOGY

# 1 Microbiology and medicine

*D. Greenwood and M. R. Barer*

## KEY POINTS

- Microbes are too small to be seen directly and special methods are needed to investigate them. In daily life and in clinical practice we are forced to use our imagination to understand how our behaviour influences and is influenced by them.
- Infections and microbes were considered as separate phenomena until the late nineteenth century when Pasteur reconciled previous observations on the physical requirements for the transmission of infection with the nature of microbes and established the necessity of a chain of transmission in infection.
- Some infections can be prevented by interrupting transmission and/or by immunization.
- The role of specific microbes in specific infective conditions may be established by propagating the microbe in pure laboratory culture and subsequently reproducing the disease in a suitable model.
- Molecular biology has opened up new ways of identifying microbes and establishing causality in infection.
- Transmission of infection is related to the *reservoir, immediate source* and *mode of transmission* of the causal agent.
- Approximately $10^{14}$ bacterial, fungal and protozoan cells live on and in healthy human bodies. Most are harmless or even beneficial. Those that cause disease in otherwise healthy individuals are termed *pathogens*. The *normal microbiota* constitutes the reservoir and immediate source for *endogenous* infection. Infections in which the source of the causal organism is external are termed *exogenous* infections.
- Many infections can now be treated with antimicrobial agents that possess *selective toxicity*. None the less, infection remains the most common cause of morbidity and premature death in the world.

Read this paragraph, then close your eyes and think through the following: inside your intestines, in your mouth and on your skin, there reside more than $100\,000\,000\,000\,000$ microbial cells – 100-fold more than the number of cells that make up the human body. We are not conscious of these companions any more than we are conscious of passing them round every time we shake hands, speak or touch a surface. Inoculation with just one microbe of the wrong type in the wrong way may kill you, yet we tolerate and indeed thrive on constant appropriate exposure to this unseen world.

Because microbes are generally hidden from our senses, an appreciation of microbiology and infection demands imagination. Our forebears who established the discipline lavished imagination on the problems they studied. Sadly it is that lack of imagination that now underpins serious problems such as hospital-acquired infection and antibiotic resistance.

Hard-won advances in microbiology have transformed the diagnosis, prevention and cure of infection and have made key contributions to improved human health and a doubling in life expectancy. The conquest of epidemic and fatal infections has sometimes seemed so conclusive that infections may be dismissed as of minor concern to modern doctors in wealthy countries. However, infection is far from defeated. In resource-poor countries, an estimated 10 million young children die each year from the effects of infectious diarrhoea, measles, malaria, tetanus, diphtheria and whooping cough alone. Many other classical scourges, such as tuberculosis, cholera, typhoid and leprosy, continue to take their toll. Although we have the potential to prevent nearly all of these deaths, political and social issues constantly hinder progress, and more effective and economic means of delivery provide a constant challenge.

Even in wealthy nations, infection is still extremely common: at least a quarter of all illnesses for which patients consult their doctors in the UK are infective and around one in ten patients acquire infection while in hospital, sometimes with multiresistant organisms. Global communications and changes in production systems, particularly those affecting food, can have a profound effect on the spread of infectious disease. The emergence of human immunodeficiency virus (HIV), new-variant Creutzfeldt–Jakob disease (CJD), severe acute respiratory syndrome (SARS), avian and most recently so-called swine influenza illustrate the need for continued vigilance.

The relative freedom of wealthy societies from fatal infections has been won through great struggles, which are all too easily forgotten. As generations grow up without the experience of losing friends and relatives through infection, so the balance of perceived risk and benefit looks different. So now, in addition to the old threats which are ever present, we constantly face pressure to drop or modify measures such as public immunization. A historical understanding of infection is as important in maintaining and improving the present status as is knowledge of contemporary progress.

## AN OUTLINE HISTORY OF MICROBIOLOGY AND INFECTION

### Micro-organisms and infection

Infection and microbiology followed different strands of development for centuries (Fig. 1.1). We tend to map this story against the recorded efforts of prominent individuals, though many others doubtless contributed.

Ideas of infection and epidemics were recorded by Hippocrates, but it was nearly 2000 years before Girolamo Fracastoro (1483–1553) proposed in his classic tome 'De Contagione' that 'seeds of contagion' (as opposed to spirits in the ether) might be responsible. Quite separately, the early microscopists began to make observations on objects too small to be seen by the naked eye. Foremost among these was the Dutchman Antonie van Leeuwenhoek (1632–1723). With his remarkable home-made and hand-held microscope, he found many micro-organisms in materials such as water, mud, saliva and the intestinal contents of healthy subjects, and recognized them as living creatures ('animalcules') because they swam about actively. That he saw bacteria as well as the larger microbes is known from his measurements of their size ('one-sixth the diameter of a red blood corpuscle').

Before the discipline of microbiology was formally established in the second half of the nineteenth century, three key aspects of infection were

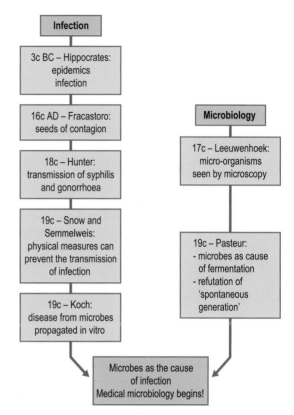

**Fig. 1.1**  Timelines for the history of infection and microbiology.

brought into stark relief by publicly acknowledged demonstrations:

1. John Hunter (1728–1793) inoculated secretions from sores around a prostitute's genitals into a penis (his own according to some sources) and demonstrated a *physical reality to the transmission of infection*, in this case syphilis and gonorrhoea (the prostitute had both, leading to a mistaken belief that the distinctive symptoms were manifestations of the same disease).
2. Edward Jenner (1749–1823) adapted the long-established oriental practice of variolation (inoculation with material from a mild case of smallpox) for the prevention of smallpox, by showing that cowpox was as effective and safer. The procedure, termed *vaccination* (Latin vacca = cow) established the concept of *immunization* in Europe.
3. John Snow (1813–1858) showed that, by preventing access to a water source epidemiologically linked to a cholera outbreak, further infections could be terminated. This established that *physical measures could prevent the transmission of infection*, a point further

illustrated by Ignaz Semmelweis (1818–1865) in Vienna and others who showed that fatal streptococcal infections (puerperal fever) affecting mothers following childbirth could be substantially reduced if those attending the birth applied simple hygienic measures.

Later two towering figures, Louis Pasteur (1822–1895) and Robert Koch (1843–1910), played central roles in establishing the microbial causation of infectious disease. The brilliant French chemist Louis Pasteur crushed two prevailing dogmas: that the fermentation responsible for alcohol formation was a purely chemical process (by demonstrating that the presence of living micro-organisms was essential), and that life could be spontaneously generated (by showing that nutrient solutions remained sterile if microbes were excluded). Refutation of spontaneous generation established unequivocally that all life must come from progenitors of the same species and, therefore, the need for a *chain of transmission* where infection is concerned. Pasteur made many other seminal contributions, including the identification of several causal agents of disease and the recognition that microbes could be rendered less capable of causing disease (less *virulent*) or *attenuated* by artificial subculture. He used the principle of attenuation to develop a successful vaccine against anthrax for use in animals. It was the influence of Pasteur's work that inspired the British surgeon Joseph Lister (1827–1912) to establish *antisepsis*, aimed at destroying the micro-organisms responsible for infection during surgery.

The other great founding father of medical microbiology, Robert Koch, came to microbiology through medicine. Working originally as a country doctor in East Prussia, he established the techniques required to isolate and propagate pure cultures of specific bacteria. His numerous contributions include establishment of the bacterial causes of anthrax, tuberculosis and cholera. He also formulated more precisely proposals first put forward by one of his mentors, Jacob Henle (1809–1885), describing how specific microbes might be recognized as the cause of specific diseases. These principles, often referred to as *Koch's postulates*, are used to substantiate claims that a particular organism causes a specific ailment. They require that:

- The organism is demonstrable in every case of the disease.
- It can be isolated and propagated in pure culture in vitro.
- Inoculation of the pure culture by a suitable route into a suitable host should reproduce the disease.
- The organism can be re-isolated from the new host.

For various reasons, universal application of the postulates is impossible and greater subtleties in establishing causal relationships in infection are now recognized. Austin Bradford Hill (1897–1991) developed a sophisticated algorithm to recognize a biological gradient of association; most recently an approach to determining the role of specific molecules in pathogenesis has been enshrined in 'molecular Koch's postulates'.

Organisms for which Koch's postulates and later modifications have been fulfilled are clearly capable of inducing disease and are designated as *pathogens* to distinguish them from the vast majority of *non-pathogenic* micro-organisms. It should be emphasized that fulfilment of the postulates and the diagnostic process in which a given patient's illness is attributed to a known pathogen are profoundly different processes. In the former, many experiments are done to provide robust scientific evidence, whereas in the latter circumstantial evidence is obtained, which, in the light of experience, identifies a particular micro-organism as the most likely cause of the illness.

In the century following Pasteur and Koch's work, the list of specific human pathogens has extended to include several hundred organisms. Early on, fungal and protozoan pathogens were recognized, as were macroscopic agents including parasitic worms and insects. Technological breakthroughs, including tissue culture and electron microscopy, were required to enable recognition of viruses. In the early days, viral pathogens were termed filterable agents, because they passed through filters designed to retain bacteria. In many cases pathogens of insects, animals or even plants were described before their medical equivalents were recognized.

Many further advances in technology through the twentieth century provided more precise understanding of the nature and function of microbes. The revolution in molecular biology that followed the elucidation of the structure of DNA by James Watson, Francis Crick, Maurice Wilkins and Rosalind Franklin in 1953 ultimately enabled a leap forward in analytical capability. For three decades this did not radically change the understanding of microbes and infection. However, almost exactly a century after Pasteur and Koch initiated what has been called the 'golden era of bacteriology', three interconnected breakthroughs once again altered the perspective:

1. The recognition, principally by the American molecular biologist Carl Woese, that ribosomal ribonucleic acid (rRNA), which has essentially the same core structure in all cells, carries unique signatures indicating its evolutionary

relationships. It transpires that all cellular forms of life can be classified according to the DNA sequence encoding their rRNA (rDNA). Determination of this sequence provides a means of identifying all microbes and has led to the discovery of a previously unsuspected third 'domain' of life, the *Archaea* (see Ch. 2).

2. Technological advances made possible by molecular genetics. The molecular basis for the pathogenesis of infection now enables recognition of the specific roles of individual genes and their products in both the pathogen and the host. This offers the promise of new approaches to treatment and prevention of infection. The discovery of mobile genetic elements that convey genes from one organism to another (see Ch. 6) confronted our biological sense of what makes up an individual. Mobile bacterial genes encoding antibiotic resistance present a major problem to the practice of medicine.

3. The development of ultra-sensitive means of detecting specific DNA or RNA sequences and the development, by Kary Mullis, of the polymerase chain reaction (PCR) in 1986. The analytical capacity of nucleic acid amplification techniques offers the prospect that it may be possible to diagnose microbial disease routinely by these methods. However, there are many challenges to be met before this shift away from detection of micro-organisms by isolation in laboratory cultures can be accepted.

Our capacity to exploit these breakthroughs has been enhanced enormously by the development of DNA sequencing by the double Nobel Laureate Fred Sanger in Cambridge. Most recently, advances in DNA analytical technologies offer real prospect that rapid sequence analyses will be performed in clinical diagnostic labs. This type of analysis has the potential to transform our insights into the epidemiology of infection and the ongoing evolution of the microbes that cause disease.

## Hygiene, treatment and prevention of infection

The work of Snow, Semmelweis, Lister and others led to an appreciation of the benefits of hygiene in the prevention of infection. Nursing practices rooted in almost obsessive cleanliness became the norm and *aseptic* practice (avoidance of contact between sterile body tissues and materials contaminated with live micro-organisms) was introduced to supplement the use of antisepsis. Before the advent of antibiotics,

hygiene was a matter of life and death; institutes of hygiene were established around the world. When treatment of infection later became reliable and routine, hygiene standards were often allowed to drop, leading to present problems, notably with hospital-acquired infection.

The discovery of phagocytic cells and humoral immunity (antibodies) as natural defence mechanisms at the end of the nineteenth century led to a re-assessment of the response to infection. One outcome was the use of antibodies produced in one host for the protection of another *(serum therapy)*. This produced some spectacular successes, notably in the life-saving use of antitoxin in diphtheria and tetanus. Unfortunately these foreign proteins often caused hypersensitivity reactions *(serum sickness)* and few diseases responded reliably to serum therapy. Nevertheless, the capacity of the immune system to achieve *selective toxicity*, and observations by the brilliant German doctor Paul Ehrlich (1854–1915) that dyes used to stain infected tissues selectively labelled parasites in preference to host tissues, contributed to the notion that systemic chemotherapy might be achievable.

In 1909 Ehrlich and his colleagues introduced the arsenical drug Salvarsan for the treatment of syphilis, but it fell short of his ideal of a *magic bullet* that would destroy the parasite without harming the host. A more important breakthrough than Ehrlich's came in 1935 with the publication of a paper by Gerhard Domagk (1895–1964) of the German dyestuffs consortium, IG Farbenindustrie. Domagk described the remarkable activity against streptococci of a dye derivative, prontosil, which turned out to owe its activity to a sulphonamide substituent previously unsuspected of antibacterial activity. Earlier, in 1928, Alexander Fleming had accidentally discovered the antibacterial properties of a fungal mould *Penicillium notatum*, but he was unable to purify the active component or exploit the therapeutic potential of his discovery. This was left to a team of scientists at Oxford led by the Australian experimental pathologist Howard Florey (1898–1968), heralding the start of the antibiotic era – the most important therapeutic development of the twentieth century.

Meanwhile, in America, the Ukrainian-born soil microbiologist Selman Waksman (1888–1973) undertook a systematic search for antibiotic substances produced by soil micro-organisms that achieved its greatest success in 1943 with the discovery of streptomycin by one of his PhD students, Albert Schatz (1920–2005). The hunt for antibiotics intensified after the Second World War, yielding chloramphenicol, tetracyclines and many other natural, synthetic and semi-synthetic antibacterial compounds. Progress in the development of antiviral, antifungal and antiparasitic compounds has been much slower, despite the fact that two effective antiprotozoal drugs, quinine (cinchona bark) and emetine (ipecacuanha root), and some natural anthelminthic agents have been recognized for centuries. Therapeutic choice in nonbacterial infection consequently remains severely limited, although the human immunodeficiency virus (HIV) pandemic has stimulated much work in the antiviral field that has been rewarded with significant success. Meanwhile, the explosion of knowledge in immunology has renewed hopes that it may be possible to manipulate immunological processes triggered by infection to the benefit of the host.

## SOURCES AND SPREAD OF INFECTION

To adequately grasp the ways in which the microbial world intersects with human lives it is necessary to understand different microbial lifestyles and the degree to which they depend on human beings. Thus there are some pathogens for which an association with man is essential in order for them to propagate, whereas for others human association is of little significance compared with their propagation in other species or environments. Microbes that depend on human beings are *obligate parasites.* A few actually need to cause disease to propagate themselves; these are termed *obligate pathogens.* In most cases, disease is accidental, or even detrimental, to the microbe's long-term survival. Viruses that cause disease in man are obligate parasites, although they often cause inapparent, subclinical or *asymptomatic* infection. Many viruses rely on infecting a particular host species. Smallpox was eradicated, not only because of the availability of an effective vaccine, but also because man was the only host. Some bacteria, fungi, protozoa and helminths are also species-specific. Among bacteria, the agent of tuberculosis, which is harboured by one-third of humanity, has an absolute requirement to cause disease for its natural transmission to continue.

Since Pasteur established the need for a chain of transmission in infection, it has been possible to fit the sources and spread of infection into a relatively simple framework. All infection recently transmitted has an *immediate source* and reaches the newly infected individual via one or more specific *mode(s) of transmission.* Behind these events, the organism, which of course does not care how we choose to classify it or its activities, lives and propagates in its natural

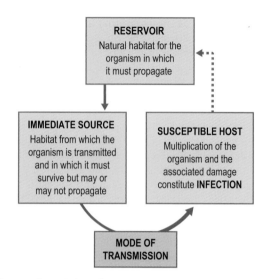

**Fig. 1.2** Reservoir, immediate source and mode of transmission in infection.

habitat(s). These may or may not be the same as the immediate source but, in considering the control of infection, the natural habitat of the causal organism constitutes the *reservoir of infection.* These points are illustrated in Figure 1.2. Elimination of the organism from the reservoir will lead to eradication of the infection, whereas elimination from the immediate source, if this is distinct from the reservoir, provides one means by which control of infection can be achieved.

The mode of transmission can involve: other infected individuals in the case of *contagious* infections; food in the case of foodborne infections; water in waterborne infection; aerosol generation by an infected individual; or contamination of an inanimate object *(fomites)* such as medical equipment or bed linen. The possible sources and modes of transmission of infection are enormous, and new variants are continually being recognized. Engagement of all healthcare workers in recognizing and controlling these hazards is a vital part of medical practice. Fortunately, most infections are transmitted by well recognized pathways (Table 1.1), and these must be clearly understood and learnt.

In the public mind, most infection is seen as contagious, but a large proportion of infections result from *endogenous infection* with a bacterium or fungus that is normally resident in the patient concerned. These resident organisms constitute the *normal microbiota* of the host (the term 'normal flora' cannot be considered appropriate any longer as it denotes plant life and does not reflect the relationships between microbes

**Table 1.1** Examples of reservoirs, sources and modes of transmission

| Infective disease | Agent of infection | Reservoir | Immediate source | Mode of transmission |
|---|---|---|---|---|
| Sore throat | *Streptococcus pyogenes*[a] (bacterium) | Human upper respiratory tract | Human upper respiratory tract | Exogenous: airborne droplets |
| Oral thrush | *Candida albicans* (fungus) | Most human mucosal surfaces | Normal microbiota of oral mucosa | Endogenous: overgrowth in antibiotic-treated or immunocompromised patient |
| Tetanus | *Clostridium tetani* (bacterium) | Soil or animal intestine | Any environment contaminated with soil or animal faeces | Exogenous: penetrating injury |
| Syphilis | *Treponema pallidum* (bacterium) | Infected human beings | Patients with genital ulcers or secondary syphilis | Exogenous: sexual contact |
| Yellow fever[b] | Yellow fever virus (virus) | Monkeys | Usually infected human beings, occasionally monkeys | Exogenous: mosquito-borne |
| AIDS | Human immunodeficiency virus (virus) | Infected human beings | Usually human blood | Exogenous: mainly blood-borne and by sexual contact |
| Toxoplasmosis[b] | *Toxoplasma gondii* (protozoon) | Cats | Undercooked meat or contact with areas contaminated by cat faeces | Exogenous: ingestion |

[a]One of many causes of sore throat.
[b]Example of a zoonosis.
AIDS, acquired immune deficiency syndrome.

and other organisms). These abundant fellow travellers generally cause infection when they get into the wrong place, often as a result of traumatic wounds (including surgery) or other types of impairment of the host's ability to prevent the spread of organisms to sites where they may cause mischief. Disturbance of the normal microbiota by antibiotics may also allow unaffected *opportunist* pathogens from the endogenous microbiota or the environment to cause infection.

In the case of endogenous infection, the reservoir and source of infection are the same and transmission is unnecessary. When infection comes from an external source it is termed *exogenous infection* and the reservoir reflects the natural habitat of the organism. Where other animals constitute that habitat, the infection is termed a *zoonosis*. In many countries bacteria, protozoa, helminths and viruses are commonly transmitted by insects or other arthropods and the conditions they cause are classified as *vector-borne* diseases.

Study of the ecology and transmission of disease, including infectious disease, is the province of the important public health discipline of *epidemiology*.

Important tools include surveillance of the *prevalence* (total cases in a defined population at a particular time) and *incidence* (number of new cases occurring during a defined period) of disease. Knowledge of the ways in which micro-organisms spread and cause disease in communities has produced vital insights that can be used to inform effective control programmes in hospitals and the wider community. Monitoring of the prevalence and incidence of infection on an institutional, local, national or global basis can similarly help in the formulation of policies that reduce the impact of specific infections (monitoring of influenza virus variants to forestall global pandemics is a good example) or of drug-resistant micro-organisms such as those causing malaria, tuberculosis or staphylococcal infections. The World Health Organization and other national or international surveillance agencies carry out much of this important work and deserve full support. For, make no mistake, despite antibiotics, immunization and – for the fortunate – improved living conditions and effective health services, infection will remain the most common cause of sickness and premature death for the foreseeable future.

## RECOMMENDED READING

Brock TD, editor: *Milestones in Microbiology*, Washington, DC, 1999, American Society for Microbiology.

Bulloch W: *The History of Bacteriology*, Oxford, 1938, Oxford University Press.

Collard P: *The Development of Microbiology*, Cambridge, 1976, Cambridge University Press.

Cox FEG, editor: *Illustrated History of Tropical Diseases*, London, 1996, Wellcome Trust.

Foster WD: *A History of Medical Bacteriology and Immunology*, London, 1970, Cox and Wyman.

Greenwood D: *Antimicrobial Drugs: Chronicle of a Twentieth Century Medical Triumph*, 2008, Oxford University Press.

Grove DI: *A History of Human Helminthology*,. Oxford, 1990, CAB International, Wallingford.

Mann J: *The Elusive Magic Bullet: The Search for the Perfect Drug*, Oxford, 1999, Oxford University Press.

Waterson AP, Wilkinson L: *An Introduction to the History of Virology*, Cambridge, 1978, Cambridge University Press.

Zinsser H: *Rats, Lice and History*, London, 1935, Routledge.

## Websites

United Nations Children's Fund: The State of the World's Children 2009. http://www.unicef.org/sowc09/

World Health Organization: Infectious diseases. http://www.who.int/topics/infectious_diseases/en/

# 2

# Morphology and nature of micro-organisms

*M. R. Barer*  ·

## KEY POINTS

- Agents of infection include cellular organisms belonging to two of the three recently defined *domains* of life, the *Bacteria* and the *Eukarya*. The latter include fungi and protozoa. The subcellular entities *viruses, viroids* and *prions* also cause infection but depend on host cells and tissues for propagation.
- Bacterial and eukaryotic micro-organisms can be detected by light microscopy, whereas electron microscopy is required for viruses. Adult stages of multicellular eukaryotic agents of infection or infestation, such as *helminths* (worms) and insects, are generally visible to the naked eye.
- Most pathogenic bacteria can be recognized as either *Gram-positive* or *Gram-negative* after staining. These properties reflect, respectively, the relatively thick *peptidoglycan* layer and the thin peptidoglycan plus outer membrane cell wall structures possessed by cells belonging to these two groups.
- The mycobacteria, which include the global pathogens causing tuberculosis and leprosy, have a different staining property, described as *acid fast*.
- In addition to the cell wall, key bacterial structures with biological and medical significance include the *nucleoid, inclusion granules* and *spores* within the cell, and *flagella, fimbriae* or *pili*, and *capsules* on the cell surface.
- Bacterial *endospores* are highly resistant bacterial cells that result from a differentiation process in some Gram-positive bacteria.
- Viruses are obligate intracellular parasites that use the host cell's machinery to replicate. They contain a nucleic acid core comprising DNA or RNA (not both) in single- or double-stranded form.
- The core is surrounded by a protein *capsid* comprising multiple *capsomeres*; an envelope derived from the host cell membrane surrounds the capsid of some viruses.

Micro-organisms are beyond doubt the most successful forms of life; they have been here longest, they are the most numerous and their distribution defines the limits of the biosphere, encompassing environments previously thought incapable of sustaining life. Here, we are concerned with the tiny fraction of micro-organisms that form associations with human beings and these encompass the cellular entities, *bacteria, archaea, fungi* and *protozoa,* and the subcellular entities, viruses, viroids and prions. Whether the last three can be considered organisms or even living entities is a matter for debate. None the less, their transmissible nature, the immune responses they provoke and our inability to detect them with the naked eye place them firmly within the province of medical microbiology. The first two of these criteria also require us to consider some multicellular macroscopically visible organisms (members of the *helminths*) as agents of infection (see Ch. 63). Most of this chapter is concerned with bacteria. The subcellular entities are introduced briefly and the remaining medically significant groups are considered in more specialized chapters.

Medical microbiology has been founded on recognizing micro-organisms that are associated with human disease. This recognition has relied predominantly on two techniques:

- microscopy
- propagation in laboratory cultures.

Over the last quarter of the 20<sup>th</sup> century, it became possible to detect, describe and differentiate micro-organisms by biochemical and genetic methods, and this had two profound effects on microbiology. First, due largely to the work of Carl Woese (see Ch. 1), it is now possible to make a reasonable assessment of the evolutionary relationships between micro-organisms, a task that previously could be achieved for macro-organisms only by examining fossil records (micro-organisms have not left interpretable fossils). Woese's approach led to the recognition of a whole

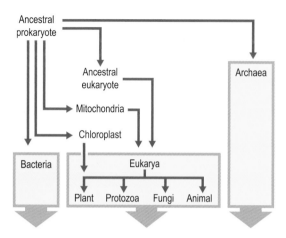

**Fig. 2.1** Diagram illustrating proposed evolutionary pathways from a putative common ancestral prokaryote to the present. The Archaea were not recognized as a separate lineage until Woese's work.

'new' *domain* (a group ranking above kingdom level) of cellular organisms, the *Archaea,* and a fundamental review of microbial classification (Fig. 2.1). Second, we have now amassed an enormous body nucleotide sequence and other molecular data describing microbes. Complete genome sequences are available for all the major bacterial and viral pathogens and most of the pathogenic protozoa and fungi. At the time of writing, the US National Center for Biotechnology Information provides access to 1356 bacterial genomes and, given that current technologies allow the raw data for a complete genome to be generated, within a day. We can stop counting now as it will soon be easier to obtain a complete sequence than subject a new strain of an isolate to a typing analysis. Thus morphology and cultural characteristics are regarded by many as secondary characteristics in the context of classification and identification, while molecular detection methods are steadily encroaching on microscopy and culture in clinical laboratories. Indeed genomic information has repeatedly revealed that some bacteria have structures that have not been revealed by conventional laboratory studies. The capsule (see below) of *Campylobacter jejuni* provides one prominent example of this.

We are currently in a transitional, information gathering phase. Molecular descriptions and detection methods are coming to dominate our view of the microbial world. However, at present it must be emphasized that the morphological classification provides a basic structure that is understood by clinicians and will remain as a basis for communication, at least in the medium term. Moreover, although this will change, light and fluorescence microscopy remain

competitively cheap and rapid compared with molecular methods as means of providing information relevant to the clinical management of infection. Finally, the discipline of medical microbiology requires the understanding of the basic structural properties and physiology of micro-organisms to underpin our approach to infections.

## PROKARYOTIC AND EUKARYOTIC CELLS

Micro-organisms are microscopic in size and are usually unicellular. The diameter of the smallest body that can be resolved and seen clearly with the naked eye is about 100 μm. All medically relevant bacteria are smaller than this and a microscope is therefore necessary to see individual cells. When propagated on solid media, bacteria (and fungi) form macroscopically visible structures comprising at least $10^8$ cells, which are known as *colonies.*

Woese's insights provided for the first time a coherent view of the evolutionary pathways behind the diversity of all living organisms. In particular, a satisfactory explanation is offered for the existence and diversity of *prokaryotic* and *eukaryotic* cells, and all living forms are seen to fall within three *domains* of life: the *Bacteria,* the *Archaea* and the *Eukarya.* Although the first two of these are prokaryotes (organisms without a membrane-bound nucleus), the *Archaea* share many characteristics with the *Eukarya.* This division is of practical significance, as the earlier the point of divergence, the greater the difference in metabolic properties between the present-day representatives of the two lineages. These differences can be exploited by directing treatments at processes unique to the target organism. Some key differences between the three domains of life are summarized in Table 2.1.

## ANATOMY OF THE BACTERIAL CELL

The principal structures of a typical bacterial cell revealed by long established methods are shown in Figure 2.2. Over the last two decades, developments in genetic manipulation combined with advances in fluorescence and electron microscopy have opened up our understanding of microbial cytology, to the point where many key macromolecular assemblies can be described in great and dynamic detail. Some of these will be mentioned below but, for the most part, this account is rooted in well established descriptions.

The cytoplasm is bounded peripherally by a very thin, elastic and semi-permeable cytoplasmic (or

**Table 2.1**  General characteristics of cellular micro-organisms in the three domains of life

| | Prokaryotes | | Eukaryotes |
|---|---|---|---|
| Domains | Bacteria | Archaea | Eukarya |
| Major groups (examples only) | Gram positives, Proteobacteria | *Methanococcus, Thermococcus* | Fungi, entamoebae, ciliates, flagellates |
| Cell diameter | ≈1 μm | ≈1 μm | ≈10 μm |
| Membrane-bound organelles | − | − | + (e.g. mitochondria, nucleus, Golgi, etc.) |
| Chromosomes | Single, closed circular | Single, closed circular | Multiple, linear |
| Introns | Very Rare | Rare | Common |
| Transcription/translation | Coupled | Coupled | Compartmentalized |
| mRNA | Very labile | Very labile | Stable and labile |
| Ribosomes | 70S | 70S | 80S |
| Protein synthesis inhibited by: | | | |
|   Chloramphenicol | + | − | − |
|   Diphtheria toxin | − | + | + |
| Peptidoglycan cell wall | + | − | − |

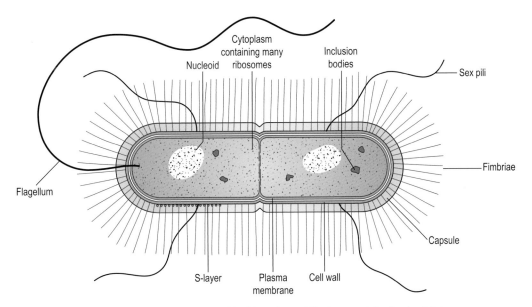

**Fig. 2.2**  Diagram illustrating the key features of bacterial cells. The S-layer is a variably demonstrated ordered protein layer.

plasma) membrane (a conventional phospholipid bilayer). Outside, and closely covering this, lies the rigid, supporting *cell wall*, which is porous and relatively permeable. Cell division occurs by the development of constrictions mediated by the assembly of an actin-like protein, FtsZ. The constrictions proceed from the periphery inwards and, in some cases, produce a transverse cell wall known as a *septum* or *cross-wall*.

The exact pattern of cell division and the structures associated with the cell wall and cytoplasmic membrane (collectively the cell envelope) combine to produce the cell morphology and characteristic patterns of cell arrangement. The recognition of

these features by oil-immersion light microscopy remains of great practical value in making presumptive identifications of bacteria associated with human infections. Bacterial cells may have two basic shapes, spherical (*coccus*) or rod shaped (*bacillus*); the rod-shaped bacteria show variants that are comma shaped (*vibrio*), spiral (*spirillum* and *spirochaete*) or filamentous (Fig. 2.3).

The *cytoplasm* is a predominantly aqueous environment packed with ribosomes and numerous other protein and nucleotide–protein complexes. The cytoplasmic contents are not normally visible by light microscopy, which can only resolve objects more than 0.2 μm in diameter. Although bacterial cytoplasm has

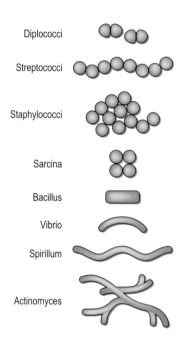

Fig. 2.3 The shapes and characteristic groupings of various bacterial cells.

Diplococci

Streptococci

Staphylococci

Sarcina

Bacillus

Vibrio

Spirillum

Actinomyces

**Fig. 2.4** Thin section of a dividing bacillus showing cell wall, cytoplasmic membrane, ribosomes, a developing cross-wall and a mesosome, a membranous structure now generally considered to be an artifact or reflecting some form of cell damage. Magnification ×50 000. By courtesy of Dr PJ Highton and the editors of *Journal of Ultrastructure Research*.

traditionally been viewed as devoid of structure, it is now clear that, like eukarya, bacteria have an extensive cytoskeletal network which, in different genera, include structures corresponding to eukaryotic actin, tubulin and intermediate filaments (e.g. MreB, FtsZ and crescentin, respectively). The importance of these is emerging in determining cell shape, division and spore formation (see below). As predicted in the previous edition of this book, antimicrobials targeting these functions, specifically Ftz, have recently been described.

Some larger structures such as spores or *inclusion bodies* of storage products such as volutin (polyphosphate), lipid (e.g. poly-β-hydroxyalkanoate or triacylglycerol), glycogen or starch occur in some species under specific growth conditions. Specialized labelling techniques (generally requiring fluorescence imaging) enable visualization of the nuclear material or *nucleoid* and other structures (e.g. the forming cell division annulus). Figure 2.4 is an electron micrograph of a thin section of a dividing bacterial cell. Outside the cell wall there may be a protective gelatinous covering layer called a *capsule* or, when it is too thin to be resolved with the light microscope, a *microcapsule*. Soluble large-molecular material may be dispersed by the bacterium into the environment as *loose slime*. Some bacteria bear, protruding outwards from the cell wall, one or more kinds of protein-based filamentous appendages called *flagella*, which are organs of locomotion, and hair-like structures termed *fimbriae* or *pili*, which, via specific receptor–ligand interactions at their tip, mediate adhesion.

## Bacterial nucleoid

The genetic information of a bacterial cell is mostly contained (with a few exceptions) in a single, long molecule of double-stranded DNA, which can be extracted in the form of a closed circular thread about 1 mm long. The cell solves the problem of packaging this enormous macromolecule by condensing and looping it into a *supercoiled* state. As well as the chromosome, the bacterium may contain one or more additional fragments of *episomal* (extrachromosomal) DNA, known as *plasmids*. Bacteria are essentially haploid organisms with only one allele of each gene per cell, although there may be multiple copies of chromosomes and plasmids. Unlike the mitotic or meiotic divisions of eukaryotic cells, chromosomal segregation in bacteria at the time of cell division (or fission) does not involve structures that can be resolved by light microscopy. None the less, the speed at which replication can occur (cell divisions more frequently than one every 15 min in some cases) and the simultaneous requirement for multiple rounds of chromosome replication in one cell provide a mind-boggling challenge for the segregation machinery. (Imagine unravelling two 1 m threads inside a 1 mm sphere!)

The bacterial nucleoid lies within the cytoplasm and is associated with several nucleoid-associated proteins

(NAPs). Although these were originally referred to as histone-like, they are not structurally related and they function in the cytoplasm rather than within a membrane-bound nucleus. The NAPs such as H-NS and IHF exert important influences on prokaryotic gene expression (see Chapters 4 and 6). The cytoplasmic location of the nucleoid means that as DNA-dependent RNA polymerase makes RNA, ribosomes may attach and initiate protein synthesis on the still attached (nascent) messenger RNA. Synthesis of mRNA and protein (transcription and translation) are therefore seen to be directly coupled in bacteria. In contrast, complete transcripts in eukaryotic cells have to be spliced (to remove the non-coding introns) and capped with polyadenine (this rarely occurs with bacterial mRNA) before the post-transcriptionally modified message is translocated to the cytoplasm.

## Ribosomes

Bacterial ribosomes are slightly smaller (10–20 nm) than those of eukaryotic cells and they have a sedimentation coefficient of 70S, being composed of a 30S and a 50S subunit (cf. 40S and 60S in the 80S eukaryotic counterparts). They may be seen with the electron microscope, and number tens of thousands in growing cells. Multiple ribosomes attach to single mRNA molecules to form *polysomes*. It was the nucleotide sequencing of DNA encoding small-subunit ribosomal RNA (rDNA) that led Woese to postulate the evolutionary pathways shown in Figure 2.1. Essentially all cellular organisms can now be classified at least down to genus level by their small-subunit rRNA (SSrRNA) nucleotide sequences. Subsequently it was recognized that, as growing cells contain so many ribosomes, it should be possible to detect unique identifying (or determinative) SSrRNA sequences by complementary in-situ hybridization with fluorescently labelled oligonucleotide probes. Indeed, it is now possible to apply this approach to natural samples and this has enabled recognition of bacteria that have never been grown in laboratory culture. Finally it should be noted that two key organelles in eukaryotes, mitochondria and chloroplasts, both contain 70S ribosomes. When the SSrRNA-encoding genes on the circular chromosomes of these organelles were sequenced, their original free-living bacterial origin was clearly indicated and the proposed endosymbiotic route by which they became organelles confirmed.

## Cytoplasmic membrane

The bacterial cytoplasmic membrane is 5–10 nm thick and consists mainly of phospholipids and proteins. Its structure can be resolved in some ultra-thin sections examined by electron microscopy. *Membranes* generally appear in suitably stained electron microscope preparations as two dark lines about 2.5 nm wide, separated by a lighter area of similar width. Integral, transmembrane, and peripheral or anchored proteins occur in abundance and perform similar functions to those described in eukaryotes (e.g. transport and signal transduction). A key feature differentiating prokaryotic cytoplasmic membranes from those of eukaryotes is their multifunctional nature. Thus, while in eukaryotic cells the endoplasmic reticulum and Golgi apparatus are involved in protein secretion, packaging and processing, and the mitochondrial inner membrane is the site of electron transport and oxidative phosphorylation, all of these functions must be performed by one membrane in prokaryotes. It is hardly surprising that prokaryotic cell membranes are relatively protein rich, allowing relatively little space for phospholipids.

## Cell wall

The cell wall (Figs 2.5 & 2.6) lies immediately external to the cytoplasmic membrane. It is 10–25 nm thick, strong and relatively rigid, though with some elasticity, and openly porous, being freely permeable to solute molecules smaller than 10 kDa in mass and 1 nm in diameter. It is strong but elastic, and supports the weak cytoplasmic membrane against the high internal osmotic pressure (25 and 5 atm in Gram-positive and Gram-negative cells respectively) and maintains the characteristic shape of the bacterium in its coccal, bacillary, filamentous or spiral form.

Except under defined osmotic conditions, cell survival is dependent on the integrity of the cell wall. If the wall is weakened or ruptured, the cytoplasm may swell from osmotic inflow of water and burst the weak cytoplasmic membrane. This process of lethal disintegration and dissolution is termed *lysis*.

The chemical composition of the cell wall differs considerably between different bacterial species, but in all species the main strengthening component is *peptidoglycan* (syn. *mucopeptide* or *murein*). Peptidoglycan is composed of *N*-acetylglucosamine and *N*-acetylmuramic acid molecules linked alternately in a chain (Fig. 2.7). This heteropolymer forms a single molecular continuous sac external to the cytoplasmic membrane (described as the murein sacculus). The thickness of the peptidoglycan layer turns out to be of great practical importance in differentiating medically significant bacteria. In the late nineteenth century a Danish physician, Christian Gram, immortalized himself by devising a staining procedure that we now

**Fig. 2.5** Electron micrograph and diagrams illustrating the basis for the Gram reaction in bacteria.

know distinguishes bacteria with a thick (Gram-positive) and a thin (Gram-negative) murein sacculus (see Fig. 2.5). The traditional classification of bacteria is fundamentally rooted in this dichotomy, which has, fortunately, largely been supported by rRNA-based classification.

The rapid (<5 min) Gram-stain procedure remains a cornerstone of day-to-day practice in detecting and identifying bacteria in clinical laboratories. *Gram's stain* distinguishes bacteria as 'Gram-positive' or 'Gram-negative', according to whether or not they resist decolouration with acetone, alcohol or aniline oil after staining with a triphenyl methane dye, such as crystal violet, and subsequent treatment with iodine. The Gram-positive bacteria resist decoloura-tion and remain stained a dark purple colour. The Gram-negative bacteria are decolorized, and are then counterstained light pink by the subsequent applica-tion of safranin, neutral red or dilute carbol fuchsin. In routine diagnostic work a Gram-stained smear is often the only preparation examined microscopically, as it shows clearly the general morphology of the bacteria as well as revealing their Gram reaction. It should be noted that characteristically Gram-positive

species may sometimes appear Gram-negative under certain conditions of growth, especially in ageing cultures on nutrient agar or after exposure to antibiotics.

The *N*-acetylmuramic acid units of peptidoglycan each carry a short peptide, usually consisting of L-alanine, D-glutamic acid, either *meso*-diaminopimelic acid (in Gram-negative bacteria) or L-lysine (in Gram-positive bacteria) and D-alanyl-D-alanine. The wall is given its strength by cross-links that form between adjacent strands. These may be formed directly between the *meso*-diaminopimelic acid or L-lysine of one strand and the penultimate D-alanine of the next, or (the usual form in Gram-positive organisms) through an interpeptide bridge composed of up to five amino acids; in either case, the terminal D-alanine is lost in the cross-linking reaction (Fig. 2.8). Several antibiotics interfere with the construction of the cell wall peptidoglycan (see Ch. 5).

The bacterial cell wall also contains other com-ponents whose nature and amount vary with the species. Many Gram-positive bacteria contain rela-tively large amounts of *teichoic acid* (a polymer of ribitol or glycerol phosphate complexed with sugar

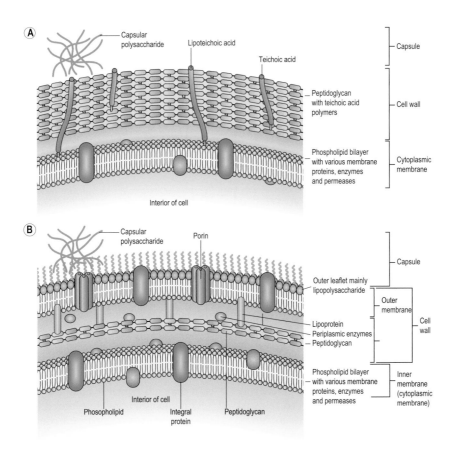

**Fig. 2.6**   The envelope of (A) the Gram-positive cell wall and (B) the Gram-negative cell wall.

**Fig. 2.7**   The basic building block of bacterial cell wall peptidoglycan. *N*-acetylmuramic acid is derived from *N*-acetylglucosamine by the addition of a lactic acid unit. Each *N*-acetylmuramic acid molecule is substituted with a pentapeptide; an *N*-acetylglucosamine molecule is joined to the muramylpentapeptide within the cell membrane and the unit is transferred to growth points in the existing peptidoglycan, where adjacent strands are cross-linked. (See also Fig. 2.8.)

residues) interspersed with the peptidoglycan; some of this material (*lipoteichoic acid*) is linked to lipids buried in the cell membrane.

Electron microscopy reveals that Gram-negative bacteria possess a second *outer membrane* external to the peptidoglycan layer. This is essentially another unit membrane in which the outer leaflet is largely composed of a molecule referred to as lipopolysaccharide (LPS). Like the cytoplasmic membrane, this membrane contains many associated proteins whose functions include selective permeability (porins) and attachment (adhesins). The outer membrane confers several important properties on Gram-negative bacteria:

- It protects the peptidoglycan from the effects of lysozyme (a natural body defence substance that cleaves the link between *N*-acetylglucosamine and *N*-acetylmuramic acid (see Fig. 2.7).
- It impedes the ingress of many antibiotics.

*Staph. aureus*      *Esch. coli*

**Fig. 2.8** Schematic representation of the peptidoglycan of a representative Gram-positive organism (*Staphylococcus aureus*) and a representative Gram-negative organism (*Escherichia coli*). Note that in the Gram-positive bacterium cross-linking occurs through a peptide bridge (pentaglycine in *Staph. aureus*), whereas direct cross-linking occurs in *E. coli*. In both cases the terminal D-alanine is lost. Not all peptides are engaged in cross-linking in *E. coli*, and carboxypeptidases remove redundant D-alanine residues. NAG, N-acetylglucosamine; NAMA, N-acetylmuramic acid; *m*-DAP, meso-diaminopimelic acid.

Components of the LPS, in particular the core structure, lipid A, form endotoxin, which, when released into the bloodstream, may give rise to endotoxic shock (see Ch. 13).

In addition to the basic Gram stain-related properties outlined above, a third type of cell envelope is characteristic of mycobacteria, a group that includes the causal agents of tuberculosis and leprosy. Mycobacteria are related to Gram-positive bacteria, though they can rarely be demonstrated as such. The peptidoglycan layer is covalently linked on its outer aspect to arabinogalactan, which is itself substituted with unique lipids known as *mycolic acids*. These β-hydroxy fatty acids consist of 60 to 90 carbon residues and, together with non-covalently linked free lipids, form an extremely hydrophobic external layer. This layer has some properties in common with the Gram-negative outer membrane (indeed, porins have recently been detected therein). The whole envelope structure confers the property of *acid-fast staining* by methods such as the Ziehl–Neelsen (ZN) and phenol–auramine procedures.

The ZN method is of great value in the detection of the tubercle bacillus and other mycobacteria. The mycolic acids referred to above provide a barrier to simple aqueous stains, but when permeability is altered by heating or phenol (or both), concentrated solutions of basic fuchsin, and the fluorescent dyes auramine and rhodamine, can produce well-stained cells that subsequently resist decolorization by strong acid in alcohol. Any decoloured non-acid-fast organisms are counterstained in a contrasting colour with methylene blue or malachite green. Modifications of the ZN method are also useful for the demonstration of bacterial endospores and organisms such as *Nocardia* spp. and cysts of some protozoa, notably *Cryptosporidium* spp.

The recognition that some bacterial genera have two boundary lipid layers while others have one has led to the recommendation that the descriptive term, diderm (two skin) be applied to Gram-negative bacteria and to a number of other groups, such as the mycobacteria. In this nomenclature bacteria with a single lipid boundary such as conventional Gram-positive bacteria, are referred to as monoderms.

The cell envelope is a highly dynamic structure in growing bacterial cultures. Its components are subject to rapid turnover (synthesis, assembly, disassembly and degradation) and there is busy molecular traffic in and out of the cytoplasm. Although the diagrammatic and photographic representations here give it a somewhat monolithic and immutable character, the envelope and other surface structures can change very rapidly (within minutes) in response to environmental signals. The cell surface receives and transmits many signals from the surrounding environment, including those involving other bacteria, particularly those belonging to the same strain. This latter phenomenon is known as *quorum sensing* and appears to be important in regulating gene expression in groups of bacteria.

The structures involved in the molecular traffic through the cell envelope are the subject of intense investigation. In particular, the outward secretion of proteins attracts much current interest. At least seven distinct processes have been identified; all involve impressive macromolecular complexes anchored in the cytoplasmic membrane. Of particular interest here are the *type III secretion systems* in Gram-negative bacteria. The fully assembled multiprotein complex spans the cytoplasmic membrane, the periplasmic space, the murein sacculus and the outer membrane, and in some cases projects from the cell surface into an adjacent host (human) cell. These impressive delivery systems are capable of injecting *effector molecules* into the host cell and thereby subvert the latter's function to the advantage of the microbe.

## Extracellular polysaccharides: capsules, microcapsules and loose slime

Many bacteria have been demonstrated to possess a more or less continuous but relatively amorphous layer external to the Gram-negative and Gram-positive envelopes described above. Although these are detected quite readily in some bacteria grown under laboratory conditions, they are somewhat ephemeral in others. These structures appear to be important in mediating contact with potentially hostile environments and may be subject to strict environmental control.

When this layer is fully hydrated and resolvable by light microscopy, it is called a *capsule* (Fig. 2.9). When it is narrower, and detectable only by indirect, serological means or by electron microscopy, it may be termed a *microcapsule*. The capsular gel consists

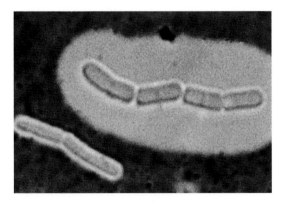

**Fig. 2.9** *Bacillus megaterium*. A chain of bacilli with a large capsule, and a pair with a very small capsule. Wet film with India ink, ×3500.

largely of water and has only a small content (e.g. 2%) of solids. In most species, the solid material is a complex polysaccharide, although in some species its main constituent is polypeptide.

*Loose slime*, or *free slime*, is an amorphous, viscid, colloidal material that is secreted extracellularly by some bacteria. In bacteria that also possess a demonstrable capsule, the slime is generally similar in chemical composition and antigenic character to the capsular substance. When slime-forming bacteria are grown on a solid culture medium, the slime remains around the bacteria as a matrix in which they are embedded, and its presence confers on the growths a watery and sticky 'mucoid' character. The slime is freely soluble in water and, when the bacteria are grown or suspended in a liquid medium, it passes away from them and disperses through the medium.

All of these features appear to have some role in interactions with the external environment. In some cases capsules have been shown to protect against phagocytosis, the lytic action of complement and bacteriophage invasion. In at least three instances antibodies directed against capsular antigens have been shown to protect against infection and, indeed, capsular preparations are used in several vaccines. Capsules also appear to have a role in protecting cells against desiccation. The production of extracellular polysaccharides in general provides a matrix within which *biofilm* formation can take place.

## S-layers

A rather more structured (paracrystalline) protein layer has been demonstrated in some bacteria. This S-layer can be shown by electron microscopy and appears to share at least some functional properties with capsules.

## Flagella and motility

Motile bacteria possess filamentous appendages known as *flagella* (singular, *flagellum*), which act as organs of locomotion. The flagellum is a long, thin filament, twisted spirally in an open, regular waveform. It is about 0.02 μm thick and is usually several times the length of the bacterial cell. It originates in the bacterial cytooplasm and the structure projects through the cell envelope. According to the species, there may be one, or up to 20, flagella per cell. In elongated bacteria the arrangement of the flagella may be *peritrichous*, or *lateral*, when they originate from the sides of the cell, or *polar*, when they originate from one or both ends. Where several occur on a cell, they may function coiled together as a single 'tail'. The external portion of a flagellum is essentially a polymer of a single protein, *flagellin*, whereas the basal region inserted into the cytoplasmic membrane comprises multiple subunits that anchor and power the organ. In a remarkably elegant manner, the flagellar motor is powered directly (as opposed to indirectly via adenosine triphosphate) by the proton gradient created across the cytoplasmic membrane by electron transport. In *Escherichia coli*, alternation between the anticlockwise and clockwise motion of the flagella effects, respectively, linear or tumbling motility. The intervals between these two patterns are modulated by chemical signals in the environment and the end result is that the bacterium shows *chemotactic behaviour* (movement towards or away from certain stimuli).

Flagella are invisible in ordinary light microscope preparations, but may be shown by the use of special staining methods, and in special circumstances by dark-ground illumination. Because of the difficulties of these methods, the presence of flagella is commonly inferred from the observation of motility. They can be demonstrated easily and clearly with the electron microscope, usually appearing as simple fibrils without internal differentiation (Fig. 2.10). In some preparations the flagellum appears as a hollow tube formed of helically twisted fibrils, and the flagella of some bacteria (e.g. vibrios) have an outer sheath. In the spirochaetes the flagellum is located in the periplasm and hence is referred to as an endo-flagellum, and this presumably underpins their characteristic spiral motion.

Motility is clearly important to many bacteria and probably serves mainly to place the cell in environments favourable to growth and free from noxious influences. In some cases possession of flagella is thought to contribute to the pathogenesis of disease.

## Fimbriae and pili

Many bacteria possess filamentous appendages called *fimbriae* or *pili*. These terms are often used interchangeably, although the latter was originally reserved for structures involved in genetic exchange between bacteria (*sex pili*; see below). Fimbriae are far more numerous than flagella (e.g. 100–500, being borne peritrichously by each cell), and are much shorter and only about half as thick (e.g. varying from 0.1 to 1.5 µm in length and having a uniform width between 4 and 8 nm). They do not have the smoothly curved spiral form of flagella and are mostly more or less straight. They cannot be seen with the light microscope but are clearly seen with the electron microscope in preparations (see Fig. 2.10). The molecular structure of pili has been studied extensively and reveals many features required to span the bacterial cell envelope that are common to different bacterial groups and difference cells structures.

Multiple types (e.g. types 1 and 2, P type, etc.) of fimbriae have been recognized according to their dimensions, antigenic and phenotypic properties. Until recently it was thought that they were confined to Gram-negative bacteria but now they have been demonstrated in many Gram-positive bacteria. In medical and veterinary contexts, fimbriae are recognized to be important in mediating adhesion between the bacterium and host cells (classically this was recognized in the phenomenon of haemagglutination, a property of type 1, mannose-sensitive pili). In contrast, *sex pili* are structurally similar to other fimbriae but are longer and confer the ability to attach specifically to other bacteria that lack these appendages. Sex pili initiate the process of conjugation (see Ch. 6); they also act as receptor sites for certain bacteriophages described as being 'donor specific'.

It should be noted that fimbriae are not the only means by which bacteria can be involved in specific adhesion events. *Non-fimbrial adhesins* (generally proteins or glyco-proteins) are also important in

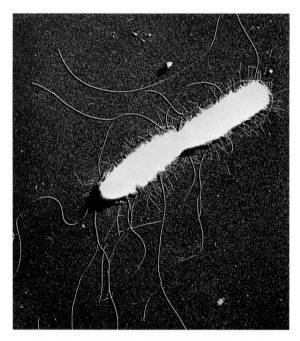

**Fig. 2.10** *Salmonella enterica* serotype Typhi. Dividing bacillus from log-phase culture bears about 15 long wavy flagella and more than 100 short fimbriae. Note the dense (white) protoplast shrunken away from the cell wall. Whole bacillus dried and shadow-cast. Electron micrograph, ×16 000. From Duguid JP, Wilkinson JF 1961 Environmentally induced changes in bacterial morphology. *Symposia of the Society for General Microbiology* 11: 69–99.

this regard. Receptor-specific interactions are very important in infective disease, as they are thought to determine much of the tissue tropism of the pathological process.

## Importance of microbial surface structures in infection

The structures described have significance for the function of bacteria and their identification by clinical microbiologists, but the surface structures of all micro-organisms (not just bacteria) are of critical importance in the process of infection. They are vital in initiating the contact that occurs during the encounter and establishment of infection (see Ch. 13). Moreover, in addition to substances secreted by micro-organisms, surface structures are exposed to the actions of the innate and adaptive immune systems (see Ch. 8) and, among pathogens, their composition, variability and function reflect these selection pressures and provide opportunities for immunization.

## THE BACTERIAL 'LIFE CYCLE'

Multicellular organisms have long been recognized to pass through many different stages. These may include many immature forms (cf. the larval stages of helminth parasitic worms) or dormant forms (e.g. plant seeds). Even protozoa and fungi may show multiple developmental stages. In contrast, bacteria have been viewed as growing (*vegetative*), stationary or dead. With the exception of spore-forming genera (see below), because they do not undergo morphological differentiation, bacterial cells have been considered essentially uniform in their properties. As indicated above, it is now recognized that all bacteria adapt extensively and rapidly to their environment. This adaptation takes place at both phenotypic (gene expression) and genotypic (genetic complement and arrangement) levels. It seems clear that there are many more physiological states in which bacteria can exist than previously acknowledged and that these states may influence the capacity of the immune system and antimicrobial agents to eliminate them. In particular, the possibility that non-sporulating bacteria are capable of dormancy (a reversible state of metabolic shutdown) has attracted much interest. Spore formation, however, is the key paradigm of differentiation and dormancy in bacteria.

The different forms taken on by organisms at different stages in the life cycle are of course important in their recognition. The range of basic cellular forms of bacteria was mentioned above. It is difficult to

generalize, but important to mention that bacterial cell morphology does alter with the physiological state. Characteristically, the cells of bacteria that are growing rapidly are larger than their non- or slowly growing counterparts. Although this does not alter basic coccal morphology, it may make bacilli appear more intermediate (cocco-bacillary) or spherical (coccoid) in shape. Bacilli exposed to certain noxious influences (notably some antibiotics) may produce extended forms that are sometimes described as filamentous. Bacteria that are characterized as essentially filamentous produce a mat of intertwining filaments known as a mycelium (one characteristic form of fungal growth). This form of growth is also associated with fragmentation in which coccal forms may be released, and this results in highly *pleomorphic* cultures. All of these alternative growth forms are undoubtedly under the influence of environmental signals, although their identities have yet to be determined in most cases.

## Bacterial spores

Some bacteria, notably those of the genera *Bacillus* and *Clostridium*, develop a highly resistant resting phase or *endospore*, whereby the organism can survive in a dormant state through a long period of starvation or other adverse environmental conditions (resuscitation of spores several thousand years old has been claimed). The process does not involve multiplication: in *sporulation*, each vegetative cell forms only one spore, and in subsequent *germination* each spore gives rise to a single vegetative cell. Geneticists have viewed sporulation as a paradigm of a simple differentiation process, and the key molecular processes required in *Bacillus subtilis* are now understood in great detail. In the face of sporulation stimuli, classically starvation or transition from growth to stationary phase, a programme of sequential expression of specific genes is triggered. The end result is a morphologically distinct structure, the endospore, within the *mother cell*.

In unstained preparations the spore is recognized within the parent cell by its greater refractility. It is larger than lipid inclusion granules and is often ovoid, in contrast to the spherical shape of the lipid granules. Mature ungerminated spores are 'phase bright' when viewed by phase-contrast microscopy; immature or germinated spores are 'phase dark'. When mature, the spore resists coloration by simple stains, appearing as a clear space within the stained cell. Spores are slightly acid-fast and may be stained differentially by a modification of the ZN method. The appearance of the mature spores varies according to the species, being spherical, ovoid or elongated, occupying a terminal,

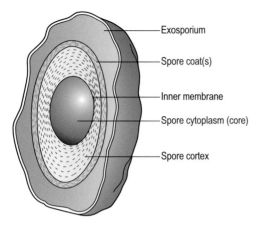

**Fig. 2.11** Cross-section of a bacterial spore. The core is surrounded by the inner spore membrane. The cortex, a laminated structure, is protected by a more resistant layer or multiple layers forming the spore coat. In some cases, a loose outer covering (exosporium) can be defined.

Labels in figure:
- Exosporium
- Spore coat(s)
- Inner membrane
- Spore cytoplasm (core)
- Spore cortex

subterminal or central position, and being narrower than the cell, or broader and bulging it. Spores of some species have an additional, apparently loose, covering known as the *exosporium* (Fig. 2.11).

Spores are much more resistant than the vegetative forms to exposure to disinfectants, drying and heating. Thus, application of moist heat at 100–120°C or more for a period of 10–20 min may be needed to kill spores, whereas heating at 60°C suffices to kill vegetative cells. In the dry state, or in moist conditions unfavourable to growth, spores may remain viable for many years. The marked resistance of spores has been attributed to several factors in which they differ from vegetative cells: the impermeability of their cortex and outer coat, their high content of calcium and dipicolinic acid, their low content of water, and their very low metabolic and enzymic activity.

Reactivation of the spore is termed *germination* and it should be noted that this is not just a reversal of the process by which the spore was formed. Germination of the spore occurs in response to specific stimuli that are generally related to external conditions favourable to growth. It is irreversible and involves rapid degradative changes. The spore successively loses its heat resistance and its dipicolinic acid; it loses calcium, it becomes permeable to dyes and its refractivity changes. Spores that have survived exposure to severe adverse influences such as heat are much more exacting than normal spores in their requirements for germination. For this reason, specially enriched culture media are used when testing the sterility of materials, such as surgical catgut, that have been exposed to disinfecting procedures. In the process of germination, the spore swells,

its cortex disintegrates, its coat is broken open and a single vegetative cell emerges.

The initiation of germination (*activation*) is incompletely understood. It is clear that the state of dormancy of spores may be altered by various treatments, such as transient exposure to heat at 80°C, so that germination can then proceed more rapidly in the individual cells or more completely in a spore population. Activation is distinct from germination and is reversible if germination does not proceed.

After germination, cell growth leading up to the formation of the first vegetative cell and before the first cell division is referred to as *outgrowth*. The conditions required for successful outgrowth may differ markedly from those that allow germination.

## Conidia (exospores)

Some of the mycelial bacteria (*Actinomycetales*) and many filamentous fungi form *conidia*, resting spores of a kind different from endospores. The conidia are borne *externally* by abstriction from the ends of the parent cells (conidiophores), and are disseminated by the air or other means to fresh habitats. They are not especially resistant to heat and disinfectants.

## Pleomorphism and involution

During growth, bacteria of a single strain may show considerable variation in size and shape, or form a proportion of cells that are swollen, spherical, elongated or pear shaped. This pleomorphism occurs most readily in certain species (e.g. *Streptobacillus moniliformis* and *Yersinia pestis*) in ageing cultures, on artificial medium and especially in the presence of antagonistic substances such as penicillin, glycine, lithium chloride, sodium chloride in high concentrations, and organic acids at low pH. The abnormal cells are generally regarded as degenerate or *involution* forms; some are non-viable, whereas others may grow and revert to the normal form when transferred to a suitable environment. In many cases the abnormal shape seems to be the result of defective cell wall synthesis and produces a grotesquely swollen cell, comparable to a spheroplast (see below), that later usually bursts and lyses.

## Spheroplasts, protoplasts and L-forms

If bacteria have their cell walls removed or weakened while they are held in a solution of sufficient osmolarity to prevent them taking up water by osmosis, they may escape being lysed and, instead, may become converted into viable spherical bodies. If all the cell wall material has been removed from them, the spheres are *free protoplasts*. If they remain enclosed by an intact, but weakened, residual cell wall, they are called *spheroplasts*. Protoplasts and spheroplasts are osmotically sensitive; they vary in size with the osmotic pressure of the suspending medium and, if the medium is much diluted, they swell up and perish by lysis. In contrast to these laboratory generated forms (which may be made deliberately for research or biotechnological applications), *L-forms* of bacteria may arise spontaneously and are also cell wall deficient. There is much controversy about the contribution of L-forms to infection. They are difficult to demonstrate as they do not stain with Gram or acid-fast methods and may not propagate in vitro. In common with another controversial area in bacteriology, the 'nanobacteria', L-forms may pass through standard bacteria-stopping filters.

## THE NATURE AND COMPOSITION OF VIRUSES

### Structure

The basic infectious particle of a virus is known as the *virion*. In the simplest viruses this consists of nucleic acid and a surrounding coat of protein called the *capsid*. Some viruses are enclosed within an *envelope*, derived from host cell membranes but modified by the inclusion of viral glycoproteins. The capsid is composed of distinct morphological units or *capsomeres*, which are assembled from viral proteins. Depending on the arrangement of these proteins, the capsomeres may be spherical, cylindrical or ring-like in appearance. The *nucleocapsid* is the combination of nucleic acid and capsid. The arrangement of the capsomeres around the nucleic acid determines the *symmetry* of the virion. When the capsomeres are applied directly to the helical nucleic acid, a coil-like structure with the appearance of a hollow tube is formed. Viruses with this arrangement are said to have *helical symmetry*. Most helical viruses enclose the nucleocapsid within an envelope and thus do not have a rigid appearance. The other major type is shown by the viruses with *icosahedral symmetry* (Fig. 2.12), in which the capsomeres are arranged as if lying on the faces of an icosahedron with 20 equilateral triangular faces and 12 corners or apices (Fig. 2.13). Capsomeres on the faces and edges of this figure are called hexons, as they always link with six adjacent capsomeres; those positioned at the apices are the pentons, as they always join to five capsomeres. Viruses with icosahedral symmetry have a rigid structure and, under the electron

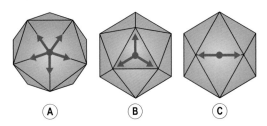

**Fig. 2.12** An icosahedron viewed along its (A) five-fold, (B) three-fold and (C) two-fold axes of symmetry.

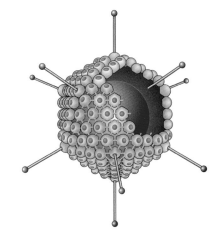

**Fig. 2.13** Icosahedron of an adenovirus. The core of DNA is represented by a circular mass. Some of the pentamers at the 12 vertices have been indicated with protruding fibres and terminal knobs. The remaining 240 hexamer capsids are, for the most part, shown as compressed into hollow spheres linked to one another by divalent bonds. The hexagonal shape of a few of the capsomeres is seen in the centre of the diagram.

microscope, have a characteristic hexagonal outline with triangular faces. However, if the diameter of the virion is less than about 50 nm the particle will appear spherical. Many viruses with icosahedral symmetry are enclosed by an outer envelope. The poxviruses are large and complex, and do not show either type of symmetry; they are referred to as complex. The size of virions varies considerably, from 25–300 nm, in different families (Fig. 2.14).

### Viral nucleic acid

The most common types of nucleic acid in viruses of human beings are single-stranded RNA and double-stranded DNA. However, both double-stranded RNA and single-stranded DNA occur in the reoviruses and parvoviruses, respectively. The genomes of RNA viruses may be present as a single strand as in paramyxoviruses, or as two copies as in the

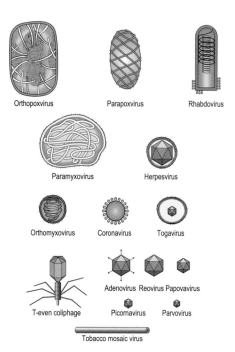

Orthopoxvirus

Parapoxvirus

Rhabdovirus

Paramyxovirus

Herpesvirus

Orthomyxovirus

Coronavirus

Togavirus

T-even coliphage

Adenovirus Reovirus Papovavirus

Picornavirus

Parvovirus

Tobacco mosaic virus

**Fig. 2.14** Morphology of viruses.

retroviruses, or exist as a specific number of fragments as in the orthomyxoviruses and reoviruses. Circular molecules of DNA are present in the virions of papovaviruses and hepadnaviruses. The amount of nucleic acid in virions is constant for a particular virus but shows considerable variation; thus the genome can vary from 5 kilobase pairs in parvoviruses to 375 kilobase pairs in the largest poxviruses.

## Virion enzymes

Several viruses carry essential enzymes in the virion. As discussed in Chapter 7, an RNA-dependent RNA polymerase or transcriptase is an essential component of the virion in several virus families, including the negative-strand RNA viruses. Among DNA viruses only the poxviruses carry a DNA-dependent RNA polymerase. The hepadnaviruses have a virion polymerase complex that has some similarity to the reverse transcriptase complex found in the retroviruses.

## Viral proteins

Analysis of the proteins produced in a cell during viral infection shows that some are essential components of the virion; these are the structural proteins and include capsid proteins and enzymes as well as basic core proteins that may be necessary to package the nucleic acid within the capsid. Other proteins such as enzymes are needed for the production of viral components but are not part of the virion; these are the non-structural proteins. The essential steps of virus attachment and penetration of the host cell are known to depend on regions of the outer capsid, such as the apical fibres and knobs of adenoviruses, or on parts of the envelope glycoproteins of viruses, such as influenza A and B and the human immunodeficiency virus.

## Viroids, defective viruses and prions

Our concept of the organismal nature of infectious agents is stretched to the limit by these infective entities. Viroids are essentially circular RNA molecules that have been associated with several plant diseases; they do not encode proteins or possess a capsid. The hepatitis delta agent has some features in common with viroids and defective viruses (viruses that need the help of another virus for the formation of infectious particles). In the case of the delta agent these features result in an infective agent that can be transmitted in parallel with hepatitis B.

Prions are proteinaceous infective agents that are responsible for the transmissible spongiform encephalopathies (see Ch. 60). An increase in the number of prion proteins in a new host seems to result from the capacity of the introduced protein to induce abnormal conformational changes in a closely related host protein, rather than by replication. Accumulation of the protein in the induced conformation produces the characteristic pathology of the disease.

## RECOMMENDED READING

Blair DF: How bacteria sense and swim, *Annual Review of Microbiology* 49:489–522, 1995.

Cabeen MT, Jacobs-Wagner C: Skin and bones, the bacterial cytoskeleton, cell wall, and cell morphogenesis, *Journal of Cell Biology* 179:381–387, 2007

Frey D, Oldfield RJ, Bridger RC: *A Colour Atlas of Pathogenic Fungi*, London, 1979, Wolfe Medical.

Li Z, Jensen GJ: Electron cryotomograpy: a new view into microbial ultrastructure, *Current Opinion in Microbiology* 12:333–340, 2009.

Madeley CR, Field AM: *Virus Morphology*, ed 2, Edinburgh, 1988, Churchill Livingstone.

Moat AG, Foster JW: *Microbial Physiology*, ed 4, New York, 2002, Wiley-Liss.

Neidhardt FC, Ingraham JL, Schaechter M: *Physiology of the Bacterial Cell: A Molecular Approach*, Sunderland, MA, 1990, Sinauer.

Nikaido H, Vaara M: Molecular basis of bacterial outer membrane permeability, *Microbiological Reviews* 49:1–32, 1985.

Olds RJ: *A Colour Atlas of Microbiology*, London, 1975, Wolfe Medical.

Proft T, Baker EN: Pili in Gram negative and Gram positive bacteria – structure, assembly and their role in disease, *Cellular and Molecular Life Sciences* 66:613–635, 2009.

Wadhams GH, Armitage JP: Making sense of it all: Bacterial chemotaxis, *Nature Reviews in Molecular Cell Biology* 5:1024–1037, 2004.

## Websites

CELLS alive! http://www.cellsalive.com/

Tree of Life Web Project. http://tolweb.org/tree/

University of California, Berkeley. More on bacterial morphology. http://www.ucmp.berkeley.edu/bacteria/bacteriamm.html

# 3 Classification, identification and typing of micro-organisms

*T. L. Pitt and M. R. Barer*

## KEY POINTS

- Taxonomy is the classification, nomenclature and identification of microbes (algae, protozoa, slime moulds, fungi, bacteria, archaea and viruses). The naming of organisms by genus and species is governed by an international code.
- Bacteria can be separated into two major divisions by their reaction to Gram's stain, and exhibit a range of shapes and sizes from spherical (cocci) through rod shaped (bacilli) to filaments and spiral shapes.
- In clinical practice, bacteria are classified by macroscopic and microscopic morphology, their requirement for oxygen, and activity in phenotypic and biochemical tests.
- Various diagnostic test systems are used to detect specific bacteria in clinical systems, including specific gene probes, reaction with antibodies in ELISA formats, immunofluorescence and, increasingly, PCR-based technology.
- Different bacterial species often exhibit different population structures, highly diverse (panmictic) or relatively uniform (clonal) depending mainly on the frequency of gene recombination (from external sources).
- Typing of bacterial isolates is necessary for epidemiological investigations in outbreaks and for surveillance, and a variety of phenotypic and genetic methods has evolved for the identification of strains.

Micro-organisms may be classified in the following large biological groups:

1. Algae
2. Protozoa
3. Slime moulds
4. Fungi
5. Bacteria
6. Archaea
7. Viruses.

The algae (excluding the blue–green algae), the protozoa, slime moulds and fungi include the larger *eukaryotic* (see Ch. 2) micro-organisms; their cells have the same general type of structure and organization as that found in plants and animals. The bacteria, including organisms of the mycoplasma, rickettsia and chlamydia groups, together with the related blue–green algae, comprise the smaller micro-organisms, with the form of cellular organization described as *prokaryotic*. The archaea are a distinct phylogenetic group of prokaryotes that bear only a remote ancestral relationship to other organisms (see Ch. 2). As the algae, slime moulds and archaea are not currently thought to contain species of medical or veterinary importance, they will not be considered further. Blue–green algae do not cause infection, but certain species produce potent peptide toxins that may affect persons or animals ingesting polluted water.

The viruses are the smallest of the infective agents; they have a relatively simple structure that is not comparable with that of a cell, and their mode of reproduction is fundamentally different from that of cellular organisms. Even simpler are *viroids*, protein-free fragments of single-stranded circular RNA that cause disease in plants. Another class of infectious particles are *prions*, the causative agents of fatal neurodegenerative disorders in animals and man. These are postulated to be naturally occurring host cell membrane glycoproteins that undergo conformative changes to an infectious isoform (see Ch. 60).

## TAXONOMY

*Taxonomy* consists of three components: *classification, nomenclature* and *identification*. Classification allows the orderly grouping of micro-organisms, whereas nomenclature concerns the naming of these organisms and requires agreement so that the same name is used unambiguously by everyone. Changes in nomenclature may give rise to confusion and are subject to internationally agreed rules. In clinical practice, micro-biologists are generally concerned with identification – the correct naming of isolates according to agreed systems of classification. These components, together with taxonomy, make up the overarching discipline of *systematics*, which is concerned with evolution, genetics and speciation of organisms, and is commonly referred to as *phylogenetics*.

Protozoa, fungi and helminths are classified and named according to the standard rules of classification and nomenclature that have been developed following the pioneering work of the eighteenth century Swedish botanist Linnaeus (Carl von Linné). Large subdivisions (class, order, family, etc.) are finally classified into individual *species* designated by a Latin binomial, the first term of which is the *genus*, e.g. *Plasmodium* (genus) *falciparum* (species). Occasionally it is useful to recognize a biological variant with particular properties: thus, *Trypanosoma* (genus) *brucei* (species) *gambiense* (variant) differs from the variant *T. brucei brucei* in being pathogenic for man.

Bacteria are similarly classified, but bacterial diversity encompasses more variety than all the rest of cellular life put together and the natural capacity of bacteria for genetic and phenotypic variation and adaptation make rigid classifications difficult. To date, identification has predominantly been performed by the use of keys that allow the organization of bacterial traits based on growth or activity in systems that test their biochemical properties. Some tests are definitive of a genus or species, for example the universal production of catalase enzyme and cytochrome c, respectively, by *Staphylococcus* spp. and *Pseudomonas aeruginosa*. Other characters may be unique to individual species and serve to differentiate them from organisms with closely similar biochemical activity profiles. Some bacteria do not grow in the laboratory (leprosy bacillus, treponemes), and identification by genetic methods may be necessary. As the technologies for genetic analysis become more readily applicable in clinical labs, so they and other rapid analytical methods, such as those based on mass spectrometry, are coming to replace the traditional biochemical methods to achieve identification. The taxonomic ranks used in the classification of bacteria are (example in parentheses):

- Kingdom (Prokaryotae)
- Division (Gracilicutes)
- Class (Betaproteobacteria)
- Order (Burkholderiales)
- Family (Burkholderiaceae)
- Genus (*Burkholderia*)
- Species (*Burkholderia cepacia*).

Some genera, such as *Acinetobacter*, have been subdivided into a number of genomic species by DNA homology analysis. Some are named and others are referred to only by a number. Many of the genomic species cannot be differentiated with accuracy by phenotypic tests. Another subgenus grouping in current usage recognizes species complexes, which are differentiated into genomovars by polyphasic taxonomic methods. A good example of this is the *B. cepacia* complex of organisms, which includes a very diverse group of organisms ranging from strict plant to human pathogens.

At present no standard classification of bacteria is universally accepted and applied, although *Bergey's Manual of Determinative Bacteriology* is widely used as an authoritative source. Bacterial nomenclature is governed by an international code prepared by the International Committee on Systematic Bacteriology and published as *Approved Lists of Bacterial Names* in the *International Journal of Systematic and Evolutionary Microbiology*; most new species are also first described in this journal, and a species is considered to be validly published only if it appears on a validation list in this journal.

The International Committee on Taxonomy of Viruses (ICTV) classifies viruses and publishes its reports in the journal *Archives of Virology*. Latin names are used wherever possible for the ranks family, subfamily and genus, but at present there are no formal categories higher than family and binomial nomenclature is not used for species. Viruses do not lend themselves easily to classification according to Linnaean principles, and vernacular names still have wide usage among medical virologists. Readers are referred to the standard work on virus taxonomy *Classification and Nomenclature of Viruses* and the ICTV database website.

## METHODS OF CLASSIFICATION

### Adansonian or numerical classification

In most systems of bacterial classification, the major groups are distinguished by fundamental characters such as cell shape, Gram-stain reaction and spore formation; genera and species are usually distinguished by properties such as fermentation reactions, nutritional requirements and pathogenicity. The relative 'importance' of different characters in defining major and minor groupings is often purely arbitrary. The uncertainties of arbitrary choices are avoided in the Adansonian system of taxonomy. This system determines the degrees of relationship between strains by a

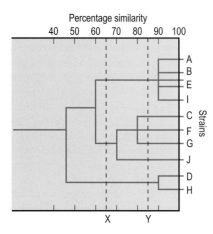

**Fig. 3.1** Hierarchical taxonomic tree (*dendrogram*) prepared from similarity matrix data. The dashed lines X and Y indicate levels of similarity at which separation into genera and species might be possible.

statistical coefficient that takes account of the widest range of characters, all of which are considered of equal weight. It is clear, of course, that some characters, for instance cell shape or Gram-stain reaction, represent a much wider and permanent genetic commitment than other characters which, being dependent on only one or a few genes, may be unstable. For this reason, the Adansonian method is most useful for the classification of strains within a larger grouping that shares major characters.

By scoring a large number of phenotypic characters it is possible to estimate a *similarity coefficient* when shared positive characters are considered or a *matching coefficient* when both negative and positive shared characters (matches) are taken into account. This numerical taxonomy is best performed on a computer that can calculate degrees of similarity for a group of different organisms; these data are displayed as a *similarity matrix* or a dendrogram tree (Fig. 3.1) (see also Owen 2004 in Recommended reading list).

## DNA composition

The hydrogen bonding between guanine and cytosine (G–C) base pairs in DNA is stronger than that between adenine and thymine (A–T). Thus, the melting or denaturation temperature of DNA (at which the two strands separate) is determined primarily by the G + C content. At the melting temperature, the separation of the strands brings about a marked change in the light absorption characteristics at a wavelength of 260 nm, and this is readily detected by spectrophotometry. There is a very wide range in the G + C

component of bacterial DNA, varying from about 25–80% mol in different genera. However, for any one species, the G + C content is relatively fixed, or falls within a very narrow range, and this provides a basis for classification.

## DNA homology

Another approach to classification is to arrange individual organisms into groups on the basis of the *homology* of their DNA base sequences. This exploits the fact that double strands re-form (anneal) from separated strands during controlled cooling of a heated preparation of DNA. This process can be readily demonstrated with suitably heated homologous DNA extracted from a single species, but it can also occur with DNA from two related species, so that hybrid pairs of DNA strands are produced. These hybrid pairings occur with high frequency between complementary regions of DNA, and the degree of hybridization can be assessed if labelled DNA preparations are used. Binding studies with messenger RNA (mRNA) can also give information to complement these observations, which provide genetic evidence of relatedness among bacteria. Organisms with different G + C ratios are unlikely to show significant DNA homology. However, organisms with the same, or close, G + C ratios do not necessarily show homology. A novel real-time polymerase chain reaction (PCR) (see pp. 31 and 79–80) has been described for estimation of G + C content.

## Ribosomal RNA sequencing

The structure of ribosomal RNA (rRNA) appears to have been highly conserved during the course of evolution, and close similarities in nucleotide sequences reflect phylogenetic relationships. Advances in technology have made nucleotide sequencing relatively simple, and the rDNA sequences (and other genes) of most medically important bacterial species are available from a number of internet sites. Far fewer full-length gene sequences are known for 23S rRNA than for 16S rRNA and 16S–23S internal transcribed sequences. In practice the DNA of the test organism is extracted and amplified by PCR using universal primers. The DNA sequence of the product is determined and the sequence compared against databases to find the closest fit. It is generally accepted that sequence similarity between 0.5% and 1.0% (with the type species) is required for the identification of an unknown organism, and less than 97% similarity is a common cut-off point for the differentiation of species. However, different species of *Mycobacterium* may exhibit more than 97% similarity in rDNA sequence. Commercial systems are available for bacterial species identification (MicroSeq; Applied Biosystems, Foster City, California, USA).

Nucleotide sequence variation in ribosomal genes is sometimes insufficient to discriminate between closely related species. Other candidate genes have been explored but the *recA* gene, which encodes a protein essential for repair and recombination of DNA, appears to be one of the best suited for phylogenetic analysis in that it defines evolutionary trees consistent with those observed for rRNA genes. Additional housekeeping genes used for phylogenetic studies include *rpoB* (RNA polymerase), *groEL* (heat shock protein) and *gyrB* (DNA gyrase), among others.

## CLASSIFICATION IN CLINICAL PRACTICE

The identification of micro-organisms in routine practice requires a pragmatic approach to taxonomy. The primary purpose of the names used is to communicate amongst the clinical and public health teams so that appropriate management of individuals and groups can be implemented. Unfortunately, as we learn more about the interrelatedness of microbes, largely through genome sequence data, certain reallocation and renaming becomes necessary in order to sustain a coherent relationship with our basic understanding. Table 3.1 outlines a simple, but practical, classification scheme in which organisms are grouped according to a few shared characteristics; as far as possible these have been reconciled with the relatively recently established phylogenetic nomenclature. Within these groups, organisms may be further identified, sometimes to species level, by a few supplementary tests. Protozoa, helminths and fungi can often be definitively identified on morphological criteria alone (see appropriate chapters).

## Protozoa

These are non-photosynthetic unicellular organisms with protoplasm clearly differentiated into nucleus and cytoplasm. They are relatively large, with transverse diameters mainly in the range of 2–100 μμm. Their surface membranes vary in complexity and rigidity from a thin, flexible membrane in amoebae, which allows major changes in cell shape and the protrusion of pseudopodia for the purposes of locomotion and ingestion, to a relatively stiff pellicle in ciliate protozoa, preserving a characteristic cell shape. Most free-living and some parasitic species capture, ingest and digest internally solid particles of food material; many protozoa, for instance, feed on bacteria. Protozoa, therefore, are generally regarded as the lowest forms of animal life, although certain flagellate protozoa are closely related in their morphology and mode of development to photosynthetic flagellate algae in the plant kingdom. Protozoa reproduce asexually by binary fission or multiple fission (*schizogony*), and some also by a sexual mechanism (*sporogony*).

**Table 3.1** Simplified classification of some cellular micro-organisms of medical importance

| Common group name | Normal genus names |
| --- | --- |
| **Eukaryotes** | |
| **Protozoa** | |
| Sporozoa | *Plasmodium, Isospora, Toxoplasma, Cryptosporidium* |
| Flagellates | *Giardia, Trichomonas, Trypanosoma, Leishmania* |
| Amoebae | *Entamoeba, Naegleria, Acanthamoeba* |
| Other | *Babesia, Balantidium* |
| **Fungi** | |
| Mould-like | *Epidermophyton, Trichophyton, Microsporum, Aspergillus* |
| Yeast-like | *Candida* |
| Dimorphic | *Histoplasma, Blastomyces, Coccidioides* |
| True yeast | *Cryptococcus* |
| | |
| **Prokaryotes** | |
| **Bacteria** | |
| Actinobacteria | (High G+C Gram positives) |
| | *Actinomyces, Streptomyces, Corynebacterium, Nocardia, Mycobacterium, Micrococcus* |
| Firmicutes | (Low G+C Gram positives) |
| Gram-positive bacilli | *Listeria, Bacillus, Clostridium\*, Lactobacillus\*, Eubacterium\** |
| Gram-positive cocci | *Staphylococcus, Streptococcus, Enterococcus* |
| Gram-negative cocci\*\* | *Veillonella\*, Mycoplasma* |
| Proteobacteria | (a very large group with 5 sub-divisions) |
| Gram-negative cocci | *Neisseria, Moraxella* |
| Gram-negative bacilli | Enterobacteria – *Escherichia, Klebsiella, Proteus, Salmonella, Shigella, Yersinia* |
| | Pseudomonads – *Pseudomonas, Burkholderia, Stenotrophomonas* |
| | *Haemophilus, Bordetella, Brucella, Pasteurella* |
| | *Rickettsia, Coxiella* |
| Gram-negative curved and spiral bacilli | *Vibrio, Spirillum, Campylobacter, Helicobacter* |
| Bacteroidetetes | *Bacteroides\*, Prevotella\** |
| Spirochaetes | *Borrelia, Treponema, Brachyspira, Leptospira* |
| Chlamydia | *Chlamydia* |

\*Anaerobic organism.
\*\*Exceptions in a predominantly Gram-positive group.

The most important groups of medical protozoa are the *sporozoa* (malaria parasites, etc.), amoebae and flagellates (see Ch. 62).

## Fungi

These are non-photosynthetic organisms that possess relatively rigid cell walls. They may be saprophytic or parasitic, and take in soluble nutrients by diffusion through their cell surfaces.

*Moulds* grow as branching filaments (*hyphae*), usually 2–10 μm in width, which interlace to form a meshwork (*mycelium*). The hyphae are coenocytic (i.e. have a continuous multinucleate protoplasm), being either non-septate or septate with a central pore in each cross-wall. Moulds reproduce by the formation of various kinds of sexual and asexual spores that develop from the vegetative (feeding) mycelium, or from an aerial mycelium that effects their air-borne dissemination (see Ch. 61).

*Yeasts* are ovoid or spherical cells that reproduce asexually by budding and also, in many cases, sexually, with the formation of sexual spores. They do not form a mycelium, although the intermediate *yeast-like fungi* form a pseudo-mycelium consisting of chains of elongated cells. The *dimorphic fungi* produce a vegetative mycelium in artificial culture, but are yeast-like in infected lesions. The higher fungi of the class *Basidiomycetes* (mushrooms), which produce large fruiting structures for aerial dissemination of spores, are not infectious for human beings or animals, although some species are poisonous.

## Bacteria

The main groups of bacteria are mostly distinguished by microscopic observation of their morphology and staining reactions. The Gram-staining procedure, which reflects fundamental differences in cell wall structure, separates most bacteria into two great divisions: *Gram-positive bacteria* and *Gram-negative bacteria* (see Ch. 2). Where bacteria can be Gram stained the cell shape and clustering are of practical value in identification. However, at this point the relationship of the older, largely phenotypic, classification system to the newer DNA sequence-based phylogenetic classification, which reflects the evolutionary relationships between groups, begins to break down and anomalies are apparent. Nonetheless, practical identification schemes used in clinical labs rely heavily on recognizing whether bacteria are Gram positive or negative, bacillary or coccal in shape, able to grow aerobically or anaerobically (see Ch. 4) and whether they form spores.

The major phylogenetic groupings of medically significant *bacteria* are:

- *Actinobacteria*, these are also recognised as Gram-positve bacteria with a high G + C content, many of which are capable of filamentous growth with true branching and which may produce a type of mycelium. Many members of this group do not stain well with the Gram method and, importantly, they include the mycobacteria which can be recognized with acid fast stains (see Ch. 2).
- *Firmicutes*, low G + C Gram-positive bacteria including bacilli, some of which are spore formers and cocci; the group includes most of the medically significant Gram-positives. Two groups that have presumably lost their Gram-positivity, *Veillonella* and *Mycoplasma* are included here.
- *Proteobacteria*, a very large of group of Gram-negative bacteria (bacilli and cocci) with five subdivisions (alpha, beta, gamma, delta and epsilon).
- *Bacteroidetes*, Gram-negative anaerobes.
- *Spirochaetes*, possessing cells with a tight spiral shape and an internal flagellum.
- *Chlamydiae*, which are strict intracellular parasites.

### Actinobacteria

These include antibiotic producing bacteria and a small number of highly significant pathogens.

- *Actinomyces.* Gram-positive, non-acid-fast, tend to fragment into short coccal and bacillary forms and not to form conidia; anaerobic (e.g. *Actinomyces israelii*).
- *Streptomyces.* Vegetative mycelium does not fragment into short forms; conidia form in chains from aerial hyphae (e.g. *Streptomyces griseus*).
- *Mycobacterium.* Acid-fast; Gram-positive, but does not readily stain by the Gram method; usually bacillary, rarely branching; make mycolic acids (e.g. *Mycobacterium tuberculosis*).
- *Nocardia.* Similar to *Actinomyces*, but aerobic and mostly acid-fast; make mycolic acids (e.g. *Nocardia asteroides*).
- *Corynebacterium.* Pleiomorphic (variably shaped) Gram-positive bacilli; make mycolic acids (e.g. *Corynebacterium diphtheriae*).

### Firmicutes

- *Streptococcus.* Gram-positive cocci, mainly adherent in chains due to successive cell divisions

**3**

occurring in the same axis (e.g. *Streptococcus pyogenes*); sometimes predominantly diplococcal (e.g. *Streptococcus pneumoniae*).
- *Staphylococcus.* Gram-positive cocci, mainly adherent in irregular clusters due to successive divisions occurring irregularly in different planes (e.g. *Staph. aureus*).
- *Mycoplasma and ureoplasma.* Pleiomorphic cocci that do not make peptidoglycan.
- *Veillonella.* Gram-negative; generally very small cocci arranged mainly in clusters and pairs; anaerobic (e.g. *Veillonella parvula*).
- *Gram-positive spore-forming bacilli.* The key medically relevant genera here the genera *Bacillus* and *Clostridium* (anaerobic). They are Gram positive, but liable to become Gram negative in ageing cultures. The size, shape and position of the spore may assist recognition of the species, for example the bulging, spherical, terminal spore ('drumstick' form) of *Clostridium tetani*.
- *Gram-positive non-sporing bacilli.* These include several genera. *Erysipelothrix* and *Lactobacillus* are distinguished by a tendency to grow in chains and filaments, and *Listeria* by flagella that confer motility.

## Proteobacteria

Gram-negative bacteria.

- *Alphaproteobacteria.* Include the cell dependent *Rickettsia* group, the facultatively intracellular *Brucella* group and the *Bartonella* group.
- *Betaproteobacteria.* Neisseria – cocci, mainly adherent in pairs and slightly elongated at right angles to axis of pairs (e.g. *Neisseria meningitidis*). Burkholderia – bacilli (*Burkholderia pseudomallei*).
- *Gammaproteobacteria.* Bacilli including the enterobacteria (*Escherichia coli*), and the genera *Pseudomonas*, *Legionella* and the curved vibrios (e.g. *Vibrio cholera*).
- *Deltaproteobacteria.* No medically significant bacteria.
- *Epsilonproteobacteria.* Curved and loosely spiral bacilli including the genera *Helicobacter* and *Campylobacter*.

## Bacteroidetes

Gram-negative non-sporing anaerobic bacilli.

- *Bacteroides*, *Prevotella* and *Porphyromonas* are major genera.

## Spirochaetales

These organisms differ from the other groups in being slender flexuous spiral filaments that, unlike the spirilla, are motile without possession of flagella. The staining reaction, when demonstrable, is Gram negative. The different varieties are recognized by their size, shape, waveform and refractility, observed in the natural state in unstained wet films by dark-ground microscopy. Genera of medical importance include *Borrelia*, *Treponema* and *Leptospira*.

## Chlamydiae

Chlamydiae have a complex intracellular cycle (e.g. *Chlamydia trachomatis*).

## Viruses

Viruses usually consist of little more than a strand of DNA or RNA enclosed in a simple protein shell known as a *capsid*. Sometimes the complete nucleocapsid may be enclosed in a lipoprotein envelope derived largely from the host cell. Viruses are capable of growing only within the living cells of an appropriate animal, plant or bacterial host; none can grow in an inanimate nutrient medium. The viruses that infect and parasitize bacteria are termed *bacteriophages* or *phages*. A simple classification of the viruses that are involved in human disease is shown in Table 3.2.

## IDENTIFICATION OF MICRO-ORGANISMS

Precise or *definitive* identification of bacteria is time consuming, contentious and best carried out in specialized reference centres. For most clinical purposes, clear, rapid guidance on the likely cause of an infection is required and, consequently, microbiologists usually rely on a few simple procedures, notably microscopy and culture, backed up, when necessary, by a few supplementary tests to achieve a *presumptive* identification. Microscopy is the most rapid test of all, but culture inevitably takes at least 24 hours, sometimes longer. More rapid tests are constantly being sought, and antigen detection methods and genetic detection methods are now well established (see below).

Most specimens for bacteriological examination, whether from human beings, animals or the environment, contain mixtures of bacteria, and it is essential to obtain *pure cultures* of individual isolates before embarking on identification. Non-cultural methods, such as antigen or nucleic acid based detection, do not

**Table 3.2** Principal types of virus causing human disease

| Type of virus | Examples |
|---|---|
| **RNA viruses** | |
| Orthomyxoviruses | Influenza A, B and C viruses |
| Paramyxoviruses | Parainfluenza viruses, mumps virus, measles virus, respiratory syncytial virus, Hendra virus, Nipah virus, human metapneumovirus |
| Rhabdoviruses | Rabies virus |
| Arenaviruses | Lassa virus |
| Filoviruses | Marburg and Ebola viruses |
| Togaviruses | Many arboviruses, rubella virus |
| Flaviviruses | Yellow fever virus, Dengue virus, Japanese encephalitis virus, West Nile virus, hepatitis C virus |
| Bunyaviruses | Hantaan virus |
| Coronaviruses | Human coronavirus, 229E (group 1), OC43 (group 2), NL63 (group 1-like novel corona viruses), SARS (zoonosis) |
| Caliciviruses | Norwalk-like viruses, hepatitis E virus |
| Picornaviruses | Enteroviruses: poliovirus (3 types), echovirus (31 types), Coxsackie A virus (24 types), Coxsackie B virus (6 types), enterovirus types 68–71, hepatitis A virus (type 72), rhinovirus, many serotypes |
| Retroviruses | Human immunodeficiency virus types 1 and 2, human T-lymphotropic virus types I and II |
| Reoviruses | Rotaviruses |
| **DNA viruses** | |
| Poxviruses | Variola, vaccinia, molluscum contagiosum virus, Orf virus |
| Herpesviruses | Herpes simplex virus types 1 and 2, varicella-zoster virus, cytomegalovirus, Epstein–Barr virus, human herpesvirus types 6, 7 and 8 |
| Adenoviruses | Many serotypes |
| Papovaviruses | JC virus, BK virus, human papillomavirus |
| Hepadnaviruses | Hepatitis B virus |
| Parvoviruses | B 19 virus, new human parvovirus |

SARS, severe acute respiratory syndrome.

have this disadvantage; however, they do have the potential limitation of being highly specific so that the investigator must know beforehand what it is necessary to look for.

## Microscopy

Morphology and staining reactions of individual organisms generally serve as preliminary criteria to place an unknown species in its appropriate biological group. A Gram-stain smear suffices to show the Gram reaction, size, shape and grouping of the bacteria, and the arrangement of any endospores. An unstained wet film may be examined with dark-ground illumination in the microscope to observe the morphology of delicate spirochaetes; an unstained wet film, or 'hanging-drop', preparation is examined with ordinary bright-field illumination for observation of motility. Capsules surrounding bacterial cells are demonstrated by 'negative staining' with India ink; the capsules remain unstained against the background of ink particles. To identify mycobacteria, or other acid-fast organisms, a preparation is stained by the Ziehl–Neelsen method or one of its modifications (see p. 16). The microscopic characters of certain organisms in pathological specimens may be sufficient for presumptive identification, for example tubercle bacilli in sputum, or *T. pallidum* in exudate from a chancre. However, many bacteria share similar morphological features, and further tests must be applied to differentiate them.

## Cultural characteristics

The appearance of colonial growth on the surface of a solid medium, such as nutrient agar, is often very characteristic. Attention is paid to the diameter of the colonies, their outline, their elevation, their translucency (clear, translucent or opaque) and colour. Changes brought about in the medium (e.g. haemolysis in a blood agar medium) may also be significant. The range of conditions that support growth is characteristic of particular organisms. The ability or inability of the organism to grow in the presence (aerobe) or absence (anaerobe) of oxygen, in a reduced oxygen atmosphere (micro-aerophile) or in the presence of carbon dioxide, or on media containing selective inhibitory factors (e.g. bile salt, specific antimicrobial agents, or low or high pH) may also be of diagnostic significance (see Table 4.1).

## Biochemical reactions

Species that cannot be distinguished by morphology and cultural characters may exhibit metabolic differences that can be exploited. It is usual to test the ability of the organism to produce acidic and gaseous end-products when presented with individual carbohydrates (glucose, lactose, sucrose, mannitol, etc.) as the sole carbon source. Other tests determine whether the bacterium produces particular end-products (e.g. indole or hydrogen sulphide) when grown in suitable culture media, and whether it possesses certain enzyme activities, such as oxidase, catalase, urease, gelatinase or lecithinase. Traditionally, such tests have been performed selectively and individually according to the recommendations of standard guides, such as the invaluable *Cowan and Steel's Manual for the Identification of Medical Bacteria*. However, today most diagnostic laboratories use commercially prepared microgalleries of identification tests which, though expensive, combine simplicity and accuracy. Test kits are now available for a number of different groups of organisms, including enterobacteria, staphylococci, streptococci and anaerobes. Other kits facilitate the testing of carbon source utilization, the assimilation of specific substrates and the enzymes produced by an organism.

On occasion, more elaborate procedures may be used for the analysis of metabolic products or whole-cell fatty acids. Indeed, a fully automated, fatty acid-based identification system, which combines high-resolution gas chromatography and pattern recognition software, is widely used to identify a variety of aerobic and anaerobic bacterial species. New profiles are added to a computerized database, thus increasing the sensitivity of the system. Mass spectrometric methods show promise for rapid identification, particularly matrix-assisted laser desorption ionization time-of-flight (MALDI-TOF) mass spectrometry. This offers the analysis of whole bacterial cultures for unique mass spectra from charged macromolecules by rapid, high-throughput testing with a rapidly growing database.

## INDIRECT IDENTIFICATION METHODS

### Gene-targeted analyses

These are fragments of DNA that recognize complementary sequences within micro-organisms (see p. 79). Binding is detected by tagging the DNA with a radioactive label, or with a reagent that can be developed to give a colour reaction, such as biotin. By selecting DNA fragments specific for features characteristic of individual organisms, gene probes can be tailored to the rapid identification of individual species in clinical material. The disadvantages of this approach are that the organism itself may be dead and a viable isolate is not made available for subsequent tests of susceptibility to antimicrobial agents, toxin production or epidemiological investigation.

Culture and preliminary identification of bacteria in the laboratory is time consuming and relatively labour intensive. Bacteria may also be uncultivable, slow growing, or fastidious in nutrient requirements. Nucleic acid techniques for the detection and identification of bacteria have evolved against this background; today numerous commercially available systems have been developed and many are in use in diagnostic laboratories. The technologies fall into three basic groups:

1. Target amplification by PCR, transcription-mediated amplification, nucleic acid sequence-based amplification, etc.
2. Probe amplification using ligase chain reaction or Q-beta replicase.
3. Signal amplification, as in branched DNA assay.

It is possible to detect the presence of an increasing number of species either by PCR of universal or specific gene targets or by hybridization with specific probes. As with conventional methods, nucleic acid technology has its limitations, the most frequent being contamination of a sample by post-amplification products. Other factors include operator skill, primer design, stringency of assay, presence of inhibitory compounds in the specimen and the ubiquity of the organism sought. The latter is fundamental to the interpretation of results as many bacterial pathogens occur naturally as commensals in certain body sites. The new technologies do, however, offer a considerable advantage over phenotypic methods in terms of sensitivity, and many optimized PCR systems claim to be able to detect as few as two to ten bacteria per millilitre of specimen, which is far below the threshold of conventional culture.

Nucleic acid assays for antimicrobial resistance genes are also in use and development. A recently described innovation may have the potential to detect, identify the species, subtype the organism and identify resistance genes on microscope slide smears. The technique uses peptide nucleic acid (PNA, pseudopeptides) with DNA binding capacity. The PNA molecules have a polyamide backbone instead of the sugar phosphate of DNA and RNA, and nucleotide bases attached to this backbone are able to hybridize by specific base pairing with complementary DNA or RNA sequences. PCR amplification of target genes on conventionally stained microscope smears is also possible, and this accelerates the prospect of very rapid and sensitive test methods limited only by the specificity of the primer for the target.

The availability of numerous prokaryotic genomic sequences has enabled the development of high-density oligonucleotide arrays which consist of many thousands of different probes. These arrays are constructed by in-situ oligonucleotide synthesis on a glass support by photolithography or other methods. Hybridization of the prelabelled target nucleic acids to the bound probe is detected directly with fluorescein or radioactive ligands, or indirectly using enzyme conjugates. Areas of application for high-density arrays include DNA sequencing, strain genotyping, identifying gene functions, location of resistance genes, changes in mRNA expression and phylogenetic relatedness. Arrays with selected gene targets have recently been developed in an Eppendorf tube format. The chip is embedded in the bottom of the tube and carries optimized sets of oligonucleotide probes specific for certain organisms or for antimicrobial resistance genes or virulence factors. In this way chips can be customized for individual bacteria or groups of bacteria. All stages of the assay – sample preparation from agar-grown colonies, PCR amplification, hybridization, conjugation with reporter molecule and detection by automated image recording – are carried out in a single tube within 6–8 hours.

A widely used development is that of real-time PCR, which combines sample amplification with a means for detection of the specific product by fluorescence so that both steps take place conveniently in a single reaction tube. The system has significant advantages over conventional PCR in terms of rapidity, simplicity and number of manual procedures; contamination is effectively eliminated by the tube being closed after amplification. The DNA product may be detected with a fluorescent dye, or increased specificity obtained with hybridization with fluorescence-labelled sequence-specific oligonucleotide probes. Quantification of the target DNA is also possible with this system, allowing estimation of viral or bacterial numbers in a specimen (see p. 79–80).

Fluorescence in-situ hybridization (FISH) directed to the multiple copies of 16S ribosomal RNA has also been used to detect bacteria directly in clinical specimens. This technique utilizes probes specific for target organisms in the sample without the need for culture and allows quantification of the cell count and morphology. Sensitivity and specificity vary according to the probe used, but if the probe is optimized it can rival conventional culture methods.

## Antibody reactions

Species and types of micro-organism can often be identified by specific serological reactions. These depend on the fact that the serum of an animal immunized against a micro-organism contains antibodies specific for the homologous species or type that react in a characteristic manner (e.g. agglutination or precipitation) with the particular micro-organism. Such simple in-vitro tests have been used for many years in microbiology, notably in the formal identification of presumptive isolates of pathogens (e.g. salmonellae) from clinical material. The specificity and range of antibody tests have been greatly improved by the availability of highly specific *monoclonal antibodies*. These are produced by the *hybridoma* technique in which individual antibody-producing spleen cells are

fused with 'immortal' tumour cells in vitro. The progeny of these hybrid cells produce only the type of antibody appropriate to the spleen cell precursor (see p. 125).

## Latex agglutination

By adsorbing specific antibody to inert latex particles, a visible agglutination reaction can be induced in the presence of homologous antigen. This principle can be applied in reverse to detect serum antibodies. Latex-based kits are widely used for serological grouping of organisms and detection of toxins produced by bacteria during growth.

## Enzyme–linked immunosorbent assay

In enzyme-linked immunosorbent assay (ELISA), a specific antibody is attached to the surface of a plastic well and material containing the test antigen is added. After washing, the presence of the antigen is detected by addition of more of the specific antibody, this time labelled with an enzyme that can initiate a colour reaction when provided with the appropriate substrate. The intensity of the colour change is related to the amount of antigen bound. The ELISA method may also be used in the reverse manner for the quantitative detection of antibodies, by adsorbing purified antigen to the well before adding test serum; in this case the enzyme-linked system used to detect the antigen–antibody reaction is a labelled anti-human globulin. In immunoglobulin (Ig) M antibody capture ELISA (MAC-ELISA), widely used in virological diagnosis for the detection of IgM, anti-human μ-chain antibody (usually raised in goats) is bound to the well. The test serum is added, and any IgM binds to the capture reagent; after washing, purified antigen (e.g. rubella antigen) is added, and this can be detected with an appropriate labelled antibody.

## Haemagglutination and haemadsorption

Certain viruses, notably the influenza viruses, have the property of attaching to specific receptors on the surface of appropriate red blood cells. In this manner the virus particles act as bridges linking the red cells in visible clumps. In tissue culture, such haemagglutinins may appear on the surface of cells infected with a virus. If red cells are added to the tissue culture, they adhere to the surface of infected cells, a phenomenon known as *haemadsorption*. Red blood cells can also be coated with specific antibody so that they agglutinate in the presence of the homologous virus particle in a

**Table 3.3** Panmictic versus clonal populations

|  | Reproduction | Recombination | Allele arrangement | Mutation | Selective pressures |
|---|---|---|---|---|---|
| Panmictic | Sexual* | Frequent | Segregated | Normal | Natural selection |
| Clonal | Asexual | Rare | Non-random association | Normal | Environmental |

*Refers to recombination between genetic elements from different organisms in bacteria.

manner similar to that described for latex agglutination above.

## Fluorescence microscopy and immunofluorescence

When certain dyes are exposed to ultraviolet light, they absorb energy and emit visible light; that is, they fluoresce. Tissues or organisms stained with such a dye and examined with ultraviolet light in a specially adapted microscope are seen as fluorescent objects; for example, auramine can be used in this way to stain *Mycobacterium tuberculosis*. Antibody molecules can be labelled by conjugation with a fluorochrome dye such as fluorescein isothiocyanate (which fluoresces green) or rhodamine (orange–red). When fluorescent antibody is allowed to react with homologous antigen exposed at a cell surface, this *direct immunofluorescence* procedure affords a highly sensitive method for the identification of the particular antigen. For this procedure it is necessary to have a specific antibody conjugate for each antigen; however, unconjugated antibody can be used and the reaction then detected by the addition of an antiglobulin conjugate, which will react with any antibody from the species in which the antibody was raised.

## Immuno–polymerase chain reaction

This technique arose out of the fusion of antibody technology with PCR methods with the aim of enhancing the capability of antigen detection systems. In immuno-PCR, a linker molecule with bispecific binding affinity for DNA and antibodies is used to attach a DNA molecule (marker) to an antigen–antibody complex. This produces a specific antigen–antibody–DNA conjugate. The attached DNA marker can be amplified by PCR with appropriate primers, and the presence of amplification products shows that the marker DNA is attached to antigen–antibody complexes, indicating the presence of antigen. The enhanced sensitivity of immuno-PCR achieved over ELISA is reported to be in excess of $10^5$, theoretically allowing as few as 580 antigen molecules ($9.6 \times 10^{-22}$ moles) to be detected.

## TYPING OF BACTERIA

Different bacterial species often exhibit different population structures. Some species are characterized by highly diverse populations at one extreme and closely similar members at the other. The frequency of recombination of chromosomal genes (see Ch. 6) is considered the major determinant of a population structure of a given species, and this frequency ranges from absent to low to very high. Highly recombining populations are termed *panmictic*, in contrast to *clonal* populations where recombination is infrequent (Table 3.3). Species such as *Neisseria gonorrhoeae* and *Haemophilus influenzae* are naturally transformable, that is, they are able to take up DNA (foreign and native) from their environment, and their populations are characterized by a high frequency of recombination, segregation of alleles and relatively low mutation. In clonal populations such as *Salmonella enterica,* recombination is rare and there is non-random association of alleles in a background of limited genetic exchange. Mutations occur as a result of natural and selective pressures, but these are not sufficient to disrupt the clonal lineage and daughter cells continue to resemble the ancestral parent. Bacterial clones are therefore not identical to their parents but display a number of characteristics in common with their ancestors. Many species are characterized by considerable genetic diversity but with clonal expansion of a subpopulation. Some of these clones may be transient, although others may persist and spread nationally and globally.

By *typing* we identify a recognizable subdivision of a species that serves as a reference marker against which other isolates of the same species can be compared. A population of bacteria presumed to descend from a single bacterium, as found in a natural habitat, in primary cultures from the habitat, and in subcultures from the primary cultures, is called a *strain.* Each primary culture from a natural source is called an *isolate*. The distinction between strains and isolates may be important; for example, cultures of typhoid bacilli isolated from ten different patients should be regarded simply as ten different *isolates* unless epidemiological or other evidence indicates that the patients have been infected from a common source with the same *strain*. The ability to discriminate between similar strains may be of great epidemiological value in tracing sources or modes of spread of infection in a community or hospital ward, and various typing methods have been devised. Strains may be distinguishable only in minor characters and it is usually simpler to establish differences between isolates from a common source than unequivocally to prove their identity. Demonstration of an identical response by a single reproducible typing method is not proof that two strains are the same. However, the confidence with which similarity can be inferred is greatly increased if more than one typing method is used.

Typing may inform different levels of epidemiological investigation, ranging from micro-epidemiology (local investigation), macro-epidemiology (regional, national, international) to population structure analysis (evolution of strains and global patterns of spread). The data derived may assist in the control of infection by excluding sources, identifying carriers and establishing the prevalence of individual strains. Common reasons for microbial typing are to identify common or point sources, discriminate between mixed strain infections, distinguish re-infection from relapse, and occasionally to identify a type and disease association (e.g. *Escherichia coli* O157 and haemolytic uraemic syndrome, skin and throat types of group A *Str. pyogenes*, etc.).

Typing methods should be reproducible both in the laboratory and clinically. The former is easily established by repeated tests on a sample of experimental strains, but should also be established in vivo by examining multiple pairs of isolates from single sources to determine the stability of the strain characteristics probed by the typing method used. A typing method should also discriminate adequately and clearly between different populations and be comprehensive, that is, assign most populations to a type. The typing data should be in a format that is easily assimilated into databases and should be able to be incorporated into the national picture to inform other workers in the field. Very few, if any, single typing methods will meet these criteria and hence there is a need to utilize different methods, preferably directed at unlinked targets and always in the context of an epidemiological investigation.

## Biotyping

Biochemical test reactions that are not universally positive or negative within a species may define *biotypes* of the species, and these may be efficient strain markers. In practice biotyping is often less discriminatory than other strain typing methods and may be unstable because of loss of the property. Differences among strains may also be detected by variations in sensitivity to fixed concentrations of chemicals such as heavy metals, a process known as *resistotyping*. The nutritional requirements of the isolate (amino acids) for growth may also be used to define the *auxotype* of an isolate.

## Serotyping

Many surface structures of bacteria (lipopolysaccharide and outer membrane, flagella, capsule, etc.) are antigenic, and antibodies raised against them can be used to group isolates into defined *serotypes*. Some species are characterized by numerous antigenic types and serotyping for these species is highly discriminatory, whereas for others conservation of antigen epitopes renders serotyping of little value for epidemiological purposes. Members of the species *Salmonella enterica* are defined by their somatic and flagellar serotypes (see Ch. 24). Capsular antigens may be associated with pathogenicity of the organism, and many vaccines protect the individual against infection by stimulating antibodies to capsular antigen epitopes. Agglutination of bacterial suspensions with rabbit antibodies is the most commonly used method for typing, but other techniques such as precipitation in agar gels, ELISA and capsular swelling (Fig. 3.2) may be used.

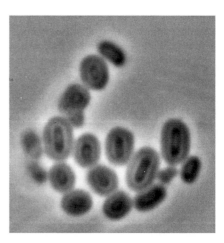

**Fig. 3.2** Capsular swelling reaction of *Klebsiella pneumoniae*. Antibody adsorbed to capsule alters the refractive index, allowing visualization of the capsule around the cell within.

## Phage typing

Bacteria often show differential susceptibility to lysis by certain bacteriophages. The phage adsorbs to a specific receptor on the bacterial surface and injects its DNA into the host. Phage DNA may become stably integrated into the bacterial chromosome and this state is referred to as *lysogeny*; phages capable of this are called *temperate phages*. In lysogeny, a small proportion of host cells express the phage genes, and some cell lysis and liberation of phage progeny occurs. Alternatively, the phage DNA may enter a replicative cycle, leading to the death of the host and the production of new phage particles. These *lytic* or *virulent* wild phages lyse the bacterium at the end of the replicative cycle and release a large number of daughter phage particles that infect neighbouring cells.

This process leads to visible inhibition of the growth of the host cells (Fig. 3.3). The *phage type* of the culture is identified according to the pattern of susceptibility to a set of lytic and/or temperate phages. Lytic phages may be readily recovered from sewage, waste and river water, and temperate phages may be released from a lysogenic strain by induction with ultraviolet radiation or chemical mutagens.

The critical factors governing the interpretation of phage typing results are discrimination and reproducibility. If the system is both highly discriminatory and reproducible, any differences in lysis patterns of isolates will indicate that they represent different strains.

**Fig. 3.3** Phage-mediated lysis of red pigmented strain of *Serratia marcescens.*

Schemes that utilize adapted phages (a single phage propagated in different strains) that are specific for a particular receptor site such as the Vi polysaccharide of *Salmonella enterica* serotype Typhi are relatively reproducible, and minor differences are significant and reproducible. On the other hand, a phage set comprising random unrelated phages may adhere to a number of different receptor sites and have different biological properties, and so is unlikely to be highly reproducible but may be adequately discriminating. This lack of stability results in the definition of broad phage groups rather than defined types, and is the case for *Staph. aureus* where at least two strong lytic reactions have to be present in the patterns of isolates before they can be termed distinct strains.

## Bacteriocin typing

Bacteriocins are naturally occurring antibacterial substances, elaborated by most bacterial species, that are active mainly against strains of the same genus as the producer strain. Bacteriocin typing may define the spectrum of bacteriocins produced by field strains, or the sensitivity of these strains to bacteriocins of a standard panel of strains. Patterns of production or susceptibility to bacteriocins allow the division of species into *bacteriocin types*.

## Protein typing

Bacteria manufacture thousands of proteins that can be visualized by electrophoresis in acrylamide gels in the presence of a strong detergent. The proteins separate according to molecular size and, after staining with a dye, the pattern of bands from each isolate can be compared. This system has been used successfully to type many bacterial and fungal species, but lacks reproducibility. Investigation of microbial populations by gel electrophoresis of metabolic enzymes, which can then be detected by specific substrates, has also in the past been applied widely for clonal analysis within species.

## Restriction endonuclease typing

*Restriction endonucleases* are a family of enzymes that each cut DNA at a specific sequence recognition site, which may be rare or frequent in the DNA of the species being examined. The frequency with which an enzyme cuts in a particular species is dependent on the oligonucleotide sequence, the frequency of the restriction site, and the percentage G + C content of the species. For example, the recognition site of enzyme *Sma*I is 5′-CCC↓GGG-3′ (↓ site of cleavage) and this cuts infrequently in the AT-rich genome of *Staph. aureus*, whereas enzyme *Xba*I (5′-T↓CTAGA-3′) is a rare cutter in most Gram-negative species with a high GC content. Both plasmid and chromosomal DNA can be analysed by this means. Frequent-cutting endonucleases generate numerous small fragments that can be resolved by conventional electrophoresis in agarose gel and detected by staining with a dye. The resolution of conventional agarose gel electrophoresis does not exceed 20 kb and optimal separation in standard length gels is achieved between 1 and 15 kb.

The large DNA fragments produced by infrequent-cutting enzymes need to be separated in special electrical fields with a pulsed current (*pulsed-field gel electrophoresis*; PFGE). In this technique, bacteria are encased in an agarose plug (to minimize shearing of DNA) and the cells are digested with proteinase K enzyme before the DNA is digested with the enzyme. By introducing a pulse or change in the direction of the electric field, fragments as large as 10 Mb can be separated. The time taken by fragments to reorient to the alternate electric field is proportional to their molecular size and where they migrate in the electric field. The most widely used apparatus is the contour-clamped homogeneous electric field (CHEF), which has 24 electrodes arranged in a hexagonal array. Run times are often of the order of 30–40 hours, but shorter, more rapid, protocols have been described. A number of factors influence the quality of results, including DNA quality and concentration, agarose concentration, voltage and pulse times, and buffer strength and temperature.

Interpretation of PFGE profiles can be problematic. For some species the criteria of Tenover (see recommended reading list) can be applied to establish the significance of differences in banding profiles of strains. As a rule of thumb, isolates from an incident under investigation that show no difference in profiles can be considered indistinguishable, those with one to three band differences as closely related, four to six bands as possibly related, and seven or more band differences as indicating distinct strains. However, this rule should be applied with a degree of caution as some species (e.g. *Enterococcus faecium*) can exhibit significant variation (six to ten band differences) apparently within members of the same clone. A number of computer-assisted analysis packages are available that calculate coefficients of similarity between strains and represent these as dendrograms (Fig. 3.4). Two commonly employed coefficients, the Jaccard and Dice, use the number of concordant bands in profiles and the total number of possible band positions to calculate the percentage similarity between the isolates. The Pearson coefficient gives the advantage that specific band positions do not have to be defined. A cut-off point of 85% similarity is often used but, as for the band difference rule, this should be set by experiment with related and unrelated strain sets.

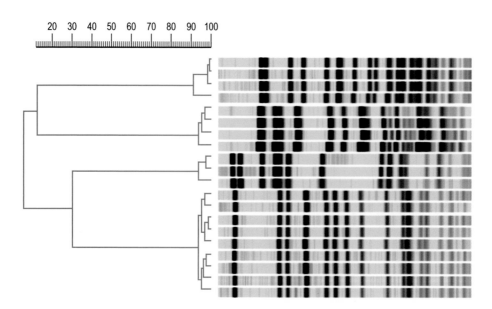

**Fig. 3.4** Pulsed-field gel electrophoresis profiles of *Xba*I digests of DNA of *Ps. aeruginosa* isolates. Dendrogram shows relative percentage similarity of profiles calculated with Pearson's coefficient.

## Gene probe typing

DNA probes (see above) for strain typing consist of cloned specific, random or universal sequences that can detect restriction site heterogeneity in the target DNA. The detection of variation in rDNA gene loci is the basis of *ribotyping*, and this method has been universally applied to the typing of various species. Other commonly used probes are *insertion sequences* (lengths of DNA involved in transposition; see Ch. 6) that may define clonal structures of populations.

## Polymerase chain reaction typing

PCR is a technique that allows specific sequences of DNA to be amplified. Multiple copies of regions of the genome defined by specific oligonucleotide primers are made by repeated cycles of amplification under controlled conditions. Such methods can be used to study DNA from any source. Several variations on the PCR theme have been described, and use of these techniques continues to expand and develop. PCR-mediated DNA fingerprinting makes use of the variable regions in DNA molecules. These may be variable numbers of tandem repeat regions or areas with restriction endonuclease recognition sequences. To perform PCR typing, it is necessary to know the sequences of the bordering regions so that specific oligonucleotide primers can be synthesized. Primers may be specific for a known sequence or be random. Random primers are extensively used in the techniques of *random amplification of polymorphic DNA* (RAPD) and *arbitrarily primed PCR* (AP-PCR). Both of these approaches have problems with reproducibility as a result of false priming, faint versus sharp bands and variation in electrophoretic migration of products. Repetitive sequence-based PCR (rep-PCR) indexes variation in multiple interspersed repetitive sequences in intergenic regions dispersed throughout the genome. An automated, standardized rep-PCR system has proven useful for strain typing of a number of species and is reported to give similar discrimination to PFGE (Bacterial Barcodes, Houston, Texas, USA). Amplified fragment length polymorphism is a DNA sequence-based technique that combines restriction endonuclease digestion with PCR. Incorporation of a fluorescent label and the use of a capillary DNA sequencer allows optimal standardization of reproducibility and resolution of single base-pair differences between genomes.

## Multilocus sequence typing

This technique indexes allelic variation in several housekeeping genes by nucleotide sequencing rather than indirectly from the electrophoretic mobilities of their gene products, as was the case with its parent technique, multilocus enzyme electrophoresis. Housekeeping genes are not subject to selective forces as are variable genes and they diversify slowly. Multiple genes (usually seven) are employed to overcome the effects of recombination in a single locus, which might distort the interpretation of the relationship of the strains being compared. Multilocus sequence typing (MLST) can rightly be referred to as definitive genotyping as sequence data are unambiguous and databases of allelic profiles of isolates of individual species are accessible via the internet. The level of discrimination of MLST depends on the degree of diversity within the population to generate alleles at each locus, but some highly uniform species such as *M. tuberculosis* are not amenable to analysis by the technique. Recently, increased discrimination has been sought in virulence-associated genes necessary for survival and spread of the organism on the basis that these genes are exposed to frequent environmental changes and thus provide a higher degree of sequence variation. Intergenic regions of selected genes are amplified by PCR and a 500-bp internal fragment sequenced to identify allelic polymorphisms.

A variant of MLST termed multilocus restriction typing introduces restriction digestion of amplified housekeeping genes and removes the need for sequencing. The restriction fragment length polymorphisms (RFLPs) can be sorted into type patterns and reveal population structures similar to those with MLST.

## Variable number tandem repeat analysis

Variable number tandem repeats (VNTRs) are short nucleotide sequences (20–100 bp) that vary in copy number in bacterial genomes. They are thought to arise through DNA strand slippage during replication and are of unknown function. Separate VNTR loci are identified from published sequences and are often located in intergenic regions and annotated open reading frames. Primers are designed to amplify five to eight loci and the products sequenced to generate a digital profile. VNTR typing is rapid and reproducible, and relatively simple to perform. Improved discrimination may be achieved by identification of more loci but there is debate about their stability over time.

## Whole genome based typing

The advent of new high throughput DNA sequencing methods is ushering in a new era in which it is becoming feasible to compare and type bacteria based on entire genome sequence data. These massively parallel sequencing technologies produce relatively short nucleotide sequence reads but on such a scale that these can be assembled into a sequence matched against those obtained from previous isolates of that organism. This enables a genome-wide comparison to be made and a more or less definitive evolutionary relationship to be established to other contemporaneous and historical isolates. The costs of such analyses are rapidly becoming competitive with traditional typing methods. Such analyses have the potential to transform medical bacteriology by producing unambiguous epidemiological information and by identifying genetic elements such as those encoding antibiotic resistance and significant antigens under selection pressures.

## RECOMMENDED READING

Barrow GI, Feltham RKA, editors: *Cowan and Steel's Manual for the Identification of Medical Bacteria*, ed 3, Cambridge, 1993, Cambridge University Press.

Garrity GM, editor: *Bergey's Manual of Systematic Bacteriology*, ed 2, New York, 2005 Springer.

Kaufmann ME: Pulsed-field gel electrophoresis. In Woodford N, Johnson AP, editors: *Methods in Molecular Medicine*, Vol. 15: *Molecular Bacteriology: Protocols and Clinical Applications*, Totowa, NJ, 1998, Humana Press, pp 33–50.

Murray PR, Baron EJ, Jorgensen JH, et al, editors: *Manual of Clinical Microbiology*, ed 8, Washington, DC, 2003, ASM Press.

Owen RJ: Bacterial taxonomics: finding the wood through the phylogenetic trees, *Methods in Molecular Biology* 266:353–384, 2004.

Schleifer KH: Classification of *Bacteria* and *Archeaea*: Past, present and future, *Systematic and Applied Microbiology* 32:533–542, 2009.

Spratt BG, Feil EJ, Smith NH: Population genetics of bacterial pathogens. In Sussman M, editor: *Molecular Medical Microbiology*, San Diego, 2002, Academic Press, pp 445–484.

Tenover FC, Arbeit RD, Goering RV, et al: Interpreting chromosomal DNA restriction patterns produced by pulsed-field gel electrophoresis: criteria for strain typing, *Journal of Clinical Microbiology* 33: 2233–2239, 1995.

Van Regenmortel MHV, Fauquet CM, Bishop DHL, editors: *Virus Taxonomy. Classification and Nomenclature of Viruses*. San Diego, 2000, Academic Press.

Woese CR: Interpreting the universal phylogenetic tree, *Proceedings of the National Academy of Sciences of the USA* 97:8392–8396, 2000.

### Websites

Genotyping database at Oxford University. http://www.mlst.net/

National Center for Biotechnology information for rRNA sequence analysis. http://www.ncbi.nlm.nih.gov/Genbank/

Ribosomal differentiation of medical microorganisms for rRNA sequence analysis. http://www.ridom-rdna.de/

Universal virus database of the International Committee on Taxonomy of Viruses. http://www.ictvdb.org/

# 4 Bacterial growth, physiology and death

*M. R. Barer*

## KEY POINTS

- Bacterial growth and multiplication is of practical value in the detection and identification of pathogens, and is generally a necessary component of infection.
- Bacteria divide asexually through a process of *binary fission*, passing through *lag, exponential* and *stationary* phases of *planktonic* growth in broth cultures. Bacterial growth can also be recognized in *sessile* form as *colonies* or *biofilms*. A given bacterial strain may have profoundly different physiological properties in each of these growth states.
- Recovery of pure bacterial cultures was greatly enhanced by the development of solidified agar media. Different medium designs enable *selection, enrichment, identification or defined* growth conditions.
- Different bacteria have evolved to grow and survive in widely differing habitats and these define their potential reservoirs and sources of infection. The growth atmospheres required by different bacteria are an important defining characteristic, and *obligate*

*aerobes, obligate anaerobes, micro-aerophilic* and *facultative* organisms are recognized.
- Bacterial viability is generally recognized and quantified by detecting growth of single cells into colonies in colony-forming unit (cfu) counts. Discrepancies between cfu counts and the number of cells seen by microscopy have led to recognition that many cells in natural samples do not form colonies.
- Bacteria may die through senescence in stationary cultures, through genetically programmed or prophage-induced cell death, or as result of external noxious influences such as antibiotics or the deliberate processes of *sterilization* and *disinfection*.
- Sterilization involves the destruction of all propagating biological entities, whereas disinfection involves a reduction in microbial load to an acceptable level. Both processes can be achieved by application of *moist and dry heat, ionizing radiation, filtration, gaseous chemical agents* and *liquid chemical agents*.

Most of what we know about bacteria derives from their growth. Their ability to propagate may be seen as a supreme achievement that enables them to attain enormous populations at rates that are breathtaking from a human perspective. These properties underpin their capacity for change by mutation and the rapidity with which some infections develop.

Bacterial growth involves both an increase in the size of organisms and an increase in their number. Whatever the balance between these two processes, the net effect is an increase in the total mass (*biomass*) of the culture. Medical microbiologists have traditionally concentrated on the number of individuals in growth studies. Whether this emphasis on cell number is appropriate remains uncertain; none the less, it will be adopted here, as the number of individual bacteria involved is important in the course and outcome of infections and in the measurement of the effects of antibiotics.

Students of medicine may be surprised and even dismayed to hear that organisms as small as bacteria have a physiology. However, the complement of enzymes and the biochemical and biophysical processes occurring in a prokaryotic cell at any one time represent the product of genetic and biochemical control mechanisms that are every bit as sophisticated and tightly regulated as those in eukaryotic cells. Moreover, the recognition and definition of the mechanisms by which bacteria sense and adapt to nutritional and noxious stimuli in their environments have provided insights that are likely to translate into medically significant advances in the foreseeable future.

In some sense asexual organisms such as bacteria appear to be immortal, but bacterial death or loss of viability occurs in many natural settings. This has practical consequences, as only viable bacteria can initiate infections and most microscopic, molecular and immunological detection methods do not differentiate between live and dead organisms. Of course, we often need to assess the lethal effects of antibiotics and processes aimed at *sterilization, disinfection* and *antisepsis*. The practical approach to assessing the effects of antibiotics is introduced in Chapter 5, but the principles of sterilization and disinfection are introduced here.

Although this chapter discusses growth and physiology only from a bacteriological perspective, some of the principles are also applicable to fungi, particularly yeasts. The central difference between their growths is that cell division is generally achieved in bacteria by *binary fission* to produce identical offspring that cannot be distinguished as parents and progeny, whereas fungi divide by budding in the case of yeast growth and hyphal septation in the mould form. In contrast, the principles of sterilization and disinfection refer to all infective agents. Their application is considered further in Chapter 68.

## BACTERIAL GROWTH

When placed in a suitable nutritious environment and maintained under appropriate physical and chemical conditions, a bacterial cell begins to grow; when it has manufactured approximately twice the amount of component materials that it started with, it divides. The range of specific components that define 'suitable' and 'appropriate' for all known bacteria (and *Archaea*) is so broad that it actually defines the global biosphere (those environments that can sustain life), and includes temperatures and pressures present at the opening of hydrothermal vents on the ocean floor to the outer reaches of the atmosphere. Although these conditions do not regularly occur in man, they serve to illustrate that no part of the body or medical device with which it may come in contact is too difficult for bacteria to colonize and that bacteria may lurk in surprising environmental niches. Conversely, the conditions required for some organisms to grow are so precise that, so far, we have not been able to reproduce them in artificial laboratory media. This applies to some well known organisms such as the agents of leprosy and syphilis, but also to many other potential pathogens about which we are beginning to learn through molecular methods that do not depend on growth. In fact, it is estimated that we have not yet isolated more than 1%

of all the bacterial species that exist, and it is almost certain that there are many medically important organisms among the 'as yet uncultivated' micro-organisms.

As the central technique in bacteriology, growth in the laboratory has been used to serve many different purposes. From the clinical perspective, growth is used for detection and identification, and for the assessment of antibiotic effects, whereas scientific and industrial objectives are often served by growth in bulk to obtain sufficient biomass for detailed biochemical analysis and to produce the desirable products of the brewing and biotechnology industries.

## Types of growth

In the laboratory, bacterial growth can be seen in three main forms:

1. By the development of *colonies*, the macroscopic product of 20–30 cell divisions of a single cell.
2. By the transformation of a clear broth medium to a turbid suspension of $10^7$–$10^9$ cells per mL.
3. In *biofilm* formation, in which growth is spread thinly (300–400 μm thick) over an inert surface and nutrition obtained from a bathing fluid.

In natural systems only biofilms, such as those that develop on the surfaces of intravascular cannulae, appear to function in a manner comparable to biofilms produced in the laboratory, whereas colonies, the other form of *sessile* growth, rarely reach macroscopic dimensions. Turbid liquid systems caused by *planktonic* growth of a single organism are also a rarity in nature. Single organism infections affecting normally sterile sites in the body are one exception to this, whereas most natural microbial communities are complex assemblies of micro-organisms competing, and in many cases co-operating, to exploit the local resources. However, in spite of these unrepresentative features, pure growth of single organisms in *monocultures* to produce macroscopic colonies or high cell densities in broth offer great practical advantages and remain central techniques.

While much has been learned about the nature of bacteria by studying them in lab cultures, it is clear that they change their properties in different patterns of growth and non-growth, and in response to their environment. Thus, when we try to treat or immunize by targeting properties revealed in standard lab cultures, we often fail because the organism is not expressing those properties. This is particularly the case for bacteria in biofilms and in non-replicating states.

**Fig. 4.1**  Phases of growth in a broth culture.

## Growth phases in broth culture

Bacterial growth in broth has been studied in great detail and has provided a framework within which the growth state or growth phase of any given pure culture of a single organism can be placed; these phases are summarized in the idealized *growth curve* shown in Figure 4.1. When growth is initiated by inoculation into appropriate broth conditions, the number of cells present appears to remain constant for the *lag phase*, during which cells are thought to be preparing for growth. Increase in cell number then becomes detectable, and its rate accelerates rapidly until it is established at the maximum achievable rate for the available conditions. This is known as the *exponential phase*, because the number of cells is increasing exponentially with time. To accommodate the astronomic changes in number, the growth curve is normally displayed on a logarithmic scale, which shows a linear increase in log cell number with time (hence the older term, *log phase*). This log-linear relationship is sufficiently constant for a given bacterial strain under one set of conditions that it can be defined mathematically, and is often quoted as the *doubling time* for that organism. Doubling times have been measured at anything between 13 min for *Vibrio cholerae* and 24 h for *Mycobacterium tuberculosis*. On this basis it is not surprising that cholera is a disease that can kill within 12 h, whereas tuberculosis takes months to develop. A further consequence is that, when specimens are submitted to diagnostic laboratories for the detection of these organisms by culture, a result is usually available for *V. cholerae* the next day, whereas several weeks are required for conventional culture of *M. tuberculosis*.

It is often difficult to grasp fully the scale of exponential microbial growth; the message may be strengthened by considering that the progeny of a lecture theatre containing 150 students would exceed the global population of humanity ($6 \times 10^9$) within 8.5 h if they were able to breed like *Escherichia coli*!

Exponential growth cannot be sustained indefinitely in a closed (*batch*) system with limited available nutrients. Eventually growth slows down, and the total bacterial cell number reaches a maximum and stabilizes. This is known as the *stationary* or *post-exponential phase*. At this stage it becomes important to know what method has been used to determine the growth curve. If a direct method that assesses the total number of cells present is used then the count remains constant. Such methods include counting cells in a volumetric chamber observed by microscopy, electronic particle counters and measurement of turbidity. If, however, the growth potential of the individual cells present in the culture is assessed by taking regular samples, making tenfold dilutions of these and inoculating them on to agar, the number of *colony-forming units* (cfu) per unit volume can be determined at each sample time. Although such cfu counts closely parallel the results obtained by direct counting methods in the exponential and early stationary phases, a divergence begins to emerge towards the end of the latter; the total cell number remains constant whereas the colony count declines. This marks the beginning of the final, *decline phase*, in the sequence of growth states that can be observed in broth. The discrepancy between the total and cfu counts is conventionally held to represent the death of cells because of nutrient exhaustion and accumulation of detrimental metabolic end-products. However, there is some doubt concerning this interpretation (see below).

As noted above there has been increased interest in the properties of bacteria in non-growing states. While there are many different systems for studying non-replicating bacteria and their separate relevance to infection is argued, one phenomenon is of particular interest as it illustrates their capacity for adaptation based on mutation. The growth advantage in stationary phase (GASP) phenomenon is now well established and illustrates that while total cell numbers in a population may remain constant or decline, multiple genetic variants arise, some of which come to dominate the population. The genes and polymorphisms that lead to the growth advantage have been informative in improving our understanding of survival and competition under nutrient limited conditions.

The study of bacterial growth in broth provides a valuable point of reference to which practical, experimental and routine diagnostic procedures are often related. For example, the length of the lag phase and rates of exponential growth in different circumstances are used to make predictions and contribute to safety standards for storage in the food industry. An important feature to emerge is that cultures inoculated with cells prepared at different stages in the growth curve yield different results. The exponential phase is the most reproducible and readily identified, and is therefore used most frequently. It can be extended in an open system known as *continuous culture* using a *chemostat* in which cells of a growing culture are harvested continuously and nutrients replenished continuously. Chemostat studies have provided very detailed information on the chemistry of microbial growth and the way in which different organisms convert specific substrates into biomass. The extraordinary efficiency of this process has made natural and genetically manipulated microbes a powerful resource for the biotechnology industry.

In contrast to growth in broth, far less is known about the state of the bacteria in a mature macroscopic colony on an agar plate. Such a colony presents a wide range of environments, from an abundance of oxygen and nutrients at the edge to almost no oxygen or nutrients available to cells in the centre. It is likely that all phases of growth are represented in colonies, depending on the location of a particular cell and the age of the culture. Although in practice colonies can be used reliably to inoculate routine tests of antimicrobial susceptibility in clinical laboratories, they cannot be considered a defined starting point for experimental work because they comprise such a heterogeneous population of cells. In fact, colonies are complex and dynamic communities in which cells at different locations can show startlingly different phenotypes. In spite of its complexity, the capacity for and quality of colonial growth of specific organisms on specialized media is central to the laboratory description of medically important bacteria.

## MEDIA FOR BACTERIAL GROWTH

The media used in a medical diagnostic bacteriology laboratory have their origins, for the most part, back in the 'golden age of bacteriology' in the late nineteenth and early twentieth centuries. A vast amount of experience and knowledge has accrued from their use and, apart from better standardization and quality control in their production, little has changed in their basic design. The objectives of early medium design were to grow pathogenic bacteria, separate them from other organisms present in samples and, ultimately, differentiate their phenotypic properties so that they

could be identified. A critical development was the introduction of solidifying agents, most particularly the largely indigestible polysaccharide extract of seaweed known as agar. Alternative solidifying agents include gelatine and egg albumen. Before the development of solid media, pure cultures could be achieved only by dilution of inocula so that only one growing cell or clump of cells was present at the initiation of growth, a very laborious and unreliable procedure. In contrast, solid media in Petri dishes provided a growth substrate on to which mixed cultures could be inoculated and, provided the population density could be made low enough to allow development of well separated colonies, the different organisms present could be differentiated and subsequently separated into pure cultures.

## Media used for isolation and identification of pathogens

The central features of media in medical bacteriology are:

1. a source of protein or protein hydrolysate, often derived from casein or an infusion of brain, heart or liver obtained from the nearest butcher
2. control of pH in the final product (after sterilization)
3. a defined salt content.

Early media often included blood or serum in an attempt to reproduce nutritional features present in the human body. Growth of some pathogens was found to be dependent on such supplements, and it was recognized that these relatively *fastidious* or *nutritionally exacting* organisms were dependent on *growth factors*. The identity of many of the growth factors is now known (e.g. haemin and several coenzymes), but blood often remains their most convenient source.

### Selective and indicator media

Tremendous ingenuity has gone into designing growth media that provide information relevant to patient management as early as possible. There are two main approaches, both of which depend on adding supplements to the basal medium. *Selective media* contain substances such as bile salts or antibiotics that inhibit the growth of some organisms but have little or no effect on the organisms for whose isolation they were designed. They are essential for samples containing a normal microbial flora such as faeces. The inclusion of components or specific reagents that show whether the bacteria possess a particular biochemical property characterizes an *indicator medium*. Such media are critical to the rapid presumptive identification of isolates. Combinations of selective and indicator supplements in agar media have led to formulations with some remarkably elegant differential properties that effectively colour-code the colonies according to their biochemical properties and restrict growth to a desired range of organisms. Broth indicator media tend to be much simpler, as they generally require a pure inoculum of a single organism and reveal only one property per formulation. Broth media with selective properties are usually referred to as *enrichment media* as they change the balance of organisms inoculated in favour of the desired range of organisms, thereby enriching them.

## Media for laboratory studies

Most of the objectives of a clinical diagnostic laboratory can be fulfilled with the range of media outlined above. However, the composition of these media is not defined, and this poses problems for some investigations, including the detailed analysis of antibiotic action. Wherever possible, such investigations are based on a *defined* or *synthetic medium* where every chemical component is carefully regulated. In genetic experiments use is often made of a *minimal medium* in which every component is required for the growth of the organism under investigation, so that if one component is removed growth cannot occur. Minimal media also prevent the growth of mutants that have additional nutritional requirements to those of the parent strain. For some organisms, particularly those that can grow outside the human body, minimal media may comprise as little as an ammonium salt to provide nitrogen, a carbon source, which in some cases can be as simple as methane or carbon monoxide, trace amounts of iron and other essential elements, and pH adjustment to within an appropriate range. Defined and minimal media generally have to be developed for small groups of closely related organisms and should not be used for other organisms.

Relatively well defined media are preferred, even for routine antibiotic tests, because quantitative aspects of bacterial biochemistry, growth and susceptibility to noxious stimuli can be influenced substantially by minor changes in medium composition. The use of fully defined media has underpinned almost all of what we know about bacterial physiology. Rather curiously, however, it is well recognized that defined media are often suboptimal for the recovery of bacteria from environments in which they have been stressed. This may reflect the support provided to injured bacteria by complex media. Defined media

can really be optimized only for bacteria in a single physiological state, whereas complex media have greater potential to cope with the diversity of states present in natural samples.

## BACTERIAL PHYSIOLOGY

The complement of processes that enable an organism to occupy and thrive in a particular environment places certain requirements on its physiology. Traditional descriptions of bacterial groups emphasize features that place a microbe in particular ecological niches. Thus we have *acidophiles* for organisms such as *Lactobacillus* spp. that grow at lower pH levels than most other organisms, and *halophiles* for organisms that grow at high salt concentrations. The environments that can be colonized by a pathogen are, of course, critical in determining its reservoirs and potential modes of transmission. More recently it has been recognized that individual bacteria are not restricted to a single physiological state. Rather, they respond to environmental stimuli and undergo *adaptive responses* that confer improved capacity for survival in adverse conditions. All of these properties sustain the *viability* of the organism. However, it has become apparent that our ability to measure viability by conventional means may be inadequate.

The specific means by which a particular organism obtains energy and raw materials to sustain its growth (its nutritional type) and the physical conditions it requires reflect its fundamental physiological characteristics. Placing an organism into the groups defined by these characteristics is an important step in its conventional classification.

## Nutritional types

Traditionally, all living organisms have been divided into two nutritional groups: *heterotrophs* and *autotrophs*. The former depend on the latter to produce organic molecules by fixing carbon dioxide, predominantly by photosynthesis. Bacterial metabolism is now recognized to be so diverse that it cannot be encompassed by these two terms. Three basic features are used in the present terminology: the *energy source*, the *hydrogen donors* and the *carbon source*.

Energy for adenosine triphosphate (ATP) synthesis may be obtained from light in a *phototrophic* organism and from chemical oxidations in the case of a *chemotrophic* organism. The hydrogen donor type characterizes an organism as an *organotroph* if it requires organic sources of hydrogen and as a *lithotroph* if it can use inorganic sources (e.g. ammonia or hydrogen sulphide). Finally, the terms autotroph and heterotroph are reserved for the carbon source; the former can fix carbon dioxide directly whereas the latter require an organic source. In general, only the energy and hydrogen donor designations are referred to routinely by combining the two terms. Hence we refer to *chemo-organotrophs* (the vast majority of currently recognized medically important organisms) and *chemolithotrophs* (e.g. some *Pseudomonas* spp.). Surprisingly, there are even some *photolithotrophs* with medical significance; the cyanobacteria are now known to produce many toxins that can affect man.

## Physical conditions required for growth

All living organisms use oxidation to transfer energy to compounds that participate in their internal biochemical and biophysical processes. Oxidation of a molecule is equivalent to the removal of hydrogen, and requires another molecule to receive electrons in the process. In *aerobic* respiration the final electron recipient in the oxidation process is molecular oxygen (i.e. $O_2$), whereas under *anaerobic* conditions (in the absence of oxygen) most medically important organisms use an organic molecule as the final electron recipient, and the oxidative process is referred to as *fermentation*. There are also some forms of anaerobic respiration that use inorganic electron acceptors such as nitrates. Respiration in this context is generally used to denote involvement of a membrane-associated electron transport chain in the oxidation. In the early period of development of life on Earth there was no oxygen in the atmosphere; thus, at this time, all bacteria were *anaerobes*. Subsequently, following the development of photo-autotrophic organisms,

atmospheric oxygen became abundant, and organisms capable of using oxygen evolved.

Although aerobic metabolism is a more efficient means of obtaining energy than anaerobiosis, it is not without its cost. Some oxidation–reduction (redox) reactions occurring in the presence of oxygen commonly result in the formation of the reactive superoxide ($O_2^-$) and hydroxyl ($OH^-$) radicals as well as hydrogen peroxide ($H_2O_2$), all of which are highly toxic. To cope with this, aerobic organisms or *aerobes* have developed two enzymes that detoxify these molecules. *Superoxide dismutase* converts superoxide radicals to hydrogen peroxide ($2 O_2^- + 2H^+ \rightarrow H_2O_2 + O_2$), whereas *catalase* converts hydrogen peroxide to water and oxygen in the reaction $2 H_2O_2 \rightarrow H_2O + O_2$. Possession or lack of these enzymes has the important consequence of defining the atmosphere necessary for growth and survival of different organisms. Moreover, when produced in large amounts, the enzymes also provide protection for pathogenic organisms against the reactive oxygen intermediates deliberately produced as a defence mechanism by phagocytic cells.

### Growth atmosphere

These oxygen-related features underpin the major practical grouping of bacteria according to their atmospheric requirements (Table 4.1). Thus, *strict* or *obligate aerobes* require oxygen, usually at ambient levels ($\approx$20%), and *strict* or *obligate anaerobes* require the complete absence of oxygen. Many organisms exhibit intermediate properties: *facultative anaerobes* generally grow better in oxygen but are still able to grow well in its absence; *micro-aerophilic* organisms require a reduced oxygen level ($\approx$5%); *aerotolerant*

**Table 4.1**    Key descriptive terms used to categorize bacteria according to their growth requirements

| Descriptive term | Property | Example |
|---|---|---|
| **Growth atmosphere** | | |
| Strict (obligate) aerobe | Requires atmospheric oxygen for growth | *Pseudomonas aeruginosa* |
| Strict (obligate) anaerobe | Will not tolerate oxygen | *Bacteroides fragilis* |
| Facultative anaerobe | Grows best aerobically, but can grow anaerobically | *Staphylococcus* spp., *E. coli*, etc. |
| Aerotolerant anaerobe | Anaerobic, but tolerates exposure to oxygen | *Clostridium perfringens* |
| Micro-aerophilic organism | Requires or prefers reduced oxygen levels | *Campylobacter* spp., *Helicobacter* spp. |
| Capnophilic organism | Requires or prefers increased carbon dioxide levels | *Neisseria* spp. |
| **Growth temperature** | | |
| Psychrophile | Grows best at low temperature (e.g. <10°C) | *Flavobacterium* spp. |
| Thermophile | Grows best at high temperature (e.g. >60°C) | *Bacillus stearothermophilus*[a] |
| Mesophile | Grows best between 20–40°C | Most bacterial pathogens |

[a]Not a pathogen; its spores are very heat resistant and are used for testing the efficiency of heat sterilization.

*anaerobes* have a fermentative pattern of metabolism but can tolerate the presence of oxygen because they possess superoxide dismutase. Many medically important organisms are facultative anaerobes. There is a mixture of aerobic and anaerobic micro-environments in the human body, and the capacity to replicate in both is clearly advantageous. For obvious reasons, strict anaerobes are particularly associated with infection of tissues where the blood supply has been interrupted.

Among the various physical requirements for the growth of different bacterial groups, atmosphere assumes particular importance because, in practice, agar cultures from most clinical specimens are set up aerobically and anaerobically. Thus, when growth is first inspected after overnight incubation, the isolates can readily be differentiated into strict aerobes, anaerobes and facultative anaerobes according to the conditions under which they have grown. Various atmospheric conditions can also be obtained in broth media. If the medium is unstirred, strict aerobes tend to grow on the surface, micro-aerophiles just under the surface and anaerobes in the body of the medium away from the surface. Growth of anaerobes is often improved by the addition of a reducing agent such as cysteine or thioglycollate to mop up any free oxygen.

### Growth temperature

The other significant physical condition for bacterial growth from the medical perspective is temperature (see Table 4.1). Pathogens that actually replicate on or in the human body must be able to grow within the temperature range of 20–40°C, and are generally referred to as *mesophiles*. Organisms that can grow outside this range are either *psychrophiles* (cold loving) or *thermophiles* (heat loving). The former may be capable of growth in food or pharmaceuticals stored at normal refrigeration temperatures (0–8°C), whereas the latter can be a source of proteins with remarkable thermotolerant properties, such as *taq* polymerase, the key enzyme used in the polymerase chain reaction. Organisms such as the leprosy bacillus that prefer lower growth temperatures are often associated with skin and superficial infections, whereas organisms that grow in the colon (often a few degrees warmer than normal body temperature) can grow well up to 44°C.

### Extremophiles

Some bacteria require ostensibly bizarre physical conditions for growth. For example, barophiles isolated from the ocean floor may require enormous pressures

before they can replicate. Such organisms are often referred to as *extremophiles*. The properties of these organisms serve to remind us that microbes have the potential to occupy any environmental niche where energy and nutrition are available. It should be noted that most extremophiles actually turn out to belong to the Archaea (see Ch. 2).

### Bacterial metabolism

Although some bacteria are able to obtain their resources for growth in ways that seem alien to us, the core of their metabolism is essentially very similar to that of mammalian cells. The basic details of glycolysis, the tricarboxylic acid cycle, oxidative phosphorylation, ATP biosynthesis and amino acid metabolism are constant although some notable minor differences occur. Variations in the pathways that feed into and flow from these core processes are readily detected by what are loosely termed *biochemical tests* in medical laboratories. These detect traits such as the ability to use individual carbohydrate sources to produce acid and the possession of specific enzymes.

The common nature of central catabolic and anabolic pathways in bacteria and multicellular organisms reflects the economy of biology and evolution. Processes that work well cannot be outcompeted and tend to be preserved in the genetic stock. Thus, many of the specific enzymes involved in bacterial metabolism show remarkable levels of conservation in their amino acid sequences across very substantial distances in evolutionary terms. DNA sequencing has enabled the identification of *molecular families* of proteins with a common evolutionary origin. In addition to the metabolic enzymes, it has been recognized that many transport proteins responsible for importing and exporting specific substrates into and out of the bacterial cytoplasm are closely related in their structure and mode of function to those present in mammalian cells. Of course, because bacteria generally have only one cell compartment in which to operate, the location of these proteins is often different; for example, as they have no mitochondria, the cytoplasmic membrane contains the components of the electron transport chain, and the proton gradient across the inner mitochondrial membrane is generated across the cytoplasmic membrane instead. This feature actually means that bacteria can perform some energy-requiring processes at the cell surface, notably flagellar rotation (motility), by directly exploiting the proton gradient rather than consuming ATP.

Aside from its role in identification and intrinsic biological interest, bacterial metabolism has real consequences for humans. In direct terms, the resident microbiota have consequences in human health and disease. For example, the bacteria in dental plaque produce acid when presented with certain carbohydrate sources, and this acid is responsible for tooth decay; on the positive side, bacteria in the intestines deconjugate bile salts and thereby contribute to the enterohepatic circulation. It seems likely that the importance of such bioconversions will be recognized increasingly in the future. In particular, the role of bacteria in recovering nitrogen excreted into the colon in marginal human nutritional states and metabolic activity leading to the formation of carcinogens or other biologically active molecules are both areas where there is much room for further work. The totality of microbes (and their genomes) within the human body is referred to as the *microbiome.* The application of high throughput nucleotide sequencing to directly determine the range of microbes and microbial genes present in different areas of the body is opening up fascinating new insights into the way in which microbial genes and their expression can interact with humans to produce health or disease. The recent proposal that particular patterns of microbes in the human colon can predispose to obesity is a particularly striking example of this.

Human beings are also indirectly affected by microbial metabolism. At one level, the chemistry of our environment has been shaped extensively by microbes; the original development of oxygen in our atmosphere, the availability of elemental sulphur and the flow of nitrogen are all critically dependent on microbial metabolism. Exploitation of microbial metabolism in industry has, of course, given us ethanol, and many of the other alcohols and acids that result from fermentation have commercial value. Finally, bacteria have been used to combat the deleterious effects of environmental pollution in the process referred to as *bioremediation.*

## Adaptive responses in bacteria

The extent to which bacteria respond to environmental stimuli was originally recognized by monitoring gross phenotypic, biochemical and behavioural changes. Much of the genetic basis for how bacteria change their phenotypes was established in the 1960s and 1970s following on from the paradigm established for β-galactosidase regulation in *E. coli* by Jacob and Monod. The scale and rapidity (major changes can be seen in seconds) of bacterial responses became apparent through the 1980s and 1990s as the use of global analytical approaches that attempt to characterize the instantaneous expression of every gene the organism carries became established. At the translational level,

the use of two-dimensional gel electrophoresis and, more recently, sophisticated forms of mass spectrometry have underpinned the so-called *proteomic* approach. This technique reveals and separates most of the several hundred proteins that are being synthesized by a pure culture at a particular time. The catalogue of different proteins detected represents those proteins that the organism requires to function in the circumstances from which the sample was drawn. Assays of this type have shown that different sets of proteins are made in the exponential and stationary phases of the growth cycle and, indeed, in response to almost any environmental change. This finding underpins the recognition of just how different the phenotype of a single organism can be in different physiological states and reinforces the need to define the inoculum used in laboratory experiments. More recently the development of DNA arrays has enabled global analysis of responses at the transcriptional level by detecting messenger RNA (mRNA) molecules relating to every gene in the organism in a single analysis. The complement of RNA species present in an organism at a given time is referred to as the *transcriptome.* The basic features of the comparative protein and mRNA analyses are outlined in Figure 4.2.

The comprehensive analyses achieved by transcriptome and proteome analyses followed on from the recognition that global genome analyses and comparisons or *genomics* (see Ch. 6) have the potential to explain many – some would say most – biological and medical phenomena. The complexities linking genotype to phenotype remain overwhelming in most instances; none the less, we have now entered an era where global analyses of mRNA, proteome and metabolic function (recently termed 'metabolomics') are being addressed enthusiastically in an integrative computational approach pooling data from different analyses in what has been termed the 'systems biology' approach.

The effects of specific sublethal but noxious stimuli on gene expression are the subject of intense current study. Each different stimulus leads to an adaptive *stress response,* which is to some extent specific to the stimulus applied. Heat shock (the effects of raising temperature to 45°C and above for a few minutes) has been studied most extensively. The newly synthesized proteins elicited in this response are referred to as *heat shock proteins.* When the amino acid sequences of the principal heat shock proteins were determined, they were found to belong to a molecular family now recognized in all prokaryotic and eukaryotic cells. Apart from their role in improving the ability of bacteria to survive heat shock, these proteins, by virtue of their similarity to analogous host cell antigens, seem to be

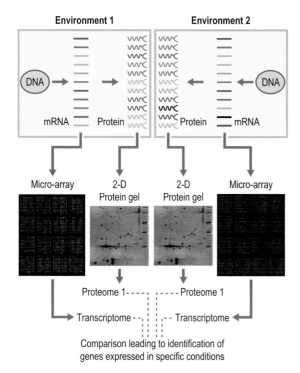

Environment 1          Environment 2

DNA → mRNA    Protein          Protein    mRNA ← DNA

Micro-array    2-D              2-D        Micro-array
               Protein gel      Protein gel

Proteome 1- - - - -  - - - - Proteome 1

Transcriptome - - -   - - Transcriptome

Comparison leading to identification of
genes expressed in specific conditions

**Fig. 4.2** Global strategies for identifying differentially expressed genes. Analysis at both mRNA and protein levels is preferred as there may be differences between the two. Individual spots on the two-dimensional (2-D) gels may be identified as specific gene products by mass spectrometry. Transcriptome analysis requires a representation of all the genes concerned in a DNA array and therefore needs prior knowledge (ideally a complete sequence) of the genome of the organism to be tested. These two global approaches provide a broad picture of the physiology of the organism under study.

involved in initiating autoimmune damage and immune dysfunction. A very important feature of the stress response in bacteria is that many of the stimuli used are prominent aspects of the stresses applied by the human immune system to an invading pathogen. Thus, acid stress is provided by the stomach and the hostile environment of phagolysosomes includes both oxidative and pH stress.

The information built up from studying stress responses has made it possible to identify sets of proteins that are made in response to several different stresses and those that appear exclusive to one stress. Together with other approaches, this has allowed recognition of *global regulatory systems* or *networks* within bacteria that are responsible for differential gene expression under different circumstances. The hierarchy of specific control mechanisms involved has spawned two important new terms, *stimulon* and *regulon*. A stimulon denotes all the genes whose expression is increased or decreased by a specific external stimulus, whereas a regulon refers to all the genes under the influence of a specific regulatory protein. A regulon may affect several operons (see Ch. 6), and there may be many regulons in one stimulon.

Regulatory networks have been identified in almost every area of bacterial physiology. Thus, in addition to the stimuli cited above, osmotic stress, cold shock, nutrient limitation (separate responses for carbon, nitrogen and phosphate), anaerobic and many other stimulons are recognized. These control systems are responsible for making sure the organism synthesizes only those proteins appropriate to its current circumstances. Particularly important medical examples of this are the regulation of proteins concerned with an organism's progress in an infection (virulence factors) and those made in response to sub-lethal levels of antibiotics. Equally important from the scientific perspective is the recognition that chemicals secreted by an organism can themselves act as regulatory stimuli to individuals of the same species in a way analogous to the pheromones released by insects.

Although it is still important to recognize that different organisms are particularly adapted to special environmental niches with descriptive terms such as mesophile, acidophile and halophile, the discovery of adaptive responses in bacteria has pushed us into an uncertain period where much of what has been established about the tolerance of micro-organisms to noxious stresses will have to be re-examined. Furthermore, as the extent to which bacteria modulate their phenotype according to their circumstances is now clear, the need for caution in concluding that any property detected in the laboratory is significant in a natural infection is unavoidably obvious.

## Bacterial defence against noxious chemicals

The features outlined above all contribute to the well-being of bacteria. In the natural world micro-organisms encounter many chemicals that could cause their destruction and, in their 3.5 billion years on earth they have evolved numerous protective mechanisms. In clinical practice these are recognized as *biochemical mechanisms of antibiotic resistance*, and four basic categories are recognized:

1. *Preventing access:* achieved by low cell envelope permeability or efflux pumps affecting the chemical concerned.
2. *Destruction:* achieved by enzymes that modify or degrade the chemical.
3. *Lack of target:* many chemicals that damage bacteria work through specific targets. The target

may be absent or be altered by mutation (see Ch. 6).
4. *Bypass of target:* in some cases an alternate or modified pathway can be used.

These mechanisms may be *intrinsic* to the organism concerned or they may be *acquired* through mutation or gene transfer (see Ch. 6).

Not all resistance to noxious molecules is mediated by the mechanisms listed above. In certain non-replicating states and in biofilms, bacteria classified as sensitive to certain agents by standard tests become resistant particularly to the lethal action of the agent concerned. This *phenotypic resistance* or *tolerance* appears to be a significant factor in the recalcitrance of certain chronic infections to antibiotic treatment and the survivors against antibiotic exposures that might reasonably be expected to be effective from conventional susceptibility tests are termed *persisters*. It is important to appreciate that these survivors are no more antibiotic-resistant than their forebears.

## Bacterial viability

A central feature of the general and adaptive physiology of bacteria is the capacity to preserve the viability of a particular organism. There is, however, a persistent problem – how do we define viability in practical terms? Traditionally, the operational definition of the capacity of a cell to form a colony on an appropriate agar medium (the colony or cfu count) has been almost universally accepted. It is also often expressed as the proportion of cells within a population that are capable of forming colonies. This has been used extensively in recognizing the *cidal* (lethal) and *static* (growth inhibitory) activities of antibiotics. In the former case, cfu counts decline, and in the latter they remain constant. However, it must be emphasized that viability is not a clearly measurable property. At the individual level it expresses the expectation that, in a suitable environment, a particular cell has the capacity to grow and undergo binary fission and that its progeny will have the same potential. The key assumption is that colony counts provide an accurate measure of viability.

The central problem can be stated as follows: it is self-evident that if a bacterial cell produces a colony it must have been viable, but to what extent is it true that a cell that fails to do this is non-viable or dead? Immediately contradictions to this proposal can be identified. The bacterial pathogens, such as *Mycobacterium leprae* and *Treponema pallidum*, which cannot be induced to form colonies on available agar media, are clearly viable. Similarly, all the 'as yet uncultivated

organisms' (possibly as many as 99% of all bacterial species) are clearly able to propagate themselves. They simply have not been sporting enough to do it on our laboratory media. A further exception is the phenomenon of bacterial recovery from injury (e.g. cold or osmotic shock) in which colony counts can be shown to rise in the absence of cell division.

It is possible that some organisms that are readily cultivable may be able to switch to a physiological state in which they cannot be induced to form colonies. A popular terminology for cells in this putative state is *viable but non-culturable* (VBNC).

Epidemiological and laboratory evidence provide some support for the existence of a VBNC state. In particular, the occurrence of several infectious diseases acquired from environmental sources, notably cholera, is at variance with our ability to recover the causal organisms from the implicated source. Environmental studies have demonstrated cells with immunological properties compatible with those of the cholera vibrio while failing to recover the organism in culture, and laboratory studies have indicated that the organism can persist in a non-culturable form. There is also evidence that non-culturable forms may revert to their 'normal' culturable state.

A major attraction of the VBNC hypothesis is that it may resolve a number of important mysteries in medical microbiology. In general, these are situations in which we know the organism must be present but are unable to culture it. This is particularly so with diseases such as tuberculosis that have latent phases.

The most significant problem for the VBNC hypothesis is that it has not been defined in physiological, biochemical or genetic terms. On the face of it, one might expect transition to the VBNC state to result from an adaptive response such as those described in the previous section. Alternatively, transition might be the result of a programme of gene expression such as that observed in spore formation or starvation. From this standpoint the stationary and decline phases in the growth cycle outlined above (when spore formation is induced in sporulating bacteria) may represent the initiation of and transition to a non-culturable phase rather than loss of viability (the traditional view). In spite of their popularity, these ideas must presently be viewed as interesting speculations for which there is circumstantial but no conclusive evidence.

Measurement of viability has been of great practical value in medical microbiology. Colony counts performed to investigate the action of antibiotics and other disruptive influences such as heat, and those performed at different stages during experimental infections in animal models of human infections, have provided a wealth of valuable information. Moreover, there is no reason to doubt that this approach will continue to be extremely useful.

None the less, it is necessary to maintain a clear view of the limitations of bacterial culture as a measure of the organisms present in a sample and of their viability. Studies often use the term 'viability' when in fact growth on agar or in broth was measured, and confusion would be prevented if the terms 'culturability' and 'colony counts' were used instead.

We are now entering an era in which many diagnostic and investigational techniques may be replaced by molecular detection procedures. The fact that signals based on such techniques may come from culturable, dead and potentially VBNC cells should be recognized. Unravelling these three possibilities presents ample challenge for medical and non-medical microbiologists alike.

## Bacterial death

Notwithstanding the problems outlined in the previous section, the ability to recognize and quantify bacterial death is of great practical significance in the practice of medicine. At present, except in highly defined circumstances, the cfu count remains the cornerstone for such measurements. In natural systems where no actively noxious environmental conditions pertain, if bacterial growth ceases, as in the stationary phase described above, after a variable period of time depending on the conditions and the organism concerned, then cfu counts begin to decline. In some cases this may lead to complete loss of viability, whereas in others a stable but lower cfu count is established. For example, *E. coli* appears to survive indefinitely in buffered salt solutions, the constant lysis of dying cells apparently providing for a balancing level of cell replication. Even after adaptation to starvation or other conditions leading to stasis, the rate at which viability is lost seems to follow a well defined pattern. Cells in stasis are clearly getting older and this provides a bacterial correlate of senescence. Although the study of bacterial cell senescence is relatively new, it is emerging that cumulative oxidative damage to cell proteins and other key macromolecules is one critical determinant of survival. This observation fits very well with the observation that one can often recover higher cfu counts of stressed facultative organisms on media containing catalase or other reagents that provide protection against reactive oxygen intermediates or following incubation under micro-aerophilic conditions.

It is not widely appreciated that many (probably all) bacteria carry genes encoding for programmed cell death. While several mechanisms are involved, these are distinct from the process of apoptosis that occurs in eukaryotic cells. These systems were first identified as toxin–antitoxin pairs functioning to maintain particular genes in the bacterial cell. However, it now seems likely that their occurrence cannot be explained solely on this basis and that, over time, they become integrated into the regulatory networks of the cell, particularly in controlling growth rate under certain conditions. It should be noted that the activation of latent prophages (see Ch. 6) constitutes another endogenous mechanism by which bacteria can initiate their own demise.

In addition to killing bacteria with antibiotics, medical practice is frequently concerned with decontaminating locations and materials that have been in contact with infectious patients. Moreover, the safe practice of surgery, parenteral administration of therapy, and the preparation of media and sampling materials for bacteriological studies all require the reduction or complete elimination of bacteria from key locations and devices. Although the methods applied to remove live bacteria may be checked with tests of biological efficacy, the relatively predictable rate of decline achieved with specific methods and target organisms enables safe practice. Because the cfu count is relatively convenient, it has been used in the establishment of most methodologies. However, removal or destruction of all infective agents is necessary to achieve sterility, and tests directed to all of these are required to some extent in establishing safe practice.

## STERILIZATION AND DISINFECTION

### Key definitions

*Sterilization.* The inactivation of all self-propagating biological entities (e.g. bacteria, viruses, prions) associated with the materials or areas under consideration.

*Disinfection.* The reduction of pathogenic organisms to a level at which they no longer constitute a risk.

*Antisepsis.* Term used to describe disinfection applied to living tissue such as a wound.

### Methods used in sterilization and disinfection

In practice, all processes of sterilization have a finite probability of failure. By convention, an article may be regarded as sterile if it can be demonstrated that there is a probability of less than one in a million of there being viable micro-organisms on it. As will be seen below, the level of microbial killing achieved by applying a particular method is dependent on the intensity with which the method is applied and its duration. Five main approaches are used.

*Heat.* The only method of sterilization that is both reliable and widely applicable is heating under carefully controlled conditions at temperatures above 100°C to ensure that bacterial spores are killed. There is some concern that even this temperature is insufficient to destroy prions. Shorter applications of lower temperatures, such as in pasteurization can effectively remove specific infection hazards.

*Ionizing radiation.* Both β-(electrons) and γ-irradiation (photons) are employed industrially for the sterilization of single-use disposable items such as needles and syringes, latex catheters and surgical gloves, and in the food industry to reduce spoilage and remove pathogens. Ultraviolet irradiation can be used to cut down the level of contamination, but is generally too mild to achieve sterility.

*Filtration.* Filters are used to remove bacteria and all larger micro-organisms from liquids that are liable to be spoiled by heating, for instance blood serum and antibiotic solutions in which contamination with filter-passing viruses is improbable or unimportant. Industrial scale filtration is used widely to reduce bacterial load and remove cysts of protozoa that are not killed by chlorination in the production of drinking water.

*Gaseous chemical agents.* Ethylene oxide is used mainly by industry for the sterilization of plastics and other thermolabile materials that cannot withstand heating. Formaldehyde in combination with subatmospheric steam is used more commonly in hospitals for reprocessing thermolabile equipment. Both processes carry toxic and other hazards for the user and the patient. Formaldehyde vapour on its own is used widely to decontaminate rooms and laboratory equipment.

*Liquid chemical agents.* Use of liquids such as glutaraldehyde is generally the least effective and most unreliable method. Such methods should be regarded as 'high-grade disinfection' only, to be applied when no other sterilization method is available, for example for heat-labile fibreoptic instruments such as flexible endoscopes. Various chemicals with antimicrobial properties are used as disinfectants. They are all liable to be inactivated by excessive dilution and contact with organic materials such as dirt or blood, or a variety of other materials. Nevertheless, they may provide a convenient method for environmental disinfection and other specific applications.

## Choice of method

The choice of method of sterilization or disinfection depends on:

- the nature of the item to be treated
- the likely microbial contamination
- the risk of transmitting infection to patients or staff in contact with the item.

Choice is based on an assessment of risk according to different categories of patient (e.g. immunocompromised), the equipment involved and its application. The selection of sterilization, disinfection or simple cleaning processes for individual items of equipment and the environment should be agreed as part of the infection control policy of a hospital (see Ch. 69). The preferred option wherever possible, for both sterilization and disinfection, is heat rather than chemicals. This relates not only to the antimicrobial efficacy but to safety considerations, which are more difficult to control in some chemical processes. Wherever chemicals are to be used for disinfection and sterilization, the safety of persons involved directly or indirectly in the procedure must be considered. It should be remembered that all sterilizing and disinfecting agents have some action on human cells. No method should be assumed to be safe unless appropriate precautions are taken.

## Measurement of microbial death

Every method used must be validated to demonstrate the required degree of microbial kill. With heat sterilization and irradiation, a biological test may not be required if the physical conditions are sufficiently well defined and controlled.

When micro-organisms are subjected to a lethal process, the number of viable cells decreases exponentially in relationship to the extent of exposure. If the logarithm of the number of survivors is plotted against the lethal dose received (e.g. time of heating at a particular temperature), the resulting curve is described as the *survivor curve*. This is independent of the size of the original population and is approximately linear. The linear survivor curve is an idealized concept and, in practice, minor variations, such as an initial shoulder or final tail, occur (Fig. 4.3).

### D value

The *D value* or *decimal reduction value* is the dose required to inactivate 90% of the initial population. From Figure 4.3, it can be seen that the time (dose) required to reduce the population from $10^6$ to $10^5$ is

**Fig. 4.3** Rate of inactivation of an inoculum of bacterial spores showing the decimal reduction time (*D* value) at 100°C and the nonlinear 'shoulder and tail' effects.

the same as the time (dose) required to reduce the population from $10^5$ to $10^4$, that is, the *D* value remains constant over the full range of the survivor curve. Extending the treatment beyond the point at which there is one surviving cell does not give rise to fractions of a surviving cell but rather to a statement of the probability of finding one survivor. Thus, by extrapolation from the experimental data, it is possible to determine the lethal dose required to give a probability of less than $10^{-6}$, which is required to meet the pharmacopoeial definition of 'sterile'. Note that in preparations intended for mass use, if the probability of a single live organism in a batch from which 10 million doses are to be administered is $10^{-6}$, then it is likely that around ten people will receive doses containing live organisms! Another consequence recognizable from Figure 4.3 is that the greater the number of microbes in the material to be sterilized, the longer the required exposure time. Thus, where efficient decontamination is the target, thorough cleansing can reduce the microbial load by several orders of magnitude and dramatically reduce both the time required and the level of certainty that sterility or adequate disinfection has been achieved.

## Resistance to sterilization and disinfection

Many common factors affect the ability of microorganisms to withstand the lethal effects of sterilization or disinfection processes. Factors specific to individual processes are considered in the description of those processes. In general, vegetative bacteria and viruses are more susceptible, and bacterial spores the most resistant, to sterilizing and disinfecting agents. However, within different species and strains of species there may be wide variation in intrinsic resistance. For example, within the Enterobacteriaceae, *D* values at 60°C range from a few minutes (*E. coli*) to 1 h (*Salmonella enterica* serotype Senftenberg). The typical *D* value for *Staphylococcus aureus* at 70°C is less than 1 min, compared with 3 min for *Staph. epidermidis*. However, an unusual strain of *Staph. aureus* has been isolated with a *D* value of 14 min at 70°C. Such variations may be attributed to morphological or physiological changes such as alterations in cell proteins or specific targets in the cell envelope affecting permeability.

Inactivation data obtained for one micro-organism should not be extrapolated to another; thus it should not be assumed that bactericidal disinfectants are also potent against viruses. The inactivation data for scrapie, bovine spongiform encephalopathy and Creutzfeldt–Jakob disease (CJD) suggest that prions are highly resistant agents, requiring six times the normal heat sterilization cycle (134°C for 18 min). This has led to requirements for the mandatory use of disposable instruments that are in direct contact with brain or other nervous tissue (including the retina) or tonsils where the risk of exposure to the prion causing CJD is high.

Owing to the adaptive processes described above, the conditions under which the micro-organisms were grown or maintained before exposure to the lethal process have a marked effect on their resistance. Organisms grown under nutrient-limiting conditions are typically more resistant than those grown under nutrient-rich conditions. Resistance usually increases through the late logarithmic phase of growth of vegetative cells and declines erratically during the stationary phase. Finally bacterial endospores, formed principally by *Bacillus* and *Clostridium* species, are relatively resistant to most processes. Similarly, fungal spores are more resistant than the vegetative mycelium, although they are not usually as resistant as bacterial spores. Bacterial spores were used to define the sterilization processes in current use, and preparations of bacterial spores (biological indicators) are used to monitor the efficacy of ethylene oxide sterilization, in which physical monitoring is inadequate. In general, disinfection processes have little or no activity against bacterial spores.

The micro-environment of the organism during exposure to the lethal process has a profound effect on its resistance. Thus, micro-organisms occluded in salt have greatly enhanced resistance to ethylene oxide; the presence of blood or other organic material will reduce the effectiveness of hypochlorite solution.

## Sterilization by moist heat

Moist heat is much more effective than dry heat because hydrated proteins can be denatured with less energy than dehydrated semi-crystalline proteins. Further, where steam is used, its condensation delivers the latent heat of vaporization to the surface concerned. It is therefore necessary that all parts of the load to be sterilized are in direct contact with the water molecules in steam. Sterilization requires, in most cases, exposure to moist heat at 121°C for 15 min.

Moist heat sterilization requires temperatures above that of boiling water. Such conditions are attained under controlled conditions by raising the pressure of steam in a pressure vessel (*autoclave*). At sea level, boiling water at atmospheric pressure (1 bar) produces steam at 98–100°C, whereas raising the pressure to 2.4 bar increases the temperature to 125°C, and at 3.0 bar to 134°C. Conversely, at subatmospheric pressures, including those at higher altitude, water boils at lower temperatures.

Steam is non-toxic and non-corrosive, but for effective sterilization it must be *saturated*, which means that it holds all the water it can in the form of a transparent vapour. It must also be *dry*, which means that it does not contain water droplets. When dry saturated steam meets a cooler surface it condenses into a small volume of water and liberates the latent heat of vaporization. The energy available from this latent heat is considerable; for example, 6 L of steam at a temperature of 134°C (and a corresponding pressure of 3 bar absolute) will condense into 10 mL of water and liberate 2162 J of heat energy. By comparison, less than 100 J of heat energy is released to an article by the sensible heat from air at 134°C.

Steam at a higher temperature than the corresponding pressure would allow is referred to as *super-heated steam,* and behaves in a similar manner to hot air. Conversely, steam that contains suspended droplets of water at the same temperature is referred to as *wet steam* and is less efficient. The presence of air in steam affects the sterilizing efficiency by changing the pressure–temperature relationship.

As can be seen from the foregoing, sterilization by moist heat requires delivery of steam at exactly the right temperature and pressure, and for the right time. This places considerable demands on the engineering and maintenance of autoclaves, and in critical situations such as provision of sterile materials for clinical practice their performance must be monitored continually and precisely. Physical measurements of temperature, pressure and time with thermometers and pressure gauges are recorded for every load, and periodic detailed tests are undertaken with temperature-sensitive probes (thermocouples) inserted into standard test packs. Biological indicators comprising dried spore suspensions of a reference heat-resistant bacterium, *Bacillus stearothermophilus*, are no longer considered appropriate for routine testing, although spore indicators are essential for low-temperature gaseous processes in which the physical measurements are not reliable.

## Sterilization by dry heat

Dry heat is believed to kill micro-organisms by causing a destructive oxidation of essential cell constituents. Killing of the most resistant spores by dry heat requires a temperature of 160°C for 2 h. This high temperature causes slight charring of paper, cotton and other organic materials.

Incineration is an efficient method for the sterilization and disposal of contaminated materials at a high temperature. It has a particular application for pathological waste materials, surgical dressings, sharp needles and other clinical waste. Red heat is achieved by holding inoculating wires, loops and points of forceps in the flame of a Bunsen burner until they are red hot.

Hot air sterilizers are used to process materials that can withstand high temperatures for the length of time needed for sterilization by dry heat, but that are likely to be affected by contact with steam. Examples include oils, powders, carbon steel microsurgical instruments and empty laboratory glassware. The overall cycle of heating up and cooling may take several hours.

## Disinfection by chemicals

Chemicals used in the environment or on the skin (*disinfectants* or *antiseptics*) cannot be relied on to kill or inhibit all pathogenic micro-organisms. The distinction between disinfectants and antiseptics is not clear-cut; an antiseptic can be regarded as a special kind of disinfectant that is sufficiently free from injurious effects to be applied to the surface of the body, though not suitable for systemic administration. Some would restrict the term *antiseptic* to preparations applied to open wounds or abraded tissue, and prefer the term *skin disinfection* for the removal of organisms from the hands and intact skin surfaces.

The efficacy of a particular method of chemical disinfection is heavily dependent on the concentration and stability of the agent; the number, type and accessibility of micro-organisms; the temperature and pH; and the presence of organic (especially protein) or other interfering substances.

In general, the rate of inactivation of a susceptible microbial population in the presence of an antimicrobial chemical is dependent on the relative concentration of the two reactants, the micro-organism and the chemical. The optimum concentration required to produce a standardized microbial effect in practice is described as the *in-use* concentration. Care must always be taken in preparing an accurate in-use dilution of concentrated product. Accidental or arbitrary overdilution may result in failure of disinfection.

The velocity of the reaction depends on the number and type of organisms present. In general, Gram-positive bacteria are more sensitive to disinfectants than Gram-negative bacteria; mycobacteria and fungal spores are relatively resistant, and bacterial spores are highly resistant. Enveloped or lipophilic viruses are relatively sensitive, whereas hydrophilic viruses such as poliovirus and other enteroviruses are less susceptible. Although difficult to test in vitro, there is evidence that hepatitis B virus is more resistant than other viruses (including human immunodeficiency virus) and most vegetative bacteria to the action of chemical disinfectants and heat.

Glutaraldehyde is highly active against bacteria, viruses and spores. Other disinfectants, such as hexachlorophane, have a relatively narrow range of activity, predominantly against Gram-positive cocci. Some disinfectants are more active or stable at a particular pH value; although glutaraldehyde is more stable under acidic conditions, use at a higher pH (8.0) improves the antimicrobial effect.

Disinfectants may be inactivated by hard tap water, cork, plastics, blood, urine, soaps and detergents, or another disinfectant. Information should be sought from the manufacturer or from reference authorities to confirm that the disinfectant will remain active in the circumstances of use.

Maintenance of effective disinfection in large healthcare facilities is a major challenge requiring management skills and technical understanding in equal measure. The selection of appropriate disinfectants and maintaining standards in practice is supported by the development of local disinfection policies. These points are considered further in Chapter 68.

## RECOMMENDED READING

Barer MR, Harwood CR: Bacterial viability and culturability, *Advances in Microbial Physiology* 41:94–138, 1999.

Block SS, editor: *Disinfection, Sterilization and Preservation*, ed 5, Philadelphia, 2000, Lea and Febiger.

Finkel SE: Long-term survival during stationary phase: evolution and the GASP phenotype, *Nature Reviews Microbiology* 4:113–119, 2006.

Hall-Stoodley L, Stoodley P: Evolving concepts in biofilm infections, *Cellular Microbiology* 11:1034–1043, 2009.

Moat AG, Foster JW: *Microbial Physiology*, ed 4, New York, 2002, Wiley-Liss.

Musser JM, Deleo FR: Toward a genome-wide systems biology analysis of host–pathogen interactions in group A streptococcus, *American Journal of Pathology* 167:1461–1472, 2005.

Neidhardt FC, Ingraham JL, Schaechter M: *Physiology of the Bacterial Cell: A Molecular Approach*, Sunderland, MA, 1990, Sinauer.

Roszaak DB, Colwell RR: Survival strategies of bacteria in the natural environment, *Microbiological Reviews* 51:365–379, 1987.

Russell AD, Hugo WB, Ayliffe GAJ, editors: *Principles and Practice of Disinfection, Preservation and Sterilisation*, ed 3, Oxford, 1998, Blackwell Scientific.

### Websites

LabWork. Bacterial growth curve. http://www.microbiologybytes.com/LabWork/bact/bact1.htm

# 5 | Antimicrobial agents

*D. Greenwood and W. L. Irving*

## KEY POINTS

- Most antimicrobial agents are active only against bacteria; smaller numbers of antifungal, antiviral, antiprotozoal and anthelminthic agents are available.
- Antimicrobial agents used in clinical medicine do not affect spores of bacteria or fungi, or latent viruses.
- The largest group of antibacterial agents are β-lactam compounds (penicillins, cephalosporins, etc.), most of which are semi-synthetic derivatives of naturally occurring antibiotics. Members of this group have widely different properties.
- Other widely used antibacterial agents include aminoglycosides, tetracyclines, macrolides, glycopeptides and quinolones.
- Most antifungal agents are suitable only for topical application. Agents used for systemic therapy of fungal infection include amphotericin B, certain azole derivatives, griseofulvin and terbinafine.
- The largest groups of antiviral compounds are the antiretroviral (anti-HIV) and the anti-herpes agents, such as aciclovir, that act on nucleic acid synthesis.
- Combinations of three or more antiretroviral drugs can effectively keep HIV levels in the circulation down below the limit of detection.
- Most antiparasitic agents have specific activity against particular protozoa or helminths, although some have broader activity.
- Routine antibiotic sensitivity testing is useful in the case of common bacterial pathogens. The disc diffusion method is commonly used.

Antimicrobial agents are used not only to treat bacterial diseases, but also infections with viruses, fungi, protozoa and helminths. These drugs have transformed the management of infectious disease, but none is free from unwanted side effects, and microbial resistance is a constant threat. Consequently, they must be used with discretion and understanding of their individual properties. The treatment of individual infections is dealt with in the appropriate chapters. The general strategy of antimicrobial chemotherapy, which is crucial to the control of antimicrobial drug resistance, is covered in Chapter 67.

*Antibiotics* are naturally occurring microbial products; synthetic compounds such as sulphonamides, quinolones, nitrofurans and imidazoles should strictly be referred to as *chemotherapeutic agents*. However, as some antibiotics can be manufactured synthetically whereas others are the products of chemical manipulation of naturally occurring compounds (*semi-synthetic antibiotics*), the distinction is ill defined. Nowadays the term *antibiotic* is used loosely to describe agents (mainly, but not exclusively, antibacterial agents) employed to treat systemic infection. Antimicrobial substances that are too toxic to be used other than in topical therapy or for environmental decontamination are referred to as *antiseptics* or *disinfectants* (see Ch. 4).

## ANTIBACTERIAL AGENTS

The principal types of antibacterial agent are listed in Table 5.1. Because there are so many, it is convenient to group them according to their site of action.

### Inhibitors of bacterial cell wall synthesis

As most bacteria possess a rigid cell wall that is lacking in mammalian cells (see Ch. 2, p. 13), this structure is a prime target for agents that exhibit *selective toxicity*, the ability to inhibit or destroy the microbe without harming the host. However, the bacterial cell wall can also prevent access of agents that would otherwise be effective. Thus, the complex outer envelope of Gram-negative bacteria is impermeable to large hydrophilic molecules, which may be prevented from reaching an otherwise susceptible target.

**Table 5.1**   Principal types of antibacterial agent (other than agents used exclusively in mycobacterial infection)

| Agent | Site of action | Usual activity[a] against: | | | | | |
|---|---|---|---|---|---|---|---|
| | | Staphylococci | Streptococci | Enterobacteria | *Pseudomonas aeruginosa* | *Mycobacterium tuberculosis* | Anaerobes |
| Penicillins | Cell wall | +R | + | V | V | – | +[b] |
| Cephalosporins | Cell wall | + | + | + | V | – | +[b] |
| Other β-lactam agents | Cell wall | V | V | + | V | – | V |
| Glycopeptides | Cell wall | + | + | – | – | – | +[c] |
| Tetracyclines | Ribosome | +R | +R | +R | – | – | +R |
| Chloramphenicol | Ribosome | + | + | + | – | – | – |
| Aminoglycosides | Ribosome | + | – | + | V | V | – |
| Macrolides | Ribosome | + | + | – | – | – | + |
| Lincosamides | Ribosome | + | + | – | – | – | + |
| Fusidic acid | Ribosome | + | + | – | – | + | + |
| Oxazolidinones | Ribosome | + | + | – | – | – | – |
| Streptogramins | Ribosome | + | +[d] | – | – | – | |
| Rifamycins | RNA synthesis | + | + | + | – | + | + |
| Sulphonamides | Folate metabolism | +R | +R | +R | – | – | – |
| Diaminopyrimidines | Folate metabolism | + | + | +R | – | – | – |
| Quinolones | DNA synthesis | V | V | + | V | V | – |
| Nitrofurans | DNA synthesis | – | – | + | – | – | + |
| Nitroimidazoles | DNA synthesis | – | – | – | – | – | + |

[a]Usual spectrum of intrinsic activity
[b]Poor activity against anaerobes of the *Bacteroides fragilis* group.
[c]Poor activity against most Gram-negative anaerobes.
[d]Poor activity against *Enterococcus faecalis*.
+, active; –, inactive; V, variable activity among different agents of the group. +R indicates that acquired resistance is very common.

Inhibitors of bacterial cell wall synthesis act on the formation of the peptidoglycan layer (Fig. 5.1). Bacteria that lack peptidoglycan, such as mycoplasmas, are resistant to these agents.

## β-Lactam agents

Penicillins, cephalosporins and other compounds that feature a β-lactam ring in their structure fall into this group (Fig. 5.2). All of these compounds bind to proteins situated at the cell wall–cell membrane interface. These *penicillin-binding proteins* are involved in cell wall construction, including the cross-linking of the peptidoglycan strands that gives the wall its strength. Opening of the β-lactam ring by hydrolytic enzymes, collectively called *β-lactamases*, abolishes antibacterial activity. Many such enzymes are found in bacteria. Those elaborated by Gram-negative enteric bacilli are particularly diverse in their activity and properties. Most prevalent are the so-called *TEM β-lactamases* (TEM-1, TEM-2, etc.), numerous forms of which have evolved under selective pressure of β-lactam antibiotic use. Gram-negative bacteria able to produce enzymes that inactivate many different β-lactam antibiotics – so-called *extended-spectrum β-lactamases* (ESBLs) – sometimes become endemic in hospitals, causing serious problems, especially in patients in high-dependency units.

*Penicillins.* The original penicillin, benzylpenicillin (penicillin G; often called simply 'penicillin') exhibits unrivalled activity against staphylococci, streptococci, neisseriae, spirochaetes and certain other organisms. However, resistance, normally due to the production of β-lactamase, has undermined its activity against staphylococci and, to a lesser extent, gonococci. Bacteria, including staphylococci and pneumococci, that exhibit reduced susceptibility to penicillin by a non-enzymic mechanism are also encountered. Benzylpenicillin revolutionized the treatment of infection caused by some of the most virulent bacterial pathogens, but it also suffers from several shortcomings:

- breakdown by gastric acidity when given orally
- very rapid excretion by the kidney
- susceptibility to penicillinase (β-lactamase)
- restricted spectrum of activity.

Further development of the penicillin family has been directed towards improving these properties. Crucial to this was the discovery that removal of the

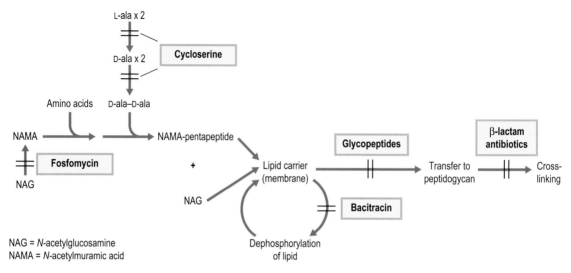

**Fig. 5.1**   Formation of bacterial cell wall peptidoglycan, showing the sites of action of inhibitors of the process.

phenylacetic acid side-chain left intact the core struc-ture, 6-aminopenicillanic acid, the starting point for the numerous semi-synthetic penicillins that have been produced. Among the most important penicillins that followed the introduction of benzylpenicillin are:

- phenoxymethylpenicillin (penicillin V), which can be given orally
- procaine penicillin, a long-acting salt of benzylpenicillin
- flucloxacillin, dicloxacillin and oxacillin, compounds resistant to staphylococcal β-lactamase
- ampicillin and amoxicillin, which are active against some enterobacteria
- ticarcillin, azlocillin and piperacillin, which are active against *Pseudomonas aeruginosa*.

Penicillins other than flucloxacillin and its relatives are inactivated by staphylococcal β-lactamase. *Methicillin-resistant Staphylococcus aureus* (MRSA; a term that has persisted although methicillin is now virtually obsolete) owe their resistance to alterations in the target penicillin-binding proteins; they are resistant to all penicillins and to all other β-lactam antibiotics with the exception of certain new cepha-losporins (see below).

Ampicillin is sometimes administered as an esteri-fied *prodrug*, a formulation providing improved absorption in the gut, where it releases the active ingredient into the circulation.

*Cephalosporins.*   Cephalosporins are close cousins of the penicillins, but the β-lactam ring is fused to a six-membered dihydrothiazine ring rather than the five-membered thiazolidine ring of penicillins. The additional carbon carries substitutions that may alter the pharmacological behaviour of the molecule, and sometimes its antibacterial activity. Some cepha-losporins (e.g. cefalotin [formerly called cephalothin] and cefotaxime) carry an acetoxymethyl group on the extra carbon. This can be removed by hepatic enzymes to yield a less active derivative, but it is doubtful whether this has any therapeutic significance. Other cephalosporins (e.g. cefamandole, cefoperazone and the oxa-cephem, latamoxef) possess a methyltetrazole substituent. Use of compounds with this feature has been associated with hypoprothrombinaemia and bleeding in some patients.

Cephalosporins are generally stable to staphylo-coccal penicillinase (though they are differentially susceptible to hydrolysis by the various types of enterobacterial β-lactamase), but they lack activity against enterococci. They exhibit a broader spectrum than most penicillins and are less prone to cause hypersensitivity reactions. Among the most impor-tant cephalosporins in therapeutic use are:

- cefalexin, cefradine and cefaclor, which can be given orally
- cefuroxime and cefoxitin, which are stable to many β-lactamases
- cefotaxime and ceftriaxone, which combine β-lactamase stability with high intrinsic activity
- cefpodoxine (as the proxetil prodrug) and cefixime, which combine stability to enterobacterial β-lactamases with oral absorption

**Fig. 5.2** Examples of different types of molecular structure among β-lactam antibiotics.

- ceftazidime and cefpirome, which additionally exhibit good activity against *Ps. aeruginosa*
- ceftobiprole and ceftaroline, which are active against MRSA.

*Other β-lactam agents.* Various agents with diverse properties share the structural feature of a β-lactam ring with penicillins and cephalosporins (see Fig. 5.2):

- *Carbapenems* (e.g. imipenem, meropenem and ertapenem) have a broad spectrum of activity, embracing most Gram-positive and Gram-negative aerobic and anaerobic bacteria. Imipenem is inactivated by a dehydropeptidase in the human kidney, and is co-administered with a dehydropeptidase inhibitor, cilastatin.
- The *oxa-cephem* latamoxef is a broad-spectrum β-lactamase-stable compound.

- The *monobactam*, aztreonam, is a monocyclic compound with a spectrum that is restricted to aerobic Gram-negative bacteria.
- The *clavam*, clavulanic acid, exhibits poor antibacterial activity, but has proved useful as a β-lactamase inhibitor when used in combination with β-lactamase-susceptible compounds such as amoxicillin (co-amoxiclav) and ticarcillin.
- The *sulphones*, sulbactam and tazobactam, also act as β-lactamase inhibitors and are marketed in combination with ampicillin (or cefoperazone) and piperacillin, respectively.

## Glycopeptides

Vancomycin and teicoplanin are large molecules that are unable to penetrate the outer membrane of Gram-negative bacteria, and the spectrum is consequently restricted to Gram-positive organisms. Their chief importance resides in their action against Gram-positive cocci with multiple resistance to other drugs. Enterococci and staphylococci, including MRSA, that exhibit resistance or reduced sensitivity to glycopeptides are being reported more frequently. Other glycopeptides are under development.

## Other inhibitors of bacterial cell wall synthesis

- Fosfomycin is a simple phosphonic acid antibiotic used mainly for the treatment of urinary tract infection. Resistance arises readily in vitro.
- Bacitracin is active against Gram-positive bacteria, but is too toxic for systemic use. It is found in many topical preparations, and is also used in the laboratory in the presumptive identification of haemolytic streptococci of Lancefield group A (see pp. 184 and 195).
- Isoniazid and some other compounds used to treat tuberculosis interfere with the formation of the mycolic acids of the mycobacterial cell wall.
- Cycloserine is an analogue of D-alanine used occasionally against multiresistant strains of *Mycobacterium tuberculosis*.

## Inhibitors of bacterial protein synthesis

Bacterial ribosomes are sufficiently different from those of mammalian cells to allow selective inhibition of protein synthesis. Most agents that act at this level are true antibiotics (or derivatives thereof) produced by *Streptomyces* species or other soil organisms. Some have an effect in eukaryotic cells, which have mitochondrial ribosomes similar to those of bacteria (see p. 13).

## Tetracyclines

These are broad-spectrum agents with important activity against chlamydiae, rickettsiae, mycoplasmas and, surprisingly, malaria parasites, as well as most conventional Gram-positive and Gram-negative bacteria. They prevent binding of amino-acyl transfer RNA (tRNA) to the ribosome and inhibit, but do not kill, susceptible bacteria. The various members of the tetracycline group are closely related and differ more in their pharmacological behaviour than in antibacterial activity. Doxycycline and minocycline are in most common use. Resistance has limited the value of tetracyclines against many Gram-positive and Gram-negative bacteria, but rickettsiae, chlamydiae and mycoplasmas are usually susceptible. Tigecycline (a *glycylcycline*) retains activity against many bacteria resistant to other tetracyclines.

## Chloramphenicol

Chloramphenicol also possesses a very broad antibacterial spectrum. It acts by blocking the growth of the peptide chain. Use of chloramphenicol has been limited because of the occurrence of a rare but fatal side effect, aplastic anaemia.

## Aminoglycosides

Streptomycin, the first antibiotic to be discovered by random screening of soil organisms, is predominantly active against enterobacteria and *M. tuberculosis*. Like other members of the aminoglycoside family it has no useful activity against streptococci, anaerobes or intracellular bacteria. The group also has in common a tendency to damage the eighth cranial nerve (ototoxicity) and the kidney (nephrotoxicity).

The chief properties of aminoglycosides are shown in Table 5.2. They inhibit formation of the ribosomal initiation complex and also cause misreading of messenger RNA (mRNA). They are bactericidal compounds, and some, notably gentamicin and tobramycin, exhibit good activity against *Ps. aeruginosa*. Such compounds have been used widely, often in combination with β-lactam antibiotics, with which they interact synergistically, in the 'blind' treatment of sepsis in immunocompromised patients. Resistance may arise from ribosomal changes (streptomycin) or alterations in drug uptake. However, it is more often caused by bacterial enzymes that phosphorylate, acetylate or adenylate exposed amino or hydroxyl groups. Enzymic resistance consequently affects the various aminoglycosides differentially, depending on the possession of exposed groups that can be attacked by the enzyme

**Table 5.2** Summary of the important differential properties of aminoglycoside antibiotics

| Aminoglycoside | Activity against: | | Relative susceptibility to inactivation by bacterial enzymes | Relative degree of: | |
| | *Pseudomonas aeruginosa* | *Mycobacterium tuberculosis* | | Ototoxicity | Nephrotoxicity |
| --- | --- | --- | --- | --- | --- |
| Amikacin | + | + | ± | ++ | + |
| Gentamicin | + | − | ++ | ++ | ++ |
| Kanamycin | − | + | ++ | ++ | ++ |
| Neomycin | − | ± | ++ | +++ | ++ |
| Netilmicin | + | − | + | + | + |
| Streptomycin | − | + | ++ | +++ | ± |
| Tobramycin | + | − | ++ | ++ | ++ |

involved. Amikacin is resistant to most of the common enzymes.

## Macrolides

Macrolide antibiotics have a large macrocyclic lactone ring substituted with some unusual sugars. They act by interfering with the translocation of mRNA on the bacterial ribosome. They are used mainly as antistaphylococcal and antistreptococcal agents, though some have wider applications. They have no useful activity against enteric Gram-negative bacilli. The original macrolide, erythromycin, is unstable in gastric acid and is usually administered orally as the stearate salt or as an esterified *pro-drug* (pharmacological preparations that improve absorption and deliver the active drug into the circulation). Salts suitable for intravenous administration are also available. Certain other macrolides, notably clarithromycin, offer improved pharmacological properties.

The macrolactone ring of most macrolides is composed of 14 atoms, but others have a 16-membered structure. These include spiramycin, which has some useful activity against the protozoan parasite, *Toxoplasma gondii*.

Some macrolides feature structural changes in the macrocyclic ring: in azithromycin, a compound distinguished by good tissue penetration and a long terminal half-life, the ring has been expanded by inclusion of a nitrogen atom to form an *azalide*; in telithromycin, a compound that retains activity against macrolide-resistant Gram-positive cocci, a keto function has been introduced to produce a *ketolide*.

## Lincosamides

The original lincosamide antibiotic, lincomycin, has been superseded by a derivative, clindamycin, that is better absorbed after oral administration and is more active against the organisms within its spectrum.

These include staphylococci, streptococci and most anaerobic bacteria, against which clindamycin exhibits outstanding activity. Enthusiasm for the use of clindamycin has been tempered by an association with the occasional development of severe diarrhoea, which sometimes progresses to a life-threatening pseudomembranous colitis (see *Clostridium difficile*, p. 254).

Lincosamides bind to the 50S ribosomal subunit at a site closely related to that at which macrolides act. Inducible resistance to macrolides caused by enzymic modification of the ribosomal binding site also renders the cells resistant to lincosamides (and streptogramins; see below), but only in the presence of macrolides, which alone are able to act as inducers.

## Fusidic acid

The structure of fusidic acid is related to that of steroids, but the antibiotic is devoid of steroid-like activity. It blocks factor G, which is involved in peptide elongation. Fusidic acid has an unusual spectrum of activity that includes corynebacteria, nocardia and *M. tuberculosis*, but the antibiotic is usually regarded simply as an antistaphylococcal agent. It penetrates well into bone and has been used widely (generally in combination with a β-lactam antibiotic to prevent the selection of resistant variants) in the treatment of staphylococcal osteomyelitis.

## Linezolid

Linezolid is an oxazolidinone. It is a narrow-spectrum anti-Gram-positive agent which acts by preventing the formation of the ribosomal initiation complex. It is used exclusively against MRSA and other Gram-positive cocci resistant to older agents. There is some evidence that it may be of use in drug-resistant tuberculosis.

## Streptogramins

This is the collective name for a family of antibiotics that occur naturally as two synergistic components. They were formerly used mainly in animal husbandry, although one member of the group, pristinamycin, is available in some countries as an antistaphylococcal agent. Use was limited by poor solubility, but derivatives suitable for parenteral administration, quinupristin and dalfopristin, have been developed. The combination exhibits bactericidal activity against most Gram-positive cocci, but has poor activity against *Enterococcus faecalis.*

## Mupirocin

This is an antibiotic, produced by *Pseudomonas fluorescens*, that blocks incorporation of isoleucine into proteins. Its useful activity is restricted to staphylococci and streptococci; as it is inactivated when given systemically, it is used only in topical preparations.

## Inhibitors of nucleic acid synthesis

A number of important antibacterial agents act directly or indirectly on DNA or RNA synthesis.

## Sulphonamides and diaminopyrimidines

These agents affect DNA synthesis because of their role in folic acid metabolism. Folic acid is used in many one-carbon transfers in living cells, including the conversion of deoxyuridine to thymidine. During this process the active form of the vitamin, tetrahydrofolate, is oxidized to dihydrofolate, and this must be reduced before it can function in further reactions.

Sulphonamides are analogues of *para*-aminobenzoic acid, and prevent the condensation of this compound with dihydropteridine during the formation of folic acid. Diaminopyrimidines, which include the broad-spectrum antibacterial agent trimethoprim and the antimalarial compounds pyrimethamine and cycloguanil (the metabolic product of proguanil), prevent the reduction of dihydrofolate to tetrahydrofolate. Sulphonamides and diaminopyrimidines thus act at sequential stages of the same metabolic pathway and interact synergistically, although in bacterial infections trimethoprim is generally sufficiently effective, and less toxic, when used alone.

Sulphonamides are broad-spectrum antibacterial agents, but resistance is common and the group also suffers from problems of toxicity. The numerous sulphonamides exhibit similar antibacterial activity, but differ widely in their pharmacokinetic behaviour. They have largely been replaced by safer and more active agents, although the combination of sulfamethoxazole with trimethoprim (co-trimoxazole) is still used. Sulfadoxine or sulfadiazine combined with pyrimethamine are used in malaria and toxoplasmosis, respectively.

## Quinolones

These drugs act on the α subunit of DNA gyrase. Their properties allow them to be categorized roughly into three groups (Table 5.3). Nalidixic acid and its early congeners are narrow-spectrum agents active only against Gram-negative bacteria. Their use is virtually restricted to urinary tract infection, although they have also been used in enteric infections. Later quinolones, such as ciprofloxacin and ofloxacin, which are 6-fluoro derivatives and are described as *fluoroquinolones*, display much enhanced activity and a broader spectrum, although activity against some Gram-positive cocci, notably *Streptococcus pneumoniae*, is unreliable. Continued development has produced compounds that lack the latter defect and, in some cases, exhibit further broadening of the spectrum and improved pharmacokinetic properties.

**Table 5.3** Principal types of quinolone antibacterial agent

| Narrow-spectrum compounds[a] | Broad-spectrum compounds[b] | Compounds with further enhanced spectrum[c] |
|---|---|---|
| Cinoxacin | Ciprofloxacin | Clinafloxacin |
| Nalidixic acid | Enoxacin | Gemifloxacin |
| Oxolinic acid | Levofloxacin | Moxifloxacin |
| Pipemidic acid | Lomefloxacin | Sparfloxacin |
| | Norfloxacin | |
| | Ofloxacin | |

[a]Spectrum restricted to enteric Gram-negative bacilli.
[b]Improved activity against *Pseudomonas aeruginosa* and Gram-positive cocci.
[c]Further improved activity against Gram-positive cocci and some anaerobes.

Quinolones are quite well absorbed when given orally and are widely distributed throughout the body. Extensive metabolization may occur, particularly with nalidixic acid and the older derivatives. Ciprofloxacin and other fluoroquinolones are used widely despite certain problems of toxicity, and resistance is becoming more prevalent.

### Nitroimidazoles

Azole derivatives feature prominently among antifungal, antiprotozoal and anthelminthic agents. Those that exhibit antibacterial activity are 5-nitroimidazoles. At low redox ($E_h$) values they are reduced to a short-lived intermediate that causes DNA strand breakage. Because of the requirement for low $E_h$ values, 5-nitroimidazoles are active only against anaerobic (and certain micro-aerophilic) bacteria and anaerobic protozoa. The representative of the group most commonly used clinically is metronidazole; similar derivatives include tinidazole, and nimorazole.

### Nitrofurans

The most familiar nitrofuran is nitrofurantoin, an agent used exclusively in urinary tract infection. Other derivatives, including furazolidone, which is used in enteric infections, are marketed for a variety of purposes in some parts of the world. These compounds probably act on DNA through a reduced metabolite, in a manner analogous to that of the nitroimidazoles.

### Rifamycins

This group of antibiotics is characterized by excellent activity against mycobacteria, although other bacteria are also susceptible; staphylococci in particular are exquisitely sensitive. These compounds act by inhibiting transcription of RNA from DNA. Rifampicin, the best known member of the group, is used in tuberculosis and leprosy. Wider use has been discouraged on the grounds that it might inadvertently foster the emergence of resistance in mycobacteria. Rifapentine has similar properties, but exhibits a longer plasma half-life. Rifabutin (ansamycin) is used in infections caused by atypical mycobacteria of the avium-intracellulare group (see Ch. 19).

## Miscellaneous antibacterial agents

### Polymyxins

Polymyxin B and colistin (polymyxin E) act like cationic detergents to disrupt cell membranes. They exhibit potent antipseudomonal activity, but toxicity has limited their usefulness, except in topical preparations and bowel decontamination regimens. If systemic use is contemplated, a sulphomethylated derivative, colistin sulfomethate, is preferred.

### Daptomycin

Daptomycin is a semi-synthetic lipopeptide antibiotic with activity against Gram-positive cocci. It has a role in the treatment of infections caused by multiresistant organisms.

### Antimycobacterial agents

As well as streptomycin and rifampicin (see above), various agents are used exclusively for the treatment of mycobacterial infection. These include isoniazid, ethambutol and pyrazinamide, which are commonly found in antituberculosis regimens, and diaminodiphenylsulfone (dapsone) and clofazimine, which are used in leprosy. Cycloserine and $p$-aminosalicylic acid (PAS), which were formerly used in tuberculosis, have now been largely abandoned except for drug-resistant tuberculosis. Some fluoroquinolones and macrolides exhibit activity against certain mycobacteria, and may have a role in treatment.

## ANTIFUNGAL AGENTS

Although fungi cause a wide variety of infections, relatively few agents are available for treatment, especially for the systemic therapy of serious mycoses. Superficial fungal infections of the skin and mucous membranes can often be treated with topical agents, including *polyenes*, such as nystatin, or *azole* derivatives, of which many (clotrimazole, miconazole, econazole, etc.) are marketed as vaginal pessaries and creams. For dermatophyte infections of the nails, oral therapy with griseofulvin or the allylamine derivative terbinafine is peculiarly suitable, as these agents are deposited in newly formed keratin.

Serious systemic disease caused by yeasts and other fungi is often treated with the polyene, amphotericin B, which is extremely toxic. Newer formulations of the drug, in which it is complexed with liposomes or lipids, are better tolerated. The pyrimidine analogue 5-fluorocytosine is active against many types of yeast, and is used in combination with amphotericin B in severe systemic yeast infections. Anidulafungin, caspofungin and micafungin are members of the *echinocandin* class of agents They are active against various fungi, including *Candida, Aspergillus* and

**Table 5.4**  Summary of the spectrum of activity of antifungal agents

| Agent | Candida albicans | Cryptococcus neoformans | Dermatophytes | Aspergillus fumigatus | Dimorphic fungi |
|---|---|---|---|---|---|
| Amphotericin B | + | + | – | + | + |
| Echinocandins | + | – | – | + | +[b] |
| Flucytosine | + | + | – | – | – |
| Griseofulvin | – | – | + | – | – |
| Imidazoles | + | + | + | – | + |
| Nystatin[a] | + | – | + | – | – |
| Terbinafine | – | – | + | +[b] | +[b] |
| Triazoles | + | + | + | (+)[c] | + |

[a]For topical use only.
[b]Clinical efficacy not yet established.
[c]Itraconazole, posaconazole and voriconazole are active against *A. fumigatus*, but fluconazole is not.

*Histoplasma* spp. and *Pneumocystis jirovecii* (formerly *P. carinii*), a fungus long thought to be a protozoon.

Azole derivatives exhibit the broadest spectrum of activity, embracing yeasts, filamentous fungi and dimorphic fungi, but few are suitable for systemic use. Those that are include the 2-nitroimidazole ketoconazole, and the triazoles fluconazole, itraconazole, posaconazole and voriconazole. The latter three exhibit useful activity against *Aspergillus fumigatus*. Fluconazole is well distributed after oral administration, and has been used successfully in systemic yeast infections, including cryptococcal meningitis.

The spectrum of activity of the common antifungal compounds is shown in Table 5.4. Most act by interfering with the integrity of the fungal cell membrane, either by binding to membrane sterols (polyenes) or by preventing the synthesis of ergosterol (azoles and allylamines). Echinocandins interfere with β-glucan synthesis in the fungal cell wall. Use in individual fungal diseases is considered in Chapter 61.

## ANTIVIRAL AGENTS

Compared with the number of agents available for the treatment of bacterial infection, there are relatively few antiviral agents. However, an increasing number are effective in the treatment and prophylaxis of a range of viral diseases. Those antiviral agents in clinical use are presented in Table 5.5 for agents used for diseases other than human immunodeficiency virus (HIV) infection, and in Table 5.6 for the equally long list of antiretroviral agents.

About half of all the antiviral agents presently available are nucleoside (or nucleotide) analogues, which are phosphorylated within cells to an active triphosphate and inhibit viral DNA synthesis. Some important antiviral compounds, representing a range of molecular structures, are illustrated in Figure 5.3.

## Nucleoside analogues

### Inhibitors of herpesvirus DNA polymerases

The most widely used antiviral agent, aciclovir (and the related penciclovir), is first phosphorylated to the monophosphate by a virus-encoded thymidine kinase produced in cells infected by the herpes simplex virus (HSV) or by varicella-zoster virus (VZV). Subsequent phosphorylation steps are completed by cellular kinases to form aciclovir triphosphate. This competes with the natural substrate for the viral DNA polymerase, becomes incorporated into the viral DNA chain and inhibits further DNA polymerase activity (Fig. 5.4). Aciclovir lacks a 3'-hydroxyl group on its acyclic side-chain, and therefore it cannot form a phosphodiester bond with the next nucleotide due to be added to the growing herpesvirus DNA chain, which is terminated prematurely. The lack of cellular toxicity of aciclovir is a consequence of three selective features:

1. Initial phosphorylation takes place only in virus-infected cells.
2. As phosphorylation within virally-infected cells reduces the intracellular concentration of free aciclovir, more drug will diffuse into the cell from the extracellular space, thereby resulting in concentration of drug specifically within virally-infected cells.
3. Aciclovir triphosphate inhibits viral (not cellular) DNA polymerase.

Aciclovir has an established record in the treatment of HSV and VZV disease, as prophylaxis against HSV reactivation after transplantation, and in the long-term suppression of recurrent genital herpes. Valaciclovir and famciclovir are oral pro-drug formulations of aciclovir and penciclovir, respectively. They provide improved systemic drug levels and require less frequent administration.

**Table 5.5** Antiviral agents in clinical use for infections other than human immunodeficiency virus

| Compound | Mode of action | Indication |
|---|---|---|
| **Anti-herpesvirus agents** | | |
| Aciclovir | Nucleoside analogue | Herpes simplex; varicella-zoster |
| Cidofovir | Nucleotide analogue | Cytomegalovirus retinitis |
| Famciclovir | Pro-drug of penciclovir | Herpes simplex; varicella-zoster |
| Fomivirsen | Antisense oligonucleotide | Cytomegalovirus retinitis |
| Foscarnet | Inhibition of DNA polymerase | Cytomegalovirus; aciclovir-resistant herpes simplex or varicella-zoster |
| Ganciclovir | Nucleoside analogue | Cytomegalovirus |
| Penciclovir | Nucleoside analogue | Herpes simplex; varicella-zoster |
| Valaciclovir | Pro-drug of aciclovir | Herpes simplex; varicella-zoster |
| Valganciclovir | Pro-drug of ganciclovir | Cytomegalovirus |
| **Anti-influenza agents** | | |
| Amantadine (and rimantadine) | Viral uncoating | Influenza A |
| Oseltamivir | Neuraminidase inhibitor | Influenza A and B |
| Zanamivir | Neuraminidase inhibitor | Influenza A and B |
| **Anti-hepatitis agents** | | |
| Adefovir | Nucleotide analogue | Chronic hepatitis B |
| Boceprevir | NS3 Protease inhibitor | Chronic hepatitis C |
| Entecavir | Nucleoside analogue | Chronic hepatitis B |
| Interferon-$\alpha$ | Immunomodulator | Chronic hepatitis B and C |
| Lamivudine | Nucleoside analogue | Chronic hepatitis B |
| Telaprevir | NS3 Protease inhibitor | Chronic hepatitis C |
| Telbivudine | Nucleoside analogue | Chronic hepatitis B |
| Tenofovir | Nucleotide analogue | Chronic hepatitis B |
| **Other antiviral agents** | | |
| Ribavirin | Nucleoside analogue | Respiratory syncytial virus; hepatitis C |

**Table 5.6** Antiretroviral agents in clinical use

| Type of agent | Drug names |
|---|---|
| Nucleoside analogue reverse transcriptase inhibitor | Abacavir, didanosine, emtricitabine, lamivudine, stavudine, zalcitabine, zidovudine |
| Nucleotide analogue reverse transcriptase inhibitor | Tenofovir |
| Non-nucleoside reverse transcriptase inhibitor[a] | Delavirdine, efavirenz, etravirine, nevirapine |
| Protease inhibitor | Atazanavir, amprenavir (and fosamprenavir), darunavir, indinavir, lopinavir (formulated with ritonavir), nelfinavir, ritonavir, saquinavir, tipranavir |
| Fusion inhibitor | Enfuvirtide[a] |
| Entry inhibitor | Maraviroc[b] |
| Integrase inhibitor | Raltegravir |

[a]Active against only HIV-1.
[b]Active against only those HIV strains which use CCR5 co-receptors.

Ganciclovir, which exhibits preferential activity against another herpesvirus, cytomegalovirus (CMV), is activated by a CMV protein kinase encoded by the viral gene UL97 in CMV-infected cells, but there is also considerable phosphorylation in uninfected cells, and ganciclovir is much more toxic than aciclovir, particularly to the bone marrow. Ganciclovir also exhibits antiviral effects against human herpesviruses HHV-6 and HHV-7, which do not respond to aciclovir. Valganciclovir is an oral pro-drug formulation providing a much improved systemic concentration of ganciclovir after oral administration.

Cidofovir is a nucleoside phosphonate and therefore does not require activation. It is converted in cells into the diphosphate, which inhibits CMV DNA polymerase. It shows activity against a range of DNA viruses, but its main clinical use is for CMV retinitis. It is not absorbed orally, has a very-long half-life (2 weeks), and is nephrotoxic.

Aciclovir

Zidovudine

Ribavirin

Amantadine

Foscarnet

Nevirapine

**Fig. 5.3** Molecular structures of some antiviral compounds.

dATP

dTTP

dCTP

+

ACV → ACVMP → ACVDP → ACVTP

Viral thymidine kinase

Phosphorylation by cell enzymes

Viral DNA polymerase

vDNA

• Incorporated into viral DNA
• Premature chain termination
• Viral DNA synthesis halted
• Viral DNA polymerase irreversibly inactivated

**Fig. 5.4** Mode of activation and action of aciclovir (ACV). ACVMP, aciclovir monophosphate; ACVDP, aciclovir diphosphate; ACVTP, aciclovir triphosphate; dATP, deoxyadenosine triphosphate; dTTP, deoxythymidine triphosphate; dCTP, deoxycytidine triphosphate; vDNA, viral deoxyribonucleic acid.

These antiviral agents inhibit only replicating herpesvirus and do not eliminate the latent virus. Reduced susceptibility is occasionally found in isolates of HSV, VZV or CMV, usually derived from severely immunocompromised hosts who have been receiving prolonged antiviral therapy. Clinically significant antiviral resistance arises from mutations in the viral DNA polymerases which no longer bind the antiviral triphosphate derivatives, or, in the case of CMV, mutations in the UL97 gene such that the virus cannot phosphorylate ganciclovir.

## Other inhibitors of viral RNA or DNA synthesis

Ribavirin is a nucleoside analogue that has no useful anti-herpes activity, but is used in a nebulized form in the treatment of respiratory syncytial virus infection and intravenously for Lassa fever. It is also used orally in combination with interferon for the treatment of chronic hepatitis C. Its mechanism of action is unclear, but the wide antiviral spectrum it exhibits, particularly in vitro, suggests that it may interfere with the processing of virally-derived mRNA.

The nucleoside analogues lamivudine, entecavir and telbivudine, and the nucleotide analogues adefovir and tenofovir (used as pro-drugs, adefovir dipivoxil and tenofovir disoproxil, respectively) all inhibit the reverse transcriptase activity of hepatitis B virus (HBV), thereby reducing virus replication. These drugs differ in their potency and also in the genetic barrier to development of resistance within the viral enzyme, with entecavir and tenofovir being classified as highly potent drugs with the least likelihood of emergence of resistance.

There is great interest in the development of new antiviral drugs directed against various targets within hepatitis C virus, including the NS5b RNA-dependent

RNA polymerase enzyme. However, the first directly acting agents, licensed in late 2011, for the treatment of HCV infection are the NS3 protease inhibitors telaprevir and boceprevir.

## Non-nucleoside anti-herpes agents

Foscarnet, a pyrophosphate analogue, inhibits nucleic acid synthesis without requiring any activation, and is an important agent for treatment of cytomegalovirus or of other herpesvirus infections that have become resistant to aciclovir or ganciclovir through mutations in the viral DNA polymerase or protein kinase genes. It is poorly absorbed orally, and exhibits nephrotoxicity. Fomivirsen is an antisense oligonucleotide that inhibits translation of mRNA into proteins. It has limited use as a local treatment for CMV retinitis.

## Agents that block viral uncoating

Amantadine, a symmetrical amine compound, has long been known to inhibit influenza A virus replication. Amantadine (and its derivative, rimantadine) blocks an ion channel formed by the integral membrane protein (M2) of influenza A (but not influenza B) virus, preventing uncoating of the virus within cells. Resistance arises rapidly through mutations in the M2 gene.

## Neuraminidase inhibitors

Zanamivir and oseltamivir are agents specifically designed to block the action of the influenza virus enzyme neuraminidase by occupying the catalytic site. They act on all influenza viruses. Neuraminidase is found on the surface of influenza virus, and these compounds act to prevent release of newly-formed viral particles from the cell surface, reducing the spread of influenza viruses locally. Zanamivir is taken by inhalation into the oropharynx; oseltamivir is the oral pro-drug form of a similar agent.

## Interferons

Interferons, naturally occurring antiviral compounds produced by mammalian cells in response to viral infection, are now manufactured by genetic recombination. Interferon-α (given by either subcutaneous or intramuscular injection) is used to treat chronic infection with hepatitis B and C viruses. The mode of action of interferon-α is complex, producing an antiviral state in cells to which it binds, and interfering with the production of virus in those cells (see Ch. 10). However, interferons also act through immune modulation, upregulating the expression of major histocompatibility complex (MHC) molecules on cell surfaces. This is a significant part of the action in clearing chronic hepatitis B.

Modification of interferon by addition of polyethylene glycol – *peginterferon* – results in sustained effects after just one dose per week. This agent appears to offer an effective treatment for chronic hepatitis C, a common form of chronic hepatitis, when combined with oral ribavirin.

## Antiretroviral agents

The HIV pandemic has generated an enormous interest in potential antiviral agents. Seven classes of drugs are now generally available, acting variously to inhibit viral nucleic acid synthesis, viral protein synthesis, viral entry, and integration of the DNA provirus into the host genome (see Table 5.6). All inhibit only replicating HIV and do not eliminate the integrated proviral DNA.

The use of multiple drugs in combination antiretroviral therapy (cART, previously known as 'highly active antiretroviral therapy' or HAART; see Ch. 55) may result in such suppression of HIV replication that virus is undetectable in the circulation. The use of cART prevents the development of immune deficiency in infected patients, and may also result in immune reconstitution in patients who have already developed the acquired immunodeficiency syndrome (AIDS).

Emergence of resistant mutants has been a problem with all classes of anti-HIV agent, and has stimulated developments in the field of antiviral susceptibility testing.

### Nucleoside and nucleotide reverse transcriptase inhibitors

The earliest anti-HIV agent, zidovudine (azidothymidine), and several other compounds, including didanosine (dideoxyinosine), zalcitabine (dideoxycytidine; now rarely used), lamivudine and stavudine, are nucleoside analogues. New additions include abacavir and emtricitabine, and a nucleotide analogue, tenofovir. They are activated (phosphorylated) by cellular enzymes and inhibit the reverse transcriptase function of the viral polymerase of HIV-1 or HIV-2, with many terminating the chain of proviral DNA. Phosphorylation rates vary in different cell types, and between resting and replicating cells.

Unlike aciclovir, these nucleoside analogues are associated with some toxicity as there is less selectivity in their activation and action:

- Initial phosphorylation is by cellular kinases.
- Some inhibition of cellular (mitochondrial) DNA polymerase occurs.

### Non-nucleoside reverse transcriptase inhibitors

These compounds, which include nevirapine, delavirdine (no longer widely available), efavirenz and etravirine inhibit only HIV-1. They bind directly, without activation, away from the catalytic site of reverse transcriptase, but exert a structural change that inhibits its action. They are not incorporated into the DNA chain.

### HIV protease inhibitors

These compounds act at a late stage in the viral cycle by interfering with the cleavage of essential polyprotein precursors. The numerous derivatives now available are listed in Table 5.6.

### HIV fusion inhibitors

Only one example of this class of antiretroviral agents is presently available: enfuvirtide. This drug is a homologue of the short peptide sequence active in fusion of the HIV-1 envelope to the cell membrane after attachment, and it inhibits that final stage of the entry process. The drug has to be given by subcutaneous injection, and its use is reserved for patients who have limited options for treatment. It is not active against HIV-2.

Other inhibitors of the HIV entry process are under development, including drugs that block the co-receptors for attachment. Cellular as well as viral factors will influence the success of this approach.

### HIV entry inhibitors

Initial binding of HIV to CD4 molecules present on the target cell surface is followed by binding to one of a number of secondary receptors, the most commonly used of which is CCR5, a chemokine receptor. Maraviroc is a drug which binds specifically to CCR5, thereby preventing access of viral particles to this molecule.

### HIV integrase inhibitors

Once viral RNA has been reverse transcribed into a DNA form (known as the provirus), integration of the provirus into the host cell genome is mediated by a viral integrase enzyme. The latest antiretroviral drugs to have been developed are integrase inhibitors, acting to prevent this step in the viral life cycle.

## ANTIPARASITIC AGENTS

The choice of agents for the treatment of protozoal and helminthic infections remains extremely limited. Part of the problem is that protozoa and helminths are very varied, reflecting diverse solutions to the problems of their specialized parasitic existence. Consequently, there are few 'broad-spectrum' antiprotozoal or anthelminthic agents, although some compounds exhibit a surprising range of activity. Thus the antiprotozoal nitroimidazoles, such as metronidazole, are active against *Entamoeba histolytica, Trichomonas vaginalis* and *Giardia lamblia* (see Ch. 62); benzimidazoles, such as mebendazole and albendazole, act against most intestinal nematodes; praziquantel not only exhibits good activity against all human schistosomes but also includes other trematodes and tapeworms in its spectrum (see Ch. 63). Most remarkably of all, ivermectin is active not only against many filarial worms and some intestinal roundworms but also against ectoparasites such as the scabies mite.

Antimicrobial agents commonly used against pathogenic protozoa and helminths are shown in Tables 5.7 and 5.8, respectively.

## ANTIMICROBIAL SENSITIVITY TESTS

To establish the activity of an antimicrobial agent, micro-organisms are tested for their ability to grow in the presence of suitable concentrations of the drug. Bacteria are the simplest to test and, in practice, routine sensitivity testing is usually reserved for the common, easily grown, bacterial pathogens. Tests of mycobacteria, fungi, viruses and some other organisms are available in certain laboratories and reference units. Genotypic assays for mutations associated with antiviral resistance are becoming more widely available in specialist virology centres. Similarly, genotypic assays that detect resistance mutations affecting antituberculosis therapy are available through reference centres.

### Antibacterial agents

Potency of antibacterial agents is often expressed as the *minimum inhibitory concentration* (MIC): the lowest concentration of the agent that prevents the development of visible growth of the test organism during overnight incubation. Serial dilutions of the agent are prepared in a suitable broth or agar medium, and a standard inoculum of the test organism is

**Table 5.7** Principal agents used against the major protozoan parasites of man

| Species | Agent |
|---------|-------|
| *Cryptosporidium parvum* | Nitazoxanide |
| *Entamoeba histolytica* | Metronidazole<br>Diloxanide furoate<br>(Emetine) |
| *Giardia lamblia* | Metronidazole<br>(Mepacrine) |
| *Leishmania* spp. | Sodium stibogluconate<br>Amphotericin B<br>Miltefosine |
| *Plasmodium* spp. | Chloroquine<br>Quinine<br>Pyrimethamine<br>Proguanil<br>Mefloquine<br>Halofantrine<br>Artemisinin and its derivatives |
| *Toxoplasma gondii* | Pyrimethamine + sulfadiazine |
| *Trichomonas vaginalis* | Metronidazole |
| *Trypanosoma brucei* ssp. *rhodesiense* and *gambiense* | Eflornithine[a]<br>Melarsoprol<br>(Suramin)<br>(Pentamidine) |
| *Trypanosoma cruzi* | (Benznidazole) |

Compounds in parentheses are of limited value.
[a]Not active against *T. brucei rhodesiense*.

**Table 5.8** Spectrum of activity of the principal anthelminthic agents

| Agent | Active against |
|-------|----------------|
| Benzimidazoles[a] | Intestinal nematodes |
| Diethylcarbamazine | Filarial worms |
| Ivermectin | *Onchocerca volvulus;* other filariae |
| Levamisole | Hookworms; *Ascaris lumbricoides* |
| Niclosamide | Tapeworms |
| Metrifonate | *Schistosoma haematobium* |
| Oxamniquine | *Schistosoma mansoni* |
| Piperazine | *Ascaris lumbricoides; Enterobius vermicularis* |
| Praziquantel | *Schistosoma* spp.; other trematodes; tapeworms |
| Pyrantel pamoate | *A. lumbricoides; E. vermicularis;* hookworms |
| Trivalent antimonials | *Schistosoma* spp. |

[a]Include mebendazole, tiabendazole and albendazole.

added. If agar is used, many different isolates can be tested at the same time by spot inoculation of the plate. Broth dilution MIC titrations have the advantage that the *minimum bactericidal concentration* (MBC) can additionally be estimated by subculture of dilutions of the antibiotic above that in which inhibition has occurred overnight. The MBC is usually taken as the lowest concentration capable of reducing the original inoculum by a factor of 1000, for example from $10^5$ colony-forming units (cfu)/mL to $10^2$ cfu/mL or below. To establish the rate of killing, the number of viable organisms in broth cultures is measured at timed intervals after addition of appropriate concentrations of the antibiotic.

Antibiotic titrations are too laborious for the routine assessment of antibiotic activity in clinical practice, although a truncated form of the method, in which isolates are tested at agreed *break points* of sensitivity or resistance, is sometimes used. A common alternative method is the *disc diffusion test*. The culture to be examined is seeded confluently, or semiconfluently, over the surface of an agar plate, and paper discs individually impregnated with different antibiotics are spaced evenly over the inoculated plate. Antibiotic diffuses outwards from each disc into the surrounding agar and produces a diminishing gradient of concentration. On incubation, the bacteria grow on areas of the plate except those around the drugs to which they are sensitive. The width of the *zone of inhibition* is a rough measure of the degree of sensitivity to the drug. A highly standardized version of the disc diffusion method, the *Bauer–Kirby test*, is favoured in the USA and some other countries.

Characteristics of the growth medium (such as pH or the presence of antagonizing substances), the size of the bacterial inoculum and the conditions of the test may influence the results of sensitivity tests. In disc methods, the size of the inhibition zone is additionally affected by the diffusion characteristics of the antibiotic. It is therefore important that suitable control organisms are tested in parallel in all tests of antibiotic susceptibility. In *Stokes' method*, control is achieved by placing antibiotic discs at the interface between inocula of the test and control bacteria on the same plate. In this way the zone of inhibition obtained with the test organism can be compared directly with that of a known control, and variations in the cultural conditions or in disc content can be avoided.

## Antiviral agents

Tests for antiviral susceptibility are still far from routine, being readily available only through reference or specialist laboratories. Experience with these assays is steadily increasing, and the clinical benefits of measuring antiviral susceptibility are gradually being established.

The detection of mutations associated with drug resistance is now a routine procedure in the management of HIV infection. Some reference laboratories have built up a great deal of experience with in-house sequencing of HIV genes and have generated large databases, which are shared on an international basis to allow for prediction of reduced susceptibility. Expert opinion on the significance of the mutations may usefully guide therapeutic decisions and is invaluable for selection of therapeutic combinations.

### Phenotypic assays

Phenotypic assays measure the inhibitory effect of the antiviral agent on the clinical virus isolate. The plaque reduction assay for inhibition of HSV by aciclovir is one example. An effect is usually considered to be significant when virus replication or product formation is reduced by 50% compared to that found with no drug (50% inhibitory concentration: $IC_{50}$).

For HIV assays, inhibition of replication in cultures of peripheral blood mononuclear cells is preferred. There are also recombinant virus assays in which HIV genes of interest from the test isolate are put into a laboratory strain to provide a cheaper, faster assay.

### Genotypic assays

These tests detect the presence of known resistance-associated mutations in viral genes (e.g. HIV reverse transcriptase or protease, or HBV polymerase), from which reduced susceptibility is predicted. Some of these assays are available in commercial kit format, for example:

- a line probe assay by reverse hybridization of amplified viral fragments with a panel of oligonucleotides
- an automated sequencing programme detecting mutations in reverse transcriptase and protease genes.

Genotypic assays are more commonly used than phenotypic ones, being simpler, safer and less costly for routine use.

## ASSAY OF ANTIMICROBIAL DRUGS

In most clinical circumstances in which antimicrobial agents are used it is not usually necessary to measure the concentrations achieved in blood or other body fluids (see Ch. 67). Such measurements are needed, however, during the development of a new agent to establish the pharmacokinetic behaviour of the drug.

Various techniques are available, including microbiological methods in which the antibiotic-containing material and known dilutions of the drug are titrated in parallel against a susceptible indicator organism. Analytical techniques such as high-pressure liquid chromatography may also be used.

In the few cases in which assays are needed in clinical practice, notably during treatment with aminoglycosides, immunochemical methods are often used with commercially available instrumentation.

With regard to antiviral drug assays, concerns over toxic levels of aciclovir or ganciclovir arise on occasion, and these can be measured. Therapeutic drug monitoring is also practised in relation to HIV therapy, mainly to test for compliance with the onerous regimens necessary in the management of this chronic condition.

RECOMMENDED READING

De Clercq E: In search of a selective therapy of viral infections, *Antiviral Research* 85:19–24, 2009.

Finch RG, Davey PG, Wilcox MH, Irving WL: *Antimicrobial Chemotherapy*, ed 6, Oxford, 2012, Oxford University Press.

Finch RG, Greenwood D, Norrby SR, Whitley RJ: *Antibiotic and Chemotherapy: Anti-infective Agents and their Use in Therapy*, ed 9, London, 2010, Saunders, Elsevier.

Franklin TJ, Snow GA: *Biochemistry and Molecular Biology of Antimicrobial Drug Action*, ed 6, New York, 2005, Springer.

Grayson ML, Crowe SM, McCarthy J, et al: *Kucers' The Use of Antibiotics: A Clinical Review of Antibacterial, Antifungal and Antiviral Drugs*, ed 6, London, 2010, Hodder Arnold.

Lorian V, editor: *Antibiotics in Laboratory Medicine*, ed 5, Baltimore, 2005, Lippincott, Williams & Wilkins.

Volberding P, Deeks SG: Antiretroviral therapy and management of HIV infection, *Lancet* 376:49–62, 2010.

### Websites

National electronic library of infection. Bugs & drugs on the web. http://www.antibioticresistance.org.uk/

United States National Library of Medicine and National Institutes of Health. Antibiotics. http://www.nlm.nih.gov/medlineplus/antibiotics.html

World Health Organization. Essential Medicines and Pharmaceutical Policies. http://www.who.int/medicines/en/

# 6 Bacterial genetics

K. J. Towner

## KEY POINTS

- The properties of a bacterial cell are defined by the information encoded in its double-stranded DNA genetic complement and its interaction with the environment. The single circular chromosome that, in most cases, comprises the *genome*, carries most of this, but much additional information resides within extrachromosomal elements known as *plasmids.*
- Plasmids and several other mobile genetic elements, including *bacteriophages, transposons* and other *integron*-based entities, render the bacterial genetic complement highly susceptible to variation by the addition of new genes. Such elements are often organized into *pathogenicity islands* or *resistance islands* and may affect the medical significance of bacterial strains when the genes they encode affect antibiotic susceptibility or virulence.
- Mobile genetic elements are transferred between related bacteria through the processes of *transformation, conjugation* and *transduction.*
- Bacterial genomes are also susceptible to change through mutation, in which the primary nucleotide sequence of one or more genes or regulatory elements is altered. Because bacterial replication produces very large cell numbers, the possibilities for generation and survival of advantageous mutations (commonly at frequencies of $10^{-7}$–$10^{-10}$), such as those conferring resistance to antibiotics, are of practical significance.
- These forms of *genotypic variation* should be distinguished from *phenotypic variation*, as the former are heritable whereas the latter are not, and reflect changes in gene expression and, in the case of *phase variation*, genetic rearrangements leading to altered expression patterns without changing the cell's genetic complement.
- Knowledge of the genetic complement of bacteria enables their specific detection, typing and recognition of key aspects of genotypic variation by the application of specific gene (hybridization) probes and by the use of targeted DNA amplification technologies such as the *polymerase chain reaction (PCR)*. The possibility of rapid detection (hours) of many different targets has been enhanced by the development of *real-time PCR*.

## GENETIC ORGANIZATION AND REGULATION OF THE BACTERIAL CELL

All properties of a bacterial cell, including those of medical importance such as virulence, pathogenicity and antibiotic resistance, are determined ultimately by the genetic information contained within the cell *genome*. This information is normally encoded by the specific sequence of nucleotide bases comprising the DNA of the cell. There are four common nucleotide bases in DNA: adenine, guanine, cytosine and thymine; it is the linear order in which these bases are arranged that determines the properties of the cell. With only a few exceptions, most of the genetic information required by the bacterial cell is arranged in the form of a single circular double-stranded chromosome. It is worth noting that the main bacterial chromosome is not a completely stable structure, but can exhibit quite dynamic reorganization following the insertion or deletion of *transposons, integrons* and *genomic islands* (see below) under fluctuating environmental and selective conditions. In *Escherichia coli* the chromosome is about 1300 μm long and occurs in an irregular coiled bundle lying free in the cytoplasm. The DNA is not associated with histone proteins as it is in eukaryotic cell chromosomes, although there are many DNA binding proteins involved in regulation of gene expression, including several proteins referred to as histone-like.

In addition to the single main chromosome, bacterial cells may also carry one or more small circular extrachromosomal elements termed *plasmids*. Plasmids replicate independently of the main chromosome in the cell. Although dispensable, they often carry supplementary genetic information coding for beneficial properties (e.g. resistance to antibiotics) that enable the host cell to survive under a particular set of environmental conditions.

A third source of genetic information in a bacterial cell can be provided by the presence of certain types of bacterial virus, *bacteriophages*. Bacteriophages consist essentially of just a protein coat enclosing the virus genome and, because they are unable to multiply in the absence of their bacterial host, generally they are lethal to their host cell. In some instances, they can enter a potentially long-term state of controlled replication, *lysogeny*, within the bacterial cell without causing lysis. In such a state the bacteriophage genome is referred to as a *prophage* and effectively becomes a temporary part of the total genetic information available to the cell and may consequently bestow additional properties on the cell.

Not all genetic material consists of double-stranded DNA. Some bacteriophages contain single-stranded molecules of either DNA or RNA, which can be either circular or linear in configuration. The genetic elements under consideration here, including bacteriophages, plasmids and members of the domain *Bacteria*, vary in size by more than three orders of magnitude, from about 3–5000 kilobases (kb) (Table 6.1).

## Processes leading to protein synthesis

The character of a bacterial cell is determined essentially by the specific polypeptides that comprise its enzymes and other proteins. The DNA acts as a template for the *transcription* of RNA by RNA polymerase for subsequent protein production within the cell. In the transcription process the specific sequence of nucleotides in the DNA determines the corresponding sequence of nucleotides in the messenger RNA (mRNA). This, in turn, is then *translated* into the appropriate sequence of amino acids by ribosomes. Finally, the sequence of amino acids in the resulting polypeptide chain determines the configuration into which the polypeptide chain folds itself, which in many cases determines the enzymic properties of the completed protein. A segment of DNA that specifies the production of a particular polypeptide chain is called a *gene*, and the processes of transcription and translation leading to protein synthesis are collectively termed the *central dogma* of molecular biology. These processes are illustrated schematically in Figure 6.1.

## Gene regulation

Most bacteria contain enough DNA to code for the production of between 1000 and 3000 different polypeptide chains – 1000 to 3000 different genes. However, during normal bacterial life, some polypeptides will be required only at particular stages, whereas others will be needed only when the cell is provided with a new or unusual growth substrate, or is confronted with a new challenge, such as an antibiotic. Thus, many antibiotic resistance mechanisms found in bacteria are *inducible* (see below). Protein production is an energy-intensive process, and therefore the expression of many genes is controlled actively within the cell to prevent wasteful energy consumption.

In bacteria the process of gene expression is regulated mainly at the transcriptional level, thereby conserving the energy supply and the transcription–translation apparatus. This is achieved by means of regulatory elements that either inhibit or enhance the rate of RNA chain initiation and termination for a particular gene. Numerous complex regulatory chain mechanisms are involved in coordinating the many biochemical reactions that proceed inside a cell, but related genes involved in a common regulatory system are often clustered on the bacterial chromosome. Such functional clusters are known as *operons*, of which the most well known example is the lactose operon of *E. coli* (Fig. 6.2).

For transcription to occur as the first stage in protein synthesis, RNA polymerase has to attach to

**Table 6.1** Examples of prokaryotic genetic elements

| Genetic element | Type | Configuration | Size (kb) |
|---|---|---|---|
| **Bacterial chromosome** | | | |
| *Escherichia coli* | DNA | ds circular | $3.8 \times 10^3$ |
| *Bacillus subtilis* | DNA | ds circular | $2.0 \times 10^3$ |
| **Plasmids** | | | |
| R300B | DNA | ds circular | 9.0 |
| RK2 | DNA | ds circular | 60.0 |
| **Bacteriophages** | | | |
| MS2 | RNA | ss linear | 3.6 |
| ΦPH174 | DNA | ss circular | 5.4 |
| T7 | DNA | ds linear | 40.4 |

ss, single-stranded; ds, double-stranded.

**Fig. 6.1** The central dogma of molecular biology.

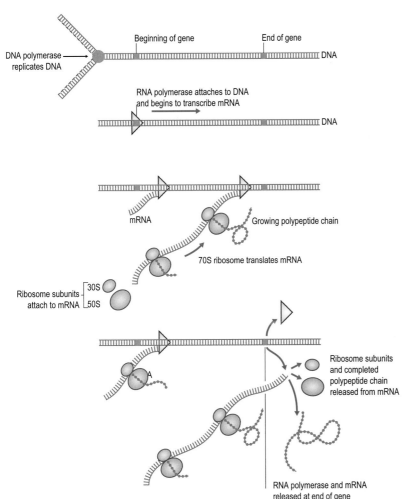

DNA polymerase replicates DNA

Beginning of gene

End of gene

DNA

RNA polymerase attaches to DNA and begins to transcribe mRNA

DNA

mRNA

Growing polypeptide chain

70S ribosome translates mRNA

Ribosome subunits attach to mRNA

30S

50S

Ribosome subunits and completed polypeptide chain released from mRNA

RNA polymerase and mRNA released at end of gene

DNA at a specific *promoter* region and transcribe the DNA in a fixed direction. This process can be switched off by the attachment of a *repressor* molecule to a specific region of the DNA, known as the *operator*. This lies between the promoter and the structural gene(s) being transcribed; the repressor then blocks the movement of the RNA polymerase molecule so that the genes downstream are not transcribed.

The repressor is often an allosteric molecule with two active sites. One recognizes the operator region so that the repressor can bind to it to prevent transcription. The other recognizes an *inducer* molecule. When the inducer is present, it binds to the repressor and alters simultaneously the binding specificity at the other site, so that the repressor no longer binds to the operator and transcription can resume.

There are many different variations on this basic regulatory system. For example, a repressor may be normally inactive, but activated by the end-product of a biosynthetic pathway; thus, only when the end-product is present in adequate concentration will the repressor combine with the operator and switch off transcription of the operon. Alternatively, regulation of certain operons involves proteins that bind to the DNA and assist RNA polymerase to initiate transcription. These are just a few examples, and other regulatory systems display both minor and major differences. Finally, it should be stressed that prokaryotic gene regulation frequently involves interwoven regulatory circuits that respond to a variety of different stimuli. As noted in Chapter 4, these networks of genes are organized into functional units known as *stimulons* when they respond to a particular stimulus

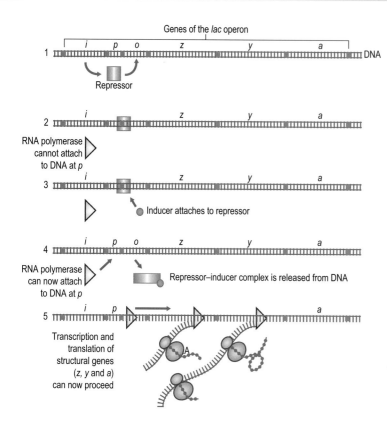

**Fig. 6.2**   The *lac* operon of *Escherichia coli*. (1) The *lac* repressor is produced from the *i* gene. (2) Binding of the repressor to the operator site (*o*) prevents transcription of the genes *z* (β-galactosidase), *y* (galactoside permease) and *a* (transacetylase). (3) The inducer (lactose, or a closely related derivative) can bind specifically to the repressor. (4) The repressor molecule is thereby altered at its operator-binding site and the repressor–inducer complex is released from the DNA. (5) RNA polymerase can now attach to the promoter site (*p*) and transcribe the structural genes of the *lac* operon. Note that, in bacteria, several genes may be transcribed into a single *polycistronic* mRNA molecule.

and *regulons* when they are regulated by a single protein.

## MUTATION

As bacteria reproduce by asexual binary fission, the genome is normally identical in all of the progeny. However, one of the fundamental requirements for evolution is that, although gene replication must normally be completely accurate to ensure stability, there must also be occasional variation to produce new or altered characters that might be of selective value to the organism. Rare inaccuracies in the DNA replication process produce a slightly altered nucleotide sequence in one of the progeny cells. Such a mutation is heritable and will be passed on stably to subsequent generations. Mutations may not produce any observable effect on the structure or function of the corresponding protein, but in a small proportion of cases an enzyme with altered specificity for substrates, inhibitors or regulatory molecules may be produced. This is the kind of mutation that is most likely to be of evolutionary value to an organism; indeed, many examples of acquired antibiotic resistance have been shown to

be of this type. Other mutations may alter a gene so that a non-functional protein is formed; if this protein is essential to the cell then the mutation will be lethal.

As a mutation may occur in any one of the several thousand genes of the cell, and different mutations in the same gene may produce different effects in the cell, the number of possible mutations is very large. Particular mutations occur at fairly constant rates, normally between one per $10^4$ and one per $10^{10}$ cell divisions. As a large bacterial colony contains at least $10^9$ cells, even a 'pure' bacterial culture will contain many thousands of different mutations affecting many of the genes in the cell. Some of these mutations will be viable and could be selected by particular environmental conditions during subculture. For the same reason, in an infected patient, a variety of mutants will appear spontaneously in the population that grows from the few bacteria originally entering the body. Such mutations may enhance the ability of an organism to cause infection, for example by conferring antibiotic resistance, enhanced virulence or altered surface antigens. In such a situation, cells with the mutation will rapidly outgrow cells without the mutation, so that selection of the mutant cells occurs and they soon become the predominant type.

## Phenotypic variation

The properties of a bacterial cell at a particular time are referred to as the *phenotype* of the cell. These properties are determined not only by its genome (*genotype*), but also by its environment. *Phenotypic variation* occurs when the *expression* of genes is changed in response to the environment, for instance by the induction or repression of synthesis of particular enzymes. Such changes in gene expression underpin the differentiation process involved in sporulation (see p. 19), the differing phenotypes observed during different growth phases and under different growth conditions (p. 40) and the physiological *adaptive* responses of bacteria (p. 46). The distinction between genotypic mutation and phenotypic variation is critical; the former is heritable and maintained through changes in environmental conditions, whereas the latter is reversible, being dependent on environmental conditions and altering when these change. Phenotypic variation is therefore not a form of mutation.

## Types of mutation

Mutations can be divided conveniently into *multisite mutations*, involving extensive chromosomal rearrangements such as inversions, duplications and deletions, and *point mutations*, which are defined as only affecting one, or very few, nucleotides. The structure of DNA is such that point mutations can be divided into one of three basic types (Fig. 6.3):

1. substitution of one nucleotide for another
2. deletion of one or more nucleotides
3. insertion of one or more nucleotides.

Mutations occur spontaneously during replication of DNA, but most are corrected immediately by the editing apparatus of the cell. Occasional mutations, particularly those conferring a selective advantage to the cell, will be inherited stably by the progeny, but secondary mutations can occasionally restore the original nucleotide sequence. It is important to distinguish this relatively rare event of *back-mutation* from the separate process of *phase variation*, which is readily reversible and occurs with relatively high frequency in either direction, for example once per $10^3$ cell divisions. The variation of certain Gram-negative bacteria between a fimbriate and a non-fimbriate phase, and the variation of flagellar antigens in *Salmonella enterica* serotypes, are examples of phase variation. These seem to involve special genetic regions that are specifically inverted to yield alternative gene products and different phenotypes. In some cases it is known that promoters initiate RNA transcription in different directions to give a flip-flop type of action. The number of such switching systems is probably quite limited, but they have value to the organism in providing a mechanism to switch to a reversible alternative, as opposed to an irreversible change.

Mutations may occur in any gene, but many individual mutations are lethal. Other mutations affect gene products that are essential only under particular cultural conditions. The detailed function and regulation of processes in the bacterial cell can often be analyzed only by searching systematically for mutations that affect each separate step in a process. Thus, mutations can be found that produce increased resistance to almost any antimicrobial agent, and the study of such mutants is an essential step in understanding the modes of action of antibiotic agents and mechanisms of resistance to them.

# GENE TRANSFER

A change in the genome of a bacterial cell may be caused either by a mutation in the DNA of the cell or result from the acquisition of additional DNA from an external source. DNA may be transferred between bacteria by three mechanisms:

1. transformation
2. conjugation
3. transduction.

Each of these mechanisms probably occurs at a low frequency in nature and may therefore be of value in bacterial evolution. It is important to note that acquisition by bacteria of new properties following gene transfer or mutation is only significant if the new genetic end-product is subject to favourable selection

**Fig. 6.3** Examples of types of mutation. The top sequence represents a portion of the wild-type chromosome from which the different mutational rearrangements shown below are derived.

by the conditions under which the bacteria are growing.

## Transformation

Most species of bacteria are unable to take up exogenous DNA from the environment; indeed, most bacteria produce nucleases that recognize and break down foreign DNA. However, bacteria in some genera, notably pneumococci, *Haemophilus influenzae* and certain *Bacillus* species, have been shown to be capable of taking up DNA either extracted artificially or released by lysis from cells of another strain. Cells are *competent* for transformation only under certain conditions of growth, usually in late log phase or, in *Bacillus* species, during sporulation. However, bacterial geneticists have also developed treatments by means of which organisms can be made artificially competent.

Once a piece of DNA has entered the cell by transformation, it has to become incorporated into the existing chromosome of the cell by a process of *recombination* in order to survive. This is a complex molecular process for which the transformed DNA must have been derived from a closely related strain, as pieces of DNA can normally recombine with the chromosome only when there is a high degree of nucleic acid similarity (*homology*).

Any gene may be transferred by transformation, as any fragment of a donor chromosome may be taken up by the recipient cells. However, a piece of DNA introduced into a cell by transformation will normally be relatively short, and will contain only a very small number of genes. For this reason, transformation is of limited use for studying the organization of genes in relation to one another (*genetic mapping*; see below).

## Conjugation

Conjugation is a process by which one cell, the *donor* or male cell, makes contact with another, the *recipient* or female cell, and DNA is transferred directly from the donor into the recipient. Certain types of plasmids carry the genetic information necessary for conjugation to occur. Only cells that contain such a plasmid can act as donors; those lacking a corresponding plasmid act as recipients.

Transfer of DNA between cells by conjugation requires direct contact between donor and recipient cells. Plasmids capable of mediating conjugation carry genes coding for the production of a 1–2-μm long protein appendage, termed a *pilus*, on the surface of the donor cell. The tip of the pilus attaches to the surface of a recipient cell and holds the two cells together so that DNA can pass into the recipient cell. It is probable, but not absolutely certain, that transfer actually occurs through the pilus; alternatively, the pilus could act simply as a mechanism by which the donor and recipient cells are drawn together. Different types of pilus are specified by different types of plasmid and can therefore be used as an aid to plasmid classification.

In the vast majority of cases, the only DNA transferred during the conjugation process is the plasmid that mediates the process. It is thought that one strand of the circular DNA of the plasmid is nicked open at a specific site and the free end is passed into the recipient cell. The DNA is replicated during transfer so that each cell receives a copy. As donor ability is dependent upon having a copy of the plasmid, the recipient strain becomes converted into a donor, able to conjugate with further recipients and convert them in turn. In this way a plasmid may spread rapidly through a whole population of recipient cells; this process is sometimes described as infectious spread of a plasmid.

### Mobilization of chromosomal genes by conjugation

Many different types of plasmid have the ability to transfer themselves. Some (but not all) plasmids also have the ability to mobilize the chromosomal genes of bacteria. The first reported plasmid of this type was the 'F factor' (fertility factor) of *E. coli*. Cells that contain the F plasmid free in the cytoplasm (*$F^+$ cells*) have no unusual characteristics apart from the ability to produce F pili and to transfer the F plasmid to *$F^-$ cells* by conjugation. In a very small proportion of $F^+$ cells, the F plasmid becomes inserted into the bacterial chromosome. Once inserted, the entire chromosome behaves like an enormous F plasmid, and hence chromosomal genes can be transferred in the normal manner to a recipient cell at a relatively high frequency. Such cultures are termed *high-frequency recombination* (Hfr) strains.

It is important to emphasize that the F plasmid system is confined to *E. coli* and other closely related enteric bacteria. However, many other plasmids are capable of mediating conjugation, and sometimes chromosome mobilization, not only in *E. coli* but also in other bacteria. For example, plasmid RP4 and its relatives have been used to mediate conjugation in a wide range of Gram-negative bacteria, and there have been reports of conjugation systems in Gram-positive bacteria, such as *Enterococcus faecalis*, and several *Streptomyces* species.

## Transduction

The third known mechanism of gene transfer in bacteria involves the transfer of DNA between cells by bacteriophages. Most bacteriophages carry their genetic information (the phage genome) as a length of double-stranded DNA coiled up inside a protein coat. Other phages are known in which the phage genome consists of single-stranded DNA or RNA but, as far as is known, transducing phages all contain double-stranded DNA. Two major types of transduction are known to occur in bacteria: *generalized* and *specialized* transduction. In both types, bacterial genes are occasionally and accidentally incorporated into new phage particles. When such a phage particle subsequently infects a second bacterial cell, the DNA that enters the cell includes a short segment of chromosome from the original host. Bacterial genes have been *transduced* by the phage into the second cell. Genes can be transduced only between fairly closely related strains, as particular phages usually attack only a limited range of bacteria. As well as chromosomal genes, transducing bacteriophages may also pick up and transfer plasmid DNA. As an example, the penicillinase gene in staphylococci is usually located on a plasmid, and it may be transferred into other staphylococcal strains by transduction.

### Lysogenic conversion

The presence of prophage DNA constitutes a genetic alteration to the host cell. Usually only the phage repressor gene is expressed, but in certain cases it can be demonstrated that other genes are also expressed by the host cell. For example, *Corynebacterium diphtheriae* produces diphtheria toxin only when it is lysogenized by β phage; the toxin is specified by one of the phage genes. This process is termed *lysogenic conversion*. It is probable that the production of many toxins by staphylococci, streptococci and clostridia is also dependent upon lysogenic conversion by specific bacteriophages. In such cases, lysogenic conversion not only gives the cell superinfection immunity, but also actively influences the virulence of the bacterium for humans.

## PLASMIDS

### Properties encoded by plasmids

As described above, plasmids are circular extra-chromosomal genetic elements that may encode a variety of supplementary genetic information, including the information for self-transfer to other cells by conjugation. Not all plasmids can transfer themselves, but *non-conjugative* plasmids can be *mobilized* by other conjugative plasmids present in the same donor cell. Apart from this optional transfer ability, all bacterial plasmids contain the basic genetic information necessary for self-replication and segregation into daughter cells at cell division. Plasmids seem to be ubiquitous in bacteria; many encode genetic information for such properties as resistance to antibiotics, bacteriocin production, resistance to toxic metal ions, production of toxins and other virulence factors, reduced sensitivity to mutagens, or the ability to degrade complex organic molecules.

## Plasmid classification

Because of the vast range of plasmids, it is necessary to have a means of classification so that their distribution and epidemiology can be studied. Plasmids can be grouped initially according to the properties that they encode, but other physical and genetical methods are needed to study their spread and distribution.

As all plasmids are relatively small structures that are normally separate from the bacterial cell chromosome, it is possible to isolate them from the chromosome by centrifugation and electrophoresis techniques that allow the sizes of different plasmids to be compared directly. Plasmids of similar size that confer identical phenotypes on host cells can be compared by generating *restriction endonuclease fingerprints* from purified plasmid DNA. A restriction endonuclease is an enzyme that cuts the DNA molecule at, or near to, a specific nucleotide sequence to produce discrete DNA fragments that can be separated by gel electrophoresis. The pattern ('fingerprint') of fragments produced is dependent on the distribution of the specific DNA sequences recognized by the enzyme. Closely related plasmids will produce the same, or very similar, fingerprints, whereas unrelated plasmids will produce different fingerprints. Restriction endonucleases of different specificities may be needed to generate distinctive fingerprints.

An initial genetic test will distinguish groups of plasmids that are self-transmissible from those that are not. Linked with the question of transferability is the question of host range; for example, some groups can be transferred only between members of the enterobacteria, other groups can be transferred from the enteric bacteria to the *Pseudomonas* family, whereas others can be transferred between almost any Gram-negative bacteria. Similar host range relationships exist among plasmids of Gram-positive bacteria.

Once the host range of a plasmid has been determined, plasmids may be classified by *incompatibility testing*. This method relies on the fact that closely related plasmids are unable to coexist stably in the same bacterial cell. Plasmids that are sufficiently closely related to interfere with one another's replication in this manner are said to be *incompatible* and to belong to the same *incompatibility group*. In contrast, unrelated plasmids can coexist stably and are therefore said to belong to different incompatibility groups. Recent developments in molecular biology enable the incompatibility group of a plasmid to be determined from the DNA sequence of its replicase (*rep*) gene as opposed to the original more time-consuming process of testing the stability of pairs of plasmids in a bacterial cell.

A final method for plasmid classification involves the use of specific virulent bacteriophages. All members of the same plasmid incompatibility group produce the same type of pilus for conjugation. For some incompatibility groups, specific virulent bacteriophages have been isolated that will adhere only to the type of pilus produced by that particular group of plasmids. Lysis by such a phage shows that a particular type of pilus is being produced, which in turn allows the identification of the group to which the plasmid contained in the cell belongs.

### Plasmid epidemiology and distribution

Some plasmid groups have been identified in many different countries of the world, whereas others have so far been found only in a single bacterial species isolated from a solitary ecological niche. There seem to be two major ways in which plasmids spread:

1. by direct transfer from one bacterium to another in a particular micro-environment
2. by being carried in a particular host from one environment, such as a hospital, to another.

The epidemiological tracing of these pathways requires identification not just of the plasmids involved but also typing of their host bacterial strains (see Ch. 3).

### TRANSPOSONS, INTEGRONS AND GENOMIC ISLANDS

As mentioned above, the main bacterial chromosome can exhibit quite dynamic reorganization following the insertion or deletion of transposons, integrons and genomic islands under fluctuating environmental and selective conditions. *Transposons* are linear pieces of DNA, often including genes for antibiotic resistance (see below), that can migrate between unrelated plasmids and/or the bacterial chromosome independently of the normal bacterial recombination processes. *Integrons* form an essential 'building block' of many transposons and allow the rapid formation and expression of new combinations of genes in response to selection pressures. A detailed description of the properties of these elements lies outside the scope of this text (see Recommended Reading), but suffice it to say that these elements seem to provide the primary mechanism for 'foreign' gene capture and dissemination, certainly among Gram-negative bacteria. It is also now recognized that transposons and integrons (as well as other genes) can often be found inserted into the main bacterial chromosome at specific sites where they form *genomic islands* of 'foreign' genetic material. Depending on the precise genes contained in these islands, they can also be referred to as *pathogenicity islands* or *resistance islands*. In some cases, the collection of genes contained in such islands can form a highly mobile structure. For example, highly mobile superantigen-encoding pathogenicity islands can be found in *Staph. aureus*; these are characterized by a specific set of phage-related functions that enable them to use the phage reproduction cycle for their own transduction across quite large phylogenetic distances.

### GENETIC MAPPING

The location of genes with reference to one another and to their respective control regions by mapping techniques is an essential part of genetic analysis. Historically, this required the transfer of genetic material between different mutants, initially by conjugation to locate the approximate position of an unknown gene on the chromosome or a plasmid, followed by fine structure mapping with generalized transduction.

A more modern approach that can be used for all bacterial genera makes use of molecular techniques allowing the sequencing of whole genomes (see *Genomics*, below), followed if appropriate by the isolation, cloning and nucleotide sequencing of individual genes. Once a particular gene or sequence of DNA has been selected and analyzed, it is possible to label it and use the gene as a *probe* in hybridization experiments. Alternatively, it is possible to synthesize a small stretch of nucleotides, termed an *oligonucleotide*, from within the overall gene sequence for use as a probe. *Hybridization* is a process in which two single strands of nucleic acid come together to form a stable double-stranded molecule. As long as the sequence of bases is complementary on each strand, the two strands will bind together by the formation of hydrogen bonds. Oligonucleotide probes are normally only 10–40 bases in length, and can be synthesized and chemically labelled by automated instruments designed specifically for this purpose. The labelled probe can then be used in hybridization experiments with relatively large fragments ('fingerprints') generated from the entire bacterial chromosome with rare-cutting restriction endonucleases. The probe will hybridize only to the chromosomal DNA fragment containing the original gene from which the probe was derived, and will therefore indicate the precise physical location of the original gene in relation to other known genes and control regions. Thus, it is now possible to elucidate the relationship between gene structure and function in the cell at the most fundamental molecular level.

## GENETIC BASIS OF ANTIBIOTIC RESISTANCE

All of the properties of a micro-organism are determined ultimately by genes located or inserted either on the main chromosome or on plasmids or on lysogenic bacteriophages. With regard to antibiotic resistance, it is important to distinguish between *intrinsic* and *acquired* resistance. Intrinsic resistance is dependent upon the natural insusceptibility of an organism. In contrast, acquired resistance involves changes in the DNA content of a cell, such that the cell acquires a phenotype (i.e. antibiotic resistance) that is not inherent in that particular species.

### Intrinsic resistance

Organisms that are naturally insensitive to a particular drug will always exist. The most obvious determinant of bacterial response to an antibiotic is the presence or absence of the target for the action of the drug. Thus, polyene antibiotics such as amphotericin B kill fungi by binding tightly to the sterols in the fungal cell membrane and altering the permeability of the fungal cell. As bacterial membranes do not contain sterols they are intrinsically resistant to this class of antibiotics. Similarly, the presence of a permeability barrier provided by the cell envelopes of Gram-negative bacteria is important in determining sensitivity patterns to many antibiotics. Intrinsic resistance is usually predictable in a clinical situation and requires an informed and judicious choice of appropriate antimicrobial therapy.

### Acquired resistance

An ongoing problem of antimicrobial chemotherapy has been the appearance of resistance to particular drugs in a normally sensitive microbial population. An organism may lose its sensitivity to an antibiotic during a course of treatment. In some cases the loss of sensitivity may be slight, but often organisms become resistant to clinically achievable concentrations of a drug. Once resistance has appeared, the continuing presence of an antibiotic exerts a *selective pressure* in favour of the resistant organisms. Three main factors affect the frequency of acquired resistance:

1. the amount of antibiotic that is being used
2. the frequency with which bacteria can undergo spontaneous mutations to resistance
3. the prevalence of plasmids able to transfer resistance from one bacterium to another.

### *Chromosomal mutations*

Random spontaneous mutations occur continuously at a low frequency in all bacterial populations, and some mutations may confer resistance to a particular antibiotic. The rate at which these mutations occur is not normally influenced by presence of the antibiotic, but in the presence of the drug the resistant mutant can survive, grow and eventually become the predominant, or only, member of the population. The degree of resistance conferred by chromosomal mutation depends on the biological consequences of the mutation. With *single large-step mutations*, the drug target is altered by mutation so that it is totally unable to bind a drug, although it can still carry out its normal biological functions sufficiently well to permit the continued survival of the cell. This type of mutation occurs with nalidixic acid and rifampicin. More commonly, the target is altered so that it can no longer bind a drug as efficiently, although it still has some residual affinity. In such a case a higher concentration of antibiotic would be required to produce the same antimicrobial effect: the *minimum inhibitory concentration* (MIC) of the antibiotic for the organism would be increased. Once a slightly resistant organism has been produced, additional mutational events – each conferring an additional small degree of resistance – can eventually lead to the production of organisms that are highly resistant. This is called the *multistep pattern of resistance*. Spontaneous chromosomal mutation is of clinical importance in tuberculosis, in which mutants resistant to any single drug (e.g. streptomycin, rifampicin or isoniazid) are likely to be present in the patient before the start of treatment. If only one drug is given to the patient, the few resistant mutant bacteria will multiply and eventually cause a relapse of the disease. Combined therapy with several drugs to which the organism is sensitive is used in the treatment of tuberculosis, so that each drug kills the few mutants that are resistant to the other. The frequency with which double or triple mutations occur spontaneously in the same cell is so low as to be clinically insignificant.

There are many other examples of chromosomal mutations to antibiotic resistance that have assumed clinical importance. Bacterial enzymes called β-lactamases are commonly responsible for resistance to penicillins, cephalosporins and related antibiotics that contain a β-lactam ring (see Ch. 5). Mutations in the genes controlling the production of chromosomally encoded β-lactamases in Gram-negative bacteria can result in overproduction of these enzymes and consequent resistance to the cephalosporin antibiotics normally regarded as stable to β-lactamase.

Chromosomal mutations leading to antibiotic resistance are in many cases just as important clinically as the types of transferable resistance described in the next section.

### Transferable antibiotic resistance

Of the three modes of gene transfer in bacteria, plasmid-mediated conjugation is of greatest significance in terms of drug resistance. Plasmids conferring resistance to one or more unrelated groups of antibiotics (R plasmids) can be transferred rapidly by conjugation throughout the population.

R plasmids were first demonstrated in Japan in 1959, when it was shown that resistance to several antibiotics could be transferred by conjugation between strains of Shigella and E. coli. Many surveys since then in all parts of the world have shown that R plasmids are common and widespread.

The way in which R plasmids are built up in vivo probably varies from case to case, but it is clear that simple transfer factors can pick up resistance genes and combine them with non-transmissible resistance plasmids to produce complex transmissible R plasmids that encode resistance to as many as eight or more different antimicrobial drugs. This process of plasmid evolution is accelerated considerably by the involvement of transposons and integrons (see above). R plasmids can transfer themselves into a wide range of commensal and pathogenic bacteria. Once resistance to an antibiotic appears in any one of these species, the process of transposition assists the dissemination of the responsible gene between different R plasmids and subsequent distribution to other

bacterial species. As described above, integrons form an essential 'building block' of many transposons and allow the rapid formation and expression of new combinations of antibiotic resistance genes in response to selection pressures. These, in turn, can be assembled into resistance islands that can be found inserted into the bacterial chromosome. For example, antibiotic resistance in several Salm. enterica serovars that cause gastrointestinal disease in humans is caused by the presence in the chromosome of a set of related genomic islands carrying a class 1 integron, which carries the resistance genes. Salmonella genomic island 1 (SGI1), the first island of this type, was found in Salm. enterica serovar Typhimurium DT104 isolates, which are resistant to ampicillin, chloramphenicol, florfenicol, streptomycin, spectinomycin, sulphonamides and tetracycline. Several Salmonella serovars and Proteus mirabilis have since been shown to harbor SGI1 or related islands carrying various sets of resistance genes and some distinct groups have emerged. SGI1 is an integrative mobilizable element and can be transferred experimentally into Escherichia coli.

As the prevalence of multiple-resistance R plasmids carrying transposons and integrons continues to increase, infections caused by a wide range of pathogens become more difficult to treat. In addition, R plasmids can also carry genes, for example for toxin production, that confer increased virulence on a bacterial cell. Thus, use of antibiotics may select for bacteria carrying plasmids that confer not only multiple drug resistance but also increased pathogenicity.

## Control of antibiotic resistance

The major cause of the spread of genes conferring antibiotic resistance is the selection pressure brought about by the increased, and often indiscriminate, use of antibiotics in man and animals. Plasmid-encoded drug resistance is increased by the widespread use of antibiotics in animal husbandry, where antibiotics are used as animal feed supplements and whole animal populations may be treated, rather than an individual subject as occurs in medical practice. When R plasmids are present, the mass use of antibiotics fails to prevent the spread of resistance and selects R plasmids in the gut microbiota of the whole population of animals. Such R plasmids, evolved in farm animals, have the potential to spread to human commensal bacteria, followed by transfer to more important human pathogens.

It is important to minimize the use of antibiotics as much as possible and to reduce the chance of cross-infection. Rational use of antibiotics and sensible restriction of their availability in man and animals could prevent further spread of R plasmids and perhaps reduce their incidence. Some R plasmids are unstable and tend to lose resistance genes when the selection pressure is removed. R plasmids are also lost spontaneously from a small proportion of cells in a culture, as plasmid replication and segregation are not always precisely synchronous with chromosome replication and segregation. Cells that lose an R plasmid may have a slight metabolic advantage and may slowly outgrow drug-resistant organisms. Moreover, R plasmids that evolve in one species may be unstable in another or may transfer themselves to other organisms much less efficiently. Similarly, organisms that are adapted to the gut of a calf, pig or chicken may not establish readily in human beings. Such factors may help to contain the spread of R plasmids.

**Fig. 6.4** Schematic outline of the polymerase chain reaction (PCR). Each cycle in the exponential reaction consists of three steps: (i) heat denaturation, typically at 94°C, to dissociate double-stranded (ds) DNA; (ii) annealing of primers (▭) at a temperature determined empirically for each individual PCR; (iii) elongation at an optimal temperature for thermostable polymerase activity, typically 72°C for *Taq* polymerase.

## APPLICATIONS OF MOLECULAR GENETICS

### Specific gene probes

Every properly classified species must, by definition, have somewhere on its chromosome a unique DNA sequence that distinguishes it from every other species. If this sequence can be identified, a specific labelled DNA probe (see above) can be used in a hybridization reaction to recognize pathogen-specific DNA released from clinical samples. Initial isolation of the infecting pathogen is not necessary and, consequently, DNA probes can be used to detect pathogens that cannot be cultured easily in vitro.

DNA probes have already been used successfully to identify a wide variety of pathogens, from simple viruses to pathogenic bacteria and parasites. Probes have also been developed that can recognize specific antibiotic resistance genes, so that antimicrobial susceptibility of an infecting organism can be determined directly without primary isolation and growth. Commercial kits incorporating DNA probes are now available to detect a range of bacteria and viruses.

### Nucleic acid amplification technology

In the *polymerase chain reaction* (PCR) a thermostable DNA polymerase and two specific oligonucleotide primers are used to produce multiple copies of specific nucleic acid regions quickly and exponentially (Fig. 6.4). The specificity of the reaction is controlled by the oligonucleotide primers that direct replication of the intervening 'target' region. In an exponential reaction, the target sequence is amplified a million-fold or more within a few hours. Although PCR is the most widely used method, other amplification techniques for DNA and RNA molecules are available. Once an amplification reaction has occurred, a variety of manual and automated methods is available to detect the amplified product, of which the simplest is to identify the product by size after electrophoresis and migration on an agarose gel. For many diagnostic applications, the simple visualization of an amplification product of characteristic size is a significant result, because it indicates the presence of the target DNA sequence in the original sample, but confirmation of sequence identity by specific hybridization tests is often required.

Amplification offers an exquisitely sensitive approach to the detection and identification of specific microorganisms in a variety of sample types. Potentially, a characteristic DNA or RNA sequence from a single virus particle or bacterial cell can be amplified to detectable levels within a very short period of time. The method has received particular attention for detecting the presence of low numbers of bacteria or virus particles in clinical and environmental specimens. For example, although a diagnostic antibody response may take up to 8 weeks to develop in an individual infected with human immunodeficiency virus (HIV), specific HIV sequences can be detected in a few hours by PCR, even if present at only 1 part per 100 000 human genome equivalents.

### Real-time amplification

It is the detection process that discriminates real-time amplification from conventional PCR assays. The possibility of detecting the accumulation of amplification product in real time as the PCR progresses has been made possible by the labelling of primers, oligonucleotide probes (*oligoprobes*) or amplicons with molecules capable of fluorescing in the reaction tube. These fluorescent labels produce a change in signal at a specific wavelength following direct interaction with, or hybridization to, the amplicon. The signal produced is related to the amount of amplicon present at the end of each cycle and increases as the amount of specific amplicon increases (see Recommended Reading). Commercially available robotic nucleic acid extraction systems, combined with rapid thermal cyclers and instrumentation (e.g. LightCycler®, TaqMan®) capable of detecting and differentiating multiple amplicons, make real-time PCR an attractive and viable proposition for the routine diagnostic laboratory. Real-time PCR assays have been extremely useful for studying microbial agents of infectious disease. The greatest impact to date has been in the field of virology, where real-time assays have been used to rapidly detect a range of viruses in human specimens and to monitor quantitatively viral loads and response to antiviral therapy. Benefits to the patient can also be seen in bacteriology, where rapid detection of bacterial pathogens and/or antibiotic resistance genes can help to ensure the appropriate use of antibiotics, reduce the duration of hospital stay and minimize the potential for resistant strains of bacteria to emerge. Recent developments in real-time PCR have suggested a future in which rapid identification, quantification and typing of a range of microbial targets in single multiplex reactions will become commonplace, although it is not clear whether current resource-limited clinical microbiology services will be enabled to introduce these improved new technologies on a wide scale.

## Molecular typing of micro–organisms

Typing of micro-organisms is increasingly important for studying cross-infection and epidemiological relationships, particularly during outbreaks of nosocomial infection (see Ch. 69). Molecular fingerprinting methods are now the most commonly used techniques for assessing the relatedness of individual bacterial isolates in epidemiological studies. These techniques can be used to study any organism from which DNA can be prepared and offer the possibility of a unified approach to microbial typing that can be applied immediately to a new epidemiological problem with no prior knowledge of the organisms being investigated (see Ch. 3).

A complete DNA sequence forms the ultimate reference standard for identifying micro-organisms and their sub types. Increasing numbers of micro-organisms are now being sequenced and the knowledge gained is of immense value for research purposes. However, even with rapid automated sequencing techniques, it is highly unlikely that routine diagnostic laboratories will ever have the facilities or resources to sequence all their isolates of clinical or epidemiological interest routinely. One possibility might involve the sequencing of small relatively conserved regions of the genome that can provide diagnostic information, and such techniques for sequencing genes encoding 16S ribosomal RNA are sometimes used presumptively to identify 'unknown' or unculturable isolates derived from clinical specimens.

Recent developments in automation and sequencing chemistries have resulted in the development of a typing technique termed *multilocus sequence typing* (MLST). The technique relies on the analysis of sequence variation in a relatively small set of 'housekeeping genes' (usually about seven) that are present in all isolates of a particular bacterial species. The genes selected for analysis should be widely separated on the chromosome and should not be adjacent to genes that may be under selective pressure. Specific primers are designed that amplify c. 500-bp fragments of these genes, which are then sequenced to determine naturally occurring variation. The sequences can be compared with those already contained in worldwide databases in order to analyse both global and local epidemiology. MLST schemes and databases are already available for more than 40 bacterial species, including *Neisseria meningitidis, Streptococcus pneumoniae, Staphylococcus aureus* and *Haemophilus influenzae*. This is a powerful new approach for the characterization of micro-organisms, as it provides unambiguous data that are electronically portable between laboratories and can be used for global epidemiological studies.

## Genomics

Entire genome sequences for pathogenic micro-organisms are increasingly becoming available. It is becoming increasingly apparent that many species of bacteria exhibit significant variability among strains in terms of pathogenicity and ecological flexibility. As described above, such differences reflect the dynamic nature of the bacterial genome, which is now considered to be composed of a relatively invariable 'core genome' (comprising the basic gene complement forming much of the main chromosome) and a highly variable 'accessory genome' (comprising plasmids, bacteriophages, transposons, integrons and genomic islands, some or all of which may also be integrated into the main chromosome). Such structures may play an important role in bacterial evolution. For example, *Vibrio cholerae* contains a large chromosomal structure with integron characteristics that harbours several hundred gene cassettes, as well as a large second structure which has variously been referred to as a second chromosome, a megaplasmid or a chromid. This second chromosome also carries a gene capture system (termed the integron island) and host 'addiction' genes that are typically found on plasmids. It therefore appears that these structures represent a very efficient system by which bacteria can scavenge foreign genes that may confer increased fitness in particular environmental niches.

New methods for obtaining genome-wide mRNA expression data mean that a global view of changes in gene expression patterns in response to physiological alterations or manipulations of transcriptional regulators can also now be obtained. An alternative approach for identification and typing is already available that involves the use of *DNA microarrays* (sometimes called '*DNA chips*'). These consist of a very large number of evenly spaced spots of DNA fixed to a microscope slide. Each spot is a unique DNA fragment transferred by a gridding robot from multi-well plates on to the slide. Such DNA chips may become commercially available and could then be hybridized in diagnostic laboratories with DNA extracts from 'unknown' isolates to yield distinctive patterns of hybridization on the slide. Such patterns would be readily amenable to computerized analysis and comparison with electronic databases. More advanced chips are 'nanolaboratories', in that nanotechnology can be used to perform PCR, chromatography, electrophoresis and other techniques on a single chip. Some chips allow multiplexed systems, so that several techniques can be used simultaneously with several samples. Microarrays have already been used to investigate genetic expression, polymorphisms and antibiotic resistance in pathogens such as *Mycobacterium tuberculosis, E. coli, S. aureus* and *Helicobacter pylori*, not only in the context of epidemiological research, but also as a rapid diagnostic method for use with critically ill patients. Such techniques are not yet used routinely in diagnostic laboratories, but this is the beginning of a new molecular era for the diagnosis and treatment of infectious diseases, and these approaches offer the possibility of a very important shortcut to early diagnosis and treatment. The fundamental strategy of the current era of genomics is to move from studying single genes to the simultaneous study of a large number of interacting genes and their corresponding proteins. At the time of writing, this technology is still in the process of gradual development for routine use, but may ultimately revolutionize diagnostic microbiology in the twenty-first century.

## RECOMMENDED READING

Dijkshoorn L, Towner KJ, Struelens M, editors: *New Approaches for the Generation and Analysis of Microbial Typing Data*, Amsterdam, 2001, Elsevier.

Erlich HA: *PCR Technology – Principles and Applications of DNA Amplification*, New York, 1989, Stockton Press.

Goering RV: The molecular epidemiology of nosocomial infection: past, present and future, *Reviews in Medical Microbiology* 11:145–152, 2000.

Hall RM: Salmonella genomic islands and antibiotic resistance in Salmonella enterica, *Future Microbiology* 5:1525–1538, 2010.

Hall RM, Collis CM: Antibiotic resistance in Gram-negative bacteria: the role of gene cassettes and integrons, *Drug Resistance Updates* 1:109–119, 1998.

Innis MA, Gelfand DH, Sninsky JJ, White T: *PCR Protocols – A Guide to Methods and Applications*, San Diego, 1990, Academic Press.

Kung VL: The accessory genome of Pseudomonas aeruginosa, *Microbiology and Molecular Biology Reviews* 74:621–641, 2010.

Mackay IM: Real-time PCR in the microbiology laboratory, *Clinical Microbiology and Infection* 10:190–212, 2004.

Mazel D, Davies J: Antibiotic resistance in microbes, *Cellular and Molecular Life Sciences* 56:742–754, 1999.

Novick RP, Christie GE, Penadés JR: The phage-related chromosomal islands of Gram-positive bacteria, *Nature Reviews Microbiology* 8:541–551, 2010.

Rowe-Magnus DA, Mazel D: Resistance gene capture, *Current Opinion in Microbiology* 2:483–488, 1999.

Rowe-Magnus DA, Guèrout A-M, Mazel D: Super-integrons, *Research in Microbiology* 150:641–651, 1999.

Spratt BG: Multilocus sequence typing: molecular typing of bacteria pathogens in an era of rapid DNA sequencing and the internet, *Current Opinion in Microbiology* 2:312–316, 1999.

Summers DK: *The Biology of Plasmids*, Oxford, 1996, Blackwell.

Tenover FC: Diagnostic deoxyribonucleic acid probes for infectious diseases, *Clinical Microbiology Reviews* 1:82–101, 1988.

## Websites

PubMLST (Multilocus Sequence Typing). http://pubmlst.org/

# 7 Virus–cell interactions

*M. Norval*

## KEY POINTS

- Viruses are completely dependent on the host cell for their replication.
- A part of the *capsid* (in the case of *non-enveloped viruses*) or *envelope* (in the case of *enveloped viruses*) binds to a specific receptor or receptors on the host cell to initiate entry of the virus into the cell.
- The interaction of viruses with cells can result in:
  - *production* of new virus particles with or without lysis of the host cells
  - *abortive infection*
  - *latency*
  - *transformation*.
- In the productive replication cycle, the sequential stages are *attachment* (adsorption), *entry* (penetration) into the cytosol, *uncoating*, synthesis of *viral macromolecules* (mRNA, proteins and genomes), *assembly* of new viral particles, *morphogenesis* and *release*.
- In latency, the virus persists as its genome, with limited expression of selected viral genes, sometimes as RNA only.
- In viral transformation, the virus persists as its genome, with expression of selected viral proteins that induce the host cell to behave like a tumour cell.

Viruses are totally dependent on the cells they infect to provide the energy, metabolic intermediates and most (in some cases all) of the enzymes required for their replication. With advances in the techniques of molecular virology, crystallography and modelling, together with the classical methods of electron microscopy, titration and biochemical assay, it has become possible to study virus–cell interactions to a sophisticated level. The picture that has emerged, and is still emerging, is a fascinating one, as viruses are found to associate with, and affect, cells in a wide variety of ways. The range of possible interactions is indicated in Table 7.1. It is possible to divide these into three broad categories that show considerable overlap:

1. Viruses that infect and replicate within cells causing the cells to lyse when the progeny virions are released. This is called a *cytolytic cycle*; the infection is productive and the cell culture demonstrates *cytopathic effects*, which are often characteristic of the infecting virus. The host cells are termed *permissive*. In some instances viruses are produced from the infected cells but the cells are not killed by the process: that is, the infection is *productive* but *non-cytolytic*, and may become *persistent*.
2. Viruses that infect cells but do not complete the replication cycle. The infection is thus called *abortive* or *non-productive*. Abortive infections can be due to a mutation in the virus so that some essential function is lost, or to the production of defective interfering particles, or to the action of interferons. It may be possible to manipulate the conditions in vitro to obtain a *steady state* or *persistent* infection in which infected and uninfected cells coexist and there is some, generally limited, virus production.
3. Viruses that enter cells but are not produced by the infected cell. The virus is maintained within the cell in the form of DNA, which replicates in association with the host cell DNA. The host cell is termed *non-permissive* and the infection is *non-productive*. Occasionally this type of interaction results in *transformation*, where the cell exhibits many of the properties of a tumour cell. In other cases a *latent infection* ensues in which little or no viral gene expression is found, no viral replication occurs and the cell retains its normal properties.

**Table 7.1**   The range of virus-cell interactions

| Type of infection/effect on cells | Comment |
|---|---|
| Cytolytic | Virus produced |
| Non-cytolytic (persistent) | Virus produced |
| Abortive | Virus not produced |
| Abortive (persistent) | Virus produced |
| Latency (persistent) | Viral nucleic acid present |
| Transformation (persistent) | Viral nucleic acid present |

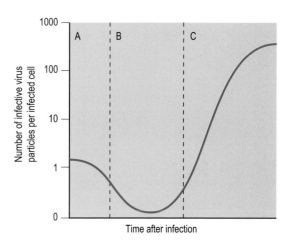

**Fig. 7.1**   Lytic growth cycle of a virus. Samples are removed from the infected culture at intervals and assayed for the total content of virus. Phase A, adsorption; phase B, eclipse; phase C, assembly and release.

## THE CYTOLYTIC OR CYTOCIDAL GROWTH CYCLE

Although there are large differences in the details of the lytic growth cycle depending on the virus studied, and to some extent on the host cell, certain features are common, and a simplified description is given first. The quantitative aspects of virion production were determined initially using bacteriophages, but have now been ascertained for many animal viruses growing in vitro in cell culture. A one-step growth curve is obtained when samples are removed from an infected cell culture at intervals and assayed for the total content of infectious virus after artificial lysis of the cells (Fig. 7.1).

In the early part of the cycle, virus particles come into contact with the cells, and may then *attach* or *adsorb* to them. This marks the start of the *eclipse phase*. The virion then *enters* or *penetrates* into the host cell and is partially *uncoated* to reveal the viral genome. *Macromolecular synthesis* of viral components follows. This can often be divided into *early* and *late phases* separated by the replication of the viral nucleic acid. Early messenger RNA (mRNA) is first transcribed and translated into proteins. These are frequently non-structural proteins and enzymes required to undertake nucleic acid synthesis and the later stages of replication. Viral nucleic acid is then produced, followed by late mRNA transcription and translation. Most proteins synthesized at this stage are structural ones, and will make up part of the final virion. The eclipse phase ends with the *assembly* and *release* of newly formed virus particles. The cycle is shown in diagrammatic form in Figure 7.2, and can vary from as little as 8 h for some picornaviruses to more than 40 h for human cytomegalovirus, a herpesvirus.

### Attachment (adsorption)

The initial interaction is by random collision and depends on the relative concentrations of virus particles and cells. Under in vitro conditions, the ionic composition of the culture medium is an important factor as both viruses and cells are negatively charged at neutral pH and thus tend to repel one another. The presence of cations, such as $Mg^{2+}$, helps to promote close contact. Adsorption then takes place through *specific binding sites* on the virus and *receptors* on the plasma membrane of the cell. It is largely a temperature- and energy-independent process. Viruses vary widely in the range of cells to which they can adsorb, depending on the nature of the sites to which they attach and how widespread they are among cells of different types, tissues and species. The presence of the receptor determines whether the cell will be susceptible to the virus, but the cells must also be *permissive*: that is, for successful production of new virions, they need to contain the range of intracellular components required by the virus for its replication. The ability of a virus to enter and replicate in a particular cell type is called tissue or cell *tropism*.

Many cellular receptors are protein in nature but they can also be composed of carbohydrate or lipid. There is considerable interest in identifying receptors for particular viruses, as the attachment step is a potential target for antiviral therapy and could aid in the understanding of viral pathogenesis. Specific receptors for selected viruses have been described, but have frequently been disputed. Newer techniques involving monoclonal antibodies, molecular cloning and gene transfer have helped to resolve these issues. It has become apparent that more than one type of receptor molecule may be required by the majority of viruses to complete the entry stage of the replication cycle. Indeed it is likely that there is a complex

**Fig. 7.2** A simplified viral replication cycle showing a hypothetical virus particle (1) attaching to the surface of a susceptible cell (2), entering into the cell (3), being uncoated (4), undergoing early transcription and translation (5), then replication of the viral nucleic acid (6), late transcription and translation (7), and, finally, assembly of new virus particles (8) and release from the cell (9).

interaction between different functional domains of the virus and several receptor arrays. First there is the 'true' attachment step whereby the virus binds to the cell receptor, and then entry itself may involve a further set of receptors called *co-receptors* or *post-binding receptors*, acting either in succession or in parallel. These interactions frequently induce conformation changes in the surface proteins of the virus, exposing hidden domains that are required for the entry step (see next section). This more complicated view of the initial contact between the virus and the cell suggests that the binding receptor may not be the only determinant of tropism, and the adsorption process may be influenced by factors such as virus strain, cell type and even the multiplicity of infection.

In Table 7.2, examples of viruses whose cellular receptors have been identified are shown.

## Entry (penetration)

Entry occurs immediately after attachment and, unlike adsorption, requires energy and does not occur at 0°C. The speed of this stage of the replication cycle varies between different viruses, some penetrating into cells in less than a second and others taking several minutes. In addition, the efficiency of the process varies from 50% of attached viruses entering successfully to less than 0.1%. Entry is complex and, despite much study, it is still not clear exactly what the steps are for the majority of viruses.

For viruses with envelopes, penetration is accomplished by membrane fusion catalysed by fusion proteins in the viral envelope. The fusions proteins that mediate entry have been divided into two categories. *Class I fusion proteins* include influenza haemagglutinin protein, human immunodeficiency virus (HIV) gp120 and paramyxovirus fusion protein. They are all cleaved into two pieces during synthesis, are found as trimeric spikes protruding from the surface of the viral particles and contain a fusion peptide characteristically composed of 20 hydrophobic amino acids. In some cases, for example HIV, fusion occurs at the cell surface at neutral pH with the activation energy being provided by receptor binding. In other cases, for example influenza virus, receptor-mediated endocytosis occurs. Receptors with adsorbed virus move together (patch) to pits coated with *clathrin* before moving into the cytosol to form small uncoated vesicles, which then fuse together as endosomes. A proton pump in the endosome lowers the pH to about 5. This acidic pH triggers the conformational change leading to the fusion of the viral and endosomal membranes, releasing the nucleocapsid into the cytosol. The endosomes combine with lysosomes, which eventually degrade any viral components contained within. This process is outlined in Figure 7.3. *Class II fusion proteins* are found in Flaviviruses (e.g. yellow fever virus, hepatitis C virus) and Togaviruses (e.g. rubella). They have different structural features from the class I fusion proteins, consisting of heterodimers. In the acidic endosome following receptor-mediated endocytosis, reorganization of the protein takes place with formation of active homotrimers and insertion of a hydrophobic fusion loop into the target membrane.

Viral entry via endocytosis can be independent of clathrin and dependent instead on *caveolae* or *lipid rafts*. These are areas of the membrane that

**Table 7.2**  Examples of viral receptors and co-receptors

| Virus | Receptor |
|---|---|
| Coxsackievirus A21 | CD55 (decay-accelerating protein), ICAM-1 |
| Epstein–Barr virus | CD21 (complement receptor), HLA Class II, various integrins |
| Foot and mouth disease virus | Sialic acid, various integrins |
| Herpes simplex virus type 1 | Heparan sulfate, herpesvirus entry-mediator A, nectin 1 and 2,various integrins |
| Human immunodeficiency virus type 1 | CD4, chemokine receptors (CCR5, CXCR4) |
| Influenza virus A | Sialic acid |
| Lassa virus | β-dystroglycan |
| New World haemorrhagic fever arenaviruses | Transferrin receptor 1 |
| Rabies virus | Nicotinic acetylcholine receptor, CD56 (neuronal cell adhesion molecule), low affinity nerve growth factor receptor |
| Respiratory syncytial virus | Heparan sulfate, ICAM-I |
| Rhinovirus | ICAM-I (majority of strains), low density lipoprotein receptor (minority of strains) |
| Rotavirus | Sialic acid, various integrins, heat shock protein 70 |
| Severe acute respiratory syndrome coronavirus | Angiotensin-converting enzyme 2 |

CD, cluster of differentiation; HLA, human leukocyte antigen; ICAM, intercellular adhesion molecule.

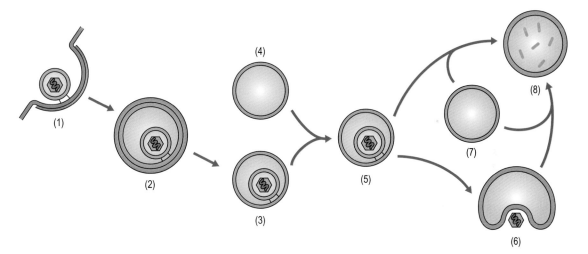

**Fig. 7.3**  Receptor-mediated endocytosis and entry of an enveloped virus. The virus attaches to specific receptors on the cell membrane (1) that patch at coated pits before being pinched off to form vesicles (2). These lose their coat (3) and fuse with other vesicles (4) to form endosomes (5). At the acid pH of endosomes, fusion of the viral envelope and the endosome membrane occurs, releasing the virus into the cytosol (6). (7) Fusion of the endosome with lysosomes leads to the final degradation of viral components and their return to the surface (8).

are rich in cholesterol and sphingolipids. Penetration into the cytosol occurs through the endoplasmic reticulum.

For many non-enveloped viruses, the mechanism by which they deliver their genomes across the host cell membrane in the absence of fusion is poorly understood. Recent findings indicate that such viruses may undergo programmed conformational changes following attachment, resulting in capsid disassembly and the release of small membrane-interacting peptides. These breach the membrane, thus allowing the viral genome to enter the cell.

## Uncoating

Uncoating can take place at several stages and sites in the cell and, generally, is not a well understood process. Some viruses undergo conformational changes on attachment that result in the opening of the capsid and release of selected viral proteins and viral nucleic acid into the cell. For example, crystallography studies of picornaviruses have revealed that the myristic acid groups at one end of the VP4 structural protein interact with the host membrane; this causes VP4 and the viral genome to exit from the capsid through a channel and to enter the cytosol. Enveloped viruses that enter by receptor-mediated endocytosis may be affected by the low pH in the endosome and the action of lysosomal enzymes. Uncoating can also take place in the cytosol or at the nuclear membrane. Reoviruses never fully uncoat, the viral genome remaining within a recognizable capsid structure. Poxviruses become uncoated in two stages. In the first, the outer layers and lateral bodies are removed within endosomal vesicles using host enzymes, and the core lies in the cytosol. Poxviruses carry their own DNA-dependent RNA polymerase, and this enzyme is used in the second stage to transcribe mRNA, which is translated into a special uncoating protein; this enables the final release of viral DNA from the core.

The final step in the complex uncoating process involves transport of the capsid (or the viral genome with, in some instances, viral enzymes and proteins) to the correct site in the cell to commence synthesis of the macromolecules that will comprise the new virions. Although details are not available for many viruses, it is clear that microtubules and microtubule-dependent motors are frequently involved in the transport. Some viruses stay in the cytosol for the remainder of their replication (e.g. poliovirus), but others proceed towards the nucleus where they are uncoated at the nuclear membrane before entry into the nucleus (e.g. herpesviruses) or enter the nucleus intact (e.g. papillomaviruses). Targeting to the nucleus depends on nuclear localization sequences found on the surface of the capsids. To gain access to the nucleus, the virus or its genome can either enter when the cell is undergoing mitosis (when the nuclear membrane is temporarily absent) or, more commonly, be delivered directly into the nucleoplasm though nuclear pore complexes.

## Synthesis of viral components

The nucleic acid in viruses is either single or double stranded, circular or linear, in one piece or segmented. In addition, viruses vary enormously in their complexity, ranging from those with nucleic acid sufficient to code for only a few proteins, such as the papovaviruses, up to those coding for several hundred proteins, such as the poxviruses. Although every virus has a unique method of replicating and has a strict temporal control on the synthesis of components, each must present functional mRNA to the cell, so that new virally encoded polypeptides and nucleic acid can be synthesized using the normal cellular processes. Thus, only viruses that contain DNA and replicate in the nucleus can use solely cellular enzymes for

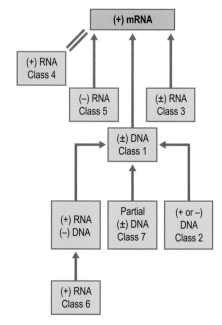

**Fig. 7.4** Division of animal viruses into seven classes, based on mechanisms of transcription.

transcription and translation. All other viruses must synthesize their mRNA by processes other than those found in uninfected cells. Seven different classes, six of which were first described by Baltimore in 1970, can be distinguished (Fig. 7.4). Conventionally in the scheme, nucleic acid of the same polarity or sense as mRNA is called 'positive' (+), and that of the opposite polarity or anti-sense is called 'negative' (-). Rather than be exhaustive, one or two illustrative examples from each class will now be described.

### Class 1: Double-stranded DNA viruses

This comprises a very large group of viruses that contain double-stranded DNA in a linear form (e.g. herpesviruses, adenoviruses and poxviruses) or a circular form (e.g. papovaviruses). The poxviruses can be separated from the others, as their replication takes place entirely in the cytoplasm and they can code for all the factors required for their own transcription and genomic replication. In the remaining double-stranded DNA viruses, replication occurs in the nucleus and is dependent to some extent on host cell factors. Herpes simplex virus is used as an example (Fig. 7.5).

After uncoating at the nuclear pore, the viral nucleic acid enters the nucleus and, using the normal host cell mechanisms of transcription and translation, three groups of viral polypeptides are synthesized in a strict temporal fashion. They are called immediate early (α),

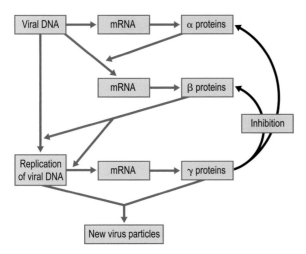

Fig. 7.5 Diagram of macromolecular synthesis during the replication of herpes simplex virus.

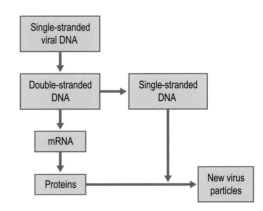

Fig. 7.6 Diagram of parvovirus replication.

early (β) and late (γ). A component in the virus particle (α-transcription initiation factor [α-TIF], a γ protein), acting as a transactivator, induces the transcription of the first set of mRNAs. A second component of the viral tegument called virion host shut-off protein (VHS) inhibits host cell macromolecular synthesis, and all the metabolic energy of the cell is turned towards the production of new virus particles. The genes coding for the α, β and γ proteins have been mapped on the genome and, whereas the β and γ genes tend to be scattered, the α genes are located together. Among the early gene products are thymidine kinase and a virus-specific DNA polymerase. Most of the late proteins are structural proteins that inhibit the synthesis of the α and β proteins. Between β and γ protein synthesis, new viral DNA begins to be made, probably by circularization using a rolling circle model.

## Class 2: Single-stranded DNA viruses

Parvoviruses comprise the sole family in this group. They are small, with DNA of about 5 kilobases. Some parvoviruses contain DNA of '–' polarity, and grow only in rapidly dividing cells; others contain either '+' or '–' DNA, and depend on coinfection with a helper virus for their replication. Parvoviruses use the cellular DNA polymerases to make the viral genome double stranded, called the replicative form. Priming is by the viral nucleic acid itself forming a loop at the 3′ terminus. This is followed by displacement of the parental DNA strand and synthesis of more DNA complementary to the template strand. Messenger RNAs are made using the appropriate DNA strand

as the template, and are translated into viral proteins (Fig. 7.6).

## Class 3: Double-stranded RNA viruses

This group includes the reoviruses and rotaviruses. All members have segmented genomes and each RNA segment codes for a single polypeptide. Replication of viral nucleic acid, transcription and translation occur solely in the cytoplasm without nuclear involvement at any stage. Each infectious virus carries its own RNA-dependent RNA polymerase, an enzyme unique to some RNA viruses and not found in uninfected cells. It enables the transcription of one strand (-) into mRNAs, which are subsequently translated into viral proteins. The transcription is thus asymmetric and conservative: that is, only mRNAs are formed and the parental duplex is not broken apart. Each mRNA is later encapsidated and copied once to form double-stranded molecules (Fig. 7.7). Several hours pass between the '+' and '–' strands of the new virus particles being synthesized. Thus the replication of the double-stranded DNA and RNA viruses is very different.

## Class 4: '+' single-stranded RNA viruses

This class comprises a large group of viruses containing RNA of the same polarity as mRNA. Because they code for all the proteins required during replication, the viral RNA extracted from the virions is infectious by itself. Poliovirus falls into this category, and is used as an example (Fig. 7.8). Macromolecular synthesis of viral components occurs entirely in the cytoplasm.

After entry of poliovirus into the cell, the viral RNA binds to ribosomes, acts as mRNA and is

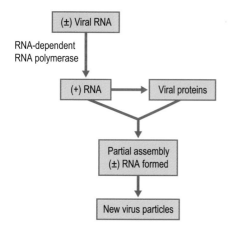

**Fig. 7.7** Diagram of double-stranded RNA virus replication.

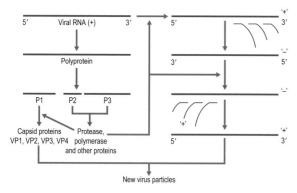

**Fig. 7.8** Diagram of poliovirus replication.

translated in its entirety into one large polypeptide. This is then proteolytically cleaved to give the products RNA polymerase and protease enzymes and new capsid proteins. Using the polymerase enzyme, '–'-strand RNA is synthesized with the genomic RNA as the template, and a temporary double-stranded RNA is formed, called the replicative intermediate. The replicative intermediate consists of complete '+' RNA and numerous partially completed '–' strands. When the '–' strands are ready, they can be used as templates to make more '+'-strand RNA. This is required as genomic RNA for assembly into new virus particles and for transcription into more viral proteins.

At the same time as viral replication, host cell protein synthesis and RNA synthesis are inhibited. Initiation of translation of cellular mRNA requires the participation of a cap-binding protein at the 5′ end. Poliovirus induces the cleavage of this protein, and thus halts the synthesis of cellular proteins. The RNA genome of poliovirus does not have such a

**Fig. 7.9** Diagram of influenza virus replication.

cap although it has a small protein, called VPg, at the 5′ end. A special region near the 5′ end of the genome directs cap-independent initiation of protein synthesis.

Complex interactions between viral and cellular proteins are thought to determine how much viral RNA is used for new virus particles or is translated into protein. The capsid of poliovirus consists of 60 copies of each of four proteins, VP1, VP2, VP3 and VP4, forming the icosahedron. One of the first cleavages of the polyprotein produces VP1, which is then broken into VP0, VP3 and VP1. Finally, on assembly, VP0 is cleaved into VP4 and VP2, a process catalysed by VP0 itself.

## Class 5: '–' single-stranded RNA viruses

Viruses of this group have single-stranded RNA of '–' polarity and must carry their own RNA transcriptase complex to be infectious, as the normal cellular enzymes are unable to replicate RNA. Influenza virus is an example (Fig. 7.9). It contains eight segments of '–'-strand RNA, plus the RNA transcriptase complex within each virus particle.

After entry into the cell by receptor-mediated endocytosis, transcription to viral mRNA occurs in the nucleus. Influenza virus is the only '–'-strand RNA virus to replicate in the nucleus. To initiate transcription, a nucleotide sequence of about 10–13 bases, found at the 5′ end of the cellular mRNAs and already capped, is used. This is cleaved from cellular mRNAs by an endonuclease activity of the viral RNA transcriptase complex. Thus, all the viral mRNAs have a 5′-terminal segment of the host cell mRNA.

Once the mRNAs have been generated, they are translated into polypeptides. Each genomic segment produces one mRNA, translated into one polypeptide except in two instances where, by RNA splicing of the original transcript, more than one mRNA is produced and therefore more than one protein. Unlike the transcription of mRNAs, the production of '+'-strand RNAs, required as intermediates to make the progeny

'–'-strand RNAs, proceeds without the need for primers.

There is much trafficking of viral polypeptides in the cell; the haemagglutinin, neuraminidase and $M_2$ protein are inserted in the plasma membrane, and the $M_1$ protein below this point on the membrane, whereas the nucleocapsid assembles around the viral RNAs in the nucleus.

## Class 6: Retroviruses

Viruses of this group are unique as they contain single-stranded RNA (in the form of two identical subunits), yet they replicate via an integrated double-stranded DNA stage. Retroviruses are the only such family and the virus particles contain a reverse transcriptase complex, with RNA-dependent DNA polymerase activity, from which the name 'retrovirus' is derived. This enzyme is not found in uninfected cells.

After entry, synthesis of DNA complementary to the viral RNA occurs using the reverse transcriptase, originating at a primer binding site near the 5′ end of the viral genome. The primer is a specific transfer RNA (tRNA) and varies from one retrovirus to another (e.g. tRNAlys in HIV). Transcription proceeds towards the 5′ end, and is probably continued by a jump across to the 3′ end of the same molecule. In addition to RNA-dependent DNA polymerase activity, the reverse transcriptase complex has ribonuclease (RNAase) H activity, that is, it is able to digest RNA from a DNA–RNA hybrid (Fig. 7.10). The resulting single-stranded DNA is then made double stranded, using the reverse transcriptase as enzyme and starting from a purine-rich sequence. Thus, a linear double-stranded DNA form is produced, first found in the cytoplasm.

The viral RNA has a short sequence of about 12–235 bases repeated at each end. During replication there is generation of a longer repeat sequence, from 250–1000 nucleotides, at both ends of the DNA molecule. This is called the *long terminal repeat*; it contains the enhancer and promoter sequences controlling the expression of the viral genome as well as the sequence for the initiation of transcription. The linear double-stranded DNA is able to circularize, and is found in this form in the nucleus.

The next step is integration of the circular DNA into the host cell DNA. This is catalysed by an integrase carried by the virion. It is thought that the circular viral DNA is cleaved leaving staggered ends, and the cellular DNA similarly, to allow insertion of the viral DNA into the cellular DNA; the viral DNA is now called a *provirus*. The site of insertion is not

**Fig. 7.10** Diagram of retrovirus replication.

thought to be specific. The provirus is co-linear with the original viral genome, and is always flanked by a 4–6-base pair direct repeat of the host DNA; this repeat is also found flanking transposons. The integrated state is a stable one and, as the DNA of the cell is replicated during cell growth, so the viral DNA is also replicated. Integration can result, on occasion, in cell transformation (see below).

The replication cycle is completed using the normal cellular RNA polymerase II to synthesize viral RNA and viral mRNAs, which are translated into polyproteins and processed into the final proteins found in the virus particle. A viral protease is responsible for many of these cleavages. The control of this stage is complex.

## Class 7: Partial double-stranded DNA viruses

Hepadnaviruses are unique among the animal viruses in containing partial double-stranded DNA and replicating via an RNA intermediate, as shown in Figure 7.11. One example of this group is hepatitis B virus.

The first stage in the replication cycle is the production, in the nucleus, of fully double-stranded DNA, followed by the synthesis of single-stranded positive-sense RNA using the cellular DNA-dependent RNA polymerase. The RNA is transported into the cytoplasm and translated into the core protein, which encapsidates the RNA, together with newly synthesized viral RNA-dependent DNA polymerase (reverse

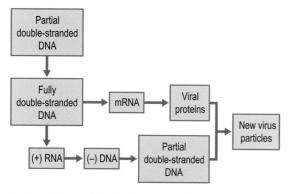

**Fig. 7.11**  Diagram of hepatitis B virus replication.

**Fig. 7.12**  Budding of retroviruses. ×70 000.

transcriptase). Then, using this enzyme, a complementary negative strand of DNA is made, while the RNA is degraded. The DNA is next transcribed into positive-sense DNA, and is found as partial double-stranded DNA in the new virus particles.

## Assembly and release

After synthesis of viral proteins and viral nucleic acid, there is a stage of assembly called *morphogenesis*. Generally the components that will constitute the new virions are produced in high quantities, and the assembly process is probably rather inefficient. Assembly is followed by *release* of virus particles, the productive phase of the infection. The release is either through *cell lysis*, as used by many non-enveloped viruses, or through *budding*, in most cases without cell death, as used by many enveloped viruses. Recently some non-enveloped DNA viruses have been shown to code for a small basic regulatory protein (the agnoprotein) whose function is to act as a *viroporin*, resulting in membrane permeabilisation and the subsequent release of the newly synthesized virus particles. There is also evidence for active release without cell lysis for other non-enveloped viruses, perhaps via vesicles resembling autophagosomes that contain the newly synthesized viruses. In some cases, viruses can be transferred directly from the infected cell to the neighbouring cells, thus avoiding any exposure to the extracellular environment or to the immune response of the host. The transfer could be through tight junctions or at sites of synaptic contact.

Viruses that are released by killing the cell depend on the cell disintegrating to let them out. Here, morphogenesis may occur spontaneously once the capsid proteins have been made, the specificity depending on the amino acid sequence of the proteins. Thus the structural proteins of the viruses can

form capsomeres by themselves, which then aggregate to form the procapsid, a structure without nucleic acid. Often there is proteolytic cleavage of a capsid protein to form the final virus particle, as has been described above for poliovirus. Details regarding the precise nature of the interaction between the nucleic acid and the structural proteins that make up the capsid are uncertain, despite extensive study. It is possible that the viral nucleic acid is inserted into the procapsid through a pore, or it might cause a structural reorientation of the procapsid, thereby becoming internalized. Alternatively, the capsomeres may accumulate around a condensed core of nucleic acid as the nucleic acid is being synthesized. Some evidence for specific viral components or cellular proteins, called scaffolding proteins, assisting the assembly process has been obtained.

The other major method of assembly and release is by budding. This can take place through the plasma membrane, thus releasing the virions from the cell (e.g. orthomyxoviruses and retroviruses; Fig. 7.12), or through internal membranes, such as the inner nuclear membrane in the case of the herpesviruses (Fig. 7.13B), followed by fusion of the vesicles containing the viruses with the plasma membrane. Envelope glycoproteins specified by the virus are synthesized by essentially the same mechanism as cellular membrane glycoproteins. The viral proteins destined to become envelope proteins contain a sequence of 15–30 hydrophobic amino acids, known as the signal sequence. This sequence binds the growing polypeptide chain to a receptor on the cytoplasmic side of the rough endoplasmic reticulum and enables its passage through the membrane. Glycosylation occurs in the lumen of the rough endoplasmic reticulum, and the proteins are transported to the Golgi apparatus. There they are further glycosylated and acylated before transport to the plasma membrane, the direction probably

**Fig. 7.13** Effects of viruses on cells. (A) Light microscopy of a skin lesion due to herpesvirus infection, showing cell fusion and intranuclear inclusions (Cowdry type A). ×60. (B) Electron micrograph of a cell infected with herpes simplex virus. Assembly of capsids within nucleus and enveloped virus between layers of nuclear membrane. ×9000. (C) Type A (accumulation of viral protein) and type B (virus factory) inclusions (identified as A and B, respectively) in the cytoplasm of a poxvirus-infected cell. V, virus; N, the cell nucleus. ×700.

determined by a sorting signal in the polypeptide sequence. In some cases, the signal directs the viral glycoprotein to one surface of the cell only; for example, orthomyxoviruses bud only from the outer (apical) surface of epithelial cells, whereas rhabdoviruses bud only from the inner (basal) surface. The viral glycoproteins are very important in terms of antigenicity as the hydrophilic domains protrude from the surface of the cell, with the N terminus being furthest away, and change the surface structure significantly. They remain anchored in the membrane via a hydrophobic domain near the carboxyl (C) terminus. After insertion into the membrane, the viral glycoproteins accumulate together to form oligomers; at the same time the host cell glycoproteins move away. At the C terminus of the viral glycoproteins, there is frequently a short hydrophilic sequence that remains inside the cell and is assumed to interact with the internal components of the virus during assembly. Lipid rafts function as microdomains for the accumulation of many viral glycoproteins, and may also

initiate the actual budding sequence. It is not known how the nucleocapsids are directed to the assembly site. Once there, they are engulfed by the membrane; this process requires bending of the membrane, leading to its outward curvature. In the case of the class I fusion proteins described above, a final cleavage of the glycoprotein is required to make the virus infectious. For example, the haemagglutinin $H_0$ of influenza virus is cleaved into two peptides, $HA_1$ and $HA_2$, linked by disulphide bridges. The bud is completed by the fusion of the two apposing membranes, and it finally separates from the plasma membrane of the host to become a new infectious virus. For retroviruses, budding occurs by highjacking a cellular pathway that normally creates vesicles that bud into late endosomal compartments called multivesicular bodies. These viruses then exit through the plasma membrane or via exosomes. During or shortly after budding, the viral protease enzyme cleaves at specific sites within precursor proteins to produce the proteins found in the mature virus particles.

Several thousand virus particles can be produced per infected cell, although this number varies considerably with virus type and host cell type. The budding viruses tend to be released slowly over several hours, whereas the lytic ones are released together. Only a few of the newly formed virus particles are infectious, as indicated by a high ratio of particles to infectious virions. Presumably most do not have the correct complement of proteins, enzymes or viral nucleic acid, or have been assembled incorrectly.

Evidence has accumulated to indicate that, for some viruses at least, perturbation of the normal cell metabolism during replication can stimulate cell death by *apoptosis*. Several virus-specific factors have been identified as inducers of apoptosis, such as by causing DNA strand breaks in the case of a parvovirus, by stabilization of the tumour suppressor gene product p53 in the case of Epstein–Barr virus, or by receptor signalling in the case of HIV. The advantage to the virus could be that the spread of the infection is enhanced as the entire cellular contents, including progeny viruses, are packaged into membrane-bound apoptotic bodies that are then taken up by adjacent cells. In contrast, other viral proteins have been revealed that block or delay apoptosis, presumably until sufficient progeny viruses have been produced within the cells. In this case, the factors target specific stages of the apoptotic pathway. For example, caspases are inhibited during poxvirus infections, the action of interferon is downregulated during influenza virus infections and p53 is destroyed during some human papillomavirus infections. Therefore the susceptibility of the host cell to apoptosis depends on the acute death pathways in the cell itself and the range of apoptotic modulators induced by the infecting viruses.

## Microscopy of infected cells

It is possible to observe effects on the host cell microscopically. Firstly, there may be morphological changes called *inclusion bodies* in the infected cell, seen by altered staining characteristics. The inclusion bodies are nuclear or cytoplasmic and vary in their composition. They can consist of viral factories in which morphogenesis occurs, crystalline arrays of virus particles ready for release, overproduction of a particular viral protein or proteins, or some aberrant cellular structure, such as clumped chromatin. Virally encoded non-structural proteins are likely to be involved in forming the matrix of these structures and in recruiting viral components to them. Some examples of inclusion bodies are shown in Figure 7.13. Secondly, the cells may be killed by the viral infection. There are several possible reasons for this, including factors produced by the virus that induce apoptosis (see above). It is likely that the accumulation of viral structural proteins is toxic for the cells in some cases. In addition, some viruses, such as herpes simplex virus and the poxviruses, inhibit host cell macromolecular synthesis from an early stage in the replication cycle, leading to structural and functional damage. Plasma membrane function and permeability change, and lysosomal membranes begin to break down, allowing leakage of the contents with degradative activity into the cytoplasm. There may also be marked effects on the cytoskeleton. These changes lead to a *cytopathic effect*, seen clearly in cell culture. It can take several forms, one of the most common being *cell rounding* and subsequent detachment from the solid surface (Fig. 7.14B). Another is the formation of a *syncytium*, whereby the membranes of adjacent infected cells fuse and a giant cell is formed containing many nuclei (Fig. 7.13A and 7.14C). In some cases, the nuclei fuse to make hybrid cells, a property that has been exploited in monoclonal antibody production.

## NON-CYTOCIDAL PRODUCTIVE INFECTIONS

Some viruses are able to infect cells productively but the cells are not killed by the replication process.

**Fig. 7.14** Cytopathic effects: (A) uninfected fibroblast cells; (B) Cell rounding due to herpes simplex virus; (C) Syncytium formation or cell fusion due to respiratory syncytial virus. All unstained. ×65.

Viruses that are released by budding frequently come into this category. The cell type used for the infection is critical and, presumably, any inhibitory effect of the virus on the cellular metabolism does not take place. This type of interaction may lead to a *persistent infection* in which infected cells and viruses coexist over a long period of time. There will, however, be antigenic changes in the infected cells, often the insertion of viral glycoproteins in the plasma membrane. This can be exploited for the detection of a virus; for example, when influenza virus is cultured in monkey kidney cells, virus is produced from the cells but there is no immediate cytopathic effect. However, there is insertion of viral haemagglutinin into the plasma membrane during replication. Thus, when red blood cells of certain species are added to the infected cells, they adhere to the haemagglutinin and can be seen microscopically. This phenomenon is called *haemadsorption*.

## ABORTIVE (NON–PRODUCTIVE) INFECTIONS

Some viruses are unable to infect cells because they cannot adsorb to them; the cells are therefore called *resistant*. In other cases viruses are able to infect cells but are not produced from them; such infection is called *non-productive* or *abortive*, and the cells are *non-permissive*. Often there is a block at one stage of the replication cycle owing to the absence of a cellular function essential for viral replication. This can also occur in a permissive cell if the viral genome itself is *defective* in some way, so that the replication cannot be completed. This can happen in two ways:

1. The virus is too small to code for all the proteins required for replication. An example is provided by the adeno-associated viruses belonging to the Parvoviridae family. They are unable to replicate on their own but depend on a second 'helper' virus infecting the same cell and providing the essential function that they lack. Adenoviruses act as the helper viruses and are thought to activate transcription of the parvovirus genome in the infected cell.
2. Abortive infections can arise as a result of viral mutation. In fact, only a few amino acid substitutions in selected proteins of the virus can change the nature of a lytic infection. In some cases the non-productive infection can be converted into a persistent one, in which new virus particles are synthesized; three examples are given below.

## Temperature-sensitive mutants

Here the wild-type virus has mutated to produce a variant – a temperature-sensitive mutant – that lacks an essential gene function at the *non-permissive temperature*, normally above 38°C. This is thought to be due to the thermal instability of the secondary or tertiary structure of a particular protein. The temperature can be lowered, generally to below 35°C, to a level called permissive, where the defect is no longer functional and the infection becomes productive. However, temperature-sensitive mutants tend to be less cytopathic than the wild type, even at permissive temperatures, probably because they synthesize less mRNA and protein. Thus, within a cell culture, a persistent infection can result with a balance between infected and uninfected cells together with virus production. Temperature-sensitive mutants have been used to identify the gene responsible for a particular replication step and to map where functions lie on the viral genome. It is possible to place these mutants into complementation groups where, at the non-permissive temperature, the defect in one temperature-sensitive mutant is compensated for by a second one with a defect in a different gene.

## Defective interfering particles

It has been known for many years that, when cells are infected at high multiplicity, there will be a number of virus particles among the progeny with genomes shorter than normal, containing at least one deletion – so-called *defective interfering particles*. These particles cannot replicate themselves, although they are able to infect new cells. However, they can replicate in the presence of helper virus, often the parental virus, which compensates for the lack of a particular gene or gene cluster. The defective particles retain an origin of replication and the ability to form capsids. One of their important properties is that they *interfere* with the replication of normal parental viruses because, first, less time and energy are required to replicate the defective genome compared with the full-length genome and, second, the transcriptase complex has a greater affinity for the defective genome than the full-length one. Hence defective interfering particles, as their numbers increase, have a greater and greater effect on the replication of parental virus. It is possible to obtain an in vitro cell culture in which infected and uninfected cells together with infectious virus and defective particles are in balance for a prolonged period of time. Thus a steady state exists and the infection is persistent.

## Abortive infections maintained by interferons

The final example of abortive infections arises from the action of *interferons* in infected cell cultures. Interferons are produced from virally infected cells and can protect other cells from attack by viruses. These molecules, of α or β type, inhibit various stages of the viral replication cycle, especially polypeptide synthesis (see Ch. 10 for details). In cell culture, persistent infections can be obtained when the antiviral effects of interferons protect sufficient cells from the cytolytic effects of viral replication to allow cells and viruses to coexist.

It should be noted that some viruses can mutate so that they replicate poorly, if at all, in some cell types in vitro and in vivo, or they replicate normally but are less virulent in vivo. These mutated strains are described as *attenuated* and are the basis of most live viral vaccines. For example, the three serotypes used in the Sabin poliovirus vaccine have attenuating mutations in the non-coding regions of the viral RNA, leading to a failure to replicate in the brain and less efficient replication than the wild-type strains at the primary site of infection in the gut. Attenuation can be achieved by culturing the viruses repeatedly in cells other than those of the normal host or by culturing at non-physiological temperatures.

## LATENCY

Latency represents a type of persistence whereby the virus is present in the form of its genome only and there is limited expression of viral genes. The genome is found either integrated into the host cell chromosome or as a circular non-integrated episome. It is maintained throughout cell division when the host cell replicates. Latent infections are more common with DNA viruses than RNA viruses, perhaps because no mechanisms exist to maintain RNA for long periods of time intracellularly. One example of latency is provided by Epstein–Barr virus, which persists in B lymphocytes as episomal viral DNA with limited transcription of viral genes, probably around 11 protein products being expressed. These ensure maintenance of the viral genome in dividing cells, prevent apoptosis of the host cells, and help to evade immune responses. For herpes simplex virus, latency occurs in neuronal cells with the viral genome being maintained in the nucleus as an episome. All the lytic genes are switched off but one set of transcripts, the latency-associated transcripts (LATs), is abundantly expressed. The LATs can inhibit apoptosis and thus contribute to persistence of the virus. However, whether viral gene expression is substantially prevented by the action of the LATs or by the immune response of the host, such as via the local production of interferons and cytokines, is uncertain. Specific stimuli can trigger the reactivation of the virus from the latent state, and the infection becomes productive with the appearance of new virions.

## TRANSFORMATION

In this type of virus–cell interaction, the virus infects the cell non-productively and is found in the form of viral DNA, either integrated in the host cell DNA or unintegrated, or in both states. The properties of the cells are changed dramatically, a process called *transformation*. Transformed cells have similar properties to tumour cells, and a detailed study of the mechanism of viral transformation has led to increased understanding of the molecular basis of cancer. Only members of some virus families are able to transform cells. These include herpesviruses, adenoviruses, hepadnaviruses, papovaviruses and poxviruses of the DNA viruses, and, of the RNA viruses, only retroviruses. The type of cell infected and the species are also important. It should be noted that transformation is a rare event: at most only 1 in $10^5$ cells infected by a particular virus will become transformed.

Some of the main properties of transformed cells that distinguish them from normal cells are listed below:

- loss of contact inhibition of growth
- can grow to high saturation density
- less requirement for serum factors
- indefinite number of cell divisions
- expression of viral antigens
- absence of fibronectin
- fetal antigens often present
- changes in agglutinability by plant lectins
- induction of tumours in experimental animals.

One of the most striking changes is the loss of contact inhibition of growth, whereby cells that normally grow in an ordered fashion beside their neighbours and stop dividing when they touch one another now grow on top of each other and lose their orientation with respect to each other (Fig. 7.15). As a result they reach much higher densities. They have less requirement for serum factors in the medium and can be cultured in suspension without being attached to a solid surface (anchorage independent). Normal cells have a limited number of cell divisions, called the *Hayflick limit*, that they can undergo in vitro before

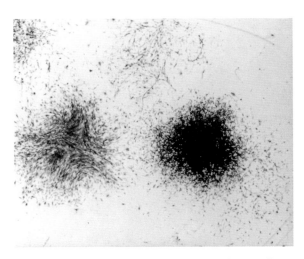

**Fig. 7.15** Colonies of human embryo fibroblasts growing normally (left) and following viral transformation (right).

apoptosis; for example, the Hayflick limit for cells taken from a human fetus is around 60 divisions. Transformed cells no longer have this limit and thus can grow and divide indefinitely. There are many changes in the surface properties of transformed cells. Often viral-specific antigens are found, particularly ones synthesized early in the replication cycle. Fibronectin, a surface glycoprotein thought to be important in keeping cells together in a tissue or organ, is no longer found. Commonly fetal antigens are expressed, and the agglutinability of cells by plant lectins changes, demonstrating alterations in the distribution of membrane glycoproteins. Finally, some transformed cells form tumours when injected into susceptible animals. Often these animals have to be immunocompromised in some way before tumours are produced, or the cells inserted into an immunologically protected site, such as the cheek pouch of the hamster. In addition, it is important to appreciate that by no means all transformed cells will form tumours. It is thought that there are degrees of transformation and that several stages have to be completed before the cells are fully transformed and equivalent to malignant tumour cells. Viral transformation may represent only the first step or a single step in such a pathway. There are no in vitro markers that determine the degree of transformation; thus the potential ability of the transformed cell to produce tumours in experimental animals cannot be predicted, as yet.

All of the viruses that cause transformation in vitro have a similar interaction with the host cell (Fig. 7.16). The initial stages are exactly as described above for the productive infections. There is attachment, entry, uncoating and, in most but not all cases, selected viral genes are expressed as proteins, giving the cell new antigenic properties. At this stage the viral nucleic acid becomes integrated in the host cell DNA, probably not at a specific site, or it circularizes and is maintained in a non-integrated episomal form in the nucleus. The association is a stable one, so that when the host cell DNA is replicated, the viral nucleic acid is also replicated and the number of viral genome copies per cell remains constant over many cell generations. Thus, transformation is a heritable alteration. With some viruses, such as Epstein–Barr virus and the papovaviruses, the whole viral genome is normally integrated, whereas with others, such as herpes simplex virus and adenoviruses, only part of the viral genome is integrated and the remainder is lost.

Recent work in this area has concentrated on the molecular events surrounding transformation and in analysing the functions of the viral proteins found in transformed cells. Two examples of transforming viruses, one RNA and the other DNA, are described briefly below to illustrate the approaches taken. Both are associated with human tumours.

The first is human T lymphotropic or T cell leukaemia virus type I (HTLV-I), a retrovirus, which is found in CD4$^+$ T cells of patients with adult T cell leukaemia. It is able to transform CD4$^+$ lymphocytes in vitro with integration of the DNA provirus. Genetic analysis has revealed that the viral genome can code for several non-structural proteins, including one of special interest called Tax, an oncoprotein of molecular weight 40 kDa. This protein, which has no cellular homologue, is able to activate transcription in the long terminal repeat of the integrated virus. Tax also affects the transcription of a remarkable number of cellular genes that are involved in cell cycle control and the cellular response to DNA damage. In short, it functions in a complex manner to promote cell proliferation, to accumulate DNA damage with the loss of genomic integrity, and to inhibit apoptosis. However, it is unlikely that Tax expression alone leads to the end-point of leukaemia and further, so far unexplained, molecular events occurring over a period of several years, are probably necessary.

The second example is human papillomavirus type 16 (HPV-16), found as integrated DNA in many cases of carcinoma of the cervix. In vitro this virus is able to transform most types of human epithelial cells, including keratinocytes. The viral proteins responsible for transformation are the products of two genes, *E6* and *E7*, which are found in cervical tumour cells. The interaction between E6 and E7 oncoproteins and their cellular targets is required to maintain the malignant phenotype. Both proteins have multiple functions but

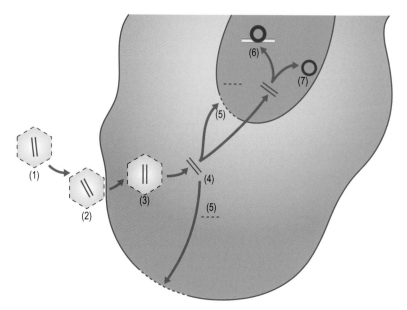

**Fig. 7.16** Simplified diagram showing the events of viral transformation. The hypothetical virus (1) attaches (2), enters (3), is uncoated (4), and usually some early viral proteins are synthesized (5) followed by integration of the viral genome in the host cell DNA (provirus) (6) or formation of a circular non-integrated genomic DNA (episome) (7).

it is probably most important that E6 interacts with p53, and E7 with retinoblastoma protein, thereby inactivating them. As both p53 and retinoblastoma protein act as cellular growth-suppressing proteins, loss of their functions is likely to lead to transformation. In addition, integration of the viral genome normally involves the disruption of the *E2* gene, the product of which is required to stop transcription of the E6 and E7 promoters, and therefore the continued expression of the E6 and E7 proteins results. Further properties of the E6 and E7 proteins include the inhibition of apoptosis, overriding of cell cycle controls, chromosome destabilisation and, in vivo, various mechanisms to evade local immune responses.

RECOMMENDED READING

Cann AJ: *Principles of Molecular Virology*, ed 4, London, 2005, Academic Press.

de la Torre JC, Oldstone MBA: Anatomy of viral persistence: mechanisms of persistence and associated diseases, *Advances in Virus Research* 46:311–343, 1996.

Flint SJ, Enquist LW, Racaniello VR, Skalka AM: *Principles of Virology*, ed 3, Washington, 2009, ASM Press.

Knipe DM, Howley PM, Griffin DE, et al: *Field's Virology*, ed 3, Philadelphia, 2007, Lippincott Williams & Wilkins.

Marsh M, Helenius A: Virus entry: open sesame, *Cell* 124:729–740, 2006.

Mettenleitur TC: Herpesvirus assembly and egress, *Journal of Virology* 76:1537–1547, 2002.

Munger K, Howley PM: Human papillomavirus immortalization and transformation functions, *Virus Research* 89:213–228, 2002.

Nayak DP, Hui EK-W, Barman S: Assembly and budding of influenza virus, *Virus Research* 106:147–165, 2004.

Radke K, Dohner K, Sodeik B: Viral interactions with the cytoskeleton: a hitchhiker's guide to the cell, *Cellular Microbiology* 8:387–400, 2006.

Wagner EK, Bloom DC: Experimental investigation of herpes simplex latency, *Clincial Microbiology Reviews* 10:419–443, 1997.

Whittaker GR, Kann M, Helenius A: Viral entry into the nucleus, *Annual Review of Cell and Developmental Biology* 16:627–651, 2000.

## Websites

Microbiology Bytes: Virus Replication. http://www.microbiologybytes.com/virology/3035Replication.html

Oregon Health & Science University, Microbiology: Virus Attachment and Entry. http://www.ohsu.edu/microbiology/courses/mbim608/Entrylecture1.pdf

University of South Carolina School of Medicine, Microbiology and Immunology On-line: Basic Virology: Replication of Viruses. http://pathmicro.med.sc.edu/mhunt/replicat.htm

# PART 2
## INFECTION AND IMMUNITY

# 8 Immunological principles: Antigens and antigen recognition

*J. Stewart*

## KEY POINTS

- The immune system recognizes molecules known as antigens. Recognition provokes a response that may be immediate and relatively non-specific (*innate immunity*) or may develop over time and become progressively more specific (*acquired immunity*).
- Antigens generally comprise multiple epitopes, each eliciting separate but specific immune responses that, in acquired immunity, may be mediated by *antibodies* (*humoral immunity*) or by T lymphocytes, which are responsible for *cell-mediated immunity*.
- Antibodies (also called *immunoglobulins*) are glycoproteins with a heterodimeric structure based on heavy (H) and light (L) chains. By genetic recombinations in the cells responsible for antibody synthesis (B lymphocytes), highly polymorphic (variable) regions are generated within H and L chains. H and L chains are brought together such that binding specificity for an enormous range of epitopes is achieved.
- Five main heavy chain types give rise to the five different immunoglobulin classes: IgG, IgA, IgM, IgE and IgD (in descending order of their relative abundance in human serum). The different classes serve different functions.
- Molecules that elicit innate immune responses display pathogen-associated molecular patterns that are recognized by pattern recognition receptors.
- In acquired immunity, antigens that elicit a humoral response are recognized by immunoglobulin molecules on B lymphocytes.
- Antigen recognition leading to cell-mediated immunity depends on T lymphocyte receptors. These are activated by epitopes resulting from intracellular processing of antigens. These epitopes are presented to T cells in combination with major histocompatibility complex (MHC) molecules on the surface of host cells.
- The two major effectors of cell-mediated immunity are T lymphocyte subsets termed CD4 and CD8 cells; these are, respectively, stimulated by epitopes presented in the context of MHC class II and class I molecules.

An antigen is any substance capable of provoking the lymphoid tissues of an animal to respond by generating an immune reaction directed specifically at the inducing substance and not at other unrelated substances. The response is not to the entire molecule but to individual chemical groups within it that have a specific three-dimensional shape. The specificity of the response to these *antigenic determinants* or *epitopes* is an important characteristic of immune responses. The reaction of an animal to contact with antigen, called the *acquired immune response*, takes two forms: first, the *humoral* or *circulating antibody response* and, second, the *cell-mediated response*, and their characteristics are described in Chapter 9. Most

of the information available on the specificity of the immune response comes from studies of the interaction of circulating antibody with antigen. An antibody directed against an epitope of a particular molecule will react only with this determinant or other very similar structures. Even minor chemical changes in the conformation of the epitope markedly reduce the ability of the original antibody to react with the altered material.

The term 'antigen', referring to substances that either act as stimulants of the immune response or react with antibody, is used rather loosely by immunologists. Use is made of the functional classification of antigens into:

- substances that are able to generate an immune response by themselves, which are termed immunogens
- molecules that are able to react with antibodies but are unable to stimulate their production directly.

The latter substances are often low molecular weight chemicals, termed *haptens*, that react with preformed antibodies but become immunogenic only when attached to large molecules, called *carriers*. The hapten forms an epitope on the carrier molecule that is recognized by the immune system and stimulates the production of antibody. In other words, the ability of a chemical grouping to interact with an antibody is not sufficient to stimulate an immune response. As we will see later, when discussing the sites on molecules recognized by cells of the immune system, all antigens can be considered to be composed of haptens on larger carrier structures. By convention, the term 'immune response' was used to refer to the acquired immune system and innate immunity was considered to be a rather non-specific, although relatively effective, defence against infection. In the past few years it has become evident that components of the innate immune system recognize a set of molecular signatures that have been termed *pathogen-associated molecular patterns* through pattern recognition receptors on the surface of cells and on secreted molecules (see Ch. 9).

## GENERAL PROPERTIES OF ANTIGENS

A substance that acts as an antigen in one species of animal may not do so in another if it is represented in the tissues or fluids of the second species. This underlines the requirement that an antigen must be a foreign substance to elicit an immune response. For example, egg albumen, although an excellent antigen in rabbits, fails to induce an antibody response in fowl. The more foreign and evolutionarily distant a substance is from a particular species, the more likely it is to be a powerful antigen.

A widely recognized requirement for a substance to be antigenic in its own right, without having to be attached to a carrier molecule, is that it should have a molecular weight in excess of 5000 Da. It is, however, possible to induce an immune response to substances of lower molecular weight. For example, glucagon (molecular weight of 3800 Da) can stimulate antibody production, but only if special measures are taken such as the use of an *adjuvant* which gives an additional stimulus to the immune system. Very large

proteins, such as the crustacean respiratory pigment haemocyanin, are very powerful antigens and are used widely in experimental immunology. Polysaccharides vary in antigenicity; for example, dextran with a molecular weight of 600 000 Da is a good antigen, whereas dextran with a molecular weight of 100 000 Da is not.

Some low molecular weight chemical substances appear to contradict the requirement that an antigen be large. Among these are picryl chloride, formaldehyde and drugs such as aspirin, penicillin and sulphonamides. These substances are highly antigenic, particularly when applied to the skin. The reason for this appears to be that such materials form complexes by means of covalent bonds with tissue proteins. The complex of such a substance, acting as a hapten, with a tissue protein acting as a carrier, forms a complete antigen. This phenomenon has important implications in the development of certain types of hypersensitivity (see Ch. 9).

## ANTIGENIC DETERMINANTS

The immune system does not recognize an infectious agent or foreign molecule as a whole, but reacts to structurally distinct areas: antigenic determinants or epitopes. Thus, exposure to a micro-organism will generate an immune response to many different epitopes. The antiserum produced will contain different antibodies reactive with each determinant. This will ensure that an individual is protected from the micro-organism by producing a response to at least a few of the possible determinants. If the host reacted only to the organism as a whole, then failure to react to this one site would have dire consequences: it would not be able to eliminate the pathogen. Certain antibodies may react with an epitope composed of residues that can also be part of two other epitopes recognized by different antibodies (Fig. 8.1).

A response to antigen involves the specific interaction of components of the immune system, antibodies and lymphocytes, with epitopes on the antigen. The lymphocytes have receptors on their surface that

**Fig. 8.1** Overlapping epitopes. Two epitopes (1 and 2) on an antigen induce the formation of three antibodies (A, B and C).

function as the recognition units; on B lymphocytes surface-bound immunoglobulin is the receptor, and on T lymphocytes the recognition unit is known as the T cell receptor. The interaction between an antibody (or cell-bound receptor) and antigen is governed by the complementarity of the electron cloud surrounding the determinants. The overall configuration of the outer electrons, not the chemical nature of the constituent residues, determines the shape of the epitope and its complementary *paratope* (the part of the antibody or T cell receptor that interacts with the epitope). The better the fit between the epitope and the paratope, the stronger the non-covalent bonds formed and consequently the higher the affinity of the interaction.

Antigenic determinants have to be topographical, that is, composed of structures on the surface of molecules, and can be constructed in two ways. They may be contained within a single segment of primary sequence or assembled from residues far apart in the primary sequence but brought together on the surface by the folding of the molecule into its native conformation. The former are known as *sequential* epitopes, and those formed from distant residues are *conformational* epitopes. The majority of antigenic structures recognized by antibodies depend on the tertiary configuration of the immunogen (conformational), whereas T cell epitopes are defined by the primary structure (sequential).

## ANTIGENIC SPECIFICITY

Foreignness of a substance to an animal can depend on the presence of chemical groupings that are not normally found in the animal's body. Arsenic acid, for example, can be chemically introduced into a protein molecule and, as a hapten, acts as a determinant of antigenic specificity of the molecule. There are many examples in which antibodies are able to distinguish subtle chemical differences between molecules. Thus, antisera can distinguish between glucose and galactose, which differ only by the interchange of a hydrogen atom and a hydroxyl group on one carbon atom.

The ability of antibody (or T cell receptors) to form a high-affinity interaction with an antigen depends on intermolecular forces, which act strongly only when the two molecules come together in a very precise manner. The better the fit, the stronger the bond. An antibody molecule directed against a particularly shaped antigenic determinant might be able to react with another similar but not quite identical determinant, as shown in Figure 8.2. This type of

**Fig. 8.2** Specificity and cross-reactions. Antibody produced in response to an antigen that contains epitope 1 will also combine with epitope 2.

cross-reaction does occur, but the strength of the bond between the two molecules is diminished in the case of the less well fitting determinant.

A common source of confusion concerning the specificity of antibodies arises when an antibody to a particular antigen is found to be capable of combining with an apparently unrelated antigen. For example, glucose residues are present in many different types of molecule, and an antibody that binds to a glucose determinant in antigen X-glucose would be likely to react with the glucose group in antigen Y-glucose, provided the two determinants were equally accessible. The antibody directed against the glucose determinant is not a non-specific type of antibody but is simply reacting with an identical chemical determinant in another antigen molecule.

In laboratory practice, cross-reactivity is often found between antisera to certain bacterial antigens and antigens present on cells such as erythrocytes. Antigens shared in this way are known as *heterophile antigens*. The best known of the heterophile antigens is the Forssman antigen, which is present on the red cells of many species as well as in bacteria such as pneumococci and salmonellae. Another heterophile antigen is found in *Escherichia coli* and human red cells of blood group B individuals. These cross-reactivities are probably responsible for the generation of antibodies found in individuals of a certain blood group that bind to the red blood cells of individuals of a different blood group. These antibodies are known as *isohaemagglutinins* because they are able to bind the red blood cells and clump them together (i.e. cause agglutination).

## IMMUNOGLOBULINS

Towards the end of the nineteenth century, von Behring and Kitasato in Berlin found that the serum of an appropriately immunized animal contained specific neutralizing substances, or antitoxins. This was the first demonstration of the activity of what

**Table 8.1** Physicochemical properties of human immunoglobulins

| | Immunoglobulin isotype | | | | |
|---|---|---|---|---|---|
| | IgA[a] | IgD | IgE | IgG | IgM[b] |
| Mean serum concentration (mg/dL) | 300 | 5 | 0.005 | 1400 | 150 |
| Mass (kDa) | 160 | 184 | 188 | 160 | 970 |
| Carbohydrate (%) | 7–11 | 9–14 | 12 | 2–3 | 12 |
| Half-life (days) | 6 | 3 | 2 | 21 | 5 |
| Heavy chain | $\alpha$ | $\delta$ | $\varepsilon$ | $\gamma$ | $\mu$ |

The immunoglobulin serotype is determined by the type of heavy chain present. The different characteristics observed are also controlled by the heavy chain. Variation within a class gives rise to subclasses.
[a]IgA is also found as a dimer, and in secretions IgA is present in dimeric form associated with a protein known as secretory component.
[b]Data for IgM as a pentamer.

are now known as *antibodies* or *immunoglobulins*. Antibodies are:

- glycoproteins
- present in the serum and body fluids
- induced when immunogenic molecules are introduced into the host's lymphoid system
- reactive with, and bind specifically to, the antigen that induced their formation.

The liquid collected from blood that has been allowed to clot is known as *serum*. It contains many different molecules but no cells or clotting factors. If serum is prepared from an animal that has been exposed to an antigen, it is known as an *antiserum* as it will contain antibodies reactive to the inducing antigen.

There are five distinct *classes* or *isotypes* of immunoglobulins: IgG, IgA, IgM, IgD and IgE. They differ from one another in terms of size, charge, carbohydrate content and, of course, amino acid composition (Table 8.1). Within certain classes there are subclasses that vary slightly in structure and function. These classes and subclasses can be differentiated from one another serologically, using antibody. If antibody from one species is injected into another species they will induce the formation of antibodies that can be used to differentiate between different isotypes.

## Antibody structure

All antibody molecules have the same basic four-chain structure composed of two light chains and two heavy chains (Fig. 8.3). The light chains (molecular weight 25 000 Da) are one of two types designated $\kappa$ and $\lambda$, and only one type is found in any one antibody molecule. The heavy chains vary in molecular weight from 50 000 to 70 000 Da, and it is these chains that determine the isotype. They are designated $\alpha$, $\delta$, $\varepsilon$, $\gamma$ and $\mu$ for the respective classes of immunoglobulin

**Fig. 8.3** Basic structure of an immunoglobulin molecule. See text for details.

(Table 8.1). The individual chains are held together by disulphide bridges and non-covalent interactions.

When individual light chains are studied, they are found to comprise two distinct areas or *domains* of approximately 110 amino acids. One end of the chain is identical in all members of the same isotype, and is termed the constant region of the light chain, $C_L$. The other end shows considerable sequence variation, and is known as the variable region, $V_L$. The heavy chains are also split into domains of approximately the same size, the number varying between the five types of heavy chain. One of these domains will show considerable sequence variation ($V_H$), whereas each of the others ($C_H$) are identical for the same domain of the same isotype. The tertiary structure generated by the combination of the $V_L$ and $V_H$ regions determines the shape of the antigen-combining site or paratope. As the two light and two heavy chains of any one antibody molecule are identical, each antibody unit has two identical paratopes, situated at the amino (N)-terminal end of the molecule, that recognizes the antigen. The carboxyl (C)-terminal end of the antibody is the same for all members of the same class or subclass, and is involved in the biological activities of the molecule. The area of the heavy chains between the $C_H1$ and $C_H2$ domains contains a varying number of interchain disulphide bonds and is known as the *hinge region*. A number of enzymes cleave immunoglobulins at distinct points to generate different peptide fragments. Using these enzymes, antibodies can be divided into a Fab region ('fragment antigen binding') containing the paratope and an Fc region ('fragment crystallizable') that is similar for all antibodies of the same isotype.

Despite the differences between the various isotypes, as shown in Table 8.1, all antibody molecules are composed of the same basic unit structure, with the Fab portion containing the antigen-recognizing paratope and the Fc region carrying out the activities that protect the host (i.e. effector functions). The differences seen in the Fc region of the various heavy chains are responsible for the different biological activities of the antibody isotypes.

## IgG

This is the major immunoglobulin of serum, making up 75% of the total and having a molecular weight of 150 000 Da in man. Four subclasses are found in man – IgG1, IgG2, IgG3 and IgG4 – that differ in their relative concentrations, amino acid composition, number and position of interchain disulphide bonds, and biological function. IgG is the major antibody of the secondary response (see Ch. 9) and is found in both the serum and tissue fluids.

## IgA

In man, most of the serum IgA occurs as a monomer, but in many other mammals it is found mostly as a dimer. The dimer is held together by a J chain, which is produced by the antibody-producing plasma cells. IgA is the predominant antibody class in seromucous secretions such as saliva, tears, colostrum, and at mucosal–epithelial surfaces in the respiratory, gastrointestinal and genitourinary secretions. This secretory IgA (sIgA) is always in the dimeric form and is composed of two basic four-chain units (two light chains and two heavy chains), a J chain and the

**Fig. 8.4** Transport of secretory IgA. J, J chain; S, secretory component.

secretory component. The secretory component is part of the molecule that transports the dimer produced by a submucosal plasma cell to the mucosal surface (Fig. 8.4). It facilitates passage through the epithelial cells and protects the secreted molecule from proteolytic digestion. There are two subclasses of IgA: IgA1 and IgA2.

## IgM

IgM is a pentamer of the basic unit with μ heavy chains and a single J chain. Because of its large size, this isotype is confined mainly to the intravascular pool, and is the first antibody type to be produced during an immune response.

## IgD

Many circulating B cells have IgD present on their surface, but IgD accounts for less than 1% of the circulating antibody. It is composed of the basic unit with Δ heavy chains. The protein is very susceptible to proteolytic attack and therefore has a very short half-life in serum.

## IgE

The IgE is present in extremely low levels in serum. However, it is found on the surface of mast cells and basophils, which possess a receptor specific for the Fc part of this molecule.

## Antigen binding

The variability in amino acid sequence in the variable domains of light and heavy chains is not found over their entire length but is restricted to short segments. These segments show considerable variation, and are termed *hypervariable regions*. Hypervariable regions contain the residues that make direct contact with the antigen, and are referred to as *complementarity determining regions*. Although the remaining *framework* residues do not come into direct contact with the antigen, they are essential for the formation of the correct tertiary structure of the variable domain and maintenance of the integrity of the binding site. In both light and heavy chains there are three complementarity determining regions that, in combination, form the paratope.

The antigen and antibody are held together by various individually weak non-covalent interactions. However, the formation of a large number of hydrogen bonds and electrostatic, van der Waals' and hydrophobic interactions leads to a considerable binding energy. These attractive forces are active only over extremely short distances, and therefore the epitope and paratope must have complementary structures to enable them to combine. If the electron clouds overlap or residues of similar charge are brought together, repulsive forces will come into play. The balance of attraction against repulsion will dictate the strength of the interaction between an antibody and a particular antigen, that is, the affinity of the antibody for the antigen.

## Antibody diversity

It is now known that an antigen selects from the available antibodies those that can combine with its epitopes. It therefore follows that an individual must have the capacity to produce an extremely large number of different antibodies to cope with the vast array of different antigens present in the environment.

### Immunoglobulin variability

The paratope is produced by the complementarity determining regions of the light and heavy chains generating a specific three-dimensional shape. Any light chain can join with any heavy chain to produce a different paratope. Thus, theoretically, with $10^4$ different light chains and $10^4$ different heavy chains, $10^8$ different specificities could be generated.

The germline DNA is the structure of the gene as it is inherited. All cells in the body contain all the inherited genes, but different genes become active in different cells at different times. The functional immunoglobulin genes within B lymphocytes, the cells that differentiate to antibody-producing plasma cells, are formed by gene rearrangements and recombinations. These events give rise to the production of different variable domains in each B lymphocyte. Once a functional gene has been constructed, no other rearrangements are allowed to take place within this cell. This dictates that one particular cell will produce antibodies with an identical antigen-combining site, and is known as *allelic exclusion*. There is evidence that the gene segments for the variable region of immunoglobulins are particularly susceptible to mutations. This can lead to subtle changes in specificity and/or affinity that are important as an immune response develops (see Ch. 9).

When a B lymphocyte is first stimulated by antigen it produces IgM. As the immune response develops, the class of antibody changes. However, the immunoglobulin produced will have the same variable domain and therefore bind to the same antigen. All that is altered, or *switched*, is the heavy-chain constant region. Thus the progeny of a single B cell will produce different immunoglobulin isotypes as the response to a particular antigen develops, but each will have the same paratope.

## Secreted and membrane immunoglobulins

At different stages in its development a B cell produces immunoglobulins that have to be inserted into the membrane or secreted. The membrane-bound immunoglobulin is used as the antigen receptor of the B cell, and a cell that binds antigen through this molecule will then secrete immunoglobulin of the same specificity. The only difference between the two types of antibody is to be found at the C terminus, where the membrane form has an additional part, the transmembrane portion.

## Antibody function

Knowledge gained from the structural studies discussed above has gone some way towards an understanding of the biological activities of the immunoglobulin molecule.

The primary function of an antibody is to bind the antigen that induced its formation. Apart from cases where this results in direct neutralization (e.g. inhibition of toxin activity or of microbial attachment), other effector functions must be generated. The binding of antigen is mediated by the Fab portion,

**Table 8.2** Biological properties of human immunoglobulins

| Function | IgA | IgD | IgE | IgG1 | IgG2 | IgG3 | IgG4 | IgM |
|---|---|---|---|---|---|---|---|---|
| Neutralize | ++ | − | − | + | + | + | + | +++ |
| Complement fixation | ±[a] | − | − | ++ | + | +++ | − | +++ |
| Binding to phagocytes | ±[b] | − | − | +++ | ± | +++ | + | − |
| Binding to mast cells | − | − | +++ | − | − | − | + | − |
| Enter tissues | − | − | − | + | + | + | + | − |
| Placental transfer | − | − | − | + | ± | + | + | − |
| Protects mucosal surfaces | + | − | − | − | − | − | − | − |

These activities are determined by the Fc portion of the molecules.
[a]IgA activates the alternative pathway.
[b]Receptors for the Fc portion of IgA have been found on neutrophils and alveolar macrophages.

and the Fc region controls the biological defence mechanisms. For every antibody the paratope is different, and different epitopes will therefore be recognized. However, for every antibody of the same isotype, the heavy-chain constant domains are the same, and they therefore all perform the same functions (Table 8.2).

## Neutralization

Because antibodies are at least divalent, they can form a complex with multivalent antigens. Depending on the physical nature of the antigen these *immune complexes* exist in various forms (Fig. 8.5). If the antibody is directed against surface antigens of particulate material such as microorganisms or erythrocytes, *agglutination* will occur. This results in a clump or aggregate that isolates the potential pathogen, stops its dissemination and stimulates its removal by other mechanisms. If the antigen is soluble, the size of the complex will determine its physical state. Small complexes remain soluble, whereas large complexes form *precipitates*.

As might be expected from knowledge of the structure of IgM, its ten combining sites make it a very efficient agglutinating antibody molecule. Rabbit IgM has been shown to be more than 20 times as active as IgG in bringing about bacterial agglutination. Because of its size, IgM is confined largely to the bloodstream and probably plays an important role in protecting against blood invasion by micro-organisms. Certain sites on micro-organisms are critical to the establishment of an infection. Antibody bound to these sites interferes with attachment processes and can, therefore, stop infection by the microbe. The binding of an antibody to functionally important residues in toxins neutralizes their harmful effects.

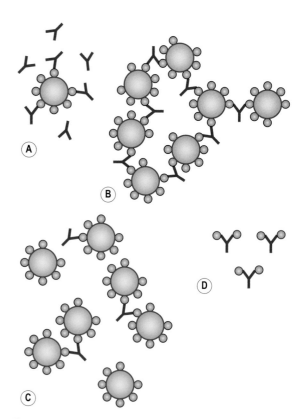

**Fig. 8.5** Immune complex formation: (A) Antibody excess; (B) Equivalence; (C) Antigen excess; (D) Monovalent antigen. At antigen or antibody excess, small complexes are formed. Between these two extremes, large complexes are formed that are maximal at equivalence. Antibody cannot agglutinate an antigen with a single epitope.

## Complement activation

Activation of the complement system is one of the most important antibody effector mechanisms. The complement cascade is a complex group of serum proteins that mediate inflammatory reactions and cell lysis, and is discussed more fully in Chapter 9. The Fc portion of certain isotypes (see Table 8.2), once antigen has been bound, will activate complement; this requires that C1q, a subunit of the first complement component, cross-links two antibody Fc portions. For this to happen the two regions must be in close proximity. It has been calculated that a single IgM molecule is 1000 times more efficient than IgG. This is because two IgG molecules must be close together for complement activation. A large number of IgG molecules would be required for this to occur if the epitopes were spread. Not all isotypes activate complement, presumably because they do not have the required amino acid sequence, and therefore tertiary structure, in the Fc portion. C1q binds to residues in the $C_H3$ domain of IgM and the $C_H2$ domain of IgG. Some isotypes, when interacting with antigen, can activate the alternative pathway of complement that does not use C1 but gives rise to the same biological activities.

### Cell binding and opsonization

The Fc portion of certain immunoglobulin isotypes is able to interact with various cell types (see Table 8.2). Antibodies specific for particular antigens, such as bacteria, play a valuable role by binding to the surface and making the antigen more susceptible to phagocytosis and subsequent elimination. This process is known as *opsonization*, and again is mediated by the Fc portion of the antibody. A specific conformation on the Fc region of certain isotypes is recognized by Fc receptors on the surface of the phagocyte. The important residues are in the $C_H2$ domain near the hinge region. Individually, the interactions are not strong enough to signal the uptake of the antibody molecule; therefore, free immunoglobulin is not internalized. However, when an antigen is coated by many antibody molecules, summation of all the interactions stimulates phagocytosis or other effector mechanisms.

Certain phagocytic cells have receptors for activated complement components – *complement receptors*. If the binding of antibody to the antigen activates the complement cascade, various complement components are deposited on the antigen–antibody complex. Phagocytic cells that have receptors for these complement components then ingest the complexes.

The above-mentioned processes require that the antibody is first complexed with antigen. However, certain cell types can bind free antibody. Mast cells and basophils have Fc receptors that are specific for IgE. These cells perform a protective function but are also involved in the hypersensitivity reactions

described in Chapter 9. In man, IgG has the ability to cross the placenta and reach the fetal circulation. This is a passive process involving specific Fc receptors. This route is limited to primates, whereas, in ruminants, immunoglobulin from colostrum is absorbed through the intestinal epithelium. Another Fc-mediated mechanism, already described, is the selective transport of IgA into mucosal secretions.

## ANTIGEN RECOGNITION

The immune system has evolved to protect us from potentially harmful material but it must not respond to self molecules. Two separate recognition systems are present:

- humoral immunity
- cell-mediated immunity.

Antibody is the recognition molecule of humoral immunity. This glycoprotein is produced by plasma cells and circulates in the blood and other body fluids. Antibody is also present on the surface of B lymphocytes. The interaction of this surface immunoglobulin with its specific antigen is responsible for the differentiation of these cells into antibody-secreting plasma cells. Antibody molecules, whether free or on the surface of a B cell, recognize free native antigen.

This contrasts dramatically with the situation in cell-mediated immunity; the T lymphocyte antigen receptor binds only to fragments of antigen that are associated with products of the major histocompatibility complex (MHC). T cell recognition of antigen is said to be MHC restricted. These MHC products are present on the surface of cells; therefore T cells recognize only cell-associated antigens. This MHC-restricted recognition mechanism has evolved because of the functions carried out by T lymphocytes. Some T cells produce immunoregulatory molecules, lymphokines, some of which influence the activities of host cells and others directly kill infected or foreign cells. Therefore, it would be inefficient or dangerous to produce these effects in response to either free antigen or antigen sitting idly on some cell membrane. The joint recognition of MHC molecules and antigen ensures that the T cell makes contact with antigen on the surface of the appropriate target cell.

### B cell receptor

Antibody is found free in body fluids and as a transmembrane protein on the surface of B lymphocytes (i.e. surface immunoglobulin), where it acts as the B cell antigen receptor. The antibody present on the surface of the B cell is exactly the same molecule as is secreted when the cell develops into a plasma cell, except for the extreme C-terminal end as described above. It should be noted that the molecules present on the cell surface are present as monomers even though they are secreted in a polymeric form.

## T cell receptor

The complex on T lymphocytes that is involved in antigen recognition is composed of a number of glycoprotein structures. Some of these molecules have been named systematically by CD (cluster of differentiation) nomenclature using antibodies. These generic names are used in preference to other symbols sometimes found in the literature.

The T cell antigen receptor is a heterodimer composed of an α and β or a γ and δ chain. Each chain contains a variable and constant domain, transmembrane portion and cytoplasmic tail. The variable domain folds to form a paratope that interacts with antigenic peptides associated with MHC molecules on the cell surface. The majority of T cells use the α–β heterodimer in antigen recognition. The role of cells that possess the γ–δ molecules is unknown, but they may be involved in the immune response to particular types of antigens at specific anatomical sites. The T cell receptor is the molecule that is responsible for the recognition of specific MHC–antigen complexes, and is different for every T cell. Genetic rearrangements of germline genes, similar to those seen in B cells, produce functional T cell receptors.

CD3 is present on all T cells and is non-covalently linked to the T cell receptor. The CD3 complex is thought to be involved in signal transduction, leading to cell activation, when a ligand binds to the T cell receptor. CD4 and CD8 are mutually exclusive molecules. They are present on T cells that are restricted in their recognition of antigen by MHC class II and class I molecules, respectively. Owing to their almost exclusive correlation with a specific MHC class, it is thought that these molecules bind to non-polymorphic determinants on the MHC molecules.

## MAJOR HISTOCOMPATIBILITY COMPLEX

The MHC is the part of the genome that codes for molecules that are important in immune recognition, including interactions between lymphoid cells and other cell types. It is also involved in the rejection of allografts. The MHCs of a number of species have been studied, although most is known about those of the mouse and man.

The gene complex contains a large number of individual genes that can be grouped into three classes on the basis of the structure and function of their products. The molecules coded for by the genes are sometimes referred to as *MHC antigens* because they were first defined by serological analysis (i.e. using antibodies).

The MHC of man is known as *human leucocyte group A* (HLA), and in mice it is referred to as *histocompatibility 2* (H2).

### Gene organization

The genes that code for the HLA molecules are found on the short arm of chromosome 6. They are arranged over a region of between 2000 and 4000 kilobases in size, containing sufficient DNA for more than 200 genes. The MHC genes are contained within regions known as A, B, C and D (Fig. 8.6).

*MHC class I molecules* consist of two non-covalently associated polypeptide chains. A single gene that codes for the larger chain is present in the A, B and C regions, whereas the smaller chain, known as $β_2$-microglobulin, is coded for elsewhere in the genome.

*MHC class II molecules* are composed of two chains, both of which are coded for within the D region. There are three class II molecules, DP, DQ and DR.

The class III genes are grouped together in a region between D and B. These genes code for a number of complement components and cytokines, but most have nothing to do with the immune system.

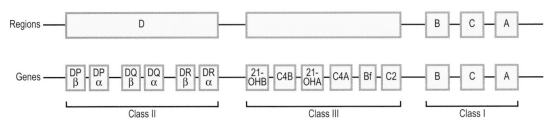

**Fig. 8.6** Human MHC gene map.

## MHC antigen structure and distribution

The MHC class I molecule is a dimer composed of a glycosylated transmembrane protein, of molecular weight 45 000 Da, coded for within the MHC, linked to a smaller protein, $\beta_2$-microglobulin (Fig. 8.7A). The globular protein formed by these two peptides is present on the surface of all human nucleated cells,

except neurones. $\beta_2$-Microglobulin is required for the processing and expression of MHC-encoded molecules on the cell membrane. The MHC-encoded class I glycoprotein folds into three globular domains ($\alpha_1$, $\alpha_2$ and $\alpha_3$) held in place by disulphide bonds and non-covalent interactions. These globular domains are found on the outer surface of the cell. There is a short cytoplasmic tail and a transmembrane portion. $\beta_2$-Microglobulin is non-covalently associated with the $\alpha_3$ domain.

The MHC class II molecules consist of two polypeptide chains ($\alpha$ and $\beta$) held together by non-covalent interactions (Fig. 8.7B). They have a much more limited cellular distribution, being limited to the surface of certain cells of the immune system. In man, they are normally found on dendritic cells, B lymphocytes, macrophages, monocytes and activated T lymphocytes. Each chain is composed of two extracellular domains, a transmembrane portion and a cytoplasmic tail.

These two types of molecule are folded into domains of a similar overall structure to immunoglobulin and, along with other molecules of the immune system involved in recognition processes, are thought to have evolved from a common ancestral molecule. A number of members of this *immunoglobulin supergene family* are depicted in Figure 8.8. MHC class II molecules, some interleukin receptors and Fc receptors are also included in the family.

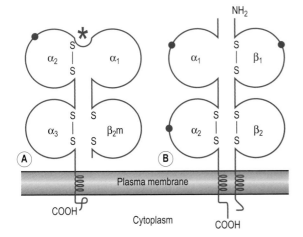

**Fig. 8.7**  Structure of MHC class I and class II molecules. Schematic representation of (A) class I and (B) class II molecules as found in the plasma membrane. $\beta_2$m, $\beta_2$-microglobulin; •, carbohydrate moieties; *, antigen-binding cleft.

**Fig. 8.8**  The immunoglobulin supergene family. A number of molecules involved in the immune system display striking similarities in overall structure. Regions similar to immunoglobulin domains are shown as circles; those related to variable and constant domains are designated V and C, respectively.

The MHC antigens of each class have a similar basic structure. However, fine structural differences can be detected in the $\alpha_1$ and $\alpha_2$ domains of class I molecules and in $\alpha_1$ and $\beta_1$ domains of class II molecules. These domains form a cleft on the outermost part of the molecules in which antigen fragments are found. The variations found are due to differences in the amino acid sequence and can be detected serologically. The variable residues give rise to different three-dimensional shapes on the MHC molecules. This, in turn, influences the selection of which antigen fragments can bind to a particular MHC molecule.

There are, therefore, many different forms of these molecules that can be identified in a population – they are highly *polymorphic*. Thus, it is highly unlikely that two individuals will have exactly the same MHC antigens. The MHC molecules of a particular individual can be given a designation using tissue-typing reagents. So, each chromosome of an individual will contain the genes that code for an A, B, C, DP, DQ and DR molecule. As the MHC genes are co-dominant, the products of both alleles are expressed on the cell surface. All of the nucleated cells in the body therefore express multiple copies of two HLA-A, two HLA-B and two HLA-C molecules. On certain cell types there will also be HLA-DP, -DQ and -DR molecules that were inherited from both parents.

## Function

The MHC class I and II molecules are essential for immune recognition by T lymphocytes which can bind to antigens only when associated with these molecules. The different classes of molecule are involved in antigen recognition by different T cell types or subsets:

- T lymphocytes that have CD4 molecules on their surface recognize antigen in association with MHC class II molecules.
- T lymphocytes that have CD8 molecules are restricted by MHC class I molecules.

The T lymphocyte subsets perform different functions, but the division is not absolute. The one thing

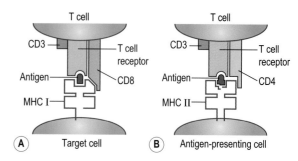

**Fig. 8.9** Molecules involved in T cell recognition. (A) Antigen fragments that associate with class I molecules are recognized by T cells that have the CD8 molecule. (B) Antigen fragments that associate with MHC class II are recognized by T cells that have the CD4 molecule on their surface.

that they have in common is that they recognize, through their T cell receptor complex (CD3, CD4 or CD8, TCR), antigen fragments in association with MHC molecules (Fig. 8.9). In general terms:

- CD4-positive (CD4$^+$) cells produce molecules, lymphokines, that stimulate and support the production of immune system cells.
- CD8$^+$ cells are involved in the destruction of virally infected cells (see Ch. 9) and the destruction of tissue grafts from MHC-incompatible donors.

CD4$^+$ cells produce molecules that stimulate the growth and differentiation of cells. These molecules are most effective over short distances, as they will be more concentrated. This happens when the two cells involved are actually joined together or in close proximity. The stimulation of CD4$^+$ T cells by antigen fragments on the surface of a responsive cell, or on a cell in the vicinity of a responsive cell, greatly increases the effectiveness of the messenger molecules produced by the T cell. In cell-mediated cytotoxicity the CD8$^+$ T cell has to bind to the infected cell so that the correct cell is killed. Therefore, the correct functioning of T lymphocytes requires direct contact with other cells. This interaction is mediated through T cell receptor recognition of antigen bound to MHC molecules on the host cell surface.

---

RECOMMENDED READING

Abbas AK, Lichtman AH, Pillai S: *Cellular and Molecular Immunology*, ed 6, Philadelphia, 2007, Saunders.
Janeway CA: How the immune system recognizes invaders, *Scientific American* Sept:41–47, 1993.

### Website

Kimball's Biology Pages. http://biology-pages.info

# 9 Innate and acquired immunity

*J. Stewart*

---

## KEY POINTS

- The cells of the immune system are divided into lymphoid and myeloid lineages. The former include T lymphocytes and their subsets identified by CD markers, B lymphocytes and natural killer (NK) cells. The myeloid lineage includes the neutrophils, eosinophils and basophils as well as the monocyte/macrophage series and platelets.
- Innate immunity depends on physical, physiological and chemical barriers to infection, on the response to injury and on detection of pathogen-associated molecular patterns (PAMPs) by pattern recognition receptors (PRRs). Phagocytic cells and the enzyme cascade known as *complement* are key effectors responding to PAMPs and components of *acute inflammation*.
- Acquired immunity depends on specific recognition of antigens either directly by antibodies on the surface of B cells or through presentation of processed antigens in the context of MHC molecules by host cells to T cells. In contrast to innate immunity, on re-exposure the responses are faster, more vigorous and more specific.
- Acquired immune responses are driven by the availability of antigen. As they mature, only cells with high-affinity receptors for the antigen are stimulated to divide. The expanded clones of antigen-specific cells are said to have resulted from *clonal selection*.
- Lymphocytes are activated by antigen and the appropriate combination of *cytokines*, signalling molecules secreted by other lymphocytes and by macrophages.
- Humoral acquired immunity leads to antigen-antibody complexes that neutralize key aspects of microbial activity either directly or through the activation of complement, *opsonization* and directed cytotoxicity.
- Cell-mediated immunity generates cytotoxic T lymphocytes (CD8⁺), which directly kill cells containing intracellular pathogens, and helper T cells (CD4⁺), which secrete lymphokines that stimulate other effector aspects of immunity.
- Inherited and acquired defects in the immune system lead to immunodeficiencies that make individuals more susceptible to certain infections.
- Damage due to immune reactions may reflect attempts to eliminate micro-organisms or self antigen-directed (*autoimmune*) reactions.

---

The environment contains a vast number of potentially infectious organisms – viruses, bacteria, fungi, protozoa and worms. Any of these can cause damage if they multiply unchecked, and many could kill the host. However, the majority of infections in the normal individual are of limited duration and leave little permanent damage. This fortunate outcome is due largely to the *immune system*.

The immune system is split into two functional divisions. *Innate immunity* is the first line of defence against infectious agents, and most potential pathogens are checked before they establish an overt infection. If these defences are breached, the acquired immune system is called into play. *Acquired immunity* produces a specific response to each infectious agent, and the effector mechanisms generated normally eradicate the offending material. Furthermore, the adaptive immune system remembers the particular infectious agent and can prevent it causing disease later.

## THE IMMUNE SYSTEM

The immune system consists of a number of organs and several different cell types. All cells of the immune system – tissue cells and white blood cells or *leucocytes* – develop from pluripotent stem cells in the bone marrow. These haemopoietic stem cells also give rise to the red blood cells or *erythrocytes*. The production of leucocytes is through two main pathways of differentiation (Fig. 9.1). The *lymphoid* lineage produces T lymphocytes and B lymphocytes. Natural killer (NK) cells, also known as large granular lymphocytes, also develop from lymphoid progenitors. The *myeloid* pathway gives rise to mononuclear phagocytes, monocytes and macrophages, and granulocytes, basophils, eosinophils and neutrophils, as well as platelets and mast cells. Platelets are involved in blood clotting and inflammation, whereas mast cells are similar to basophils but are found in tissues.

### Lymphoid cells

Lymphocytes make up about 20% of the white blood cells present in the adult circulation. Mature lymphoid cells are long lived and may survive for many years as memory cells. These mononuclear cells are heterogeneous in size and morphology. The typical small lymphocytes comprise the T and B cell populations. The larger and less numerous cells, sometimes

referred to as large granular lymphocytes, contain the population of NK cells. Cells within this population are able to kill certain tumour and virally infected cells (natural killing) and destroy cells coated with immunoglobulin (antibody-dependent cell-mediated cytotoxicity).

Morphologically it is quite difficult to distinguish between the different lymphoid cells and impossible to differentiate the subclasses of T cell. As these cells carry out different processes, they possess molecules on their surface unique to that functional requirement. These molecules, referred to as cell markers, can be used to distinguish between different cell types and also to identify cells at different stages of differentiation. The different cell surface molecules have been systematically named by the CD (cluster of differentiation) system; some of those expressed by different T cell populations are shown in Table 9.1. These CD markers are identified using specific monoclonal antibodies (see p. 125). The presence of these specific antibodies on the cell surface is then visualized using labelled antibodies that recognize the first antibody.

### Myeloid cells

The second pathway of development gives rise to a variety of cell types of different morphology and function.

#### Mononuclear phagocytes

The common myeloid progenitor in the bone marrow gives rise to *monocytes*, which circulate in the blood and migrate into organs and tissues to become *macrophages*. The human blood monocyte is larger than a lymphocyte and usually has a kidney-shaped nucleus. This actively phagocytic cell has a ruffled membrane and many cytoplasmic granules. These *lysosomes* contain enzymes and molecules that are

**Fig. 9.1** Cells of the immune system.

| Table 9.1 | Major T lymphocyte markers | |
|---|---|---|
| Marker | Distribution | Proposed function |
| CD2 | All T cells | Adherence to target cell |
| CD3 | All T cells | Part of T cell antigen-receptor complex |
| CD4 | Helper subset ($T_H$) | MHC class II-restricted recognition |
| CD7 | All T cells | Unknown |
| CD8 | Cytotoxic subset ($T_C$) | MHC class I-restricted recognition |
| CD, cluster of differentiation; MHC, major histocompatibility complex. | | |

involved in the killing of microorganisms. Mononuclear phagocytes adhere strongly to surfaces and have various cell membrane receptors to aid the binding and ingestion of foreign material. Their activities can be enhanced by molecules produced by T lymphocytes, called *lymphokines*. Macrophages and monocytes are capable of producing various complement components, prostaglandins, interferons and *monokines* such as interleukin (IL)-1 and tumour necrosis factor. Lymphokines and monokines are collectively known as *cytokines*.

## Granulocytes

*Granulocytes* are short-lived cells; days, compared to macrophages, which may survive for months or years. They are classified as *neutrophils, eosinophils* and *basophils* on the basis of their histochemical staining. The mature forms have a multilobed nucleus and many granules. Neutrophils constitute 60–70% of the leucocytes, but also migrate into tissues in response to injury or infection.

**Neutrophils.** These are the most abundant circulating granulocyte. Their granules contain numerous microbicidal molecules and the cells enter the tissues when a chemotactic factor is produced, as the result of infection or injury.

**Eosinophils.** Eosinophils are also phagocytic cells, although they appear to be less efficient than neutrophils. They are present in low numbers in a healthy individual (1–2% of leucocytes), but their numbers rise in certain allergic conditions. The granule contents can be released by the appropriate signal, and the cytotoxic molecules can then kill parasites that are too large to be phagocytosed.

**Basophils.** These cells are found in extremely small numbers in the circulation (<0.2%) and have certain characteristics in common with tissue *mast cells*. Both cell types have receptors on their surface for the Fc portion of immunoglobulin (Ig) E, and cross-linking of this immunoglobulin by antigen leads to the release of various pharmacological mediators. These molecules stimulate an inflammatory response. There are two types of mast cell: one is found in connective tissue and the other is mucosa associated. Mast cells and basophils are both derived from bone marrow, but their developmental relationship is not clear.

## Platelets

Platelets are also derived from myeloid progenitors. In addition to their role in clotting, they are involved in inflammation.

**Table 9.2** Characteristics and determinants of innate and acquired immunity

| Innate immunity | Acquired immunity |
|---|---|
| Broad specificity | Specific |
| No change with repeat exposure | Memory |
| Mechanical barriers | |
| Bactericidal substances | |
| Natural flora | |
| **Humoral** | |
| Acute-phase proteins | Antibody |
| Interferons | |
| Lysozyme | |
| Complement | |
| **Cell-mediated** | |
| Natural killer cells | T lymphocytes |
| Phagocytes | |

## INNATE IMMUNITY

The healthy individual is protected from potentially harmful micro-organisms in the environment by a number of effective mechanisms, present from birth, that do not depend upon prior exposure to any particular microorganism. The innate defence mechanisms show broad specificity in the sense that they are effective against a wide range of potentially infectious agents. The characteristics and constituents of innate and acquired immunity are shown in Table 9.2.

## FEATURES OF INNATE IMMUNITY

The components of the innate immune system recognize structures that are unique to microbes. These include complex lipids and carbohydrates such as peptidoglycan of bacteria, lipopolysaccharides of Gram-negative bacteria, lipoteichoic acid in Gram-positive bacteria and mannose-containing oligosaccharides found in many microbial molecules. Other microbial specific molecules include double-stranded RNA found in replicating viruses and unmethylated CpG sequences in bacteria. Therefore, the innate immune system is able to recognize non-self structures and react appropriately but does not recognize self structure, so the potential of autoimmunity is avoided. The microbial products recognized by the innate immune system, known as pathogen-associated molecular patterns (PAMPs), are essential for survival of the micro-organisms and cannot easily be discarded or mutated. Different classes of micro-organism express different PAMPs that are recognized by different

**Table 9.3** Examples of pathogen-associated molecular patterns (PAMPs) and pattern recognition receptors (PRRs) in innate immunity

| PAMP | Source | PRR | Response |
|---|---|---|---|
| Sugars (mannose) | Microbial glycoproteins and glycolipids | Mannose receptors | Phagocytosis |
| | | Mannose-binding protein | Complement activation |
| | | Lectin-like receptors | Phagocytosis |
| N-formylmethionyl peptides | Bacterial protein synthesis | N-formylmethionyl peptides receptors | Chemotaxis and phagocyte activation |
| Phosphorylcholine | Microbial membranes | C-reactive protein | Complement activation |
| Lipoarabinomannan | Yeast cell wall | Toll-like receptor 2 | |
| Lipoteichoic acid | Gram-positive bacterial cell wall | Toll-like receptor 2 | Macrophage activation |
| Lipopolysaccharide | Gram-negative bacterial cell wall | Toll-like receptors 4 and 2 | Cytokine production |
| Unmethylated CpG necleotides | Bacterial DNA | Toll-like receptor 9 | |
| dsRNA | Replicating viruses | Toll-like receptor 3 | Type 1 interferon production |

dsRNA, double-stranded ribonucleic acid.

pattern recognition receptors (PRRs) on host cells and circulating molecules (Table 9.3). One group of PRRs that are still being characterized are the Toll-like receptors. Mammalian Toll-like receptors are expressed on different cell types that are components of the innate defences, including macrophages, dendritic cells, neutrophils, mucosal epithelial cells and endothelial cells. Recognition of microbial components by these receptors leads to a variety of outcomes, including cytokine release, inflammation and cell activation.

Innate defences act as the initial response to microbial challenge and can eliminate the micro-organism from the host. However, many microbes have evolved strategies to overcome innate defences, and in this situation the more potent and specialized acquired immune response is required to eliminate the pathogen. The innate immune system plays a critical role in the generation of an efficient and effective acquired immune response. Cytokines produced by the innate immune system signal that infectious agents are present and influence the type of acquired immune response that develops.

## DETERMINANTS OF INNATE IMMUNITY

### Species and strains

Marked differences exist in the susceptibility of different species to infective agents. The rat is strikingly resistant to diphtheria, whereas the guinea-pig and man are highly susceptible. The rabbit is particularly susceptible to myxomatosis, and human beings to syphilis, leprosy and meningococcal meningitis. Susceptibility to an infection does not always imply a lack

of resistance to disease caused by the micro-organism. For example, although man is highly susceptible to the common cold, the infection is overcome within a few days. In some diseases, it may be difficult to initiate the infection, but once established the disease can progress rapidly, implying a lack of resistance. For example, rabies occurs in both human beings and dogs but is not readily established as the virus does not ordinarily penetrate healthy skin. Once infected, however, both species are unable to overcome the disease. Marked variations in resistance to infection have been noted between different strains of mice, and it is possible to breed, by selection, rabbits of low, intermediate and high resistance to experimental tuberculosis.

### Individual differences and influence of age

The role of heredity in determining resistance to infection is well illustrated by studies on tuberculosis in twins. If one homozygous twin develops tuberculosis, the other twin has a three in one chance of developing the disease, compared with a one in three chance if the twins are heterozygous. Sometimes genetically controlled abnormalities are an advantage to the individual in resisting infection as, for example, in a hereditary abnormality of the red blood cells (sickling). These red blood cells cannot be parasitized by *Plasmodium falciparum*, thus conferring a degree of resistance to malaria in affected individuals.

Infectious diseases are often more severe in early childhood and in young animals; this higher susceptibility of the young appears to be associated with immaturity of the immunological mechanisms affecting the ability of the lymphoid system to deal with and react to foreign antigens. This is also the time when infectious agents are encountered for the first time (primary exposure), and a memory-acquired immune response cannot be called upon to aid elimination. In certain viral infections (e.g. polio and chickenpox), the clinical illness is more severe in adults than in children. This may be due to a more active immune response producing greater tissue damage. In the elderly, besides a general waning of the activities of the immune system, physical abnormalities (e.g. prostatic enlargement leading to stasis of urine) or long-term exposure to environmental factors (e.g. smoking) are common causes of increased susceptibility to infection.

## Hormonal influences and sex

There is decreased resistance to infection in those with diseases such as diabetes mellitus, hypothyroidism and adrenal dysfunction. The reasons for this decrease have not yet been clarified but may be related to enzyme or hormone activities. It is known that glucocorticoids are anti-inflammatory agents, decreasing the ability of phagocytes to ingest material. They also have beneficial effects by interfering in some way with the toxic effects of bacterial products such as endotoxins.

There are no marked differences in susceptibility to infections between the sexes. Although the overall incidence and death rate from infectious disease are greater in males than in females, both infectious hepatitis and whooping cough have a higher morbidity and mortality in females.

## Nutritional factors

The adverse effects of poor nutrition on susceptibility to certain infectious agents are not now seriously questioned. Experimental evidence in animals has shown repeatedly that inadequate diet may be correlated with increased susceptibility to a variety of bacterial diseases, associated with decreased phagocytic activity and leucopenia. In the case of viruses, which are intracellular parasites, malnutrition may have an effect on virus production, but the usual outcome is enhanced disease as a result of impaired immune responses, especially the cytotoxic responses.

## MECHANISMS OF INNATE IMMUNITY

## Mechanical barriers and surface secretions

The intact skin and mucous membranes of the body afford a high degree of protection against pathogens.

In conditions where the skin is damaged, such as in patients with burns and after traumatic injury or surgery, infection can be a serious problem. The skin is a resistant barrier because of its outer horny layer consisting mainly of keratin, which is indigestible by most micro-organisms, and thus shields the living cells of the epidermis from micro-organisms and their toxins. The relatively dry condition of the skin and the high concentration of salt in drying sweat are inhibitory or lethal to many micro-organisms.

The sebaceous secretions and sweat of the skin contain bactericidal and fungicidal fatty acids, which constitute an effective protective mechanism against many potential pathogens. The protective ability of these secretions varies at different stages of life, and some fungal 'ringworm' infections of children disappear at puberty with the marked increase of sebaceous secretions.

The sticky mucus covering the respiratory tract acts as a trapping mechanism for inhaled particles. The action of cilia sweeps the secretions, containing the foreign material, towards the oropharynx so that they are swallowed; in the stomach the acidic secretions destroy most of the micro-organisms present. Nasal secretions and saliva contain mucopolysaccharides capable of blocking some viruses.

The washing action of tears and flushing of urine are effective in stopping invasion by micro-organisms. The commensal micro-organisms that make up the natural bacterial flora covering epithelial surfaces are protective in a number of ways:

- Their very presence uses up a niche that cannot be used by a pathogen.
- They compete for nutrients.
- They produce byproducts that can inhibit the growth of other organisms.

It is important not to disturb the relationship between the host and its indigenous flora.

Commensal organisms from the gut or bacteria normally present on the skin can cause problems if they gain access to an area that they do not normally populate. An example of this is urinary tract infection resulting from the introduction of *Escherichia coli*, a gut commensal, by means of a urinary catheter. Some commensal organisms possessing low virulence (see p. 173) that are provided with the circumstances by which to cause infections may be referred to as *opportunistic pathogens*. Infections with these opportunists are quite widespread, often appearing as a result of medical or surgical treatment that breaches the innate defences or reduces the host's ability to respond.

## Humoral defence mechanisms

A number of microbicidal substances are present in the tissue and body fluids. Some of these molecules are produced constitutively (e.g. lysozyme), and others are produced in response to infection (e.g. acute-phase proteins and interferon). These molecules all show the characteristics of innate immunity: there is no recognition specific to the micro-organism beyond the distribution of the molecule(s) detected, and the response is not enhanced on re-exposure to the same antigen.

### Lysozyme

This is a basic protein of low molecular weight found in relatively high concentrations in neutrophils as well as in most tissue fluids, except cerebrospinal fluid, sweat and urine. It functions as a mucolytic enzyme, splitting sugars off the structural peptidoglycan of the cell wall of many Gram-positive bacteria and thus causing their lysis. It seems likely that lysozyme may also play a role in the intracellular destruction of some Gram-negative bacteria. In many pathogenic bacteria the peptidoglycan of the cell wall appears to be protected from the access of lysozyme by other wall components (e.g. lipopolysaccharide). The action of other enzymes from phagocytes or of complement may be needed to remove this protection and expose the peptidoglycan to the action of lysozyme.

### Basic polypeptides

A variety of basic proteins, derived from tissues and blood cells, have some antibacterial properties. This group includes the basic proteins called spermine and spermidine, which can kill tubercle bacilli and some staphylococci. Other toxic compounds are the arginine- and lysine-containing proteins protamine and histone. The bactericidal activity of basic polypeptides probably depends on their ability to react non-specifically with acid polysaccharides at the bacterial cell surface.

### Acute-phase proteins

The concentration of acute-phase proteins rises dramatically during an infection. Microbial products such as endotoxin can stimulate macrophages to release IL-1, which stimulates the liver to produce increased amounts of various acute-phase proteins, the concentrations of which can rise over 1000-fold. One of the best characterized acute-phase proteins is *C-reactive protein*, which binds to phosphorylcholine residues in the cell wall of certain micro-organisms. This complex is very effective at activating the classical complement pathway. Also included in this group of molecules are $\alpha_1$-antitrypsin, $\alpha_2$-macroglobulin, fibrinogen and serum amyloid A protein, all of which act to limit the spread of the infectious agent or stimulate the host response.

### Interferon

The observation that cell cultures infected with one virus resist infection by a second virus (viral interference) led to the identification of the family of antiviral agents known as *interferons*. A number of molecules have been identified; $\alpha$- and $\beta$-interferons (see Ch. 5) are part of innate immunity, and $\gamma$-interferon is produced by T cells as part of the acquired immune response (see Ch. 10).

## Complement

The existence of a heat-labile serum component with the ability to lyse red blood cells and destroy Gram-negative bacteria has been known since the 1930s. The chemical complexity of the phenomenon was not appreciated by early workers, who ascribed the activity to a single component, called complement. Complement is in fact composed of a large number of different serum proteins present in low concentration in normal serum. These molecules are present in an inactive form but can be activated to form an enzyme cascade: the product of the first reaction is the catalyst of the next and so on.

Approximately 30 proteins are involved in the complement system, some of which are enzymes, some are control molecules and others are structural proteins with no enzymatic activity. A number of the molecules involved are split into two components (a and b fragments) by the product of the previous step. There are two main pathways of complement activation, the alternative and classical, that lead to the same physiological consequences:

- opsonization
- cellular activation
- lysis.

The two pathways use different initiation processes. Component C3 forms the connection between the two pathways, and the binding of this molecule to a surface is the key process in complement activation.

### Classical pathway

The classical pathway of activation leading to the cleavage of C3 is initiated by the binding of two or more of the globular domains of the C1q component

**Fig. 9.2** Complement activation: classical and alternative pathways. Enzymatic reactions are indicated by thick arrows. I.C., immune complex.

of C1 to its ligand: immune complexes containing IgG or IgM and certain micro-organisms and their products. This causes a conformational change in the C1 complex that leads to the auto-activation of C1r. The enzyme C1r then converts C1s into an active serine esterase that acts on the thioester-containing molecule C4 to produce C4a and a reactive C4b (Fig. 9.2). C4a is released and some of the C4b becomes attached to a surface. C2 binds to the surface-bound C4b, becomes a substrate for the activated C1 complex, and is split into C2a and C2b. The C2b is released, leaving C4b2a – the classical pathway C3 convertase. This active enzyme then generates C3a and the unstable C3b from C3. A small amount of the C3b generated binds to the activating surface and acts as a focus for further complement activation. Activation of the classical pathway is regulated by C1 inhibitor and by a number of molecules that limit the production of the 'C3 convertase'.

The so-called *lectin pathway* is initiated by mannose-binding lectin (a secreted PRR) attaching to the surface of a micro-organism. This leads to the production of C4b2a and the generation of C3b on the activating surface.

## Alternative pathway

Intrinsically, C3 undergoes a low level of hydrolysis of an internal thioester bond to generate C3b. This

molecule complexes, in the presence of $Mg^{2+}$ ions, with factor B, which is then acted on by factor D to produce C3bBb. This is a 'C3 convertase', which is capable of splitting more C3 to C3b, some of which will become membrane bound.

The initial binding of C3b generated by either the classical or the alternative pathway leads to an amplification loop that results in the binding of many more C3b molecules to the same surface. Factor B binds to the surface-bound C3b to form C3bB, the substrate for factor D – a serine esterase – which is present in very low concentrations in an already active form. The cleavage of factor B results in the formation of the C3 convertase, C3bBb, which dissociates rapidly unless it is stabilized by the binding of properdin (P), forming the complex C3bBbP. This convertase can cleave many more C3 molecules, some of which become surface bound. This amplification loop is a positive feedback system that will cycle until all the C3 is used up unless it is regulated carefully.

## Regulation

The nature of the surface to which the C3b is bound regulates the outcome. Self cell membranes contain a number of regulatory molecules that promote the binding of factor H rather than factor B to C3b. This results in the inhibition of the activation process. On non-self structures the C3b is protected, as regulatory proteins are not present, and factor B has a higher affinity for C3b than factor H at these sites.

Thus the surface of many micro-organisms can stabilize the C3bBb by protecting it from factor H. In addition, another molecule, properdin, stabilizes the complex. The deposition of a few molecules of C3b on to these surfaces is followed by the formation of the relatively stable C3bBbP complex. This C3 convertase will lead to more C3b deposition. Immune complexes composed of certain immunoglobulins (e.g. IgA and IgE) also function as protected sites for C3b and activate complement by the alternative pathway. Poor activation surfaces are made more susceptible to deposition by the presence of antibody that generates C3b by the classical pathway.

## Membrane attack complex

The next step after the formation of C3b is the cleavage of C5 (Fig. 9.3). The 'C5 convertases' are generated from C4b2a of the classical pathway and C3bBb of the alternative pathway by the addition of another C3b molecule. These membrane-bound trimolecular complexes selectively bind C5 and cleave it to give fluid-phase C5a and membrane-bound C5b. The

**Fig. 9.3** Membrane attack complex.

formation of the rest of the membrane attack complex is non-enzymatic. C6 binds to C5b, and this joint complex is released from the C5 convertase. The formation of C5b67 generates a hydrophobic complex that inserts into the lipid bilayer in the vicinity of the initial activation site. Usually this is on the same cell surface as the initial trigger, but occasionally other cells may be involved. Therefore 'bystander' lysis can take place, giving rise to damage to surrounding tissue. There are a number of proteins present in body fluids to limit this potentially dangerous process by binding to fluid-phase C5b67. C8 and C9 bind to the membrane-inserted complex in sequence, resulting in the formation of a lytic polymeric complex containing up to 20 C9 monomers. A small amount of lysis can occur when C8 binds to C5b67, but it is the polymerized C9 that causes the most damage.

## Functions

The activation of complement by either pathway gives rise to C3b and the generation of a number of factors that can aid in the elimination of foreign material.

The complete insertion of the membrane attack complex into a cell will lead to membrane damage and lysis, probably by osmotic swelling. Some thin-walled pathogens, such as trypanosomes and malaria parasites, are killed by complement-mediated lysis. Some Gram-negative bacteria can be killed by complement in conjunction with lysozyme. However, complement-mediated lysis is of limited importance as a bactericidal mechanism compared with phagocyte destruction of bacteria. Inherited deficiencies of the terminal components are associated with infection by gonococci and meningococci, which can survive inside neutrophils and for which complement-mediated killing is important.

Phagocytic cells have receptors for certain complement components that facilitate the adherence of complement-coated particles. Therefore, complement is an *opsonin*, and in certain circumstances this attachment may lead to phagocytosis.

Two of the molecules released during the complement cascade, C3a and C5a, have potent biological activities. These molecules, known as *anaphylatoxins*, trigger mast cells and basophils to release mediators of inflammation (see below). They also stimulate neutrophils to produce reactive oxygen intermediates, whereas C5a on its own is a chemo-attractant and acts directly on vascular endothelium to cause vasodilatation and increased vascular permeability.

## Cells

### Phagocytes

Micro-organisms entering the tissue fluids or bloodstream are rapidly engulfed by *neutrophils* and *mononuclear phagocytes*. In the blood the latter are known as *monocytes*, whereas in the tissues they differentiate into *macrophages*. In connective tissue they are known as *histiocytes*, in kidney as *mesangial cells*, in liver as *Kupffer cells*, in bone as *osteoclasts*, in brain as *microglia*, and in the spleen, lymph node and thymus as the *sinus-lining macrophages*.

The essential features of these cells are that they:

- are actively phagocytic
- contain digestive enzymes to degrade ingested material

- are an important link between the innate and acquired immune mechanisms.

Part of their role in regard to acquired immunity is that they can process and present antigens, and produce molecules that stimulate lymphocyte differentiation into effector cells.

The role of the phagocyte in innate immunity is to engulf particles (phagocytosis) or soluble material (pinocytosis), and digest them intracellularly within specialized vacuoles. The macrophages present in the walls of capillaries and vascular sinuses in spleen, liver, lungs and bone marrow serve an important role in clearing the bloodstream of foreign particulate material such as bacteria. So efficient is this process that the repeated finding, generally by sensitive broth culture, of a few bacteria or yeasts in the bloodstream usually indicates that there is a continuing release of micro-organisms from an active focus such as an abscess or the heart valve vegetations found in bacterial endocarditis.

The ability of macrophages to ingest and destroy micro-organisms can be impaired or enhanced by depression or stimulation of the phagocyte system. Some microorganisms, such as mycobacteria and brucellae, can resist intracellular digestion by normal macrophages, though they may be digested by 'activated' ones.

## Chemotaxis

For phagocytic cells to be effective, they must be attracted to the site of infection. Once they have passed through the capillary walls they move through the tissues in response to a concentration gradient of molecules produced at the site of damage. These chemotactic factors include:

- products of injured tissue
- factors from the blood (C5a)
- substances produced by neutrophils and mast cells (leukotrienes and histamine)
- bacterial products (formyl-methionine peptides).

Neutrophils respond first and move faster than monocytes.

## Phagocytosis

Phagocytosis involves:

- recognition and binding
- ingestion
- digestion.

Phagocytosis may occur in the absence of antibody, especially on surfaces such as those of the lung alveoli

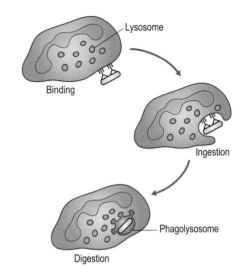

**Fig. 9.4** Stages in phagocytosis.

and when inert particles are involved. Cell membranes carry a net negative charge that keeps them apart and stops autophagocytosis. The hydrophilic nature of certain bacterial cell wall components stops them passing through the hydrophobic membrane. To overcome these difficulties the phagocytes have receptors on their surface that mediate the attachment of particles coated with the correct ligand. Phagocytes have receptors for the Fc portion of certain immunoglobulin isotypes and for some components of the complement cascade. The presence of these molecules, or *opsonins*, on the particle surface markedly enhances the ingestion process and, in some cases, digestion. Whether mediated by specific receptors or not, the foreign particle is surrounded by the cell membrane, which then invaginates and produces an *endosome* or *phagosome* within the cell (Fig. 9.4).

The microbicidal machinery of the phagocyte is contained within organelles known as *lysosomes*. This compartmentalization of potentially toxic molecules is necessary to protect the cell from self-destruction and produce an environment where the molecules can function efficiently. The phagosome and lysosome fuse to form a *phagolysosome* in which the ingested material is killed and digested by various enzyme systems.

Ingestion is accompanied by enhanced glycolysis and an increase in the synthesis of proteins and membrane phospholipids in the phagocyte. After phagocytosis there is a respiratory burst consisting of a steep rise in oxygen consumption. This is accompanied by an increase in the activity of a number of enzymes and leads to the reduction of molecular oxygen to various highly reactive intermediates, such as the superoxide anion ($O_2^{.-}$), hydrogen peroxide ($H_2O_2$), singlet oxygen ($O^.$) and the hydroxyl radical ($OH^.$). All of these chemical species have microbicidal activity and are termed oxygen-dependent killing mechanisms. The superoxide anion is a free radical produced by the one-electron reduction of molecular oxygen; it is very reactive and highly damaging to animal cells, as well as to micro-organisms. It is also the substrate for superoxide dismutase, which generates hydrogen peroxide for subsequent use in microbial killing. Myeloperoxidase uses hydrogen peroxide and halide ions, such as iodide or chloride, to produce at least two bactericidal systems. In one, halogenation (incorporation of iodine or chlorine) of the bacterial cell wall leads to death of the organism. In the second mechanism, myeloperoxidase and hydrogen peroxide damage the cell wall by converting amino acids into aldehydes that have antimicrobial activity.

Within phagocytes there are several oxygen-independent mechanisms that can destroy ingested material. Some of these enzymes can damage membranes. For example, *lysozyme* and *elastase* attack peptidoglycan of the bacterial cell wall, and then hydrolases are responsible for the complete digestion of the killed organism. The cationic proteins of lysosomes bind to and damage bacterial cell walls and enveloped viruses, such as herpes simplex virus. The iron-binding protein *lactoferrin* has antimicrobial properties. It complexes with iron, rendering it unavailable to bacteria that require iron for growth. The high acidity within phagolysosomes (pH 3.5–4.0) may have bactericidal effects, probably resulting from lactic acid production in glycolysis. In addition, many lysosomal enzymes, such as acid hydrolases, have acid pH optima. There are significant differences between macrophages and neutrophils in the killing of micro-organisms. Although macrophage lysosomes contain a variety of enzymes, including lysozyme, they lack cationic proteins and lactoferrin. Tissue macrophages do not have myeloperoxidase but probably use catalase to generate the hydrogen peroxide system. Normal macrophages are less efficient killers of certain pathogens, such as fungi, than neutrophils. The microbicidal activity of macrophages can, however, be greatly improved after contact with products of lymphocytes, known as lymphokines.

Once killed, most micro-organisms are digested and solubilized by lysosomal enzymes. The degradation products are then released to the exterior.

## Natural killer (NK) cells

NK cells recognize changes on virus-infected cells and destroy them by an extracellular killing mechanism. They recognize changes in the level of MHC class I molecules on cell membranes of cells infected with certain viruses. If the NK cell binds to an uninfected host cell, the presence of normal levels of MHC class I molecules leads to inhibition of the killing mechanisms. However, certain viruses, such as herpesviruses, evade the adaptive immune system by interfering with the production of MHC class I molecules. This leads to a reduced level of MHC class I molecules on the infected cell membrane and no inhibition of the killing mechanisms which involve the NK cell producing molecules that damage the membrane of the infected cell leading to its destruction.

Natural killing is a function of several different cell types. This activity is performed by cells described as large granular lymphocytes and also by cells with T cell markers, macrophage markers and others that do not have the characteristics of any of the main cells of the immune system. Natural killing is present without previous exposure to the infectious agent and shows all the characteristics of an innate defence mechanism. NK cells have also been implicated in host defence against cancers by a mechanism similar to that used to combat virus infection. Natural killing is enhanced by interferons that appear to stimulate the production of NK cells and also increase the rate at which they kill the target cells.

## Eosinophils

Eosinophils are granulocytes with a characteristic bi-lobed nucleus and cytoplasmic granules. They are present in the blood of normal individuals at very low levels (<1%), but their numbers increase in patients with parasitic infections and allergies. They are not efficient phagocytic cells, although their granules contain molecules that are toxic to parasites. Large parasites such as helminths cannot be internalized by phagocytes and therefore must be killed extracellularly. Eosinophil granules contain an array of enzymes and toxic molecules active against parasitic worms. The release of these molecules must be controlled so that tissue damage is avoided. The eosinophils have specific receptors, including Fc and complement receptors, that bind the labelled target (i.e. antibody or complement-coated parasites). The granule contents are then released into the space between the cell and the parasite, thus targeting the toxic molecules onto the parasite membrane.

## Temperature

The temperature preference of many micro-organisms is well known, and it is therefore apparent that temperature is an important factor in determining the innate immunity of an animal to some infectious agents. It seems likely that the pyrexia that follows so many different types of infection can function as a protective response against the infecting micro-organism. The febrile response in many cases is controlled by IL-1 produced by macrophages as part of the immune response.

## Inflammation

A number of the above factors are responsible for the process of *acute inflammation*. This is the reaction of the body to injury, such as invasion by an infectious agent, exposure to a noxious chemical or physical trauma. The signs of inflammation are redness, heat, swelling, pain and loss of function. The molecular and cellular events that occur during an inflammatory reaction are:

- vasodilatation
- increased vascular permeability
- cellular infiltration.

These changes are brought about mainly by chemical mediators (Table 9.4), which are widely distributed in a sequestered or inactive form throughout the body and are released or activated locally at the site of inflammation. After release they tend to be inactivated rapidly, to ensure control of the inflammatory process.

There is increased blood supply to the affected area owing to the action of vasoactive amines, such as histamine and 5-hydroxytryptamine, and other mediators stored within mast cells. These molecules are released:

- as a consequence of the production of the anaphylatoxins (C3a and C5a) that trigger specific receptors on mast cells
- following interaction of antigen with IgE on the surface of mast cells
- by direct physical damage to the cells.

Other mediators, such as bradykinins and prostaglandins, are produced locally or released by platelets. The vasodilatation causes increased blood supply to the area, giving rise to redness and heat. The result is an increased supply of the molecules and cells that can combat the agent responsible for the initial trigger.

The same molecules, vasoactive amines, prostaglandins and kinins, increase vascular permeability, allowing plasma and plasma proteins to traverse the endothelial lining. The plasma proteins include immunoglobulins and molecules of the clotting and complement cascades. This leaking of fluid causes swelling (oedema), which in turn leads to increased tissue tension and pain. Some of the molecules themselves, for example prostaglandins and histamine, stimulate the pain responses directly. The inflammatory exudate has several important functions. Bacteria often produce tissue-damaging toxins that are diluted

| Table 9.4 Mediators of inflammation | | |
|---|---|---|
| Mediator | Main source | Function |
| Histamine[a] | Mast cells, basophils | Vasodilatation, increased vascular permeability, contraction of smooth muscle |
| Kinins (e.g. bradykinin) | Plasma | Vasodilatation, increased vascular permeability, contraction of smooth muscle, pain |
| Prostaglandins | Neutrophils, eosinophils, monocytes, platelets | Vasodilatation, increased vascular permeability, pain |
| Leukotrienes | Neutrophils, mast cells, basophils | Vasodilatation, increased vascular permeability, contraction of smooth muscle, induction of cell adherence and chemotaxis |
| Complement components (e.g. C3a, C5a) | Plasma | Cause mast cells to release inflammatory mediators; C5a is a chemotactic factor |
| Plasmin | Plasma | Breaks down fibrin, kinin formation |
| Cytokines | Lymphocytes, macrophages | Chemotactic factors, colony-stimulating factors, macrophage activation |

[a]In rodents, 5-hydroxytryptamine (serotonin) is present in mast cells and basophils.

by the exudate. The presence of clotting factors results in the deposition of fibrin, creating a physical obstruction to the spread of bacteria. The exudate is drained continuously by the lymphatic vessels, and antigens, such as bacteria and their toxins, are carried to the draining lymph node where immune responses can be generated.

The production of chemotactic factors, including C5a, histamine, leukotrienes and molecules specific for certain cell types, attracts phagocytic cells to the site. The increased vascular permeability allows easier access for neutrophils and monocytes, and the vasodilatation means that more cells are in the vicinity. The neutrophils arrive first and begin to destroy or remove the offending agent. Most are successful but a few die, releasing their tissue-damaging contents to increase the inflammatory process. Mononuclear phagocytes arrive on the scene to finish off the removal of the residual debris and stimulate tissue repair.

When the swelling is severe there may be loss of function to the affected area. If the offending agent is quickly removed, the tissue will soon be repaired. The inflammatory process continues until the conditions responsible for its initiation have been resolved. In most circumstances this occurs fairly rapidly, with an acute inflammatory reaction lasting for a matter of hours or days. If, however, the causative agent is not easily removed or is reintroduced continuously, chronic inflammation will ensue with the possibility of tissue destruction and complete loss of function.

## ACQUIRED IMMUNITY

Micro-organisms that overcome or circumvent the innate non-specific defence mechanisms or are administered deliberately (i.e. active immunization) come up against the host's second line of defence: *acquired immunity*. To give expression to this acquired form of immunity it is necessary that the antigens of the invading microorganism come into contact with cells of the immune system (macrophages and lymphocytes) and thereby initiate an immune response specific for the foreign material. The cells that respond are pre-committed, because of their surface receptors, to respond to a particular epitope on the antigen. This response takes two forms, *humoral* and *cell mediated*, which usually develop in parallel. The part played by each depends on a number of factors, including the nature of the antigen, the route of entry and the individual who is infected.

Humoral immunity depends on the appearance in the blood of antibodies produced by plasma cells.

The term 'cell-mediated immunity' was originally coined to describe localized reactions to organisms mediated by T lymphocytes and phagocytes rather than by antibody. It is now used to describe any response in which antibody plays a subordinate role. Cell-mediated immunity depends mainly on the development of T cells that are specifically responsive to the inducing agent, and is generally active against intracellular organisms.

Specific immunity may be acquired in two main ways:

1. induced by overt clinical infection or inapparent clinical infection
2. deliberate artificial immunization.

This is *active acquired immunity*, and contrasts with *passive acquired immunity*, which is the transfer of preformed antibodies to a non-immune individual by means of blood, serum components or lymphoid cells.

Actively acquired immunity is long lasting, although it may be circumvented by antigenic change in the infecting micro-organism. Passively acquired immunity provides only temporary protection. Passive immunity may be transferred to the fetus by the passage of maternal antibodies across the placenta.

## TISSUES INVOLVED IN IMMUNE REACTIONS

For the generation of an immune response, antigen must interact with and activate a number of different cells. In addition, these cells must interact with one another. The cells involved in immune responses are organized into tissues and organs in order that these complex cellular interactions can occur most effectively. These structures are collectively referred to as the *lymphoid system*, which comprises lymphocytes, epithelial and stromal cells arranged into discrete capsulated organs or accumulations of diffuse lymphoid tissue. Lymphoid organs contain lymphocytes at various stages of development and are classified into primary and secondary lymphoid organs.

The primary lymphoid organs are the major sites of lymphopoiesis. Here, lymphoid progenitor cells develop into mature lymphocytes by a process of proliferation and differentiation. In mammals, T lymphocytes develop in the thymus, and B lymphocytes in the bone marrow and fetal liver. It is within the primary lymphoid organs that the lymphocytes acquire their repertoire of specific antigen receptors in order to cope with the antigenic challenges that the individual receives during its life. It is also within these tissues that self-reactive lymphocytes are eliminated to protect against autoimmune disease.

The secondary lymphoid organs create the environment in which lymphocytes can interact with one another and with antigen, and then disseminate the effector cells and molecules generated. Secondary lymphoid organs include lymph nodes, spleen and mucosa-associated lymphoid tissue (e.g. tonsils and Peyer's patches of the gut). These organs have a characteristic structure that relates to the function they carry out, with areas composed of mainly B cells or T cells.

## DEVELOPMENT OF THE IMMUNE SYSTEM

In man, lymphoid tissue appears first in the thymus at about 8 weeks of gestation. Peyer's patches are distinguishable by the fifth month, and immunoglobulin-secreting cells appear in the spleen and lymph nodes at about 20 weeks. From this time onwards, IgM and IgD are synthesized by the fetus (Fig. 9.5). At birth the infant has a blood concentration of IgG comparable to that of the maternal circulation, having received IgG but not IgM via the placenta. The rate of synthesis of IgM in the infant increases rapidly within the first few days of life but does not reach adult levels until about a year. Serum IgG does not reach adult levels until after the second year, and IgA takes even longer. There is an actual drop in the level of IgG from birth due to the decay of maternal antibody, with the lowest levels of total IgG at around 3 months of age. This corresponds to an age of marked susceptibility to a number of infections. Cell-mediated immunity can be stimulated at birth, but these reactions may not be as powerful as in the adult.

## LYMPHOCYTE TRAFFICKING

Lymphocytes differentiate and mature in the primary lymphoid organs and then enter the blood lymphocyte pool. B cells are produced in the bone marrow and mature there before proceeding via the circulation to the secondary lymphoid organs. T cell precursors leave the bone marrow and mature in the thymus before migrating to the secondary lymphoid organs. Once in the secondary lymphoid tissues, the lymphocytes do not remain there but move from one lymphoid organ to another through the blood and lymphatics (Fig. 9.6). One of the main advantages of this *lymphocyte recirculation* is that during the course of a natural infection the continual trafficking of lymphocytes enables many different lymphocytes to have access to the antigen.

Only a very small number of the lymphocytes will recognize a particular antigen. Pathogens can enter

**Fig. 9.5** Immunoglobulin levels in the fetus and neonate. Adult levels of the major isotypes are shown as normal ranges with mean serum levels.

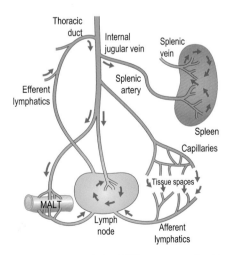

**Fig. 9.6** Lymphocyte recirculation. MALT, mucosa-associated lymphoid tissue.

the body by many routes, but must be carried from the site of infection to the secondary lymphoid tissues where they are localized and concentrated on the dendritic processes of macrophages or on the surface of antigen-presenting cells. If the infection is in the tissues, antigen is carried in the lymphatics to the draining lymph node. Under normal conditions there is a continuous active flow of lymphocytes through lymph nodes, but when antigen and antigen-reactive cells enter there is a temporary shut-down of the exit. Thus, antigen-specific cells are preferentially retained in the node draining the source of the antigen. This is partly responsible for the swollen glands (lymph nodes) that can sometimes be found during an infection. Microbes present on mucosal surfaces are taken up by specialized cells known as M cells, and are then delivered to the mucosa-associated lymphoid tissues such as the tonsils and Peyer's patches. Blood-borne antigens are trapped in the spleen. The passage of lymphocytes through an area where antigen has been localized facilitates the induction of an immune response. Lymphocytes with appropriate receptors bind to the antigen and become activated. Once activated, the lymphocytes mature into effector cells. In the case of B lymphocytes they become plasma cells and secrete antibody. T lymphocytes leave the secondary lymphoid tissue and return to the site of infection to destroy the infectious agent.

There is evidence for non-random migration of lymphocytes to particular lymphoid compartments. For example, lymphocytes that home to the gut are selectively transported across endothelial cells of venules in the intestine. It appears that lymphocytes have specific molecules on their surface that preferentially interact with endothelial cells in different anatomical sites. A lymphocyte that was initially stimulated by antigen in a Peyer's patch will migrate to the draining lymph node, respond, and memory cells will be produced. It is important that these memory cells migrate back to the area where the same pathogen might be encountered again. Therefore, they are found preferentially in the mucosa-associated lymphoid tissue.

## CLONAL SELECTION

During their development in the primary lymphoid tissues both T and B lymphocytes acquire specific cell surface receptors that commit them to a single antigenic specificity. For T cells this receptor remains the same for its life, but the surface immunoglobulin on B cells can be modified as a result of somatic mutations. In the B cell this is mirrored in the modification of the antibody produced by the cell on exposure to its specific antigen. The lymphocytes are activated when they bind specific antigen and then proliferate, differentiate and mature into effector cells.

The lymphocytes reactive to any particular antigen are only a small proportion of the total pool. Therefore, antigen binds to the small number of cells that can recognize it and selects them to proliferate and mature so that sufficient cells are formed to mount an adequate immune response. A cell that responds to an antigenic trigger and proliferates will give rise to cells with a genetically identical makeup (i.e. *clones*). This phenomenon is therefore known as *clonal selection*.

Lymphocyte receptors, generated in the primary lymphoid tissues, are created in a random fashion, so there is no reason why some could not recognize 'self' molecules. An obviously important attribute of the immune system is that it is able to discriminate between 'self' and 'non-self'. During development, any lymphocyte with a receptor that binds strongly to self molecules is eliminated.

## CELLULAR ACTIVATION

When an individual is exposed to foreign material, selected lymphocytes respond. B lymphocytes proliferate and differentiate into antibody-producing plasma cells and memory cells. T lymphocytes are stimulated to become effector cells that can directly eliminate the foreign material or produce molecules that help other cells to destroy the pathogen. The type (immunity or tolerance) and magnitude of the response, if generated, depends on a number of factors, including the nature, dose and route of entry of the antigen, and the individual's genetic make-up and previous exposure to the antigen.

The first stage in the production of effector cells and molecules is activation of the resting cells. This involves various cellular interactions with maturation of the response, leading to a co-ordinated, efficient production of effector T cells, immunoglobulin and memory cells.

Cross-linking of the B cell antigen receptor, surface immunoglobulin, is the initial trigger for activation. When this happens, a number of biochemical changes are instigated. These changes probably act through protein kinases that cause the synthesis of RNA and ultimately immunoglobulin production. In some cases this is all that is required to stimulate antibody production. However, for the majority of antigens this initial cross-linking is not enough, and molecules produced by T cells are also required.

## Thymus-independent antigens

A number of antigens will stimulate specific immunoglobulin production directly. These T-independent antigens are of two types: *mitogens* and certain large molecules.

Mitogens are substances that cause cells, particularly lymphocytes, to undergo cell division (i.e. proliferation). Certain glycoproteins, called lectins, have mitogenic activity. These molecules have specificity for sugars; they bind to the cell surface and activate all responsive cells. The response to the mitogens is therefore polyclonal, as lymphocytes of many different specificities are activated. However, at low concentrations these mitogens do not cause polyclonal activation but can lead to the stimulation of specific B cells. Lipopolysaccharide is an example of a B cell mitogen.

Some large molecules with regularly repeating epitopes, for instance polymers of D-amino acids and simple sugars such as pneumococcal polysaccharide and dextran, can interact directly with the B cell surface immunoglobulin. They may also be held on the surface of specialized macrophages in secondary lymphoid tissues, and the B cells interact with them there. The multiple repeats of the epitope interact with a large number of surface immunoglobulin molecules; the signal that is generated is sufficient to stimulate antibody production.

The immune response generated to these antigens tends to be similar on each exposure, that is, IgM is the main antibody and the response shows little memory. This suggests that class switch and memory production require additional factors (products of T lymphocytes).

## Thymus-dependent antigens

Many antigens do not stimulate antibody production without the help of T lymphocytes. These antigens first bind to the B cell, which must then be exposed to T cell-derived lymphokines (helper factors) before antibody can be produced. For the second activation signal (i.e. help) to be targeted effectively at the B cell, the T and B cells must be in direct contact. For this to happen, the B and T cell epitopes must be linked physically. However, T cells only recognize antigen that has been processed and presented in association with products of the major histocompatibility complex (MHC), so it is impossible for native antigen to form a bridge between surface immunoglobulin and the T cell receptor. The B cell binds to its epitope on free antigen, but there is no site on this molecule to which the T cell can bind, because it requires antigen associated with MHC products. The answer to this problem can be seen when the requirements for antigen presentation in T cell recognition are considered.

## Antigen processing and presentation

The development of an antibody response to a T-dependent antigen requires that the antigen becomes associated with MHC class II molecules (i.e. *processed*) and expressed on the cell surface (i.e. *presented*) in a form that helper T cells can recognize.

All cells express MHC class I molecules, but class II molecules are confined to cells of the immune system – the antigen-presenting cells. These cells present antigen to MHC class II-restricted T cells (the CD4-positive [CD4$^+$] population) and therefore play a key role in the induction and development of immune responses. Within lymph nodes, different antigen-presenting cells are found in each of the main areas (Table 9.5).

There are a large number of antigen-presenting cells in the body, most of which constitutively express MHC class II molecules. Other cells, such as T lymphocytes and endothelium, can be induced to express MHC class II molecules by suitable stimuli such as lymphokines. The relative importance of each type depends on whether a primary or secondary response is being stimulated and on the location. The most studied antigen-presenting cells are the macrophages and dendritic cells. However, it is now apparent that in certain situations B cells may be important antigen-presenting cells. The relative importance of B cells

| Table 9.5 | Antigen-presenting cells in the lymph nodes | |
|---|---|---|
| Area | Antigen-presenting cell | Antigen |
| Subcapsular marginal sinus | Marginal zone macrophage | T-independent antigens |
| Follicles and B cell areas | Follicular dendritic cells | Antigen-antibody complexes |
| Medulla | Classical macrophages | Most antigens |
| T cell areas | Interdigitating dendritic cells | Most antigens |

becomes greatest during secondary responses, especially when the antigen concentration is low. Here the B cells can specifically engulf antigen via their surface immunoglobulin. In a primary response, specific B cells are at a low frequency and their receptors are of low affinity; in this situation macrophages and dendritic cells are probably most important.

The key feature of all antigen-presenting cells is that they can ingest antigen, degrade it and present it, in the context of MHC class II molecules, to T cells. The antigen is taken into the antigen-presenting cells and enters the endocytic pathway. Before it is destroyed completely, peptide fragments are taken to a structure called the *compartment for peptide loading*. MHC class II molecules are synthesized within the endoplasmic reticulum and are also transported to the compartment for peptide loading, where they associate with the processed antigen. The MHC class II molecule with the bound peptide is then transported to the cell surface.

## T cell activation

The activation of resting $CD4^+$ T cells requires two signals. The first is antigen in association with MHC class II molecules, and the second is the *co-stimulatory signal*. The generation of the first of these signals has just been discussed (i.e. antigen presentation). The second signal is delivered by the same antigen-presenting cell that gave the first signal. The co-stimulatory signal is mediated by the interaction of a molecule on the antigen-presenting cell engaging with its receptor on the T cell. The best characterized pairing is B7 on the antigen-presenting cell and CD28 on the T cell.

When both of these signals are generated, biochemical changes occur within the T cell, leading to RNA and protein synthesis. The responsive cells progress through the cell cycle from the $G_0$ to the $G_1$ phase. The cells start to express IL-2 receptors and produce IL-2, a T cell growth factor that causes the expansion of the responsive T cell population. IL-2 was originally thought to be the only T cell growth factor, but it is now known that IL-4 and IL-1 can support T cell growth, although they are not as potent. After about 2 days, IL-2 synthesis stops, whereas IL-2 receptors remain for up to a week if the cell is not reactivated. Therefore, there is a built-in limitation on T cell growth and clonal expansion. When stimulated, T cells secrete IL-2, which interacts with IL-2 receptors to mediate growth. This can be in an '*autocrine*' fashion if the same cell that released the IL-2 is stimulated. If the responding cell is in the vicinity of the producer, the stimulation is in a '*paracrine*' manner.

IL-2 is not present at detectable levels in the blood; therefore no '*endocrine*' activity is involved (i.e. action at a distant site). The end-result is the production of a large number of activated $CD4^+$ T lymphocytes.

The other main type of T lymphocyte is the $CD8^+$ T cell. Antigen recognition by these cells is restricted by MHC class I molecules. Again, these cells require two signals to be activated: (1) antigen fragment in association with MHC class I and (2) the co-stimulatory signal. A cell that 'sees' both of these signals responds by clonal expansion and differentiation into a fully active effector T cell.

## B cell activation

Mitogens and T-independent antigens have an inherent ability to drive B cells into division and differentiation. T-dependent responses rely on T cells and their products to control the antibody class, affinity and memory. The first cells to be activated are $CD4^+$ T cells that recognize the antigen in association with MHC class II molecules (see above). These cells respond to the signal of the antigen fragment–MHC complex, and produce a variety of lymphokines that act on B cells.

As far as B cell development is concerned, the antigen-stimulated cells develop under the influence of IL-4 (previously known as B cell stimulation factor), which is produced by closely adherent T cells. IL-5 and IL-6 then bring the cells to a state of full activation with terminal differentiation into an immunoglobulin-producing plasma cell. All this happens within a germinal centre of a lymph node secondary follicle that has evolved to facilitate the necessary cellular and molecular interactions.

Therefore, for both B and T cell activation, two stimuli are required:

1. The recognition of antigen makes sure that only those cells that will be effective against the foreign material are recruited.
2. The provision of the co-stimulatory signal has evolved to control the process and aid discrimination of 'self' and 'non-self'.

## HUMORAL IMMUNITY

### Synthesis of antibody

On exposure to antigen, antibody production follows a characteristic pattern (Fig. 9.7). There is a lag phase during which antibody cannot be detected. This is the time taken for the interactions described above to take place and for antibody to reach a level that can be

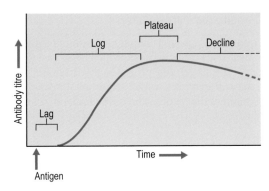

**Fig. 9.7**  Pattern of antibody production following antigen exposure.

**Fig. 9.8**  Primary and secondary antibody response. The level of serum IgM and IgG detected with time after primary immunization (day 0) and challenge (day 300) with the same antigen.

measured. There is then an exponential rise in the antibody level or titre. This log phase is followed by a plateau with a constant level of antibody, when the amount produced equals the amount removed. The amount of antibody then declines, owing to the clearing of antigen–antibody complexes and the natural catabolism of the immunoglobulin.

If the response is to a T-dependent antigen, the B cells can switch to the production of another isotype; for example, in a primary response IgM gives way to IgG production. This process is under the control of T cells, as the class of antibody produced depends on signals from the T cell. At some point, again under the control of T cells, a proportion of the antigen-reactive cells develop into memory cells. These cells react if the epitope is encountered again.

There are a number of differences in the reaction profile on second and subsequent exposures to an antigen compared with the primary response (Fig. 9.8). There is a shortened lag and an extended plateau and decline. The level and affinity of antibody

produced are much increased, and antibody is mostly of the IgG isotype. Some IgM is generated, but it will follow the same pattern as in the primary response.

When first introduced, the antigen selects the cells that can react with it. However, before antibody is produced the B cell must differentiate into a plasma cell, involving the interactions already described. The B cells that are stimulated in the primary response synthesize IgM. With time, class switch will occur in some of the B cells, leading to the production of other isotypes. Somatic mutations occur, giving rise to *affinity maturation* through selection of cells bearing high-affinity receptors as the amount of antigen in the system falls. Memory cells are also produced. An equilibrium is reached whereby there is a balance between the amount of antibody synthesized and the amount used. Various mechanisms then come into play to turn off the response when it is no longer needed (see below). The simplest is the removal of the stimulant (antigen). Thus the production of antibody is stopped and there is a natural decline in antibody levels.

On subsequent exposure the responding cells (i.e. memory cells) are at a different level of activation and are present at an increased frequency. Therefore, there is a shorter lag before antibody can be detected; the main isotype is IgG. The level of antibody produced is ten or more times greater than during the primary response. The antibody is present for an extended period and has a higher affinity for antigen due to affinity maturation. As is seen in Figure 9.8, some IgM is also produced during a secondary response. This immunoglobulin is produced by the activation of B cells that were not present in the lymphocyte pool on the previous exposure but have developed since. The development of these cells follows the characteristics of a primary response, and they will give rise to a secondary response if the antigen is encountered again.

## Monoclonal antibodies

When an antigen is introduced into the lymphoid system of a mouse, all the B cells that recognize epitopes on the antigen are stimulated to produce antibody. The serum of the immunized animal is known as a polyclonal antiserum, as it is the product of many clonally derived B cells. Even when highly purified antigen is used, the antiserum produced will contain a number of antibodies that react to the antigen and others that interact with antigens encountered naturally by the animal during this time. It is extremely difficult to purify the antibodies of interest from this complex mixture, but it is possible to fuse single plasma cells with a myeloma (a tumour) cell line to form a hybridoma that will grow in tissue culture. These cells will all be identical and therefore secrete the same antibody, a *monoclonal antibody*.

Human monoclonal antibodies are potentially of value in patient treatment. As starting material, peripheral blood or secondary lymphoid tissue such as tonsils have been used. It is impossible, for ethical reasons, to expose human subjects to most of the antigenic material that would be required to induce useful antibodies. Therefore, cells are only available from patients with certain diseases, such as tumours, infections and autoimmune diseases, or from individuals who have received immunizations.

All the molecules in a monoclonal antibody preparation have the same isotype, specificity and affinity, in contrast to the polyclonal antiserum produced by the inoculation of antigen into an experimental animal. In addition, the same polyclonal antiserum can never be reproduced, not even when using the same animal. However, monoclonal antibodies are defined reagents that can be produced indefinitely and on a large scale. They provide a standard material that can be used in studies ranging from the identification and enumeration of different cell types to blood typing and diagnosis of disease. They are also used increasingly in attempts to treat and prevent disease.

## CELL-MEDIATED IMMUNITY

Specific cell-mediated responses are mediated by two different types of T lymphocyte. T cells that have the CD8 molecule on their surface recognize antigen fragments in association with MHC class I molecules on a target cell and cause cell lysis. MHC class II-restricted recognition is seen with T cells that have the CD4 marker. These cells secrete lymphokines when stimulated by the antigen–MHC class II complex. CD4+ T cells are involved in two main activities:

1. Cell-mediated reactions, as the lymphokines can aid in the elimination of foreign material by recruiting and activating other leucocytes and promoting an inflammatory response.
2. The generation and control of an immune response, as some of the lymphokines produced are growth and differentiation factors for T and B cells.

The other cell types, NK cells and phagocytes, that can participate in cell-mediated defence mechanisms have been described.

## Cell-mediated cytotoxicity

Certain subpopulations of lymphoid and myeloid cells can destroy target cells to which they are closely bound. The stages and processes involved are similar for the different cell types, although the molecules that mediate the recognition of the target by the effector differ.

### Cytotoxic T lymphocytes

Cytotoxic T cells (Tc cells) are small T lymphocytes derived from stem cells in the bone marrow. These cells mature in the thymus. Most cells that mediate MHC-restricted cytotoxicity are CD8+, and therefore recognize antigen in association with MHC class I antigens. Some are CD4+, and therefore MHC class II restricted.

### MHC-unrestricted cytotoxic cells

A number of partially overlapping cell populations are able to carry out MHC-unrestricted killing. These include NK cells, lymphokine-activated killer (LAK) cells and killer (K) cells.

Most cells that have the capacity to perform natural killing have the morphology of large granular lymphocytes and a broad target range. Receptors on the NK cell recognise structures on host cells and will kill the host cell unless inhibitory receptors are engaged by MHC class I molecules. Therefore NK cells are involved in the destruction of host cells with low levels of MHC class I molecules, e.g. cells infected with certain viruses and some cancer cells. NK cells have been shown to produce a number of cytokines, including γ-interferon.

Several types of cell are able to destroy foreign material by antibody-dependent cell-mediated cytotoxicity. The cells that carry out this activity have a receptor for the Fc portion of immunoglobulin and are therefore able to bind to antibody-coated targets.

### Lytic mechanism

Three distinct phases have been described in cell-mediated cytotoxicity (Fig. 9.9):

- binding to target
- rearrangement of cytoplasmic granules and release of their contents
- target cell death.

Once the effector–target conjugate has been formed, the cytoplasmic granules appear to become

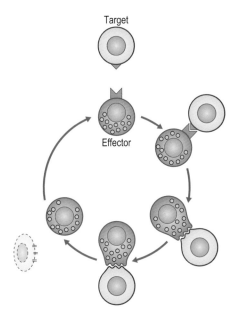

Target

Effector

**Fig. 9.9** Mechanism of cell-mediated cytotoxicity. The effector cell has a receptor that is able to bind to a target cell that possesses the appropriate ligand (▲).

rearranged and concentrated at the side of the cell adjacent to the target. The granule contents are then released into the space between the two cells. There are at least three different types of molecule stored within the granules that can cause cell death. T cells and NK cells contain perforin, which is a monomeric protein related to the complement component C9. In the presence of $Ca^{2+}$ ions the monomers bind to the target cell membrane and polymerize to form a transmembrane pore. This upsets the osmotic balance of the cell and leads to cell death. The granules also contain at least two serine esterases that may play a role in destroying the target cell. Several other toxic molecules are produced by cytotoxic cells, including tumour necrosis factor (TNF)-α, lymphotoxin (TNF-β), γ-interferon and NK cytotoxic factor. The process is unidirectional, with only the target cell being destroyed. The effector cell can then move on and eliminate another target cell.

## Lymphokine production

The other arm of cell-mediated immunity is dependent on the production of lymphokines from antigen-activated T lymphocytes. These molecules, produced in an antigen-specific fashion, can act in an antigen-non-specific manner to recruit, activate and regulate effector cells with the potential to combat infectious agents.

The first documented reference to the production of lymphokines is credited to Robert Koch in 1880. Injection of purified antigen (tuberculin) into the skin of immune individuals produced a reaction that peaked within 24–72 h. The response was characterized by reddening and swelling, and accompanied by the accumulation of lymphocytes, monocytes and basophils. Because of the time course of the reaction, this response has become known as *delayed-type hypersensitivity* (DTH), and the cells responsible were called delayed-type hypersensitivity T lymphocytes ($T_{DTH}$ or $T_D$ cells). These cells are identical to the helper T ($T_H$) cell subset as far as antigen recognition is concerned. $CD4^+$ T cells, usually still referred to as $T_H$ cells, are therefore capable of mediating both helper activities and so-called delayed hypersensitivity reactions by producing lymphokines. Although the term 'delayed hypersensitivity' suggests a disease process, the production of lymphokines has a physiological function, and only in some situations do pathological consequences occur.

Cytokines are biologically active molecules released by specific cells that elicit a particular response from other cells on which they act. A number of these regulatory molecules produced by lymphocytes (lymphokines) and monocytes (monokines) are shown in Table 9.6. The responses caused by these substances are varied and interrelated. In general, cytokines control the growth, mobility and differentiation of lymphocytes, but they also exert a similar effect on other leucocytes and some non-immune cells.

The exact signals and mechanisms controlling the activation of T cells and the release of lymphokines are not known. The balance between the different lymphokines produced determines the response generated. $CD4^+$ T cells can be divided into two main types depending on the profile of lymphokines they secrete. The $T_H2$ subset produces IL-4 and IL-5, which act on responsive B cells with antibody production as the main feature of the response. The $T_H1$ subset secretes mainly IL-2 and γ-interferon. The production of IL-2 stimulates T cell growth, whereas γ-interferon has multiple effects, including macrophage activation.

## Role of macrophages

Macrophages are able to carry out a remarkable array of different functions (Fig. 9.10). They play a key role in several aspects of cell-mediated immunity, being involved at the initiation of the response, as antigen-presenting cells, and as effector cells having microbicidal and tumoricidal activities. They also produce a number of cytokines (or more precisely monokines)

**Table 9.6** Examples of some cytokines that are of importance in the immune system

| Cytokine | Main source | Target | Main effects |
|---|---|---|---|
| IL-1 | Macrophages<br>Endothelial cells<br>Some epithelial cells | T lymphocytes<br>Tissue cells | Fever<br>Inflammation<br>T cell activation<br>Macrophage activation<br>Stimulates acute-phase protein production |
| IL-2 | T lymphocytes | T lymphocytes<br>NK cells<br>B lymphocytes | T cell proliferation |
| IL-4 | $T_H2$ cells<br>Mast cells | B lymphocytes<br>T lymphocytes<br>Mast cells | Stimulates proliferation, differentiation and class<br>  switch in B cells<br>Differentiation and proliferation of $T_H2$ cells<br>Mast cell growth |
| IL-8 | Macrophages<br>Endothelial cells | Neutrophils | Chemotaxis |
| IL-13 | $T_H2$ cells | Macrophages | Inhibits macrophage activation and activities |
| TNF-$\alpha$ | Macrophages<br>T lymphocytes | Macrophages<br>Tissue cells | Fever<br>Inflammation<br>Macrophage activation<br>Stimulates acute-phase protein production<br>Kills certain tumour cells |
| Type I IFN ($\alpha$ and $\beta$) | Virus-infected cells | Tissue cells | Antiviral effect<br>Induction of MHC class I<br>Antiproliferative effects<br>Activation of NK cells |
| IFN-$\gamma$ | T lymphocytes ($T_H1$ and $T_c$)<br>NK cells | Leucocytes and tissue cells | Macrophage activation<br>Induction of MHC class I and II<br>Antibody class switch<br>Antiviral effect |
| GM-CSF | T lymphocytes<br>Macrophages<br>Endothelial cells<br>Fibroblasts | Immature and committed progenitor<br>  cells in bone marrow | Stimulates growth and differentiation of<br>  myelomonocytic cells<br>Macrophage activation |

Many of the molecules detailed above act synergistically to produce their biological effects.
GM-CSF, granulocyte–macrophage colony-stimulating factor; IL, interleukin; IFN, interferon; MHC, major histocompatibility complex; NK, natural killer; TNF, tumour necrosis factor.

that function as regulatory molecules. These monokines contribute to inflammation and fever, and affect the functioning of other cells. Macrophages can also produce various enzymes and factors that are involved in reorganization and repair following tissue damage. However, as they contain many important biological molecules, they can themselves cause damage if these enzymes and factors are released inappropriately.

Many of these activities are enhanced in macrophages that have been 'activated' by exposure to lymphokines, such as γ-interferon produced by T cells. Macrophage activation is a complex process that probably occurs in stages, with different effector functions being expressed at different stages. Macrophages from different sites in the body show different characteristics; they are heterogeneous and have different activation requirements.

γ-Interferon is a powerful macrophage-activating molecule that increases the uptake of antigens by an enhanced expression of Fc and complement receptors; the activities of intracellular enzymes involved in killing are also raised. As γ-interferon causes an

**Fig. 9.10** The central role of macrophages.

increase in MHC class II expression, there will be an enhanced presentation of antigen to CD4$^+$ T cells. This leads to the production of more lymphokines and more effective elimination of the offending material.

CD4$^+$ T cells secrete the lymphokines that activate macrophages. Therefore, the presentation of antigen by an antigen-presenting cell leads to the production of lymphokines by T$_H$1 cells *specific* for the antigen involved. The lymphokines produced then activate any responsive macrophage in the vicinity of the responding cells. The activation process appears to depend on the presence of a number of lymphokines that act synergistically to induce activation. For example, pure IL-2, IL-4 or γ-interferon is unable to induce resistance to infection, but if γ-interferon is combined with any of the others then resistance is observed.

Macrophages and monocytes themselves are capable of producing a number of important cytokines. These monokines include:

- IL-1
- IL-6
- various colony-stimulating factors
- TNF-α.

TNF-α and IL-1, acting independently and together, have effects on many leucocytes and tissues. TNF-α is responsible for the tumoricidal activity of macrophages but is also implicated in the elimination of certain bacteria and parasites. It has a synergistic effect with γ-interferon on resistance to a number of viral infections.

## GENERATION OF IMMUNE RESPONSES

As discussed above, the generation of humoral and cell-mediated responses requires the recognition of antigen, by the responding cell, as the first signal and a co-stimulation second signal. T$_H$ cells, as has been emphasized, recognize antigen fragments only when in association with MHC class II molecules. The distribution of MHC class II molecules is limited, in normal situations, to certain cells of the immune system: the antigen-presenting cells. In certain circumstances non-lymphoid cells can present antigens if they are induced to express MHC class II molecules. To stimulate a T$_H$ cell the antigen must be taken into the cell and re-expressed on the surface in association with MHC class II molecules. As the T cell antigen receptor recognizes antigen fragments bound to the MHC molecules, the antigen-presenting cell must also be able to process the antigen. MHC class I- and class II-restricted recognition by CD8$^+$ and CD4$^+$ T cells requires antigen processing. The pathways that lead to association of an antigen fragment with a particular restriction element are not fully understood.

Immune responses are generated in secondary lymphoid tissues, such as lymph nodes. As a number of cells and molecules must all interact, the architecture of the secondary lymphoid tissue has evolved for the efficient induction of an immune response. In a secondary immune response the cells involved are at a different stage of activation: they are memory cells, having already been exposed to antigen. Therefore, the growth factor signals may not be so critical, although antigen in association with MHC class II molecules is still required. In this situation B cells are important as antigen-presenting cells.

CD8$^+$ T cells, as we have seen, recognize antigen fragments associated with MHC class I molecules. All cells have MHC class I molecules on their surface and are therefore expected to be capable of presenting antigen fragments to cytotoxic T cells, which are, for the most part, MHC class I restricted. The antigen fragments derived from endogenously synthesized molecules, for instance from a virus, are produced at a site distinct from the endocytic vesicles where exogenous antigens are processed.

At or around the site of protein synthesis, endogenously produced antigen fragments become associated with the newly produced MHC class I molecules. The MHC class II molecule picks up internalized antigen within the compartment for peptide loading (CPL), as it moves to the cell surface. In this compartment, antigen fragments cannot bind to the MHC class I molecules because these molecules have already associated with endogenously produced antigenic fragments within the endoplasmic reticulum and never go to the CPL. Thus the site where the antigen is processed determines whether it will associate with MHC class I or class II molecules. This separation of processing pathways explains why CD4$^+$ and CD8$^+$ T cells are involved in the destruction of exogenous and endogenous antigens, respectively.

If a particular antigen does not become associated with either MHC class I or class II molecules, no T-dependent immune response will be directed against that antigen. As MHC class II molecules are involved in the initiation of immune responses by presenting antigen fragments to T$_H$ cells, they can control whether or not a response takes place. It has been clearly shown that the level of an immune response to a particular antigen is controlled by the MHC class II molecules. The genes that code for these molecules (MHC class II genes) have therefore been referred to as *immune response genes*.

It should be obvious that if an antigen cannot associate with the MHC class II molecules of an individual then no immune response will be generated. As the MHC molecules are polymorphic, the cells of some individuals will present, and therefore respond to, certain antigen fragments, whereas cells from other individuals will not. Fortunately, more than one antigenic fragment can be generated from each pathogen; otherwise individuals who did not respond to the particular sequence would be vulnerable to that micro-organism. In addition, individuals have at least six different MHC class II genes and there is therefore an increased chance that some fragments will bind to at least one of their MHC class II molecules. Variations in the levels and specificity of response occur in individuals who have different MHC class II molecules and have therefore produced different MHC–antigen complexes on their cells.

Immune response gene effects can also be controlled at the level of the T cell receptor. If an individual does not have a T cell with a receptor that recognizes a particular antigen–MHC complex, no response will be generated. The T cell receptor repertoire is generated in the thymus, where the genes of the immature T cells are rearranged to give rise to a functioning receptor. T cells that cross-react too strongly with self molecules are deleted, as are cells whose receptors do not interact with self MHC molecules. Therefore, T cells that interact weakly with MHC molecules are selected to mature and leave the thymus. When these cells later come across an antigen–MHC complex, the presence of antigen strengthens the weak T cell receptor–MHC interaction, leading to a stimulatory signal being transmitted to the T cell. If, for some reason, T cells that respond to a particular MHC–antigen configuration have been deleted, suppressed or not formed, no immune response will be generated to that antigen. There is what is known as a 'hole' in the T cell repertoire.

## CONTROL OF IMMUNE RESPONSES

An antigen can induce two types of response: immunity or tolerance. Tolerance is the acquisition of non-reactivity towards a particular antigen. The generation of immunity or tolerance depends largely on the way in which the immune system first encounters the antigen. Once the immune system has been stimulated, the cells involved proliferate and produce a response that eliminates the offending agent. It is then important to dampen down the reacting cells; various feedback mechanisms operate to bring this about.

### Role of antigen

The primary regulator of an immune response is the antigen itself. This makes sense, as it is important to initiate a response when antigen enters the host and once it has been eliminated it is wasteful, and in some cases dangerous, to continue to produce effector mechanisms.

### Role of antibody

Many biological systems are controlled by the product inhibiting the reaction once a certain level has been reached. This type of negative feedback is seen with antibody, which may act by blocking the epitopes on the antigen so that it can no longer stimulate the cell through its receptor.

As antibody levels rise there is competition between free antibody and the B cell receptor. Consequently, only those B cells that have a receptor with a high affinity for antigen will be stimulated and therefore produce high-affinity antibody. For this reason antibody feedback is thought to be an important driving force in affinity maturation.

### Regulatory T cells

T$_H$ cells control the generation of effector cells by producing helper factors. However, the factors that stimulate the expansion of B and T cell numbers do not work indefinitely. Maturation factors are also produced that control terminal differentiation into effector cells. Under the influence of these latter lymphokines, the action of the proliferation factors is inhibited mainly by making the effector cell unresponsive to their effects.

Other T lymphocytes have been described that provide negative signals to the immune system. Certain regulatory T cells limit the development of antibody-producing cells and effector T cells. The activity of these cells can involve both the production of soluble factors and direct cell–cell interactions.

## TOLERANCE

Two forms of tolerance can be identified: *natural* and *acquired* tolerance. The non-response to self molecules is due to natural tolerance. If this tolerance breaks down and the body responds to self molecules, an autoimmune disease will develop. Natural tolerance appears during fetal development when the immune system is being formed. In experimental animals the introduction of foreign material at the time of birth leads to tolerance. Acquired tolerance arises when a potential immunogen induces a state of unresponsiveness to itself. This has consequences for host defences, as the presence of a tolerogenic epitope on a pathogen may compromise the ability of the body to resist infection.

An antigen can induce different effects on the two arms of the immune system. During an infection the host is exposed to a variety of antigenic determinants on a micro-organism. These epitopes are present at differing concentrations and possibly at different times during the infection. The epitopes can act as either immunogens or tolerogens. Therefore, it is possible that the antibody response to a particular antigen may be quite pronounced while the cell-mediated response may be lacking, or vice versa. Alternatively, both arms of the immune response may be stimulated or tolerized.

Generally, high doses of antigen tolerize B cells, whereas minute doses given repeatedly tolerize T cells. For acquired tolerance to be maintained, the tolerogen must persist or be administered repeatedly. This is probably necessary because of the continuous production of new T and B cells that must be made tolerant.

Several mechanisms play a role in the selective lack of response to specific antigens. As each lymphocyte has a receptor with a single specificity, the elimination of a specific cell will render the individual tolerant to the epitope it recognizes and leave the rest of the repertoire untouched. This mechanism relies on self molecules interacting with the receptor and causing their elimination. It is proposed that during lymphocyte development the cell goes through a phase in which contact with antigen leads to death or permanent inactivation. Immature B cells encountering antigen for the first time are particularly susceptible to tolerization in the presence of low doses of antigen. The requirement for two signals in the stimulation of B cells and the generation of effector T cells can give rise

to tolerance. Both cell types require stimulation via the antigen receptor and 'help' from a specific T cell. If the helper factors are not produced, the responding cells will be functionally deleted. Therefore, the elimination of self-reactive T cells in the thymus during T cell maturation is an important step in maintaining a state of tolerance. Tolerance can also be induced by active suppression. Some T cells are capable of inducing unresponsiveness by acting directly on B cells or other T cells. These regulatory T cells can be antigen-specific and probably produce signals that actively suppress cells capable of responding to a particular antigen.

It was originally thought that unresponsiveness to self was controlled by the elimination of all self-reactive cells before they matured. This cannot be true, as self-reactive B cells are found in normal adult animals. It is thought that these B cells are controlled by a lack of T cell help, that is, $T_H$ cells have been eliminated.

## IMMUNODEFICIENCY

The immunologically competent cells of the lymphoid tissues derived from, renewed by and influenced by the activities of the thymus, bone marrow and other lymphoid tissues can be the subject of disease processes. The deficiency states seen are either due to defects in one of the components of the system itself, or secondary to some other disease process affecting the normal functioning of some part of the lymphoid tissues. Deficiency of one or more of the defence mechanisms can be inherited, developmental or acquired. The types of infections and diseases seen in patients with immunodeficiencies relate to the role the affected component plays in the normal situation. An individual whose immune system has been depressed in any of these ways is said to be *immuno-compromised*. The compromised host is prone to infectious diseases that the normal individual would easily eradicate or not succumb to in the first place. Some examples of predisposing factors are given in Table 9.7.

### Defective innate defence mechanisms

Defects in phagocyte function take two forms:

1. Where there is a quantitative deficiency of neutrophils that may be congenital (e.g. infantile agranulocytosis) or acquired as a result of replacement of bone marrow by tumour cells or the toxic effects of drugs or chemicals.

**Table 9.7** The compromised host

| Predisposing factor | Effect on immune system | Type of infection |
| --- | --- | --- |
| Immunosuppression for transplant or cancer | Diminished cell-mediated and humoral immunity | Lung infections, bacteraemia, fungal infections, urinary tract infections |
| Viral immunosuppression (e.g. measles, human immunodeficiency virus, Epstein–Barr virus) | Impaired function of infected cells | Secondary bacterial infections, opportunistic pathogens |
| Tumour of immune cells | Replacement of cells of the immune system | Bacteraemia, pneumonia, urinary tract infections |
| Malnutrition | Lymphoid hypoplasia Decreased lymphocytes and phagocyte activity | Measles, tuberculosis, respiratory infections, gastro-intestinal infections |
| Breakdown of tissue barriers (e.g. surgery, burns, catheterization) | Breach innate defence mechanisms | Bacterial infections, opportunistic pathogens |
| Inhalation of particles due to employment or smoking | Damage to cilia, destruction of alveolar macrophages | Chronic respiratory infections, hypersensitivity reactions |

2. Where there is a qualitative deficiency in the functioning of neutrophils which, while ingesting bacteria normally, fail to digest them because of an enzymatic defect.

Characteristic of these diseases is a susceptibility to bacterial and fungal, but not viral or protozoan, infections. Among the enzyme deficiency disorders are *chronic granulomatous disease* and the *Chédiak–Higashi syndrome*.

The complement system can also suffer from certain defects in function leading to increased susceptibility to infection. The most severe abnormalities of host defences occur, as would be expected, when there is a defect in the functioning of C3. Severe deficiency or absence of C3 is associated with increased susceptibility to infection, particularly septicaemia, pneumonia, meningitis, otitis and pharyngitis.

## Defective acquired immune defence mechanisms

### Primary immunodeficiencies

Primary deficiencies in immunological function can arise through failure of any of the developmental processes from stem cell to functional end cell. A complete lack of all leucocytes is seen in *reticular dysgenesis* due to a defect in the development of bone marrow stem cells in the fetus. A baby born with this defect usually dies within the first year of life from recurrent, intractable infections. Defects in the development of the common lymphoid stem cell give rise to severe

combined immunodeficiency. Both T and B lymphocytes fail to develop, but functional phagocytes are present.

There are several types of B cell defect that give rise to hypogammaglobulinaemias, that is, low levels of γ-globulins (antibodies) in the blood. Deficiency of immunoglobulin synthesis is almost complete in X-linked infantile hypogammaglobulinaemia (*Bruton's disease*). Male infants suffer from severe, chronic, bacterial infections once maternal antibody has disappeared. There is an absence, or deficiency, of all five classes of serum immunoglobulin. Therefore, the defect is thought to be caused by the absence of B cell precursors or their arrest at a pre-B cell stage. Cell-mediated immune mechanisms function normally and the patients seem to be able to handle viral infections relatively well.

Partial defects in immunoglobulin synthesis have been described affecting one or more of the immunoglobulin classes. In the *Wiskott–Aldrich syndrome*, which is inherited as an X-linked recessive character, there are low levels of IgM but IgA and IgE levels are raised. Patients are susceptible to pyogenic infections, along with recurrent bleeding and eczema. The bleeding is due to reduced platelet production (thrombocytopenia), and the allergy-related eczema is linked to the increased IgE levels. In patients with *dysgammaglobulinaemia* there is a deficiency in only one antibody class. Some patients have reduced levels of IgA whereas the other isotypes are normal. These patients have an increased incidence of infections in the upper and lower respiratory tracts, where IgA is normally protective.

Individuals with T cell defects tend to have more severe and persistent infections than those with antibody deficiencies. A lack of T lymphocytes is often associated with abnormal antibody levels, as $T_H$ cells are involved in the generation and control of humoral immunity. Patients with T cell defects suffer from viral, intracellular bacterial, fungal and protozoan infections rather than acute bacterial infections. In the *DiGeorge syndrome* (congenital thymic aplasia) the person is born with little or no thymus. Individuals who survive develop recurrent and chronic infections, including pneumonia, diarrhoea and yeast infections, once passive maternal immunity has waned.

### Secondary immunodeficiencies

Acquired deficiencies can occur secondarily to a number of disease states or after exposure to drugs and chemicals.

Deficiency of immunoglobulins can be brought about by excessive loss of protein through diseased kidneys or via the intestine in protein-losing enteropathy. Malnutrition and iron deficiency can lead to depressed immune responsiveness, particularly in cell-mediated immunity. Medical and surgical treatments such as irradiation, cytotoxic drugs and steroids often have undesirable effects on the immune system. Viral infections are often immunosuppressive. For example, measles, human immunodeficiency and other viruses infect cells of the immune system.

In contrast to the deficiency states just described, raised immunoglobulin levels are found in certain disorders of plasma cells due to malignant proliferation of a particular clone or group of plasma cells. In these conditions, such as chronic lymphocytic leukaemia and multiple myeloma, malignant clones each produce one particular type of antibody. There is usually a decreased synthesis of normal immunoglobulins and an associated deficiency in the immune response to acute bacterial infections. These B lymphoproliferative disorders contrast with the situation in *Hodgkin's disease*, a reticular cell neoplasm in which the patients show defective cell-mediated immunity and are susceptible to viruses and intracellular bacteria.

## HYPERSENSITIVITY

Immunity was first recognized as a resistant state that followed infection. However, some forms of immune reaction, rather than providing exemption or safety, can produce severe and occasionally fatal results. These are known as *hypersensitivity reactions* and result from an excessive or inappropriate response to an antigenic stimulus. The mechanisms underlying these deleterious reactions are those that normally eradicate foreign material, but for various reasons the response leads to a disease state. When considering each of the four hypersensitivity states it is important to remember this fact and consider the underlying defence mechanism and how it has given rise to the observed immunopathology.

Various classifications of hypersensitivity reactions have been proposed; probably the most widely accepted is that of Coombs and Gell. This recognizes four types of hypersensitivity that are considered in turn.

### Type I: anaphylactic

If a guinea-pig is injected with a small dose of an antigen such as egg albumin, no adverse effects are noted. If a second injection of the same antigen is given intravenously after an interval of about 2 weeks, a condition known as *anaphylactic shock* is likely to develop. The animal becomes restless, starts chewing and rubbing its nose, begins to wheeze, and may develop convulsions and die. The initial injection of antigen is termed the sensitizing dose, whereas the second injection causes anaphylactic shock. Such a reaction is seen in human beings after a bee sting or injection of penicillin in sensitized individuals. Localized reactions are seen in patients with hay fever and asthma. In all of these situations the host responds to the first injection by producing IgE, and it is the level of IgE produced to a particular antigen that determines whether an anaphylactic reaction will occur on re-exposure to the same antigen. Asthma results from a similar response in the respiratory tract.

The biologically active molecules that are responsible for the manifestations of type I hypersensitivity are stored within mast cell and basophil granules or are synthesized after cell triggering. The signal for the release or production of these molecules is the cross-linking of surface-bound IgE by antigen. The release of these molecules, vasoactive amines and chemotactic factors, is responsible for the symptoms of type I hypersensitivity. IgE has been implicated in the control of parasitic worms; the importance of this is discussed in Chapter 11.

### Type II: cytotoxic

Type II reactions are initiated by the binding of an antibody to an antigenic component on a cell surface. The antibody is directed against an epitope, which can be a self molecule or a drug or microbial product passively adsorbed on to a cell surface. The cell that is covered with antibody is then destroyed by the immune system. A variety of infectious diseases caused by salmonellae and mycobacteria are associated with haemolytic anaemia. There is evidence, particularly in studies of salmonella infection, that the haemolysis is due to an immune reaction against bacterial endotoxin that becomes coated on to the erythrocytes of the patient.

## Type III: immune complex

As discussed above, when a soluble antigen combines with antibody the size and physical form of the immune complex formed depends on the relative proportions of the participating molecules and is affected by the class of antibody. Monocytes and macrophages are very efficient at binding and removing large complexes. These same cell types can also eliminate the smaller complexes made in antibody excess, but are relatively inefficient at removing those formed in antigen excess. Type III hypersensitivity reactions appear when there is a defect in the systems involving phagocytes and complement that remove immune complexes, or when the system is overloaded and the complexes are deposited in tissues. This latter situation occurs when antigens are never completely eliminated, as with persistent infection with an organism, autoimmunity and repeated contact with environmental factors.

The tissue damage that results from the deposition of immune complexes is caused by the activation of complement, platelets and phagocytes – in essence, an acute inflammatory response. In general, the degree and site of damage depend on the ratio of antigen to antibody. At equivalence or slight excess of either component, the complexes precipitate at the site of antigen injection or production and a mild, local type III hypersensitivity reaction occurs (e.g. the *Arthus reaction*). In contrast, the complexes formed in large antigen excess become soluble and circulate, causing more serious systemic reactions (e.g. *serum sickness*), or eventually deposit in organs, such as skin, kidneys and joints. The type of disease and its time course depends on the immune status of the individual.

The local release of antigens from an infectious organism can cause a type III reaction. A number of parasitic worms, although undesirable, cause little or no damage. However, if the worm is killed it can become lodged in the lymphatics, and the inflammatory response initiated by antigen–antibody complexes causes a blockage of lymph flow. This leads to the condition of elephantiasis in which enormous swellings can occur. In some cases of tuberculosis,

sarcoidosis, leprosy and streptococcal infections, vascular inflammatory lesions are seen mainly in the legs. These are variously referred to as *erythema nodosum, nodular vasculitis* and *erythema induratum*, and may be due to the deposition of immune complexes and the development of an Arthus reaction.

In systemic disease the clinical manifestations depend on where the immune complexes form or lodge – skin, joints, kidney and heart being particularly affected.

Drugs such as penicillin and sulphonamides can cause type III reactions. The most susceptible patients develop rashes (urticarial, morbilliform or scarlatiniform), pyrexia, arthralgia, lymphadenopathy and perhaps nephritis some 8–12 days after being given the drug. It is likely that similar events occur in many bacterial and viral infections (see Chs 12 and 10, respectively).

## Type IV: cell-mediated or delayed

This form of hypersensitivity can be defined as a specifically provoked, slowly evolving (24–48 h), mixed cellular reaction involving lymphocytes and macrophages. The reaction is not brought about by circulating antibody but by sensitized lymphoid cells. This type of response is seen in a number of allergic reactions to bacteria, viruses and fungi, in contact dermatitis and in graft rejection. The classical example of this type of reaction is the tuberculin response that is seen following an intradermal injection of a purified protein derivative (see p. 216) from tubercle bacilli in immune individuals. An indurated inflammatory reaction in the skin appears about 24 h later and persists for a few weeks. In humans the injection site is infiltrated with large numbers of mononuclear cells, mainly lymphocytes, with about 10–20% macrophages. Most of these cells are in or around small blood vessels. The type IV hypersensitivity state arises when an inappropriate or exaggerated cell-mediated response occurs.

Cell-mediated hypersensitivity reactions are seen in a number of chronic infectious diseases caused by myco-bacteria, protozoa and fungi. Because the host is unable to eliminate the micro-organism, the antigens persist and give rise to a chronic antigenic stimulus. Thus, continual release of lymphokines from sensitized T cells results in the accumulation of large numbers of activated macrophages that can become epithelioid cells. These cells can fuse together to form giant cells. Macrophages express antigen fragments on their surface in association with MHC class I and II molecules, and are therefore the targets of $T_C$ cells and stimulate more lymphokine production. This whole process leads to tissue damage with the formation of a *chronic granuloma* and resultant cell death.

Penicillin sensitization is a common clinical complication following topical application of the antibiotic in ointments or creams. This and other substances that cause contact sensitivity are not themselves antigenic and become so only in combination with proteins in the skin. The Langerhans cells of the epidermis are efficient antigen-presenting cells favouring the development of a T cell response. These cells pick up the newly formed antigen in the skin and transport it to the draining lymph node where a T cell response is stimulated. Here, the specific T cells are stimulated to mature, and then return to the site of entry of the offending material and release their lymphokines. In a normal situation these would help to eliminate a pathogen, but in this case the continual or subsequent exposure to the foreign material leads to an inappropriate response. The reaction site is characterized by a mononuclear cell infiltrate peaking at 48 h. The clinical symptoms in these contact dermatitis lesions include redness, swelling, vesicles, scaling and exudation of fluid (i.e. eczema).

## AUTOIMMUNITY

A fundamental characteristic of the immune system of an animal is that it does not, under normal circumstances, react against its own body constituents. Mechanisms, as we have seen, exist that allow the immune system to tolerate self and destroy non-self. Occasionally these mechanisms break down and autoantibodies are produced.

Genetic factors appear to play a role in the development of autoimmune diseases and there is a strong association between several autoimmune diseases and particular HLA (human leucocyte group A)

specificities, suggesting that immune response gene effects may be involved.

There are a number of examples where potential auto-antigenic determinants are present in exogenous material. These preparations may provide a new carrier, a T cell-stimulating determinant that provokes autoantibody formation. The encephalitis sometimes seen after rabies vaccination with the older vaccines is thought to result from a response directed against the brain that is stimulated by heterologous brain tissues present in the vaccine.

Micro-organisms are a source of cross-reacting anti-gens, sharing antigenic determinants with tissue components. This may be an important way of inducing autoimmunity. The group A streptococcus, which is closely associated with rheumatic fever, shares an antigen with the human heart. Heart lesions are a common finding in rheumatic fever, and anti-heart antibody is found in just over 50% of patients with this condition. Nephritogenic strains of type 12 group A streptococci carry surface antigens similar to those found in human glomeruli, and infection with these organisms has been associated with the development of acute nephritis. Some of the immunopathology seen in Chagas' disease has been attributed to a cross-reaction between *Trypanosoma cruzi* and cardiac muscle.

Autoimmunity can be induced by bypassing T cells. Self-reactive cells can be stimulated by polyclonal activators that directly activate B cells. A number of micro-organisms or their products are potent polyclonal activators; however, the response that is generated tends to be IgM and to wane when the pathogen is eliminated. Bacterial endotoxin, the lipopolysaccharide of Gram-negative bacteria, provides a non-specific inductive signal to B cells, bypassing the need for T cell help. A variety of antibodies are present in infectious mononucleosis, including autoantibodies, as a result of the polyclonal activation of B cells by Epstein–Barr virus.

RECOMMENDED READING

Abbas AK, Janeway CA: Immunology: improving on nature in the twenty-first century, *Cell* 100:129–138, 2000.
Abbas AK, Lichtman AH, Pillai S: *Cellular and Molecular Immunology*, ed 6, Philadelphia, 2007, Saunders.
Murphy K, Travers P, Walport M: *Janeway's Immunobiology*, ed 6, London, 2008, Garland Science.
Staros EB: Innate immunity: new approaches to understanding its clinical significance, *American Journal of Clinical Pathology* 123:305–312, 2005.

### Websites

CELLS alive! http://www.cellsalive.com/
Cytokines & Cells Online Pathfinder Encyclopaedia (COPE). http://www.copewithcytokines.de/
Microbiology and Immunology On-line. University of South Carolina School of Medicine. http://pathmicro.med.sc.edu/book/immunol-sta.htm

# 10 Immunity in viral infections

*J. Stewart*

## KEY POINTS

- *Interferons* provide a key innate defence to viral infection. Their overall effect is to inhibit viral replication.
- Antibodies act on extracellular virus to prevent establishment of infection. In view of their intracellular replication, viruses are particularly targeted by cell-mediated immunity.
- Many of the symptoms and signs of virus infection reflect immune responses to viral antigens (immunopathology) rather than direct damage due to viral replication.
- Many viral infections induce a temporary immune suppression rendering the host susceptible to bacterial infection, whereas others such as HIV produce a more permanent effect.
- There are many vaccines that protect against viral infections. Smallpox has been eradicated by vaccination and other eradications are feasible.

The host response to an invading virus depends on the characteristics of the infectious agent and where it is encountered. In many cases viral infections are sub-clinical, that is, symptomless. A vast array of host defence mechanisms work in a concerted way to protect the individual from viruses and to eliminate them if an infection occurs. In several instances, virus-induced immune responses may have immunopathological consequences.

## THE RESPONSE TO VIRAL INFECTIONS

### Interferons

At the time of the discovery of interferon in 1957, the term was used to identify a factor produced by cells in response to viral infection that protected other cells of the same species from attack by a wide range of viruses. It is now clear that this activity is mediated by members of a family of regulatory proteins.

In man, as in a number of other species, there are three main interferons:

1. α-Interferon (IFN-α), produced mainly by peripheral blood mononuclear cells
2. β-Interferon (IFN-β), produced predominantly by fibroblasts
3. γ-Interferon (IFN-γ), a lymphokine produced in response to a specific antigenic signal.

IFN-α and IFN-β are known as type 1 interferons and are considered part of the innate defences whereas IFN-γ is referred to as type 2 interferon.

There is only one gene for IFN-β and one for IFN-γ, but there are at least 18 different IFN-α genes coding for 14 functional proteins. All the IFN-α genes are closely related and clustered on chromosome 9, close to the IFN-β gene; the IFN-γ gene is on chromosome 12. The production of interferons is under strict inductional control. IFN-α and IFN-β are produced in response to the presence of viruses and certain intracellular bacteria. Double-stranded RNA may be the important inducer acting through Toll-like receptors (see p. 112) to signal the production of type 1 interferons. IFN-γ, which has an extensive role in the control of immune responses, is produced by antigen-activated T lymphocytes and natural killer (NK) cells (see pp. 127–8).

To exert their biological effects these molecules must interact with cell surface receptors. IFN-α and IFN-β share a common receptor, whereas IFN-γ binds to its own specific receptor. After binding to the cell surface receptors, interferons act by rapidly and transiently inducing or upregulating some cellular genes and downregulating others. The overall effect is to inhibit viral replication and activate host defence mechanisms.

The antiviral activity is mediated by the interferon released from a virus-infected cell binding to a neighbouring cell and inducing the synthesis of

**Fig. 10.1** Proposed mechanisms of a induction of synthesis of interferon (IFN)-α and IFN-β, and b production of resistance to virus infection. 2,5-A, 2′,5′-oligoadenylate; dsRNA, double-stranded ribonucleic acid; eIF, eukaryotic initiation factor; MHC, major histocompatibility complex; mRNA, messenger RNA; NK, natural killer cells.

interferon-stimulated cells as a result of inhibition of ribosome assembly. The 2,5-A synthetase is strongly induced in human cells by all three types of interferon and forms 2′,5′-linked oligonucleotides of adenosine from adenosine triphosphate (ATP). These oligonucleotides activate a latent cellular endonuclease that degrades both messenger and ribosomal RNA, with a resultant inhibition of protein synthesis. The requirement for the presence of dsRNA for the full expression of these responses safeguards uninfected cells from the damaging effects of the enzymes. Apart from these well characterized changes, many other changes occur in cells treated with interferons. Some viral proteins can inhibit the interferon response.

Some effects of interferon are virus-specific. The Mx protein induced in mice by IFN-α/-β is specifically involved in the resistance to influenza virus infection. There is a related protein in human cells, and it is possible that some of the other interferon-induced proteins may confer resistance to specific virus types. Resistance of IFN-γ-treated cells to the parasite *Toxoplasma gondii* is associated with induction of the enzyme indolamine dioxygenase, which catabolizes the essential amino acid tryptophan. However, interferons have effects on host cell growth and differentiation. Interferons, particularly IFN-α and IFN-β, are potent inhibitors of normal and malignant cell growth. A number of clinical trials have shown that IFN-α is active against some human cancers, especially those of haemopoietic origin.

Interferons are able to modify immune responses by:

- altering the expression of cell surface molecules
- altering the production and secretion of cellular proteins
- enhancing or inhibiting effector cell functions.

One of the main ways in which interferons control immune responses is by the induction or enhancement of major histocompatibility complex (MHC)-encoded molecules.

Class I MHC genes are upregulated by all types of interferon, as is the production of β₂-microglobulin. IFN-γ induces and increases the expression of MHC class II antigens. In addition, interferons can induce or enhance the expression of Fc receptors and receptors for a number of cytokines. These activities increase the efficiency of antigen recognition and lead to a more effective immune response.

Interferons have also been implicated in the control of B cell responses. When added in vitro or in vivo they can suppress or enhance primary or secondary antibody responses, depending on the dose and time of addition. The regulatory effects seem to be on the

antiviral proteins (Fig. 10.1). Interferons are extremely potent in this function, acting at femtomolar ($10^{-15}$M) concentrations. They can inhibit many stages of the virus life cycle – attachment and uncoating, early viral transcription, viral translation, protein synthesis and budding. Many new proteins can be detected in cells exposed to interferon, but major roles have been proposed for two enzymes that inhibit protein synthesis: 2′,5′-oligoadenylate synthetase (2,5-A synthetase) and a protein kinase. The activity of both of these enzymes is dependent on double-stranded RNA (dsRNA) provided by viral intermediates in the cell. The protein kinase is responsible for the phosphorylation of histones and the protein synthesis initiation factor eIF2. This leads to the inhibition of protein synthesis within

B cells themselves, on increased antigen presentation and through an effect on regulatory T cells.

A number of immune effector cells act by killing infected target cells. The cytotoxicity of macrophages, neutrophils, T cells and NK cells is enhanced by interferons. IFN-$\gamma$ produced by T lymphocytes is capable of activating macrophages to kill intracellular bacteria. This lymphokine has all the activities of the molecule that used to be known as macrophage-activating factor (MAF). NK cells are able to destroy a range of syngeneic, allogeneic and xenogeneic cells in an MHC-unrestricted fashion (see below). All three types of interferon increase NK cell activity in vitro and in vivo, not only by recruiting pre-NK cells to become actively lytic but also by increasing the spectrum of cells lysed. The mechanisms by which interferons make cells cytotoxic are not clear, but it is of interest that interferons can stimulate the production of cytotoxins such as TNF.

TNF has also been reported to have several antiviral activities similar to those of IFN-$\gamma$, but working through a different pathway. However, if both TNF and IFN-$\gamma$ are added together, a synergistic effect is seen. If TNF is added to cells after viral infection, it can lead to their destruction even though the cells are normally resistant to TNF. This effect is also synergistic with IFN-$\gamma$. Certain viruses have been shown to trigger the release of TNF from mononuclear cells, and it seems likely that this cytokine is an important host response to viral infections.

Certain cell-mediated reactions are also part of the innate defences against viral infection. NK cells recognize a variety of cell surface molecules and changes in the level of expression of MHC class I molecules on the infected cells leads to expression of lytic activity. A number of viruses, especially those causing latent infections, evade immune recognition by interfering with the MHC class I processing pathway. Cells infected with these viruses do not display MHC class I molecules on their surface and are therefore not recognized by cytotoxic T cells. However, the infected cells are recognized by NK cells. The formation of a close conjugate between the NK cell and the target induces the effector cell to produce molecules that lead to the death of the infected cell by apoptosis. Antibodies that recognize NK cells have been used to deplete these cells in mice. It was found that the treated mice were more susceptible to murine cytomegalovirus than were normal mice. Natural killing may form a first-line defence against viral attack, most importantly by herpesviruses, before the acquired immune response is generated. Natural killing is increased by interferons (both the number of effector cells and their killing potential) and, therefore, these two innate defence mechanisms appear to work together to protect the host from viral infection.

The interferon response is rapid and helps to protect the host until acquired responses develop. Interferons induce a febrile response and this may also be important in inhibiting viral growth in some infections with viruses that have a low ceiling temperature for growth.

## Acquired immunity

The response to viral antigens is almost entirely T cell dependent. Immunodeficiencies involving T cells are always characterized by markedly enhanced susceptibility to viral infections. However, this tells us little about the effector mechanisms involved, as T cells are required for both antibody production and cytotoxic reactions.

The viral epitopes to which the immune system responds have been studied to give an insight into the mechanisms involved in the host response to these pathogens and also to aid in the development of better vaccines. The recognition of viral antigens is similar to that for all foreign material. B cells and immunoglobulin are able to combine with exposed epitopes, and processed viral fragments presented in the context of MHC molecules are recognized by T cells.

Antigen-specific B cells can act as antigen-presenting cells and thereby generate an immune response. B cells present antigen to T cells and in return are stimulated by growth and differentiation molecules. Intramolecular help may explain hapten–carrier effects. The uptake of an intact virion means that the B cell is able to present peptides derived from internal proteins to T cells (Fig. 10.2). Thus, a B cell that is specific for a surface antigen can receive help from a T cell specific for another molecule as long as it is present within the same particle – intrastructural help.

In most cases, exogenous virus proteins (i.e. those derived from an extracellular virus and taken into a cell) are presented in the context of MHC class II molecules and stimulate $T_H$ cells. Cells that are supporting viral replication express virus-derived peptides in association with MHC class I molecules (the endogenous pathway). The fact that some endogenously produced viral proteins are presented in the context of MHC class II molecules suggests that there can be some overlap between the MHC class I and class II pathways.

### Humoral immunity

There are several ways in which antibody against viral components can protect the host. Antibodies cannot enter cells, and therefore are ineffective against latent viruses and those that spread directly from cell to cell.

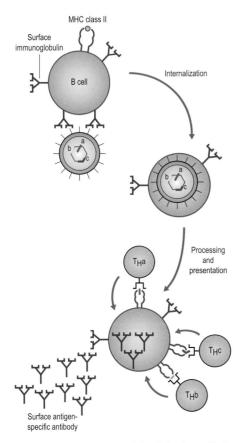

**Fig. 10.2** Intrastructural T cell help. A B cell that is specific for a surface component of a virus binds the virus through its receptor, surface immunoglobulin. The virus contains three potential T cell epitopes (a, b and c) within its nucleocapsid. The entire virus can be internalized, and all viral polypeptides will be processed and fragments re-expressed in association with MHC class II molecules (presentation) on the B cell surface.

They do, however, bind to extracellular viral epitopes. These epitopes can be on intact virions or on the surface of infected cells. The binding of antibody to free virus can inhibit a number of processes essential to virus replication. Antibodies can block binding to the host cell membrane, and thus stop attachment and penetration. The immunoglobulins IgG and IgM have this important function in serum and body fluids, and IgA can neutralize viruses by a similar mechanism on mucosal surfaces. Antibody can also work at stages after penetration. Uncoating, with its release of viral nucleic acid into the cytoplasm, can be inhibited if the virion is covered by antibody.

Antibody can also cause aggregation of virus particles, thus limiting the spread of the infectious particles and forming a complex that is readily phagocytosed. Complement can aid in the neutralization process by opsonizing the virus or directly lysing enveloped

viruses. In certain cases complement alone can inactivate viruses. Some retroviruses have a protein that can act as a receptor for C1q, and other viruses have been reported to activate the alternative pathway. In some infections, viral proteins remain on the surface of the cell after entry or become associated with the cell membrane during replication. Antibodies against these molecules can cause cell lysis by the classical pathway, but an intact alternative pathway is necessary to amplify the initial triggering by the antibody-dependent pathway. In certain situations antibody-mediated reactions are not always of benefit (see below). Antibodies are also capable of modulating or stripping viral antigens from the cell surface, allowing the infected cell to avoid destruction by other effector mechanisms.

Viral infections, particularly those caused by entero-viruses, are frequent and severe when humoral immunity is impaired, as in certain inherited immunodeficiency states. In Bruton-type deficiencies, poliomyelitis may develop after vaccination with the live virus vaccine; meningo-encephalitis, caused by echovirus and coxsackie-virus, may also be seen. In many situations, viruses seem able to escape the humoral defence mechanisms. Some viruses become latent (e.g. herpesviruses) and are reactivated despite the presence of circulating antibody, as they can pass directly from cell to cell. Other escape mechanisms include antigenic variation in which the antigenic structure of the virus (e.g. influenza type A) changes so that antibodies formed to the previous strain are no longer effective.

In viral infections the efficiency of antibody depends largely on whether the virus passes through the bloodstream outside host cells to reach its target organ. Poliovirus crosses the intestinal wall, enters the bloodstream to cause a cell-free viraemia, and passes to the spinal cord and brain where it replicates. Small amounts of antibody in the blood can neutralize the virus before it reaches its target cells in the nervous system.

In comparison, in viral diseases such as influenza and the common cold the viruses do not pass through the bloodstream. These infections have a short incubation period, their target organ being at the site of entry into the body, namely the respiratory mucous membranes. In this type of infection a high level of antibody in the blood is relatively ineffective in comparison with its effect on blood-borne viruses. In this case the antibody must be present in the mucous secretions at the time of infection. There are very low levels of IgG or IgM in secretions, but IgA has been shown to be responsible for most of the neutralizing activity present in nasal secretions against rhinoviruses and other respiratory tract viruses.

One consequence of this is that conventional immunization methods using killed virus or viral subunits, which produce high levels of circulating antibody, are unlikely to be effective against viruses that attack the mucous membranes. Some considerable effort is being directed at developing methods for stimulating local production of IgA in the mucous membranes themselves. Live virus vaccines are effective in this respect, and the intranasal administration of a live-attenuated influenza virus vaccine is an attempt to overcome this problem. The high degree of immunity provided by the oral polio vaccine is due in part to locally produced antibody in the gut neutralizing the virus before it attaches to cell receptors to cause infection. The presence of IgA against polio has been demonstrated in faeces, duodenal fluid and saliva. There is evidence to suggest that parenteral administration of a killed virus may give rise to a secretory IgA response if the individual has previously been exposed to the virus or has received an oral-attenuated vaccine. So there appears to be a link between the systemic immune system and local mucosal immunity.

Humoral immunity does play a major protective role in polio and a number of other viral infections, and is probably the predominant form of immunity responsible for protection from reinfection. Passively administered antibody can protect against several human infections, including measles, hepatitis A and B, and chickenpox, if given before or very soon after exposure. Immunity to many viral infections is lifelong. This may occur because antibodies are boosted by occasional re-exposure to the virus.

### Cell-mediated immunity

The destruction of virus-infected cells is an important mechanism in the eradication of virus from the host. Antibody can neutralize free virions, but once these agents have entered the cell other strategies are employed. The destruction of an infected cell before progeny particles are released is an effective way of terminating a viral infection. For this process to occur the immune system must recognize the infected cell, and various types of effector cell have evolved to mediate these processes.

As viral proteins are synthesized within the cell some of these molecules are processed into small peptides. These endogenously produced antigen fragments become associated with MHC class I molecules, and this complex is then transported to the cell surface where it acts as the recognition unit for cytotoxic T ($T_C$) lymphocytes. Most $T_C$ cells have a receptor that binds to fragments of the virus sitting in the cleft of an MHC class I molecule. This T cell also

has the CD8 molecule on its surface. Some $T_C$ cells are restricted in their recognition of antigen by MHC class II molecules and therefore have the CD4 molecule. Once these $T_C$ cells have bound to the infected cell they release molecules that induce apoptosis.

Many viruses, such as poliovirus and papillomavirus, replicate and produce fully infectious particles inside the cell. These viruses are liberated from the infected cell as it disintegrates. However, other viruses do not wait for the cell to die but are released by a process of budding through the cell membrane. During their replication, virus-encoded molecules (viral antigens) are inserted into the host cell membrane, and the nucleocapsid becomes associated with these molecules. The virus particle finally acquires an envelope as it is released. Such viruses include herpesviruses, alphaviruses, flaviviruses, retroviruses, hepadnaviruses, orthomyxoviruses and paramyxoviruses. Viral antigens often appear on the cell surface very early in the replicative cycle, many hours before progeny virus is liberated. In cells infected with herpes simplex virus, as many as five different viral glycoproteins appear on the cell surface. In other virus infections, such as those caused by poxviruses and papovaviruses, the viral particles are not released by budding, but viral antigens appear on the cell surface. These molecules, including those that are not incorporated into the released virion, can therefore act as signals indicating the presence of virus within a cell. If antibody binds to these cell surface viral antigens, the infected cell can be destroyed by antibody-dependent cell-mediated cytotoxicity. The effector cells have an Fc receptor that recognizes the Fc portion of immunoglobulin bound to viral antigens present on the infected cell surface. This interaction brings the two cells close together, and toxic molecules are released on to the target cell membrane, causing cell death.

$CD4^+$ and $CD8^+$ T cells can produce various lymphokines when stimulated by antigen, including molecules that are active in the elimination of virus (e.g. IFN-$\gamma$ and TNF), and others that generally increase the effectiveness of the immune system by attracting cells to the site of infection, stimulating the production of more cells and supporting their growth. Macrophages are activated, leading to enhanced microbicidal activities and the production of monokines.

### Induction of an immune response

The precise nature of the acquired immune reactions that are generated in response to infection depends to a great extent on the site of infection, type of virus, previous exposure to the agent and the genetic make-up of the host. Both humoral and cell-mediated responses are produced to all infections. The importance of genetic factors is illustrated by the severe *X-linked recessive lymphoproliferative syndrome* in which fatal infectious mononucleosis results from the unrestricted replication of Epstein–Barr virus, as affected males have reduced numbers of normal lymphocytes.

The virus or viral components entering the peripheral tissues or being produced there are carried to the draining lymph node either free in the lymph or in cells such as Langerhans' cells. Once in the secondary lymphoid tissues the free virus is taken up by macrophages and processed; viral peptides associate with MHC class II molecules and are transported to the cell surface. Langerhans' cells that enter the lymph node become interdigitating cells and present viral peptides, associated with MHC class II molecules, on their surface. A $T_H$ cell will bind to the peptide–MHC class II complex, expand clonally and produce helper factors. The proportions of the different lymphokines produced determines the type and level of the response generated. B cells will enter the node, and those that bind antigen are stimulated into antibody production. Other T cells will enter the lymph node. If these cells have a receptor that interacts with an antigen fragment–MHC class I complex, they will respond to the growth factors present in the node and proliferate and mature into effector $T_C$ cells. After a time, the products of the immune response leave the node to circulate round the body and localize at the site of infection. As the response progresses the pathogen is eliminated, the tissue repaired and memory cells generated. Finally, when all of the antigen has been eliminated, the immune response is terminated. In some instances virus-induced immune responses may have immunopathological consequences.

## IMMUNOPATHOLOGY

Viruses have evolved a multitude of mechanisms for exploiting weaknesses in the host immune system and avoiding – sometimes actually subverting – immune mechanisms. Some viruses are so successful in avoiding host defences that they persist in the host indefinitely, sometimes in a latent form without producing disease.

One of the most important strategies developed by viruses is to infect cells of the immune system itself. The effect of this is often to disable the normal functioning of the cell type that has been infected. Many common human viruses, including rubella, mumps, measles and herpes viruses, infect cells of the immune system, as does human immunodeficiency virus (HIV).

The consequences of viral infection of cells of the immune system have been categorized in two ways:

1. Infections that cause temporary immune deficiency to unrelated antigens and sometimes to the antigens of the infecting virus. It is known that infection with influenza, rubella, measles and cytomegalovirus predisposes to bacterial and other infections. This is sometimes associated with depressed immunoglobulin synthesis and interference with the antimicrobial functions of phagocytes.
2. Permanent depression of immunity to unrelated antigens and occasionally to antigens of the infecting virus. Acquired immune deficiency syndrome is an example of such a disease, where the patient becomes susceptible to otherwise harmless protozoa, bacteria, viruses and fungi.

Viruses have also developed other mechanisms to avoid the immune system. These include:

- antigenic variation
- release of antigens
- production of antigens at sites that are inaccessible to the immune system.

Viruses that cannot enter and replicate within phagocytic cells will be destroyed if they are engulfed by a neutrophil or macrophage. As neutrophils are short-lived cells they do not usually give rise to progeny virus. On the other hand, monocytes and macrophages are long-lived cells and can be responsible for disseminating a virus throughout the body. Viruses that do replicate within macrophages must escape from the phagosome very rapidly before it fuses with the lysosome. Reovirus infection of macrophages is actually helped by the lysosomal enzymes, which initiate 'uncoating' of the virus and therefore enhance viral replication.

A virus is relatively safe from immune destruction as long as it remains within the cell and allows only very low or no viral antigen expression on the infected cell membrane. This is what happens in latent infections where herpes simplex or varicella-zoster virus is present in the dorsal root ganglion.

Antibody can actually remove viral antigens from cell membranes, as cross-linking of antigens on the cell surface can lead to their internalization by capping. Here the antigens complexed with the antibody are drawn to one pole of the cell and internalized or shed into the surrounding tissue. Capping occurs on brain cells infected with measles virus in subacute sclerosing panencephalitis. Viruses that move from cell to cell without entering the extracellular fluid can also escape the action of antibodies, as can those passed from cell to cell by cell division.

A number of infections continually shed virus into external secretions, such as saliva, milk or urine. As long as the infected cell forms virus only on the luminal surface of the mucosa, cells of the immune system and antibody will be unable to destroy the infected cell. IgA present in the secretions may neutralize the virus, but this class of antibody does not activate complement efficiently, so the cell will not be lysed. A similar situation applies to epidermal infections with wart virus. The infected cell is keratinized and about to be released from the surface of the body before any virus or viral antigens are produced. The infected cell is therefore isolated from the host's immune cells.

During the course of an infection various antibodies are formed against different epitopes on a virus. These antibodies are of differing affinities and also stimulate different effector functions. Antibodies against some of the epitopes will neutralize the virus, but other antibodies will be against unimportant epitopes or be of an ineffective isotype that may fail to neutralize the virus, and may actually aid in its infectivity by allowing uptake of virus–antibody complexes via Fc receptors or cause tissue damage through immune complex disease. Soluble antigens liberated from infected cells may 'mop up' free antibody so that it can no longer interact and destroy extracellular virus. Whether the small particles present in the serum of patients and carriers with hepatitis B virus infections function in this way is not known, although patients in the prodromal phase may suffer from rash, myalgia and arthralgia. Polyarteritis nodosa and glomerulonephritis can also occur, all suggestive of immune complex formation.

Susceptibility to infection is generally greater in the very young and very old because of a weaker immune response. However, the immunopathology tends to be less severe. In the very young, infections can spread rapidly and prove fatal without the clinical and pathological changes seen in adults. Latent infections are kept under control by the immune system, and in older people the infections show an increased incidence of activation (e.g. zoster, or shingles). Immunological immaturity makes the neonate highly susceptible to many viral infections. Maternally derived antibody provides passive protection for 3–6 months, after which time the infant is at risk of infection; respiratory and alimentary tract infections are frequent.

Physical and physiological differences may also contribute to age-related disease susceptibility. Respiratory infections in old age are probably a bigger problem than in young adults because of weaker respiratory muscles and a poorer cough reflex. In the young the airways are narrower and more easily blocked by secretions and exudate. Infants, because of their low body-weight, show signs of distress from loss of fluid and electrolytes, so that fever, vomiting and diarrhoea tend to be very serious at this time of life. Often the reasons for the differences between infants and adults are not known. Respiratory syncytial virus causes severe illness in the early months of life with croup, bronchiolitis and bronchopneumonia, despite the presence of maternal IgG. In adults the virus usually causes a mild upper respiratory tract infection.

Certain viral infections produce a milder disease in children than in adults (e.g. varicella, mumps, poliomyelitis and Epstein–Barr virus infections). Varicella often causes pneumonia in adults, and mumps may involve the testes and ovaries after puberty, giving rise to orchitis and oophoritis. Epstein–Barr virus is excreted in saliva, and in developing countries most individuals are infected early in life, usually asymptomatically. In developed countries where childhood infection is less common, first infection may be delayed to adolescence or early adulthood, when salivary exposure occurs during kissing. In this age group, Epstein–Barr virus infection gives rise to glandular fever. It is not clear why these infections are more severe in adults, but it may be linked to the more powerful immune defences giving rise to immunopathological sequelae in adults.

There are also age-related differences in the incidence of infections. It is not surprising that most infections are most common in childhood when the individual is exposed to the micro-organisms for the first time.

## Antigenic variation

A micro-organism can avoid the acquired immune response by periodically changing the structure of molecules that are recognized by the host immune system. The immune system selects the variants by not being able to mount an immune response against them before they are shed. The micro-organism will only be able to change a component in a way that does not alter the functioning of the molecule. The molecules involved can be active enzymes, recognition molecules or structural proteins. HIV shows considerable variation in parts of the envelope glycoprotein within a given individual.

The significance of antigenic variation is well illustrated by influenza viruses. Here changes in the surface glycoproteins are linked to the occurrence of epidemics of infection (see Ch. 49).

With influenza virus the infection is localized to the respiratory tract where the principal protection against reinfection is secretory IgA. The virus-specific IgA still present at the mucosal surface a few years after infection can protect against the original infecting virus but may be insufficient to deal with an antigenic variant despite antigenic overlap. Thus, in effect, IgA levels become a selective pressure, which will allow infection by the mutant, and antigenic drift occurs. The very short incubation period (1–3 days) is more rapid than the secondary antibody response so that the IgA levels cannot be boosted in time to abort infection.

Antigenic variation is likely to be an important viral adaptation for overcoming host immunity in long-lived species such as humans where there is a need for multiple reinfection of the same individual if the virus is to survive and the virus is unable to become latent. In shorter-lived animals such as mice and rabbits a susceptible population appears quickly enough to maintain the infectious cycle.

## Persistence of virus

Certain viruses give rise to a persistent infection, which is held in check as long as the immune system remains intact.

Chickenpox is a persistent infection characterized by latency in that there is apparent recovery from the original infection but the virus can reappear later in life when a localized eruption, shingles, results. Other herpesviruses, cytomegalovirus and Epstein–Barr virus also persist after infection. If the carrier's immune system remains intact, there will be no evidence of disease. However, cytomegalovirus causes many problems in immunosuppressed patients. The polyomavirus, JC, usually causes asymptomatic infections, but in the immunosuppressed it has been found in areas of destruction in the central nervous system; the disease is progressive multifocal leucoencephalopathy.

In other persistent infections, the immune system contributes to the pathology of the disease, often over a period of years. Thus, in subacute sclerosing panencephalitis, persistence of measles virus in neurones triggers their destruction by the host's immune system. Similarly, the chronic active hepatitis seen in those carriers of hepatitis B who continue to produce virions appears to be caused by a $T_C$ cell response to viral antigens present in the hepatocyte membrane. In both examples, several years may elapse before symptoms appear.

## VACCINES

Natural infection with a virus is an extremely effective means of giving lifelong immunity from the disease. In most cases, where there is one virus type, this means that second attacks are extremely rare. The memory of the immune system ensures that, for these infections, a secondary response can be generated before the virus has time to cause the disease. The level of immunity needed to protect an individual depends on the incubation period of the virus and its life cycle. For viruses with very short incubation periods, a high level of protective immunity must be present before exposure to the infective agent. In the case of a virus with a long incubation period (10–20 days), the immune system has time to generate a protective response.

It is also important to consider the type of immune response that will be protective against different viruses. If antibody gives protection then steps must be taken to ensure that the material to be used for immunization contains the correct epitopes. A denatured antigen will not generate antibodies that can combine with the native virus. Sometimes the chemical treatment of the antigen may destroy important components. Thus the original killed measles virus vaccine did not contain the fusion protein. As a result, vaccinees suffered enhanced disease when exposed to the virus as viral replication and spread could occur in the presence of antibody to the other viral proteins. If T cell immunity is important, the vaccine must be in a form that will give rise to peptides in the correct compartment of the cell to produce antigen fragments in association with MHC-encoded products. It will have to associate with the MHC class II molecules to generate help and with MHC class I molecules to stimulate effector cell formation. For antibody production, T cell help is also required. Therefore, for an antibody response, a killed vaccine may be sufficient but, when T cell immunity is required, a live-attenuated vaccine is needed.

Vaccination has been responsible for the elimination of smallpox and for reducing the incidence of other viral diseases. It should be possible to control many viral diseases, but with some the problem is more difficult. New technologies and a better understanding of the immune system are helping with this task.

---

RECOMMENDED READING

---

Mims C, Nash A, Stephen J: *Mims' Pathogenesis of Infectious Disease*, ed 5, London, 2001, Academic Press.

### Website

All the virology on the www. http://www.virology.net/ garryfavwebindex.html

# 11 Parasitic infections: Pathogenesis and immunity

*J. Stewart*

## KEY POINTS

- Parasites cause disease by diverse mechanisms including mechanical damage, physiological disturbance, tissue destruction and immunopathology.
- Some parasitic worm infestations are associated with raised levels of IgE and eosinophilia. These responses may provide some protection.
- Some parasites may evade immune responses by seclusion away from the immune system, by antigenic variation, by acquiring host-derived molecules or by immunosuppression.
- Despite major efforts, particularly those directed towards malaria, there are no available effective vaccines against parasitic infections.

By convention the term 'parasitic diseases' refers to those caused by protozoa, worms (helminths) and arthropods (insects and arachnids). Such parasites affect many hundreds of millions of people in tropical parts of the world and are responsible for many severe and debilitating diseases (see Chs 62–64).

These infections are associated with a broad spectrum of effects. Some are due to the parasites themselves and others are a consequence of the host response to the invader. The nature and extent of the pathological effects are dependent upon the site and mode of infection, and also on the level of the parasite burden.

The development of protective immunity to such parasites is more complicated than that to bacteria and viruses because of the complicated life cycles of the parasites involved.

## PATHOGENIC MECHANISMS

As with other infectious agents, the site occupied by a parasite is important. A host will survive with a large number of lung flukes (*Paragonimus* spp.) in the lungs but infection in the brain may cause far more serious effects. The severity of disease depends not only on the degree of infection but also on the physiological state of the host. A lowering of general health, due to malnutrition for example, predisposes to more serious consequences following infection by parasites.

### Mechanical tissue damage

Physical obstruction of anatomical sites leading to loss of function can be a major component of the diseases caused by parasites. The intestinal lumen can be blocked by worms such as *Ascaris lumbricoides* or tapeworms, and filarial parasites (*Wuchereria bancrofti* and *Brugia malayi*) can obstruct the flow of lymph through lymphatics.

Intestinal infection with the tapeworm *Taenia solium* is usually of little consequence, but the eggs may develop into larvae (cysticerci) in humans, causing cysticercosis. The cysticerci can be found in muscle, liver, eye or, most dangerously, the brain. Hydatid cysts, the larval stage of the dog tapeworm (*Echinococcus granulosus*) in man, may reach volumes of 1–2 L, and such masses can cause severe damage to an infected organ.

### Physiological effects

Large numbers of *Giardia* spp. covering the walls of the small intestine can lead to malabsorption, especially of fats. Competition by parasites for essential nutrients leads to host deprivation. Thus depletion of vitamin $B_{12}$ by the tapeworm *Diphyllobothrium latum* sometimes leads to pernicious anaemia. Other forms of anaemia result from blood loss, especially in hookworm infection, and from red blood cell destruction in malaria.

Some parasites produce metabolites that may have profound effects on the host. *Trypanosoma cruzi* secretes a neurotoxin that affects the autonomic nervous system. Malaria parasites are thought to produce a metabolite with vasoconstrictor activity.

## Tissue damage

The presence of parasites can result in the release of proteolytic enzymes that damage host tissues. Ulceration of the intestinal wall occurs in amoebic dysentery, and trophozoites (the active, motile forms of a protozoan parasite) can penetrate deep into the wall of the intestine to reach the blood and hence the liver, lungs and brain where secondary amoebic abscesses may occur. The skin damage caused by skin-penetrating helminths, such as *Strongyloides stercoralis* and hookworms, can also permit entry of other infectious agents.

The host reaction to parasites and their products can evoke immunological reactions that may lead to secondary damage to host tissues. This is seen in schistosomiasis, where the host response to parasite eggs in tissues leads to the formation of a granuloma with subsequent tissue destruction through fibrosis. Other types of hypersensitivity reaction can be generated in various parasitic infections (see below).

## IMMUNE DEFENCE MECHANISMS

The large size of parasites means that they display more antigens than bacteria or viruses to the immune system. When the parasite has a complicated life cycle, some of these antigens may be specific to a particular stage of development. Parasites have evolved to be closely adapted to the host, and most parasitic infections are chronic and show a degree of host specificity. For example, the malaria parasites of man, birds and rodents are confined to their own particular species. An exception to this is *Trichinella spiralis*, which is able to infect many animal species.

In the natural host there is no single defence mechanism that acts in isolation against a particular parasite. In turn the parasite will have evolved a number of strategies to evade elimination. In general terms, cell-mediated immune mechanisms are more effective against intracellular protozoa, whereas antibody, with the aid of certain effector cells, is involved in the destruction of extracellular targets. Again, because of the life cycles of some parasites, either cell-mediated

or humoral immunity may be of greater importance at different states of their development.

## Innate defences

Several of the innate or natural defence mechanisms that are active against bacteria and viruses are also effective against parasitic infections. The physical barrier of the skin protects against many parasites but is ineffective against those transmitted by a blood-feeding insect. In addition, other parasites, such as schistosomes, have evolved active mechanisms for penetrating intact skin. Certain individuals are genetically less susceptible to certain parasites. Thus, individuals with the sickle cell trait have a genetic defect in their haemoglobin that causes a mechanical distortion in their erythrocytes. This somehow leads to the destruction of intracellular malaria parasites. The Duffy blood group antigen is the attachment site for one of the plasmodium parasites. Individuals who lack this determinant are therefore protected from malaria caused by *Plasmodium vivax*.

Several other non-specific host defence mechanisms are involved in the control of parasitic infections. These include direct cellular responses by monocytes, macrophages and granulocytes, and by natural killer cells. The byproducts of acquired immune reactions enhance the antiparasitic activity of these cells. For example, certain protozoan parasites infect macrophages. In particular, *Leishmania* spp. are obligate parasites of mononuclear phagocytes, and are completely dependent upon macrophages, where they survive in the phagolysosome. The parasite appears to be able to survive within non-stimulated resident macrophages, whereas they are destroyed in activated macrophages.

Complement, through activation by the alternative pathway, is active against a number of parasites, including adult worms and active larvae of *T. spiralis* and schistosomula of *Schistosoma mansoni*. The spleen is thought to be active in the elimination of intracellular parasites, as its filtering of infected erythrocytes is thought to remove intracellular plasmodium.

### Macrophages

Macrophages play an important role in the elimination and control of parasitic protozoa and worms. They secrete monokines, such as interleukin (IL)-1, tumour necrosis factor and colony-stimulating factors that affect not only T cells and antibody production but also granulocytes. However, other monokines, for instance prostaglandins, are immunosuppressive. Macrophages are also phagocytic cells and function as such in the elimination of parasites. In the same way as in the eradication of other infectious agents, opsonins greatly enhance this process. Once internalized, the parasite is killed, by oxygen-dependent and -independent mechanisms, and digested. Many of the molecules produced by macrophages are cytotoxic, and when produced in close proximity to a parasite will kill it. Specific antibody, immunoglobulin (Ig) G and IgE, can mediate the attachment of the macrophage to the surface of parasites that are too large to internalize but are vulnerable to antibody-dependent cell-mediated cytotoxicity. Acting as antigen-presenting cells, they can aid elimination by helping in the initiation of an immune response.

In addition to lymphokines some products of parasites themselves, such as those produced by *Tryp. brucei* and the malaria parasite, can cause macrophage activation. These may be direct effects or result from the production of monokines such as tumour necrosis factor.

In some parasitic infections the immune system is unable to eradicate the offending organism. The body reacts by trying to isolate the parasite within a granuloma. In this situation there is chronic stimulation of those T cells specific for antigens on the parasite. The continual release of lymphokines leads to macrophage accumulation, release of fibrogenic factors, stimulation of granuloma formation and, ultimately, fibrosis. Granuloma formation around schistosome eggs can occur in the liver, and this response is thought to benefit the host by isolating host cells from the toxic substances produced by the eggs. It can, however, lead to pathological consequences if the damage to the liver leads to loss of liver function.

## Granulocytes

Neutrophils and eosinophils are thought to play a role in the elimination of protozoa and worms. The smaller parasites can be phagocytosed and destroyed by both oxygen-dependent and -independent processes. The phagocytic capacity of neutrophils is superior to that of eosinophils. Both cell types possess receptors for the Fc portion of immunoglobulin and for various complement components, so the presence of opsonins increases phagocytosis. Extracellular destruction of large parasites can occur by antibody-dependent cell-mediated cytotoxicity.

Neutrophils are attracted to sites of inflammation and will clear the offending parasite. They have been reported to be more effective than eosinophils at eliminating several species of nematode, including *T. spiralis*, although the relative importance of the two cell types may depend on the class of antibody present.

Eosinophilia and high levels of IgE are characteristics of many parasitic worm infections. It has been suggested that eosinophils are especially active against helminths, and IgE-dependent degranulation of mast cells has evolved to attract these cells to the site where the parasite is localized. The eosinophilia is T cell dependent and the lymphokines that induce production of the cells also cause an increase in their activation state. These effector cells are attracted to the site by chemotactic factors produced by mast cells (see below). Once at the site they degranulate in response to perturbation of their cell membrane induced by antibodies and complement bound to the surface of the parasite. The toxic molecules are therefore released on to the surface of the target and cause its destruction.

### Mast cells

The mediators stored and produced by mast cells play an important role in eliminating worm infections. Parasite antigens cause the release of mediators from mast cells; these molecules induce a local inflammatory response. Chemotactic factors are produced and attract eosinophils and neutrophils. Thus the IgE-dependent release of mast cell products helps in expulsion of the worm. The number of mucosal mast cells rises during a parasitic worm infestation due to a T cell-dependent process.

### Platelets

Platelet activation results in the release of molecules that are toxic to various parasites, including schistosoma, *Toxoplasma gondii* and *Tryp. cruzi*. The release process does not require antibody, although IgE-dependent cytotoxicity is possible, but seems to involve acute-phase proteins. The cytotoxic potential of platelets is enhanced by various cytokines, including γ-interferon and tumour necrosis factor.

## Acquired immunity

An individual with a parasitic infection mounts a specific response against the invading parasite. These immune reactions generate antibody and effector T cells directed against specific parasite antigens. Memory B and T cells are also produced. For a number of reasons, described below, much acquired immunity is ineffective in protecting the host against recurrent infection. However, in certain cases, such as amoebiasis and toxoplasmosis, immunity to reinfection is fairly complete. In schistosomiasis, the presence of surviving adult forms protects against further

**Table 11.1**  Humoral defence mechanisms against parasite infections

| Mechanism | Effect | Parasite |
|---|---|---|
| Neutralization | Blocks attachment to host cell | Protozoa |
| | Acts to inhibit evasion mechanisms of intracellular organisms | Protozoa |
| | Binding to toxins or enzymes | Protozoa and worms |
| Physical interference | Obstructs orifices of parasite | Worms |
| | Agglutination | Protozoa |
| Opsonization | Increases clearance by phagocytes | Protozoa |
| Cytotoxicity | Complement-mediated lysis | Protozoa and worms |
| | Antibody-dependent cell-mediated cytotoxicity | Protozoa and worms |

infections. However, this may be an effect of the parasite and not of the host.

## Antibody

The specific immune response to parasites leads to the production of antibody. Infection by protozoan parasites is associated with the production of IgG and IgM. With helminths there is, in addition, the synthesis of substantial amounts of IgE. IgA is produced in response to intestinal protozoa, such as *Entamoeba histolytica* and *Giardia lamblia*.

In addition to these specific T-dependent responses, a non-specific hypergammaglobulinaemia is present in many parasitic infections. Much of this non-specific antibody is the result of polyclonal B cell activation by released parasite antigens acting as mitogens. This response is ineffective at counteracting the parasite and can enhance the pathogenicity by causing the production of autoantibodies, and may actually lead to a diminished specific response due to B cell exhaustion. It has also been reported that some parasite molecules are T cell mitogens. This could lead to the generation of autoreactive T cells or activation of suppressor responses.

There are a number of mechanisms by which specific antibody can provide protection against and control parasitic infections (Table 11.1). As with viral infections, antibody is effective only against extracellular parasites and where parasite antigens are displayed on the surface of infected cells. Antibody can neutralize parasites by combining with various surface molecules, blocking or interfering with their function. The binding of antibody to an attachment site stops the infection of a new host cell. The agglutination of blood parasites by IgM may occur, leading to the prevention of spread, as in the acute phase of infection with *Tryp. cruzi*. Toxins and enzymes produced by certain parasites add to their pathogenicity, and antibodies that inhibit these molecules protect the host from damage and also affect the infection process

directly. Intracellular parasites have evolved a number of mechanisms that allow them to survive in this environment. Antibodies against the molecules that aid the parasite in these activities, for instance to escape from endosomes or inhibit lysosomal fusion, lead to removal of the intruder by the phagocyte. Parasitic worms are multicellular organisms with defined anatomical features that are responsible for functions such as feeding and reproduction. Antibodies that block particular orifices (e.g. oral and genital) interfere with critical physiological functions and may cause starvation or curtail reproduction.

Antibodies can bind to the surface of parasites and cause direct damage, or interact with complement leading to cell lysis. Antibody also acts as an opsonin and hence increases uptake by phagocytic cells. In this context, complement activation leads to enhanced ingestion due to complement receptors. Macrophage activation leads to the expression of increased Fc and complement receptors, so phagocytosis is enhanced in the presence of macrophage-activating factors. Phagocytes play an important role in the control of infections by *Plasmodium* spp. and *Tryp. brucei*.

Antibody-dependent cell-mediated cytotoxicity has been shown to play a part in infections caused by a number of parasites, including *Tryp. cruzi, T. spiralis, S. mansoni* and filarial worms. The effector cells – macrophages, monocytes, neutrophils, eosinophils and natural killer cells – bind to the antibody-coated parasites by their Fc and complement receptors. Close apposition of the effector cell and the target is necessary because the toxic molecules produced are non-specific and may damage host cells. A major basic protein from eosinophils damages the tegument of schistosomes and other worms, causing their death. It appears that different cell types and immunoglobulin isotypes are active against different developmental stages of parasites. Eosinophils are more effective at killing newborn larvae of *T. spiralis* than other cells, whereas macrophages are very effective against microfilariae.

## T cells

The importance of T cells in counteracting protozoan infections has been shown using nude (athymic) or T cell-depleted mice, which have a reduced capacity to control trypanosomal and malarial infections. The transfer of spleen cells, especially T cells, from immune animals gives protection against most parasitic infections. The type of T cell that is effective depends on the parasite. CD4$^+$ T cells transfer protection against *Leishmania major* and *L. tropica*, and may be necessary for the elimination of other parasites. The intracellular parasite of cattle, *Theileria parvum*, is destroyed by cytotoxic T (T$_C$) cells.

CD4$^+$ T cells may act by providing help in antibody production, but they also secrete various lymphokines that interact with other effector cells. CD8$^+$ cells may be cytotoxic in certain situations, but these cells also produce a variety of lymphokines. IL-2 production has been shown to be deficient during parasitic infections, such as malaria and trypanosomiasis. Administration of IL-2 to mice infected with *Tryp. cruzi* reduces parasitaemia and increases survival.

Colony-stimulating factors (e.g. IL-3 and granulocyte–monocyte colony-stimulating factor) are also produced by activated T cells. These molecules act on myeloid progenitors in the bone marrow, causing increased production of neutrophils, eosinophils and monocytes. They also increase the activity of these cells; the monocytosis and splenomegaly in malaria are caused by these T cell-derived molecules. The accumulation of macrophages in the liver as granulomata in schistosomiasis and the eosinophilia that is characteristic of worm infestations are also T cell-dependent phenomena.

In certain cases the production of lymphokines may have adverse effects. *Leishmania* infects macrophages, and the release of molecules that stimulate the production of more host cells may potentiate the infection.

γ-Interferon does not inhibit or kill parasites directly, although multiplication of the liver stages of the malaria parasite is inhibited by γ-interferon, possibly through interaction with its receptor on the surface of hepatocytes. γ-Interferon is a potent macrophage activation factor and is probably involved in the resistance and elimination of intracellular parasites, such as *Toxoplasma gondii* and *Leishmania* spp. Activated macrophages are more effective killers and can destroy intracellular parasites before they establish themselves within the cell.

## EVASION MECHANISMS

All animal pathogens, including parasitic protozoa and worms, have evolved effective mechanisms to avoid elimination by host defence systems (Table 11.2).

## Seclusion

Many parasites inhabit cells or anatomical sites that are inaccessible to host defence mechanisms. Those that attempt to survive within cells avoid the effects of antibody but must possess mechanisms to avoid destruction if the cell involved is capable of destroying them. *Plasmodium* spp. inhabit erythrocytes, whereas toxoplasmas are less selective and infect non-phagocytic cells as well as phagocytes. A number of different ways of avoiding destruction in macrophages have evolved. *Leishmania donovani* amastigotes are able to survive and metabolize in the acidic environment (pH 4–5) found in phagolysosomes, and *Tox. gondii* is able to inhibit the fusion of lysosomes with the parasite-containing phagosome.

*L. major* has a similar escape mechanism by attaching to a phagocyte complement receptor (CR1) that

---

**Table 11.2** Parasite escape mechanisms

| Escape mechansim | Organisms |
|---|---|
| Intracellular habitat | Malaria parasites, trypanosomes and *Leishmania* spp. |
| Encystment | *Toxoplasma gondii* and *Trypanosoma cruzi* |
| Resistance to microbicidal products of phagocytes | *Leishmania donovani* |
| Masking of antigens | Schistosomes |
| Variation of antigen | Trypanosomes and malaria parasites |
| Suppression of immune response | Most parasites (e.g. malaria parasites, *Trichinella spirolis* and *Schistosoma monsoni*) |
| Interference by antigens | Trypanosomes |
| Polyclonal activation | Trypanosomes |
| Sharing of antigens between parasite and host (molecular mimicry) | Schistosomes |
| Continuous turnover and release of surface antigens of parasite | Schistosomes |

does not trigger the respiratory burst. Activation of the complement system by protozoan parasites seems to be a common mechanism for achieving attachment to target cells. *Tryp. cruzi* trypomastigotes can infect T cells of both the CD4 and CD8 subsets, and may be similar to retroviruses in using receptor molecules on the T cell surface for penetration.

The effectiveness of macrophages in the elimination of *Tryp. cruzi* depends upon the stage of development of the parasite. Trypomastigotes are able to escape from the phagocytic vacuole and survive in the cytoplasm, whereas epimastigotes do not escape and are killed. Macrophages are also the preferred habitat of *Leishmania* spp., which multiply in the phagolysosome where they are resistant to digestion.

In an immune host these evasion mechanisms are less effective because of the presence of antibody and lymphokines. The ability to resist complement destruction also appears to be important. For example, *L. tropica* is easily killed by complement and causes only a localized self-healing lesion in the skin, whereas a disseminating, often fatal, disease is seen with *L. donovani*, which is ten times more resistant to complement killing. Large parasites such as helminths cannot infect individual cells; however, they can still achieve anatomical seclusion. *T. spiralis* larvae avoid the immune system by encysting in muscle; intestinal nematodes live in the lumen of the intestine.

## Evasion

Parasites may avoid recognition by:

• Antigenic variation
• Acquiring host-derived molecules.

African trypanosomes have the capacity to express more than 100 different surface glycoproteins. By producing novel antigens throughout their lives, these parasites continuously evade the immune system. By the time the host has mounted a response against each new antigen, the parasite has changed again. Plasmodia pass through several discrete developmental stages, each with its own particular antigens. A similar situation is seen in certain helminths such as *T. spiralis*. As a result, each new stage of the lifecycle is seen by the host as a 'new' infective challenge.

A number of parasites are known to adsorb host-derived molecules on to their surface. This is thought to mask their own antigens and enable them to evade immunological attack.

Parasitic protozoa and worms also use devices to avoid immune destruction. Certain parasites retain a surface coat, or glycocalyx, that blocks direct exposure of its surface antigens.

## Immunosuppression

Parasites are not always able to evade detection and many have evolved mechanisms to suppress or divert immune reactions. Some parasites produce or generate molecules that act against cells of the immune system. Thus, the larvae of *T. spiralis* produce a molecule that is cytotoxic to lymphocytes, and schistosomes can cleave a peptide from IgG, thereby decreasing its effectiveness. During many parasitic infections a large amount of antigenic material is released into the body fluids, and this may inhibit the response to or divert the response away from the parasite. High antigen concentrations can lead to tolerance by clonal exhaustion or clonal deletion. The immune complexes formed can also inhibit antibody production by negative feedback via Fc receptors on plasma cells. Many of these released molecules are polyclonal activators of T and B cells. This leads to the production of non-specific antibody, impairment of B cell function and immunosuppression. It has also been proposed that many parasites can cause unresponsiveness by activating immune suppressor mechanisms.

In many cases the immunosuppression has been attributed to macrophage dysfunction associated with antigen overload or the presence of intracellular parasites. In addition to the non-specific immunosuppression there can be parasite-specific effects. Mice infected by *Leishmania* spp. show antigen-specific depression of lymphokine production. As this genus inhabits macrophages and is partly controlled by activation of these cells by lymphokines, the effect is a diminished response against the pathogen.

Schistosomes have a receptor for part of the antibody molecule. They also release several proteases that cleave antibody molecules and release products that prevent macrophage activation. A schistosome-derived inhibitory factor suppresses T cell activity and is believed to allow other parasites to survive the effects of T cells and may explain the inefficiency of cytotoxic T cells in damaging the parasite.

When tested in a lymphocyte proliferation assay, peripheral blood lymphocytes of patients infected with *Plasmodium falciparum* are unresponsive to antigen prepared from the parasite, and in nearly 40% of the patients this persists for more than 4 weeks. Patients infected with *P. falciparum* show a suppression of lymphocyte reactivity that is not related to the degree of parasitaemia or severity of the clinical illness. The depressed lymphocyte reactivity is associated with a loss of both CD4$^+$ and CD8$^+$ lymphocytes from the peripheral blood. Once the parasite has been cleared, the response returns to normal. An even more sophisticated strategy has been evolved by *Leishmania mexicana* and *L. donovani*, which use IL-2 to stimulate their own growth. Mammalian epidermal growth factor has also been shown to stimulate the growth of certain trypanosomes in vitro.

## IMMUNOPATHOLOGY

The immune response to parasites is aimed at eliminating the organisms, but many of the host reactions have pathological effects.

The IgE produced in parasitic worm infections can have severe effects on the host if it stimulates excessive mast cell degranulation (type I hypersensitivity). Anaphylactic shock can occur if a cyst ruptures and releases vast amounts of antigenic material into the circulation of a sensitized individual. Asthma-like symptoms occur in *Toxocara canis* infections when larvae of worms migrate through the lungs.

The polyclonal B cell activation seen with many parasitic infections can give rise to autoantibodies. In trypanosomiasis and malaria antibodies against red blood cells, lymphocytes and deoxyribonucleic acid (DNA) have been detected. Host antigens incorporated into the parasite, as an immune evasion mechanism may stimulate autoantibody production by giving rise to T cell help and overcoming tolerance. In Chagas' disease about 20% of individuals develop progressive cardiomyopathy and neuropathy of the digestive tract that is believed to be autoimmune in nature. These effects are thought to result from cross-reactivity between antibody or T cells responsive to *Tryp. cruzi* and nerve ganglia.

Immune complex-mediated disease occurs in malaria, trypanosomiasis, schistosomiasis and onchocerciasis. The deposition of immune complexes in the kidney is responsible for the nephrotic syndrome of quartan malaria.

Enlargement of the spleen and liver in malaria, trypanosomiasis and visceral leishmaniasis is associated with increased numbers of macrophages and lymphocytes in these organs. The liver, renal and cardiopulmonary pathology of schistosomiasis is related to cell-mediated responses to the worm eggs. Symptoms similar to those seen in endotoxaemia induced by Gram-negative bacteria are found in the acute stages of malaria.

The non-specific immunosuppression discussed above may explain why individuals with parasite infections are especially susceptible to bacterial and viral infections.

## VACCINATION

No effective vaccine for humans has so far been developed against parasitic protozoa and worms, mainly because of the complex parasite life cycles and their sophisticated adaptive responses. As protection depends in many cases on both antibody and cell-mediated reactions, a vaccine must induce long-lived B and T cell immunity. In addition, because recognition by T cells is genetically restricted, the vaccine preparation must stimulate T cells from most haplotypes, preferably without suppressor epitopes. Because of the immunopathology seen in many parasite infections, antigens that induce a potentially damaging response must be avoided.

A much better understanding of the biological mechanisms underlying the natural history of parasitic diseases is required before it will be possible to control these globally important diseases.

RECOMMENDED READING

Mims C, Nash A, Stephen J: *Mims' Pathogenesis of Infectious Disease,* ed 5, London, 2001, Academic Press.

**Website**

DPDx. Parasites & Health. http://www.dpd.cdc.gov/dpdx/HTML/ Para_Health.htm

# 12 Immunity in bacterial infections

*J. Stewart*

## KEY POINTS

- Phagocytosis and complement activation are key innate defences against bacterial infections associated with acute inflammation.
- Antibodies are notably effective against bacterial cell surface and extracellular virulence factors such as toxins. Cell-mediated immunity is essential for defence against intracellular bacteria.
- Intracellular survival and growth provides one means of immune evasion for bacteria.
- Bacterial lipoplysaccharide and a number of other cell wall components can elicit uncontrolled innate immune responses that are potentially fatal to the host in the form of *septic shock*.

Modern medical science has managed to subdue many of the classical infectious diseases, but has helped to create new ones that result from interference with normal host defence mechanisms, consequent upon medical and surgical procedures such as chemotherapy, catheterization, immunosuppression and irradiation. Infections that develop in this way are known as *iatrogenic* (physician-induced) diseases.

It is important to differentiate infection from disease. A host may be infected with a particular micro-organism and be unaware of its presence. If the microbe reproduces itself to such an extent that toxic products or sheer numbers of organisms begin to harm the host, a disease process has developed. Potentially pathogenic bacteria such as pneumococci, streptococci and salmonellae are found in the nose, throat or bowel; this is known as the carrier state and is a source of infection to other individuals. These bacteria may also cause disease in the carrier if they enter a vulnerable tissue.

## HOST DEFENCES

Few organisms can penetrate intact skin, and the various other innate defence mechanisms are extremely efficient at keeping bacteria at bay. When bacteria do gain access to the tissues, the ability of the host to limit damage and eliminate the microbe depends on the generation of an effective immune response against microbial antigens. In most cases the host defences are directed against external components and secreted molecules. Bacteria are surrounded by a cytoplasmic membrane and a peptidoglycan cell wall. Associated with these basic structures there can be a variety of other components such as proteins, capsules, lipopolysaccharide or teichoic acids. There are also structures involved in motility or adherence to the cells of the host (see Ch. 2). These are some of the components to which the immune system directs its response. In general, peptidoglycan is attacked by lysosomal enzymes, and the outer lipid layer of Gram-negative bacteria by cationic proteins and complement. Specific antibodies can bind to flagella or fimbriae, affecting their ability to function properly, and can inactivate various bacterial enzymes and toxins. Antibodies therefore interfere with many important bacterial processes but, ultimately, phagocytes are needed to destroy and remove the bacteria (Fig. 12.1). In some situations cell-mediated responses are required.

### Inflammation

Having successfully avoided the innate immune mechanisms that protect the individual (mechanical barriers, antibacterial substances and phagocytosis, described in Chapter 9), a bacterium starts to proliferate in the tissues. The presence of bacteria-specific molecules is recognized by pattern recognition receptors, leading to cytokine release. These cytokines, along with tissue-damaging toxic bacterial products,

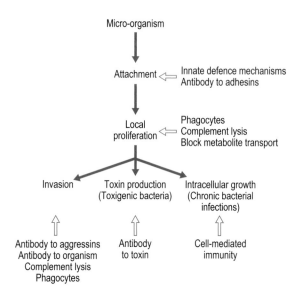

Micro-organism

↓

Attachment ⟸ Innate defence mechanisms
Antibody to adhesins

↓

Local
proliferation ⟸ Phagocytes
Complement lysis
Block metabolite transport

Invasion ← Toxin production
(Toxigenic bacteria) → Intracellular growth
(Chronic bacterial
infections)

⇑ Antibody to aggressins
Antibody to organism
Complement lysis
Phagocytes

⇑ Antibody
to toxin

⇑ Cell-mediated
immunity

**Fig. 12.1** Scheme showing the progress of infection and immunological defence mechanisms.

trigger an inflammatory reaction. The resulting increase in vascular permeability leads to an exudation of serum proteins, including complement components, antibodies and clotting factors, as well as phagocytic cells. The phagocytes are attracted to the site of inflammation by chemotactic factors. Anaphylatoxins generated by complement activation further increase vascular permeability and encourage exudation of fluid and cells at the site of inflammation. Many of these mediators also cause vasodilatation, thereby increasing blood flow to the area.

Many types of micro-organism (e.g. staphylococci and streptococci) are dealt with effectively by the phagocytes. The intensity and duration of the inflammatory process that is stimulated depends on the degree of success with which the micro-organism initially establishes itself. This, in turn, depends on the extent of the injury, the amount of associated tissue damage and the number and type of micro-organisms introduced. A localized abscess may arise at the site of infection.

If bacteria are not eliminated at the site of entry and continue to proliferate, they pass via the tissue fluids and lymphatics to the draining lymph node, where a specific acquired immune response is generated. The antibody and effector cells generated will leave the node to return to the area of infection to eliminate the bacteria. Some capsulate micro-organisms, such as pneumococci, are able to resist phagocytosis and are not dealt with effectively until large amounts of antibody have been made. These 'mop up' the released

capsular polysaccharide, and phagocytosis occurs. Other micro-organisms produce exotoxins, and effective immunity to exotoxins requires the development of specific antibodies against the toxin (i.e. *antitoxin*).

The types of infection described above are usually referred to as *acute* infections, and contrast with the protracted or *chronic* infections usually induced by bacteria that have adapted to survive within the cells of the host. Included among these are tuberculosis and leprosy, brucella infections and listeriosis. In these infections, cell-mediated immunity plays a predominant part in the final elimination of the micro-organism.

## Humoral immunity

The attachment of a micro-organism to an epithelial surface is a prerequisite for the development of an infectious process (see p. 159). A first line of attack by antibody could be to inhibit colonization by stopping attachment.

The immunoglobulin IgA can stop colonization of the mucosal surface if it interferes with the attachment molecules (*adhesins*) present on the bacterial surface. IgA does not activate complement very efficiently; therefore, an inflammatory reaction is not stimulated. Damage to the gut wall during an inflammatory reaction would allow the entry of many potential pathogens into vulnerable tissues.

Many micro-organisms owe their pathogenic abilities to the production of *exotoxins*. Among diseases dependent on this type of mechanism are diphtheria, cholera, tetanus and botulism. Antibodies acquired by either immunization or previous infection, or given passively as antiserum, are able to *neutralize* bacterial toxins.

Many bacterial exotoxins are enzymes, and protective antibody can prevent interaction of the enzyme with its substrate. The antibody can bind directly to the active site of the enzyme or to adjacent residues and inhibit by steric hindrance. Antibody may also act by stopping activation of a zymogen into an active enzyme, interfere with the interaction between the toxin and its target cell, or bind to a site on the molecule, causing a conformational change that destroys the enzymatic activity.

The direct binding of antibody to a bacterium can interfere with normal bacterial functioning in numerous ways. Antibody can kill bacteria on its own or in conjunction with host factors and cells. To survive and multiply, bacteria must ingest nutrients and ions mainly by specific transport systems. Antibodies that affect the activity of specific transport systems will deprive the bacteria of their energy supply and other essential chemicals. Some bacteria are invasive, moving into the tissues aided by enzymes that they produce. Invasion can also be inhibited by antibody that attaches to the flagella of the micro-organism in such a way as to affect its motility. Antibodies can agglutinate bacteria, and formation of the aggregate will impede spread of the organism.

In addition, the formation of an immune complex of bacteria and antibody will stimulate phagocytosis and complement activation.

When a particle is coated with antibody, a large number of Fc portions are exposed to the outside. This increases the chance that the particle will be held in contact with the phagocyte long enough to stimulate phagocytosis. The interaction of multiple ligands increases the overall affinity of the binding and, if antibody and complement components are present on the same particle, the binding is even stronger.

The bacteria are internalized and attacked by the oxygen-dependent and oxygen-independent killing mechanisms within the phagocyte. Phagocytes are also responsible for the removal and digestion of bacteria that have been killed extracellularly. Bacteria are susceptible to the lytic action of complement, which may be activated by bacterial components. The presence of antibody on the bacterial cell surface further stimulates the activation of complement. In certain circumstances, antibodies in conjunction with other bactericidal molecules lead to more efficient bacterial destruction. Gram-negative organisms are normally resistant to the action of lysozyme, probably because of the lipopolysaccharide component of the cell. The action of antibody and complement is thought to expose the underlying cell wall, which is then attacked by the lysozyme.

## Cell-mediated immunity

Ultimately, all bacteria will be engulfed by a phagocyte, either to be killed or removed after extracellular killing. The host defence mechanisms of macrophages and monocytes can be enhanced by various activating stimuli, including microbial products such as the muramyl dipeptide found in many cell walls and trehalose dimycolate from *Mycobacterium tuberculosis*. The chemotactic formylmethionyl peptides have been shown to increase the activities of various macrophage functions. The linkage of chemotaxis to activation has the advantage that the cell being attracted to the site of tissue injury will be better equipped to deal with the insult. Endotoxins present in the cell wall of Gram-negative bacteria and various carbohydrate polymers, such as β-glucans, are potent macrophage activators.

The immune system is also active in the production of macrophage-activating factors. In particular, lymphokines, produced by T lymphocytes, are often required to potentiate bacterial clearance both by attracting phagocytes to the site of infection and by activating them. The most important activator is γ-interferon, although tumour necrosis factor and colony-stimulating factors have also been implicated (see Ch. 9). All T lymphocytes produce some lymphokines when stimulated, and the balance of the different factors produced dictates the effect on surrounding cells. The overall effect of the lymphokines is to increase the effectiveness of host defence mechanisms, but if these molecules are produced in excess or to an inappropriate signal then a type IV hypersensitivity reaction can occur.

## EVASION

Once a micro-organism becomes established in the tissues, having escaped the innate defence mechanisms, it can often make use of a number of evasion strategies that protect it from the immune reactions of the host. Pathogenic bacteria produce a rather ill-defined group of bacterial products called *aggressins* and *impedins*, possession of which is associated with virulence (see Ch. 13). If antibody to such substances is present, the pathogenicity of the micro-organism is likely to be reduced.

## Intracellular bacteria

Bacteria that can survive and replicate within phagocytic cells are at an advantage as they are protected from host defence mechanisms. Some micro-organisms reside intracellularly only transiently, whereas others spend most, if not all, of their life inside cells. An intracellular lifestyle demands potent evasion mechanisms to survive this hostile environment. Some bacteria, such as *Mycobacterium leprae*, have become so accustomed to their intracellular environment that they can no longer live in the extracellular space.

*Listeria monocytogenes*, the causative agent of listeriosis, can survive and multiply in normal macrophages, but is killed within macrophages activated by lymphokines released from T lymphocytes. Listeriosis is most commonly seen in immunocompromised patients, pregnant women and neonates, in whom a lack of adequate T cell-derived macrophage-activating factors is probably the critical factor. *Salmonella* spp. and *Brucella* spp. can also survive intracellularly. Mycobacteria have a waxy cell wall that is very hydrophobic. This external surface is very resistant to lysosomal enzymes and persists for a long time even when the bacteria have been killed. In addition, these micro-organisms have evolved other strategies to evade destruction. *M. tuberculosis* secretes molecules that inhibit lysosome/phagosome fusion, and *M. leprae* can escape from the phagosome and grow in the cytoplasm. The cell wall of both of these bacteria contains lipoarabinomannan, which blocks the effects of γ-interferon on macrophages.

T lymphocytes represent the major host defence against intracellular pathogens. In many cases the bacteria themselves do not directly harm the host: the pathogenesis is caused by the immune response. After invasion of the host, intracellular bacteria are taken up by macrophages, evade intracellular killing and multiply. During intracellular replication some microbial molecules are processed and presented on the surface of the infected cell in association with major histocompatibility complex (MHC) gene products. The exact nature of the microbial molecules and the processing mechanism are not known. The processing appears to produce mainly antigen fragments in association with MHC class II molecules. This complex on the cell surface is recognized by specific CD4$^+$ T cells, which are stimulated to release lymphokines. These molecules in turn activate the macrophage so that the intracellular bacteria are killed.

It has also been proposed that peptides derived from the bacteria can become associated with MHC class I molecules. This complex leads to destruction of the infected cell by CD8$^+$ T cells. These cells also produce lymphokines that can aid in the elimination of the infection. The lymphokines produced attract blood monocytes to the site and activate them. If these newly recruited cells take up the released mycobacteria they are more likely to destroy them as they will be in an activated state. The accumulation of macrophages also causes the formation of a granuloma, which will prevent dissemination of the bacteria to other sites in the body. As conditions for the survival of the pathogens become less suitable, they stop replicating and die. Some intracellular bacteria infect cells that are unable to destroy them. In this situation a more aggressive immune response may be needed to remove the pathogen and this can cause pathogenic damage unless kept under control (see below).

## IMMUNOPATHOLOGY

The immune response to an organism leads to some tissue damage through inflammation, lymph node swelling and cell infiltration. Sometimes the damage caused by the immune system is very severe, leading to serious disease and death. Rheumatic fever can follow group A streptococcal infections of the throat and is believed to be due to antibodies formed against a streptococcal cell wall component cross-reacting with cardiac muscle or heart valve. Myocarditis develops a few weeks after the throat infection and can be restimulated if the patient is reinfected with different streptococci.

Immune complex disease (type III hypersensitivity) is frequently associated with bacterial infection. Infective endocarditis caused by staphylococci and streptococci is associated with circulating complexes of antibody and bacterial antigen. Detection of these complexes can be helpful in diagnosis, but they may lead to joint and kidney lesions, vasculitis and skin rashes. Immune complexes may play a role in the pathogenesis of leprosy, typhoid fever and gonorrhoea.

### Effects of endotoxin

Endotoxin interacts with cells and molecules of inflammation, immunity and haemostasis.

- Fever is induced by interleukin-1, produced by the liver in response to endotoxin, acting on the temperature-regulating hypothalamus.
- The action of lipopolysaccharide on platelets and activation of Hageman's factor causes disseminated intravascular coagulation with ensuing ischaemic tissue damage to various organs.
- Septic shock occurs during severe infections with Gram-negative organisms when bacteria or lipopolysaccharide enter the bloodstream.

Endotoxin acts on neutrophils, platelets and complement to produce, both directly and through mast cell degranulation, vasoactive amines that cause hypotension. The mortality rate is very high.

Recognition of endotoxin through Toll-like receptor 4 (see p. 111–112) causes macrophages to produce large quantities of potent cytokines such as interleukin-1, tumour necrosis factor and colony-stimulating factors. Endotoxin also causes polyclonal activation of B cells and can stimulate natural killer cells and other cell types to produce γ-interferon. A substantial part of the pathogenesis of endotoxin shock is probably due to the production of these molecules by cells of the immune system. In small amounts, endotoxin may actually be beneficial to the host, but when present in excess the results can be disastrous.

## Mycobacterial disease

Activated macrophages secrete a variety of biologically active molecules, including:

- proteases
- tumour necrosis factor
- reactive oxygen intermediates that are harmful to the surrounding tissue.

Tissue destruction is an inevitable side effect of this important mechanism of resistance. In the acute phase of a response this is likely to be tolerated; however, in the case of resistant organisms such as mycobacteria, the process may become chronic and the tissue destruction extensive. Mycobacterial components are still able to stimulate a response after the bacterium has been killed, because they persist for a long time, adding to the tissue damage.

There is evidence that lysis of infected cells may also occur. At first sight this may appear beneficial. Such a direct effect may be particularly relevant in the case of obligate intracellular pathogens such as *M. leprae*. Release into the hypoxic centre of a productive granuloma may also be fatal for *M. tuberculosis*, which is highly sensitive to low oxygen pressures. The same cytolytic event may also result in microbial discharge from the granuloma into surrounding capillaries or alveoli, and hence facilitate dissemination to other parts of the body or to other individuals. Lysis of infected cells causes tissue destruction, the severity of the effects depending on the importance of the tissue involved. *M. leprae* infects the Schwann cell, an irreplaceable component of the peripheral nervous system. Although the presence of *M. leprae* does not appear to affect the host cell to any extent, the presence of activated macrophages releasing toxic molecules or direct lysis by cytotoxic cells constitutes a major pathological mechanism in leprosy.

If the leprosy bacillus is released from a lysed nonphagocytic cell to be engulfed by an activated macrophage, the bacterium will be eliminated. Therefore, macrophage activation and target cell lysis can be beneficial as well as detrimental to the host.

The cell-mediated response that has the potential to eliminate these infections will give rise to type IV hypersensitivity reactions if the antigen is not removed efficiently. Chronic production of lymphokines causes granuloma formation, which with time can lead to fibrosis and loss of organ function. This type of response is particularly prevalent in patients with tuberculosis.

RECOMMENDED READING

Mims C, Nash A, Stephen J: *Mims' Pathogenesis of Infectious Disease*, ed 5, London, 2000, Academic Press.

**Website**

Todar's Online Textbook of Bacteriology. http://www.textbookofbacteriology.net/index.html

# 13 Bacterial pathogenicity

*D. A. A. Ala'Aldeen and K. G. Wooldridge*

## KEY POINTS

- Opportunist pathogens require a defect in host defence before they cause disease, whereas primary pathogens affect otherwise healthy individuals. The possession of virulence determinants generally differentiates pathogens from non-pathogens and, in turn, their number and potency separate opportunist from primary pathogens.
- Expression of virulence determinants is carefully regulated and may involve a form of chemical communication between bacteria known as *quorum sensing.*
- Adhesins are often involved the establishment of an infection. Bacterial adhesion may be mediated by fimbrial or non-fimbrial adhesins and generally involves interactions with host cell surface receptors or surface associated proteins such as fibronectin.
- Invasive pathogens gain entry and spread either by subverting host uptake mechanisms or by tissue disruption. Once established, pathogens must deploy a variety of mechanisms to avoid host defences.
- Multiplication within host tissues requires specific mechanisms to gain essential nutrients such as iron. Many pathogens make *siderophores* that compete with the host's high-affinity iron transport and storage systems.
- Host damage may be direct, via the release of toxins, or indirect, via the effects of the host's innate and adaptive immune responses (immunopathology).
- Endotoxins and exotoxins are recognized. Endotoxin is synonymous with the lipopolysaccharide or lipo-oligosaccharide of Gram-negative bacteria, and sufficient amounts elicit a cascade of responses leading to endotoxic shock.
- Exotoxins are proteins that cause damage or dysfunction by signalling at host cell membranes (type I), by damaging membranes (type II) or by entering target cells and directly altering function (type III).

Pathogenicity, or the capacity to cause disease, is a relatively rare quality among microbes. It requires the attributes of *transmissibility* or communicability from one host or reservoir to a fresh host, *survival* in the new host, *infectivity* or the ability to breach the new host's defences, and *virulence*, a variable that is multifactorial and denotes the capacity of a pathogen to harm the host. Virulence (see Ch. 14) in the clinical sense is a manifestation of a complex parasite–host relationship in which the capacity of the organism to cause disease is considered in relation to the resistance of the host.

## TYPES OF BACTERIAL PATHOGEN

Bacterial pathogens can be classified into two broad groups, *opportunists* and *primary pathogens*. Both groups have a broad spectrum of virulence capabilities, hence their overlap. In addition, some pathogens are capable of infecting a wide range of host species; such pathogens are referred to as *zoonoses*, whereas other non-zoonotic pathogens are highly adapted to a single species or a closely related group of species. Both zoonotic and non-zoonotic pathogens can be either opportunist or primary pathogens and organisms which exist as harmless commensals in one species may be pathogens in a second species.

### Opportunistic pathogens

These rarely cause disease in individuals with intact immunological and anatomical defences. Only when such defences are impaired or compromised, as a result of congenital or acquired disease, by the use of immunosuppressive therapy or surgical techniques, are these bacteria able to cause disease. Many opportunistic pathogens (e.g. coagulase-negative staphylococci) are part of the normal human flora, carried on the skin or mucosal surfaces where they cause no harm and may actually have a beneficial effect by preventing colonization by other potential pathogens. However, the introduction of these organisms into anatomical sites where they are not normally found, or removal of competing bacteria by the use of broad-spectrum antibiotics, may allow their localized multiplication and subsequent development of disease.

## Primary pathogens

These bacteria are capable of establishing infection and causing disease in previously healthy individuals with intact immunological defences. However, they may more readily cause disease in individuals with impaired defences.

The above classification is applicable to the vast majority of pathogens. However, there are exceptions and variations within both categories of bacterial pathogens. Different strains of any bacterial species can vary in their genetic make-up and virulence. For example, the majority of *Neisseria meningitidis* strains are harmless commensals and are considered to be opportunistic bacteria; however, some hypervirulent clones of the organism can cause disease in the previously healthy individual. Conversely, people vary in their genetic make-up and susceptibility to invading bacteria, including meningococci.

## Zoonoses and non-zoonotic pathogens

Some pathogens are found in a variety of animals and may be transferred to humans coming into contact with animals directly or indirectly. Familiar examples would include *Escherichia coli* O157, which are often found in association with cattle and other animals without causing apparent disease in these animals, but can cause gastrointestinal illness, as well as serious complications such as haemolytic uremic syndrome (HUS) when it infects man. By contrast, some pathogens are highly adapted to their host. For example, the pathogenic Nesseria species *N. meningitidis* and *N. gonorrhea* have only ever been isolated from human hosts and are not capable of infecting or initiating disease in other animals under normal circumstances.

## VIRULENCE DETERMINANTS

Both opportunistic and primary pathogens possess *virulence determinants* or *aggressins* that facilitate pathogenesis. Possession of a single virulence determinant is rarely sufficient to allow the initiation of infection and production of pathology. Many bacteria possess several virulence determinants, all of which play some part at various stages of the disease process. In addition, not all strains of a particular bacterial species are equally pathogenic. For example, although six separate serotypes of encapsulated *Haemophilus influenzae* are recognized, serious infection is almost exclusively associated with isolates of serotype b. Moreover, even within serotype b isolates, 80% of serious infections are caused by six of more than 100 clonal types.

Different strains of a pathogenic species may cause distinct types of infection, each associated with possession of a particular complement of virulence determinants. Different strains of *E. coli*, for example, cause several distinct gastrointestinal diseases, urinary tract infections, septicaemia, meningitis and a range of other minor infections (see Ch. 26).

## Expression and analysis of virulence determinants

Many pathogens produce an impressive armoury of virulence determinants in vitro. However, relatively early in the study of pathogenesis, it was appreciated that a knowledge of the behaviour of the pathogen in vivo is crucial to an understanding of virulence.

Animal models have been used to compare the virulence of naturally occurring variants differing in the expression of a particular determinant, and have provided much useful information. While some pathogens do not thrive or produce disease in typically available animal models, progress is being made in constructing better models by genetically manipulating the animals, for example, to express human receptors and other proteins important in human infection. Nevertheless, not all human clinical syndromes can be reproduced in animals, and extrapolation from animal studies to man can be misleading. Furthermore, the possibility that observed differences in virulence may be due to additional cryptic phenotypic or genotypic variations cannot always be excluded. Molecular techniques have been used to construct *isogenic* mutants of bacteria that differ only in the particular determinant of interest, and these constructs have allowed more detailed analysis of the role of such components in pathogenesis. More recently, comparative analysis of bacterial genome sequences have revealed the extent of genetic variation, as well as genetic mobility among bacterial strains.

Most studies of bacterial virulence determinants are by necessity performed in model systems in vitro. However, growth conditions in vitro differ significantly from those found in tissues, and as the expression of many virulence determinants is influenced by environmental factors, it is essential that such studies use cultural conditions that mimic as closely as possible those found in the host and that, where possible, confirmatory evidence is obtained that the phenomena observed actually occur during human infection.

Genetic studies have shown that expression of several different virulence determinants in a single bacterium is sometimes regulated in a coordinated fashion. Iron limitation, the situation encountered in host tissues, is one environmental stimulus that coordinately increases the production of many bacterial proteins, including virulence determinants such as haemolysin of *E. coli* and diphtheria toxin of *Corynebacterium diphtheriae*. In other bacteria, such as *Staphylococcus aureus* and *Pseudomonas aeruginosa*, some virulence determinants are expressed exclusively or maximally during the stationary phase of growth. Expression of these factors is associated with the production of inducer molecules or pheromones in the bacterial culture that accumulate as the bacteria grow until a threshold level is reached and gene expression is triggered – a process known as *quorum sensing*. The ability to regulate production of virulence determinants may save energy in situations in which expression is not required (e.g. in the environment) and quorum sensing may be important in establishing a sufficiently large population of bacteria in tissue to guarantee survival of the infecting organism. It is also clear that most organisms express some proteins only when in direct contact with host cells.

Molecular studies have also allowed mechanisms of transmission of virulence determinants to be investigated (see Ch. 6). Virulence determinants encoded by genomic DNA sequences, plasmids, bacteriophages and transposons have been reported. It is interesting that, in nature, these genetic elements can move between related organisms, transfer genes encoding virulence factors (e.g. toxins) horizontally, and transform the recipient bacteria to more adapted or more virulent pathogens. Apart from these genetic elements, there are other mechanisms by which some bacteria can exchange virulence genes. For example, neisseriae recognize and take up DNA fragments that contain specific sequences (uptake sequences) and incorporate them into their own genomes. In this way they can either vary the structure of an existing gene or, in the process, acquire a new set of genes. The genomes of many bacterial pathogens have been fully sequenced. The data reveal that several bacteria have acquired very large stretches of foreign DNA (often called pathogenicity islands) that contain virulence-related genes. This further demonstrates that the microbial population consists of a vibrant, kinetic and highly interactive community. In this community, bacteria evolve continuously and new

pathogens, or old pathogens with newly acquired capabilities, may emerge as a result.

## Establishment of infection

Potential pathogens may enter the body by various routes, including the respiratory, gastrointestinal, urinary or genital tract. Alternatively, they may enter tissues directly through insect bites, or by accidental or surgical trauma to the skin. Many opportunistic and several primary pathogens are carried as part of the normal human flora, which acts as a ready source of infection in the compromised host. For many primary pathogens, however, transmission to a new host and establishment of infection are more complex processes. Transmission of respiratory pathogens, such as *Bordetella pertussis*, may require direct contact with infectious material, as the organism cannot survive for any length of time in the environment. Sexually transmitted pathogens such as *Neisseria gonorrhoeae* and *Treponema pallidum* have evolved further along this route, and require direct person-to-person mucosal contact for transmission. Man is the only natural host for these pathogens, which die rapidly in the environment. The source of infection may be individuals with clinical disease or subclinically infected *carriers*, in whom symptoms may be absent or relatively mild either because the disease process is at an early stage or because of partial immunity to the pathogen.

In contrast, for many gastrointestinal pathogens such as *Salmonella, Shigella* and *Campylobacter* species, the primary source is environmental, and infection follows the ingestion of contaminated food or water. Many of these organisms also infect other animals, often without harmful effect, and these act as a *reservoir of infection* and source of environmental contamination (see Ch. 1).

## Colonization

For many pathogenic bacteria, the initial interaction with host tissues occurs at a mucosal surface and colonization – the establishment of a stable population of bacteria in the host – normally requires adhesion to the mucosal cell surface. This allows the establishment of a focus of infection, which may remain localized or may subsequently spread to other tissues. Adhesion is necessary to avoid innate host defence mechanisms such as peristalsis in the gut and the flushing action of mucus, saliva and urine which removes nonadherent bacteria. For invasive bacteria, adhesion is an essential preliminary to penetration through tissues. Successful colonization also requires that

**Table 13.1** Examples of fimbriae produced by Gram-negative pathogens

| Designation | Bacterium |
| --- | --- |
| Common (type 1)[a] | Enterobacteriaceae |
| | Uropathogenic *Escherichia coli* |
| CFA I, CFA II (CS1, CS2, CS3) E8775 (CS4, CS5, CS6) | Enterotoxigenic *E. coli* from humans |
| K88 | |
| K99 | } Enterotoxigenic *E. coli* from animals |
| F41 | |
| Pap-G, Prs-G | Uropathogenic *E. coli* |
| P fimbriae | } Pyelonephritogenic *E. coli* |
| X-adhesins (S, M) | |
| N-methylphenylalanine fimbriae | *Pseudomonas, Neisseria, Moraxella, Bacteroides, Vibrio* species |

See text for abbreviations and explanation.
[a]Mannose-sensitive fimbriae.

bacteria are able to acquire essential nutrients, such as iron, for growth.

## Adhesion

Adhesion involves surface interactions between specific receptors on the mammalian cell membrane (carbohydrates, proteins or glycolipids) and *ligands* (usually proteins or glycoproteins) on the bacterial surface. The presence or absence of specific *receptors* on mammalian cells contributes significantly to tissue specificity of infection. Non-specific surface properties of the bacterium, including surface charge and hydrophobicity, also contribute to the initial stages of the adhesion process. Several different mechanisms of bacterial adherence have evolved, all utilizing specialized cell surface organelles or macromolecules that help to overcome the natural forces of repulsion that exist between the pathogen and its target cell.

## Fimbrial adhesins

Electron microscopy of the surface of many Gram-negative and some Gram-positive bacteria reveals the presence of numerous thin, rigid, rod-like structures called *fimbriae*, or *pili*, that are easily distinguishable from the much thicker bacterial flagella (see p. 18). Fimbriae are involved in mediating attachment of some bacteria to mammalian cell surfaces. Different strains or species of bacteria may produce different types of fimbriae, which can be identified on the basis of antigenic composition, morphology and receptor specificity (Table 13.1). A broad division can be made between fimbriae, in which adherence in vitro is inhibited by D-mannose (*mannose-sensitive fimbriae*) and those unaffected by this treatment (*mannose-resistant fimbriae*).

The antigenic composition of fimbriae can be complex. For instance, two fimbrial antigens called colonization factor antigen (CFA) I and II have been detected in enteropathogenic *E. coli* strains. CFA-II consists of three distinct fimbrial antigens designated as coli surface (CS) antigens 1, 2 and 3. Another *E. coli* strain, E8775, has been found to produce three other CS antigens, CS4, CS5 and CS6. Pyelonephritogenic *E. coli* isolates produce a group of adhesins called X-adhesins; two fimbrial types designated S and M on the basis of receptor specificity have been identified in this group. The genes encoding a second type of fimbrae, the Chaperone Usher (CU) fimbriae, also found in *E. coli*, are found as multiple homologous, and often cryptic, variants, potentially with specificities for different carbohydrate receptors.

The evolutionary significance of such heterogeneity may be that the ability of an individual bacterium to express several different types of fimbriae allows different target receptors to be used at different anatomical sites of the infected host. In vitro, production of fimbriae is influenced by cultural conditions such as incubation temperature and medium composition, which may switch off the production of fimbriae or induce a phase change from one fimbrial type to another.

For some fimbriae the association with infection is clear. Thus the K88 fimbrial antigen is clearly associated with the ability of *E. coli* K88 to cause diarrhoea in pigs; pigs lacking the appropriate intestinal receptors are spared the enterotoxigenic effects of *E. coli* strains of this type. In many other instances the association between production of fimbriae and infection remains putative at present. Production of fimbriae is controlled by either chromosomal or plasmid genes.

The structure of one of these fimbrial types – *type 1* or *common fimbriae* – has been studied in detail. These consist of aggregates of a structural protein subunit called *fimbrillin* (or *pilin*) arranged in a regular helical array to produce a rigid rod-like structure 7 nm in diameter, with a central hole running along its length.

A highly conserved minor protein, located at both the tip and at intervals along the length of the fimbriae, mediates specific adhesion. Type 1 fimbriae bind specifically to D-mannose residues. Their role in vivo remains controversial; however, they may be involved in the pathogenesis of urinary tract infections.

Other Gram-negative bacteria, including those of the genera *Pseudomonas, Neisseria, Bacteroides* and *Vibrio*, produce fimbriae that share some homology, especially in the amino-terminal region of the fimbrillin subunits (the so-called *N-methylphenylalanine fimbriae*). These fimbriae have been shown to act as virulence determinants for *Ps. aeruginosa* and *N. gonorrhoeae*.

### Non-fimbrial adhesins

Non-fimbrial adhesins include protein or polysaccharide structures that are surface exposed on the bacterial cell and/or secreted. Protein-based adhesins include the filamentous haemagglutinin of *B. pertussis*, a mannose-resistant haemagglutinin from *Salmonella enterica* serotype Typhimurium and a fibrillar haemagglutinin from *Helicobacter pylori*. Outer membrane proteins are involved in the adherence of many, if not most, pathogenic bacteria.

Exopolysaccharides present on the surface of some Gram-positive bacteria are also involved in adhesion. For example, *Streptococcus mutans*, which is involved in the pathogenesis of dental caries, synthesizes a homopolymer of glucose that anchors the bacterium to the tooth surface and contributes to the matrix of dental plaque. Actinomyces may adhere to other oral bacteria – a process called *co-aggregation*. Teichoic acid and surface proteins of coagulase-negative staphylococci mediate adherence of the bacterium to prosthetic devices and catheters, contributing to increasing numbers of hospital-acquired infections. Continued growth following attachment to these biomaterials may result in formation of a *biofilm* (see Ch. 4), which may hinder successful antibiotic treatment by restricting access of drugs to the bacterium.

Flagella act as adhesins in *Vibrio cholerae* and *Campylobacter jejuni*. Bacterial motility is also thought to be important in chemotaxis of these organisms and *H. pylori* towards intestinal cells, and in penetration of these bacteria through the mucous layer during colonization.

### Binding to connective tissue proteins

Binding of pathogenic bacteria to a number of connective tissue proteins, including laminin, vitronectin and collagen, have been described. The best-studied of these host proteins is fibronectin, a complex multifunctional glycoprotein found in plasma and associated with mucosal cell surfaces, where it promotes numerous adhesion functions. Many pathogenic bacteria bind fibronectin at the bacterial surface, and for some organisms fibronectin has been shown to act as the cell surface receptor for bacterial adhesion. In *Streptococcus pyogenes*, lipoteichoic acid mediates attachment of the bacterium to the amino terminus of the fibronectin molecule. Attachment of *S. aureus* to cell surfaces also involves the amino terminus of fibronectin, but the bacterial ligand appears to be protein in this instance. *T. pallidum* also binds fibronectin. The significance of the interaction with fibronectin in the pathogenesis of syphilis and many other bacterial diseases needs further clarification.

### Consequences of adhesion

In addition to preventing loss of the pathogen from the host, adhesion induces structural and functional changes in mucosal cells, and these may contribute to disease. For example, adherence of enteropathogenic *E. coli* (EPEC) to epithelial cells induces rearrangements of the cell cytoskeleton causing loss of microvilli and localized accumulation of actin, without subsequent invasion of the host cell. In contrast, adherence of *H. pylori* to gastric epithelial cells causes enhanced production of the pro-inflammatory chemokine interleukin (IL)-8, which contributes to gastric pathology. In both cases, these changes involve the induction of intracellular signalling pathways triggered after binding of the bacteria to specific receptors on the epithelial cell surface. Adhesion of bacteria to mammalian cells may also induce changes in bacterial gene expression.

### Invasion

Once attached to a mucosal surface, some bacteria exert their pathogenic effects without penetrating the tissues of the host: toxins, other aggressins and induction of intracellular signalling pathways mediate tissue damage at local or distant sites. For a number of pathogenic bacteria, however, adherence to the mucosal surface represents but the first stage of the invasion of tissues. Examples of organisms that are able to invade and survive within host cells include mycobacteria and those of the genera *Salmonella*,

*Shigella, Escherichia, Yersinia, Legionella, Listeria, Campylobacter* and *Neisseria*. Cell invasion confers the ability to avoid humoral host defence mechanisms and potentially provides a niche rich in nutrients and devoid of competition from other bacteria. However, the survival of bacteria in professional phagocytes, such as macrophages or polymorphonuclear leucocytes, depends on subverting intracellular killing mechanisms that would normally result in microbial destruction (see below). For some bacteria (e.g. *Neisseria meningitidis*), penetration through or between epithelial cells allows dissemination from the initial site of entry to other body sites.

### Uptake into host cells

The initial phase of cellular invasion involves penetration of the mammalian cell membrane; rather than eliciting mechanisms for host cell penetration themselves, many intracellular pathogens induce phagocytic processes in the host cell to gain access.

Shigellae invade colonic mucosal cells but rarely penetrate deeper into the host tissues. Inside the cell, they are surrounded by a membrane-bound vesicle derived from the host cell. Soon after entry, this vesicle is lysed by the action of a plasmid-encoded haemolysin (haemolysis is just one way of detecting a membrane-damaging toxin), and the bacteria are released into the cell cytoplasm. *Listeria monocytogenes* produces a heat shock protein with a similar function, termed *listeriolysin*. Once free in the cell cytoplasm, shigellae multiply rapidly with subsequent inhibition of host cell protein synthesis. Several hours later the host cell dies, and bacteria spread to adjacent cells where the process of invasion is repeated.

Other bacteria remain within membrane-bound vesicles but modify these cellular compartments, preventing them from maturing and fusing with lysosomes. The pathogenic Neisseria, for example, elaborate a secreted toxin, immunoglobulin A protease, which in addition to cleaving immunoglobulin A during colonization of the mucosa (see below), is also capable of cleaving a key endocytic vesicle protein, LAMP1, which is responsible for acidification of the endosome. In this way the intracellular pathogen modifies the environment within the vesicle to favour its own survival. Most salmonellae proceed through the superficial layers of the gut and invade deeper tissues, in particular cells of the reticulo-endothelial system such as macrophages. Salmonellae also occupy a host-derived vesicle that does not lyse. In this case several vesicles coalesce to form large intracellular vacuoles. These vacuoles traverse the cytoplasm to reach the opposite side of the cell and initiate spread to adjacent cells and deeper tissues. Although invasion of host cells is essentially a bacterium-directed but a host-mediated process, the active participation of the bacterium and novel bacterial protein synthesis is needed.

### Role of cell receptors

The availability of specific receptors defines the types of host cell that are involved. As a result, some pathogens can invade a wide range of cell types, whereas others have a more restricted invasive potential. Specific host receptors for some of the invasive pathogens have been identified. For example, *Legionella pneumophila* and *Mycobacterium tuberculosis* adhere to complement receptors on the surface of phagocytic cells. A specific receptor for *Yersinia pseudotuberculosis* belongs to a family of proteins termed *integrins* that form a network on the surface of host cells to which host proteins such as fibronectin can bind. Mimicry of the amino acid sequence (Arg-Gly-Asp) of fibronectin that mediates attachment to the integrins may represent a common mechanism of effecting intracellular entry. The ability to utilize integrins may not be restricted to intracellular bacteria. The filamentous haemagglutinin of *B. pertussis* may use the fibronectin integrin to mediate attachment in the respiratory tract.

A number of bacterial pathogens capable of crossing the blood–brain barrier, including *N. meningitidis*, *Haemophilus influenza* and *Streptococcus pneumonia*, as well as a number of neurotropic viruses and prions, have been shown to bind to the laminin receptor protein, suggesting that binding to this host receptor protein confers a neurotropism on these pathogens.

## Survival and multiplication

To cause disease, most micro-organisms must survive on an epithelial surface, within a mucosal lumen or within host tissues and, at some stage multiply. Survival depends to a large extent on the organism's ability to avoid, evade or resist host defences. Multiplication depends on acquiring all of the nutrients necessary for growth; the most extensively studied nutritional challenge to pathogens is iron acquisition.

## Avoidance of host defence mechanisms

Colonization by bacterial pathogens, particularly of normally sterile areas of the body, results in the induction of specific and non-specific humoral and cell-mediated immune responses designed to eradicate the organism from the site of infection. Products of the organism that are not normally found within sterile tissues of the host may be chemotactic for phagocytic cells that are attracted to the site. Moreover, complement components may directly damage the bacterium and release peptides chemotactic for phagocytic cells. Other humoral antibacterial factors include lysozyme and the iron chelators transferrin and lactoferrin. Lysozyme is active primarily against Gram-positive bacteria but potentiates the activity of complement against Gram-negative organisms. Transferrin and lactoferrin chelate iron in body fluids, and reduce the amount of free iron to a level below that necessary for bacterial growth.

Pathogenic bacteria have evolved ways of avoiding or neutralizing these highly efficient clearance systems. As most of the interactions between the bacterium and the immune effectors involve the bacterial surface, resistance to these effects is related to the molecular architecture of the bacterial surface layers.

## Capsules

Many bacterial pathogens need to avoid phagocytosis; production of an extracellular capsule is the most common mechanism by which this is achieved. Virtually all the pathogens associated with meningitis and pneumonia, including *H. influenzae, N. meningitidis, E. coli* and *S. pneumoniae*, have capsules, and non-capsulate variants usually exhibit much reduced virulence. Most capsules are polysaccharides composed of sugar monomers that vary among different bacteria. Polysaccharide capsules reduce the efficiency of host defences in a number of ways:

1. In the absence of specific antibody to the bacterium, the hydrophilic nature of the capsule may hinder uptake by phagocytes, a process that occurs more readily at hydrophobic surfaces. This may be overcome if the phagocyte is able to trap the bacterium against a surface, a process referred to as *surface phagocytosis*.
2. Capsules prevent efficient opsonization of the bacterium by complement or specific antibody, events that promote interaction with phagocytic cells. Capsules may either prevent complement deposition completely or cause complement to be deposited at a distance from the bacterial membrane where it is unable to damage the organism.
3. Capsules tend to be weakly immunogenic and may mask more immunogenic surface components and reduce interactions with both complement and antibody. In some cases, for example serogroup B *N. meningitidis*

and serotype K1 *E. coli*, the capsular polysaccharide may mimic host polysaccharides moieties (e.g. brain sialic acid) and be seen as self antigen.

### Streptococcal M protein

The M protein present on the surface of *S. pyogenes* is not a capsule but functions in a similar manner to prevent complement deposition at the bacterial surface. The M protein binds both fibrinogen and fibrin, and deposition of this material on the streptococcal surface hinders the access of complement activated by the alternative pathway.

### Meningococcal factor H-binding protein

The complement system is a powerful weapon against bacterial pathogens, but can potentially damage host cells as well. The host must, therefore, protect itself against the damaging activities of complement. The serum glycoprotein factor H is a negative regulator of the complement system that protects host cells by binding to glycosamino glycans present on the surface of host but not to bacterial cells. It can downregulate the activity of complement and thus protect the host cell. *N. meningitidis* expresses a factor H-binding protein on its surface, which recruits this complement regulator, thus affording similar protection to the bacterial pathogen.

### Resistance to killing by phagocytic cells

Some pathogens not only survive within macrophages and other phagocytes, but may actually multiply intracellularly. The normal sequence of events following phagocytosis involves fusion of the *phagosome* in which the bacterium is contained with *lysosomal granules* present in the cell cytoplasm. These granules contain enzymes and cationic peptides involved in oxygen-dependent and oxygen-independent bacterial killing mechanisms (see p. 117).

Different organisms use different strategies for survival (Table 13.2). *M. tuberculosis* is thought to resist intracellular killing by preventing phagosome–lysosome fusion; other bacteria are able to resist the action of such lysosomal components after fusion. Some organisms stimulate a normal respiratory burst but are intrinsically resistant to the effects of the potentially toxic oxygen radicals produced. Production of catalase by *S. aureus* and *N. gonorrhoeae* is thought to protect these organisms from such toxic products. The smooth lipopolysaccharide of many bacterial pathogens is also thought to contribute to

**Table 13.2** Some strategies adopted by bacteria to avoid intracellular killing

| Species | Method |
|---------|--------|
| *Mycobaeterium tuberculosis* | Prevents phagosome–lysosome fusion |
| *Salmonella* serotype Typhi | Fails to stimulate oxygen-dependent killing |
| *Staphylococcus aureus* | Produces catalase to negate effect of toxic oxygen radicals |
| Pathogenic *Neisseria* species | Inhibits phagosome–lysosome acidification |

their resistance to the effects of bactericidal cationic peptides present in the phagolysosome.

## Antigenic variation

Variation in surface antigen composition during the course of infection provides a mechanism of avoidance of specific immune responses directed at those antigens. This strategy is most highly developed in blood-borne parasitic protozoa, such as trypanosomes, but is also exhibited by bacteria. Pathogenic *Neisseria*, for example, are capable of changing surface antigens using three highly efficient mechanisms. These are mutation of individual amino acids, phase variation (switching genes on and off) and horizontal exchange of DNA material. *N. meningitidis* can avoid the killing effect of antibodies against its major porin (PorA) by mutating amino acids and/or acquiring parts of or all of its *porA* gene from another meningococcal strain. The organism can switch off the expression of its capsule or its immunogenic proteins by shifts in the nucleotide sequence encoding them. The latter varies as a result of recombination or mutation during DNA replication.

Another mechanism of antigen variation in *Neisseria* is the genetic rearrangements demonstrated in the fimbriae. Usually only one complete fimbrillin gene is expressed, although there may be several incomplete 'silent' gene sequences present on the chromosome. Movement of parts of the incomplete gene sequences, either from within the genome of the expressing strain or from DNA released by a co-infecting strain to an expression locus, results in synthesis of a protein that may differ antigenically from the original.

The borreliae that cause relapsing fever use a similar strategy to generate antigenic variation in their outer surface proteins. Other bacteria show strain-specific antigenic variability, for example group A streptococci produce up to 75 antigenically distinct serotypes of M protein.

The capacity for variation in surface antigens allows for longer survival of an individual organism in a host and means that antibody produced in response to infection by one strain of a pathogen may not protect against subsequent challenge with a different strain of that bacterium. This makes the variable antigens elusive targets for protective antibodies, and the development of vaccines based on inhibition of attachment or generation of opsonic or bactericidal antibodies is particularly difficult for these organisms.

## Immunoglobulin A proteases

Several species of pathogenic bacteria that cause disease on mucosal surfaces produce a protease that specifically cleaves immunoglobulin A (IgA), the principal antibody type produced at these sites. These proteases are specific for human IgA isotype I. Nearly all of the pathogens causing meningitis possess an IgA protease and a polysaccharide capsule enabling them to persist on the mucosal surface and resist phagocytosis during the invasive phase of the disease.

## Serum resistance

To survive in the bloodstream, bacteria must be able to resist lysis as a result of deposition of complement on the bacterial surface. In the Enterobacteriaceae, resistance is primarily due to the composition of the lipopolysaccharide present in the bacterial outer membrane. *Smooth* colonial variants that possess polysaccharide 'O' side chains are more resistant than *rough* colonial variants that lack such side chains (see below). The side chains sterically hinder deposition of complement components on the bacterial surface. Conversely, however, some O-chain polysaccharides activate complement by an alternative pathway leading to lysis of the bacterial cell. In *N. meningitidis* group B and *E. coli* K1, sialic acid capsules prevent efficient complement activation and, in *N. gonorrhoeae,* complement binds but forms an aberrant configuration in the bacterial outer membrane so that it is unable to effect lysis.

## Iron acquisition

The concentration of free iron in body fluids and secretions is below that required for bacterial growth because it is bound (chelated) by high-affinity mammalian iron-binding proteins such as transferrin and lactoferrin. To multiply in body fluids or on mucous membranes bacterial pathogens have evolved efficient mechanisms for scavenging iron from mammalian iron-binding proteins. Bacteria such as *E. coli,*

*Klebsiella pneumoniae* and some staphylococci produce extracellular iron chelators called *siderophores* for this purpose. Others, including *Campylobacter jejuni* and *N. meningitides,* do not produce siderophores themselves but are able to obtain iron from siderophores produced by other species or use host molecules such as noradrenalin, which has siderophore-like activity, as a source of iron. In an alternative strategy pathogens including *N. meningitidis, Haemophilus parainfluenzae, H. influenzae* type b, *Staphylococcus epidermidis* and *S. aureus* have specific receptors for transferrin and/or lactoferrin, on their surfaces, and are able to bind these proteins and remove the bound iron directly from these host proteins. Production of siderophores, their cell surface receptors, and receptors for transferrin, lactoferrin and other mammalian iron-binding proteins is iron-regulated and occurs mainly under conditions of iron restriction.

Two other mechanisms of iron acquisition from mammalian iron chelators have been described. Some *Bacteroides* species remove iron by proteolytic cleavage of the chelator. In *L. monocytogenes*, reduction of the $Fe^{3+}$ ion to $Fe^{2+}$ reduces the affinity for the chelator sufficiently for it to be removed by the bacterium.

Many bacteria express receptors for binding and/or internalizing other mammalian iron-containing molecules, such as haem, haemoglobin and haemoglobin–haemopexin complexes. These mammalian molecules are located intracellularly, where they may be available to intracellular pathogens; they may also be released by bacterial haemolysins that lyse the red cells.

## Damage or dysfunction

In order for an infection to become apparent there must be sufficient host damage or dysfunction for the individual to become symptomatic. It is particularly important to appreciate that there are generally two components to this: the direct effect of the organism and the host response. In many cases a largely immune-mediated damage (immunopathology) can predominate. This may reflect an excessive innate response as in septic shock (see below), or the adaptive response as in tuberculosis (see Ch. 18). The most obvious means by which bacteria cause direct host damage or dysfunction is by the production of toxins.

## Toxins

In many bacterial infections part or all the characteristic pathology of the disease is caused by *toxins.* Toxins may exert their pathogenic effects directly on a target cell or may interact with cells of the immune system resulting in the release of immunological mediators (cytokines) that cause pathophysiological effects (see Chs 8, 9 and 12). Such effects may not always lead to the death of the target cell but may selectively impair specific functions. Substances that have toxic physiological effects on target cells in vitro do not necessarily exert the same effects in vivo, but a number of toxins have been shown to be responsible for the typical clinical features of bacterial disease.

Two broad categories of toxin have been described: *endotoxin*, which is a component of the outer membrane of Gram-negative bacteria, and *exotoxins*, which are produced extracellularly by both Gram-negative and Gram-positive bacteria.

### Endotoxin

Endotoxin, also called lipopolysaccharide or lipo-oligosaccharide, is a component of the outer membrane of Gram-negative bacteria and is released from the bacterial surface via outer membrane vesicles (blebs), which may be released from the bacterial cell surface, or by lysis and disintegration of the organism. Lipopolysaccharide is anchored into the bacterial outer membrane through a unique molecule termed *lipid A* (Fig. 13.1). Covalently linked to lipid A is an eight-carbon sugar, ketodeoxyoctonate, in turn linked to the chain of sugar molecules (saccharides) that form the highly variable O antigen structures of Gram-negative bacteria. On solid bacteriological media, bacteria carrying lipopolysaccharide with O antigen form *smooth* colonies with hydrophilic surfaces; in contrast those carrying lipopolysaccharide without the O antigen form *rough* colonies with hydrophobic surfaces.

The term *endotoxin* was originally introduced to describe the component of Gram-negative bacteria responsible for the pathophysiology of *endotoxic* shock, a syndrome with a high mortality rate, particularly in immunocompromised or otherwise debilitated individuals. Endotoxin activates complement via the alternative pathway, but most of the biological activity of the molecule is attributable to lipid A. Both endotoxin and lipid A are potent activators of macrophages, resulting in the induction of a range of cytokines involved in the regulation of immune and inflammatory responses (see Ch. 9). Although endotoxin from Gram-negative organisms remains central to our understanding of *septic shock*, other structural and secreted components of bacteria that interact with pattern recognition receptors (see Ch. 9) can contribute to the pathogenesis of this clinical syndrome. Thus the multi-system effects, often involving complement, blood clotting factor and kinin activation together

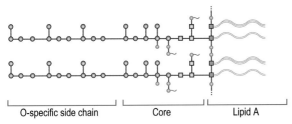

= various sugar residues

= ketodeoxyoctonate (KDO)

= glucosamine

= phosphoethanolamine

= fatty acid residues

**Fig. 13.1** Diagrammatic representation of the structure of bacterial lipopolysaccharide. After Rietschel ET, Galanos C, Lüderlitz O 1975 Structure, endotoxicity and immunogenicity of the lipid A component of bacterial lipopolysaccharide. In: Schlessinger D (ed.) *Microbiology*, pp. 307–314. American Society for Microbiology, Washington, DC.

with extensive cytokine release, should not be seen as exclusive to Gram-negative infection.

## Exotoxins

*Exotoxins*, in contrast to endotoxin, are diffusible proteins secreted into the external medium by the pathogen. Most pathogens secrete various protein molecules that facilitate adhesion to, or invasion of, the host. Many others cause damage to host cells. The damage may be physiological, for example cholera toxin promotes electrolyte (and fluid) excretion from enterocytes without killing the cells, or pathological, where the toxin (e.g. diphtheria toxin) inhibits protein synthesis and induces cell death. Exotoxins vary in their molecular structure, biological function, mechanism of secretion and immunological properties. The list of bacterial exotoxins is vast and increasing; however, they are often classified by their mode of action on animal cells:

- Type I (membrane acting) toxins bind surface receptors and stimulate transmembrane signals, and include the *super-antigenic* toxins.
- Type II (membrane damaging) toxins directly affect membranes, forming pores or disrupting lipid bilayers.
- Type III (intracellular effector) toxins translocate an active enzymatic component into the cell and modify an intracellular target molecule.

Examples of exotoxins and their effects on target cells are shown in Table 13.3. Bacteria secrete toxins and other proteins using a number of distinct mechanisms

that are understood to varying extents. Some of these systems are listed in Gram-negative bacteria as types I–VI, although this number does not reflect the total number of pathways that are known to mediate secretion of proteins across the bacterial envelope. Figure 13.2 shows the basic components of the types I and V pathways which are relatively well characterized. In type I, at least three proteins get together to form a channel through which large molecules (such as haemolysin of *E. coli*) are exported. In type V, however, a single precursor protein that consists of three domains is secreted sequentially across the inner and outer membranes. Although these latter proteins are called *autotransporters*, it is now known that both secretion steps require the activity of a number of additional cellular proteins. A typical example of an autotransporter is the IgA1 protease of *Neisseria* spp.

*Enterotoxins* cause symptoms of gastrointestinal disease, including diarrhoea, dysentery and vomiting. In some cases the disease is caused by ingestion of preformed toxin in food, but in most cases colonization of the intestine is required before toxin is made.

Cholera toxin and heat-labile toxins of enterotoxigenic *E. coli* (ETEC) do not induce inflammatory changes in the intestinal mucosa, but perturb the processes that regulate ion and water exchange across the intestinal epithelium (see Chs 26 and 30). In contrast, the enterotoxins of *Clostridium difficile, C. perfringens* type A and *Bacillus cereus* cause structural damage to epithelial cells, resulting in inflammation. Another gastrointestinal pathogen, enteropathogenic *E. coli* (EPEC), mediates damage by a process that involves secretion of a protein, Tir, directly across both bacterial membranes and the host cell membrane in a single step. Tir is subsequently inserted into the host cell membrane where it acts as a receptor for a bacterial adhesin, intimin. Binding of intimin to Tir results in phosphorylation of the latter protein; this in turn leads to a signalling cascade and cytoskeletal rearrangements within the host cell.

*B. pertussis*, the causative agent of whooping cough, produces various extracellular products, including a tracheal cytotoxin that inhibits the beating of cilia on tracheal epithelial cells, pertussis toxin, which exhibits several systemic effects, and an adenylate cyclase that interferes with phagocyte function.

Another group of toxins causes damage to subepithelial tissues following penetration and multiplication of the pathogen at the site of infection. Many of these toxins also inhibit or interfere with components of the host immune system. Membrane-damaging toxins such as staphylococcal α and β toxins,

**Table 13.3** Some effects of bacterial exotoxins

| Toxic effect | Examples |
|---|---|
| **Lethal action** | |
| Effect on neuromuscular junction | *Clostridium botulinum* toxin A |
| Effect on voluntary muscle | Tetanus toxin |
| Damage to heart, lungs, kidneys, etc. | Diphtheria toxin |
| **Pyrogenic effect** | |
| Increase in body temperature and polyclonal T cell activation | Super-antigenic exotoxins of *Staphylococcus aureus* and *Streptococcus pyogenes* (e.g. staphylococcal toxic shock syndrome toxin 1) |
| **Action on gastrointestinal tract** | |
| Secretion of water and electrolytes | Cholera and *Escherichia coli* enterotoxins |
| Pseudomembranous colitis | *Clostridium difficile* toxins A and B |
| Bacillary dysentery | Shigella toxin (Shiga toxin) |
| Vomiting | *Staphylococcus aureus* enterotoxins A–E |
| **Action on skin** | |
| Necrosis | Clostridial toxins; staphylococcal α-toxin |
| Erythema | Diphtheria toxin; streptococcal erythrogenic toxin |
| Permeability of skin capillaries | Cholera enterotoxin; *E. coli* heat-labile toxin |
| Nikolsky sign[a] | *Staphylococcus aureus* epidermolytic toxin |
| **Cytolytic effects** | |
| Lysis of blood cells | *Staphylococcus aureus* α-, β- and δ-lysins; leucocidin |
| | Streptolysin O and S |
| | *Clostridium perfringens* α and θ toxins |
| **Inhibition of metabolic activity** | |
| Protein synthesis | Diphtheria toxin; shiga toxin |

[a]Separation of epidermis from dermis.

streptolysin O and streptolysin S, and *C. perfringens* α and θ toxins inhibit leucocyte chemotaxis at subcytolytic concentrations, but cause necrosis and tissue damage at higher concentrations.

## Systemic effects of toxins

Some toxins cause damage to internal organs following absorption from the focus of infection. Included in this category are the toxins causing diphtheria, tetanus and botulism, and those associated with streptococcal scarlet fever, staphylococcal toxic shock syndrome and haemolytic uremic syndrome associated with Shiga toxin-producing enteropathogens. The diphtheria toxin, the gene for which is bacteriophage-encoded, inhibits protein synthesis in mammalian cells. Tetanus toxin, in contrast, exerts its effect by preventing the release of inhibitory neurotransmitters whose function is to prevent overstimulation of motor neurones in the central nervous system, resulting in the convulsive muscle spasm characteristic of tetanus. Diphtheria and tetanus toxins represent the sole determinant of disease and are neutralized by specific antitoxin antibody. As a result, vaccination with toxoids (formalin-inactivated toxins) derived from these toxins is highly effective (see Ch. 70).

Botulism results from the ingestion of preformed toxin produced by *Clostridium botulinum* in food contaminated with this bacterium, and is not a true infectious disease. The toxic activity is due to a family of serologically distinct polypeptide neurotoxins that prevent release of acetylcholine at neuromuscular junctions, resulting in the symptoms of flaccid paralysis. These toxins have been used clinically in treating squints and muscle spasm.

Other toxins cause disseminated multi-system organ damage. Such pathology is seen in staphylococcal *toxic shock syndrome* caused by certain strains of *S. aureus* that produce a toxin designated *toxic shock syndrome toxin 1* (TSST-1). This toxin belongs to a group of functionally related proteins collectively referred to as *superantigens*, which include the staphylococcal enterotoxins, staphylococcal exfoliative toxin and streptococcal pyrogenic exotoxin A. These molecules are potent T cell mitogens whose reactivity with lymphocytes induces cytokine release; they may

**Type I secretion**

Haemolysin secreted intact

TolC

Outer membrane

HlyD

Periplasmic space

HlyB

Inner membrane

ADP ATP ATP ADP

Haemolysin

**Autotransporters**

The functional N-terminal domain is secreted

C-terminal β domain

Signal peptide is lost

C-terminal domain forms a pore

Sec

Signal peptide

N-terminal domain

C-terminal β domain

**Fig. 13.2** Diagrammatic representation of type I and type V (autotransporter) secretion of exotoxins across the bacterial cell membrane. ADP, adenosine diphosphate; ATP, adenosine triphosphate; Hly, haemolysin; Tol, special receptor.

initiate tissue damage by mechanisms similar to those postulated to account for Gram-negative endotoxic shock (see p. 165).

## Other extracellular aggressins

Many bacteria secrete a range of enzymes that may be involved in the pathogenic processes.

*Proteus* spp. and some other bacteria that cause urinary tract infections produce *ureases* that break down urea in the urine, and the release of ammonia may contribute to the pathology. The urease produced by the gastric and duodenal pathogen *H. pylori* is similarly implicated in the virulence of the organism. *L. pneumophila* produces a metalloprotease thought to contribute to the characteristic pathology seen in legionella pneumonia.

Many other degradative enzymes, including *mucinases, phospholipases, elastases collagenases* and *hyaluronidases*, are produced by pathogenic bacteria. Many non-pathogenic bacteria and opportunistic pathogens also produce such enzymes; in most cases their role in pathogenesis requires further clarification.

An understanding of the basic mechanisms of pathogenesis is important for the design of new or improved vaccines and appropriate therapies. Such knowledge is also invaluable in the analysis of 'new' bacterial pathogens that are recognized from time to time. However, for some bacterial diseases, for example syphilis, such approaches have still not defined the mechanisms of pathogenesis or the virulence determinants involved, and new strategies employed by such successful pathogens may yet be discovered.

## RECOMMENDED READING

Alouf JE, Freer JH: *Bacterial Protein Toxins*, ed 2, London, 1999, Academic Press.
Hacker J, Hessemann J, editors: *Molecular Infection Biology: Interaction Between Microorganisms and Cells*, Hoboken, NJ, 2000, John Wiley.
Lamont R, editor: *Bacterial Invasion of Host Cells (Advances in Molecular and Cellular Microbiology)*, 2004, Cambridge University Press.
Locht C, Simonet M, editors: *Bacterial Pathogenesis: Molecular and Cellular Mechamisms*, 2012, Caister Academic Press.

Mims C, Nash A, Stephen J: *Mims' Pathogenesis of Infectious Disease*, ed 5, London, 2000, Academic Press.
Salyers AA, Whitt DD: *Bacterial Pathogenesis: A Molecular Approach*, ed 3, Washington, 2011, ASM Press.
Williams P, Ketley J, Salmond G: *Bacterial Pathogenesis*, (Vol 28), London, 1998, Academic Press.

# The natural history of infection

*M. R. Barer*

## KEY POINTS

- Symptomatic infection is a rare outcome when human beings and micro-organisms meet. None the less, some organisms, known as *obligate pathogens*, must cause disease to survive; this applies to most viral pathogens. Many bacterial pathogens appear to derive little benefit from causing infection.
- Micro-organisms that form short- or long-term associations with humans do so in a number of recognizable forms and stages, including: *entry/establishment, colonization, commensalism, spread, survival and multiplication, damage,* and *carriage.* Where these associations lead to bacterial disease, the different stages are often associated with the virulence determinants described in Chapter 13.
- Infections can generally be recognized in one of four categories: *toxin mediated, acute, subacute* and *chronic.*
- The capacity of a particular micro-organism to cause disease is known as its *virulence.* Where suitable experimental models are available, we can recognize virulence quantitatively by the ability of a low number of organisms to produce infection or death in the host population. Such measurements can be useful in identifying virulence determinants and in developing vaccines.

The purpose of this chapter is to link the basic properties of micro-organisms with the patterns of infective disease experienced in public health and clinical practice, and with the tissue and organ pathology that can be observed. Although there are numerous exceptions to the general patterns described, the intention is to give an underlying structure that can be used to make sense of the many different types of organism and the diseases they cause. The term 'natural history' is used in two senses here: first, to denote an overall biological

consideration of the life cycle of the infective agent and how this intersects with the human host and, second, to consider the process of infection from the point of the encounter between the agent and the susceptible host through to its outcome.

## MEETINGS BETWEEN HUMAN BEINGS AND MICRO-ORGANISMS

The vast majority of micro-organisms do not form stable associations with human beings. Clearly pathogens must do so, at least temporarily. However, it is worth briefly considering how important this association is to the micro-organism concerned. In some cases, humans constitute the only environment in which micro-organisms can survive (i.e. they are obligate parasites of human beings). Thus, humans are the reservoir and immediate source of the infections caused by this group (see Ch. 1). In other cases colonization or infection of human beings may be entirely incidental to the life cycle of the organism. These organisms may need to live in animals, as in the case of zoonoses, or in specific environmental reservoirs. Their life cycles in these habitats are critical to the epidemiology of the infections they cause. This biological perspective is difficult to avoid when considering the complex life cycles of parasitic protozoa and helminths, but such considerations are equally applicable to bacterial and viral pathogens.

In the previous chapter a division was made between primary and opportunistic pathogens. Here this division is maintained but the primary group is further subdivided.

### Obligate pathogens

These organisms have to cause disease in human beings in order to continue to survive and propagate. This is true for most viruses that cause human disease and for which humans are the only natural host. The major caveat to this is that the degree to which these agents cause symptomatic infections can vary over a very wide range. Thus asymptomatic infections with smallpox were virtually unknown, whereas they are very common with polio. This contributed substantially to the eradication of smallpox as it was relatively straightforward to identify where transmission was taking place. Among bacterial pathogens, *Mycobacterium tuberculosis* is a prime example of an agent that has to cause symptomatic disease in order to survive and propagate. In some cases pathogenicity reflects an early stage in the development of host-parasite relations, with pathogens evolving towards a more benign association with their host. Clearly, if a parasite kills all of its potential hosts then it has destroyed its own habitat. However, this does not always hold true. Some pathogens actually become more virulent as a means of increasing their potential to survive.

## Accidental or incidental pathogens

This term applies to many bacterial pathogens. Causing disease confers no obvious biological advantage on the organism and indeed may be a dead end. There are two groups of bacterial pathogen for which this is probably the case. The first group have their natural habitat in humans but cause disease in only a small minority; these include the major pathogens of bacterial pharyngitis (*Streptococcus pyogenes*), acute pneumonia (*Streptococcus pneumoniae*) and the principal agents of acute pyogenic meningitis (*Streptococcus pneumoniae, Neisseria meningitidis* and *Haemophilus influenzae* type b). The second group have a habitat (or reservoir) in nature but, if they encounter a susceptible host in a particular way, infection may ensue. For example, the agent of cholera, *Vibrio cholerae*, lives in brackish water and causes human disease only when ingested. *Clostridium tetani*, the agent of tetanus, probably propagates in animal gastrointestinal tracts and infects wounds contaminated by soil containing animal excreta.

## Pathogens in the environment

Whatever the method of acquisition, the organism must survive long enough to encounter a susceptible human host if it is going to cause human disease. The dynamics of pathogen survival in various environments are relevant to the control of infection. The capacities of different pathogens to survive and propagate in food and water are of particular concern, as is survival in aerosols and through desiccation and many other common environmental stresses. These

properties provide the biological basis for the transmission of infection and many opportunities for improved control of specific pathogens.

## STAGES OF INFECTION

Most infections can be broken down into a core series of steps:

- encounter
- entry and establishment
- spread
- survival and multiplication
- damage
- outcome.

It should be noted that the virulence determinants described in Chapter 13 were related to all but the first and last of these stages. Most pathogens can cause infection only via a limited set of routes (see above). Thus *Vibrio cholerae* must be ingested; it cannot cause infection if rubbed on the skin. Human immunodeficiency virus (HIV) must gain access to circulating CD4$^+$ cells via a parenteral route, and so on. Some general points concerning the passage through alternative stages of infection are made in Figure 14.1. Note that, although the simple direct pathway (A) reflects the norm for an exogenous infection, there are intermediates between this and D, endogenous infection. A single organism may be capable of following multiple routes to infection. For example, *Staphylococcus aureus* may be introduced exogenously into a wound. Around 30% of individuals are colonized with this organism at any point in time but in only one-third of these (10%) does the organism appear to be a member of the normal microbiota. Both temporary and permanent relationships may provide for endogenous infections due to *Staph. aureus*.

Many opportunistic pathogens become part of the normal microbiota before they cause infection. They may be assisted in colonizing a new host by interventions such as repeated use of antibiotics. This appears to be the case with *Pseudomonas aeruginosa*, which is resistant to most routinely used antibacterial agents, and is probably also the case for methicillin-resistant *Staph. aureus* (MRSA) and vancomycin-resistant enterococci (VRE). Most members of the normal microbiota appear to have very little capacity to cause disease. The number and identities of readily culturable bacteria varies in different parts of the body (Table 14.1) and it is clear that a 'healthy' normal microbiota provides some protection against invading pathogens. Indeed the composition of the *microbiome* of particular individuals may prove to be critical in

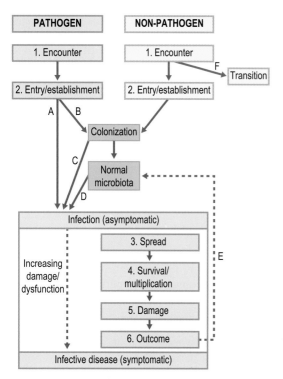

**Fig. 14.1** Pathways to and stages of infection following encounter between a host and a micro-organism. The blue sector includes the possible outcomes for a pathogen, the yellow a non-pathogen, and the green either of these. An organism detected in a diagnostic laboratory might reflect one or more of the stages identified, including transition. The possibility of transition from yellow to blue zones reflects the lack of a rigid division between pathogen and non-pathogen, and one aspect of opportunism. Detection in a diagnostic laboratory is most likely following colonization or multiplication. Infection may become apparent as a result of many different pathways: A, directly, without any colonization phase; B, many pathogens colonize first then proceed to infection either C after a brief period of colonization or D after a sustained period in which they live as *commensals* as part of the normal microbiota (progression here is not inevitable). Note that infection becomes symptomatic only when the level of damage or dysfunction is sufficient. At the end of the symptomatic infection a small number of pathogens may enter the normal microbiota (E) and the convalescent host is then described as a *carrier* for the organism concerned. F, Some organisms may simply be passing through and form no stable association with the host.

the balance between health and disease. As noted earlier, culture methods have only been able to reveal a minority of the bacterial species present in different samples and there is considerable excitement at the potential yield of a project to characterize all the organisms present by nucleic acid sequencing in the Human Microbiome Project.

The survival of humankind to the present day reflects the fact that most untreated infections are not fatal. Indeed, many human genes, particularly those concerned with the immune response, clearly reflect the selection pressure provided by infection. Before the development of antibiotics and immunization at least 50% of deaths were attributable to infection (this is still the case in many resource-poor countries). Nevertheless, owing to our inherent and highly efficient defence mechanisms, many infections resolve without medical intervention. All doctors must have some skill in recognizing those infections for which an intervention is unnecessary. This is particularly important in the case of antibiotic use because of the dangers of encouraging resistance.

## PATHOLOGICAL PATTERNS ASSOCIATED WITH INFECTION

All of the foregoing reflects a set of proposed mechanisms that, by and large, fit and make sense of the available facts concerning the epidemiology and detailed pathogenesis of infection. In this section the link to clinical practice is developed by describing the pattern of pathology directly observable in various infections. Most infections can be placed into one of four patterns:

1. Toxin mediated (mainly bacterial).
2. Acute (including acute viral syndromes and acute pyogenic bacterial infections).
3. Subacute (many virus and several 'atypical' bacterial infections).
4. Chronic (chronic viral infections, chronic granulomatous bacterial, fungal and parasitic infections).

Simply by recognizing the basic characteristics of a suspected infection against these four possibilities, the possible range of causal agents can be narrowed down substantially. Their features are summarized and exemplified from the perspective of bacterial infections in Table 14.2.

### Toxin-mediated bacterial infections

This was the first recognized pathogenic mechanism in bacterial infection and resulted in early successful therapeutic and preventive measures. When a single toxin is responsible for most of the features of an infection, the dysfunction or damage is often distant from the site of bacterial multiplication, the disease may be reproduced by administration of the pure toxin alone and it can be prevented with antibodies directed against the toxin. The clostridial diseases tetanus and botulism are toxin-mediated. In the latter

**Table 14.1** Normal human microbiota[a]

| Location[b] | Composition[c] | Abundance[d] |
|---|---|---|
| Dry skin (face, forearm) | Gram-positive anaerobes (e.g. propionibacteria) | $10^2$ |
| Moist skin (axilla, groin) | Staphylococci (esp. coagulase negative); corynebacteria; Gram-negatives rare but more frequent after prolonged hospital stay | $10^{6-7}$ |
| Oropharynx | Anaerobes; streptococci; neisseria; candida | $10^9$ |
| Small intestine | Anaerobes, lactobacilli, peptostreptocccus, porphyromonas | $10^{5-7}$ |
| Large intestine | Anaerobes, clostridium, bacteroides; enterobacteria; enterococci, candida, protozoa | $10^{9-11}$ |
| Vagina | Anaerobes, lactobacillus; streptococci, candida | $10^{8-9}$ |

[a]The term microbiota is preferred to 'flora' as the latter refers back to a period when bacteria were classified with plants.
[b]These are extremely broad. In practice each micro-niche in the body constitutes a different environment colonized with different organisms; for example, the microbiota associated with the lumen and the mucosa of the gut are different.
[c]A very rough introductory guide. Note the predominance of anaerobes.
[d]Per square centimetre of surface or gram of fluid.

**Table 14.2** Patterns in the presentation and pathology of bacterial infection

| Pattern | Examples |
|---|---|
| **Toxin–mediated disease** Pathology often distant from site of bacterial growth Protective immunity may be mediated by anti-toxin antibodies alone Disease may be fully reproduced by administering the toxin alone | Diphtheria, tetanus Staphylococcal food poisoning, cholera Pseudomembranous colitis |
| **Acute pyogenic infection** Generally rapid growing organisms Interaction with innate immune system and acute inflammation predominates Where immune damage occurs, it is 'post-infective' | Streptococcal pharyngitis Staphylococcal abscess, bacterial meningitis, lobar pneumonia, acute cystitis Post-streptococcal glomerulonephritis |
| **Subacute infection** No pattern to growth rate Site of infection may be only partially accessible to the immune system Immunopathology often in parallel with direct effects of organism | Subacute bacterial endocarditis 'Atypical' pneumonia |
| **Chronic (granulomatous)** Bacterial growth rate often moderate or slow Organisms often survive and grow intracellularly Immune damage occurs with infection – predominantly cell mediated | Tuberculosis, brucellosis (Some fungal and parasitic infections have this pattern) |

case, as in several other forms of food poisoning, ingestion of only the toxin is required, so many cases of botulism are not strictly infections. Once the pathogen has grown and produced toxin, the onset of disease can be very rapid.

It is often possible to abolish the biological activity of toxins without affecting their immunogenicity. Such *toxoids* were among the first effective immunizations against bacterial infection. Diphtheria and tetanus toxoid vaccines have controlled these infections in the UK. In life-threatening toxin-mediated disease, the administration of pre-formed antibodies can be life-saving. Antibiotics are not effective in treating established disease, but may prevent further toxin formation. In the special case of *Escherichia coli* O157 infections, however, some antibiotics actually stimulate further synthesis of toxin.

## Acute pyogenic bacterial infections

*Pyogenic* means pus inducing. Pus is composed primarily of live and dead neutrophil polymorphs. The presence of pus generally reflects an acute inflammatory process and activation of the innate immune system. The inflammatory process may be localized, as in the formation of an abscess, or more disseminated through tissue planes. Anything more than a trivial acute pyogenic infection is usually accompanied by an increase in the blood neutrophil count. The acuteness of these infections is reflected in their rapid onset. Accordingly the bacteria that cause them generally grow rapidly, producing visible colonies within 24 h of inoculation. Medical intervention is most effective when given early in infection before the development of acquired immunity, which, when successful, terminates the illness. Serological evidence of acquired immunity cannot be used in the diagnosis of infection during its acute phase. Occasionally, immunopathology occurs after the causal organism is no longer detectable in the host; classic examples are poststreptococcal glomerulonephritis and rheumatic fever. Similarly, Guillain-Barré syndrome, a paralytic disease, sometimes follows acute campylobacter infection.

Many bacteria that cause acute pyogenic infections also produce toxins. Thus there may be both acute pyogenic and toxin-mediated components to the damage and dysfunction that develops. This is particularly true of staphylococcal and streptococcal infections. The complex mixture of the pathogenic processes attributable to different virulence determinants can make the most severe of these infections very difficult to treat.

## Subacute bacterial infections

These have a more insidious onset than acute infections and are accompanied by less prominent signs of acute inflammation. Classically, bacterial endocarditis was described as subacute, although this is no longer considered a suitable catch-all term for this type of infection. Because such diseases have a more protracted course, the adaptive immune response often contributes to damage. Hence subacute forms of bacterial endocarditis are often accompanied by immune complex-mediated pathology, whereas *Mycoplasma pneumoniae* infection (a form of atypical pneumonia) may be accompanied by several different immunopathological reactions reflecting specific immune responses (see Ch. 41).

## Chronic granulomatous bacterial infections

When bacterial infections persist over months or even years they tend to elicit a pathological entity known as a *granuloma*. Granulomas are a common form of localized cell-mediated immune response directed to antigens or other foreign bodies that appear to be refractory to elimination from tissues. An ordered accumulation of lymphocytes and macrophages occurs around a central focus in a manner that, to the experienced pathologist, can be more or less

specific to the eliciting stimulus. Persisting bacterial infections, notably those due to mycobacteria (e.g. tuberculosis) and, to a lesser extent *Brucella* spp., produce chronic granulomatous infections. The agents concerned are generally slow growing and have the capacity to survive inside host cells, notably macrophages. Cell-mediated immunopathology (delayed-type hypersensitivity; see Ch. 9) is a prominent feature of these infections.

## Timing of key events in infection

As different infections proceed at different rates, the timing of the symptoms, their relation to immune responses and the ability to detect the causal agent all vary. The *incubation period*, the time between the encounter with the pathogen and the onset of symptoms, is an important practical consideration in understanding and managing infection. This is characteristic for different pathogens and can be vital in determining whether an individual is still at risk of developing disease after exposure to a particular agent. Incubation periods for the four patterns of infection discussed above are illustrated in Figure 14.2, along with the time-frames over which immune responses and presence of the pathogen are expected. A more dynamic view of individual infections is shown in Figure 14.3, in which the additional concepts of recurrent, latent and reactivated infections are illustrated. Figure 14.3 introduces the notion that the progression of an infection is related to the numbers of the pathogen. Although many other

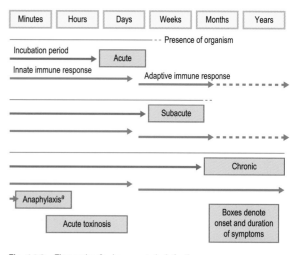

**Fig. 14.2** Timescales for key events in infection.
[a]Anaphylaxis is included for comparison and to illustrate the timescale when the adaptive immune response is primed against the antigen(s) concerned.

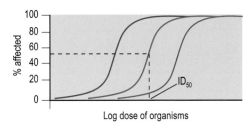

**Fig. 14.4** Quantitative relationships between organism dose and outcome in experimental infection. The organism has been administered by a single route to a uniform host population. Note that the outcome (percentage affected – which could be percentage infected, percentage who died or many other endpoints) depends on the dose. This approach allows virulence to be compared between strains of a particular micro-organism. A more virulent organism shifts the curve to the left (blue curve) and a less virulent organism to the right (red curve). Lesser or greater host resistance would, respectively, have the same effect. The approach allows for the specific recognition of virulence determinants and the effects of immunization. The dose required to produce the specified endpoint in 50% of the target population is often reproducible and can be used for statistical comparisons. The 50% infected endpoint is known as the $ID_{50}$.

Legend for Fig. 14.3:
- Asymptomatic infection
- Death
- Recovery
- - - Threshold for symptoms
- Recurrent symptoms
- Latent infection
- Reactivation

**Fig. 14.3** A model for incubation periods, progression and latency related to organism number.

factors are involved, the concept is useful because it illustrates how, in some rapidly developing infections, the interval between the onset of symptoms and death may be short. The slope of increasing pathogen numbers clearly also reflects the balance between growth of the pathogen and the efforts of the immune system to resist. Accordingly, when the immune system is suppressed, progression may be exceptionally rapid and the response must be equally so.

## VIRULENCE AND INFECTIVITY

By now it should be apparent that what makes a pathogen more or less *virulent* is, in most cases, extremely complex. None the less, when infections can be studied in animal experimental systems, virulence can be seen as a quantifiable property. As the dose administered to a group of susceptible hosts is increased, the number acquiring infections also increases in a fairly well defined dose–response relationship (Fig. 14.4). Not only does recognition of this relationship help explain why, when a group of individuals is exposed to a pathogen only some get infected, it also provides a framework for understanding the effects of immunization and immune deficiency, as well as a systematic basis for identifying individual traits that contribute to virulence and host resistance.

### RECOMMENDED READING

Burnet FM: *Natural History of Infectious Diseases*, Cambridge, 1970, Cambridge University Press.
Ewald PW: *Evolution of Infectious Disease*, USA, 1996, Oxford University Press.
Mims C, Nash A, Stephen J: *Mims' Pathogenesis of Infectious Disease*, ed 5, London, 2000, Academic Press.

Salyers AA, Wilson BA, Whitt DD: Bacterial Pathogenesis: A Molecular Approach, ed 3, Washington, DC, 2011, ASM Press.

### Websites

The Human Microbiome Project: http://commonfund.nih.gov/hmp/

# PART 3
## BACTERIAL PATHOGENS AND ASSOCIATED DISEASES

# 15 Staphylococcus

Skin infections; osteomyelitis; bloodstream infection; food poisoning; foreign body infections; MRSA

*H. Humphreys*

## KEY POINTS

- Staphylococci are commonly found on the skin of healthy individuals. *Staph. aureus* is present in the nose of 30% of healthy people but can cause infections where there is lowered host resistance (e.g. damaged skin).
- Many virulence factors have been described for *Staph. aureus*, but for most a specific role has not been determined. Exceptions include the enterotoxins, toxic shock syndrome toxin, the epidermolytic toxins and perhaps PVL, associated with community-acquired methicillin-resistant *Staph. aureus* (MRSA).
- Organisms spread from colonized sites (e.g. skin) by hands, clothing, dust and desquamation from the skin.
- MRSA is increasingly prevalent in hospitals and is emerging in the community and causes the same range of infections as methicillin-susceptible isolates.
- Flucloxacillin and vancomycin or teicoplanin are the agents of choice to treat methicillin-susceptible and methicillin-resistant *Staph. aureus* infections, respectively but newer options include linezolid and daptomycin.
- Coagulase-negative staphylococci (such as *Staph. epidermidis*) are major pathogens involving prosthetic implants such as intravascular lines or cardiac valves; the pathogenesis involves biofilm production.
- Device removal is usually required for the successful treatment of infections caused by CNS, as well as appropriate antibiotics, such as vancomycin or teicoplanin.

Sir Alexander Ogston, a Scottish surgeon, first showed in 1880 that a number of human pyogenic or pus-forming diseases were associated with a cluster-forming micro-organism. He introduced the name 'staphylococcus' (Greek: *staphyle*, bunch of grapes; *kokkos*, grain or berry), now used as the genus name for a group of facultatively anaerobic, catalase-positive, Gram-positive cocci. Staphylococci are resistant to dry conditions and high salt concentrations, and are well suited to their ecological niche which is the skin, but can survive for long periods in the environment. They may also be found as part of the normal flora of other sites such as the upper respiratory tract, and are commonly present on animals.

The major pathogen within the genus, *Staphylococcus aureus*, causes a wide range of major and minor infections in man and animals (Table 15.1) and is characterized by its ability to clot blood plasma by the action of the enzyme *coagulase*. There are at least 30 other species of staphylococci, all of which lack this enzyme. These coagulase-negative staphylococci (CNS) are skin commensals that can cause opportunistic infections especially associated with prostheses or foreign bodies (usually due to *Staph. epidermidis*), and urinary tract infections (*Staph. saprophyticus*). The presence of methicillin-resistant *Staph. aureus* (MRSA) in many hospitals and increasingly in the community has become a major public health issue, with concern expressed by patients and members of the public about the clinical implications.

## STAPHYLOCOCCUS AUREUS

### Description

*Staph. aureus* is a Gram-positive coccus about 1 μm in diameter. The cocci are usually arranged in grape-like clusters (Fig. 15.1). The organisms are non-sporing, non-motile and usually non-capsulate. When

**Fig. 15.1** Scanning electron micrograph of staphylococci in a biofilm enmeshed in exopolysaccharide (arrow). Original magnification ×15 000. (Courtesy of Dr R Bayston, University of Nottingham.)

**Table 15.1** Infections caused by *Staph. aureus*

| Pyogenic infections | Toxin-mediated infections |
| --- | --- |
| Boils, carbuncles | Scalded skin syndrome |
| Surgical site (wound) infection | Pemphigus neonatorum |
| Abscesses, e.g. spinal | Toxic shock syndrome |
| Impetigo | Food poisoning |
| Mastitis | |
| Bloodstream infections | |
| Osteomyelitis | |
| Pneumonia, e.g. ventilator-associated | |
| Endocarditis | |

**Table 15.2** Some virulence factors of *Staph. aureus*

| Virulence factor | Activity |
| --- | --- |
| **Cell wall polymers** | |
| Peptidoglycan | Inhibits inflammatory response; endotoxin-like activity |
| Teichoic acid | Phage adsorption; reservoir of bound divalent cations |
| **Cell surface proteins** | |
| Protein A | Reacts with Fc region of IgG |
| Clumping factor | Binds to fibrinogen |
| Fibronectin-binding protein | Binds to fibronectin |
| **Exoproteins** | |
| α-Lysin | |
| β-Lysin | Impairment of membrane permeability; cytotoxic effects on phagocytic and tissue cells |
| γ-Lysin | |
| δ-Lysin | |
| Panton–Valentine leucocidin | Dermo-necrotic and leucocidal |
| Epidermolytic toxins | Cause blistering of skin |
| Toxic shock syndrome toxin | Induces multi-system effects; superantigen effects |
| Enterotoxins | Induce vomiting and diarrhoea; superantigen effects |
| Coagulase | Converts fibrinogen to fibrin in plasma |
| Staphylokinase | Degrades fibrin |
| Lipase | Degrades lipid |
| Deoxyribonuclease | Degrades DNA |

grown on many types of agar for 24 h at 37°C, individual colonies are circular, 2–3 mm in diameter, with a smooth, shiny surface; colonies appear opaque and are often pigmented (golden-yellow, hence the '*aureus*'). The main distinctive diagnostic features of *Staph. aureus* are:

• Production of an extracellular enzyme, *coagulase*, which converts plasma fibrinogen into fibrin, aided by an activator present in plasma.
• Production of thermostable nucleases that break down DNA.
• Production of a surface-associated protein known as *clumping factor* or *bound coagulase* that reacts with fibrinogen.

Various commercial systems, increasingly automated, are available that rapidly identify staphylococci. They are particularly useful for screening large numbers of strains.

## Pathogenesis

*Staph. aureus* is present in the nose of 30% of healthy people and may be found on the skin. It causes infection most commonly at sites of lowered host resistance, such as damaged skin (e.g. surgical site infection) or mucous membranes (e.g. ventilator-associated pneumonia).

### Virulence factors

Recent years have seen a greater understanding of the pathogenic interaction between the host and *Staph. aureus*. Most strains possess a large number of cell-associated and extracellular factors, some of which contribute to the ability of the organism to overcome the body's defences and to invade, survive in and colonize the tissues (Table 15.2). Although the role of each factor is not fully understood individually, it is likely that they are responsible for the establishment of infection, enabling the organism to bind to connective tissue, opposing destruction by the bactericidal activities of humoral factors such as complement, and overcoming uptake and intracellular killing by phagocytes.

Neutrophils are critical in the innate immune response and the primary cellular defence against *Staph. aureus*. A multi-step process results in the mobilization of neutrophils from peripheral blood and or the bone marrow in response to a variety of factors. The staphylococcal capsule can stimulate CD4$^+$ T lymphocytes resulting in the production of chemokines that facilitate neutrophil mobilization and lipoteichoic acid in the cell wall interacts with toll-like receptors, which participate in this process. Subsequently, neutrophils use a variety of mechanisms to kill the ingested bacteria, e.g. superoxides and degranulation.

### Staphylococcal toxins

***Enterotoxins.*** Enterotoxins, types A–E, G, H, I and J, are commonly produced by up to 65% of strains of *Staph. aureus*, sometimes singly and sometimes in combination. These toxic proteins withstand exposure to 100°C for several minutes. When ingested as preformed toxins in contaminated food, microgram amounts of toxin can, within a few hours, induce the symptoms of staphylococcal food poisoning: nausea, vomiting and diarrhoea. However, enterotoxins, which are superantigens (see below) probably also play an important role in other serious staphylococcal infections, e.g. bloodstream infection (BSI), especially when accompanied by septic shock.

***Toxic shock syndrome toxin (TSST-1).*** This was discovered in the early 1980s as a result of epidemiological and microbiological investigations in the USA of *toxic shock syndrome*, a multi-system disease caused by staphylococcal TSST-1 or enterotoxin, or both. A link was established with the use of highly absorbent tampons in menstruating women, although non-menstrual cases are now as common. The absence of circulating antibodies to TSST-1 is a factor in the pathogenesis of this syndrome.

TSST-1 and the enterotoxins are now recognized as *superantigens*, that is, they are potent activators of T lymphocytes resulting in the liberation of cytokines such as tumour necrosis factor, and they bind with high affinity to mononuclear cells. These characteristics partly explain the florid and multi-system nature of the clinical conditions associated with these toxins.

***Epidermolytic toxins.*** Two kinds of epidermolytic toxin (types A and B) are commonly produced by

**Fig. 15.2** Scalded skin syndrome (toxic epidermal necrolysis). (Courtesy of Dr LG Millard, Queen's Medical Centre, Nottingham.)

strains that cause blistering diseases. These toxins induce intraepidermal blisters at the granular cell layer. Such blisters range in severity from the trivial to the distended blisters of *pemphigus neonatorum*. The most dramatic manifestation of epidermolytic toxin is the *scalded skin syndrome* in small children, where the toxin spreads systemically in individuals who lack neutralizing antitoxin. Extensive areas of skin are affected, which, after the development of a painful rash, slough off; the skin surface resembles scalding (Fig. 15.2).

***Panton-Valentine leukocidin (PVL).*** This toxin was recognized some decades back but its potential contribution to the clinical manifestations and outcome have been increasingly described in the context of community-acquired MRSA (CA-MRSA). As the name suggests PVL can adversely affect cells, resulting in leucopenia, but animal studies do not suggest high virulence. Nonetheless, epidemiological data in many countries reveal an association between necrotizing pneumonia and some complicated skin and soft tissue infections (cSSTI) caused by PVL-positive strains of CA-MRSA.

### Epidemiology
#### Sources and acquisition of infection

***Infected lesions.*** Large numbers of staphylococci are disseminated in pus and dried exudate discharged from large infected wounds, burns and secondarily infected skin lesions, and in sputum coughed from the lung of patients with pneumonia. Direct contact is the most important mode of spread, but airborne dissemination may also occur. Cross-infection is an important method of spread of staphylococcal disease, particularly in hospitals, and scrupulous hand hygiene is essential in preventing spread. Food handlers may similarly introduce enterotoxin-producing food poisoning strains into food.

***Healthy carriers.*** *Staph. aureus* grows harmlessly on the moist skin of the nostrils in about 30% of healthy persons, and the perineum is also commonly colonized. Organisms are spread from these sites into the environment by the hands, clothing, and dust consisting of skin squames and cloth fibres. Some carriers, called *shedders*, disseminate exceptionally large numbers of staphylococci.

During the first day or two of life most babies become colonized in the nose and skin by staphylococci, and transmission from babies to nursing mothers, who then develop mastitis, is well described.

***Animals.*** Animals may disseminate *Staph. aureus* and so cause human infection, e.g. milk from a dairy cow with mastitis, causing staphylococcal food poisoning.

***Environment.*** Although not spore forming, staphylococci may remain alive in a dormant state for several months when dried in pus, sputum, bed clothes or dust, or on inanimate surfaces such as floors. Environmental reservoirs are therefore increasingly recognized as important in hospitals in contributing to endemic MRSA. Staphylococci are fairly readily killed by heat (e.g. moist heat at 65°C for 30 min), by exposure to light and by common disinfectants, hence the emphasis on regular and effective environmental decontamination in controlling MRSA.

The acquisition of *Staph. aureus* infection may be *exogenous* (from an external source such as the environment) and more theoretically preventable and *endogenous* (from a carriage site, or minor lesion elsewhere in the patient's own body). It is important to remember that the body surfaces of human beings and animals are the main reservoir.

## Methicillin-resistant Staph. aureus (MRSA)

MRSA produces a penicillin binding protein 2a (mediated through the *mecA* gene), which is carried on the staphylococcal cassette chromosome mec (SCCmec) of which there are at least six different types recognized, and this results in resistance to all beta-lactam antibiotics. There is much debate on whether strains of MRSA are intrinsically more virulent than methicillin-susceptible isolates but it is agreed that MRSA causes the same range of infections resulting in excess healthcare costs, prolonged hospital stay and significant mortality. MRSA is endemic in hospitals globally except in Scandinavia and in the Netherlands although declining rates of MRSA BSI have been seen in recent years in the UK, France and other European countries. Vulnerable patients particularly at risk are those who have undergone major surgery and patients in the intensive care unit. Although 50–60% of patients with MRSA are merely colonized, i.e. representing asymptomatic carriage, serious infections occur such as BSI, respiratory tract and bone/joint infections. These infections are then more difficult to treat than infections caused by methicillin-susceptible isolates, and MRSA can spread easily among patients in hospital.

Community-acquired MRSA is increasing, especially in the USA, where 50% or more of *Staph. aureus* infections presenting to the Emergency Department may be methicillin-resistant. These occur often in otherwise healthy individuals with no recent healthcare contact. The production of PVL, alpha toxin and secreted proteases are implicated as particular virulence determinants. Community-acquired strains may cause the same range of infections as healthcare-associated strains such as BSI, but particularly cSSTI and severe pneumonia.

The control and prevention of MRSA involves the education of all healthcare professionals and the public, fast and reliable detection in the laboratory (including perhaps the use of molecular methods, see below), active surveillance (even universal surveillance), prompt patient isolation or cohorting when admitted to hospital, standard precautions and good professional practice by all health-care workers (including compliance with hand hygiene guidelines), effective hospital hygiene programmes and antibiotic stewardship programmes, e.g. avoidance of the excess use of cephalosporins and fluoroquinolones. Such measures have been very successful in Scandinavia and in the Netherlands where an aggressive 'search and destroy' approach involving the extensive screening of all MRSA contacts is employed.

## Laboratory diagnosis

One or more of the following specimens should be collected to confirm a diagnosis:

- *Pus* from abscesses, wounds, burns, etc. is much preferred to swabs.
- *Sputum* from patients with pneumonia (e.g. postinfluenzal or ventilator-associated pneumonia); bronchoscopic specimens, e.g. bronchoscopic lavage, are increasingly used in critically ill patients.
- *Faeces* or *vomit* from patients with suspected food poisoning, or the remains of implicated foods.

- *Blood* from patients with suspected BSI such as septic shock, osteomyelitis or endocarditis.
- *Mid-stream urine* from patients with suspected cystitis or pyelonephritis.
- *Anterior nasal* and *perineal swabs* (moistened in saline or sterile water) from suspected carriers; nasal swabs should be rubbed in turn over the anterior walls of both nostrils.

The characteristic clusters of Gram-positive cocci can often be demonstrated by microscopy, and the organisms cultured readily on blood agar and most other media within 24 h or less. The tube or slide coagulase test is performed to distinguish *Staph. aureus* from coagulase-negative species and antimicrobial susceptibility testing with cefoxitin to confirm MRSA using standard methods. Commercially-available molecular methods using the polymerase chain reaction (PCR) have been developed to reduce the time to the detection of MRSA from 48–72 h with culture to less than 12 h to facilitate earlier preventative measures. However, the results from trials with PCR to date are mixed and do not clearly indicate that this more expensive approach can assist in reducing MRSA rates in acute hospitals.

## Typing

Most staphylococcal infections are sporadic, but the identification of an outbreak strain, by determining whether all the isolates are of the same type, is an important aspect in the investigation of a source, particularly during outbreaks of MRSA. Traditionally, strains of *Staph. aureus* were differentiated into different *phage types* by observation of their pattern of susceptibility to lysis by a standard set of *Staph. aureus* bacteriophages (viruses that infect bacteria) with international agreement on the interpretation of results. However, many strains of MRSA have become non-typable with this method. Consequently, phage typing has been replaced by genotypic methods such as PCR, pulsed-field gel electrophoresis (PFGE) and gene sequencing (see Ch. 3). Multilocus gene sequence typing (MLST) defines the core genetic population structure but it has only moderate discriminatory power and is expensive. For local outbreak investigations, PFGE has been widely used and it is highly discriminatory but technically demanding. Assessing the gene encoding the staphylococcal surface protein A (*spa* typing) has become popular for typing MRSA and finally typing the *SCCmec* elements is used for the study of international MRSA transmission and evolution.

## Treatment

### Susceptibility to antibiotics

*Staph. aureus* and other staphylococci are inherently susceptible to many antimicrobial agents (Table 15.3). About 90% of strains found in hospitals are now resistant to benzylpenicillin due to the production of the enzyme penicillinase, a β-lactamase that opens the β-lactam ring. Methicillin (previously used for laboratory testing and initially when first produced for therapy), oxacillin, cloxacillin and flucloxacillin, are stable to the enzyme. Cephalosporins and β-lactamase inhibitors are also stable to penicillinase (see Ch. 5).

MRSA strains are resistant to all β-lactam agents, and often to other agents such as the aminoglycosides and fluoroquinolones. Glycopeptides (vancomycin or teicoplanin) are the agents of choice in the treatment of systemic infection with MRSA, but these agents are relatively expensive and may be toxic. Isolates of MRSA with reduced susceptibility or full resistance to glycopeptide antibiotics are uncommon, but have been detected sporadically. These isolates have either thickened cell walls (reduced susceptibility) or the *vanA* gene (fully resistant), and can be difficult to detect in the routine diagnostic laboratory.

### Choice of antibiotic for therapy

Pending receipt of susceptibility test results, the treatment of severe infections suspected to be caused by *Staph. aureus* should be started with flucloxacillin

**Table 15.3** Antibiotics and staphylococci

| Active agents | Agents lacking useful activity |
|---|---|
| Penicillins[a] (e.g. flucloxacillin) | Aztreonam |
| Cephalosporins (e.g. cefuroxime) | Polymyxins |
| Aminoglycosides[b] (e.g. gentamicin) | Mecillinam |
| Tetracyclines (e.g. doxycycline) | Nitroimidazoles |
| Macrolides (e.g. clarithromycin) | Quinolones[c] |
| Lincosamides (clindamycin) | |
| Glycopeptides (vancomycin & teicoplanin) | |
| Fluoroquinolones[c] (moxifloxacin) | |
| Rifampicin[b] | |
| Fusidic acid[b] | |
| Trimethoprim | |
| Chloramphenicol | |
| Carbapenems (e.g. meropenem) | |
| Oxazolidinones (linezolid) | |
| Lipopeptide (daptomycin) | |

[a]Resistance common (see text).
[b]Usually used in combination, for example with flucloxacillin.
[c]For categorization of quinolones, see Table 5.3 and associated text.

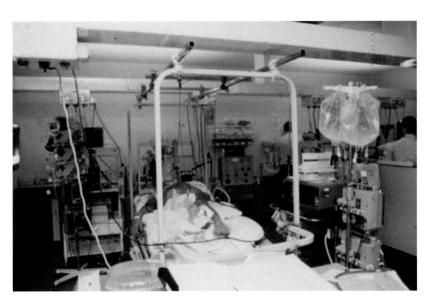

**Fig. 15.3** Patients in the intensive care unit who require multi-organ support are at particular risk of MRSA.

unless MRSA is endemic locally, in which case a glyc- opeptide such as vancomycin is indicated. Erythromy- cin, clindamycin or vancomycin (or teicoplanin) is indicated if the patient is allergic to penicillin. Fusidic acid and rifampicin are not used alone in serious infec- tions, because mutation to resistance arises readily. It is usually necessary to remove an infected source, such as a central intravascular catheter or device, e.g. artificial hip joint, or drain an abscess as part of the treatment.

Other agents have emerged in the last decade and provide alternatives for the treatment of MRSA and can also be used to treat infections caused by isolates with reduced susceptibility to the glycopep- tides. These include linezolid, which can be adminis- tered parenterally and orally and daptomycin which is bactericidal and is used to treat MRSA BSI. New agents being assessed are glycopeptide derivatives such as telavancin and anti-MRSA beta-lactams such as ceftobiprole.

Life-threatening toxin-mediated disease, such as toxic shock syndrome, requires major medical support such as intravenous fluids to prevent multi-organ failure, often best provided in the intensive care unit (Fig. 15.3).

## COAGULASE-NEGATIVE STAPHYLOCOCCI

Coagulase-negative staphylococci comprise a large group of related species commonly found on the surface of healthy persons, in whom they are rarely the cause of infection. More than 40 species are recognized. *Staph. epidermidis* accounts for about 75% of all clinical isolates, probably reflecting its pre- ponderance on the normal skin. Other important CNS include *Staph. saprophyticus* (a cause of urinary infection in young women) and *Staph. lugdunensis* (may cause severe infections like *Staph. aureus*). The emergence of CNS as major pathogens reflects the increased use of implants such as intravascular lines and cannulae, cardiac valves, artificial joints, etc and the increasing numbers of severely debilitated patients in hospitals.

### Description

Coagulase-negative staphylococci are morphologi- cally similar to *Staph. aureus* but they do not coagu- late plasma and they lack clumping factor and deoxyribonuclease. Because *Staph. epidermidis* and other CNS may contaminate clinical specimens, care has to be exercised in assessing its significance, espe- cially from superficial sites. When isolated from sites such as blood or cerebrospinal fluid, further specimens should be obtained to confirm its clinical significance.

Coagulase-negative staphylococci are opportunistic pathogens that cause infection in debilitated or com- promised patients such as premature neonates and oncology patients, often by colonizing biomedical devices such as intravascular lines. They cause par- ticular problems in:

- cardiac surgery (prosthetic valve endocarditis)
- patients fitted with cerebrospinal fluid shunts (meningitis)

- continuous ambulatory peritoneal dialysis (peritonitis)
- immunocompromised patients (e.g. bloodstream infection)
- intensive care units (multiple devices leading to septic shock).

## Pathogenesis

Adherence to the prosthetic device by the production of an exopolysaccharide intercellular adhesion (PIA) is a key step in the formation of a multi-layered biofilm, essential for the pathogenesis of device-related *Staph. epidermidis* infection. A complex array of inter-related chemical messengers controls expression of polysaccharide and drives intercellular adhesion and biofilm formation. Physiological changes in the bio-film protect *Stap. epidermidis* from the host immune defence system and restricted penetration, decreased growth rates and persistent bacterial cells as part of the biofilm often render antibiotic treatment unsuc-cessful. Consequently, there is considerable interest in the development of antimicrobial-impregnated devices such as central intravascular catheters or the use of materials that are less prone to adherence by

*Staph. epidermidis* and subsequent biofilm formation. Important factors in the pathogenesis of *Stap. sapro-phyticus* infection include a unique adhesion protein that allows it to adhere to uroepithelial cells and the production of urease. Isolates of *Staph. lugdunensis* commonly produce thermostable DNase, lipase and haemolysins, not dissimilar to *Staph. aureus*.

## Treatment

The antibiotic treatment of CNS infections is compli-cated because susceptibility is generally unpredictable. Strains resistant to penicillin, penicillinase-stable pen-icillins, gentamicin, erythromycin and chlorampheni-col are common. If a strain is the cause of systemic infection, vancomycin or teicoplanin should be used. Rifampicin in combination with a glycopeptide is occasionally useful in treating central nervous system infections or device infections associated with a biofilm. Newer agents such as daptomycin and line-zolid may have a role but clinical data is awaited to confirm their efficacy in this setting. Uncomplicated urinary tract infection caused by *Staph. saprophyticus* usually responds to trimethoprim or one of the fluoroquinolones.

### RECOMMENDED READING

Ala'Aldeen D, Hiramatsu K: *Staphylococcus aureus: Molecular and Clinical Aspects*, Chichester, 2004, Horwood Publishing.
DeLeo FR, Diep BA, Otto M: Host defense and pathogenesis in *Staphylococcus aureus* infections, *Infectious Diseases Clinics of North America* 23:17–34, 2009.
DeLeo FR, Otto M, Kreiswirth BN, Chambers HF: Community-associated meticillin-resistant *Staphylococcus aureus*, *Lancet* 375:1557–1568, 2010.
Kluytmans J, Struelens M: Meticillin resistant *Staphylococcus aureus* in the hospital, *British Medical Journal* 338:532–537, 2009.
Lowy FD: *Staphylococcus aureus* infections, *New England Journal of Medicine* 339:520–532, 1998.
McCann MT, Gilmore B, Gorman SP: *Staphylococcus epidermidis* device-related infections: pathogenesis and clinical management, *Journal of Pharmacy and Pharmacology* 60:1551–1571, 2008.

Rogers KL, Fey PD, Rupp ME: Coagulase-negative staphylococcal infections, *Infectious Diseases Clinics of North America* 23:73–98, 2009.
Working Party Report: Revised guidelines for the control of meticillin-resistant *Staphylococcus aureus* infection in hospitals, *Journal of Hospital Infection* 63(Suppl 1):S1–S44, 2006.

### Websites

European Antimicrobial Resistance Surveillance Network (EARS-Net): http://www.ecdc.europa.eu/en/activities/surveillance/EARS-Net/
UK Health Protection Agency: *Staphylococcus aureus*, http://www.hpa.org.uk/Topics/InfectiousDiseases/InfectionsAZ/StaphylococcusAureus/

# 16 Streptococcus and enterococcus

Pharyngitis; scarlet fever; skin and soft tissue infections; streptococcal toxic shock syndrome; pneumonia; meningitis; urinary tract infections; rheumatic fever; post–streptococcal glomerulonephritis

*M. Kilian*

## KEY POINTS

- *Str. pyogenes* (group A streptococcus) is among the most prevalent of human bacterial pathogens.
- *Str. pyogenes* and group C and G streptococcal infections range from sore throat, scarlet fever and superficial skin infections to invasive soft tissue infections and septicaemia.
- *Str. pyogenes* and pyogenic group C and G streptococci produce several superantigenic extracellular toxins that are involved in the pathogenesis of the rash associated with scarlet fever and streptococcal toxic shock syndrome.
- Rheumatic fever and acute glomerulonephritis are potential immune-mediated sequelae of infections with *Str. pyogenes*.
- *Str. agalactiae* (group B streptococci) causes neonatal septicaemia and meningitis.
- *Str. pneumoniae* is the principal cause of pneumonia, middle ear infections and meningitis and is one of the four most frequent causes of fatal infections worldwide.
- Commensal streptococci of the oral cavity are among the most frequent causes of subacute bacterial endocarditis.

Streptococci is the general term for a diverse collection of Gram-positive cocci that typically grow as chains or pairs (Greek: *streptos* = pliant or chain; *coccos* = a grain or berry) (Fig. 16.1). Virtually all of the streptococci that are important in human medicine and dentistry fall into the genera *Streptococcus* and *Enterococcus*. Occasional opportunistic infections are associated with other genera of streptococci, such as *Peptostreptococcus* (see Ch. 36) and *Abiotrophia* ('nutritionally variant streptococci').

Streptococci are generally strong fermenters of carbohydrates, resulting in the production of lactic acid, a property responsible for the involvement of some oral streptococci in the decalcification of teeth, i.e. dental caries, and also used in the dairy industry. Most are facultative anaerobes, although peptostreptococci are obligate anaerobes. Streptococci do not produce spores and are non-motile. They are catalase negative.

## CLASSIFICATION

The genus *Streptococcus* includes important pathogens and commensals of mucosal membranes of the upper respiratory tract and, for some species, the intestines. The genus *Enterococcus*, which is also an intestinal commensal, is related to the other streptococci, but is classified separately.

The genus *Streptococcus* includes more than 70 species. With few exceptions, the individual species are exclusively associated, as either pathogens or commensals, with man or a particular animal. The genus consists of five clusters of species (Table 16.1), each of which is characterized by distinct pathogenic potential and other properties:

- The *pyogenic* (pus generating) group includes most species that are overt human and animal pathogens.
- The *mitis* group includes commensals of the human oral cavity and pharynx, although one of the species, *Streptococcus pneumoniae*, is also one of the most important human pathogens.
- The *anginosus* and *salivarius* groups are part of the commensal microbiota of the oral cavity and pharynx.
- The *bovis* group belongs in the colon.
- The *mutans* group of streptococci colonizes exclusively the tooth surfaces of man and some animals; some species belonging to this cluster are involved in the development of dental caries.

Virtually all of the commensal species, including the enterococci, are opportunistic pathogens, primarily if

**Fig. 16.1** Scanning electron micrograph of (A) *Str. pyogenes* showing typical chain formation (original magnification ×2000) and (B) *Str. pneumoniae* showing typical diplococcus formation (original magnification ×7000). Courtesy of AP Shelton, University Hospital, Nottingham.

they gain access to the bloodstream from the oral cavity or from the gut.

## Haemolytic activity

Early attempts to distinguish between pathogenic and commensal streptococci recognized different types of reactions around colonies on blood agar plates. Colonies of streptococci belonging to the Pyogenic group are generally surrounded by a clear zone, usually several millimetres in diameter, caused by lysis of red blood cells in the agar medium induced by bacterial haemolysins. This is called *β-haemolysis* and constitutes the principal marker for potentially pathogenic streptococci in cultures of throat swabs or other clinical samples. Accordingly, the pyogenic streptococci are also referred to as *haemolytic streptococci*.

In contrast, most commensal streptococci give rise to a green discoloration around colonies on blood agar. This phenomenon is termed *α-haemolysis*, although not caused by haemolysis. The factor causing the green discoloration is hydrogen peroxide, which oxidizes haemoglobin to the green methaemoglobin.

Collectively, commensal streptococci are often called '*viridans streptococci*', which refers to their α-haemolytic property (*viridis* = green). Not quite logically, this term also includes the few streptococci, such as those of the salivarius and mutans groups, that induce neither α- nor β-haemolysis. Moreover, in common usage, the term excludes *Str. pneumoniae*, although this species is also α-haemolytic.

**Table 16.1** *Streptococcus* species of clinical importance

| Phylogenetic group | Species | Lancefield group | Type of haemolysis[a] |
|---|---|---|---|
| Pyogenic group | *Str. pyogenes* | A | β |
| | *Str. agalactiae* | B | β |
| | *Str. equisimilis* | C, G | β |
| Mitis group | *Str. pneumoniae* | O | α |
| | *Str. mitis* | O | α |
| | *Str. oralis* | Not designated | α |
| | *Str. sanguinis* | H | α |
| Anginosus group | *Str. anginosus* | C, G, F (and A) | α or β |
| | *Str. intermedius* | Not designated | α |
| Bovis group | '*Str. bovis*' | D | α or none |
| Mutans group | *Str. mutans* | Not designated | None |
| | *Str. sobrinus* | Not designated | None |

[a]On horse blood agar.

## Lancefield grouping

An important method of distinguishing between pyogenic streptococci is the serological classification pioneered by the American bacteriologist Rebecca Lancefield, who detected different versions of the major cell wall polysaccharide among the pyogenic streptococci.

This polysaccharide can be extracted from streptococci with hot hydrochloric acid and the different forms can be distinguished by precipitation with specific antibodies raised in rabbits. The polysaccharide is referred to as the group polysaccharide and

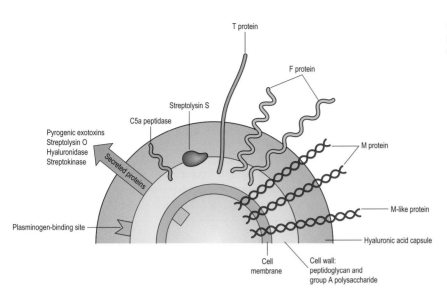

**Fig. 16.2** Schematic diagram showing the location of virulence-associated products of *Str. pyogenes*.

identifies a number of different serological groups labelled by capital letters (Lancefield groups A, B, C, etc.). Among the pyogenic streptococci, some serological groups are identical to distinct species (Table 16.1).

## STREPTOCOCCUS PYOGENES

This species, which consists of Lancefield group A streptococci, is among the most prevalent of human bacterial pathogens. It is associated exclusively with human infections. It causes a wide range of suppurative infections in the respiratory tract and skin, life-threatening soft tissue infections, and certain types of toxin-associated reactions. Some of these infections may, in addition, result in severe non-suppurative sequelae due to adverse immunological reactions induced by the infecting streptococci. A similar spectrum of infections may be caused by the closely related group C and group G streptococcis (*Str. equisimilis,* also known as *Str. dysgalactiae subspecies equisimilis*).

Some of the infections caused by *Str. pyogenes* resemble those caused by *Staphylococcus aureus*, but the clinical characteristics associated with these two groups of pyogenic cocci are often distinct. Similarities and differences can be explained by the virulence factors expressed by the two species.

## Pathogenesis

### Virulence factors

Strains of *Str. pyogenes* express a large arsenal of virulence factors involved in adherence, evasion of host immunity, and tissue damage (Fig. 16.2). Although some factors are expressed by all clinical isolates, others are variably present among *Str. pyogenes* strains. This variation is due to the horizontal transfer of virulence genes among strains, primarily by bacteriophages (transduction, see p. 75), and probably explains the temporal variations in the prevalence of severe infections and sequelae. It furthermore explains differences in the virulence of individual strains and, to some extent, the different clinical pictures that may be associated with infections due to *Str. pyogenes*. Many of the virulence factors of *Str. pyogenes* are also expressed by some of the other species of pyogenic streptococci. In some species pathogenic for animals the corresponding virulence factors are expressed in a form specifically adapted to interact with a particular host.

*Adhesion.* Interaction with host fibronectin, a matrix protein on eukaryotic cells, is considered the principal mechanism by which *Str. pyogenes* binds to epithelial cells of the pharynx and skin. The structure that recognizes host fibronectin is located on the F protein, which is one of the many proteins expressed on the surface of *Str. pyogenes* (Fig. 16.2). The interaction between the streptococcal F protein and host cell fibronectin also mediates internalization of the bacteria into host cells.

In addition to the F protein, surface-exposed lipoteichoic acid and M proteins appear to be involved in adherence to mucosal and skin epithelial cells.

*M proteins.* The ability of *Str. pyogenes* to resist phagocytosis by polymorphonuclear leucocytes is largely due to the cell-surface exposed M protein. The M protein is anchored in the cytoplasmic membrane, spans the entire cell wall, and protrudes from the cell surface as fibrils (Fig. 16.2). Some strains produce two different M proteins with antiphagocytic activity, and some an additional structurally related M-like protein. All of these proteins can bind various plasma proteins of the host, including fibrinogen, plasminogen, albumin, immunoglobulin (Ig) G, IgA, the proteinase inhibitor $\alpha_2$-macroglobulin and some regulatory factors from the complement system (factor H and C4b-binding protein). As well as masking the bacterial surface with host proteins, some of these affinities are responsible for the ability of M proteins to resist phagocytosis. Thus, factor H can destabilize the important opsonin C3b when deposited on the bacterial surface. Likewise, the C4b-binding protein inhibits surface complement deposition by stimulating degradation of both C4b and C3b.

*Str. pyogenes* can release some of the M proteins with its own cysteine protease. If shed into the circulation the M protein forms complexes with fibrinogen, which by indirect pathways induces the release of inflammatory mediators from neutrophils. This process plays an important role in the leakage of plasma into the tissues and lungs, and the ensuing low blood pressure seen in some invasive infections with *Str. pyogenes*.

Acquired resistance to infection by *Str. pyogenes* is the result of antibodies to the M protein molecule in secretions and plasma. However, as a result of genetic polymorphism in the gene encoding the M protein, the most distal part of the protein shows extensive variability among strains. As a consequence, individuals may suffer from recurrent *Str. pyogenes* infections with strains expressing different versions of the M protein. More than 150 different types of M protein have been identified by serological means and gene sequencing.

*Capsule.* Some strains of *Str. pyogenes* form a capsule composed of hyaluronic acid. Such strains grow as mucoid colonies on blood agar and are highly virulent in animal models. Although capsule production is rare among isolates from uncomplicated pharyngitis, a significant proportion of isolates from severe infections have a capsule. Like other bacterial capsules, the capsule has an antiphagocytic effect. The relative significance of the M protein and the capsule as antiphagocytic factors differs among strains.

The capsule is identical to the hyaluronic acid of the connective tissue of the host and is not immunogenic. In this way the bacteria can disguise themselves with an immunological 'self' substance.

*C5a peptidase.* The C5a peptidase, which is also found in most human pathogenic strains of *Str. agalactiae*, is present on the surface of all strains of *Str. pyogenes*. It specifically cleaves, and thereby inactivates, human C5a, one of the principal chemoattractants of phagocytic cells.

*Streptolysins.* *Str. pyogenes* produces two distinct haemolysins, termed streptolysins O (oxygen labile) and S (serum soluble), both of which lyse erythrocytes, polymorphonuclear leucocytes and platelets by forming pores in their cell membrane.

Streptolysin O belongs to a family of haemolysins found in many pathogenic bacteria. Intravenous injection into experimental animals causes death within seconds, as the result of an acute toxic action on the heart. Serum antibodies can be demonstrated after streptococcal infection, particularly after severe infections.

Streptolysin S is responsible for the β-haemolysis around colonies on blood agar plates. It can also induce the release of lysosomal contents with subsequent cell death after engulfment by phagocytes. In contrast to streptolysin O, it is not immunogenic.

*Pyrogenic exotoxins.* Most strains of *Str. pyogenes* produce one or more toxins that are called *pyrogenic* (fever generating) *exotoxins* because of their ability to induce fever. Three, designated SPE-A, SPE-B and SPE-C, have been characterized extensively, but there are several others. Purified SPE-A causes death when injected into rabbits and is the most toxic of the three, but SPE-B also causes myocardial necrosis and death in experimental animals.

The genes for SPE-A and SPE-C are transmitted between strains by bacteriophage, and stable production depends on lysogenic conversion in a manner analogous to toxin production by *Corynebacterium diphtheriae* (see p. 75). Even among strains that possess the genes, the quantity of toxin secreted varies dramatically.

SPE-A and SPE-C are also called erythrogenic toxins, as they are responsible for the rash observed in patients with scarlatina. They are genetically related to *Staph. aureus* enterotoxins and, like these, have superantigen activity. By cross-linking MHC class II molecules on antigen-presenting cells and the Vβ domain of the antigen receptor on a subset of T lymphocytes, these toxins cause comprehensive (antigen independent) activation of regulatory T lymphocytes. The result is massive release of pro-inflammatory cytokines such as interleukin (IL)-1 and IL-2, tumour necrosis factor (TNF)-α and interferon-γ. These cytokines may cause a variety of clinical signs, including inflammation, hypotensive shock and organ failure seen in some patients with severe streptococcal disease. The different clinical outcome of infections with the same *Str. pyogenes* strain appears to be due to the fact that the toxins bind preferentially to certain major histocompatibility complex (MHC) class II tissue types.

Unlike SPE-A and SPE-C, all strains of *Str. pyogenes* produce SPE-B, which is a potent cysteine proteinase capable of cleaving many host proteins.

None of the pyrogenic exotoxins is associated unambiguously with any of the clinical syndromes caused by *Str. pyogenes*. However, most isolates from episodes of severe invasive disease and toxic shock-like syndrome produce SPE-A, and the protease SPE-B appears to be responsible for the extensive tissue destruction observed in many patients with severe invasive infections, including necrotizing fasciitis.

*Hyaluronidase.* *Str. pyogenes* and several other pyogenic streptococci use a secreted hyaluronidase to degrade hyaluronic acid, the ground substance of host connective tissue. This property may facilitate the spread of infection along fascial planes. During infections, particularly those involving the skin, serum antibody titres to hyaluronidase show a significant rise.

*Streptokinase.* Streptokinase, also known as fibrinolysin, is another spreading factor. It is expressed by all strains of *Str. pyogenes* and cooperates with a surface-expressed plasminogen-binding site on the bacteria. Once host plasminogen is bound to the bacterial surface, it is activated to plasmin by streptokinase. Thus, in contrast to *Staph. aureus*, which aims at hiding behind a wall of coagulated plasma (fibrin), *Str. pyogenes* employs host plasmin to hinder the build-up of fibrin barriers. As a result, soft tissue infections due to *Str. pyogenes* are more diffuse, and often rapidly spreading, than the well localized abscesses that typify staphylococcal infections.

*Deoxyribonucleases (DNAases).* At least four distinct forms of DNAases are produced by *Str. pyogenes*. The enzymes hydrolyse nucleic acids and allows the bacteria to escape from the DNA net released from phagocytes ('neutrophil extracellular traps').

## Clinical features

Although a general decrease in the prevalence of serious infections with *Str. pyogenes* has occurred since the mid nineteenth century, there has been a resurgence in severe streptococcal infections and increased mortality due to streptococcal sepsis since the early 1980s.

The most common route of entry of *Str. pyogenes* is the upper respiratory tract, which is usually the primary site of infection and also serves as a focus for other types of infection. Spread from person to person is by respiratory droplets or by direct contact with infected wounds or sores on the skin. Not all individuals colonized by *Str. pyogenes* in the upper respiratory tract develop clinical signs of infection.

After an acute upper respiratory tract infection, the convalescent patient may carry the infecting streptococci for some weeks. Only a few healthy adults carry *Str. pyogenes* in the respiratory tract, but the carriage rate in young school children is just over 10%. It may be considerably higher before or during an epidemic.

### Non-invasive streptococcal disease

The most common infections caused by *Str. pyogenes* are relatively mild and non-invasive infections of the upper respiratory tract (*pharyngitis*) and skin (*impetigo*). In the USA more than 10 million cases of non-invasive *Str. pyogenes* infection are estimated to occur annually.

*Pharyngitis.* This is the most common infection caused by *Str. pyogenes*. Clinical signs such as abrupt onset of sore throat, fever, malaise and headache generally develop 2–4 days after exposure to the pathogen. The posterior pharynx is usually diffusely reddened, with enlarged tonsils that may show patches of grey–white exudate on their surface and, sometimes, accumulations of pus in the crypts. The local inflammation results in swelling of cervical lymph nodes. Occasionally, tonsillar abscesses develop; this is a very painful condition and potentially dangerous as the pathogen may spread to neighbouring regions and to the bloodstream.

Despite the significant symptoms and clinical signs, differentiating streptococcal pharyngitis ('*strep throat*') from viral pharyngitis is impossible without microbiological or serological examination. Culture studies show that 20–30% of cases of pharyngitis are associated with *Str. pyogenes* and *Str. equisimilis*.

*Scarlet fever.* Pharyngitis caused by certain pyrogenic exotoxin-producing strains of *Str. pyogenes* may be associated with a diffuse erythematous rash of the skin and mucous membranes (Fig. 16.3). The condition is known as *scarlet fever* or *scarlatina*. The rash develops within 1–2 days after the first symptoms of pharyngitis and initially appears on the upper chest, then spreading to the extremities. After an initial phase with a yellowish-white coating, the tongue becomes red and denuded ('*strawberry tongue*').

Between 1860 and 1870 the mean annual death rate from scarlet fever in England and Wales was close to 2500 per million of the population. Since then a steady decline in incidence has been observed. By the end of the twentieth century the number of scarlet fever cases in England and Wales had fallen below 25 per million, and death is now extremely rare.

**Fig. 16.3**    The characteristic erythematous rash on (A) tongue and (B) skin associated with scarlet fever.

**Fig. 16.4**    Impetigo. Courtesy of Dr LG Millard, Queen's Medical Centre, Nottingham.

***Skin infections.*** *Str. pyogenes* may cause several types of skin infection, sometimes in association with *Staph. aureus*. The superficial and localized skin infection, known as *impetigo* or *pyoderma*, occurs mainly in children (Fig. 16.4). It primarily affects exposed areas on the face, arms or legs. The skin becomes colonized after contact with an infected person and the bacteria enter the skin through small defects. Initially, clear vesicles develop, which within a few days become pus filled. Secondary spread is often seen as a result of scratching.

Potentially more severe is the acute skin infection *erysipelas* (*erythros* = red; *pella* = skin), which occurs in the superficial layers of the skin (cellulitis) and involves the lymphatics. The infection is characterized by diffuse redness of the skin, and patients experience local pain, enlargement of regional lymph nodes and fever. Untreated, the infection may spread to the bloodstream, and was often fatal before antibiotics became available.

### Invasive soft tissue infections

Severe, sometimes life-threatening, *Str. pyogenes* infections may occur when the bacteria get into normally sterile parts of the body. The most severe forms of invasive infections are *necrotizing fasciitis*, streptococcal *toxic shock syndrome* and *puerperal fever*, all of which are associated with bacteraemia.

Worldwide, rates of invasive infection increased from the mid 1980s to the early 1990s. In 2002, around 9000 cases of invasive *Str. pyogenes* infection occurred in the USA. Although these infections may occur in previously healthy individuals, patients with chronic illnesses such as cancer and diabetes, and those on kidney dialysis or receiving steroids, have a higher risk. Even with antibiotic treatment death occurs in 10–13% of all invasive cases: 45% of patients with toxic shock syndrome and 25% of patients with necrotizing fasciitis.

***Necrotizing fasciitis.*** This infection progresses very rapidly, destroying fat and fascia. Although *Str. pyogenes* gains entry to these tissues through the skin after trauma, often of a minor nature, the skin itself may show only minimal signs of infection and may indeed be spared (Fig. 16.5). Systemic shock and

**Fig. 16.5** Necrotizing fasciitis (A) before and (B) after surgical exploration and debridement. Courtesy of Dr M Llewelyn, reproduced with permission from Elsevier.

general deterioration occur very quickly. The disease affects the fit young person with no obvious underlying pathology, as well as the immunocompromised.

The clinical diagnosis may be difficult because *Staph. aureus* and anaerobes such as *Clostridium perfringens* can produce a similar clinical picture. Streptococci can be isolated from the blood, blister fluid and cultures of the infected area.

*Streptococcal toxic shock syndrome.* Patients with invasive and bacteraemic *Str. pyogenes* infections, and in particular necrotizing fasciitis, may develop streptococcal toxic shock syndrome. The disease, which was first described in the late 1980s, is the result of the release of streptococcal toxins to the bloodstream. A striking feature of this acute fulminating disease is severe pain at the site of initial infection, usually the soft tissues. The additional clinical signs resemble those of staphylococcal toxic shock syndrome (see p. 178) and include fever, malaise, nausea, vomiting and diarrhoea, dizziness, confusion and a flat rash over large parts of the body. Without treatment, the disease progresses to shock and general organ failure.

*Other suppurative infections.* Historically, *Str. pyogenes* has been an important cause of puerperal sepsis. However, since the introduction of antibiotic therapy, this and other suppurative infections such as lymphangitis, pneumonia and meningitis are relatively rare.

*Bacteraemia.* *Str. pyogenes* is the second most common (after *Str. agalactiae*) of the pyogenic streptococci isolated from blood cultures. Bacteraemia is seen regularly in patients with necrotizing fasciitis and toxic shock syndrome, but rarely as a complication to pharyngitis and local skin infections. Once in the blood, *Str. pyogenes* multiplies with incredible speed (doubling time 18 min), and the mortality rate approaches 40%. The potential complications include acute endocarditis leading to heart failure.

## Non-suppurative sequelae

Two serious diseases may develop as sequelae to *Str. pyogenes* infections:

1. *Rheumatic fever*, a potential sequela to pharyngitis (including scarlet fever).
2. *Acute glomerulonephritis*, which is primarily, but not exclusively, associated with skin infections.

Both are caused by immune reactions induced by the streptococcal infection. The first clinical signs appear 1–5 weeks after the infection and at a time when the bacteria may have been eradicated by the immune system or as a result of antibiotic therapy.

Clinical correlations suggest that certain forms of *psoriasis* may also be triggered by *Str. pyogenes* throat infection. Preliminary evidence supports the hypothesis that some streptococcal superantigens cause disruption of immunological tolerance of a CD8[+] T cell subset that recognizes cross-reactive epitopes on M proteins and skin keratin.

*Rheumatic fever.* This manifests as an inflammation of the joints (arthritis), heart (carditis), central nervous system (chorea), skin (erythema marginatum) and/or subcutaneous nodules. Polyarticular arthritis is the most common manifestation, whereas carditis is the most serious as it leads to permanent damage, particularly of the heart valves.

Rheumatic fever is a major cause of acquired heart disease in young people throughout the world. The incidence of rheumatic heart disease worldwide ranges from 0.5 to 11 per 1000 of the population. New cases are relatively rare in most of Europe, but increased incidences have been observed among the aboriginal populations of Australia and New Zealand, and in Hawaii and Sri Lanka. Outbreaks of rheumatic fever have also been seen in the USA.

The disease is autoimmune in nature and is believed to result from the production of autoreactive (and polyspecific) antibodies and T lymphocytes induced by cross-reactive components of the bacteria and host tissues. Therefore, repeated episodes of *Str. pyogenes* infection increase the severity of the disease. The major antigens involved are myosin, tropomyosin, laminin and keratin in the human tissues, and the group A antigen (a polymer of *N*-acetylglucosamine) in the *Str. pyogenes* cell wall in addition to epitopes on some variants of surface M proteins.

***Acute post-streptococcal glomerulonephritis.*** The clinical manifestations include:

- coffee-coloured urine caused by haematuria
- oedema of the face and extremities
- circulatory congestion caused by renal impairment.

Unlike rheumatic disease, outbreaks of post-streptococcal acute glomerulonephritis have continued to decline in most parts of the world. Regions that still exhibit a high incidence of this disease include Africa, the Caribbean, South America, New Zealand and Kuwait.

Post-streptococcal glomerulonephritis is usually referred to as an immune complex-mediated disease. However, the exact pathogenesis is not clear. Several mechanisms have been proposed, including:

- immune complex deposition in the glomeruli
- reaction of antibodies cross-reactive with streptococcal and glomerular antigens
- alterations of glomerular tissues by streptococcal products such as streptokinase
- direct complement activation by streptococcal components that have a direct affinity for glomerular tissues.

Disease is associated with a limited number of M types of *Str. pyogenes*, and there is evidence that particular variants of streptokinase are crucial nephritogenic factors.

Unlike rheumatic fever, there is a general absence of individual recurrences, suggesting that antibodies to nephritogenic factors protect against disease rather than the opposite.

## STREPTOCOCCUS AGALACTIAE

*Str. agalactiae* is equivalent to Lancefield group B streptococci. Its primary human habitat is the colon. It may be carried in the throat and, importantly, 10–40% of women intermittently carry *Str. agalactiae* in the vagina.

Previously, *Str. agalactiae* was recognized primarily as a cause of bovine mastitis (*agalactia*, want of milk). However, since 1960 it has become the leading cause of neonatal infections in industrialized countries and is also an important cause of morbidity among peripartum women and non-pregnant adults with chronic medical conditions. Among β-haemolytic streptococci, *Str. agalactiae* is the most frequent isolate from blood cultures.

### Pathogenesis

#### Virulence factors

*Str. agalactiae* produces several virulence factors, including haemolysins, capsule polysaccharide, C5a peptidase (only human pathogenic strains), hyaluronidase (not all strains), and various surface proteins that bind human IgA and serve as adhesins.

Ten different types of the capsular polysaccharide have been identified (Ia, Ib and II–IX). The serotype most frequently associated with neonatal infections is type III, whereas infections in adults are more evenly distributed over the different serotypes.

Among the haemolysins produced by *Str. agalactiae*, one, known as the CAMP factor (so-called because it was originally described by Christie, Atkins and Munch-Petersen), plays an important role in the recognition of this species in the laboratory. The CAMP factor lyses sheep or bovine red blood cells pretreated with the β-toxin of *Staph. aureus* (Fig. 16.6). Purified CAMP factor protein is fatal to rabbits when injected intravenously.

### Clinical features

#### Infection in the neonate

Two different entities are recognized:

1. *Early-onset disease*, most cases of which present at or within 12 h of birth.
2. *Late-onset disease*, presenting more than 7 days and up to 3 months after birth.

***Early-onset disease.*** This results from ascending spread of *Str. agalactiae* from the vagina into the

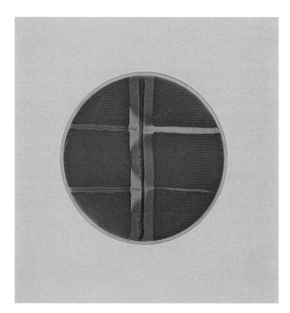

**Fig. 16.6** Blood agar culture of strains of *Str. pyogenes* (group A) (upper right), *Str. equisimilis* (group C) (lower right) and *Str. agalactiae* (group B) (upper and lower left) surrounding a vertical streak of *Staph. aureus*. The two *Str. agalactiae* strains show a positive CAMP reaction.

amniotic fluid, which is then aspirated by the infant and results in septicaemia in the infant or the mother, or both. Infants borne by mothers carrying *Str. agalactiae* may also become colonized during passage through the vagina.

Depending on the site of initial contamination, neonates may be ill at birth or develop acute and fulminating illness a few hours, or a day or two, later. The clinical symptoms include lethargy, cyanosis and apnoea; when septicaemia progresses, shock ensues and death will occur if treatment is not instituted quickly. Meningitis and pulmonary infection may be associated.

As a result of improved recognition and prompt treatment of babies with symptoms, the fatality rate has been reduced to less than 10%. However, considerable morbidity persists among some survivors, especially those with meningitis.

Risk factors for neonatal colonization and infection are:

- premature rupture of membranes
- prolonged labour
- premature delivery
- low birth-weight
- intrapartum fever.

The immune status of the mother, and hence the level of maternal IgG antibodies in the infant, appears to be more important than the degree of colonization of the mother's genital tract by *Str. agalactiae*.

It is possible that *Str. agalactiae* itself may cause premature rupture of membranes as a result of secretion of proteases and activation of local inflammation.

***Late-onset disease.*** Purulent meningitis is the most common manifestation, but septic arthritis, osteomyelitis, conjunctivitis, sinusitis, otitis media, endocarditis and peritonitis also occur. The incidence of invasive infection is higher among pre-term infants than among those born at term.

The pathogenesis is distinct from that of early-onset disease. There is usually no history of obstetric complications and the disease is unrelated to vaginal colonization in the mother. Many cases are acquired in hospital. Ward staff can be carriers of *Str. agalactiae*, and contamination of the baby may occur during nursing procedures, with subsequent baby-to-baby spread. Mastitis in the mother has also been described as a source of infection.

### Infections in the adult

Ascending spread of *Str. agalactiae* leading to amniotic infection may result in abortion, chorioamnionitis, post-partum sepsis (endometritis) and other infections (e.g. pneumonia) in the postpartum period in young, previously healthy women.

*Str. agalactiae* is also a frequent cause of infection in certain risk groups of non-pregnant adults. Disease may manifest as sepsis, pneumonia, soft tissue infections such as cellulitis and arthritis, and urinary tract infections complicated by bacteraemia. The risk factors in these patients are diabetes mellitus, liver cirrhosis, renal failure, stroke and cancer. Older age, independent of underlying medical conditions, increases the risk of invasive *Str. agalactiae* infection.

## OTHER PYOGENIC STREPTOCOCCI

*Str. suis* serotype 2 (group R streptococci) cause septicaemia and meningitis in pigs. They belong to a phylogenetic lineage separate from the other pyogenic streptococci. They occasionally infect people in contact with contaminated pork or infected pigs, and may cause septicaemia, meningitis and respiratory tract infections. Abattoir workers, butchers and, to a lesser extent, those involved in domestic food preparation are at risk.

## *STREPTOCOCCUS PNEUMONIAE*

*Str. pneumoniae*, commonly called the pneumococcus, is a member of the oropharyngeal microbiota of 5–70% of the population, with the highest isolation rate in children during the winter months. In contrast to other streptococci, *Str. pneumoniae* generally occurs as characteristic diplococci (see Fig. 16.1). Although closely related genetically to the commensal *Str. mitis* and *Str. oralis*, *Str. pneumoniae* is one of the four most frequent causes of fatal infections worldwide. It primarily causes disease of the airways and associated tissues (middle ear, paranasal sinuses, mastoids and lung parenchyma), but may spread to other sites, such as the meninges, joints, peritoneum, and endocardium.

*Str. pneumoniae* is genetically very flexible because of frequent recombination between individual strains. Gene transfer is by transformation and may result in the expression of a different capsular serotype. Experimental transfer of capsule genes in pneumococci was the basis of the original demonstration that DNA contains the genetic information in cells.

## Pathogenesis

### Virulence factors

*Capsule.* The capsular polysaccharide is a crucial virulence factor. The capsule is antiphagocytic, inhibiting complement deposition and phagocytosis where type-specific opsonic antibody is absent. A total of 91 different capsular serotypes have been identified.

The serotypes are designated by numbers, and those that are structurally related are grouped together (1, 2, 3, 4, 5, 6A, 6B, etc.). The different serotypes differ in virulence. Thus, about 90% of cases of bacteraemic pneumococcal pneumonia and meningitis are caused by some 23 serotypes.

*IgA1 protease.* Like the two other principal causes of bacterial meningitis (*Neisseria meningitidis* and *Haemophilus influenzae*), pneumococci produce an extracellular protease that specifically cleaves human IgA1 in the hinge region. This protease enables these pathogens to evade the protective functions of the principal immunoglobulin isotype of the upper respiratory tract.

*Pneumolysin.* Pneumococci produce an intracellular membrane-damaging toxin known as pneumolysin, which is released by autolysis. Pneumolysin inhibits:

- neutrophil chemotaxis
- phagocytosis and the respiratory burst

- lymphocyte proliferation and immunoglobulin synthesis.

In experimental models it induces the features of lobar pneumonia and contributes to the mortality associated with this disease.

*Autolysin.* When activated, the pneumococcal autolysin breaks the peptide cross-linking of the cell wall peptidoglycan, leading to lysis of the bacteria. Autolysis enables the release of pneumolysin and, in addition, large amounts of cell wall fragments. The massive inflammatory response to these peptidoglycan fragments is an important component of the pathogenesis of pneumococcal pneumonia and meningitis.

## Clinical features

### Predisposing factors

Most *Str. pneumoniae* infections are associated with various predisposing conditions. Although occasional clusterings of pneumococcal infections are recognized, person-to-person spread is uncommon.

Pneumonia results from aspiration of pneumococci contained in upper airway secretions into the lower respiratory tract; for example when the normal mechanisms of mucus entrapment and expulsion by an intact glottic reflex and mucociliary escalator are impaired. This situation may arise in:

- disturbed consciousness in association with general anaesthesia, convulsions, alcoholism, epilepsy or head trauma
- respiratory viral infections, such as influenza
- chronic bronchitis and other forms of chronic bronchial sepsis.

Other predisposing disease states in which pneumococcal pneumonia may be the terminal event include:

- valvular and ischaemic heart disease
- chronic renal failure
- diabetes mellitus
- bronchogenic and metastatic malignancy
- advancing age.

Immune deficiencies that predispose to pneumococcal infection include:

- hypogammaglobulinaemia
- asplenia or hyposplenism
- malignancies such as multiple myeloma.

In these conditions there is either a relative or absolute deficiency of opsonic antibody activity or an inability to induce a sufficient type-specific antibody response. *Tuftsin*, a naturally occurring tetrapeptide secreted by the spleen, also plays a role in combating pneumococcal sepsis; particularly at risk are those deficient in splenic activity:

- congenital asplenia
- traumatic removal
- functional impairment (e.g. homozygous sickle cell disease).

Human immunodeficiency virus (HIV) infection carries an increased risk of bacterial infections, including those caused by the pneumococcus, particularly in children.

Acute infections of the middle ear and paranasal sinuses occur in otherwise healthy children, but are usually preceded by a viral infection of the upper respiratory tract leading to local inflammation and swelling, and obstruction of the flow from these sites.

## Pneumonia

*Str. pneumoniae* is the most frequent cause of pneumonia. The estimated annual incidence is 1–3 per 1000 of the population, with a 5% case fatality rate. Pneumococcal pneumonia follows aspiration with subsequent migration through the bronchial mucosa to involve the peribronchial lymphatics. The inflammatory reaction is focused primarily within the alveolus of a single lobule or lobe, although multilobar disease can also occur. Contiguous spread commonly results in inflammatory involvement of the pleura; this may progress to empyema.

Pericarditis is an uncommon but well recognized complication. Occasionally, lung necrosis and intrapulmonary abscess formation occur with the more virulent pneumococcal serotypes. Bacteraemia may complicate pneumococcal pneumonia in up to 15% of patients. This can result in metastatic involvement of the meninges, joints and, rarely, the endocardium.

The mortality rate from pneumococcal pneumonia in those admitted to hospital in the UK is approximately 15%. It is increased by age, underlying disease, bloodstream involvement, metastatic infection and certain types of pneumococci with large capsules (e.g. serotype 3).

## Otitis media and sinusitis

Middle ear infections (otitis media) affect approximately half of all children between the ages of 6 months and 3 years; approximately one-third of cases are caused by *Str. pneumoniae*. Disease occurs after acquisition of a new strain to which there is no preexisting immunity. The prevalence is highest among children attending kinder garten or primary school, where there is a constant exchange of pneumococcal strains.

## Meningitis

*Str. pneumoniae* is among the three leading causes of bacterial meningitis. It is assumed that invasion arises from the pharynx to the meninges via the bloodstream, as bacteraemia usually coexists. Meningitis may occasionally complicate pneumococcal infection at other sites, such as the lung and middle ear.

The incidence of pneumococcal meningitis is bimodal and affects children less than 3 years of age and adults of 45 years and above. The fatality rates are 20% and 30%, respectively, considerably higher than those associated with other types of bacterial meningitis.

## COMMENSAL STREPTOCOCCI

### Viridans streptococci

The viridans streptococci, and in particular the species of the mitis and salivarius groups, are dominant members of the resident microbiota of the oral cavity and pharynx in all age groups. They play an important role by inhibiting the colonization of many pathogens, including pyogenic streptococci. This is achieved by two different mechanisms:

1. production of bacteriocins (see p. 35)
2. production of hydrogen peroxide (also responsible for α-haemolysis).

Most strains secrete bacteriocins. Experimental implantation of strains of *Str. salivarius* with strong bacteriocin activity prevents colonization with *Str. pyogenes* in humans.

***Mitis group.*** *Str. mitis*, *Str. oralis* and *Str. sanguinis*, among other viridans streptococci, colonize tooth surfaces as well as mucosal membranes. Because of their presence in the bacterial biofilms (dental plaque) on tooth surfaces, these species may enter the bloodstream during dental procedures such as tooth extraction or vigorous tooth cleaning, particularly when the gingival tissue is inflamed.

In healthy individuals, bacteria of such low virulence are cleared from the circulation within 1 h. However, in patients with various predisposing conditions (Table 16.2), in particular heart valve damage due to post-streptococcal rheumatic fever, the circulating streptococci may settle in a niche protected from phagocytic cells. Local growth on the surface of heart valves eventually causes scarring and functional

**Table 16.2**  Factors predisposing to infective endocarditis

| Cardiac factors | Non-cardiac factors |
| --- | --- |
| Rheumatic heart disease | Dental manipulations[a] |
| Atherosclerotic heart disease | Endoscopy |
| Congenital heart disease | Intravenous drug abuse |
| Cardiac surgery | Intravenous cannulae and shunts |
| Prosthetic heart valves | Sepsis |
| Previous endocarditis | |

[a]Procedures in which bleeding occurs.

deficiency. As the disease progresses over several months, it is referred to as *subacute bacterial endocarditis*. It is usually accompanied by intermittent fever. Disruption of bacteria from the cardiac vegetations may cause embolic abscesses in various organs, including the brain. Until endocarditis due to skin staphylococci became more prevalent as a result of intravenous drug abuse, viridans streptococci were the most frequent causes of infective endocarditis.

*Str. mitis* and *Str. oralis* are increasingly recognized as causes of often fatal septicaemias in immunocompromised patients.

**Mutans group.**  *Str. mutans* and *Str. sobrinus* exclusively colonize tooth enamel and do not occur until tooth eruption. Their proportions in the biofilm forming on tooth surfaces (dental plaque) are closely related to sugar consumption, and they are a major cause of dental caries because of their ability to produce large amounts of lactic acid even at pH values below 5.0. Like most other plaque streptococci they may cause subacute bacterial endocarditis.

**Anginosus group.**  *Str. anginosus* and *Str. intermedius,* among other species, are regular members of the commensal bacteria on tooth surfaces, in particular in the gingival crevices. They are often isolated from abscesses and other opportunistic purulent infections.

**Bovis group.**  Some of the species of this group are present in the human gut. They occasionally cause bacteraemia and subacute endocarditis. These infections are often associated with colonic carcinoma, which jeopardizes the barrier function of the intestinal wall.

## *Enterococcus* species

As indicated by the name, members of the genus *Enterococcus* have their natural habitat in the human intestines. The species most commonly associated with human disease are *E. faecalis* and *E. faecium.* The diseases with which they are associated are:

- urinary tract infection
- infective endocarditis
- biliary tract infections
- suppurative abdominal lesions
- peritonitis.

*E. faecalis* and *E. faecium* are important causes of wound and urinary tract infection in hospital patients and may cause sporadic outbreaks. Bacteraemia carries a poor prognosis as it often occurs in patients with major underlying pathology and in those who are immunocompromised.

## LABORATORY DIAGNOSIS

### Collection of specimens

The diagnosis of streptococcal infections is established by demonstrating the presence of the pathogen in throat or skin swabs, pus, blood cultures, cerebrospinal fluid (CSF), expectorates or urine according to the site of infection. In pneumococcal meningitis the CSF is often macroscopically cloudy. The cell count is usually increased markedly and shows a predominance of polymorphonuclear leucocytes. Typical Gram-positive diplococci can commonly be demonstrated, sometimes in enormous numbers, by Gram-stain examination of a CSF deposit. The appearance is often typical, and a presumptive diagnosis can be made to allow appropriate therapy to be started before the identity of the organism is confirmed by culture.

Blood cultures are of value in patients with invasive streptococcal infections. This is also the case in patients with suspected pneumococcal pneumonia, particularly when this is severe, as up to 15% of patients are bacteraemic. Detection of bacteria by direct plating or microscopy of blood is not feasible owing to their low density.

Other body sites that may merit investigation according to the clinical presentation include joint and peritoneal fluids. Tympanocentesis provides the possibility of establishing the microbial cause of otitis media, but as most of these infections settle spontaneously, or with the assistance of a few days' antibiotic treatment, tympanocentesis is not usually necessary.

### Cultivation and identification

Unlike staphylococci, streptococci lack the enzyme catalase, which releases oxygen from hydrogen peroxide. Catalase-negative Gram-positive cocci are therefore likely to be streptococci. The appearance of cocci in obvious chains (see Fig. 16.1) is another useful criterion, but the length of the chains varies with the species and conditions of growth. Optimal chain formation is seen in broth cultures. There may be marked variation in size and shape, particularly in older cultures or in direct smears from purulent exudates.

The primary cultivation medium for streptococci is blood agar, supplemented, whenever enterococci are suspected, with an agar medium (e.g. MacConkey's medium) selective for enterobacteria. Streptococci of aetiological significance usually predominate in the culture even when the sample is taken from a site with a resident microbiota.

The pyogenic streptococci are detected initially by their β-haemolytic activity. The colonies are about 1 mm in diameter and, in contrast to those of staphylococci, lack pigment. Colonies of pneumococci are α-haemolytic, smooth, and may vary in size according to the amount of capsular polysaccharide produced; those of serotypes 3 and 37 are usually larger than the rest and have a watery or mucoid appearance. During prolonged incubation, autolysis of bacteria within the flat pneumococcal colonies results in a typical subsidence of the centre ('*draughtsman colonies*').

Species identification of pyogenic streptococci is based largely on serological detection of group antigens by immune precipitation or co-agglutination techniques. An additional test that is helpful in the presumptive identification of *Str. pyogenes* is the bacitracin sensitivity test. In contrast to most other streptococci, *Str. pyogenes* is uniformly sensitive and large inhibition zones are formed round bacitracin discs on blood agar. Likewise, *Str. agalactiae* can be identified presumptively by the CAMP reaction (see Fig. 16.6).

Pneumococci are distinguished from other α-haemolytic streptococci by their characteristic sensitivity to optochin (ethylhydrocupreine). Growth of pneumococci is inhibited around an optochin disc applied to an inoculated blood agar plate. With few exceptions, other α-haemolytic streptococci are not inhibited. In doubtful cases the identity of pneumococci is confirmed by demonstrating bile solubility, autolysis or reactivity to a poly-specific antiserum ('omniserum') against capsular polysaccharides.

Other streptococci are identified by biochemical characteristics, such as the ability to ferment various carbohydrates and hydrolyse amino acids. However, some of the viridans streptococci are notoriously difficult to identify.

Enterococci are unique among the streptococci in their ability to grow on bile-containing media.

## Antigen detection

Numerous commercial kits are available for the detection of *Str. pyogenes* directly in throat swabs without cultivation. These diagnostic kits use specific antibodies to detect the group A antigen in the material on the swab. They allow practitioners to test whether a throat infection is caused by *Str. pyogenes*, but the sensitivity and specificity of individual tests vary.

## Antibody detection

Detection of antibodies against antigens of *Str. pyogenes* is an important means of establishing the diagnosis of poststreptococcal rheumatic fever and glomerulonephritis. In many cases the initiating infection in the throat or on the skin is no longer present.

Immune responses vary depending on whether the original focus is the throat or skin. Antibodies against streptolysin O (the ASO test) are used to document antecedent streptococcal infection in the throat of patients with clinical signs of rheumatic fever. A significant increase in antibody titre appears 3–4 weeks after initial exposure to the micro-organism. Detection of increased levels of serum antibodies to streptococcal hyaluronidase and DNAase B is also of diagnostic importance.

ASO estimation is unreliable in pyoderma-associated acute glomerulonephritis. A raised ASO titre is not observed in these patients, perhaps because lipids present in the skin inactivate the streptolysin O. Detection of antibodies against streptococcal DNAase B is recommended as a diagnostic tool in these patients.

## Typing of streptococci

Strains of *Str. pyogenes* can be subdivided into serological types. The most comprehensive typing scheme is based on structural differences in the highly variable surface M protein. More than 150 different M types may be distinguished with type-specific antisera or by sequence differences in the gene (*emm*) encoding the M protein. An alternative typing scheme is based on the surface protein known as the T antigen.

Apart from serving epidemiological purposes, particular M types are associated with particular types of infection. Thus, certain M types are more commonly associated with skin infections than mucosal infections. Recent increases in the rate and severity of invasive *Str. pyogenes* infections (toxic shock syndrome and necrotizing fasciitis) have been associated primarily with serotypes M-1 and M-3. Rheumatic fever is often, but not exclusively, associated with M serotypes 1, 3, 5, 6 and 18.

Pneumococci are typed on the basis of the differences in capsular polysaccharides, of which 91 have been described. The addition of India ink to a suspension of pneumococci shows the presence of the capsule as a clear halo around the organisms. Mixing a suspension of pneumococci with type-specific antisera increases the visibility of the capsule in the microscope, and is the basis of the *quellung reaction* or *capsular swelling test*. Serotyping of pneumococci is carried out mainly in reference laboratories.

Multilocus sequence typing (MLST) schemes based on allelic sequence profiles of seven housekeeping genes are available for several *Streptococcus* species and allow mapping of the global distribution of *sequence types*.

## TREATMENT

Penicillin resistance has never been detected in *Str. pyogenes*. As a result, benzylpenicillin (penicillin G) or oral phenoxymethylpenicillin (penicillin V) are the drugs of choice for treatment of infections with *Str. pyogenes*. Antibiotic sensitivity tests are currently unnecessary when that species is identified as the infecting organism. In cases of hypersensitivity to penicillin, erythromycin is usually the second choice, but resistance occurs and is common in some countries.

Treatment for 3–5 days limits the effect of severe attacks of streptococcal infection and prevents suppurative complications such as otitis media, although the streptococci are eliminated from the infected area only if treatment is continued for 10 days.

Surgery is essential to remove damaged tissue in case of necrotizing fasciitis, as antibiotic penetration of the infected area is poor. Clindamycin is preferred to penicillin because it inhibits protein synthesis, including production of exotoxin.

Most strains of *Str. agalactiae* are susceptible to penicillins, macrolides and glycopeptides.

Although streptococci are intrinsically resistant to aminoglycosides, these agents interact synergically with penicillins and the combination is often used in the treatment of streptococcal and enterococcal endocarditis.

Pneumococci and viridans streptococci are often resistant to penicillins owing to mutations in the target penicillin-binding proteins. These mutations have accumulated in strains of *Str. mitis* and *Str. oralis*, and the altered genes have subsequently been transferred by genetic transformation to *Str. pneumoniae*. High-level penicillin resistance (minimum inhibitory concentration above 2 mg/L) was first recognized in 1977 in South Africa, where it was responsible for an epidemic of pneumococcal meningitis unresponsive to penicillin. The incidence of penicillin resistance is quite variable geographically and reflects the local level of antibiotic usage.

Most pneumococcal infections with strains exhibiting intermediate-level resistance to penicillin (minimum inhibitory concentration 0.1–1 mg/L) respond to highdose therapy; an exception is meningitis, because of problems of penetration into the CSF. Penicillin resistance in pneumococci and other viridans streptococci is often linked to resistance to several other antibiotics. Resistance to erythromycin, tetracycline and chloramphenicol is not uncommon, and tolerance even to vancomycin has been reported.

The dose of penicillin necessary to treat susceptible pneumococcal infection is determined largely by pharmacological factors at the site of infection. For example, pneumococcal pneumonia responds to doses of penicillin as low as 0.3 g (0.5 mega-units) twice daily, whereas pneumococcal meningitis requires much higher doses. In patients unable to tolerate penicillin, erythromycin is the most widely used alternative agent for respiratory pneumococcal infections.

Unlike other streptococci, enterococci are intrinsically resistant to cephalosporins. Sensitivity to penicillins and other antibiotics varies widely, and clinical isolates must be tested for their susceptibility. Vancomycin resistance has been observed in enterococci and is a problem in high-dependency areas of some hospitals.

## PREVENTION AND CONTROL

### Hygienic measures

Skin infections with *Str. pyogenes* are usually associated with poor hygiene, and can to a large extent be prevented by standard hygienic measures. Late-onset neonatal infections with *Str. agalactiae* may also be prevented or significantly reduced by standard aseptic nursing procedures.

Likewise, hygiene is the most important preventive measure in relation to dental caries, which can be prevented largely by regular tooth-brushing with a fluoride-containing dentifrice combined with restricted consumption of fermentable carbohydrates, in particular sucrose.

## Chemoprophylaxis

Prophylactic use of antibiotics is relevant in some streptococcal infections. As the primary attack of rheumatic fever usually occurs during childhood, long-term penicillin prophylaxis until adulthood is recommended to reduce the risk of further attacks and further heart injury. This is not the case in patients with acute glomerulonephritis, because of the lack of recurrences.

Two different approaches are used to prevent early-onset neonatal *Str. agalactiae* infections:

1. A risk-based strategy in which women of unknown colonization status receive intrapartum antibiotic prophylaxis in case of: threatened delivery at less than 37 weeks' gestation; premature rupture of the membranes; intrapartum fever; or previous delivery of a child who developed neonatal infection
2. A screening-based approach in which all pregnant women at 35–37 weeks' gestation are screened for *Str. agalactiae* colonization in vaginal and rectal specimens. All identified carriers are offered intrapartum chemoprophylaxis. This screening-based prophylaxis is used in the USA and in many European countries and has led to a significant decline in the incidence of early onset neonatal infections due to *Str. agalactiae*. Intravenous or intramuscular penicillin is the agent of choice because its antimicrobial spectrum, narrower than that of ampicillin, reduces the likelihood of resistance developing in other bacteria and selection of other potential pathogens. Antimicrobial susceptibility testing of GBS isolates is crucial for appropriate antibiotic prophylaxis selection for penicillin-allergic women because resistance to clindamycin, the most common agent used in this population, is increasing among GBS isolates.

Patients at risk of developing infective endocarditis (see Table 16.2) should be given prophylactic antibiotics in association with dental procedures that lead to bleeding. The current international recommendations are amoxicillin 1 h before dental treatment or, in case of penicillin allergy, clindamycin. If the patient has been on long-term penicillin prophylaxis, the oral streptococci are likely to have reduced susceptibility to penicillins, and clindamycin or vancomycin is recommended as the alternative. It is imperative that patients at risk maintain healthy periodontal conditions and that the amount of dental plaque is kept to a minimum.

## Vaccines

### Pyogenic streptococci

Attempts to develop a vaccine against *Str. pyogenes* infections have been hampered by two problems:

1. The considerable antigenic diversity of the M protein and other vaccine candidate antigens.
2. The potential immunological cross-reactivity of many of the antigens with host tissue components.

Several strategies are currently being tested, including oral vaccination.

A vaccine against neonatal *Str. agalactiae* infection based on protein-conjugated type III capsular polysaccharide is being tested for use primarily in women of reproductive age. However, additional serotypes are increasingly prevalent.

### Pneumococci

Before the widespread availability of effective antimicrobial drugs the treatment of pneumococcal infections was based on the use of type-specific antiserum. This reduced the mortality rate associated with bacteraemic pneumococcal pneumonia, but not to the same extent that penicillin was subsequently shown to achieve. However, it indicated that type-specific antibody had a role in the control of pneumococcal disease and led to a variety of prototype vaccines. The vaccine that has been in use for many years contains a mixture of 23 polysaccharide serotypes chosen according to the prevalence of serotypes responsible for bacteraemic pneumococcal infection. It offers protection against 90% of isolates.

Like other vaccines based on pure polysaccharides, the immunogenicity of the multivalent vaccine is inadequate in those below 2 years of age and in those immunosuppressed as a result of malignancy, steroid therapy or other chronic disease. To overcome this problem, pneumococcal vaccines containing capsular polysaccharide coupled to a carrier protein are now available. These vaccines increase the immunogenicity of the polysaccharide by rendering the response dependent on T lymphocyte help. The current conjugate vaccines include 11–13 of the capsular polysaccharides, and are now part of the childhood vaccination programme in many countries.

Immunization is recommended for various groups at risk of pneumococcal disease, particularly those with congenital or surgical asplenia and those with hereditary haemoglobinopathies such as sickle cell disease, as pneumococcal infection can be fulminant in these patients. Vaccine efficacy is not complete and many clinicians also prescribe oral phenoxymethyl-penicillin as long-term chemoprophylaxis in this high-risk group. In some countries, including the USA and the UK, the vaccine is recommended for those over 65 years of age, with or without previous ill health, although there have been difficulties in establishing scientifically the efficacy in this group.

## RECOMMENDED READING

Carapetis JR, Steer AC, Mulholland EK, Weber M: The global burden of group A streptococcal diseases, *Lancet Infectious Diseases* 5:685–694, 2005.

Cunningham MW: Pathogenesis of group A streptococcal infections, *Clinical Microbiology Reviews* 13:470–511, 2000.

Henriques-Normark B, Blomberg C, Dagerhamn J, et al: The rise and fall of bacterial clones: Streptococcus pneumoniae, *Nature Reviews Microbiology* 6:827–837, 2008.

Kilian M; Streptococcus and Lactobacillus. In Borriello P, Murray PR, Funke G, editors: Topley and Wilson's Microbiology and Microbial Infections, Vol. 2, ed 9, London, 2005, Arnold, pp 833–881.

Llewelyn M, Cohen J: Superantigens: microbial agents that corrupt immunity, *The Lancet Infectious Diseases* 2:156–162, 2002.

Marsh PD, Martin MW: *Oral Microbiology*, ed 5, Oxford, 2009, Elsevier.

Mitchell TJ: The pathogenesis of streptococcal infections: from tooth decay to meningitis, *Nature Reviews* 1:219–230, 2003.

Reinert RR, Reinert S, van der Linden M, et al: Antimicrobial susceptibility of Streptococcus pneumoniae in eight European countries from 2001 to 2003, *Antimicrobial Agents and Chemotherapy* 49:2903–2913, 2005.

Verani JR, McGee L, Schrag SJ: Prevention of perinatal group B streptococcal disease. Revised guidelines from CDC, *Morbidity and Mortality Weekly Report* 59:1–32, 2010.

## Websites

Centers for Disease Control and Prevention: Disease listing. http://www.cdc.gov/ncidod/dbmd/diseaseinfo/

Multi Locus Sequence Typing: Schemes for streptococci and several other pathogenic bacteria. http://www.mlst.net/

# 17 Coryneform bacteria, listeria and erysipelothrix

## Diphtheria; listeriosis; erysipeloid

*J. McLauchlin and P. Riegel*

## KEY POINTS

- The genus *Corynebacterium* includes *C. diphtheriae*, which causes the toxin-mediated pharyngeal infection diphtheria. The infection has largely been controlled by widespread use of a toxoid vaccine.
- Diphtheria toxin is encoded by a lysogenic bacteriophage and has cardiac and neurotoxic effects. Non-toxigenic strains are occasionally isolated from diverse infections.
- Other medically significant corynebacteria include *C. ulcerans*, which causes exudative pharyngitis, and *C. jeikeium*, which is part of the normal skin flora and is an opportunistic pathogen of hospital (particularly neutropenic) patients.
- *Listeria* is a genus of environmental bacteria and includes *L. monocytogenes*, an important cause of disease in domestic animals, that also causes severe systemic disease in the immunosuppressed and elderly as well as the unborn or newly delivered.
- Listeriosis is transmitted predominantly by the consumption of contaminated ready-to-eat foods; the agent is able to grow in a variety of foods at refrigeration temperatures.
- *Erysipelothrix rhusiopathiae* causes economically important disease in domestic animals, notably pigs. Occasional human infections occur, and present as a cellulitis.

## CORYNEFORM BACTERIA

The term *coryneform* is used to describe aerobic, non-sporing and irregularly shaped Gram-positive rods. According to this broad definition, they include bacteria of the genus *Corynebacterium* with a typically club-shaped morphology (Greek κορσψυη = club), environmental bacteria showing coccoid forms such as *Rhodococcus*, *Gordonia* and *Brevibacterium* species, and preferentially anaerobic bacteria of the genera *Actinomyces* (see Ch. 20), *Actinobaculum*, *Arcanobacterium* and *Propionibacterium*, which exhibit some branched forms.

## CORYNEBACTERIUM DIPHTHERIAE

The major disease caused by *C. diphtheriae* is *diphtheria*, an infection of the local tissue of the upper respiratory tract with the production of a toxin that causes systemic effects, notably in the heart and peripheral nerves. Diphtheria has virtually disappeared in developed countries following mass immunization, but is still endemic in many regions of the world. Skin infections are prevalent in some countries. Non-toxigenic strains have been associated with endocarditis, meningitis, cerebral abscess and osteoarthritis throughout the world.

### Description

*C. diphtheriae*, like other members of the genus, are non-motile, non-spore-forming, straight or slightly curved rods with tapered ends. They are Gram-positive, but easily decolourized, particularly in older cultures. Cells often contain metachromatic granules (polymetaphosphate), which stain bluish-purple with methylene blue. Snapping division produces groups of cells in angular and palisade arrangements that create a 'Chinese character' effect. *C. diphtheriae* is aerobic and facultatively anaerobic, growing best on a blood- or serum-containing medium at 35–37°C with or without carbon dioxide enrichment. On agar medium containing tellurite, colonies of *C. diphtheriae* are characteristically black or grey after 24–48 h.

Biotypes of *C. diphtheriae* named *gravis*, *intermedius* or *mitis* are genomically similar variants exhibiting distinct biochemical features and cultural morphology. Bacilli of the gravis biotype are usually short, whereas those of biotype mitis are long and

**Fig. 17.1** Diphtheritic membrane on throat. From Conlon, C., Snydman, D 2000 *Mosby's Color Atlas and Text of Infectious Diseases.* Edinburgh: Mosby Elsevier. Courtesy of Nigel Day.

pleomorphic; biotype intermedius ranges from very long to short rods. In broth medium, *C. diphtheriae* biotype *gravis* forms a pellicle and a granular deposit, whereas *C. diphtheriae* biotype *mitis* produces a diffuse turbidity. The biotype *intermedius* forms no pellicle, but a fine granular deposit can be observed.

## Pathogenesis

To cause disease *C. diphtheriae* must:

• invade, colonize and proliferate in local tissues
• be lysogenized by a specific β-phage, enabling it to produce toxin.

In the upper respiratory tract, diphtheria bacilli elicit an inflammatory exudate and cause necrosis of the cells of the faucial mucosa (Fig. 17.1). The diphtheria toxin possibly assists colonization of the throat or skin by killing epithelial cells or neutrophils.

The organisms do not penetrate deeply into the mucosal tissue and bacteraemia does not usually occur. The exotoxin is produced locally and spread by the bloodstream to distant organs, with a special affinity for heart muscle, the peripheral nervous system and the adrenal glands.

*C. diphtheriae* can colonize the throats of people who have been immunized against diphtheria or who have become immune as a result of natural exposure, but usually no pseudomembrane develops.

The diphtheria toxin is a heat-stable polypeptide, composed of two fragments: A (active) and B (binding). The toxin binds to a specific receptor on susceptible cells and enters by receptor-mediated endocytosis. The A subunit is cleaved and released from the B subunit as it inserts and passes through the lysosomal membrane into the cytoplasm. Fragment A catalyses the transfer of adenosine disphosphate (ADP)-ribose from nicotinamide adenine dinucleotide (NAD) to the eukaryotic elongation factor 2,

which inhibits the function of the latter in protein synthesis. Inhibition of protein synthesis is probably responsible for both the necrotic and neurotoxic effects of the toxin. Production of toxin by lysogenized *C. diphtheriae* is enhanced considerably when the bacteria are grown in low iron conditions. Other factors such as osmolarity, amino acid concentrations and pH have a role.

The *Schick test*, an intradermal injection of stabilized diphtheria toxin, was formerly used to determine individual susceptibility to the toxin. Absence of a reaction indicates immunity. Tissue culture neutralization tests, enzyme-linked immunosorbent assay (ELISA) and passive haemagglutination assay to measure serum antitoxin levels, are now preferred. For epidemiological purposes the minimum protective level is considered to be 0.01 international units (IU) of diphtheria antitoxin per millilitre in a serum sample. A level of 0.1 IU/mL is desirable for individual protection.

Non-toxigenic strains of *C. diphtheriae* may cause pharyngitis and cutaneous abscesses. Systemic disease, including endocarditis, septic arthritis and osteomyelitis, has also been reported. *C. diphtheriae* biotype *belfanti* could be involved in the processus of a chronic atrophic rhinitis named ozena. The virulence factors of these strains remain unknown. Conversion of a non-toxigenic strain to a toxigenic strain by phage infection can occur in human populations.

## Clinical features

The incubation period of diphtheria is 2–5 days, with a range of 1–10 days. At first, patients present with malaise, sore throat and moderate fever. A thick, adherent green *pseudomembrane* is present on one or both tonsils or adjacent pharynx. In nasopharyngeal infection, the pseudomembrane may involve nasal mucosa, the pharyngeal wall and the soft palate. In this form, oedema involving the cervical lymph glands may occur in the anterior tissues of the neck, a condition known as *bullneck diphtheria*.

Laryngeal involvement leads to obstruction of the larynx and lower airways. Organisms multiply within the membranes and toxaemia is prominent. The patient is gravely ill, with a weak pulse, restlessness and confusion. Intoxication takes the form of myocarditis and peripheral neuritis, and may be associated with thrombocytopenia. Visual disturbance, difficulty in swallowing, and paralysis of the arms and legs also occur but usually resolve spontaneously. Complete heart block may result from myocarditis. Death is most commonly due to congestive heart failure and cardiac arrhythmias.

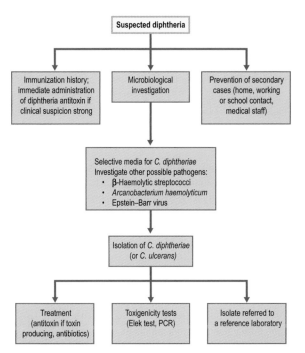

**Suspected diphtheria**

- Immunization history; immediate administration of diphtheria antitoxin if clinical suspicion strong
- Microbiological investigation
- Prevention of secondary cases (home, working or school contact, medical staff)

Selective media for *C. diphtheriae*
Investigate other possible pathogens:
- β-Haemolytic streptococci
- *Arcanobacterium haemolyticum*
- Epstein–Barr virus

Isolation of *C. diphtheriae* (or *C. ulcerans*)

- Treatment (antitoxin if toxin producing, antibiotics)
- Toxigenicity tests (Elek test, PCR)
- Isolate referred to a reference laboratory

**Fig. 17.2** Algorithm for the management of a suspected case of diphtheria. *Note:* Antitoxin treatment should not await laboratory confirmation, which may take several days. Photograph courtesy of Dr A. Efstratiou, Central Public Health Laboratory, London.

**Fig. 17.3** Elek plate for the detection of *C. diphtheriae* toxin production. Cultures are streaked horizontally, then overlaid with an antitoxin-impregnated strip. Toxin and antitoxin diffuse into the culture during incubation, and precipitin lines develop where toxin and antitoxin are present in a critical ratio. Positive reactions in test cultures are indicated by precipitin lines that arc with those produced by positive controls. The *C. diphtheriae* cultures are (top to bottom): National Collection of Type Cultures (NCTC) strain 10648 (positive control); test culture (positive); NCTC 10356 (negative control); NCTC 3984 (weak positive control); NCTC 10648 (positive control); test culture (negative); NCTC 10356 (negative control). Courtesy of Dr A Efstratiou, Health Protection Agency, London.

Cutaneous diphtheria occurs mostly in tropical countries. The lesion is usually characterized by an ulcer covered by a necrotic pseudomembrane and may involve any area of the skin. Although the organism usually produces toxin, systemic toxic manifestations are uncommon.

## Diagnosis

The diagnosis is made on clinical grounds, supported by a history of diphtheria among contacts, lack of prior immunization or travel in countries where diphtheria is endemic.

The role of the laboratory is to confirm the diagnosis by recovery of *C. diphtheriae* in culture followed by appropriate tests for detection of toxin production (Fig. 17.2). The clinician should inform the laboratory of the presumptive diagnosis of diphtheria because isolation of *C. diphtheriae* requires special media. Material for cultures should be obtained on a swab from the inflamed areas surrounding the pseudomembranes.

Direct microscopy of a smear is unreliable because *C. diphtheriae* is morphologically similar to other coryneforms. The recommended media include blood agar and a selective medium containing tellurite

and cysteine. Identification is based on carbohydrate fermentation reactions and enzymatic activities. Commercial kits such as the API Coryne strip provide a reliable identification. Matrix-assisted laser desorption/ionisation time-of-flight (MALDI-TOF) is also a reliable tool for rapid diagnosis of potentially toxigenic *Corynebacterium* species.

Toxigenicity testing is essential. Production of diphtheria toxin is demonstrated by the agar immunoprecipitation test (*Elek test*; Fig. 17.3) or by the tissue culture cytotoxicity assay, which has replaced the virulence test in guinea-pigs. The toxin gene can be detected by the polymerase chain reaction (PCR). This test shows excellent correlation with guinea-pig virulence, although there is the rare possibility of a false-positive PCR assay if the strain harbouring the *tox* gene is unable to express it. The detection of the *tox* gene by PCR directly from clinical specimens is feasible. All biotypes are potentially toxigenic. Multilocus sequence typing provides high-resolution data appropriate for the epidemiological investigation of diphtheria.

Measurement of antibodies to diphtheria toxin in serum collected before administration of antitoxin may support the diagnosis when cultures are negative. An algorithm for the management of suspect cases of diphtheria is shown in Figure 17.2.

## Treatment

If diphtheria is strongly suspected on clinical grounds, treatment should not await laboratory confirmation, which may take several days (Fig. 17.2). Diphtheria antitoxin (hyperimmune horse serum) is given, as antibiotics have no effect on preformed toxin which rapidly diffuses from the local lesions and soon becomes irreversibly bound to tissue cells. Because antitoxin neutralizes only circulating toxin, it should be administered promptly.

Treatment with parenteral penicillin or oral erythromycin eradicates the organism and terminates toxin production. *C. diphtheriae* is universally sensitive to penicillins but some strains are resistant to erythromycin, tetracyclines and rifampicin. Erythromycin may be preferred to penicillin for elimination of the bacilli from the throat, particularly in treatment of persistent carriers. Some strains are tolerant to the bactericidal action of penicillins, and treatment of complicated infections should contain an association with an aminoglycoside.

Patients should be placed in strict isolation, nursed by staff whose immunization history is documented and have daily platelet counts and electrocardiography.

## Epidemiology

Diphtheria has virtually disappeared in developed countries following mass immunization in the 1940s, but is still endemic in many regions of the world. About 50 000 cases of diphtheria occurred in the newly independent states of the former Soviet Union during 1990–1996, leading to infection in short-term visitors from western Europe. Other countries that have experienced outbreaks of diphtheria in recent years include China, Ecuador, Algeria, South-East Asia and the eastern Mediterranean. In the USA, only 45 cases were reported during 1980–1995. In 2002, one case of diphtheria was reported in the USA but more toxigenic strains were referred to North American reference laboratories. In 2003, a total of 896 cases were reported from the World Health Organization European Region; 99% were from Eastern Europe. There were 102 cases of infections caused by toxigenic corynebacteria diphtheria in the UK between 1986 and 2008: 42 *C. diphtheriae*, 59 *C. ulcerans* and one *C. pseudotuberculosis*. Five fatalities were reported, all in unvaccinated patients. Non-toxigenic strains capable of causing mild disease continue to circulate throughout the world. In European countries, carriages rates of non-toxigenic strains ranged from 0 in Ireland to 4.0 per 1000 in Turkey.

Infection is confined to man and usually involves contact with a diphtheria case or a carrier. The most important mode of spread is person-to-person transmission by aerosolized droplets when an infected person coughs, sneezes or talks, or by direct contact with skin lesions. Most clinical infections are probably contracted from carriers rather than symptomatic patients. Prolonged close contact with an infected person and intimate contact increases the likelihood of transmission.

Acquired immunity to diphtheria is due primarily to toxin-neutralizing antibody (antitoxin). Passive immunity in utero is acquired transplacentally and can last for 1 or 2 years after birth. Active immunity can probably be produced by a mild or subclinical infection in infants who retain some maternal immunity. Unimmunized children under 15 years old are most likely to contract diphtheria. The disease is also found among adults whose immunization was neglected. The mortality rate is highest among young children and in people aged over 40 years. Skin infections caused by *C. diphtheriae* may result in early development of natural immunity against the disease.

*C. diphtheriae* persists longer in skin lesions than in the tonsils or nose, and cutaneous diphtheria appears to be more contagious than respiratory diphtheria. Untreated people who are infected with the diphtheria bacillus can be contagious for up to 2 weeks, but seldom for more than 4 weeks. If treated with appropriate antibiotics, the contagious period can be limited to less than 4 days. *C. diphtheriae* can survive in the environment in dust and on dry vomits for several months, and transmission via vomits has been documented. Animal-to-man transmission and foodborne transmission by consumption of contaminated foods such as raw milk have been described, but are very rare.

## Control

High population immunity achieved through mass immunization (at least 95% coverage in children and at least 90% coverage in adults) is the most effective measure to control epidemic diphtheria. Immunization with diphtheria toxoid was first introduced in 1923. Large-scale immunization programmes introduced in the 1940s reduced the incidence of diphtheria dramatically, although the disease was not eradicated completely. Immunization schedules are discussed in Chapter 70.

Prevention of secondary cases by the rapid investigation of close contacts is essential. These investigations should include ascertainment of the immunization histories of all home and school contacts. Primary

**Table 17.1** Habitat and disease associations of corynebacteria

| Organism | Major habitat | Disease association |
|---|---|---|
| Corynebacterium diphtheriae | Throat, skin | Diphtheria (toxigenic strains), wound infections, bacteraemia, endocarditis |
| C. ulcerans | Human throat and skin / Animals: raw milk, dogs, cats | Man: diphtheria (toxigenic strains), pharyngitis and wound infection / Cattle: mastitis |
| C. pseudotuberculosis | Sheep, horses, goats | Man: lymphadenitis / Animals: abscesses and abortion |
| C. jeikeium | Skin | Bacteraemia, endocarditis; infection of foreign bodies and CSF shunts |
| C. urealyticum | Skin, urinary tract | Urinary tract infection, pyelonephritis, endocarditis |
| C. amycolatum | Man and animals | Man: bacteraemia, endocarditis, peritonitis and wound infection / Cattle: mastitis |
| C. glucuronolyticum | Urinary tract of man and animals | Urogenital tract infection |
| C. minutissimum | Skin, urinary tract | Erythrasma, bacteraemia |
| C. striatum | Respiratory tract, skin | Respiratory tract infection, wound infection, bacteraemia |
| C. pseudodiphtheriticum | Respiratory tract | Respiratory tract infection, endocarditis |
| C. kroppenstedtii | Unknown | Breast abscess, granulomatous mastitis |
| Arcanobacterium haemolyticum | Throat | Pharyngitis, skin ulcers, endocarditis |
| Rhodococcus equi | Animals, soil | Pulmonary infection and soft tissue infection |

courses of immunization or a booster are given if necessary.

## OTHER MEDICALLY IMPORTANT CORYNEBACTERIA

The non-diphtheria corynebacteria ('diphtheroids') are diverse and comprise strictly aerobic bacteria usually isolated from the environment, as well as facultative or preferentially anaerobic bacteria, which are commensals of the skin and mucous membranes. The principal species involved and the main clinical syndromes associated with infection are shown in Table 17.1.

### Corynebacterium ulcerans

C. ulcerans has been isolated from raw milk and can cause mastitis in cattle. In man, it is seen almost exclusively in cases of exudative pharyngitis, but occasional soft tissue infections occur. C. ulcerans can produce a toxin that is 95% identical to the diphtheria toxin, causing a diphtheria-like illness. It seems likely that many human infections are transmitted by a dog or cat. Therapy involves the administration of appropriate antibiotics, such as penicillins or erythromycin, and of diphtheria antitoxin in the case of diphtheria-like disease.

### Corynebacterium pseudotuberculosis

C. pseudotuberculosis is primarily an animal pathogen and rarely infects man. It causes caseous lymphadenitis in sheep and goats, and abscesses or ulcerative lymphangitis in horses. Human infections occur mainly in patients with animal contact. Infection usually presents as a subacute or chronic granulomatous lymphadenitis involving the axillary or cervical nodes, but pneumonias have been described. Some strains are lysogenized by bacteriophages of C. diphtheriae and thus produce diphtheria toxin, but no clinical cases of diphtheria-like disease have been attributed to C. pseudotuberculosis infection. Treatment requires prolonged antibiotic therapy with erythromycin, penicillins or tetracycline, and surgical drainage or excision.

### Corynebacterium jeikeium

C. jeikeium (formerly CDC coryneform group JK) is part of the normal skin flora, particularly in inguinal, axillary and rectal areas. Colonization by antibiotic-resistant strains is unusual in healthy individuals, but is common in hospital patients, particularly those who are neutropenic or receiving antibiotics. Most infections are associated with skin damaged by wounds or invasive devices. Such infections include:

- prosthetic valve endocarditis
- bacteraemia associated with infected long-term intravenous cannulae
- peritonitis in patients on peritoneal dialysis
- septicaemia and local infection following insertion of an epicardial pacemaker
- central nervous system infection in patients with ventriculoperitoneal or atrial shunts for hydrocephalus.

Most infections occur in patients in hospital for prolonged periods and who have received broad-spectrum antimicrobial therapy. Spread is through environmental contamination, the hands of ward staff or auto-infection.

### Treatment

Most isolates of *C. jeikeium* recovered from infections are highly resistant to penicillins and cephalosporins in vitro. Even with susceptible isolates, penicillin is incompletely bactericidal, but aminoglycoside-sensitive strains can be eradicated successfully with combined penicillin and aminoglycoside therapy. Systemic amoxicillin, gentamicin, rifampicin or ciprofloxacin can be used if the isolate is susceptible. Resistance to aminoglycosides and macrolides has been reported in more than 60% of isolates and resistance to fluoroquinolones is variable.

Glycopeptides are the drugs of choice for treating serious infections. *C. jeikeium* is sensitive to glycopeptides and these antibiotics are bactericidal. Combinations of vancomycin with gentamicin have been used to treat infective endocarditis. Peritonitis secondary to peritoneal dialysis and meningitis related to shunts can be treated with intra-peritoneal or intrathecal vancomycin, respectively.

### Corynebacterium urealyticum

*C. urealyticum* (formerly CDC coryneform group D-2) is a frequent skin colonizer, mainly in hospital patients. The groin, abdominal wall and axilla are most frequently colonized. This micro-organism is associated with urinary tract infections, particularly with alkaline-encrusted cystitis and pyelitis related to its strong urease production. Infection is a consequence of the use of broad-spectrum antibiotics for patients with underlying conditions that predispose to urinary tract infection. The organism may also cause pyelonephritis and is an infrequent cause of endocarditis, osteomyelitis or soft tissue infection.

Like *C. jeikeium*, *C. urealyticum* is usually highly resistant to most antimicrobial agents, except glycopeptides. Vancomycin, tetracyclines, erythromycin and norfloxacin have proven effective in treatment. Prolonged treatment with appropriate antibiotics, acidification of the urine, and removal of crusts is essential for proper management of encrusted cystitis.

### Corynebacterium amycolatum

*C. amycolatum* is a human skin commensal similar to other corynebacteria, but lacks cell wall mycolic acids.

Its biochemical characteristics are variable and it is often misidentified. Strains isolated from hospital patients may be multiresistant to antibiotics except glycopeptides. *C. amycolatum* has been reported as causing bacteraemi, endocarditis, peritonitis and wound infection.

### Corynebacterium glucuronolyticum

*C. glucuronolyticum* (syn. *C. seminale*) is most commonly isolated from men with prostatitis and urethritis, but can be also isolated from the female genital tract. It is commonly isolated from semen specimens, especially in sexually experienced men. It exhibits strong β-glucuronidase activity and some strains produce urease. It is usually sensitive to antibiotics, although tetracyclines and macrolides are the most effective in vitro.

### Corynebacterium minutissimum

*C. minutissimum* is believed to be the cause of erythrasma, a relatively common and localized infection of the stratum corneum that produces reddish-brown scaly patches in intertriginous sites. Lesions usually involve the groin, toeweb and axillae, and fluoresce coral red when examined by Wood's light. The organism can be cultured from skin scrapings, but the diagnosis is usually based on clinical aspects and the characteristic fluorescence. More serious infections have been described, including bacteraemia and breast abscess. Some infections attributed to *C. minutissimum* may have been caused by *C. amycolatum*.

*C. minutissimum* is sensitive to penicillins; susceptibility to erythromycin is variable.

### Corynebacterium striatum

This species is part of the normal flora of the nose and skin. It is a rare cause of pulmonary infection, particularly in patients with chronic obstructive airway disease or those who are intubated. Transmission to mechanically ventilated patients in an intensive care unit has been documented. It has also been isolated from blood, catheter tips, wounds, leg ulcers, peritoneal fluid, urine, semen, vaginal exudate and placental tissues. *C. striatum* is sensitive to penicillins and glycopeptides; susceptibility to aminoglycosides, ciprofloxacin, erythromycin and rifampicin is variable. Many isolates are resistant to cephalosporins.

### Corynebacterium pseudodiphtheriticum

*C. pseudodiphtheriticum* is a commensal of the human nasopharynx. It is occasionally associated with respiratory tract infections, including tracheobronchitis, necrotizing tracheitis, pneumonia and lung abscess. Most isolates come from patients with endotracheal tubes or chronic obstructive pulmonary disease. It has also been reported to cause endocarditis in patients with prosthetic valves or pre-existing valvular damage. *C. pseudodiphtheriticum* is usually susceptible to most antibiotics except erythromycin.

## Corynebacterium kroppenstedtii

*C. kroppenstedtii* was first described in 1998, after isolation of a single strain from human sputum. Later, when an association was found between corynebacterial infection and granulomatous mastitis, most of the corynebacteria were identified as *C. kroppenstedtii*. Isolation of the species requires Tween-supplemented media and prolonged incubation. *C. kroppenstedtii* is sensitive to many antibiotics including penicillins. Treatment of granulomatous mastitis is usually based on steroids, but addition of antibiotics is appropriate.

## Arcanobacterium haemolyticum

*A. haemolyticum* is phylogenetically related to *Actinomyces* spp. (see Ch. 20). It causes pharyngitis and chronic skin ulcers. Cases of cellulitis, osteomyelitis, brain abscesses and endocarditis have occasionally been described. The species produces at least two extracellular toxins, phospholipase D and a haemolysin.

Most patients are young adults who present with sore throat; some have membranous exudates and peri-tonsillar abscesses. The organism is rarely found in healthy individuals, but occurs in about 2% of symptomatic 15–25-year-olds with pharyngitis. Infection cannot be differentiated from streptococcal pharyngitis on clinical findings alone. *A. haemolyticum* is often isolated in association with streptococci of the *Streptococcus anginosus* group (see p. 194). A scarlatiniform rash occurs in half of the patients with pharyngitis, perhaps caused by a toxin genetically related to the erythrogenic toxin of *Str. pyogenes*. Erythromycin or other macrolides seem to be effective in treatment. *A. haemolyticum* is sensitive to penicillin, but treatment failure has been documented.

## Rhodococcus equi

*R. equi* is a pathogen of horses, pigs and cattle. It is a rare cause of severe pulmonary infections in patients with the acquired immune deficiency syndrome, neoplastic diseases or renal transplants. Most infections develop insidiously, with fever and respiratory symptoms difficult to distinguish from mycobacterial infection. Infections are often recurrent and refractory to treatment, and may be associated with pleural effusion and bacteraemia. The diagnosis is usually established from bronchoscopy specimens, pleural fluid cultures or blood cultures.

*R. equi* is usually sensitive to tetracyclines, macrolides, rifampicin, imipenem and vancomycin, but resistance to penicillins has been reported. Treatment includes surgical drainage when feasible and prolonged therapy with an antibiotic combination such as erythromycin and rifampicin or imipenem and vancomycin, established by in-vitro tests.

## Other coryneform bacteria

- *C. accolens* is usually recovered from respiratory specimens.
- *C. afermentans* ssp. *lipophilum* and CDC coryneform groups G and F-1 may be isolated from a variety of sources, including blood, wound, semen and urine.
- *C. argentoratense, C. propinquum, C. matruchotii* and *C. durum* have been isolated from the throat, but no pathogenic role has been demonstrated.
- *C. aurimucosum* (syn. *C. nigricans*) exhibits black-pigmented colonies. It has been isolated from genital specimens of women with complications of pregnancy.
- *C. bovis* is commonly isolated from bovine mastitis, but is rarely encountered in human infection.
- *C. macginleyi* strains have been isolated from the eye, often in association with infection.
- *C. xerosis* has been confused with *C. amycolatum* and is very rare.
- *Rothia dentocariosa* is commonly isolated from respiratory tract specimens and has been associated with endocarditis and brain abscess.
- *Turicella otitidis* and *C. auris* have been isolated from ears of healthy patients and those with ear infections.
- Several species of *Arthrobacter* and *Actinobaculum* have been recovered from patients with urinary tract infections.

## LISTERIA

Organisms of the genus *Listeria* are non-sporing Gram-positive bacilli. The genus contains eight species (*L. monocytogenes, L. seeligeri, L. ivanovii, L. welshimeri, L. grayi, L. innocua, L. marthii* and *L.*

rocourtiae), but almost all cases of human listeriosis are caused by *L. monocytogenes*. The disease chiefly affects the immunosuppressed and elderly, as well as to a lesser extent the pregnant women, unborn or newly delivered infants. Listeriosis is transmitted predominantly by the consumption of contaminated food. The majority of animal listeriosis is also due to *L. monocytogenes* but *L. ivanovii* is associated with about 10% of infections in sheep.

*Listeria* spp. grows well on a wide variety of non-selective laboratory media and some species, including *L. monocytogenes*, exhibit β-haemolysis on blood agar. These bacteria are non-motile at 37°C, but exhibit characteristic 'tumbling' motility when tested at 25°C.

## LISTERIA MONOCYTOGENES

### Description

*L. monocytogenes* is genetically similar to other *Listeria* species, but can be differentiated by phenotypic or genotypic tests. Thirteen serotypes (serovars) are recognized which can be further subdivided by a variety of phenotypic and now almost exclusively genotypic methods.

Most cases of human listeriosis are caused by serovars 4b, 1/2a and 1/2b. Large food-borne outbreaks have been caused predominantly by serovar 4b strains.

The properties of the organism favour food as an agent in transmission of listeriosis. It widespread in the environment, able to colonise places where food is produced and grows in a wide range of foods having relatively high water activities ($a_w$ >0.95) and over a wide range of temperatures (0–45°C). Growth at refrigeration temperatures is relatively slow, with a maximum doubling time of about 1–2 days at 4°C. Multiplication in food is restricted to the pH range 5–9. *L. monocytogenes* is not sufficiently heat resistant to survive pasteurization.

### Pathogenesis

*L. monocytogenes* is an intracellular parasite, and it is in this environment that the pathogen gains protection and evades some of the host's defences. However, the host has a number of strategies to deal with such parasites. Non-specific mechanisms of resistance are important as first lines of defence once the mucous membranes have been breached. Human neutrophils and non-activated macrophages can phagocytose and kill the bacteria. Protective immunity in humans probably depends on T lymphocytes, with antibodies playing little or no role.

*L. monocytogenes* enters phagocytic and non-phagocytic cells and a listerial surface protein, *internalin* (reminiscent of the M protein of *Str. pyogenes*), is involved with the initial stages of invasion on all cell types. After internalization, *L. monocytogenes* becomes encapsulated in a membrane-bound compartment. In the phagocyte, most cells in the phagocytic vacuole are probably killed. However, those surviving in the phagocytic vacuole, and those in the membrane-bound compartment of non-professional phagocytes, mediate the dissolution of the vacuole membrane by means of a haemolysin (listeriolysin O), and in addition, possibly, the action of a phospholipase C.

In the host cell cytoplasm, where bacterial growth occurs, the organism becomes surrounded by polymerized host cell actin. The ability to polymerize actin preferentially on the older pole of the listeria cell with a surface protein (ActA) subverts the host cell's cytoskeleton and confers intracellular motility to the bacterium. The resulting 'comet tail'-like structure pushes the bacterium into an adjacent mammalian cell, where it again becomes encapsulated in a vacuole. A listerial lecithinase is involved with dissolution of these membranes; the haemolysin may also contribute in this process. Intracellular growth and movement in the newly invaded cell is then repeated. The genes associated with virulaence in *L. monocytogeneces* occur as homologous in *L. ivanovii* and *L. seeligeri*.

### Clinical aspects of infection

*L. monocytogenes* principally causes intra-uterine infection, meningitis and septicaemia. The incubation period varies widely between individuals from 1 to 90 days, with an average for intra-uterine infection of around 30 days.

#### Infection in pregnancy and the neonate

Listeriosis in pregnancy is classified by fetal gestation at onset, as this correlates best with the clinical features, microbiology and prognosis. Maternal listeriosis occurs throughout gestation, but is rare before 20 weeks of pregnancy. The mother is usually previously well with a normal pregnancy. Pregnant women often have very mild symptoms (chills, fever, back pain, sore throat and headache, sometimes with conjunctivitis, diarrhoea or drowsiness), but may be asymptomatic until the delivery of an infected infant. Symptomatic women may have positive blood cultures. Cultures from high vaginal swabs, stool and midstream urine samples, together with pre- or post-natal antibody tests, are of little help in diagnosis. With the onset of fever, fetal movements are reduced, and premature labour occurs within about 1 week. There may be a transient fever during labour, and the amniotic fluid is often discoloured or stained with meconium. Culture of the amniotic fluid, placenta or high vaginal swab after delivery invariably yields a heavy growth of *L. monocytogenes*. Fever resolves soon after birth, and the vagina is usually culture negative after about 1 month. Maternal infection without infection of the foetus can occur and even progress to placental infection without ill effects for the foetus. Repeated pregnancy-associated infections are exceedingly rare, and an association between listeria carriage and habitual abortion has not been substantiated.

Although the outcome of infection for the mother is invariably benign, the outcome for the infant is more variable. Abortion, stillbirth and early-onset neonatal disease are common, depending on the gestation at infection. Neonatal infection is divided into

disease of early (<2 days old), intermediate (3–5 days old) and late (>5 days old) onset. Early neonatal listeriosis is predominantly a septicaemic illness, contracted in utero. In contrast, late neonatal infection is predominantly meningitic and may be associated with hospital cross-infection acquired from an early onset neonatal case. The main characteristics of these two forms are summarized in Table 17.2. Early-onset disease represents a spectrum of mild to severe infection, which can be correlated with the microbiological findings. Those neonates who die from infection usually do so within a few days of birth and have pneumonia, hepatosplenomegaly, petechiae, abscesses in the liver or brain, peritonitis and enterocolitis.

In late-onset neonatal disease the cerebrospinal fluid (CSF) protein content is almost always raised and the glucose level reduced. The total number of white cells is increased but the counts are variable; neutrophils usually predominate, but lymphocytes or monocytes may be the main cell type. In about 50% of Gram films, bacteria, which may resemble rods or cocci, are seen.

**Table 17.2** Characteristics of neonatal infection with *L. monocytogenes*

| | Type of infection | |
|---|---|---|
| | Early | Late |
| Onset after delivery | <2 days | >5 days |
| Maternal factors[a] | Common | Rare |
| Source of infection | Intrauterine infection acquired haematogenously from mother | Hospital-acquired from early-onset case, post-natal environment or maternally acquired during delivery |
| Signs/symptoms | Disseminated infection; Cardiopulmonary distress; Central nervous system signs; Vomiting and diarrhoea; Hepatosplenomegaly; Skin rash | Meningitis; Irritability; Poor appetite; Fever |
| Laboratory findings | Leucocytosis or leucopenia; Thrombocytopenia; Mottling on chest radiography; Increased fibrinogen | Leucocytosis; occasional radiographic changes; CSF: total protein and white cell count raised; glucose level lowered |
| Sites of isolation | Blood, superficial sites and amniotic fluid; less commonly gastric aspirate, CSF and HVS | Commonly CSF; rarely blood |
| Mortality rate | 30–60% | 10–12% |

CSF, cerebrospinal fluid; HVS, high vaginal swab.
[a]Obstetric problems; low birth-weight; maternal fever; abnormal amniotic fluid.

## Adult and juvenile infection

Adult infection is now the most common manifestation of the disease in Northern Europe and North America. In adults and juveniles the main syndromes are septicaemia and central nervous system infection. There was a dramatic increase in the incidence in listerial bacteraemia in patients over 60 years of age in Northern Europe at the start of the 21st century; the rate in this group increased almost 4-fold in England and Wales between 1990 and 2010. Most cases occur in immunosuppressed patients receiving steroid or cytotoxic therapy or with malignant neoplasms. Autoimmune disease, diabetes, alcohol related disease and immunosuppressive treatments are all risk factors for listerial infection. However, about one-third of patients with meningitis and around 10% with primary bacteraemia are apparently immunocompetent. Listeriosis in children older than 1 month is very rare, except in those with underlying disease.

## Meningitis

The clinical presentation is the same in all groups, but progression is more rapid in immunocompromised subjects. A peripheral blood leucocytosis occurs, and the CSF white blood cell count is raised. The CSF glucose level is low and the protein level is raised; a very high protein concentration may be a poor prognostic indicator. Gram stains of the CSF are often negative, and the clinical features of infection are such that it is not possible to tell listerial meningitis from meningococcal or pneumococcal infection. However, *L. monocytogenes* is isolated from blood cultures in most cases.

In the rare cases of encephalitis, cerebritis or cerebral abscesses, the CSF may be normal, but the white blood cell count is often raised mildly and the protein level is slightly increased, with a low glucose concentration. The Gram film and culture are usually negative. Blood cultures are the main source of the organism in many of these patients.

## Bacteraemia

Primary bacteraemia is more common in men than in women, and occurs most often in patients >60 years of age as well as those with haematological malignancy or a renal transplant. As compared to patients with central nervous system infections, those with listerial bacteraemia present more often with gastrointestinal symptoms, particularly those with gastric malignancies, and treatment to reduce stomach acid secretion.

## Gastroenteritis

Several food-borne outbreaks of acute gastroenteritis with fever have been described. The foods associated with these outbreaks have been diverse, but heavily contaminated by the bacterium. Symptoms develop in 1–2 days. Large numbers of *L. monocytogenes* are present in the stool, and a few patients develop serious systemic infection. The ability to cause gastroenteritis may be specific to certain strains.

## Other infections

Rarer manifestations of listeriosis include arthritis, hepatitis, endophthalmitis, pneumonia, endocarditis, cutaneous lesions and peritonitis in patients on continuous ambulatory peritoneal dialysis.

# Epidemiology

## Incidence

Most western countries report infection rates of 1–10 cases per million of the population per year. Pregnancy and neonatal disease account for about 10% of cases. Among these, 15–25% of infections lead to abortion and stillbirth, and about 70% are neonatal infections. In about 5% of maternal infections bacteraemia occurs and the foetus is not affected.

The incidence of infection increases with age so that the mean age of adult infections is over 55 years. Men are more commonly infected than women over the age of 40 years. Immunosuppression is a major risk factor for both the epidemic and sporadic forms of listeriosis and probably accounts for the increasing incidence with age. Human immunodeficiency virus disease has been reported as a predisposing factor in some areas. The peak incidence of human disease usually occurs in July, August or September. Most cases are apparently sporadic, and the patients live in urban areas without exposure to animals.

*L. monocytogenes*, like other *Listeria* species, has been isolated from numerous environmental sites, including soil, sewage, water and decaying plant material, where it can survive for more than 2 years. Although the true home of listeria is probably in the environment, these organisms are also found in excreta of apparently healthy animals, including man. Up to 5% of healthy adults may have the organism in their faeces. Faecal carriage in man probably reflects consumption of contaminated foods and is likely to be transitory.

Numerous types of raw, processed, cooked and ready-to-eat foods contain *L. monocytogenes*, usually at low levels of contamination. The tolerance of the bacterium to sodium chloride and sodium nitrite, and the ability to multiply (albeit slowly) at refrigeration temperatures makes *L. monocytogenes* of particular concern as a post-processing contaminant in long-shelf-life refrigerated foods. Even when present at high levels in foods, spoilage or taints are not generally produced. The widespread distribution of *L. monocytogenes* and the ability to survive on dry and moist surfaces favour post-processing contamination of foods from both raw product and factory sites.

### Transmission

Most cases are sporadic and in only a few is a route of infection identified. The consumption of contaminated foods is the principal route of transmission. Microbiological and epidemiological evidence supports an association with many food types (dairy, meat, vegetable, fish and shellfish) in both sporadic and epidemic listeriosis. Foods associated with transmission often show the following common features:

- able to support the multiplication of *L. monocytogenes* (relatively high water activity and near-neutral pH)
- relatively heavily contaminated (>$10^3$ *L. monocytogenes* per gram) with the implicated strain
- processed with an extended (refrigerated) shelf-life
- ready to eat and consumed without further cooking.

The food type currently most commonly associated with transmission in the UK is pre-prepared sandwiches served in hospitals.

Outbreaks of human listeriosis involving more than 100 individuals have occurred, some lasting for several years. This is likely to represent a long-term colonization of a single site in the food manufacturing environment as well as the long incubation periods shown by some patients. Sites of contamination within food processing facilities involved in human infection have included equipment, shelving, conveyor belts, condensates and drains. *L. monocytogenes* survives well in moist environments with organic material, and it is from such sites that contamination of food occurs during processing. Epidemiological typing is invaluable for the identification of common source foodborne outbreaks and for tracking the bacterium in the food chain.

Listeriosis transmitted by direct contact with the environment, infected animals or animal material is relatively rare. Papular or pustular cutaneous lesions have been described, usually on the arms and hands of farmers or veterinarians 1–4 days after attending bovine abortions. Infection is invariably mild and usually resolves without antimicrobial therapy, although serious systemic involvement has been described. Conjunctivitis in poultry workers has also been reported.

Hospital cross-infection between newborn infants occurs. Typically, an apparently healthy baby (rarely more than one) develops late-onset listeriosis 5–12 days after delivery in a hospital in which an infant with congenital listeriosis was born shortly before. The same strain of *L. monocytogenes* is isolated from both infants and the mother of the early-onset case, but not from the mother of the late-onset case. The cases are usually delivered or nursed in the same or adjacent delivery suits or neonatal units, and consequently staff and equipment (particularly respiratory resuscitation equipment) are common to both. There is little evidence of cross-infection or person-to-person transmission outside the neonatal period.

### Diagnosis and treatment

Conventional culture of blood and or CSF remain the mainstays of treatment although Gram-staining of surface swabs and of merconium stained amniotic fluid has been reported to have a very high predictive value for neonatal listeriosis during outbreaks. PCR based procedures for amplification of *L. monocytogenes*-specific DNA sequences from serum and CSF have been reported.

*L. monocytogenes* is susceptible to a wide range of antibiotics in vitro, including ampicillin, penicillin, vancomycin, tetracyclines, chloramphenicol, aminoglycosides and co-trimoxazole. There is little agreement about the best treatment, but many patients have been treated successfully with ampicillin or penicillin with or without an aminoglycoside. Cephalosporins are ineffective.

No significant change in the antimicrobial susceptibility of *L. monocytogenes* has been recognized over the past 40 years, and resistance to any of the agents recommended for therapy is unlikely.

### Prognosis

The mortality rate in late neonatal disease is about 10%. In contrast, the mortality rate in early disease is 30–60%, and about 20–40% of survivors develop sequelae such as lung disease, hydrocephalus or other neurological defects. Early use of appropriate antibiotics during pregnancy may improve neonatal survival.

The mortality rate in both adult meningitis and bacteraemia is about 20–50%. Amongst patients with meningitis, mortality is significantly less likely in patients less than 60 years of age; however the death rates are similar in these age groups in patients with bacteraemia. Between 25–75% of patients surviving central nervous system infection suffer sequelae such as hemiplegia and other neurological defects.

## ERYSIPELOTHRIX

*Erysipelothrix* is a genus of aerobic, non-sporing, non-motile, Gram-positive bacilli. The genus comprises at least three species: *E. rhusiopathiae, E. inopinata* and *E. tonsillarum. E. rhusiopathiae* causes economically important disease in domestic animals, notably pigs. Human infections from *E. rhusiopathiae* are rare, but present as a localized cutaneous infection (*erysipeloid*), which occasionally becomes diffuse and may lead to septicaemia and endocarditis. Infection is most often associated with close animal contact and usually occurs in such occupational groups as butchers, abattoir workers, veterinarians, farmers, and fish-handlers.

The organism is cultured most often from biopsies, aspirates or blood. The bacilli are short (1–2 µm), but may produce long filamentous forms resembling lactobacilli. Growth is improved by incubation in 5–10% carbon dioxide. Colonies on blood agar are α-haemolytic.

Penicillin and other β-lactam antibiotics are effective. Erythromycin and clindamycin offer suitable alternatives, but *E. rhusiopathiae* is resistant to vancomycin.

### RECOMMENDED READING

Allerberger F, Wagner M: Listeriosis: a resurgent foodborne infection, *Clinical Microbiology and Infection* 16:16–23, 2010.

Cossart P, Toledo-Arana A: Listeria monocytogenes, a unique model in infection biology: an overview, *Microbes and Infection* 10:1041–1050, 2008.

Begg N: *Manual for the Management and Control of Diphtheria in the European Region*, Copenhagen, 1994, World Health Organization.

Brooke CJ, Riley TV: Erysipelothrix rhusiopathiae: biology, epidemiology and clinical manifestations of an occupational pathogen, *Journal of Medical Microbiology* 48:789–799, 1999.

Denny J, McLauchlin J: Human Listeria monocytogenes infections in Europe: An opportunity for improved pan-European Surveillance, *Eurosurveillance* 13:pii=8082, 2008.

Efstratiou A, George RC: Microbiology and epidemiology of diphtheria, *Reviews in Medical Microbiology* 7:31–42, 1996.

Efstratiou A, Engler KH, Mazurova IK et al: Current approaches to the laboratory diagnosis of diphtheria, *Journal of Infectious Diseases* 181:S138–S145, 2000.

Farber JM, Peterkin PI: Listeria monocytogenes, a food-borne pathogen, *Microbiology Reviews* 55:476–511, 1991.

Funke G, von Graevenitz A, Clarridge JE, Bernard K A: Clinical microbiology of coryneform bacteria, *Clinical Microbiology Reviews* 10:125–159, 1997.

Lianou A, Sofos JN: A review of the incidence and transmission of Listeria monocytogenes in ready-to-eat products in retail and food service environments, *Journal of Food Protection* 70:2172–2198, 2007.

Low JC, Donachie W: A review of Listeria monocytogenes and listeriosis, *Veterinary Journal* 153:9–29, 1997.

Robson JM, McDougall R, van der Valk S et al: Erysipelothrix rhusiopathiae: an uncommon but ever present zoonosis, *Pathology* 30:391–394, 1998.

Swaminathan B, Gerner-Smidt P: The epidemiology of human listeriosis, *Microbes and Infection* 9:1236–1243, 2007.

Wagner KS, White JM, Crowcroft NS et al: Diphtheria in the United Kingdom 1986–2008: the increasing role of Corynebacterium ulcerans, *Epidemiology and Infection* 138:1519–1530, 2010.

# 18 Mycobacterium

## Tuberculosis; leprosy

*J. M. Grange*

---

## KEY POINTS

- The mycobacteria are characterized by thick lipid-rich cell walls and the 'acid-fast' staining property.
- Most of the 130 or so named mycobacterial species are environmental saprophytes, although some occasionally cause disease, notably in immunosuppressed persons. *M. tuberculosis* and *M. leprae* are obligate pathogens.
- Tuberculosis is a chronic intracellular infection characterized by granuloma formation. Most individuals (about 90%) do not develop symptomatic disease and some remain latently infected.
- The lung is the usual site of initial infection and disease, but non-pulmonary forms occur. *Post-primary* tuberculosis is characterized by gross tissue necrosis leading to pulmonary cavity formation and aerogenous infectivity
- One-third of the world's population has been infected by the tubercle bacillus and about 100 million individuals are newly infected annually.
- Diagnosis is made by clinical and radiological examination, tuberculin testing and detection of the tubercle bacillus by acid-fast staining, culture and nucleic acid-based techniques. Therapy is based on a regimen of several drugs, usually for a period of 6 months. BCG is an attenuated live vaccine; its protective efficacy varies greatly between geographical regions and its overall impact on tuberculosis control is limited.
- Multi- and extensively drug resistant tuberculosis is encountered worldwide and requires the use of an extended range of anti-tuberculosis agents for its treatment.
- *M. leprae* has never been cultivated in vitro. In leprosy, the nerves and skin are the principal sites of disease, resulting in deformities and visible lesions.
- Transmission is probably by the aerogenous route rather than by touch.
- *Tuberculoid* leprosy is characterized by excessive granuloma formation in the presence of a very small (*paucibacillary*) bacterial load, whereas *lepromatous* leprosy is characterized by a huge (*multibacillary*) bacterial load and little or no immune reactivity.
- Diagnosis is by clinical examination, microscopic detection or PCR of bacilli in skin or nasal smears and biopsies. Multidrug treatment regimens are highly effective and BCG vaccination appears to offer some degree of protection.

The name of the genus *Mycobacterium* (fungus-bacterium) is an allusion to the mould-like pellicles formed when members of this genus are grown in liquid media. This hydrophobic property is due to their possession of thick, complex, lipid-rich, waxy cell walls. A further important characteristic, also due to their waxy cell walls, is *acid-fastness*, or resistance to decolourization by a dilute mineral acid (or acid with alcohol) after staining with hot carbol fuchsin or other arylmethane dyes.

There are over 130 named species of mycobacteria, the great majority of which are environmental saprophytes, although some cause opportunist disease in humans and animals (see Ch. 19). There are, however, two human mycobacterial diseases caused by obligate pathogens – tuberculosis and leprosy. The former is caused by members of the *Mycobacterium tuberculosis* complex, strictly speaking one species, and the latter by the leprosy bacillus, *Mycobacterium leprae,* which has never convincingly been grown in vitro.

## MYCOBACTERIUM TUBERCULOSIS COMPLEX

The '*M. tuberculosis* complex' refers to a group of genetically very closely related variants of what is strictly speaking a single species. All cause *tuberculosis*, a chronic granulomatous disease affecting humans and many other mammals. The complex includes:

- *M. tuberculosis*, the predominant cause of human tuberculosis.
- *M. bovis*, the principal cause of tuberculosis in cattle and many other mammals including humans.
- *M. africanum*, which appears to be intermediate in form between the human and bovine types. It causes human tuberculosis and is found mainly in equatorial Africa. Type 1 is more common in West Africa and has several features in common with *M. bovis*; type 2 is mainly of east African origin and more closely resembles *M. tuberculosis*.
- *M. caprae*, isolated from goats and the cause of a few cases of tuberculosis in veterinary surgeons.
- *M. pinnipedi*, an uncommon pathogen of seals and a very rare cause of tuberculosis in those occupationally exposed to seals.
- *M. microti*, a rarely encountered pathogen of voles and other small mammals, but which is attenuated in humans.
- *M. canetti*, a very rare and genetically primitive member of the complex.

## DESCRIPTION

The entire genomes of *M. tuberculosis* and *M. bovis* have been sequenced. On the basis of sequencing, there is evidence that the members of the *M. tuberculosis complex (tubercle bacilli)* listed above devolved from a common progenitor by the successive loss of short chromosomal segments known as Regions of Difference (RD). The variants closest to the progenitor form are *M. canetti* and certain strains common in South India. Contrary to earlier opinion, *M. bovis* appears to have devolved from *M. tuberculosis*. A number of families or lineages are distinguishable within each species, notably *M. tuberculosis*, and one particular family, the Beijing or W/Beijing family, is spreading worldwide, is of high virulence and readily mutates to drug resistance while retaining high virulence.

Tubercle bacilli are non-motile, non-sporing, non-capsulate, straight or slightly curved rods about 3 ×

**Fig. 18.1** Fluorescent stained microcolonies of *M. tuberculosis* showing 'serpentine cord' formation.

0.3 µm in size. In sputum and other clinical specimens they may occur singly or in small clumps, and in liquid cultures they often grow as twisted rope-like colonies termed *serpentine cords* (Fig. 18.1). They are able to grow on a wide range of enriched culture media, but Löwenstein–Jensen (LJ) medium is the most widely used in clinical practice. This is an egg–glycerol-based medium to which malachite green dye is added to inhibit the growth of some contaminating bacteria and to provide a contrasting colour against which colonies of mycobacteria are easily seen. Strains of *M. bovis* grow poorly, or not at all, on standard LJ medium but grow much better on media containing sodium pyruvate in place of glycerol. Agar-based media or broths enriched with bovine serum albumin are also used, particularly in automated culture systems.

On subculture, human tubercle bacilli usually produce visible growth on LJ medium in 2–4 weeks, although on primary isolation from clinical material colonies may take up to 8 weeks to appear. Colonies are of an off-white (buff) colour and (except for the very rarely encountered *M. canetti* which has smooth colonies) usually have a dry breadcrumb-like appearance. Growth is characteristically heaped up and luxuriant or 'eugonic', in contrast to the small, flat 'dysgonic' colonies of *M. bovis*.

The optimal growth temperature of tubercle bacilli is 35–37°C, but they fail to grow at 25°C or 41°C. Most other mycobacteria grow at one or other, or both, of these temperatures.

All mycobacteria are obligate aerobes, but *M. bovis* grows better in conditions of reduced oxygen tension.

**Table 18.1** Some differential characteristics of the principal tubercle bacilli causing human disease

| Species | Atmospheric preference | Nitratase | TCH | Pyrazinamide |
|---|---|---|---|---|
| *M. tuberculosis* | Aerobic | Positive | Resistant[a] | Sensitive |
| *M. bovis* | Micro-aerophilic | Negative | Sensitive | Resistant |
| *M. bovis* BCG | Aerobic | Negative | Sensitive | Resistant |
| *M. africanum* I | Micro-aerophilic | Negative | Sensitive | Sensitive |
| *M. africanum* II | Micro-aerophilic | Positive | Sensitive | Sensitive |

[a]Strains from southern India may be sensitive.
TCH, thiophen-2-carboxylic acid hydrazide.

Thus, when incorporated in soft agar media, *M. tuberculosis* grows on the surface whereas *M. bovis* grows as a band a few millimetres below the surface. This provides a useful differentiating test. Various other differential characteristics of human tubercle bacilli are shown in Table 18.1.

Tubercle bacilli survive in milk and other organic materials and on pasture land so long as they are not exposed to ultraviolet light, to which they are very sensitive. They are also heat sensitive and are destroyed by pasteurization. Mycobacteria are susceptible to alcohol, formaldehyde, glutaraldehyde and, to a lesser extent, hypochlorites and phenolic disinfectants. They are considerably more resistant than other bacteria to acids, alkalis and quaternary ammonium compounds.

## PATHOGENESIS

The tubercle bacillus owes its virulence to its ability to survive within the macrophage rather than to the production of a toxic substance. The mechanism of virulence is poorly understood and is almost certainly multifactorial, resulting in inappropriate patterns of immune reactivity. The immune response to the bacillus is of the cell-mediated type, which, if mediated by T helper ($T_H$) cells and associated type 1 cytokines, leads to protective immunity, although the presence of $T_H2$ cells and associated cytokines facilitates tissue-destroying hypersensitivity reactions and progression of the disease process. The nature of the immune responses following infection changes with time, so that human tuberculosis is divisible into primary and post-primary forms with quite different pathological features.

### Primary tuberculosis

The site of the initial infection is usually the lung, following the inhalation of bacilli. These bacilli are

**Fig. 18.2** Tuberculous cervical lymphadenitis (scrofula) with sinus formation in an Indonesian woman.

engulfed by alveolar macrophages in which they replicate to form the initial lesion. Some bacilli are carried in phagocytic cells to the hilar lymph nodes where additional foci of infection develop. The initial focus of infection together with the enlarged hilar lymph nodes forms the *primary complex*. In addition, bacilli are seeded by further lymphatic and haematogenous dissemination in many organs and tissues, including other parts of the lung. When the bacilli enter the mouth, as when drinking milk containing *M. bovis*, the primary complexes involve the tonsil and cervical nodes (*scrofula*; Fig. 18.2) or the intestine, often the ileocaecal region, and the mesenteric lymph nodes. Likewise, the primary focus may be in the skin, with involvement of the regional lymph nodes. This uncommon type of tuberculosis, formerly termed *prosector's wart*, is principally an occupational disease of anatomists, pathologists and meat handlers.

During infection, antigens of *M. tuberculosis* are processed by antigen-presenting cells, activated by bacterial components termed adjuvants, and presented to antigen-specific T lymphocytes which undergo clonal proliferation. The activated T cells release cytokines, notably interferon-γ, which, together with calcitriol, activate macrophages (Fig. 18.3) and cause them to form a compact cluster, or granuloma, around the foci of infection (Fig. 18.4). These activated macrophages are termed *epithelioid cells* because of their microscopical resemblance to epithelial cells. Some of them fuse to form multinucleate giant cells. The centre of the granuloma contains a mixture of necrotic tissue and dead macrophages, and, because

of its cheese-like appearance and consistency, is referred to as *caseation*.

Activated human macrophages inhibit the replication of the tubercle bacilli, but their ability to kill ingested bacilli is limited. Being metabolically very active, the macrophages in the granuloma consume oxygen, and the resulting anoxia and acidosis in the centre of the lesion probably kills most of the bacilli. Granuloma formation is usually sufficient to limit the primary infection: the lesions become quiescent and surrounding fibroblasts produce dense scar tissue, which may become calcified. Programmed cell death (apoptosis) of bacteria-laden macrophages by cytotoxic T cells and natural killer (NK) cells contributes to protective immunity by generating a metabolic burst that kills tubercle bacilli.

In a minority of cases one of the infective foci progresses and gives rise to the serious manifestations of primary disease, including progressive local lesions (particularly in infants; Table 18.2), meningitis, pleurisy and disease of the kidneys, spine (*Pott's disease*) and other bones and joints. If a focus ruptures into a blood vessel, bacilli are disseminated throughout the body with the formation of numerous granulomata. This, from the millet seed-like appearance of the lesions, is known as *miliary tuberculosis*.

## Tuberculin reactivity

About 6–8 weeks after the initial infection, the phenomenon of tuberculin conversion occurs. This altered reactivity was discovered by Robert Koch while attempting to develop a remedy for tuberculosis based on *old tuberculin* – a heat-concentrated filtrate of a broth in which tubercle bacilli had been grown. Although Koch's tuberculin proved unsuccessful as a therapeutic agent, it formed the basis of the widely used tuberculin test (see below).

## Latent tuberculosis

In most infected individuals, the primary infection resolves but some residual tubercle bacilli enter a poorly understood stage of latency or dormancy. It was previously assumed that 'once infected, always infected', but as the risk of developing active tuberculosis after initial infection is highest within the first and second year, around 1% and 0.3% respectively, and much lower in subsequent years, it seems likely that tubercle bacilli are totally eliminated in many infected individuals. This is also suggested by the finding that the risk of a HIV-infected person developing tuberculosis is much higher if they are newly infected by tubercle bacilli than if they had been

**Fig. 18.3** Antigens of *M. tuberculosis* are, after priming by adjuvants, processed by the antigen-presenting cell (APC) and presented to T helper lymphocytes (T), which are activated and proliferate to form a clone. T cell-produced interferon (IFN)-γ and calcitriol activate the resting macrophages (MAC).

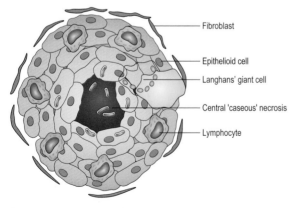

**Fig. 18.4** The granuloma of primary tuberculosis.

**Table 18.2** Stages of primary tuberculosis in childhood

| Stage | Time (from onset) | Characteristics |
|---|---|---|
| 1 | 3–8 weeks | Primary complex develops and tuberculin conversion occurs |
| 2 | 2–6 months | Progressive healing of primary complex |
| | | Possibility of pleural effusion |
| 3 | 6–12 months | Possibility of miliary or meningeal tuberculosis |
| 4 | 1–3 years | Possibility of bone or joint tuberculosis |
| 5 | 3–5 years or more | Possibility of genito-urinary or chronic skin tuberculosis |

Adapted from Miller FJW 1982 *Tuberculosis in Children.* Churchill Livingstone, Edinburgh.

**Table 18.3** Main differences between primary and post-primary tuberculosis in non-immunocompromised patients

| Characteristic | Primary | Post-primary |
|---|---|---|
| Local lesion | Small | Large |
| Lymphatic involvement | Yes | Minimal |
| Cavity formation | Rare | Frequent |
| Tuberculin reactivity | Negative (initially) | Positive |
| Infectivity[a] | Uncommon | Usual |
| Site | Any part of lung | Apical region |
| Local spread | Uncommon | Frequent |

[a]Pulmonary cases.

infected before acquiring HIV. The use of molecular fingerprinting has established that exogenous reinfection occurs far more readily than was previously thought. Long term latency may, however, occur as small numbers of reactivation tuberculosis due to *M. bovis* are encountered for several decades after effective eradication of cattle tuberculosis in a given region.

## Post-primary tuberculosis

Reactivation of dormant foci of tubercle bacilli or exogenous reinfection leads to post-primary tuberculosis, which differs in several respects from primary disease (Table 18.3). For unknown reasons, reactivation or reinfection tuberculosis tends to develop in the upper lobes of the lungs. The same process of granuloma formation occurs, but the necrotic element of the reaction causes extensive tissue destruction and the formation of large areas of caseation termed *tuberculomas*. Proteases liberated by activated macrophages soften and liquefy the caseous material, and an excess of tumour necrosis factor and other immunological mediators causes the wasting and fevers characteristic of the disease.

The interior of the tuberculoma is acidic and anoxic, and contains few viable tubercle bacilli. Eventually, however, the expanding lesion erodes through the wall of a bronchus, the liquefied contents are discharged and a well aerated cavity is formed. The atmosphere of the lung, with a high carbon dioxide level, is ideal for supporting the growth of the bacilli, and huge numbers of these are found in the cavity walls. For this reason, closure of the cavities by collapsing the lung, either by artificial pneumothorax or by excising large portions of the chest wall, was a standard treatment for tuberculosis in the pre-chemotherapy era.

Once the cavity is formed, large numbers of bacilli gain access to the sputum, and the patient becomes an open or infectious case. This is a good example of the transmissibility of a pathogen being dependent upon the host's immune response to infection. Surprisingly, about 20% of cases of open cavitating tuberculosis in the pre-therapy era resolved without treatment.

In post-primary tuberculosis, dissemination of bacilli to lymph nodes and other organs is unusual. Instead, spread of infection occurs through the bronchial tree so that secondary lesions develop in the lower lobes of the lung and, occasionally, in the trachea, larynx and mouth. Bacilli in swallowed sputum cause intestinal lesions. Secondary lesions may also develop in the bladder and epididymis in cases of renal tuberculosis. Post-primary cutaneous tuberculosis (*lupus vulgaris*) usually affects the face and neck. Untreated, it is a chronic condition leading to gross scarring and deformity. Most cases of lupus vulgaris were caused by *M. bovis* and this condition is now rarely seen in developed countries where transmission of disease from cattle rarely if ever occurs. Some cases of cutaneous tuberculosis are secondary to sinus formation between tuberculous lymph nodes and the skin (*scrofuloderma*) and other structures including bones and joints (Fig. 18.5).

### Immunocompromised individuals

People with congenital or acquired causes of immunosuppression, including the very young, the elderly and recipients of organ transplants, are at a much higher

**Fig. 18.5** Tuberculosis of the ankle with sinus formation and overlying involvement of the skin.

risk of developing tuberculosis due to reactivation of latent disease or following infection or reinfection. HIV infection has emerged as the major predisposing factor to active tuberculosis worldwide (see below). Tuberculosis acts synergistically with HIV to lower the patient's immunity and it is a defining condition for the acquired immune deficiency syndrome (AIDS). As a result, even when tuberculosis is treated effectively in HIV-positive patients, the mortality rate from other AIDS-related conditions is high, with many dying within 2 years. Cavity formation is unusual in the more profoundly immunocompromised patients, emphasizing the importance of the immune response in this pathological process. Instead, diffuse infiltrates develop in any part of the lung. In contrast to post-primary disease in non-immunocompromised individuals, lymphatic and haematogenous dissemination are common. Sometimes there are numerous minute lesions teeming with tubercle bacilli throughout the body – a rapidly fatal condition termed cryptic disseminated tuberculosis. The interval between infection and development of disease is considerably shortened in immunocompromised persons.

### The tuberculin test and other immunological tests

Although Robert Koch's attempts to use old tuberculin as a remedy for tuberculosis failed, an Austrian physician, Clemens von Pirquet, used the Koch phenomenon as an indication of bacterial 'allergy'

resulting from previous infection. Individuals with active tuberculosis were usually tuberculin positive, but many of those with disseminated and rapidly progressive disease were negative. This led to the widespread but erroneous belief that tuberculin reactivity is an indicator of immunity to tuberculosis.

Old tuberculin caused non-specific reactions and has been replaced by *purified protein derivative* (PPD). This is given by:

- intracutaneous injection (Mantoux method)
- a spring-loaded gun which fires six prongs into the skin through a drop of PPD (Heaf method)
- single-test disposable devices with PPD dried on to prongs (tine tests).

The biological activity of tuberculin is compared with international standards and activity expressed in international units (IU). In the UK, solutions of PPD for Mantoux testing are supplied as dilutions of 1 in 10 000, 1 in 1000 and 1 in 100, which correspond to 1, 10 and 100 IU in the injected dose of 0.1 mL. The standard test dose is 10 IU, but those suspected of having tuberculosis, and who are therefore likely to react strongly, may first be tested with 1 IU. Undiluted PPD is supplied for use with the Heaf gun.

The tuberculin test is widely used as a diagnostic test, although its usefulness is limited by its failure to distinguish active disease from quiescent infections and past Bacille Calmette–Guérin (BCG) vaccination and, in some regions, sensitization by environmental mycobacteria. Numerous attempts have therefore been made to develop alternative immunological tests for the disease, though with many setbacks. One promising approach, though not without problems of specificity, is the detection of interferon-γ-producing peripheral blood T cells that respond to antigens present in virulent tubercle bacilli but not environmental mycobacteria or BCG.

## LABORATORY DIAGNOSIS

The definitive diagnosis of tuberculosis is based on detection of the causative organism in clinical specimens by microscopy, cultural techniques or the polymerase chain reaction (PCR) and its various derivatives.

### Specimens

The most usual specimen for diagnosis of pulmonary tuberculosis is sputum but, if none is produced, bronchial washings, brushings or biopsies and early-morning gastric aspirates (to harvest any bacilli swallowed overnight) may be examined. Tissue biopsies are homogenized by grinding for microscopy and culture. Cerebrospinal fluid, pleural fluid, urine and other fluids are centrifuged and the deposits examined.

## Microscopy

Use is made of the acid-fast property of mycobacteria to detect them in sputum and other clinical material. In the Ziehl–Neelsen (ZN) staining technique, heat-fixed smears of the specimens are flooded with a solution of carbol fuchsin (a mixture of basic fuchsin and phenol) and heated until steam rises. After washing with water, the slide is flooded with a dilute mineral acid (e.g. 3% hydrochloric acid) and, after further washing, a green or blue counterstain is applied. Red bacilli are seen against the contrasting background colour. In some methods, the acid is diluted in 95% ethanol rather than water. This gives a cleaner background but, contrary to a common belief, it does not enable tubercle bacilli to be distinguished from other mycobacteria. Fluorescence microscopy, based on the same principle of acid-fastness, is increasingly used and is much less tiring for the microscopist. Modifications of the various staining techniques are used to examine tissue sections.

## Cultural methods

As sputum and certain other specimens frequently contain many bacteria and fungi that would rapidly overgrow any mycobacteria on the culture media, these must be destroyed. Decontamination methods make use of the relatively high resistance of mycobacteria to acids, alkalis and certain disinfectants. In the widely used *Petroff method*, sputum is mixed well with 4% sodium hydroxide for 15–30 min, neutralized with potassium dihydrogen orthophosphate and centrifuged. The deposit is used to inoculate LJ or similar media. Specimens such as cerebrospinal fluid and tissue biopsies, which are unlikely to be contaminated, are inoculated directly on to culture media. As an alternative to chemical decontamination, mixtures of antibiotics that kill fungi and all bacteria other than mycobacteria may be added to the culture media. These are used principally in the automated culture systems described below.

Inoculated media are incubated at 35–37°C and inspected weekly for at least 8 weeks. Cultures of material from skin lesions should also be incubated at 33°C. Any bacterial growth is stained by the ZN method and, if acid-fast, subcultured for further identification.

A more rapid bacteriological diagnosis is achievable by use of commercially available automated systems. Systems that detect colour changes in dyes induced by the release of carbon dioxide, or the unquenching of fluorescent dyes on the consumption of oxygen by metabolizing bacilli, have replaced the earlier radiometric method.

The first step in identification is to determine whether an isolate is a member of the *M. tuberculosis* complex. These organisms:

- grow slowly
- do not produce yellow pigment
- fail to grow at 25°C and 41°C
- do not grow on egg media containing *p*-nitrobenzoic acid (500 mg/L).

Strains differing in any of these properties belong to other species.

## Nucleic acid technology

Amplification of specific nucleic acid sequences in specimens is achievable by PCR and related techniques. Initial problems of low sensitivity, 'false-positive' reactions and cross-contamination have been largely overcome by the introduction of closed-system, isothermal techniques for amplification of species-specific 16S ribosomal ribonucleic acid (RNA). User-friendly automated systems with high sensitivity and specificity are commercially available.

Molecular techniques for fingerprinting members of the *M. tuberculosis* complex for epidemiological purposes have been developed. An early method, restriction length polymorphism (RFLP) analysis, was based on the determination of the numbers and position on electrophoretic gels and of the insertion sequence IS6110, 1 to 20 copies of which are present in most strains. Preferred methods now include spoligotyping, based on the detection of spacer oligonucleotides, short DNA sequences found around the sites of the insertion sequences, and analysis of genetic units termed mycobacterial interspersed repetitive units (MIRU), each of which each has sequential, or tandem, repeats which vary in number from species to species, proving a highly discriminative typing system for strains with few or no IS6110 insertion sequences.

## Drug susceptibility testing

Several methods have been described.

- Assessment of growth inhibition on solid media containing various dilutions of the drug, in comparison with test strains. As the methods depend on observation of visible growth, results are not available until several weeks after isolation of the organism.

- Automated systems, based on the activation or quenching of dyes by metabolic activity of the bacilli, provide results more quickly.
- Nucleic acid technology, which is even more rapid, though relatively expensive. Reverse hybridization assays for the detection of resistance to rifampicin and isoniazid are commercially available and 'in-house' assay methods for pyrazinamide and ethambutol have been described.

## TREATMENT

The antituberculosis drugs are divisible into three groups (Table 18.4):

1. Bactericidal drugs that effectively sterilize tuberculous lesions.
2. Bactericidal drugs that kill tubercle bacilli only in certain situations. Streptomycin is effective in neutral or alkaline environments, such as the cavity wall; pyrazinamide is active only in acidic environments, such as within macrophages and in dense inflammatory tissue; and isoniazid only kills actively replicating bacilli.
3. Bacteristatic drugs, which are of limited usefulness and are only used when drug resistance renders the agents in the two groups above ineffective.

Mutation to drug resistance occurs at a rate of about one mutation every $10^8$ cell divisions. Successful therapy requires the prevention of the emergence of drug-resistant strains by the simultaneous use of at least two drugs to which the organism is sensitive.

The current World Health Organization recommendations are that all new patients with tuberculosis, irrespective of site or severity of disease, and in the absence of evidence of drug resistance, should receive a 6-month course of therapy, consisting of a 2-month intensive phase of rifampicin, isoniazid, pyrazinamide and ethambutol followed by 4-month phase of rifampicin and isoniazid. Ideally, the drugs are given daily, but they may be given thrice weekly during the continuation phase or throughout, provided that all doses are given under careful supervision and that the patient is not HIV seropositive.

The response to therapy of drug-susceptible tuberculosis is divisible into three phases:

1. During the first week or two, the large numbers of actively replicating bacilli in cavity walls are killed, principally by isoniazid, but also by rifampicin and ethambutol. The patient rapidly ceases to be infectious, and prolonged hospitalization with barrier nursing is now rarely necessary.
2. In the following few weeks the less active bacilli within macrophages, caseous material and dense, acidic, inflammatory lesions are killed by pyrazinamide and rifampicin.
3. In the continuation phase any remaining dormant bacilli are killed by rifampicin during their short bursts of metabolic activity. Any rifampicin-resistant mutants that arise and start to replicate are killed by isoniazid.

Short-course regimens are usually well tolerated by the patient. Isoniazid, rifampicin and pyrazinamide are all potentially hepatotoxic, and rifampicin may cause an influenza-like syndrome, which, paradoxically, is more likely to occur when the drug is given intermittently. Rifampicin antagonizes the action of several drugs and also oral contraceptives – an important point to be considered when treating women. There is also mutual antagonism between rifampicin and the antiretroviral drugs used for HIV infection (see Ch. 55). Isoniazid may cause mild psychiatric disturbances and peripheral neuropathy, particularly in alcoholics, but these are usually preventable by prescribing pyridoxine (vitamin $B_6$). Ethambutol is toxic to the eye and, although this is rare with standard dosages, care is required; the patient should be informed of this possibility.

The emergence of drug-resistant strains is a major barrier to the control of tuberculosis. According to World Health Organization there were, in 2009, an estimated 250 000 patients (range, 230 000–270 000) with multidrug resistant tuberculosis worldwide, but only 12% were diagnosed and notified, indicating a serious need to strengthen services to address this emerging problem.

Resistance may develop during therapy (acquired resistance) with poor quality drugs or inadequate supervision, or patients may be infected with resistant

| Table 18.4 | In-vivo activity of antituberculosis drugs | |
| --- | --- | --- |
| Sterilizing | Bactericidal | Bacteristatic |
| Rifampicin | Isoniazid | Ethionamide |
| Pyrazinamide | Streptomycin | Prothionamide |
| | Ethambutol[a] | Thiacetazone |
| | Quinolones | p-Aminosalicylic acid |
| | Macrolides | Cycloserine |

[a]In early stages of therapy.

strains (initial or primary resistance). Multidrug-resistant strains are defined as those resistant to isoniazid and rifampicin, with or without resistance to additional drugs. The newer category of extensively drug resistant tuberculosis (XDR-TB) is defined as resistance to, at least, isoniazid, rifampicin, any fluroquinolone and any injectable agent. The exact incidence of XDR-TB is unknown as susceptibility testing to a wide range of drugs is not widely available but in June 2008, 49 countries reported confirmed cases.

Wherever possible, drug susceptibility tests, at least for isoniazid and rifampicin and ideally by rapid molecular methods, should be conducted on all patients who relapse after a course of standard therapy. The categories of agents for treating drug-resistant tuberculosis are listed in Table 18.5 and their use depends on local guidelines based on known resistance trends. Group 1 agents are the most effective and best tolerated; Group 2 (injectable) and Group 3 (fluroquinolone) agents are added unless resistance to them is has been demonstrated. Group 4 agents are less effective and often poorly tolerated and, like Group 5 agents, are used in cases of extensive resistance in which the previous groups would prove ineffective. With careful and caring supervision, the

majority of patients with drug resistance can be cured, although HIV seropositivity is a poor prognostic factor.

## EPIDEMIOLOGY

In 2009 there were, according to World Health Organization estimates, 9.4 million new cases of tuberculosis (range, 8.9 million–9.9 million) and 14 million prevalent cases (range, 12 million–16 million) worldwide. Most cases were in the South-East Asia (35%), African (30%) and Western Pacific regions (20%). There were an estimated 1.3 million deaths due to tuberculosis among HIV-negative people (range, 1.2 million–1.5 million) and 0.38 million deaths among HIV-positive people (range, 0.32 million–0.45 million).

Human tuberculosis is transmitted principally by inhalation of bacilli in moist droplets coughed out by individuals with open pulmonary tuberculosis. Dried bacilli in dust appear to be much less of a health hazard. The sputum of patients with positive findings on microscopy contains at least 5000 tubercle bacilli per millilitre; these patients are considerably more infectious than those who have negative findings on microscopy. Most transmission of the disease occurs within households or other environments where individuals are close together for long periods.

For epidemiological purposes, the incidence of infection by the tubercle bacillus in a community is calculated from the number of tuberculin-positive individuals in different age groups, provided they have not received BCG vaccination. The annual infection rate gives an indirect measure of the number of open or infectious individuals in the community. Although subject to many variables, a 1% annual infection rate indicates that there are around 50 infectious cases in every 100 000 members of the community. The prevalence of tuberculosis in a region is not the same as the annual infection rate, because only a minority of infected individuals develop overt disease and they often become ill several years after the initial infection.

Tuberculosis is relatively uncommon in the industrially developed nations, with an annual infection rate of 0.3–0.1% or less, but the previous decline has halted and in several countries there has been an increase in notifications since around 1990. The disease is often concentrated in certain 'hot spots', particularly deprived inner city areas. In the developing countries the annual infection rates are usually between 2% and 5%.

In many parts of the world, implementation of the World Health Organization control strategies have

| Table 18.5 WHO groups of antituberculosis agents for the treatment of multi- and extensive drug resistant tuberculosis | |
|---|---|
| Group | Antituberculosis agent |
| 1: First-line oral agents | Pyrazinamide<br>Ethambutol<br>Rifabutin |
| 2: Injectable agents | Capreomycin<br>Amikacin<br>Streptomycin<br>Kanamycin |
| 3: Fluoroquinolones | Levofloxacin<br>Ofloxacin<br>Moxifloxacin |
| 4: Oral bacteriostatic second-line agents | p-Aminosalicylic acid<br>Cycloserine<br>Terizidone<br>Ethionamide<br>Prothionamide |
| 5: Agents with unclear roles in the treatment of drug resistant tuberculosis | Clofazimine<br>Linezolid<br>Amoxycillin/clavulanate<br>Thioacetazone<br>Imipenem/cilastatin<br>High-dose isoniazid<br>Clarithromycin |

led to substantial reductions in the incidence of tuberculosis but, overall these gains have been offset by the impact of the HIV/AIDS pandemic. In 2009, 11–12% of all cases of tuberculosis were HIV related, with 80% of cases occurring in sub-Saharan Africa.

A person infected by the tubercle bacillus before acquiring HIV has an 8% annual risk of developing active tuberculosis but the risk of an HIV-infected person developing tuberculosis after infection or reinfection is much higher, approaching 100%. The interval between infection and overt disease is considerably shortened, resulting in explosive mini-epidemics in institutions where HIV-positive persons congregate. Some such mini-epidemics have involved multidrug-resistant strains, notably in the USA.

Bovine tuberculosis is spread from animal to animal, and sometimes to human attendants, in moist cough spray. About 1% of infected cows develop lesions in the udder, and bacilli excreted in the milk can then infect people who drink it. Heat treatment, or pasteurization, prevents milk-borne disease. In most developed countries, the incidence of bovine tuberculosis has been reduced drastically by regular tuberculin testing of herds and the slaughter of reactors, but the total eradication has been prevented by infection of cattle from wild animals, notably badgers in the UK and possums in New Zealand. Human disease due to *M. bovis* is very rare in developed countries and is usually the result of reactivation of old lesions. Cattle have occasionally been infected by farm workers with open tuberculosis due to *M. bovis*. The prevalence of the disease in cattle in the developing nations is poorly documented. Person-to-person spread of *M. bovis* leading to active disease is uncommon, although a few instances of such spread among HIV-positive persons have been reported. Occupational exposure to goats and seals has resulted in a few cases of tuberculosis due, respectively, to *M. caprae* and *M. pinnipedi*.

## CONTROL

Human tuberculosis is preventable:

- by the early detection and effective therapy of the open or infectious individuals in a community
- by lowering the chance of infection by reducing overcrowding
- to a limited extent, by vaccination.

Active case finding involves a deliberate search, often on a house-to-house basis or in workplaces, for suspects with a chronic cough of a month or more in duration. Merely waiting for patients with symptoms

to seek medical attention is much less effective, even when supported by education programmes. Regular chest examination by mass miniature radiography detects fewer than 15% of individuals with tuberculosis and its use is now restricted to certain high-risk situations.

The most important factors affecting the incidence of tuberculosis are socio-economic ones, particularly those leading to a reduction of overcrowding in homes and workplaces. In developing countries it is estimated that each patient with open tuberculosis infects about 20 contacts annually, whereas in Europe the corresponding figure is two or three.

## Vaccination

Bacille Calmette–Guérin (BCG) is a living attenuated vaccine derived from a strain of *M. bovis* by repeated subculture between the years 1908 and 1921. This species was selected rather than *M. tuberculosis* as the vaccine was initially intended for veterinary use. Although originally administered orally, BCG is now given by intracutaneous injection.

The protective efficacy of BCG varies enormously from country to country. Early trials in the UK indicated that administration of BCG to schoolchildren afforded 78% protection, but a major trial in south India involving individuals of all ages found no protection (Table 18.6). Several explanations have been advanced for this difference, the most likely one being prior exposure of the human population to environmental mycobacteria, which, in some regions, confer some protection, but in others induce inappropriate immune reactions that antagonize protection. For this reason, neonatal vaccination is recommended.

When BCG vaccination is introduced into a region it has an immediate impact on the incidence of the

**Table 18.6** Variations in the protective efficacy of BCG vaccinations in nine major trials

| Country or population | Age range of vaccinees (years) | Protection (%) |
|---|---|---|
| North American Indian | 0–20 | 80 |
| UK | 14–15 | 78 |
| Chicago, Illinois, USA | Neonates | 75 |
| Puerto Rico | 1–18 | 31 |
| South India (Bangalore) | All ages | 30 |
| Georgia and Alabama, USA | >5 | 14 |
| Georgia, USA | 6–17 | 0 |
| Illinois, USA | Young adults | 0 |
| South India (Chingleput) | All ages | 0[a] |

[a]Some protection demonstrated in those vaccinated neonatally on 15-year follow-up.

serious but non-infectious forms of childhood tuberculosis such as meningitis, but has little impact on the annual infection rate in the community as the smear-positive source cases arise mostly from among the older, unvaccinated, tuberculin-positive members of the community. Vaccination has not therefore proved to be an effective control measure.

Being a living vaccine, serious infections and even disseminated disease may occur in immunocompromised persons. Thus, BCG should never be given to persons known to be HIV-positive. Many attempts are currently being made to develop alternative vaccines, particularly non-viable subunit ones.

## Prophylactic chemotherapy

In true prophylactic chemotherapy, drugs are administered to uninfected individuals who are in unavoidable contact with a patient with open tuberculosis. The main example is an infant born to a mother with the disease. More usually, it refers to therapy, principally with isoniazid alone for 6–12 months, given to individuals who have been infected but show no signs of active disease. A shorter, 3-month, regimen of isoniazid and rifampicin is as effective as a 12-month course of isoniazid and with less hepatic toxicity and is advocated in the UK. An even shorter, 2-month, regimen of isoniazid, rifampicin and pyrazinamide was equally effective but was withdrawn due to severe and sometimes fatal adverse effects in HIV-positive patients. Persons co-infected with *M. tuberculosis* and HIV who are positive on tuberculin testing or the interferon-γ test are much more responsive to preventive therapy than those who are negative, and the WHO thus recommends prophylactic therapy only for the former. Other indications are for children positive on tuberculin testing or the interferon-γ test, recently converting adults exposed to a source case or with an immune suppressing condition, and those with fibrotic lung lesions suggesting untreated but healed tuberculosis.

## MYCOBACTERIUM LEPRAE

Leprosy is a particularly tragic affliction as the nature of the infection often causes severe disfigurement and deformity which, throughout history, have led to social ostracism or even total banishment from society of those suffering from the disease. The disease was long endemic in the British Isles; Robert the Bruce of Scotland was one of its victims. The last British patient to acquire the disease in this country died in the Shetland Islands in 1798. In Norway the disease persisted into the twentieth century; Armauer Hansen first described the causative organism in that country in 1873.

The current situation is cause for optimism as the number of registered patients on treatment declined from more than 10 million in 1982 to 514 718 in 2003 and 244 796 in 2009. The decline has been slower in recent years, but this may reflect a higher case detection rate. Leprosy has been eliminated from 119 out of the 122 countries in which the disease was regarded as a public health problem in 1985 and, in stark contrast to tuberculosis, resistance to therapy has not proved to be a barrier to treatment. The World Health Organization has therefore adopted a 'final push' strategy with the goal of eliminating this disease.

Leprosy is often cited as a disease of great antiquity but literary and skeletal evidence of this very characteristic disease go back no further than 500 BC. Biblical leprosy was almost certainly not the same as the disease that now bears this name. This raises the intriguing question of the ancestry of this bacillus which has no widespread animal reservoirs. Natural environmental reservoirs for a progenitor of *M. leprae*, such as amoebe, have been postulated but not convincingly demonstrated. Likewise, it has been postulated that *M. leprae* can survive in the environment, possibly in amoebe, and infect human beings.

## DESCRIPTION

*M. leprae* has never convincingly been cultivated in vitro; this has been attributed to a loss or disruption of many of the genes required for metabolism. The genome of *M. leprae* is smaller than that of cultivable mycobacteria, and about half of its genes are defective counterparts of functional ones found in other mycobacteria. In the 1970s it was shown that armadillos experimentally infected with *M. leprae* often developed extensive disease, with up to $10^{10}$ bacilli in each gram of diseased tissue. This animal has therefore provided sufficient bacilli for research projects and for the production of a skin test reagent, leprosin-A. Limited replication, yielding $10^6$ bacilli after 6–8 months, also occurs in the mouse footpad, and this has been used for testing the sensitivity of bacilli to antileprosy drugs.

Leprosy bacilli resemble tubercle bacilli in their general morphology, but they are not so strongly acid-fast. In clinical material from lepromatous patients, the bacilli are typically found within macrophages in dense clumps. A characteristic surface lipid, peptidoglycolipid-1 (PGL-1), has been extracted from *M. leprae*, and its unique carbohydrate antigenic determinant has been synthesized. Specific PCR primers for diagnostic purposes and for seeking the bacillus or its progenitor in the natural environment have been synthesized.

## PATHOGENESIS

The principal target cell for the leprosy bacillus is the Schwann cell. The resulting nerve damage is responsible for the main clinical features of leprosy: anaesthesia and muscle paralysis. Repeated injuries to, and infection of, the anaesthetic extremities leads to their gradual destruction (Fig. 18.6). Infiltration of the skin and cutaneous nerves by bacilli leads to the formation of visible lesions, often with pigmentary changes.

**Fig. 18.6**   Borderline tuberculoid leprosy. Trophic changes in the hands secondary to nerve damage, vasculitis and anaesthesia.

The first sign of leprosy is a non-specific or indeterminate skin lesion, which often heals spontaneously. If the disease progresses, its clinical manifestation is determined by the specific immune responsiveness of the patient to the bacillus, and there is a distinct immunological spectrum of the disease (Table 18.7). The points on the spectrum are:

- Hyper-reactive *tuberculoid* (TT) leprosy, with small numbers of localized skin lesions containing so few bacilli that they are not seen on microscopy and an inappropriately intense granulomatous response that often damages major nerve trunks.
- Anergic *lepromatous* (LL) leprosy, in which the skin lesions are numerous or confluent and contain huge numbers of bacilli, usually seen as clusters or globi within monocytes. Cooler parts of the body, such as the ear lobes, are particularly heavily infiltrated by bacilli (Fig. 18.7). There is no histological evidence of an immune response.
- Intermediate forms classified as borderline tuberculoid (BT), mid-borderline (BB) or borderline lepromatous (BL).

Destruction of the nasal bones may lead to collapse of the nose (Fig. 18.8). In addition, large numbers of leprosy bacilli are discharged in nasal secretions in multibacillary disease. The eye is frequently damaged by direct bacillary invasion, uveitis or corneal infection secondary to paralysis of the eyelids (Fig. 18.9). Blindness is a common and tragic complication of untreated leprosy.

Additional tissue damage in leprosy is caused by immune reactions resulting from delayed hypersensitivity (Jopling type 1 reactions) or a vasculitis associated with the deposition of antigen–antibody complexes (Jopling type 2 reactions, *erythema nodosum leprosum*) (Table 18.8). The former, which occurs in

| Table 18.7 | Characteristics of the five points on the spectrum of leprosy | | | | |
|---|---|---|---|---|---|
| Characteristic | TT | BT | BB | BL | LL |
| Bacilli seen in skin | − | ± | + | ++ | +++ |
| Bacilli in nasal secretions | − | − | − | + | +++ |
| Granuloma formation | +++ | ++ | + | − | − |
| Reaction to lepromin | +++ | + | ± | − | − |
| Antibodies to *M. leprae* | ± | ± | + | ++ | +++ |
| Main phagocytic cell | Mature epithelioid | Immature epithelioid | Immature epithelioid | Macrophage | Macrophage |
| In-vitro correlates of CMI | +++/++ | + | + | − | − |
| Type 1 reactions | − | + | + | + | − |
| Type 2 reactions | − | − | ± | ++ | |

CMI, cell-mediated immunity. See text for other abbreviations.

**Fig. 18.7** Lepromatous leprosy. Nodular swelling of face, enlargement of ear lobes and loss of eyebrows.

**Fig. 18.8** Treated lepromatous leprosy. The nodularity of the skin has resolved on treatment but the absence of eyebrows and the nasal collapse remain.

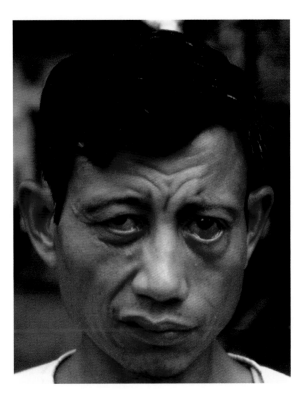

**Fig. 18.9** Tuberculoid leprosy. The only feature on presentation was paralysis of the left facial nerve, resulting in loss of the left nasolabial fold and an inability to close the eye, predisposing to corneal damage.

## LABORATORY DIAGNOSIS

The clinical diagnosis may be confirmed by histological examination of skin biopsies and by the detection of acid-fast bacilli in nasal discharges, scrapings from the nasal mucosa and *slit-skin smears*. The latter are prepared by making superficial incisions in the skin, scraping out some tissue fluid and cells, and making smears on glass slides. Smears are obtained from obvious lesions, the ear lobes and apparently unaffected skin. Secretions and skin smears are stained by the ZN method, and the number of bacilli seen in each high-power field may be recorded as the *bacillary index*; however, for usual practical purposes, patients with clinically active leprosy but in whom no bacilli are seen on slit-skin smear examination are described as having *paucibacillary* disease, and those who are positive at any site are described as having *multibacillary* disease. This is an important distinction for the selection of treatment (see below).

It is widely assumed, but unproven, that leprosy bacilli that stain strongly and evenly are viable whereas those that stain weakly and irregularly are dead. The

borderline cases (BT, BB and BL), may rapidly cause severe and permanent nerve damage, and requires urgent treatment with anti-inflammatory agents and, sometimes, surgical decompression of a greatly swollen nerve. The latter occurs at the multibacillary pole of the spectrum (BL and LL) and is principally due to deposition of antigen-antibody complexes.

**Table 18.8**   Main characteristics of the reactions in leprosy

| Characteristic | Type 1 (reversal reaction) | Type 2 (erythema nodosum leprosum) |
|---|---|---|
| Immunological basis | Cell mediated | Vasculitis with antigen-antibody complex deposition |
| Type of patient | BT, BB, BL | BL, LL |
| Systemic disturbance | No (or mild) | Yes |
| Haematological changes | No | Yes |
| Proteinuria | No | Frequently |
| Relation to therapy | Usually within first 6 months | Rare during first 6 months |

See text for explanation of abbreviations.

**Table 18.9**   WHO recommendations for multidrug therapy of leprosy

| Type of leprosy | Drug | Dose (mg) | Frequency | Total duration (months) |
|---|---|---|---|---|
| Paucibacillary | Rifampicin | 600 | Monthly, supervised | 6 |
| | Dapsone | 100 | Daily, unsupervised | |
| Multibacillary | Rifampicin | 600 | Monthly, supervised | 12 |
| | Dapsone | 100 | Daily, unsupervised | |
| | Clofazimine | 300 and 50 | Monthly, supervised | |
| | | | Daily, unsupervised | |

percentage of the former gives the *morphological index*, which declines during chemotherapy. An increase in the morphological index is a useful indication of non-compliance of the patient and the emergence of drug resistance. Where facilities exist, PCR may be used to detect *M. leprae* in clinical specimens.

## TREATMENT

Multidrug therapy based on dapsone, rifampicin and clofazimine is highly effective. The choice of regimen is determined by whether the patient has paucibacillary or multibacillary disease (Table 18.9). Clofazimine causes skin discoloration, particularly in fair-skinned people. If this results in the patient refusing the drug, a combination of rifampicin, ofloxacin and minocycline, administered monthly for 24 months for multibacillary disease, may be used instead. A single dose of rifampicin (600 mg), ofloxacin (400 mg) and minocycline (100 mg) has been advocated for the treatment of adults with single-lesion paucibacillary leprosy, although some authorities consider this to be inadequte.

The treatment of leprosy demands far more than the administration of antimicrobial agents. It is often necessary to:

- correct deformities
- prevent blindness and further damage to anaesthetic extremities
- treat reactions with anti-inflammatory drugs

- attend to the patient's social, psychological and spiritual welfare.

## EPIDEMIOLOGY

Once thought to be restricted to humans, leprosy has been reported in chimpanzees and sooty mangabey monkeys in Africa, and in free-living armadillos in Louisiana, USA. It was also thought that leprosy was transmitted by skin-to-skin contact but it now appears more likely that the bacilli are disseminated from the nasal secretions of patients with lepromatous leprosy. In addition, the blood of patients with lepromatous leprosy contains enough bacilli to render transmission by blood-sucking insects a definite, though unproven, possibility.

As in the case of tuberculosis, transmission of bacilli from patients with multibacillary leprosy to their contacts occurs readily, but only a minority of those infected develop overt disease. The infectivity of patients with paucibacillary leprosy is much lower. Leprosy often commences during childhood or early adult life but, as the incubation period is usually 3–5 years, it is rare in children aged less than 5 years.

Epidemiological studies on the prevalence and transmission of leprosy have been aided by skin test reagents, of which there are two types:

1. *Lepromins*, which are prepared from boiled bacilli-rich lepromatous lesions.

2. *Leprosins*, which are ultrasonicates of tissue-free bacilli extracted from lesions (the suffixes -H and -A are used to denote human and armadillo origins, respectively).

These reagents elicit two types of reaction:

1. The *Fernandez reaction* is analogous to tuberculin reactivity and appears in sensitized subjects 48 h after skin testing. It is best seen with leprosins.
2. The *Mitsuda reaction* is a granulomatous swelling that appears about 3 weeks after testing with lepromin. This reaction is indicative of the host's ability to give a granulomatous response to antigens of *M. leprae*, and is positive at or near the TT pole.

Skin testing is of limited diagnostic value, but is useful in epidemiological studies to establish the extent of infection in contacts and in the community, and in classifying patients according to the immunological spectrum.

## CONTROL

The most effective control measure in leprosy, as in tuberculosis, is the early detection and treatment of infectious cases. This requires that patients should attend for therapy as soon as signs of the disease appear. Unfortunately, owing to the stigma associated with the disease, many patients delay seeking treatment until they have infected many contacts and developed irreversible disfigurement and handicap. Women, in particular, are likely to conceal their disease.

No living attenuated vaccines have been prepared for *M. leprae*, but BCG vaccine seems to protect against leprosy in regions where it protects against tuberculosis, strongly suggesting that protection is induced by common mycobacterial antigens.

### RECOMMENDED READING

Britton WJ: Leprosy. In Cohen J, Powderly WG, Opal SM, editors: *Infectious Diseases*, ed 3, London, 2010, Mosby Elsevier, pp 1099–1105.

Brown T, Nikolayevskyy V, Velji P, Drobniewski F: Associations between Mycobacterium tuberculosis strains and phenotypes, *Emerging Infectious Diseases* 16:272–280, 2010.

Cole ST, Brosch R, Parkhill J, et al: Deciphering the biology of Mycobacterium tuberculosis from the complete genome sequence, *Nature* 393:537–544, 1998.

Davies PDO, Barnes PF, Gordon SB, editors: *Clinical Tuberculosis*, ed 4, London, 2008, Hodder Arnold.

Ridley DS: *Pathogenesis of Leprosy and Related Diseases*, London, 1988, Wright.

Scollard DM, Adams LB, Gillis TP, et al: The continuing challenges of leprosy, *Clinical Microbiology Review* 19:338–381, 2009.

Withington SG: Leprosy. In Cook GC, Zumla AI, editors: *Manson's Tropical Diseases*, ed 22, London, 2009, Saunders Elsevier, pp 1053–1074.

World Health Organization: *Global Tuberculosis Control 2010*, Geneva, 2010, WHO.

World Health Organization: *Multidrug and extensively drug-resistant TB (M/XDR-TB): 2010 global report on surveillance and response*, Geneva, 2010, WHO.

World Health Organization: *Treatment of Tuberculosis: Guidelines*, ed 4, Geneva, 2009, WHO.

Zumla A, Schaaf S, editors: *Tuberculosis – a Comprehensive Clinical Reference*, London, 2009, Elsevier.

### Websites

Centers for Disease Control and Prevention: Division of Tuberculosis Elimination. http://www.cdc.gov/tb/

International Federation of Anti-Leprosy Associations: http://www.ilep.org.uk/

International Leprosy Association: http://www.leprosy-ila.org/

International Union Against Tuberculosis and Lung Disease: http://www.theunion.org/

Montefiore Medical Center, New York: http://www.tuberculosis.net/

New Jersey Medical School Global Tuberculosis Institute: http://www.umdnj.edu/globaltb/home.htm

TB Alert: http://www.tbalert.org/

Tuberculosis Structural Genetics Consortium: http://www.webtb.org/

World Health Organization. A World Free of TB. http://www.who.int/tb/en/

World Health Organization. Leprosy elimination. http://www.who.int/lep/

World Health Organization. Stop TB Partnership: http://www.stoptb.org/

World Health Organization: Tuberculosis. http://www.who.int/topics/tuberculosis/en/

# 19 Environmental mycobacteria

## Opportunist disease

*J. M. Grange*

## KEY POINTS

- Environmental or non-tuberculous mycobacteria (about 130 species) are divisible into slow and rapid growers. Human disease is often opportunistic (e.g. in AIDS and chronic pre-existing lung disease) and attributable to slow growers, notably members of the *M. avium* complex.
- Infection is from the environment, and transmission control methods applied to tuberculosis are ineffective.
- Presentations include localized lymphadenitis, post-inoculation (injection or trauma) skin lesions, tuberculosis-like pulmonary lesions, solitary non-pulmonary lesions and disseminated disease.
- Lymphadenitis occurs in otherwise healthy young children (<6 years of age) and in immunosuppressed persons.
- Skin diseases include swimming pool granuloma (*M. marinum*), Buruli ulcer (*M. ulcerans*) and post-inoculation abscesses caused by various rapid growers.
- Diagnosis is based on a range of simple tests or by molecular techniques including DNA probes or specific PCR primers. Repeated detection in the face of progressive disease assists in distinguishing pathogenic association from contamination or colonization.
- Therapy depends on the causative organism and is largely empirical as few clinical trials have been conducted and drug susceptibility tests are not very reliable.

In addition to the tubercle and leprosy bacilli there are more than 130 recognized species of mycobacteria in the *List of Prokaryotic names with Standing in Nomenclature* that normally exist as saprophytes of soil and water. Termed environmental (or non-tuberculous) mycobacteria, some of these species

occasionally cause opportunist disease in animals and man. Those species described here are well-recognised human pathogens but many of the other species are rare causes of disease, especially in those with HIV disease and other causes of profound immunosuppression. Mycobacterial species are divided into *photochromogens*, which develop yellow or orange pigmentation in (or after exposure to) light, *scotochromogens*, which become pigmented in the dark, and *non-chromogens*. They are also divided into slow and *rapid growers*, with the latter species producing visible growth on Löwenstein–Jensen medium within 1 week on subculture, although growth on primary culture of clinical material often takes considerably longer. Traditionally, mycobacterial species were characterised by a range of physical and biochemical properties but molecular methods, notably determination the base sequence of the 16S ribosomal RNA, provide the 'gold standards' for speciation.

## DESCRIPTION

### Photochromogens

- *Mycobacterium kansasii*, which grows well at 37°C and is isolated principally from patients with pulmonary disease. On microscopy, it often appears elongated and distinctly beaded (Fig. 19.1).
- *M. simiae*, which, like *M. kansasii*, grows at 37°C and is occasionally involved in pulmonary disease.
- *M. marinum*, the cause of a warty skin infection known as *swimming pool granuloma* or *fish tank granuloma*. It grows poorly, if at all, at 37°C, and cultures from skin lesions should be incubated at 33°C. Microscopically, it resembles *M. kansasii*.

### Scotochromogens

Most slowly growing scotochromogens isolated from sputum or urine are of no clinical significance. These include *M. gordonae* (formerly *M. aquae*), which is

**Fig. 19.1** *Mycobacterium kansasii* in sputum, showing elongated and beaded appearance. Courtesy of Professor John Stanford.

frequently found in water and is a common contaminant of clinical material. It is, however, a rare cause of pulmonary disease. Two species are more usually associated with disease:

1. *M. scrofulaceum* is associated principally with scrofula or cervical lymphadenitis, but also causes pulmonary disease.
2. *M. szulgai*, an uncommon cause of pulmonary disease and bursitis, is a scotochromogen when incubated at 37°C but a photochromogen at 25°C.

## Non-chromogens

The most prevalent and important opportunistic pathogens are in a group known as the *M. avium* complex (MAC). This group consists of:

- *M. avium avium* (the avian tubercle bacillus), a pathogen of birds and also a cause of lymphadenitis in pigs as well as occasional disease in various other wild and domestic animals.
- *M. avium intracellulare*, principally a human pathogen but also a cause of disease in animals including pigs. Many isolates formerly included in this species are now identified as *M. avium hominissuis,* although this term has not been formally published.
- *M. avium paratuberculosis*, the cause of chronic hypertrophic enteritis or Johne's disease of cattle. There have been claims, which remain to be substantiated, that it is a cause of Crohn's disease in man. It produces little or no mycobactin, a lipid-soluble iron-binding compound essential for

growth, and this substance must be added to media used for cultivation.
- *M. avium sylvaticum*, a cause of tuberculosis in wood pigeons. Like *M. paratuberculosis* it needs mycobactin for growth.
- *M. avium lepraemurium*, the cause of a leprosy-like disease of rats, mice and cats.

Both *M. avium hominissuis* and *M. avium intracellulare* are causative agents of lymphadenitis and pulmonary disease. They are also a cause of disseminated disease in profoundly immunosuppressed patients, notably in those with the acquired immune deficiency syndrome (AIDS). Most clinical isolates are smooth and easy to emulsify and were previously typed by agglutination serology although RFLP and MIRU-VNTR (see Ch. 18) are now used.

Other non-chromogens include:

- *M. ulcerans*, a very slowly growing species that grows in vitro only at 31–34°C. Colonies are non-pigmented or a pale lemon-yellow colour. *M. ulcerans* is the cause of *Buruli ulcer*; unlike other mycobacterial pathogens it produces a toxin that causes tissue necrosis and is involved in the pathogenesis of the disease. *M. shinshuense*, a very rare cause of skin ulcers in Japan and China, is a variant of *M. ulcerans*.
- *M. xenopi*, originally isolated from a xenopus toad, is a thermophile that grows well at 45°C. It is principally responsible for pulmonary lesions in man. Most reported cases have been from London and south-east England and northern France. Two phylogenetically similar species, *M. celatum* and *M. branderi*, have been described.
- *M. malmoense* is a cause of pulmonary disease and lymphadenitis. It grows very slowly, often taking as long as 10 weeks to appear on primary culture, and is therefore likely to be missed if cultures are discarded earlier. For unknown reasons, disease due to this pathogen is increasing in several European countries. In some regions, notably northern England, it has become one of the most frequently isolated of the environmental mycobacteria from patients with pulmonary disease.
- *M. terrae* (the radish bacillus), *M. nonchromogenicum* and *M. triviale* are sometimes grouped as the *M. terrae* complex. They are very rare causes of pulmonary disease and, in the case of *M. terrae*, infections of injuries acquired while farming or gardening.
- *M. haemophilum*, characterized by its growth requirement for haem or other sources of iron, is a rare cause of granulomatous or ulcerative skin

lesions in xenograft recipients and other immunocompromised individuals, and of lymphadenitis in otherwise healthy children.

- *M. genevense*, a very slow growing organism occasionally isolated from patients infected with HIV or with other causes of immunosuppresion, from pet and zoo birds and, rarely, other animals.

## Rapid growers

Four rapidly growing non-chromogenic species are well-recognized human pathogens: *M. chelonae*, *M. abscessus*, *M. fortuitum* and *M. peregrinum*. They occasionally cause pulmonary or disseminated disease but are principally responsible for post-injection abscesses and wound infections, including corneal ulcers.

Most of the many other rapidly growing species are pigmented and, although disease due to them is exceedingly rare, they frequently contaminate clinical specimens. They are found on the genitalia and gain access to urine samples, although, contrary to a common belief, *M. smegmatis* is rarely found in this site. *M. flavescens*, which grows more slowly than other members of this group and is therefore sometimes classified as a slow grower, is an occasional cause of post-injection abscesses.

## PATHOGENESIS

Compared with tubercle bacilli, environmental mycobacteria are of low virulence and, although human beings are in regular contact with these organisms and therefore frequently infected, overt disease is uncommon except in those who are profoundly immunosuppressed. Five main types of opportunist mycobacterial disease have been described in man (Table 19.1):

1. localized lymphadenitis
2. skin lesions following traumatic inoculation of bacteria
3. tuberculosis-like pulmonary lesions
4. tuberculosis-like non-pulmonary lesions
5. disseminated disease.

## Lymphadenitis

This is caused by a number of different species that vary in relative frequency from region to region. The *M. avium* complex is the predominant cause worldwide. Earlier reports claimed a high incidence of *M. scrofulaceum*, but these strains were probably misidentified members of the *M. avium* complex. In most

**Table 19.1** Principal types of opportunist mycobacterial disease in man, and the usual causative agents

| Disease | Usual causative agent |
|---|---|
| Lymphadenopathy | *M. avium* complex |
| | *M. scrofulaceum* |
| **Skin lesions** | |
| Post-traumatic abscesses | *M. chelonae* |
| | *M. abscessus* |
| | *M. fortuitum* |
| | *M. peregrinum* |
| Swimming pool granuloma | *M. marinum* |
| Buruli ulcer | *M. ulcerans* |
| Pulmonary disease and solitary non-pulmonary lesions | *M. avium* complex |
| | *M. kansasii* |
| | *M. xenopi* |
| | *M. malmoense* |
| **Disseminated disease** | |
| AIDS related | *M. avium* complex |
| | *M. genevense* |
| Non-AIDS related | *M. avium* complex |
| | *M. chelonae* |
| | *M. abscessus* |

cases a single node, usually tonsillar or pre-auricular, is involved, and most patients are children aged less than 5 years (Fig. 19.2). Unless contra-indicated by the risk of nerve damage, excision of the node, usually performed for diagnostic purposes, is almost always curative. This disease was very rare where children were vaccinated with BCG (Bacille Calmette–Guérin) neonatally, but the incidence increased considerably in countries where such vaccination was terminated. Lymphadenitis occasionally occurs as part of a more disseminated infection, particularly in individuals with AIDS.

## Skin lesions

Three main types have been described: post-injection (and post-traumatic) abscesses, swimming pool granuloma and Buruli ulcer.

### Post-injection and post-traumatic abscesses

These are usually caused by the rapidly growing pathogens *M. abscessus*, *M. chelonae*, *M. fortuitum* and, less frequently, *M. peregrinum* and *M. flavescens*. Abscesses occur sporadically, particularly in the tropics, or in small epidemics when these bacteria contaminate batches of injectable materials. Abscesses develop within a week or so, or for up to a year or

Fig. 19.3 Keratitis due to *M. chelonae* following corneal grafting. The cornea shows a characteristic 'cracked windscreen' appearance. Reproduced by permission of Elsevier from Khooshabeh R, Grange JM, Yates MD, McCartney ACE, Casey T A 1994 A case report of *Mycobacterium chelonae* keratitis and a review of mycobacterial infections of the eye. *Tubercle and Lung Disease* 75: 377–382.

Fig. 19.2 Pre-auricular lymphadenitis due to an environmental mycobacterium in a child. Courtesy of Professor Ali Zumla, University College London.

more, after the injection. They are painful, may become quite large – up to 8 or 10 cm in diameter – and may persist for many months. Treatment is by drainage with curettage or total excision. Chemotherapy is not required unless there is local spread of disease or multiple abscesses, as may occur in insulin-injecting diabetics.

More serious lesions, also usually due to these rapidly growing pathogens, have followed surgery, particularly procedures involving insertion of prostheses such as heart valves, and corneal infections have followed ocular injuries or surgery (Fig. 19.3). Infections by *M. terrae* have occurred in farmers and others who have been injured while working with soil.

### Swimming pool granuloma

This is also known as *fish tank granuloma* and, occasionally, *fish fancier's finger*, and is caused by *M. marinum*. Those affected are mostly users of swimming pools, keepers of tropical fish and others involved in aquatic hobbies. The bacilli enter scratches and abrasions, and cause warty lesions similar to those seen in skin tuberculosis. The lesions, which usually occur on the knees and elbows of swimmers and on the hands of aquarium keepers, are usually localized, although secondary lesions sometimes appear along the line of the dermal lymphatics. This is termed *sporotrichoid spread* as a similar phenomenon occurs in

the fungus infection sporotrichosis (see Ch. 61). A few cases of disseminated disease have occurred in immunosuppressed patients, including those treated with systemic steroids.

### Buruli ulcer

This disease, caused by *M. ulcerans*, was first described in Australia, although the name is derived from the Buruli district of Uganda where a large outbreak was investigated extensively in the 1960s. Buruli ulcer has been reported in over 30 countries including Ghana, Nigeria, Congo Kinshasa, Côte d'Ivoire, Togo, Mexico, Malaysia, Papua New Guinea and Australia, and is limited to certain localities, characteristically low-lying areas subject to periodic flooding. *M. shinshuense*, a rare cause of similar lesions in Japan and China, is a variant of *M. ulcerans*. There is strong though indirect evidence that *M. ulcerans* is introduced from the environment into the human dermis by minor injuries, particularly by spiky grasses and, possibly, by biting insects. It is becoming a major public health problem in central and western equatorial Africa, where the number and severity of cases has increased; in some areas, its incidence is exceeding that of tuberculosis and leprosy. The risk of the disease is higher in those infected with HIV, in whom the disease may be more aggressive, but this is not the sole cause of the increase.

The first manifestation of the disease is a hard cutaneous nodule, which may be itchy. The nodule enlarges and develops central softening and fluctuation owing

**Fig. 19.4** Buruli ulcer. Undermined ulcer overlying the biceps and swelling of the surrounding tissues. Courtesy of Dr Alan Knell, Wellcome Tropical Institute.

to necrosis of the subcutaneous adipose tissue caused by an exotoxin, which also has immunosuppressive properties. The overlying skin becomes anoxic and breaks down, the liquefied necrotic contents of the lesion are discharged, and one or more ulcers with deeply undermined edges are thereby formed (Fig. 19.4). At this stage the lesion is teeming with acid-fast bacilli and there is no histological immunological evidence of an active cell-mediated immune response. During this anergic stage the lesion may progress to an enormous size, sometimes involving an entire limb or a major part of the trunk.

For unknown reasons, the anergic phase may eventually give way to an immunoreactive phase when a granulomatous response develops in the lesion, the acid-fast bacilli disappear and immune reactivity to antigens of *M. ulcerans* is detectable. Healing then occurs but the patient is often left with considerable disfigurement and disability caused by extensive scarring and contractures.

## Pulmonary disease

This is seen most frequently in middle-aged or elderly men with lung damage caused by smoking or exposure to industrial dusts. It also occurs in individuals with congenital or acquired immune deficiencies, malignant disease and cystic fibrosis, but a substantial minority of cases occur in persons with no apparent underlying localized or generalized disorder. The disease may be caused by many species, although the most frequent are the *M. avium* complex and *M. kansasii*. Other causative organisms in the UK are *M. xenopi* and *M. malmoense*, with the former being

more common in the south of the country and the latter in the north.

## Localized non–pulmonary disease

Localized non-pulmonary lesions resembling those seen in tuberculosis are uncommon. Disease involving the meninges, bone (including the spine) and joints, kidney and male genitalia has been described. Mycobacterial peritonitis is a serious complication of peritoneal dialysis.

## Disseminated disease

In the 1980s and early 1990s, up to a half of all persons dying from AIDS in the USA had disseminated mycobacterial disease, almost always due to the *M. avium* complex. This AIDS-related disease was also common in Europe but not in Africa. The introduction of highly active antiretroviral therapy (see Ch. 55) has led to a substantial decline in the incidence of this disease in developed nations.

The source of the causative organisms is uncertain. Some workers consider that disease is due to reactivation of dormant foci of infection acquired in childhood, whereas others argue that it results from recent infection from the environment; these explanations are not mutually exclusive. Acid-fast bacilli are readily isolated from bone marrow aspirates, intestinal biopsies, blood and faeces. A few cases of AIDS-related disseminated disease have been caused by other species, including *M. genavense*.

Disseminated disease occurs occasionally in individuals with other congenital or acquired causes of immuno-suppression, including renal transplantation. Again, the *M. avium* complex is the usual cause, but disseminated disease due to other infections, notably *M. chelonae*, has occurred in recipients of renal transplants and in other immunocompromised patients (Fig. 19.5).

## LABORATORY DIAGNOSIS

Most environmental mycobacteria can be detected microscopically and cultured on media suitable for *M. tuberculosis* (see p. 212). Great care must be taken to differentiate true disease from transient colonization or superinfection. In particular, there are no clinical or radiological characteristics that reliably differentiate pulmonary disease caused by opportunist mycobacteria from tuberculosis, and the diagnosis is therefore made by isolation and identification of the pathogen. As a general rule, a diagnosis of

**Fig. 19.5** Skin ulcer on the face due to disseminated *M. chelonae* in an immunocompromised child. Courtesy of Dr Kurt Schopfer.

opportunist mycobacterial disease may be made when a heavy growth of the pathogen is repeatedly isolated from the sputum of a patient with compatible clinical and radiological features, and in whom other causes of these features have been carefully excluded. Fibreoptic bronchoscopy is a useful aid to diagnosis as lesions may be directly biopsied.

Identification is usually undertaken by specialist reference laboratories. There is no universally recognized identification scheme, although reliance is usually placed on cultural characteristics (rate and temperature of growth and pigmentation), various biochemical reactions and resistance to antimicrobial agents. Some reference centres use HPLC to delineate the chromatographic profile of cell wall mycolic acids and some use nucleic acid-based methods including commercially available PCR primers and DNA probes and sequencing of the 16S ribosomal DNA.

## TREATMENT

Most slowly growing environmental mycobacteria are resistant to many antituberculosis drugs in vitro, although infections often respond to various combinations of these drugs. Few controlled trials of therapy for pulmonary disease caused by the *M. avium* complex and other slowly growing species including *M. xenopi*, *M. kansasii* and *M. malmoense*

have been conducted, but the available data indicate that a two-year regimen of rifampicin and ethambutol with addition of either clarithromycin or ciprofloxacin, or both if there is no clinical response after one year, is highly effective.

Similar drug regimens based on a macrolide (clarithromycin or azithromycin) and ethambutol are effective against AIDS-associated disease caused by the *M. avium* complex. There is, however, evidence that reduction of the viral load by use of antiretroviral agents contributes more to remission of such disease than antibacterial therapy.

Pulmonary and non-pulmonary disease due to the rapidly growing species *M. abscessus*, *M. chelonae*, *M. fortuitum* and *M. peregrinum*, have been treated successfully by various combinations of erythromycin, newer macrolides, sulphonamides, trimethoprim, amikacin, gentamicin, imipenem, extended-spectrum cephalosporins and fluoroquinolones. In-vitro susceptibility tests are not always a reliable guide of clinical response and some infections, notably keratitis due to *M. chelonae*, frequently relapse and require surgical intervention, despite in-vitro drug susceptibility.

*Mycobacterium marinum* disease is usually self-limiting, although chemotherapy with minocycline, co-trimoxazole or rifampicin with ethambutol hastens its resolution and surgical debridement is required if the disease involves joints or tendons. More aggressive antimicrobial therapy, usually based on rifampicin, ethambutol and clarithromycin is required for extensive and disseminated disease.

The early, pre-ulcerative, lesions of Buruli ulcer are easily treatable by excision and primary closure by suture. Ulcerated lesions require excision and skin grafting. After disappointing early results, antibiotic therapy has been shown to be effective in the majority of treated patients. The World Health Organization recommends 4 weeks of treatment with rifampicin and streptomycin, then surgery followed by 8 more weeks of antibiotic therapy, depending on clinical response.

## EPIDEMIOLOGY

Mycobacteria are widely distributed in the environment and are particularly abundant in wet soil, marshland, streams, rivers and estuaries. Some species, such as *M. terrae*, are found in soil whereas others, including *M. marinum* and *M. gordonae*, prefer free water. Many species, including potential pathogens such as the *M. avium* complex, *M. kansasii* and *M. xenopi*, are able to colonize piped water supplies. Human beings are therefore regularly exposed to mycobacteria as a result of drinking, washing, showering and inhalation of natural aerosols. Such repeated subclinical infection may induce sensitization to tuberculin and other mycobacterial skin-testing reagents. There is also evidence that contact with environmental mycobacteria profoundly affects the subsequent ability of BCG vaccine to induce protective immunity, thereby explaining the great regional differences in the efficacy of this vaccine (see p. 220).

The number of cases of disease due to environmental mycobacteria relative to cases of tuberculosis increases in regions where the latter is uncommon and declining in incidence. In addition, the absolute incidence is increasing as a result of the growing number of immunocompromised individuals, notably patients with AIDS.

A few 'epidemics' of falsely diagnosed mycobacterial pulmonary disease and urinary tract infection have resulted from the collection of sputum and urine specimens in containers rinsed out with water from taps colonized by mycobacteria. Inadequate cleaning of endoscopes has also led to mycobacterial contamination of clinical specimens and diagnostic confusion. Likewise, false-positive sputum smear examinations for acid-fast bacilli have occurred when staining reagents were prepared from contaminated water.

## CONTROL

The incidence and type of disease in any region are determined by the species and numbers of mycobacteria in the environment and the opportunities for human transmission. Unlike tuberculosis, person-to-person transmission of opportunist mycobacterial disease rarely, if ever, occurs. Thus the incidence of such disease is independent of that of tuberculosis and unaffected by public health measures designed to control the latter.

RECOMMENDED READING

Asiedu K, Scherpbier R, Raviglione M: *Buruli Ulcer. Mycobacterium ulcerans Infection*, Geneva, 2000, World Health Organization Global Buruli Ulcer Initiative.

Banks J, Campbell IA: Environmental mycobacteria. In Davies PDO, Barnes PF, Gordon SB, editors: *Clinical Tuberculosis*, ed 4, London, 2008, Hodder Arnold, pp 509–518.

Daley CL, Heifets L: Other mycobacteria causing human disease. In Schaaf HS, Zumla AI, editors: *Tuberculosis. A Comprehensive Clinical Reference*, London, 2009, Saunders Elsevier, pp 60–74.

Griffith DE, Aksamit T, Brown-Elliott BA, et al: An official ATS/IDSA statement: diagnosis, treatment, and prevention of nontuberculous mycobacterial diseases, *American Journal of Respiratory and Critical Care Medicine* 175:367–416, 2007.

Jenkins PA, Campbell IA, Banks J, et al: Clarithromycin vs ciprofloxacin as adjuncts to rifampicin and ethambutol in treating opportunist mycobacterial lung diseases and an assessment of *Mycobacterium vaccae* immunotherapy, *Thorax* 63:627–634, 2008.

Pfyffer GE, Inderlied CB: Mycobacteria. In Cohen J, Opal SM, Powderley WG, editors: *Infectious Diseases*, ed 3, London, 2010, Mosby Elsevier, pp 1777–1800.

van der Werf TS, Stienstra Y Johnson RC, et al: *Mycobacterium ulcerans* disease, *Bulletin – World Health Organization* 83:785–791, 2005.

World Health Organization: Buruli ulcer: progress report, 2004–2008, *Weekly Epidemiological Record* 83:145–154, 2008.

## Websites

Chest Medicine On-line: Environmental mycobacteria. http://priory.com/cmol/envmyco1.htm

List of Prokaryotic names with Standing in Nomenclature: http://www.bacterio.cict.fr/

World Health Organization: Buruli ulcer. http://www.who.int/buruli/en/

# 20 Actinomyces, nocardia and tropheryma

Actinomycosis; nocardiasis; Whipple's disease

*J. M. Grange*

## KEY POINTS

- Several species of *Actinomyces* cause chronic lesions characterized by multiple abscesses, granulomata, tissue destruction, extensive fibrosis and sinus formation.
- More than half of human cases occur in the cervicofacial region and often involve the jaw. Other cases occur in the thorax, abdomen and pelvis.
- Lesions may contain various concomitant organisms of doubtful significance to pathogenesis.
- Diagnosis is made by observation of the characteristic 'sulphur granules' in clinical material and by culture of the organism. Treatment is usually by prolonged penicillin-based regimens.
- Many species of *Nocardia* have been described but only a few, notably *N. asteroides*, cause human disease. Lung involvement in immunocompromised individuals predominates. Secondary abscesses, notably in the brain, occur in about one-third of patients.
- Post-inoculation cutaneous infections (primary cuteneous nocardiasis) may result in fungating tumour-like masses termed mycetomas.
- *Tropheryma whippeli*, the cause of Whipple's disease, was one of the first bacterial pathogens identified by 16S rRNA studies.
- Whipple's disease is a rare multi-system disease with principal involvement of the intestine, resulting in diarrhoea and malabsorption. The central nervous system is also often involved.

Gram-positive bacteria with branching filaments that sometimes develop into mycelia are included in the rather loosely defined order Actinomycetales. Although mostly soil saprophytes, five genera, *Actinomyces*, *Nocardia*, *Actinomadura*, *Propionibacterium* and *Bifidobacterium* (the latter two are considered briefly in Ch. 36), occasionally cause chronic granulomatous infections in animals and human beings. Members of the genera *Gordona*, *Oerskovia*, *Rothia* and *Tsukamurella* very rarely cause similar infections.

*Tropheryma whipplei*, the causative agent of Whipple's disease, has been shown to be an actinomycete on the basis of nucleic acid studies. Another genus, *Streptomyces*, is an extremely rare cause of disease, but is the source of several antibiotics. Repeated inhalation of thermophilic actinomycetes, notably *Faenia rectivirgula* and *Thermo-actinomyces* species, causes extrinsic allergic alveolitis (farmer's lung, mushroom worker's lung, bagassosis) in those who are occupationally exposed to mouldy vegetable matter.

## ACTINOMYCES

### DESCRIPTION

Actinomyces are branching Gram-positive bacilli. They are facultative anaerobes, but often fail to grow aerobically on primary culture. They grow best under anaerobic or micro-aerophilic conditions with the addition of 5–10% carbon dioxide. Almost all species are commensals of the mouth and have a narrow temperature range of growth of around 35–37°C. They are responsible for the disease known as *actinomycosis*. Three-quarters of human cases are caused by *Actinomyces israelii*. Less common causes include *A. gerencseriae*, *A. naeslundii*, *A. odontolyticus*, *A. viscosus*, *A. meyeri*, *Arachnia propionica* and members of the genus *Bifidobacterium*.

Concomitant bacteria, notably a small Gram-negative rod, *Actinobacillus actinomycetemcomitans*, but also *Haemophilus* species, fusiforms and anaerobic streptococci, are sometimes found in actinomycotic lesions, although their contribution to the

233

pathogenesis of the disease, if any, is unknown. *Act. actinomycetemcomitans* is a rare cause of endocarditis.

## PATHOGENESIS

Actinomycosis is a chronic disease characterized by multiple abscesses and granulomata, tissue destruction, extensive fibrosis and the formation of sinuses. Within diseased tissues the actinomycetes form large masses of mycelia embedded in an amorphous protein–polysaccharide matrix and surrounded by a zone of Gram-negative, weakly acid-fast, club-like structures. These clubs were once thought to consist, at least in part, of material derived from host tissue, but it now appears that they are formed entirely from the bacteria. The mycelial masses may be visible to the naked eye and, as they are often light yellow in colour, they are called *sulphur granules*. In older lesions the sulphur granules may be dark brown and very hard because of the deposition of calcium phosphate in the matrix. Various species of actinomyces may colonize diseased tissue, such as lung cancer, but sulphur granules are not seen.

The principal forms of human actinomycosis are:

- Cervicofacial infection, which accounts for more than half of reported cases; the jaw is often involved. The disease is endogenous in origin; dental caries is a predisposing factor, and infection may follow tooth extractions or other dental procedures. Men are affected more frequently than women, and in some regions the disease is more common in rural agricultural workers than in town dwellers, probably owing to lower standards of dental care in the former.
- Thoracic actinomycosis commences in the lung, probably as a result of aspiration of actinomyces from the mouth. Sinuses often appear on the chest wall, and the ribs and spine may be eroded. Primary endobronchial actinomycosis is an uncommon complication of an inhaled foreign body.
- Abdominal cases commence in the appendix or, less frequently, in colonic diverticulae.
- Pelvic actinomycosis occurs occasionally in women fitted with plastic intra-uterine contraceptive devices.
- Actinomyces have been isolated from cases of chronic granulomatous disease and should be vigorously sought in this rare condition.

The lymphatics are not usually involved, but haematogenous spread to the liver, brain and other internal organs occurs occasionally. Involvement of bone is uncommon in human actinomycosis and is usually the result of direct extension of adjacent soft tissue lesions.

## LABORATORY DIAGNOSIS

Specimens should be obtained directly from lesions by open biopsy, needle aspiration or, in the case of pulmonary lesions, by fibreoptic bronchoscopy. Examination of sputum is of no value as it frequently contains oral actinomycetes. Material from suspected cases is shaken with sterile water in a tube. Sulphur granules settle to the bottom and may be removed with a Pasteur pipette. Granules crushed between two glass slides are stained by the Gram and Ziehl–Neelsen (modified by using 1% sulphuric acid for decolorization) methods, which reveal the Gram-positive mycelia and the zone of radiating acid-fast clubs. Sulphur granules and mycelia in tissue sections are identifiable by use of fluorescein-conjugated specific antisera. In-situ PCR has been used to detect *A. israelii* in tissue biopsies.

For culture, suitable media, such as blood or brain–heart infusion agar, glucose broth and enriched thioglycollate broth, are inoculated with washed and crushed granules. Contamination is reduced by the incorporation of metronidazole and nalidixic acid or cadmium sulphate in the media. Cultures are incubated aerobically and anaerobically for up to 14 days. After several days on agar medium, *A. israelii* may form so-called *spider colonies* that resemble molar teeth. The identity may be confirmed by biochemical tests, by staining with specific fluorescent antisera or by gas chromatography of metabolic products of carbohydrate fermentation.

## TREATMENT

Actinomyces are sensitive to many antibiotics, but the penetration of drugs into the densely fibrotic diseased tissue is poor. Thus, large doses are required for prolonged periods, and recurrence of disease is not uncommon. Surgical debridement reduces scarring and deformity, hastens healing and lowers the incidence of recurrences. Prolonged penicillin-based regimens are increasingly being replaced by shorter regimens based on amoxicillin with clavulanic acid (the clavulanic acid is required because lesions are often concomitantly infected with β-lactamase-producing bacteria) or cephalosporins, especially ceftriaxone. Alternative agents include tetracyclines, macrolides, fluoroquinolones and imipenem but in-vitro sensitivity testing is unreliable. Additional drugs, including aminoglycosides and metronidazole, may be required when concomitant organisms are present.

## NOCARDIA

### DESCRIPTION

The nocardiae are branched, strictly aerobic, Gram-positive bacteria that are closely related to the rapidly growing mycobacteria. Like the latter, but unlike actinomyces, they are environmental saprophytes with a broad temperature range of growth. The properties of nocardiae and actinomycetes are compared in Table 20.1. Most isolates are acid-fast when decolorized with 1% sulphuric acid.

Many species of nocardia are found in the environment, notably in soil, and a range of species cause human opportunist disease, notably *Nocardia asteroides*, so named because of its star-shaped colonies, *N, abscessus, N. farcinica, N. brasiliensis, N. brevicatena, N. otitidiscaviarum, N. nova* and *N. transvalensis*. A wider range of species is encountered in profoundly immunosuppressed patients.

A related group of non-acid-fast species are assigned to the genus *Actinomadura*, which includes the species *Actinomadura madurae* and *A. pelletieri*, common causes of Madura foot (see below).

### PATHOGENESIS

Nocardiae, principally *N. asteroides*, are uncommon causes of opportunist pulmonary disease, which usually, but not always, occurs in immunocompromised individuals, including those receiving post-transplant immunosuppressive therapy or chemotherapy for cancer and those with acquired immune deficiency syndrome (AIDS). Corticosteroid therapy is a strong risk factor. As a result, the frequency and diversity of clinical manifestations of nocardial disease has increased over the past few decades. Pre-existing lung disease, notably alveolar proteinosis, also predisposes to nocardial disease. The infection is exogenous, resulting from inhalation of the bacilli. The clinical and radiological features are very variable and non-specific, and diagnosis is not easy. In most cases there are multiple confluent abscesses with little or no surrounding fibrous reaction, and local spread may result in pleural effusions, empyema and invasion of bones. In some cases the disease is chronic, whereas in others it spreads rapidly through the lungs. Secondary abscesses in the brain and, less frequently, in other organs occur in about one-third of patients with pulmonary nocardiasis. Acute dissemination with involvement of many organs occurs in profoundly immunosuppressed persons, notably those with AIDS. Recurrence is common in immunosuppressed patients and mortality is high.

Nocardiae also cause primary post-traumatic, post-operative or post-inoculation cutaneous infections (primary cuteneous nocardiasis). The most frequent cause is *N. brasiliensis* but some cases are caused by *N. asteroides* or other species. In the USA and the southern hemisphere, but rarely in Europe, cutaneous infections may result in fungating tumour-like masses termed *mycetomas*.

*Madura foot* is a chronic granulomatous infection of the bones and soft tissues of the foot resulting in mycetoma formation and gross deformity. It occurs in Sudan, North Africa and the west coast of India, principally among those who walk barefoot and are therefore prone to contamination of foot injuries by soil-derived organisms. A common causative organism is *Actinomadura madurae*, but Madura foot is also caused by other actinomycetes including *Streptomyces somaliensis* and by fungi (see Ch. 61).

### LABORATORY DIAGNOSIS

A presumptive diagnosis of pulmonary nocardiasis may be made by a microscopical examination of sputum. In many cases the sputum contains numerous lymphocytes and macrophages, some of which contain pleomorphic Gram-positive and weakly acid-fast bacilli, and occasional extracellular branching filaments. Nocardiae are not so easily seen in tissue biopsies stained by the Gram or modified Ziehl–Neelsen methods, but may be seen in preparations stained by the Gram–Weigert or Gomori methenamine silver methods.

**Table 20.1** Differences between the genera *Actinomyces* and *Nocardia*

| *Actinomyces* spp. | *Nocardia* spp. |
|---|---|
| Facultative anaerobes | Strict aerobes |
| Grow at 35–37°C | Wide temperature range of growth |
| Oral commensals | Environmental saprophytes |
| Non-acid-fast mycelia | Weakly acid-fast |
| Endogenous cause of disease | Exogenous cause of disease |

Nocardiae grow on blood agar, although growth is better on enriched media including Löwenstein–Jensen medium, brain–heart infusion agar and Sabouraud's dextrose agar containing chloramphenicol as a selective agent. Growth is visible after incubation for between 2 days and 1 month; selective growth is favoured by incubation at 45°C. Colonies are cream, orange or pink coloured; their surfaces may develop a dry, chalky appearance, and they adhere firmly to the medium.

Identification of species is usually undertaken in reference laboratories, with the most common technique being analysis of 16S rRNA gene sequences, a technique that has delineated over 30 species.

## TREATMENT

A widely used regimen is sulfamethoxazole with trimethoprim (co-trimoxazole) for 3–6 months, although this prolonged course often causes adverse drug reactions. In addition, some strains, especially of *N. farcinica*, are resistant to sulphonamides. An alternative regimen, particularly in severe disease, is high-dose imipenem with amikacin for 4–6 weeks. Minocycline, third generation cephalosporins, amoxicillin–clavulanate combinations and linezolid, an oxazolidinone, are also effective. Drug susceptibility testing is subject to several variables and no standardized methods have been proposed. Mycetomata due to nocardiae are much easier to treat than those due to fungi. Even long-standing cases with extensive mycetoma formation respond well to chemotherapy. Despite therapy, mortality of pulmonary and disseminated nocardiasis is high.

## *TROPHERYMA WHIPPELI*

*Whipple's disease* is a rare multi-system disease with symptoms including diarrhoea and malabsorption, often with arthralgia, lymphadenopathy and fever. The intestine is principally affected but involvement of the lung, heart and skeletal muscle also occurs. PCR studies indicate that the central nervous system is often involved, even in the absence of neurological signs and symptoms. Most cases occur in middle-aged white males. The causative organism, *Tropheryma whipplei*, has a depleted genome and was originally cultivated in human embryonic lung cells, but sequencing of the genome has permitted the development of a medium for its cultivation in vitro. The organism is an environmental saprophyte and has been detected by PCR in stool samples from healthy individuals. Diagnosis is usually made by histological examination of periodic acid–Schiff stained biopsies of the duodenum or other affected organs, immunostaining with specific antibody, electron microscopy and PCR detection. The ideal treatment, especially for relapses, has not yet been defined but a very effective regimen is a 2-week course of intravenous ceftriazone (to achieve high cerebrospinal fluid levels), followed by twice-daily cotrimoxazole for 1 year.

## RECOMMENDED READING

Ambrosioni J, Lew D, Garbino J: Nocardiosis: updated clinical review and experience at a tertiary center, *Infection* 38:89–97, 2010.

Conville PS, Murray PR, Zelazny AM: Evaluation of the integrated database network system (IDNS) SmartGene software for analysis of 16S rRNA gene sequences for identification of Nocardia species, *Journal of Clinical Microbiology* 48:2995–2998, 2010.

Freeman HJ: Tropheryma whipplei infection, *World Journal of Gastroenterology* 15:2078–2080, 2009.

Hay RJ: Nocardiasis: In Warrel DA, Firth JD, Cox TM, editors: *Oxford Textbook of Medicine*, ed 5, Oxford, 2010, Oxford University Press.

Kiska DL, Hicks K, Pettit DJ: Identification of medically relevant Nocardia species with an abbreviated battery of tests, *Journal of Clinical Microbiology* 40:1346–1351, 2002.

Lederman ER, Crum NF: A case series and focused review of nocardiosis. Clinical and microbiological aspects, *Medicine (Baltimore)* 83:300–313, 2004.

Reichenbach J, Lopatin U, Mahlaoui N, et al: Actinomyces in chronic granulomatous disease: an emerging and unanticipated pathogen, *Clinical Infectious Disease* 49:1703–1710, 2009.

Schaal KP: Actinomycosis. In Warrel DA, Firth JD, Cox TM, editors: *Oxford Textbook of Medicine*, ed 5, Oxford, 2010, Oxford University Press.

Schneider T, Moos V, Loddenkemper C, et al: Whipple's disease: new aspects of pathogenesis and treatment, *Lancet Infectious Diseases* 8:179–190, 2009.

Scott G: Actinomycosis. In Cook GC, Zumla AI, editors: *Manson's Tropical Diseases*, ed 21, London, 2003, Saunders, pp 1091–1093.

### Website

European Network on *Tropheryma whippeli* Infection: Whipple's Disease. http://www.whipplesdisease.info/

# 21 Bacillus

## Anthrax; food poisoning

*J. E. Thwaite and H. S. Atkins*

### KEY POINTS

- Bacteria belonging to the *Bacillus* genus are common environmental Gram-positive bacilli.
- *Bacillus anthracis* causes cutaneous, inhalational and ingestional anthrax.
- The pathogenicity of anthrax depends on the capsule and toxins.
- Antibiotic treatment of inhalational or ingestional anthrax is difficult.
- *B. anthracis* Sterne strain (toxin-negative) is used as an animal vaccine.
- A recombinant protein vaccine for anthrax is in development.
- *Bacillus cereus* commonly causes food poisoning.
- A *B. cereus* strain with anthrax toxin genes causes anthrax-like disease.

The genus *Bacillus* originally included all rod-shaped bacteria, but now comprises only large, spore-forming, Gram-positive bacilli that form chains and usually grow aerobically or anaerobically. They are common environmental organisms, frequently isolated in laboratories as contaminants of media or specimens. The *Bacillus* genus encompasses 70 species including *Bacillus anthracis, Bacillus cereus, Bacillus subtilis* and *Bacillus thuringiensis*. *B. anthracis*, the cause of anthrax, is the most important pathogen of the group. The organism holds a crucial place in the history of medical microbiology:

- Robert Koch's work on anthrax showed that a causative organism could be isolated from the blood of infected animals, artificially grown in pure culture and then used to reproduce the disease in animals. This led to the development of current methods of isolation and identification of bacteria, and to the formulation of *Koch's postulates* (see Ch. 1).
- Louis Pasteur showed that animals could be actively immunized by infecting them with cultures of *B. anthracis* that had been attenuated by growth at 43°C.

Although rare in the industrialized nations, the cases of anthrax in the USA caused by the contamination of mail with *B. anthracis* spores is a reminder of the potential for this pathogen to be used as a biological weapon.

*Bacillus cereus* may contaminate food, especially rice, in large numbers and is commonly implicated in episodes of food poisoning. An atypical strain of *B. cereus* has been implicated as the causative agent of an 'anthrax-like' disease in humans. Other species of *Bacillus* occasionally incriminated as human pathogens, usually in the immunocompromized.

## BACILLUS ANTHRACIS

### DESCRIPTION

*B. anthracis* is a large (4–8 × 1–1.5 μm) non-motile, sporing bacillus. The spores, which form readily when the bacterium is grown on certain artificial media, are oval, refractile and central in position. The temperature range for growth is 12–45°C (optimum 35°C); it grows on all ordinary media as typical colonies with 'ground-glass' surface appearance and a wavy margin with small projections, the so-called *medusa head* appearance. Table 21.1 lists some of the differences between *B. anthracis* and other important members of the genus *Bacillus*.

Genome sequences of multiple strains of *B. anthracis* have been determined. In addition to the chromosome, wild-type strains harbour two plasmids termed

**Table 21.1** Distinguishing properties of some important *Bacillus* species

| Property | B. anthracis | B. cereus[a] | B. subtilis | B. stearothermophilus |
|---|---|---|---|---|
| Colony size | Large | Large | Small | Small |
| Motility | – | + | + | + |
| Capsule | + | – | – | – |
| Mouse pathogenicity | +++ | + | – | – |
| Gamma phage susceptibility | + | – | – | – |
| Anaerobic growth | + | + | – | ± |
| Optimal growth temperature (°C) | 35 | 30 | 37 | 55 |

[a]Atypical strains may cause an anthrax-like disease.

pX01 and pX02, encoding the toxin and capsule, respectively. Most of the chromosomal genes of *B. anthracis* are also found in *B. cereus*. A plasmid similar to pX01 has been found in some *B. cereus* strains (see below).

## PATHOGENESIS

Anthrax is a *zoonosis* – a disease of animals transmissible secondarily to humans. Humans are relatively resistant to infection with *B. anthracis* and anthrax arises most commonly by inoculation through the skin of material from infected animals or their products. The disease is usually a consequence of the exposure of a susceptible host to spores of the bacillus. Spores are not found in host tissues, but appear on exposure of the vegetative cells to oxygen in the air. During naturally occurring disease this is the result of the leakage of infected blood and other body fluids from the corpse.

*B. anthracis* spores introduced into the body by abrasion, inhalation or ingestion are phagocytosed by macrophages and transported from the site of infection to regional lymph nodes, where the spores germinate and vegetative bacteria multiply. The bacilli then enter the bloodstream causing massive septicaemia, with up to $10^8$ colony forming units/mL of blood.

### Virulence factors

The pathogenicity of *B. anthracis* depends primarily on two major virulence factors:

1. The poly-D-glutamic acid capsule.
2. The toxin complex comprising three proteins: the *protective antigen, oedema factor* and *lethal factor.*

The *B. anthracis* capsule is composed of a high molecular weight polypeptide (poly-D-glutamic acid) capsule whose biosynthesis is encoded by the *capBCADE* operon located on the pXO2 plasmid. The capsule appears to enhance the virulence of *B. anthracis* by inhibiting the phagocytosis of vegetative cells in the extracellular environment of the lymphatic system and bloodstream. It is mainly the action of the toxin that mediates damage to the host. The three components of the tripartite toxin combine to form two binary toxins, the *oedema toxin* and *lethal toxin*, formed by association of the protective antigen with the oedema factor and lethal factor, respectively. In each case, the protective antigen binds to host cells and facilitates the entry of the associated oedema or lethal factor (Fig. 21.1).

The oedema toxin is thought to be responsible for the characteristic localised swelling associated with cutaneous anthrax. Oedema factor is a calmodulin-dependent adenylate cyclase that catalyses the production of intracellular cyclic adenosine monophosphate (cAMP) from host adenosine triphosphate (ATP), inducing interleukin (IL)-6 and inhibiting tumour necrosis factor (TNF)-α in monocytes. In addition to disrupting cytokine responses, the oedema toxin may also increase host susceptibility to infection by impairing neutrophil function. However, it is the lethal toxin that is believed to play the major role in damage to the host and death. Lethal factor is a zinc metalloprotease that inactivates mitogen-activated protein kinase kinase, particularly in macrophages. The lethal toxin stimulates macrophages to produce IL-1β and TNF-α. During infection, IL-1β accumulates within macrophages and TNF-α is released. As the concentration of lethal toxin increases later in the infection process, macrophage lysis produces a sudden release of IL-1β, causing shock and death.

Thus, the pathogenesis of anthrax is related to the sensitivity of macrophages to:

• the antiphagocytic activity of the capsule
• the adenylate cyclase activity of the oedema toxin
• the metalloprotease activity of the lethal toxin.

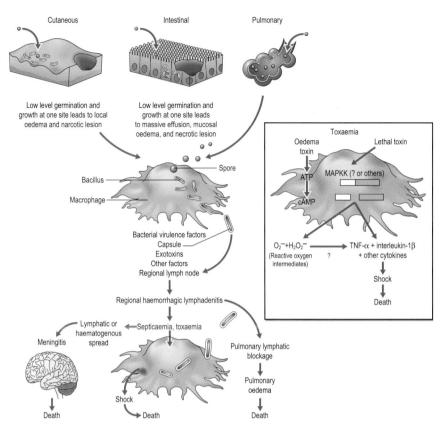

**Fig. 21.1** Pathophysiology of anthrax. *Bacillus anthracis* spores reach a primary site in the subcutaneous layer, gastrointestinal mucosa or alveolar spaces. For cutaneous and gastrointestinal anthrax, low-level germination occurs at the primary site, leading to local oedema and necrosis. Endospores are phagocytosed by macrophages, and germinate. Macrophages containing bacilli detach and migrate to the regional lymph node. Vegetative anthrax bacilli grow in the lymph node, creating regional haemorrhagic lymphadenitis. Bacteria spread through the blood and lymph and multiply, causing severe septicaemia. High levels of exotoxins are produced that are responsible for overt symptoms and death. In a small number of cases, systemic anthrax can lead to meningeal involvement by means of lymphatic or haematogenous spread. In cases of pulmonary anthrax, peribronchial haemorrhagic lymphadenitis blocks pulmonary lymphatic drainage, leading to pulmonary oedema. Death results from septicaemia, toxaemia or pulmonary complications and can occur 1–7 days after exposure. The inset shows the effects of anthrax exotoxins on macrophages. See text for explanation. ATP, adenosine triphosphate; cAMP, cyclic adenosine monophosphate; IL, interleukin; MAPKK, mitogen-activated protein kinase kinase; TNF, tumour necrosis factor. (Reproduced with permission from Dixon et al 1999. © Massachusetts Medical Society, USA.)

## CLINICAL FEATURES

### Cutaneous anthrax

The primary lesion is often described as a *malignant pustule* because of its characteristic appearance (Fig. 21.2). Coagulation necrosis of the centre of the pustule results in the formation of a dark-coloured *eschar* that is later surrounded by a ring of vesicles containing serous fluid and an area of oedema and induration, which may become extensive. In patients with severe toxic signs and widespread oedema, the prognosis is poor.

### Inhalation anthrax

This is a consequence of the inhalation of spores and is the most acute form of the disease, associated with a high mortality rate. The infectious human dose by the air-borne route is in the range of 25 000 to 55 000 spores. Although sometimes incorrectly referred to as pneumonic anthrax, the disease does not develop as a bronchopneumonia.

Inhalational anthrax carries a high mortality rate owing to the intense inflammation, haemorrhage and septicaemia that result from the multiplication of organisms in bronchi and spread to the lungs,

**Fig. 21.2** Stages in the development and resolution of cutaneous anthrax lesions: (A) As first seen; (B) On day 2 or 3; (C) On day 6. (Images kindly provided by Dr Peter Turnbull.)

lymphatics and bloodstream. The production of toxins and the considerable bacterial load that rapidly occurs in the terminal septicaemic phase produce increased vascular permeability and hypotension similar to endotoxic shock.

In the past, cases of inhalation anthrax were reported in persons working in industries handling animal skins, hides and wool, giving rise to the name of *Woolsorter's disease*. In the UK inhalational anthrax from this source was eliminated by the close control of imported wool and fleeces, and by the disinfection of suspect materials. An accident at a former Soviet Union biological weapons factory in the 1980s resulted in the release of spores into the air. In the town of Sverdlovsk, located downwind of the factory, 79 cases of human inhalation anthrax were recorded, some up to 6 weeks after exposure; even with antibiotic therapy there were 68 deaths.

## Intestinal anthrax

The intestinal form of anthrax occurs among pastoralists who may be forced through poverty to eat infected animals that have been found dead. An individual may suffer after a day or so from haemorrhagic diarrhoea, and dies rapidly from septicaemia. Often these episodes occur as small outbreaks in a family or village. Because some individuals may suffer only cutaneous lesions, the recognition of the microbial cause of the outbreak is easily made clinically.

## Meningitis

Haemorrhagic meningitis may complicate any form of anthrax infection, when the bacteraemia spreads across the blood-brain barrier to the central nervous system (CNS). A striking pathological sign of anthrax meningitis is termed the *Cardinal's cap* characterized by dark-red extensive haemorrhaging beneath the lining of the skull.

## Naturally occurring infections of animals

All mammals are susceptible to anthrax although, in general, carnivores are relatively resistant to the disease. Herbivores are highly susceptible and omnivores show an intermediate level of resistance. Disease in wild herbivores or domesticated animals is usually septicaemic and follows the ingestion of spores along with coarse vegetation or soil particles. These abrasive particles probably predispose to trauma of the mouth or intestinal tract, allowing entry of the spores into the host. More rarely infection occurs after the inhalation of dust into the respiratory tract and, as in human disease, through skin abrasions leading to malignant pustules.

Although cases of anthrax are usually localized and sporadic, there may be large outbreaks of disease in wild or domesticated livestock. In the UK, the disease is occasionally found in livestock, chiefly cattle. Disease in pigs is atypical, appearing as a chronic disease with few fatalities. Sudden death in any herbivore should be treated with suspicion, and a veterinary officer summoned to examine the carcass without a post-mortem examination. A blood slide should be taken for Gram or MacFayean's polychrome methylene blue staining. Under the Anthrax Order the animal must remain on the farm and be incinerated on site if found to be positive. Deep burial in quicklime is an alternative method of disposal, but the spores remain viable for many years and may subsequently contaminate pasture and infect grazing animals. Very large numbers of bacilli are present in the terminal stages of disease in animals so that widespread dissemination may occur on death. These highly infectious animals serve as a source of anthrax both by direct spread to another beast and by contamination of the environment.

## Infections in humans

During the period 1981–2001 there were 14 human cases of anthrax in the UK, all of which were the cutaneous form of the disease. However, in recent years there have been a number of fatal inhalation anthrax cases. The first ever drug-related outbreak of anthrax was recorded between December 2009 and February 2010, and was traced to contaminated heroin supplies. This outbreak resulted in 21 confirmed cases with 11 fatalities across Scotland, England and Germany. Furthermore, two cases of fatal inhalational anthrax (Scotland 2006 and London 2008) have been described in the UK, where the cause of the infection was attributed to the making and playing of traditional African animal hide drums. *B. anthracis* has also been associated with use as a biological weapon; in 2001 letters contaminated with anthrax spores were sent via the US postal system. The resulting anthrax exposure led to 22 anthrax infections; of which 5 were fatal.

## Animal models of disease

Various animals, including mice, guinea-pigs, rabbits and non-human primates have been used as models of human anthrax. Several strains of mice are highly susceptible to anthrax, but the response between infecting dose and morbidity is not always clear. To resolve this problem, the use of a partially attenuated strain of *B. anthracis* in mice deficient in complement C5 (e.g. A/J strain) has been proposed.

Guinea-pigs are extremely susceptible to anthrax, both by injection and by inhalation. After subcutaneous challenge the animal usually dies within 2–3 days, showing a marked inflammatory lesion at the site of inoculation and extensive gelatinous oedema in the subcutaneous tissues. Large numbers of the bacilli are present in the local lesion, and are also profusely present in the heart, blood and capillaries of the internal organs. They are especially numerous in the spleen (Fig. 21.3), which is enlarged and soft, giving rise to the description *splenic fever* in the ox and the German name for the organism – *Milzbrandbazillus* (spleen-destroying bacillus). Mice, guinea-pigs and rabbits offer models of human inhalational anthrax which, although limited by their differing physiology to the human respiratory tract, are useful for some pathogenesis studies and initial medical countermeasure efficacy studies.

Studies in non-human primates have provided significant insight into the pathogenesis of inhalational anthrax and offer a relevant animal model for the evaluation of medical countermeasures for human inhalational anthrax. The estimation of the infectious dose in man is based largely on studies in non-human primates. Small particles of less than 5 μm containing spores are deposited on the alveolar walls and taken

**Fig. 21.3** Guinea-pig spleen imprint showing typical anthrax bacilli.

up by phagocytes. These phagocytes migrate to the draining lymph nodes, which become inflamed and enlarged. Surprisingly, ungerminated spores in phagocytes can remain in these lymph nodes for at least 100 days after exposure.

## LABORATORY DIAGNOSIS

### Clinical specimens

The fully developed malignant pustule may be difficult to swab and the central necrotic area gives a poor yield. Fluid aspirated from the surrounding vesicles, when present, is more likely to yield anthrax bacilli. Specimens should be taken before antibiotic therapy has been instituted. In laboratories unfamiliar with the disease, additional precautions for staff safety need to be organized. However, the relative ease of clinical diagnosis, given the characteristic appearance and occupational exposure, often makes laboratory confirmation superfluous.

Gram's stain may show typical large Gram-positive bacilli, and culture on blood agar yields the large, flat, greyish, 'ground-glass' colonies with the characteristic 'medusa head' appearance. Staining of films from these colonies shows long chains of Gram-positive bacilli, some containing spores. Demonstration of non-motility, gelatin liquefaction, growth in straight chains and enhanced growth aerobically, as seen in the characteristic *inverted fir tree* appearance in a gelatin stab, will generally identify *B. anthracis* completely. The FDA has recently approved a diagnostic method for the differentiation of *B. anthracis* vegetative cells from other *Bacilli* based on the susceptibility of *B. anthracis* to gamma-phage.

Serological diagnosis by enzyme-linked immuno-sorbent assay (ELISA) may be of value retrospectively, but is seldom used diagnostically. For the rapid identification of bacteria and diagnosis of disease, the polymerase chain reaction should be used. Because *B. anthracis* possesses a number of unique genes, the selection of suitable gene targets is not problematic. Toxin production can be demonstrated by immunological or gene probe methods in reference laboratories.

### Environmental samples

It is occasionally necessary to isolate *B. anthracis* from potentially contaminated material such as animal hair, hides or soil. The heat treatment of aqueous extracts of these materials at 60°C for 1 h kills all except spore-forming bacteria and fungi. However, the isolation of *B. anthracis* may still be difficult because of the large number of spores of non-pathogenic *Bacillus* species found in the environment. For some soil types selective agars have been developed that allow preferential growth of *B. anthracis*.

## TREATMENT

*B. anthracis* is susceptible *in vitro* to a wide range of antimicrobial agents and many have been used successfully for the treatment of anthrax in humans. Penicillin remains the drug of choice, as β-lactamase-producing strains of *B. anthracis* are rare. Most strains are also sensitive to macrolides, aminoglycosides, tetracyclines and chloramphenicol. Ciprofloxacin (or a similar fluoroquinolone) is recommended as prophylaxis or early treatment for those considered at greatest risk of exposure following a large-scale release of anthrax spores in a deliberate attack.

The efficacy of antibiotics for the treatment of disease is dependent largely on the time at which therapy commences. Treatment with antibiotics is generally ineffective when septicaemic disease has developed and, in the later stages of disease, the general principles applied to the management of any patient in shock are more important than antimicrobial therapy. Because septicaemia develops rapidly in the case of intestinal or inhalational anthrax, these forms of the disease can be especially difficult to treat. It has been common practice to isolate patients with anthrax because of its highly infectious reputation. In fact, human-to-human spread does not occur. The use of specific antiserum is not recommended presently although, in the future, immunotherapy may play an important role in the treatment of septicaemic individuals.

## EPIDEMIOLOGY AND CONTROL

Anthrax is endemic to southern Europe, parts of Africa, Australia, Asia and North and South America. It persists in arid deserts of the Middle East, Asia, Africa, Australia and South America, with most cases reported from Iran, Turkey, Pakistan and Sudan. When the disease is established in livestock and pasture becomes heavily contaminated with spores, an *enzootic* focus is created. Occasionally the disease may erupt in large numbers of domestic animals with associated human cases. In this situation anthrax is *epizootic*. Areas in which anthrax used to be *enzootic*, such as much of Europe, have been able to control the disease by controlling livestock and animal feeds (especially bone meal), and by strict regulations on the importation of animal hides.

The ability of the bacterium to persist in the soil is a consequence of the formation of spores that are able to survive for long periods in the environment. An indication of the robustness of the spores is their ability to survive exposure to chemical disinfectants and heat. For example, the spores will resist dry heat at 140°C for 1–3 h and boiling or steam at 100°C for 5–10 min. Autoclaving at 121°C (15 lb/in$^2$) destroys them in 15 min.

Heavy contamination of soil exists in enzootic foci in many parts of the world, and spores may be recovered many years after the last known case. Artificial contamination of Gruinard Island off the northwest coast of Scotland occurred in 1942–1943 as a result of tests of a biological warfare bomb containing live anthrax spores. Even by 1979 spores could still be detected in a 3-hectare area of the island. In the 1980s the area was decontaminated by burning the vegetation and spraying with 5% formaldehyde in seawater. By 1987, the ground was declared anthrax-free and, after reseeding, sheep were able to graze safely. In enzootic areas, disinfection of soil is not a practical control measure, and pastures known to be heavily contaminated should not be used for grazing animals. The organism multiplies when the soil pH is greater than 6 and when early rain has been followed by a long dry spell. Control in animals depends upon:

- early diagnosis
- isolation and incineration of infected animals
- use of vaccines.

In countries in which the disease is relatively rare in animals, contamination with imported materials is the most common form of human infection. In general, the infectivity of *B. anthracis* for man is not of a high order, and when a case occurs in a factory spores are often widely distributed in large numbers in the dust and air. Anthrax is a recognized industrial hazard that, in the UK, is notifiable to Consultants in Communicable Disease Control and to the Health and Safety Executive. There is control on the importation of animal hides and hair, which are disinfected if considered infected. Workers at risk of exposure in the leather or wool industries, and veterinarians, may be offered immunization routinely and antibiotic prophylaxis if exposed to a known risk.

## Immunization

Live-attenuated bacilli were first used by Louis Pasteur in May 1881, when he confounded professional scepticism in a famous public demonstration of the efficacy of a live vaccine at a farm at Pouilly-le-Fort in France. The 25 sheep that were vaccinated with heat-attenuated live bacilli and then inoculated with virulent anthrax material resisted infection, whereas 22 of 25 sheep acting as controls succumbed within 48 h. Thousands of sheep, cattle and horses were subsequently vaccinated, and the mortality rate among domesticated animals fell dramatically. Later, the Sterne strain of *B. anthracis*, which lacks the pX02 plasmid, was adopted for the immunization of animals, and this vaccine is still in use today.

Live vaccines are not considered to be sufficiently safe for human use and alternative vaccines based on the anthrax toxin have been developed. The currently licensed human vaccines are based on an alum precipitate of culture supernatant fluid. Predominantly they contain protective antigen, but there are also traces of lethal factor and oedema factor, which might account for the transient side-effects experienced by some vaccinees.

New recombinant protective antigen vaccine preparations free of toxin components may give better immunity and fewer adverse reactions; several types are in clinical trials.

## BACILLUS CEREUS

## DESCRIPTION

*B. cereus* is a large Gram-positive bacillus that resembles *B. anthracis*, except that it is motile, resistant to gamma phage and lacks the poly-D-glutamic acid capsule. Like other members of the genus it is a saprophyte and frequents soil, water and vegetation. *B. cereus* closely resembles *B. anthracis* in culture, forming large, grey, irregular colonies described as 'anthracoid'. Large inocula injected into laboratory

animals may cause death but without the haemorrhagic appearance of anthrax, and blood smears do not show the characteristic pink capsule with McFadyean's polychrome methylene blue stain.

## PATHOGENESIS

*B. cereus* is most commonly associated with food poisoning, but the organism can also cause post-traumatic ophthalmitis, which requires rapid, aggressive management locally.

An atypical *B. cereus* strain capable of causing a disease that resembled inhalation anthrax has been described. This strain appears to have acquired the toxin-encoding pX01 plasmid, and a plasmid encoding a polysaccharide capsule. The capsule presumably fulfils the same role as the poly-D-glutamic acid capsule on the surface of *B. anthracis*. Preliminary animal studies suggest that the strain is as virulent as *B. anthracis*; however its origins are presently unclear.

## Food poisoning

Spores of *B. cereus* are particularly heat-resistant and most strains produce toxins. The organism is widespread in the environment and is found in most raw foods, especially cereals such as rice. Enormous numbers of organisms (up to $10^{10}$ organisms/g) may be found in contaminated food (commonly lightly cooked Chinese dishes), leading to two types of food poisoning:

1. Cases in which vomiting, occurring within 6 h of ingestion, is the main symptom. It is caused by preformed toxin, which is a low molecular weight, heat- and acid-stable peptide that can withstand intestinal proteolytic enzymes.
2. A diarrhoeal form of food poisoning, occurring 8–24 h after ingestion, similar to enteritis caused by *Escherichia coli* or *Salmonella enterica* serotypes. This is caused by enterotoxins, which, like the *Clostridium perfringens* enterotoxin, are heat labile and formed in the intestine.

## LABORATORY DIAGNOSIS

In the case of food poisoning, laboratory confirmation is easy if suspect food is available for testing. High numbers of *B. cereus*, often exceeding $10^8$ organisms/g, are sufficient to make the diagnosis in the absence of other food-poisoning bacteria. Large facultatively anaerobic Gram-positive bacilli that produce anthracoid colonies on blood agar after overnight incubation at 37°C are almost certain to be *B. cereus*. Food reference laboratories are able to confirm identification and type if necessary.

Methods for the laboratory identification of *B. cereus* strains that cause an inhalation anthrax-like disease have yet to be devised. It is likely that genetic tests will be effective in identifying these atypical strains.

## TREATMENT

Both the emetic and diarrhoeal syndromes associated with *B. cereus* are short lived and no specific treatment is needed. Most sufferers, even those with underlying conditions, seldom come to any harm. Acute symptoms last less than 24 h and recovery on a reduced diet and fluids is rapid. In comparison, the single case of inhalation anthrax-like disease caused by *B. cereus* was fatal. However, it is likely that antibiotic regimens for the treatment of anthrax would be equally effective for the treatment of disease caused by atypical strains of *B. cereus* strains.

## CONTROL

Food poisoning caused by *B. cereus* is easily prevented by proper cooling and storage of food. Ideally, all dishes should be freshly prepared and eaten. Rice, in particular, should not be stored for long periods at temperatures in excess of 10°C.

## OTHER BACILLUS SPECIES

*Bacillus subtilis, Bacillus pumilis* and *Bacillus licheniformis* have been implicated in causing food poisoning similar to that due to *B. cereus*. They do not appear to form toxins, but some strains produce antibacterial peptides, such as the antibiotic bacitracin, which may facilitate growth in the intestinal tract. *Bacillus polymyxa* is the source of the antibiotic polymyxin.

*B. cereus, B. subtilis* and, rarely, other members of the genus may be found in wounds and tissues of immuno-compromised or burned patients. These opportunist pathogens are also common contaminants of specimens and laboratory media, so that the interpretation of significance is sometimes difficult. When found in numbers in normally sterile sites, such as blood or cerebrospinal fluid, these otherwise insignificant pathogens require specific treatment. Most strains produce abundant β-lactamase, which differs from the enzyme found in staphylococci.

## STERILIZATION TEST BACILLI

*Bacillus stearothermophilus* was, until the discovery of archaebacteria in hot springs, the most heat-resistant organism known. Spores withstand 121°C for up to 12 min, and this has made the organism ideal for testing autoclaves that run on a time–temperature cycle designed to ensure the destruction of spores. Strips containing *B. stearothermophilus* are included with the material being autoclaved, and are subsequently examined by culture for surviving spores. The organism grows only at raised temperatures, typically between 50°C and 60°C; there is hardly any growth below 40°C. *Bacillus globigi*, a red-pigmented variant of *B. subtilis*, has been used to test ethylene oxide sterilizers, and *B. pumilis* has been used to test the efficacy of ionizing radiation.

RECOMMENDED READING

Beyer W, Turnbull PCB: Anthrax in animals, *Molecular Aspects of Medicine* 30:481–489, 2009.

Bottone EJ: *Bacillus cereus*, a volatile human pathogen, *Clinical Microbiology Reviews* 23:382–398, 2010.

Dricks A: The *Bacillus anthracis* spore, *Molecular Aspects of Medicine* 30:368–373, 2009.

Goossens PL: Animal models of human anthrax: The quest for the holy grail, *Molecular Aspects of Medicine* 30:467–480, 2009.

Hoffmaster AR, Ravel J, Rasko DA, et al: Identification of anthrax toxin genes in *Bacillus cereus* associated with an illness resembling inhalation anthrax, *Proceedings of the National Academy of Sciences of the USA* 101:8449–8454, 2004.

Hugh-Jones M, Blackburn J: The ecology of *Bacillus anthracis, Molecular Aspects of Medicine* 30:356–367, 2009.

Moayeri M, Leppla SH: Cellular and systemic effects of anthrax lethal toxin and edema toxin, *Molecular Aspects of Medicine* 30:439–455, 2009.

Rao SS, Mohan KVK, Atreya CD: Detection technologies for *Bacillus anthracis*: Prospects and challenges, *Journal of Microbiological Methods* 82:1–10, 2010.

Stenfors Arnesen LP, Fagerlund A, Granum PE: From soil to gut: *Bacillus cereus* and its food poisoning toxins, *FEMS Microbiology Reviews* 32:579–606, 2009.

### Website

Federal Bureau of Investigation (FBI): Anthrax links, http://www.fbi.gov/about-us/history/famous-cases/anthrax-amerithrax.

# 22 Clostridium

## Gas gangrene; tetanus; food poisoning; pseudomembranous colitis

*T. V. Riley*

## KEY POINTS

- All clostridial infections are characterized by toxin production by the infecting species.
- The major toxins produced by the species are neurotoxins affecting nervous tissue, histotoxins affecting soft tissue and enterotoxins affecting the gut.
- *C. perfringens* is the major cause of gas gangrene.
- Tetanus, particularly neonatal tetanus, is still a major public health issue in developing countries.
- Botulism occurs predominantly as a severe form of food poisoning.
- *C. difficile* is the most common cause of diarrhoea in hospital patients in the developed world.

The clostridia are Gram-positive spore-bearing anaerobic bacilli. Most species are saprophytes that normally occur in soil, water and decomposing plant and animal matter; they play an important part in natural processes of putrefaction. Some, such as *Clostridium perfringens* and *C. sporogenes*, are commensals of the animal and human gut. On the death of the host, these organisms and other members of the intestinal flora rapidly invade the blood and tissues, and initiate the decomposition of the corpse. The genus has undergone a major taxonomic revision, but this has had little impact on clostridia of medical significance.

Pathogenic species include:

- *C. perfringens, C. septicum* and *C. novyi*, the causes of gas gangrene and other infections. *C. perfringens* is also associated with a form of food poisoning.
- *C. tetani*, the cause of tetanus.
- *C. botulinum*, the cause of botulism.
- *C. difficile*, the cause of pseudomembranous colitis and antibiotic-associated diarrhoea.

Genome sequencing of the toxin-producing pathogens *C. perfringens, C. tetani, C. botulinum* and *C. difficile* has provided important data on pathogenic determinants and the regulatory events governing their expression as well as revealing the contribution of extra-chromosomal elements to a pathogenic phenotype.

## GENERAL DESCRIPTION

The clostridia are typically large, straight rods with slightly rounded ends. Pleomorphic forms, including filaments or elongated cells, club and spindle-shaped forms (*clostridium* is Latin for 'little spindle') are commonly seen in stained smears from cultures or wounds. They are Gram positive, but may appear to be Gram negative. All produce spores, which enable the organisms to survive in adverse conditions, for example in soil and dust and on skin.

Most species are obligate anaerobes: their spores do not germinate and growth does not normally proceed unless a suitably low redox potential ($E_h$) exists. A few species grow in the presence of trace amounts of air, and some actually grow slowly under normal atmospheric conditions.

Clostridia are biochemically active, frequently possessing both saccharolytic and proteolytic properties, although in varying degrees. Many species are highly toxigenic. The toxins produced by the organisms of tetanus and botulism attack nervous pathways and are referred to as neurotoxins. The organisms associated with gas gangrene attack soft tissues by producing toxins and aggressins, and are referred to as histotoxic. *C. difficile* and some strains of *C. perfringens* produce enterotoxins.

## CLOSTRIDIUM PERFRINGENS

## DESCRIPTION

*C. perfringens* is a relatively large Gram-positive bacillus (about 4–6 × 1 μm) with blunt ends. It is capsulate and non-motile. It grows quickly on laboratory media, particularly at high temperatures (approximately 42°C), when the doubling time can be as short as 8 min. It can be identified by the *Nagler reaction*, which exploits the action of its phospholipase on egg yolk medium; colonies are surrounded by zones of turbidity, and the effect is specifically inhibited if *C. perfringens* antiserum containing α-antitoxin is present on the medium. Typical food-poisoning strains produce heat-resistant spores that can survive boiling for several hours, whereas the spores of the type A strains that cause gas gangrene are inactivated within a few minutes by boiling.

## GAS GANGRENE

*C. perfringens* is the most common cause of gas gangrene, although various other species of clostridia, including *C. septicum*, *C. novyi* type A, *C. histolyticum* and *C. sordellii* are occasionally implicated, either alone or in combination. Gas gangrene is almost always a polymicrobial infection involving anaerobes and facultative organisms.

The disease is characterized by rapidly spreading oedema, myositis, necrosis of tissues, gas production and profound toxaemia occurring as a complication of wound infection. The diagnosis is made primarily on clinical grounds with laboratory confirmation.

The main source of the organisms is animal and human excreta, and spores of the causative clostridia are distributed widely. Infection usually results from contamination of a wound with soil, particularly from manured and cultivated land. However, it may be derived indirectly from dirty clothing, street dust, and even the air of an operating theatre if the ventilating system is poorly designed or improperly maintained. The skin often bears spores of *C. perfringens*, especially in areas of the body that may be contaminated with intestinal organisms.

### Pathogenesis of gas gangrene

Impairment of the normal blood supply of tissue with a consequent reduction in oxygen tension may allow an anaerobic focus to develop. The patient's condition may deteriorate rapidly with the development of severe shock (Fig. 22.1).

Crushing of tissue and the severing of arteries in accidental injuries, rough handling of tissue and over-zealous clamping during surgery, or shock waves from gunshot injuries may compromise the microcirculation in an extensive area of tissue and prejudice tissue perfusion. The presence of devitalized or dead tissue, blood clot, extravasated fluid, foreign bodies and coincident pyogenic infection are all factors that promote the occurrence of gas gangrene in a wound. The spores of the clostridia and their vegetative bacilli cannot readily initiate infection in healthy tissues, presumably because the $E_h$ is too high, and the organisms are unable to avoid destruction and clearance by

Fig. 22.1 Circumstances and events that may lead to gas gangrene.

phagocytosis. Predisposing host factors include debility, old age and diabetes.

When clostridial infection has been initiated in a focus of devitalized anaerobic tissue, the organisms multiply rapidly and produce a range of toxins and aggressins. These damage tissue by various necrotizing effects, and some have demonstrable lethal effects. They spread into adjacent viable tissue, particularly muscle, kill it, and render it anaerobic and vulnerable to further colonization, with the production of more toxins and aggressins.

- Hyaluronidase produced by *C. perfringens* breaks down intercellular cement substance and promotes the spread of the infection along tissue planes.
- Collagenase and other proteinases break down tissues and virtually liquefy muscles. The whole of a muscle group or segment of a limb may be affected.
- α-Toxin, a phospholipase C (lecithinase), is generally considered to be the main cause of the toxaemia associated with gas gangrene, although other clostridial species can produce similar manifestations.

In puerperal infections or in cases of septic abortion, the organisms may gain access from faeces-contaminated perineal skin or contaminated instruments to necrotic or devitalized tissues in the uterus or adnexa. Here they set up a dangerous and often fulminating pelvic infection, possibly with prompt invasion of the bloodstream. There may be intravascular haemolysis and anuria.

*C. perfringens* may also participate in peritoneal infections that occur as a result of extension of pathogens from the alimentary tract, as in cases of gangrenous appendicitis or intestinal obstruction or mesenteric thrombosis.

If a preparation of adrenaline (epinephrine) used for injection is contaminated with clostridial spores, the combination of an infective inoculum with the local ischaemia that follows the injection may be catastrophic. Gas gangrene may complicate surgical operations on the lower limb or hip of patients whose blood supply is inadequate to maintain oxygenation in the post-operative period.

Clostridia may be associated with less severe forms of infection without the toxaemia and aggression of gas gangrene. Moreover, potentially pathogenic anaerobes may be cultivated from a wound that never shows any sign of gas gangrene, and sometimes the laboratory isolation may be attributed to the germination of a few contaminating spores when the specimen was being processed. Thus, the onus is on the clinician to relate a laboratory report to the patient's circumstances.

Clinical clues include *crepitus*, the sponge-cake consistency caused by small bubbles of gas in adjacent tissues. In the early stages, the patient has an anxious, frightened appearance. Local pain is increased, and there is swelling of the affected tissues. Toxaemia and shock supervene, and the patient becomes drowsy and drifts into coma. Prompt diagnosis and intensive surgical and antimicrobial treatment greatly influence the patient's chance of survival and may avoid the loss of the affected limb, but all devitalized tissue must be excised (see below).

## Laboratory diagnosis

If there are sloughs of necrotic tissue in the wound, small pieces should be transferred aseptically into a sterile screw-capped bottle and examined immediately by microscopy and culture. Specimens of exudate should be taken from the deeper areas of the wound where the infection seems to be most pronounced. Gram smears are prepared. If gas gangrene exists, typical Gram-positive bacilli may predominate, often with other bacteria present in a mixed infection. However, there is usually a pronounced lack of inflammatory cells. Initiation of treatment should not await a full laboratory report and early discussion with the bacteriologist is crucial. A direct smear of a wound exudate is often of great help in providing evidence of the relative numbers of different bacteria that may be participating in a mixed infection or may merely be present as contaminants, but the distinction is not invariably easy and joint discussions are important.

## Treatment

Prompt and adequate surgical attention to the wound is of the utmost importance (Fig. 22.2).

- Sutures are removed, and necrotic and devitalized tissue is excised with careful debridement.
- Fascial compartments are incised to release tension.
- Any foreign body is found and removed.
- The wound is not resutured but is left open after thorough cleansing, and loosely packed.

Antibiotic therapy is started immediately in very high doses. This must take account of the likely coexistence of coliform organisms, Gram-positive cocci and faecal anaerobes. Accordingly, penicillin, metronidazole and an aminoglycoside may be given in combination. Alternatively, clindamycin plus an aminoglycoside or a broad-spectrum antibiotic, such as meropenem or imipenem, may be considered. Much intensive supportive therapy is needed.

**Fig. 22.2** Gas gangrene. Wound after debridement.

Enthusiastic claims have been made for the efficacy of hyperbaric oxygen therapy, but clinical trials have given conflicting results. Patients are placed in a special pressurized chamber where they breathe oxygen at 2–3 atm pressure for periods of 1–2 h twice daily on several successive days. This may limit the amount of radical surgery needed.

A polyvalent antiserum containing *C. perfringens*, *C. septicum* and *C. novyi* antitoxins was used formerly, but has been replaced by intensive antimicrobial therapy.

## Prophylaxis

### Surgical wounds

*C. perfringens* is normally present in large numbers in human faeces, and its spores are found regularly on the skin, especially of the buttocks and thighs. As clostridial spores are very resistant to most disinfectants, they are likely to survive normal pre-operative skin preparation and persist in the area of the planned incision. The numbers can be reduced by more prolonged skin preparation with the sustained action of an antiseptic such as povidone–iodine for a day or two; this procedure has a place in orthopaedic surgery.

When inevitable skin contamination is combined with circumstances that predispose to devitalization of tissue and reduced oxygen tension, a patient may be vulnerable to the development of post-operative gas gangrene. These circumstances arise when an elderly patient or a patient with vascular insufficiency undergoes major surgery to the hip or lower limb. Perioperative antimicrobial prophylaxis with penicillin is justified in such cases.

### Accidental wounds

The prevention of gas gangrene in accidentally sustained wounds must take account of the endogenous factors noted above and the exogenous sources of clostridial spores and vegetative forms in soil, on contaminated clothing, etc. In addition, there is an increased risk of anaerobic infection developing when foreign bodies such as soil, clothing, metal (nails, wire, bullets, shrapnel) and skin are driven into devitalized tissues. Prompt and adequate surgical attention is of paramount importance, but prophylactic administration of benzylpenicillin for patients presenting with serious contaminated wounds is also worthwhile. Prophylaxis may be omitted if the state of the wound and the patient's general condition are expertly and frequently monitored throughout the recovery period.

## FOOD POISONING

Carrier rates for 'typical food poisoning strains' of *C. perfringens* range from about 2% to more than 30% in different surveys across the world. These bacteria also occur in animals; thus, meat is often contaminated with heat-resistant spores. When meat is cooked in bulk, heat penetration and subsequent cooling is slow unless special precautions are taken. During the cooling period surviving spores may germinate and multiply in the anaerobic environment produced by the cooked meat. Anyone eating this will consume the equivalent of a cooked meat broth culture of the organism. The organisms are protected from the gastric acid by the protein in the meal and pass in large numbers into the intestine.

Ingestion of large numbers of viable organisms is necessary for the production of the typical disease syndrome, which is mediated by an enterotoxin that is released when sporulation occurs in the gut. Typical symptoms are abdominal cramps beginning about 8–12 h after ingestion, followed by diarrhoea. Fever and vomiting are not usually encountered and symptoms generally subside within a day or two. No specific treatment is indicated. The carrier state persists for several weeks, but this should not be regarded as an indication for exclusion from any duties, as carriers may be quite numerous in various communities.

The vehicle of infection is usually a pre-cooked meat food that has been allowed to stand at a temperature conducive to the multiplication of *C. perfringens*. Although the heat resistance of spores of typical food-poisoning strains ensures their survival in cooked foods, and presumably accounts for the association of these strains with most of the reported outbreaks of *C. perfringens* food poisoning, similar trouble can be caused by classical heat-sensitive type A strains if they gain access to food during the cooling period under conditions suitable for their subsequent multiplication.

## Laboratory diagnosis

This can be difficult as some people carry large numbers of *C. perfringens*. Diagnosis depends upon the isolation of similar strains of *C. perfringens* from the faeces of patients and from others at risk who have eaten the suspected food, and from the food itself. Numbers usually exceed $10^6$ organisms/g faeces. The isolates can be sent to a reference laboratory for special typing to prove their relatedness.

## Prevention

The occurrence of this type of food poisoning is an indictment of the catering practices concerned, as food has to be mishandled to allow the chain of events to take place. Nevertheless, *C. perfringens* is among the most common causes of food poisoning.

## COLITIS

A sporadic diarrhoeal syndrome, usually occurring in elderly patients during treatment with antibiotics, has been described. The circumstances differ substantially from those of *C. perfringens* food poisoning. A cytopathic enterotoxin can be detected in the patient's faeces.

## ENTERITIS NECROTICANS (PIGBEL)

A subgroup of *C. perfringens* type C that produces heat-resistant spores is the cause of a disease that affects New Guinea natives when they have pork feasts. The method of cooking the pork allows the clostridia to survive. When the contaminated meat is eaten along with a sweet potato vegetable that contains a proteinase inhibitor, a toxin (the β-toxin) is able to act on the small intestine to produce a necrotizing enteritis. A successful vaccination programme has reduced the incidence of pigbel dramatically.

## CLOSTRIDIUM SEPTICUM

## DESCRIPTION

The bacilli are generally large and actively motile with numerous flagella. It is one of the less exacting anaerobes and grows well at 37°C on ordinary media. Spores are readily formed and, as they develop, various pleomorphic forms arise ranging from swollen Gram-positive 'citron bodies' to obviously sporing forms in which the oval spores may be central or subterminal and are clearly bulging.

## PATHOGENESIS

*C. septicum* is one of the gas gangrene group of clostridia. It occurs harmlessly in the human intestine, but if the integrity of the gut epithelium is impaired, for instance by leukaemic infiltration, bacteraemia may occur. Cyclic or other forms of neutropenia are also associated with spontaneous, non-traumatic gas gangrene that begins with a bacteraemic phase. *Typhlitis*, a rapidly fatal terminal ileal infection and septicaemia in immunocompromised patients, is most commonly associated with *C. septicum*.

Intramuscular injection of cultures into laboratory animals produces a spreading inflammatory oedema, with slight gas formation in the tissues. Organisms invade the blood and the animal dies within a day or two. Smears from the liver show long filamentous forms and citron bodies. *C. septicum* produces several toxins (α, β, δ and ε). The α-toxin, which has lethal, haemolytic and necrotizing activity, appears to be the most important; it does not have phospholipase C activity and thus differs from the α-toxin of *C. perfringens*.

## CLOSTRIDIUM NOVYI

*C. novyi* resembles *C. perfringens* in morphology, but is larger, more pleomorphic and more strictly anaerobic; it is readily killed when vegetative cells are exposed to air. The spores are oval, central or subterminal. The organism occurs widely in soil and is associated with disease in man and animals. There are four types – A, B, C and D – distinguished on the basis of permutations of the toxins and other soluble antigens they produce. Only type A strains are of medical interest as they cause some cases of gas gangrene in man. In 2000, an outbreak of *C. novyi* type A infections among injecting heroin users killed 13 people in the UK.

*C. novyi* gas gangrene is associated with profound toxaemia. Culture filtrates are highly toxic and possess at least four active substances (α, β, δ and ε toxins) that account for the various haemolytic, necrotizing, lethal, phospholipase and lipase activities of this organism.

## CLOSTRIDIUM SPOROGENES

This clostridium is widely distributed in nature as a harmless saprophyte. Its spores may survive boiling for periods up to 6 h and the organism is often encountered in mixed cultures after preliminary heating to select heat-resistant pathogens. Although its presence in wound exudates may accelerate an established anaerobic infection by enhancing local conditions, it is not a pathogen in its own right and does not cause gas gangrene.

## CLOSTRIDIUM TETANI

### DESCRIPTION

The tetanus bacillus is a motile, straight, slender, Gram-positive rod. A fully developed terminal spore gives the organism the appearance of a drumstick with a large round end. Gram-negative forms are usually encountered in stained smears. It is an obligate anaerobe that grows well in cooked meat broth and produces a thin spreading film when grown on enriched blood agar. The spores may be highly resistant to adverse conditions, but the degree of resistance varies with the strain. Spores of some strains resist boiling in water for up to 3 h. They may resist dry heat at 160°C for 1 h, and 5% phenol for 2 weeks or more. Iodine (1%) in water is said to kill the spores within a few hours, but glutaraldehyde is one of the few chemical disinfectants that is assuredly sporicidal.

### PATHOGENESIS

As in gas gangrene (see p. 246), germination of spores and their outgrowth depend upon reduced oxygen tension in devitalized tissue and non-viable material in a wound. When infection occurs, often assisted by the simultaneous growth of facultatively anaerobic organisms in a mixed inoculum, the tetanus bacillus remains strictly localized, but tetanus toxin is elaborated and diffuses, as described below.

### Toxins

*C. tetani* produces an oxygen-labile haemolysin (tetanolysin), but the organism's neurotoxin (tetanospasmin) is the essential pathogenic product. Strains vary in their toxigenicity; some are highly toxigenic. Most strains produce demonstrable toxin after culture in broth for a few days.

The gene encoding the neurotoxin is located on a plasmid. The toxin is synthesized as a single polypeptide with a molecular weight of 150 000 Da, which undergoes post-translational cleavage into a heavy chain and a light chain linked by a disulphide bond. The estimated lethal dose for a mouse of pure tetanospasmin is 0.0001 µg. It is toxic to man and various animals when injected parenterally, but not by the oral route.

When tetanus occurs naturally, the tetanus bacilli stay at the site of the initial infection and are not generally invasive. Toxin diffuses to affect the relevant level of the spinal cord (local tetanus) and then to affect the entire system (generalized tetanus). These stages, including the intermediate one of 'ascending tetanus', are demonstrable in experimental animals, but the stages tend to merge in their clinical presentation in man.

The toxin is absorbed from the site of its production in an infective focus, but may be delivered via the blood to all nerves in the body. The heavy chain mediates attachment to gangliosides and the toxin is internalized. It is then moved from the peripheral to the central nervous system by retrograde axonal transport and trans-synaptic spread. The tendency for the first signs of human tetanus to be in the head and neck is attributed to the shorter length of the cranial nerves. In fact, descending involvement of the nervous system is seen as the tetanus toxin takes longer to traverse the longer motor nerves and also diffuses in the spinal cord.

Once the entire toxin molecule has been internalized into presynaptic cells, the light chain is released and affects the membrane of synaptic vesicles. This prevents the release of the neurotransmitter γ-aminobutyric acid. Motor neurones are left under no inhibitory control and undergo sustained excitatory discharge, causing the characteristic motor spasms of tetanus. The toxin exerts its effects on the spinal cord, brainstem, peripheral nerves, at neuromuscular junctions and directly on muscles.

### Clinical features of tetanus

Cases of tetanus have been reported in which the infection was apparently associated with a superficial abrasion, a contaminated splinter or a minor thorn prick. *Otogenic tetanus* may be attributable to over-zealous cleansing of the external auditory meatus with a small stick. In other patients, the site of infection remains undiscovered (*cryptogenic tetanus*). Tetanus infection may also occur in or near the uterus in cases of septic abortion.

*Tetanus neonatorum* follows infection of the umbilical wound of newborn infants (see below). Cases of *post-operative tetanus* have been attributed to imperfectly sterilized catgut, dressings or glove powder, and sometimes to dust-borne infection of the wound at operation.

The onset of signs and symptoms is gradual, usually starting with some stiffness and perhaps pain in or near a recent wound. In some cases the initial complaint may be of stiffness of the jaw (*lockjaw*). Pain and stiffness in the neck and back may follow. The stiffness spreads to involve all muscle groups; facial spasms produce the 'sardonic grin', and in severe cases spasm of the back muscles produces extreme arching of the back (*opisthotonos*). The period between injury and the first signs is usually about 10–14 days, but there is a considerable range. A severe case with a relatively poor prognosis shows rapid progression from the first signs to the development of generalized spasms. Sweating, tachycardia and arrhythmia, and swings in blood pressure, reflect sympathetic stimulation, which is not well understood but creates problems of management.

## TREATMENT

The patient remains conscious and requires skilled sedation and constant nursing. If generalized spasms are worrying, the patient is paralysed and ventilated mechanically until the toxin that has been taken up has decayed; this may take some weeks.

The patient is given 10 000 units of human tetanus immunoglobulin (HTIG) in saline by slow intravenous infusion. Full wound exploration and debridement is arranged, and the wound is cleansed and left open with a loose pack. Penicillin or metronidazole is given for as long as considered necessary to ensure that bacterial growth and toxin production are stopped. The antitoxin and antibiotics are given immediately, and preferably before surgical excision, but delay must be avoided.

## LABORATORY DIAGNOSIS

Gram smears of the wound exudate and any necrotic material may show the typical 'drumstick' bacilli, but this is not invariably so, and thus provides only presumptive evidence as other organisms that resemble

*C. tetani* have terminal spores. Simple light microscopy is often unsuccessful; immunofluorescence microscopy with a specific stain is possible but not generally available.

Direct culture of unheated material on blood agar incubated anaerobically is often the best method of detecting *C. tetani*. There are various other tricks that exploit the organism's motility and fine spreading growth; sometimes these are vitiated by overgrowth with *Proteus* species. Material from the wound or from a mixed sporing subculture may be heated at various temperatures and for various times to exclude non-sporing bacteria; the heated specimens are then seeded on to solid media and incubated anaerobically. Tetanus may be produced in mice by subcutaneous injection of an anaerobic culture prepared from wound material; control mice are protected with tetanus antitoxin.

## EPIDEMIOLOGY

Tetanus bacilli may be found in the human intestine, but infection seems to be derived primarily from animal faeces and soil. The organism is especially prevalent in manured soil and for this reason a wound through skin contaminated with soil or manure deserves special attention. However, tetanus spores occur very widely and are commonly present in gardens, sports fields and roads, in the dust, plaster and air of hospitals and houses, on clothing and on articles of common use.

Spores of *C. tetani* and other anaerobes may be embedded in surgical catgut and other dressings. However, the sterility of surgical catgut (prepared from the gut of cattle and sheep) is now rigorously controlled.

Tetanus ranks among the major fatal infections. During the 1980s there were between 800 000 and 1 million deaths annually from tetanus, of which 400 000 were due to neonatal tetanus. The incidence varies enormously from country to country, and is inversely related to socio-economic development and standards of living, preventive medicine and wound management. In developed countries, the reported incidence of adult and childhood tetanus is low. There is a direct relationship with fertile soil and a warm climate; thus, people living in the agricultural areas of developing tropical and subtropical countries are exposed to severe challenges associated with poor hygiene, lack of shoes, neglect of wounds and inadequate immunization.

In addition, some local customs promote the occurrence of tetanus:

- treatment of the umbilical cord stump with primitive applications that include animal dung

- tying of the umbilical cord itself with primitive ligatures
- ear-piercing and other operations performed with unsterile instruments.

Fatality rates may exceed 50% and neonatal tetanus carries a very high mortality rate. Case fatality rates can be greatly reduced to less than 10% by modern methods of treatment in specialist centres. Unfortunately, such expensive skilled help is available for only a small proportion of patients. Under-privileged people in countries with poorly developed or expensive medical services are at greatest risk, and are least likely to receive sophisticated assistance; 80% of deaths occur in Africa and Southeast Asia. A maternal vaccination campaign mounted by the United Nations Children's Fund (UNICEF) during the past 15 years has reduced the incidence of neonatal tetanus by 50%.

## PREVENTION AND CONTROL

Prompt and adequate wound toilet and proper surgical debridement of wounds are of paramount importance. There is an increased risk that tetanus spores may germinate in a wound if cleansing is delayed and if sepsis develops. Clean superficial wounds that receive prompt attention may not require specific protection against tetanus and it is unreasonable to insist that every small prick or abrasion requires protection with antitoxin or antibiotic.

Routine practice should take account of the local incidence of tetanus and the individual circumstances of the case. It is wise to recommend specific prophylaxis for a non-immunized patient with a deep wound, puncture or stab wound, ragged laceration, a wound with much bruising and any devitalized tissue, a wound that is already septic, or a bite wound or other type of wound that is likely to be heavily contaminated. Figure 22.3 shows an approach that reflects current thinking in the UK.

The need for passive immunization is avoided if the patient is known to be properly immunized against tetanus (see Ch. 70). A patient may be regarded as immune for 6 months after the first two injections, or for 5–10 years after a planned course of three injections (or a subsequent booster injection) of adsorbed tetanus toxoid. Tetanus antitoxin should not be given to immune patients, but their active immunity may be enhanced when necessary by giving a dose of tetanus toxoid at the time of injury if the circumstances justify it.

A patient is considered non-immune if there is no history of having had an injection of tetanus toxoid

**Fig. 22.3** Wound management guidelines, with special reference to the prevention of tetanus.

TT = Adsorbed tetanus toxoid    HTIG = human tetanus immunoglobulin    GP = General practitioner, family doctor or if only one injection has been given. Take care: a patient may recall having had 'a tetanus shot', but this may have been a previous dose of antitoxin for passive protection (which is transient and cannot be boosted by toxoid). If more than 6 months have elapsed after a course of two injections, or more than 10 years after a full primary course of three injections of adsorbed toxoid (or a booster injection), the patient should be regarded as non-immune. A patient is non-immune if more than 2–3 weeks have elapsed since a previous injection of equine antitoxin, or more than 6–8 weeks in the case of homologous (human) antitoxin. Non-immunity should be assumed if there is any doubt about the immunization history.

## Passive immunization with antitoxin

HTIG (homologous antitoxin) is available for passive protection and now supersedes equine antitoxin (heterologous antitoxin), which was associated with occasional adverse reactions. However, equine antiserum should not be prematurely discarded in countries that do not yet have HTIG. The prophylactic dose of HTIG is 250–500 units by intramuscular injection.

## Combined active–passive immunization

A non-immune patient receiving passive protection with HTIG after injury may be given the first dose of a course of active immunization with adsorbed toxoid at the same time, provided the injections are given from different syringes and into contralateral sites. The active immunization course must subsequently be completed.

## Antibiotic protection

The prophylactic administration of antibiotics to all cases of open wounds is not recommended, although the use of penicillin or clindamycin is justified in some cases when there is a significant risk of infection. This precaution must not replace prompt and adequate surgical wound toilet.

## CLOSTRIDIUM BOTULINUM

## DESCRIPTION

C. botulinum is a strictly anaerobic Gram-positive bacillus. It is motile and has spores that are oval and subterminal. It is a widely distributed saprophyte found in soil, vegetables, fruits, leaves, silage, manure, the mud of lakes and sea mud. Its optimal growth temperature is about 35°C, but some strains can grow and produce toxin at temperatures as low as 1–5°C.

The widespread occurrence of C. botulinum in nature, its ability to produce a potent neurotoxin in food, and the resistance of its spores to inactivation combine to make it a formidable pathogen. Spores of some strains withstand boiling in water (100°C) for several hours. They are usually destroyed by moist heat at 120°C within 5 min. Spores of type E strains (see below) are usually much less heat resistant. Insufficient heating in the process of preserving foods is an important factor in the causation of botulism. The resistance of the spores to radiation is of special relevance to food processing.

Botulinum toxin is categorized as a biothreat level A biological warfare agent. Introduction of toxin into a target population by contaminating food or water is unlikely to succeed because of logistical problems, but botulinum toxin can also cause disease by inhalation.

Carefully controlled injections of toxin are used to treat involuntary muscle disorders, and as an 'anti-aging' remedy.

## PATHOGENESIS

Botulism is a severe, often fatal, form of food poisoning characterized by pronounced neurotoxic effects. Botulinum toxins are among the most poisonous natural substances known. Seven main types of C. botulinum, designated A–G, produce antigenically distinct toxins with pharmacologically identical actions. All types can cause human disease, but types A, B and E are most common. The importance of this point is that, if antitoxin is given to a patient in an emergency, only the type-specific antitoxin will be effective.

The disease has been linked to a wide range of foods, including preserved hams, large sausages of the salami type, home-preserved meats and vegetables, canned products such as fish, liver paste, and even hazelnut purée and honey. Traditional dishes such as fish or seal flipper fermented in a barrel buried in the ground cannot be recommended by a bacteriologist! Type E strains are particularly but not invariably associated with a marine source, whereas type A and type B strains are usually associated with soil.

Foods responsible for botulism may not exhibit signs of spoilage. The pre-formed toxin in the food is absorbed from the intestinal tract. Although it is protein, intestinal proteolytic enzymes do not inactivate it. After absorption, botulinum toxin binds irreversibly to the presynaptic nerve endings of the peripheral nervous system and cranial nerves, where it inhibits acetylcholine release.

## Clinical features

The period between ingestion of the toxin and the appearance of signs and symptoms is usually 1–2 days, but it may be much longer. There may be initial nausea and vomiting. The oculomotor muscles are affected, and the patient may have diplopia and drooping eyelids with a squint. There may be vertigo and blurred vision.

There is progressive descending motor loss with flaccid paralysis but with no loss of consciousness or sensation, although weakness and sleepiness are often described. The patient is thirsty, with a dry mouth and tongue. There are difficulties in speech and swallowing, with later problems of breathing and despair. There may be abdominal pain and restlessness. Death is due to respiratory or cardiac failure.

### Wound botulism

Rare cases of wound infection with *C. botulinum* resulting in the characteristic signs and symptoms of botulism have been recorded.

### Infant botulism

The 'floppy child syndrome' describes a young child, usually less than 6 months old, with flaccid paralysis that is ascribed to the growth of *C. botulinum* in the intestine at a stage in development when the colonization resistance of the gut is poor. Some cases have been attributed to the presence of *C. botulinum* spores in honey; when the honey was given as an encouragement to feed, the ingested spores were able to germinate and produce toxin in the infant gut.

## LABORATORY DIAGNOSIS

The organism or its toxin may be detected in the suspected food, and toxin may be demonstrated in the patient's blood by toxin–antitoxin neutralization tests in mice. Samples of faeces or vomit may also yield such evidence. Take care: bear in mind that botulinum toxin is very dangerous – specialist help should be summoned and the laboratory alerted.

## TREATMENT

The priorities are:

- to remove unabsorbed toxin from the stomach and intestinal tract

- to neutralize unfixed toxin by giving polyvalent antitoxin (with due precautions to avoid hypersensitivity reactions to the heterologous antiserum)
- to give relevant intensive care and support.

## CONTROL

Great care must be taken in canning factories to ensure that adequate heating is achieved in all parts of the can contents. Home canning of foodstuffs should be avoided. The amateur preservation of meat and vegetables, especially beans, peas and root vegetables, is dangerous in inexperienced hands. Acid fruits may be bottled safely in the home with heating at 100°C, as a low pH is inhibitory to the growth of *C. botulinum*.

A prophylactic dose of polyvalent antitoxin should be given intramuscularly to all persons who have eaten food suspected of causing botulism. Injecting three doses of mixed toxoid at intervals of 2 months can produce active immunity, but the very low incidence of the disease under normal conditions does not justify this as a routine. Active immunization should be considered for laboratory staff who might have to handle the organism or specimens containing the organism or its toxin.

## CLOSTRIDIUM DIFFICILE

## DESCRIPTION

*C. difficile* is a motile Gram-positive rod with oval subterminal spores. It commonly occurs in the faeces of neonates and babies until the age of weaning, but it is not generally found in adults.

The organism produces an enterotoxin (toxin A) and a cytotoxin (toxin B); some strains produce a third, binary, toxin. It causes antibiotic-associated diarrhoea, occasionally leading to a life-threatening condition, *pseudomembranous colitis* (Fig. 22.4). There is almost always a history of previous antibiotic therapy although exposure to any agent that perturbs the gut flora, including cytotoxic drugs, may lead to infection. Clindamycin and lincomycin are associated with a particularly high risk but extended-spectrum cephalosporins are also commonly incriminated and are much more commonly used; virtually no antimicrobial drug has escaped blame. A worldwide epidemic of fluoroquinolone-resistant ribotype 027 *C. difficile* infection is probably due to excessive use of these agents.

**Fig. 22.4** Pseudomembranous colitis.

## LABORATORY DIAGNOSIS

*C. difficile* can be isolated from the faeces by enrichment and selective culture procedures. Toxin B can be detected in the patient's faeces by testing extracts against monolayers of susceptible cells, or both toxins may be demonstrated by immunological methods, such as enzyme-linked immunosorbent assay (ELISA). The sensitivity of many ELISA kits is only 50–70% and results should be interpreted with caution. Moreover, toxin A negative strains, which still cause disease and are prevalent in certain regions of the world, are not detected by some kits. Due to these issues, highly sensitive PCR (polymerase chain reaction) detection of the toxin B gene is now the favoured approach.

## TREATMENT

It is essential to discontinue the antibiotic that is presumed to have precipitated the disease and to suppress the growth and toxin production of *C. difficile* by giving oral metronidazole or vancomycin. Pseudomembranous colitis may be fatal if it is not quickly recognized and treated.

## EPIDEMIOLOGY

The organism is usually acquired from an exogenous source by a patient whose intestinal colonization resistance has been compromised by antibiotic exposure. Patients developing infection have often spent lengthy periods in hospital. Re-infection occurs in 20–50% of cases as it may take the gut 2–3 months to normalize after perturbation.

Many production and companion animals are colonized by *C. difficile* before weaning and meat and meat products in North America have been found to be contaminated by *C. difficile* spores. Although the suggestion that *C. difficile* is a common food-borne pathogen is premature, animals may be an important reservoir of disease. An apparent increase in community-acquired infection in the absence of risk factors such as antibiotic exposure, has led to suggestions that all patients with community-acquired diarrhoea should be tested for *C. difficile*.

## PREVENTION

Clinical awareness is the keynote. *C. difficile* is the most common cause of hospital-acquired diarrhoea. If a patient develops diarrhoea after at least 48 h in hospital, especially while taking antibiotics, the possibility of *C. difficile* infection must be considered. If several cases occur in a hospital unit, cross-infection should be considered as the hospital environment can become extensively contaminated with *C. difficile* spores. The existing antibiotic and infection control policies of the unit should be reviewed.

RECOMMENDED READING

Caya JG, Agni R, Miller JE: *Clostridium botulinum* and the clinical laboratorian. *Archives of Pathology and Laboratory Medicine* 128:653–662, 2004.

Crobach MJ, Dekkers OM, Wilcox MH, Kuijper EJ: European Society of Clinical Microbiology and Infectious Diseases (ESCMID): data review and recommendations for diagnosing Clostridium difficile-infection (CDI). *Clinical Microbiology and Infection* 15:1053–1066, 2009.

Farrar JJ, Yen LM, Cook T, et al: Tetanus. *Journal of Neurology, Neurosurgery & Psychiatry* 69:292–301, 2000.

Freeman J, Bauer MP, Baines S, et al: The changing epidemiology of *Clostridium difficile* infections. *Journal of Clinical Microbiology* 23:529–549, 2010.

McLauchlin J, Little C: *Hobbs' 1993 Food Poisoning and Food Hygiene*, ed 7, London, 2007, Hodder Arnold.

Popoff MR, Bouvet P: Clostridial toxins. *Future Microbiology* 4:1021–1064, 2009.

Rood JI, McClane BA, Songer JG, Titball RW: *The Clostridia – Molecular Biology and Pathogenesis*, ed 1, San Diego, 1997, Academic Press.

Shapiro RL, Hatheway C, Swerdlow DL: Botulism in the United States: a clinical and epidemiologic review. *Annals of Internal Medicine* 129:221–228, 1998.

# 23 Neisseria and moraxella

## Meningitis; septicaemia; gonorrhoea; respiratory infections

*N. J. Oldfield and D. A. A. Ala'Aldeen*

## KEY POINTS

- *Neisseria meningitidis* (meningococcus) and *N. gonorrhoeae* (gonococcus) are obligate human parasites.
- *N. meningitidis* lives commensally in the nasopharynx, is transmitted via close kissing contact, and causes disease that varies in severity from mild sore throat to meningitis, septicaemia or septicaemic shock (circulatory failure, multi-organ dysfunction and coagulopathy).
- Treatment is by intravenous administration of penicillin or ceftriaxone. Prophylactic antibiotics (e.g. rifampicin or ciprofloxacin) can be given to contacts to eradicate carriage and control outbreaks.
- Of the 13 serogroups, groups A, B, C, W-135, X and Y cause more than 90% of cases. Vaccines are available against A, C, W-135 and Y, but not group B, which is most prevalent in the developed world.
- *N. gonorrhoeae* causes the sexually transmitted disease gonorrhoea. Asymptomatic carriage in women is common, but the organism may give rise to acute salpingitis, which may be followed by pelvic inflammatory disease and a high probability of sterility if inadequately treated.
- In the UK, cephalosporins such as ceftriaxone are the drugs of choice. Use of antibiotics is limited in some countries by a high prevalence of resistance.
- Early diagnosis, effective treatment and contact tracing are key to preventing the spread of disease. There is no effective vaccine to prevent gonorrhoea.
- *Moraxella catarrhalis* is an upper respiratory tract commensal that causes lower respiratory tract infections and otitis media.

The genus *Neisseria* contains two species of clinical significance: *N. meningitidis* (meningococcus) and *N. gonorrhoeae* (gonococcus). They are Gram-negative diplococci and obligate human pathogens, typically found inside polymorphonuclear pus cells of the inflammatory exudate. Although similar in terms of morphological and cultural characteristics, they are associated with entirely different diseases:

- *N. meningitidis* causes a range of diseases embraced by the term *invasive meningococcal disease*. Most common are purulent meningitis (variously called *epidemic cerebrospinal meningitis, cerebrospinal fever* or, because of the purpuric rash that is sometimes present, *spotted fever*) and an acute septicaemic illness with a petechial rash in the presence or absence of meningitis. About one-third of cases of meningococcal disease present as septicaemia; meningitis (with or without septicaemia) accounts for most others.
- *N. gonorrhoeae* causes the sexually transmitted disease *gonorrhoea*, which most commonly presents as a purulent infection of the mucous membrane of the urethra in men and the cervix uteri in women. In the newborn the gonococcus may give rise to a purulent conjunctivitis and in young girls a vulvovaginitis. Disseminated gonococcal infection, which is recognized by a rash and evidence of blood spread, may also occur, more commonly in women.

Other members of the *Neisseria* genus are common commensals of the upper respiratory tract (which is also the reservoir of the meningococcus and, occasionally, the gonococcus) and are of low pathogenicity in the immunocompetent host. Commensal species include *N. lactamica, N. cinerea, N. subflava* (of which there are several biovars), *N. sicca, N. polysaccharea, N. mucosa* and *N. flavescens*. Several other commensal species, including *N. elongata, N. weaveri* and *N. bacilliformis*, are unusual in being rod shaped.

Moraxellae are non-fermentative organisms that may be coccoid or rod shaped. There is still uncertainty as to their taxonomic position. Some strains resemble *Acinetobacter* spp. and other glucose non-fermenters (see p. 304). The most important member of the group, *Moraxella catarrhalis* (formerly known as *Branhamella catarrhalis*), is a common commensal of the upper respiratory tract and an opportunistic pathogen associated with otitis media in children and exacerbations of chronic obstructive pulmonary disease in adults.

## NEISSERIA

### Description

*N. meningitidis* and *N. gonorrhoeae* are morphologically and culturally very similar. They are Gram-negative, oval cocci occurring in pairs with the apposed surfaces flat or slightly concave (bean shaped), and with the axis of the pair parallel and not in line as in the pneumococcus. In pus from inflammatory exudates, such as the cerebrospinal fluid (CSF) or urethral discharge, many diplococci are found in a small proportion of the polymorphonuclear cells. This is more marked with the gonococcus than with the meningococcus. Extracellular cocci also occur and there may be considerable variation in their size and intensity of staining.

Non-pathogenic neisseriae grow on ordinary nutrient media, but meningococci and gonococci require the addition of heated blood (or ascitic fluid) and incubation at 35–37°C, in a moist atmosphere containing 5–10% carbon dioxide. Growth is rather slow (more so with the gonococcus) but, grey, glistening, slightly convex colonies of 0.5–1.0 mm in diameter appear in 8–24 h. After incubation for a further 24 h, the colonies are much larger and the gonococcus, in particular, tends to have a slightly roughened surface and a crenated margin.

Colonies of meningococci and gonococci react quickly in the test for cytochrome oxidase; non-pathogenic neisseriae react more slowly. Species identification depends on carbohydrate utilization reactions. *N. gonorrhoeae* produces acid from glucose, but not maltose, whilst *N. meningitidis* produces acid from both. Commercial kits that rapidly detect pre-formed enzymes, such as aminopeptidases and β-galactosidase, are commonly used for identification.

### Genome analysis

Genome sequence analysis shows that *N. meningitidis* and *N. gonorrhoeae* are very similar, although each species has several hundred unique genes, which may explain their differing interactions with the host. Importantly, these species have evolved highly efficient ways of varying their genes and antigens, thus undermining host defence mechanisms. Diversity is generated in a number of ways including natural transformation with DNA from other cells of the same or related species and by a range of recombination- and mutation-based systems, including phase variation (reversibly switching genes on and off) and antigenic variation of expressed antigens using information from silent genetic loci. Among the key antigenically variable antigens is the PilE protein, which is the predominant constituent of the pilus, a multi-functional appendage associated with attachment to mucosal surfaces (see p. 18). Antigenic variation follows genetic recombination of the PilE expression locus (*pilE*) with one or more silent *pil* loci.

## NEISSERIA MENINGITIDIS

### Classification

Meningococci are divisible into 13 serogroups, based on antigenic differences in their capsular polysaccharides, but only six of these have significant pathogenic potential. Over 90% of worldwide invasive disease is caused by strains from serogroups A, B, C, W-135, X and Y. The serogroup is usually determined by a slide agglutination test with absorbed group-specific antisera.

Meningococcal serotypes and serosubtypes are determined by specific monoclonal antibodies raised against the antigenically hypervariable outer membrane proteins (porins) PorB and PorA. Strain identities are designated by their serogroup (e.g. B), serotype (e.g. 15) and serosubtype (e.g. P1.16). As a result of genetic variations in the antigens used for typing, and incomplete coverage of typing reagents, non-typable strains are often isolated. In these cases, the corresponding porin genes can be sequenced and classified. Immunotyping, based on antigenic variation of lipo-oligosaccharides, is sometimes carried out.

Multilocus sequence typing and multilocus enzyme electrophoresis (see p. 37) are able to distinguish numerous genotypes of meningococci. Use of these methods has established that meningococcal populations are genetically highly diverse and that only a few hypervirulent lineages, designated clonal complexes, are associated with disease worldwide. For example, the sequence types ST-32 and ST-11 complexes (formerly electrophoretic types ET-5 and ET-37) dominated the serogroup B and C strains, respectively, which caused disease in the UK and the rest of Europe in the 1980s. These dominant complexes change over time, and an increase in the incidence of disease may coincide with the introduction of a new clonal complex to a particular community.

## Pathogenesis

The natural habitat of the meningococcus is the human nasopharynx, and transmission is largely via close (intimate, kissing) contact. Acquisition may be transient, lead to asymptomatic colonization (carriage) or result in invasive disease. The carrier:case ratio varies in different outbreaks and with the strain and population surveyed. Around 5–10% of general populations are normally carriers of meningococci. In communities experiencing outbreaks of invasive meningococcal disease the carriage rate of the epidemic strain may range from 20–50% or more.

The incidence of meningococcal disease increases when:

- meningococcal strains of high virulence are encountered
- factors that increase meningococcal transmission are present
- susceptible individuals who lack bactericidal antibodies to the current strains are present in the population.

Some studies show that a sharp increase in the carrier rate of pathogenic groups of meningococci precedes the occurrence of clinical cases. Bacterial, environmental and host factors are probably all equally important in the development of disease.

### Bacterial factors

Some meningococcal strains are more able than others to cause invasive disease, although the basis for this is still unclear. Surface structures subject to phase or antigenic variation, such as capsular polysaccharide, outer membrane proteins and lipo-oligosaccharide are major virulence components. Capsule protects the meningococcus from phagocytic killing, opsonization and complement-mediated bactericidal killing in the blood. Outer membrane and pilus proteins act as adhesins, facilitating attachment to host cells, while lipo-oligosaccharide is a key mediator of the pathogenesis of fulminant sepsis and meningitis.

### Environmental factors

Environmental risk factors for carriage and disease include overcrowding, respiratory viral infections, including influenza, and damage to the upper respiratory tract caused by very low humidity, dust or trauma. Meningococcal infections tend to peak during the winter months in countries with temperate climates, but in the dry season in countries in sub-Saharan Africa. Household contacts of a case are 500 to 800 times more likely to develop meningococcal infection than the general population.

### Host factors

For largely unknown reasons, some individuals are more susceptible to infection than others and some do worse than others. The absence of bactericidal antibody in the blood is believed to be the factor most closely related to susceptibility to clinical infection. The disappearance of antibody acquired from the mother increases the risk for infants and young children. Similarly, congenital and acquired antibody deficiencies also increase risk, as does asplenia. Group-specific (anti-capsular) antibody is protective and this is the basis of the success of vaccination against meningococcal disease. Antibodies to immunogenic and surface-exposed outer membrane proteins also protect, but the range of antigens involved, and the role of non-specific defence mechanisms in preventing clinical disease, are ill understood. The complement system is important, as shown by the recurrent attacks of meningococcal infections in those with defects in the pathway.

A genetic basis of susceptibility, severity and outcome of meningococcal disease is far from clear, but studies suggest that genetic polymorphisms in key regulators of complement activation, surfactant proteins and several other proteins may increase risk.

### Pathophysiology

During meningococcal septicaemia there are signs and symptoms of circulatory failure, multi-organ dysfunction and coagulopathy. There is increased vascular permeability and vasodilatation that result in capillary leak syndrome with peripheral oedema. Loss of intravascular fluid and plasma proteins results in hypovolaemia and reduced venous return, and hence reduced cardiac output, hypotension and reduced perfusion of vital organs. Systemic hypoxia, acidosis, and gross electrolyte and metabolic impairment eventually culminate in multi-organ dysfunction. At the molecular level, the underlying pathophysiology of meningococcal sepsis is complex and involves numerous interactive cascades, including cytokine, chemokine, host cell receptors, and coagulation and complement components.

Meningococcal lipo-oligosaccharide, or more specifically its lipid A moiety, is thought to be primarily responsible for septic shock, extensive tissue damage and multi-organ dysfunction by stimulating the release of inflammatory mediators including tumour necrosis factor-α and a series of interleukins, other cytokines and major intravascular cascade systems (see Ch. 9). Levels of circulating lipo-oligosaccharide exceeding 700 ng/L are associated with fulminant septic shock, disseminated intravascular coagulation and a high fatality rate.

### Clinical manifestations

Meningococci are able to cause a wide range of clinical syndromes varying in severity from a transient mild sore throat to meningitis or acute meningococcal septicaemia, which can cause death within hours of the appearance of symptoms.

Bacteraemia with or without sepsis, meningococcal septicaemia with or without meningitis, meningo-encephalitis, chronic meningococcaemia, pneumonia, septic arthritis, pericarditis, myocarditis, endocarditis, conjunctivitis, panophthalmitis, genitourinary tract infection, pelvic infection, peritonitis and proctitis are among the diseases caused by meningococci. Meningitis and/or septicaemia are by far the most common presentations of disease. It is important to remember that the clinical picture can progress from one end of the spectrum to the other during the course of disease.

A significant number of the patients who recover end up with permanent neurological sequelae, including intellectual impairment, cranial nerve deficits and deafness due to auditory nerve damage. The mortality rate from meningococcal disease varies between 5% and 70% depending on a number of factors including the severity of disease, the speed with which it develops, the organs involved, the age and immune status of the patient, the socio-economic status, the standard of health care, and the speed with which the disease is diagnosed and antibiotics administered.

### Laboratory diagnosis

In any suspected meningococcal infection, blood culture must be undertaken; if meningitis is suspected, a lumbar puncture should be performed as soon as possible, unless there are signs of raised intracranial pressure. Typically, the CSF will contain high numbers of white blood cells, high protein levels and reduced glucose levels. Microscopic examination of the stained centrifuged deposit should be performed without delay; the presence of Gram-negative diplococci will enable urgent antibiotic therapy to be started. The CSF is also cultured on heated blood (chocolate) agar and on blood agar. In the absence of visible meningococci, glucose broth may be added to the remaining sediment of the centrifuged deposit to facilitate the isolation of very sparse organisms. Cultures are incubated overnight at 37°C in an atmosphere of 5–10% carbon dioxide. As many patients receive penicillin before admission to hospital, lumbar puncture yields more positive cultures than blood.

A rapidly positive oxidase test on any Gram-negative diplococci that are grown is strong evidence that the isolates are pathogenic neisseria. Sugar utilization tests or commercial kits are used to further differentiate species. Direct slide agglutination with specific antisera may be carried out on suspensions of colonies picked from solid medium.

Growth of the meningococcus from a normally sterile site, such as CSF or blood, is definitive evidence of disease. Rapid PCR (polymerase chain reaction) tests are useful and may be positive when early antibiotic treatment has prevented successful culture. Meningococcal capsular polysaccharide may be detected in CSF by latex agglutination.

Where facilities exist, isolates should be sent to a reference laboratory for further procedures that provide important epidemiological information.

Meningococci may be found in genital sites, and it is important to identify these organisms accurately and differentiate them from gonococci.

### Treatment

Treatment should begin at the point of first contact as soon as meningococcal disease is suspected, even before the patient is transferred to hospital or investigated. Intravenous penicillin, cefotaxime or ceftriaxone are the drugs of choice. Although these agents do not cross uninflamed meninges well, they readily pass into CSF when inflammation is present. Chloramphenicol is effective, but risks of blood dyscrasia have limited its use.

In the absence of organisms in the Gram-stained CSF deposit, it is wise to give therapy with cefotaxime or ceftriaxone, which cover *Haemophilus influenzae* and *Streptococcus pneumoniae*, the other two principal causes of meningitis in childhood after the neonatal period.

Most clinical isolates of meningococci are presently sensitive to benzylpenicillin. However, meningococci of reduced susceptibility to penicillin have been reported and it is important that accurate sensitivity testing is carried out on all isolates from clinical disease. At the end of a course of therapy with penicillin eradicative treatment with rifampicin or ciprofloxacin should be given because penicillin does not eradicate meningococci from the nasopharynx and a patient returning home as a carrier may infect others. This probably does not apply to ceftriaxone or cefotaxime, which also eradicate throat carriage.

The mortality rate in septicaemic illness may range from 14% up to 50% in some outbreaks. The rate in meningitis is about 2–7%. Bad prognostic signs are:

- the presence of coma on admission to hospital
- a rapidly coalescing purpuric rash
- signs of shock.

Occasionally in the most fulminating forms of septicaemia there may not be time for the rash to develop before death. In such cases meningococci are isolated from the blood in life or post mortem, and hemorrhagic adrenals are seen at autopsy, these being characteristic of the *Waterhouse–Friderichsen syndrome*.

## Epidemiology

Over half of cases of invasive meningococcal disease occur in the first 5 years of life. The peak prevalence of disease is in the first year and there is a smaller peak in adolescence (Fig. 23.1) The increase in immunity observed with increasing age is likely to be due to asymptomatic carriage, often for many months, of virulent or avirulent meningococci or other neisseriae. The incidence is slightly higher in men than in women. Meningococcal infections occur worldwide and are notifiable in most countries. *N. meningitidis* is the only

bacterium capable of generating epidemic outbreaks of meningitis. These occur every 5–15 years in sub-Saharan Africa; endemic disease or localized outbreaks are seen in the rest of the world.

- Serogroup A disease (ST-5 or ST-7 complexes) is most prevalent in sub-Saharan Africa (the African meningitis belt) and the Middle East, where tens of thousands of cases are reported each year.
- Serogroup B strains are dominant among pathogenic meningococci in most industrialized countries and are a major cause of sporadic or endemic disease. Prolonged outbreaks in several countries have caused significant morbidity and mortality.
- Serogroup C strains (especially ST-11 complexes) have caused epidemics (e.g. China, Africa, Brazil) and more localized outbreaks in North America and Europe. Effective vaccination has reduced the incidence of serogroup C disease in many countries.
- Serogroup W-135 is present in small numbers worldwide, but has been associated with outbreaks following the pilgrimage to Mecca (the Hajj) and is a significant cause of disease in parts of the African meningitis belt.
- Serogroup Y (ST-23 and related sequence types) has caused increased rates of disease in the USA and South America, and serogroup X has been responsible for localized outbreaks in parts of the African meningitis belt.

## Control

### Chemoprophylaxis

All household and other intimate (e.g. mouth kissing) contacts of a case should be given chemoprophylaxis to eliminate carriage. Rifampicin is the preferred drug for children, although resistance can develop rapidly. Ciprofloxacin is used widely for adolescents and adults as a single oral dose. While chemoprophylaxis is effective in contacts and in limited outbreak settings, the development of antibiotic resistance, availability of drugs, and the large size of some outbreaks mean that the prevention of disease by vaccination is often the best control strategy.

### Vaccination

Resistance to meningococcal infection is closely associated with the possession of bactericidal antibodies that may be maternal in origin or actively produced in response to carriage. Vaccines containing the native, unconjugated, group-specific capsular

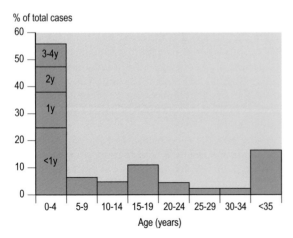

**Fig. 23.1** Age distribution of meningococcal infection (England and Wales, 2008 calendar year). (Data from the Health Protection Agency.)

polysaccharide of meningococci of groups A, C, Y and W-135 have been available since the 1970s and are good immunogens in children over 2 years. However, polysaccharide vaccines do not induce immunological memory and protection is limited to 3–5 years. Also, they have no effect on nasopharyngeal carriage and thus do not generate herd immunity.

Despite their limitations, meningococcal polysaccharide vaccines have been used extensively, most notably to help control epidemics of serogroup A disease in countries of the African meningitis belt. However, the development of protein-conjugated vaccines has changed the outlook for prevention. These vaccines are immunogenic in young children, induce immunological memory and decrease nasopharyngeal carriage. In the UK, introduction of a conjugate vaccine against serogroup C meningococci into the routine childhood immunization programme has led to significant reductions in serogroup C disease. This is partly the result of herd immunity effects, which protect unvaccinated individuals.

A low cost serogroup A specific conjugate vaccine has been introduced into some African countries. The effectiveness of this vaccine in preventing the epidemics of meningococcal disease that regularly sweep across the region is currently unclear.

Quadrivalent conjugate vaccines offering protection against serogroups A, C, W-135 and Y have also been developed but are not yet widely available.

Trials are in progress on several vaccines against group B meningococci, but it has been difficult to find a suitable immunogenic epitope. The group B capsular polysaccharide is a poor immunogen that does not induce a protective IgG response. Strategies have therefore focused on non-capsular antigens such as outer membrane proteins, vesicles and lipo-oligosaccharides. Diversity of major outer membrane structures in meningococci has limited these approaches, but genome sequence analysis to identify conserved, novel surface proteins for use in combination vaccines may allow for the future prevention of serogroup B meningococcal disease.

## NEISSERIA GONORRHOEAE

The name 'gonorrhoea' derives from the Greek words *gonos* (seed) and *rhoia* (flow), and described a condition in which semen flowed from the male organ without erection. It became apparent that gonorrhoea was associated with sexual promiscuity, one of the diseases celebrated by being named after the Roman goddess of love, Venus. Indeed, gonorrhoea is a classical venereal disease, being spread almost exclusively by sexual contact, having a short incubation period and being relatively easy to diagnose and treat. In the UK the highest infection rates are seen in men aged 20–24 years and women aged 16–19 years.

Gonococci are as antigenically heterogeneous as meningococci; many of the major cell surface antigens are shared between both species, with the exception of the capsule, which is not encoded by the gonococcus. Classically, strains are characterized by *auxotyping*, which recognizes requirements for specific nutrients, such as arginine, proline, hypoxanthine and uracil. Panels of monoclonal antibodies that recognize specific proteins are also used to divide strains into various serovars. Epidemiological typing makes use of both methods as well as newer molecular techniques, such as multi-antigen sequence typing.

## Pathogenesis

*N. gonorrhoeae* is exclusively a human pathogen, although chimpanzees have been infected artificially. It is never found as a normal commensal, but a proportion of those infected, particularly women, may remain asymptomatic. These individuals may develop systemic or ascending infection at a later stage.

Gonorrhoeal infection is generally limited to superficial mucosal surfaces lined with columnar epithelium. The areas most frequently involved are the cervix, urethra, rectum, pharynx and conjunctiva. Squamous epithelium, which lines the adult vagina, is not susceptible to infection by the gonococcus. However, the prepubertal vaginal epithelium, which has not been keratinized under the influence of oestrogen, may be infected. Hence, gonorrhoea in young girls may present as vulvovaginitis.

The most common clinical presentation is acute urethritis in the male a few days after unprotected vaginal or anal sexual intercourse. Dysuria and a purulent penile discharge make most sufferers seek treatment rapidly. A few men have relatively minor symptoms, which may disappear rapidly. Truly asymptomatic infection is rare in the active male. However, up to 5% may carry the organism without apparent distress, and this is more common with certain types of gonococci. Rectal and pharyngeal infection is less often symptomatic and may be discovered only after tracing contacts.

Endocervical infection is the most common form of uncomplicated gonorrhoea in women. Such infections are usually characterized by vaginal discharge and sometimes by dysuria. The cervical os may be erythematous and friable, with a purulent exudate. In women with vaginal infection, only half may have symptoms of discharge and dysuria. Most seek attention because of their partner's symptoms, or as part of contact tracing or screening of high-risk individuals. Local complications include abscesses in Bartholin's and Skene's glands. Rectal infections (proctitis) with *N. gonorrhoeae* occur in about one-third of women with cervical infection and are rarely symptomatic. In contrast, gonococcal proctitis in homosexual men is often symptomatic.

Asymptomatic carriage in women is common, especially in the endocervical canal. At menstruation or after instrumentation, particularly termination of pregnancy, gonococci ascend to the fallopian tubes to give rise to *acute salpingitis*, which may be followed by *pelvic inflammatory disease* and a high probability of sterility if treated inadequately. Peritoneal spread occurs occasionally and may produce a perihepatic inflammation (*Fitz-Hugh–Curtis syndrome*). Some lineages of *N. gonorrhoeae* spread more widely and give rise to disseminated gonococcal infection.

Disseminated infection is seen more commonly in women, who may present with painful joints, fever and a few septic skin lesions on their extremities (Fig. 23.2). The diagnosis of a venereal disease may not be obvious and isolation of gonococci from joint fluid, blood culture and skin aspirates requires particular

care. The organisms are invariably present in the cervix, but in many cases antibiotics have been given before the diagnosis is considered. Rarely, disseminated gonococcal infection may present as endocarditis or meningitis.

Babies born to infected women may suffer *ophthalmia neonatorum*, in which the eyes are coated with gonococci as the baby passes down the birth canal. A severe purulent eye discharge with peri-orbital oedema occurs within a few days of birth. If untreated, ophthalmia leads rapidly to blindness. It may be prevented in areas of high prevalence by the instillation of 1% aqueous silver nitrate in the eyes of newborn babies. Alternatively, topical erythromycin can be used; this has the advantage of being active against chlamydia and is less toxic than silver nitrate.

Vulvovaginitis in prepubertal girls occurs either in conditions of poor hygiene or by sexual abuse; it should always be investigated carefully and the child put in touch with social services and other professionals capable of dealing with this difficult condition.

## Laboratory diagnosis

Cultivation of *N. gonorrhoeae* from sites with few commensals, such as the male urethra, rarely presents any problems, and Gram staining of a smear is usually 95% sensitive. *N. gonorrhoeae* is intolerant of drying and temperature changes; it readily undergoes autolysis. It is a fastidious microbe, requiring humidity, 5–7% carbon dioxide and complex media for growth. Ideally, exudate is taken directly from the patient on to appropriate preheated, freshly prepared solid media and immediately placed in a carbon dioxide incubator. This is usually possible only in specialized clinics with sufficient patient numbers to justify the expense. Where there is likely to be any delay, transport media must be used to carry the material on swabs.

The combination of oxidase-positive colonies and Gram-negative diplococci provides a presumptive diagnosis. The use of gonococcal specific antibodies and carbohydrate utilization tests, with or without the detection of preformed enzymes, will give full speciation of the organism. DNA probes have also been used to detect gonococci in urethral and cervical specimens. PCR-based methods are available in some specialized laboratories.

**Fig. 23.2** Skin lesions in disseminated gonococcal infection.

## Treatment

The susceptibility of isolates of *N. gonorrhoeae* to commonly used antibiotics varies so much that regular testing is essential.

**Table 23.1** Resistance to antimicrobial agents among isolates of *N. gonorrhoeae* in the UK

| Antimicrobial agent | Percentage resistant | |
|---|---|---|
| | 2006 | 2007 |
| Penicillin | 9.5 | 24 |
| Ciprofloxacin | 27 | 28 |
| Cefixime or ceftriaxone | 0 | 0.2 |
| Azithromycin | 1.8 | 4.1 |
| Tetracycline | 37 | 60 |
| Spectinomycin | 0 | 0 |

Data from the Health Protection Agency 2007.

Penicillin, especially in slow-release intramuscular forms such as procaine penicillin, remains the preferred therapy in many parts of the world. Small decreases in susceptibility can be overcome by increasing the size of the single dose. However, by the 1970s the dose of penicillin required to cure simple acute gonorrhoea in men in some parts of the world had reached an impossibly large injection.

Strains of *N. gonorrhoeae* that are completely resistant to penicillins are now common throughout the world, although the prevalence varies from country to country. These strains possess the gene coding for the TEM-type β-lactamase commonly found in *Escherichia coli*.

Ceftriaxone or cefixime are recommended as first-line therapy in the UK, but these drugs are expensive and may not be affordable in developing countries. Alternatives to cephalosporins and penicillin include fluoroquinolones (e.g. ciprofloxacin), azithromycin, tetracyclines, co-amoxiclav and spectinomycin. Use of these antibiotics is often limited in places where inappropriate use has led to a high prevalence of resistance. Resistance, or reduced susceptibility, to most of the commonly used antibiotics is increasing in the UK (Table 23.1).

Single-dose therapy appears adequate for uncomplicated cases of acute genital gonorrhoea in men and women. There are obvious advantages to this approach in obtaining complete compliance and stopping the chain of infection. In disseminated gonococcal disease and any complicated infection, treatment for 7–10 days is necessary.

## Epidemiology and control

Acute gonorrhoea is usually easily diagnosed and treated, and was well controlled in much of the world until the 1960s. The remarkable changes in travel, migration, sexual licence and availability of oral contraceptives rapidly reversed this process so that there was an increase in gonorrhoea and non-specific genital infection (caused mainly by chlamydiae; see Chapter 39) every year until scares about the acquired immune deficiency syndrome in the 1980s temporarily halted the rise. Barrier methods of contraception, condoms in particular, greatly reduce the rate of transmission.

The keys to control of gonorrhoea are:

• rapid diagnosis
• use of effective antibiotics
• tracing, examination and treatment of contacts.

Unfortunately, in many places, inappropriate self-medication has contributed to widespread antimicrobial resistance. Inability to treat contacts ensures the spread of the disease and re-infections.

There is no effective vaccine to prevent gonorrhoea. The organism is non-capsulate and its immunogenic outer membrane proteins are antigenically variable. These, and lack of suitable animal models, have hampered vaccine development.

## MORAXELLA

Moraxellae are Gram-negative, asaccharolytic, oxidase-positive, catalase-positive short rods, coccobacilli or, in the case of *M. catarrhalis*, diplococci. They are commensals of mucosal surfaces and occasionally give rise to opportunistic infections. *M. lacunata* is occasionally encountered as a cause of 'angular' blepharoconjunctivitis.

The related genus *Kingella* contains organisms that differ from the moraxellae in being catalase-negative, glucose-fermenting coccobacilli. In common with some other Gram-negative rods, such as *Cardiobacterium hominis* and *Eikenella corrodens*, *Kingella* species (usually *K. kingae*) are sometimes found in endocarditis. They have also been implicated in joint infections.

### MORAXELLA CATARRHALIS

#### Pathogenesis

*M. catarrhalis* is a respiratory tract commensal and, as with other members of the upper respiratory tract flora such as the pneumococcus and *H. influenzae*, it can gain access to the lower respiratory tract in patients with chronic chest disease or compromised host defences. *M. catarrhalis* is commonly isolated from sputum, and a pathogenic role is suspected only when the sputum contains large numbers of pus cells and Gram-negative diplococci, and when culture yields a heavy growth of *M. catarrhalis* in the absence of other recognized respiratory pathogens. As well as causing chest infection itself, *M. catarrhalis* may also protect other respiratory pathogens from the action of penicillin or ampicillin by producing β-lactamase.

*M. catarrhalis* is also a cause of otitis media and sinusitis in children. In acute otitis media the organism is present in 15–20% of cultures of middle ear fluid presumably migrating from the nasopharynx to the middle ear via the Eustachian tube.

## Laboratory diagnosis

Sputum is examined by Gram film. In true infections, large numbers of Gram-negative diplococci may be seen dispersed between the pus cells. Sputum is cultured on media suitable for the isolation of other potential respiratory pathogens (e.g. blood agar and chocolate agar) and incubated in 5% carbon dioxide overnight. In situations in which it is held to be pathogenic, *M. catarrhalis* is predominant in culture.

*M. catarrhalis* produces rough, circular, convex colonies that can be lifted off intact with a wire loop from agar culture medium. Colonies are oxidase positive. In common with other moraxellae, they do not ferment sugars and are easily differentiated from neisseriae by the tributyrin test. Growth on nutrient agar at 22°C has been suggested as a differential characteristic, but clinically significant isolates of *M. catarrhalis* may not grow in these conditions. Tests for deoxyribonuclease and for butyrate esterase are positive. Around 90% of strains are β-lactamase positive.

## Treatment

*M. catarrhalis* is sensitive to amoxicillin, combined with clavulanic acid (co-amoxiclav) in the case of β-lactamase-producing strains, and also to cephalosporins, tetracyclines, macrolides and fluoroquinolones. No vaccine is currently available, although several are in development.

### RECOMMENDED READING

Ala'Aldeen DAA, Turner DPJ: Neisseria meningitidis. In Gillespie S, Hawkey P, editors: *Principles and Practice of Clinical Bacteriology*, ed 2, Chichester, 2006, John Wiley.

Barker RM, Shakespeare RM, Mortimore AJ, et al: Practical guidelines for responding to an outbreak of meningococcal disease among university students based on experience in Southampton, *Communicable Disease and Public Health* 2:168–173, 1999.

Bignell C: European (IUSTI/WHO) guideline on the diagnosis and treatment of gonorrhoea in adults, *International Journal of STD and AIDS* 20:453–457, 2009.

Hart CA, Thomson APJ: Meningococcal disease and its management in children, *British Medical Journal* 333:685–690, 2006.

Health Protection Agency: *The gonococcal resistance to antimicrobials surveillance programme 2008 report: Trends in antimicrobial resistant gonorrhoea*, London, 2009, Health Protection Agency.

Heath Protection Agency Meningococcus Forum: *Guidance for public health management of meningococcal disease in the UK*, London, 2006, *Health* Protection Agency.

Khatami A, Pollard AJ: The epidemiology of meningococcal disease and the impact of vaccines, *Expert Review of Vaccines* 9:285–298, 2010.

Murphy TF, Parameswaran GI: *Moraxella catarrhalis*, a human respiratory tract pathogen, *Clinical Infectious Diseases* 49:124–131, 2009.

Stephens DS, Greenwood B, Brandtzaeg P: Epidemic meningitis, meningococcaemia, and *Neisseria meningitides*, Lancet 369: 2196–2210, 2007.

### Website

Health Protection Agency: Guidelines and Advice – Meningococcal. http://www.hpa.org.uk/infections/topics_az/meningo/guidelines.htm

# 24 Salmonella

Food poisoning; enteric fever

*H. Chart*

## KEY POINTS

- There are more than 2000 different antigenic types of *Salmonella*; those pathogenic to man are serotypes of *S. enterica*.
- Most serotypes of *S. enterica* cause food-borne gastroenteritis and have animal reservoirs.
- *S. enterica* serotypes Typhi and Paratyphi cause typhoid fever.
- Typhoid and other serious systemic salmonella infections are treated with amoxicillin, co-trimoxazole, ciprofloxacin or chloramphenicol.
- Antibiotics have no place in the management of salmonella gastroenteritis unless invasive complications are suspected.
- Clean water, sanitation and hygienic handling of foodstuffs are the keys to prevention.

There are well over 2000 different antigenic types of salmonella. They were originally classified as separate species, but it is now generally accepted that they represent serotypes (serovars) of a single species, *Salmonella enterica*. Various subspecies are recognized, but most of the serotypes that infect mammals are found in a subspecies also designated *enterica*. For example, the full designation of the serotype formerly called *Salmonella enteritidis* is: *Salmonella enterica* subspecies *enterica* serotype Enteritidis. This cumbersome nomenclature is often abbreviated to *Salmonella* Enteritidis (*S.* Enteritidis) and this convention will be followed here in considering those salmonellae responsible for human infections.

Certain serotypes are a major cause of food-borne infection worldwide. Most infections are relatively benign and restricted to the intestinal tract, causing a short-lived diarrhoea, but some *S. enterica* serotypes, notably Typhi and Paratyphi, cause life-threatening systemic disease.

## DESCRIPTION

Salmonellae are typical members of the Enterobacteriaceae: facultatively anaerobic Gram-negative bacilli able to grow on a wide range of relatively simple media and distinguished from other members of the family by their biochemical characteristics and antigenic structure. Their normal habitat is the animal intestine.

### Antigens

Typical strains of *S. enterica* express two sets of antigens, which are readily demonstrable by serotyping. Long-chain lipopolysaccharide (LPS) comprises heat-stable polysaccharide commonly known as the *somatic* or '*O*' antigens. These molecules are located in the outer membrane and are anchored into the cell wall by antigenically conserved lipid A and LPS-core regions. The long-chain LPS molecules exhibit considerable variation in sugar composition and degree of polysaccharide branching, and this structural heterogeneity is responsible for the large number of serotypes. Salmonellae are usually highly motile when growing in laboratory media, and flagellar protein subunits contain the epitopes that form the basis of the flagella-based serotyping scheme generally known as the '*H*' antigens (Fig. 24.1). In most strains of *S. enterica* the flagella exhibit the property of diphasic variation, whereby one of two genetically distinct flagellar structures are expressed. When one flagellar structure is expressed it contains *phase 1* antigens, whereas when the other set is operative *phase 2* antigens are synthesized.

Certain serotypes of *S. enterica* express a surface polysaccharide, of which the Vi (virulence) antigen of *S.* Typhi is the most important example. As the polysaccharide may encapsulate the entire bacterium, antibodies designed to recognize the LPS antigens

**Fig. 24.1** Electron micrograph of *S.* Typhi. Arrow indicates the flagella that carry the 'H' antigens. Bar = 500 nm.

**Table 24.1** Antigenic structure of some representative salmonellae

| Serotype | 'O' antigens | 'H' antigens | |
|---|---|---|---|
| | | Phase 1 | Phase 2 |
| Typhi | 9, 12, [Vi] | d | – |
| Paratyphi B | 1, 4, 5, 12 | b | 1, 2 |
| Typhimurium | 1, 4, 5, 12 | i | 1, 2 |
| Enteritidis | 1, 9, 12 | g, m | 1, 7 |
| Virchow | 6, 7 | r | 1, 2 |
| Kedougou | 1, 13, 23 | i | 1, w |
| Hadar | 6, 8 | Z10 | e, n, x |
| Heidelberg | 1, 4, 5, 12 | r | 1, 2 |
| Infantis | 6, 7, 14 | r | 1, 5 |
| Newport | 6, 8, 20 | e, h | 1, 2 |
| Panama | 1, 9, 12 | l, v | 1, 5 |
| Dublin | 1, 9, 12 | g, p | – |

may be prevented from binding; this can occasionally make detection of the O antigens difficult.

The various O-antigens of salmonellae are numbered with Arabic numerals. The flagellar antigens of phase 1 are designated by lower-case letters, and those of phase 2 by a mixture of lower-case letters and Arabic numerals. The antigenic structure of any serotype of salmonella is thus expressed as an antigenic formula, which has three parts, describing the O antigens, the phase 1 H antigens and the phase 2 H antigens, in that order. The three parts are separated by colons, and the component antigens in each part by commas; for example, the distinctive antigenic formula of *S.* Enteritidis is 1, 9, 12: g, m: 1, 7.

The original Kauffmann–White scheme, which elegantly catalogued salmonellae (but named them as individual species), placed them into some 30 groups on the basis of shared O antigens, and further subdivided the groups into clusters with H antigens in common. Some salmonellae, such as *S.* Typhi (9, 12, [Vi]: d), express only one flagellar phase. Some of the commoner serotypes are shown in Table 24.1.

## Typing methods

Phage typing schemes have proved extremely useful for discriminating within strains of *S. enterica* serotypes Typhimurium, Virchow, Enteritidis and Typhi. The numbers of phages comprising the various schemes are constantly being increased to improve strain discrimination.

Characterization of strains of *S. enterica* is also assisted by determining their distinctive patterns of resistance to a range of antibiotics. For example, certain strains of *S.* Typhimurium definitive type (DT) 104 are characterized by resistance to ampicillin, chloramphenicol, aminoglycosides and co-trimoxazole.

Pulsed-field gel electrophoresis analysis, of the entire *Salmonella* genome following digestion with selected enzymes, has facilitated strain discrimination in outbreak situations.

## Host range and pathogenicity

Strains of *S. enterica* are widely distributed in nature. All vertebrates appear capable of harbouring these bacteria in their gut, and certain serotypes have also been isolated from a wide range of arthropods, including flies and cockroaches. Most animal infections seem to range from those without symptoms to those resulting in self-limiting gastroenteritis of variable severity. Some strains, such as those belonging to serotype Typhimurium, show a wide host range and can be isolated from many different animal species. A small number of strains, the *host-adapted* serotypes, are much more restricted in the species they inhabit, and show a different spectrum of illness.

Among the host-adapted serotypes, Typhi and Paratyphi A and C are rarely, if ever, isolated from animals other than man. Paratyphi B, although essentially a human pathogen, is occasionally isolated from cattle, pigs, poultry, exotic reptiles and other animals, although cycles of transmission in these hosts have not been demonstrated. Human infection with these organisms is characterized by a long incubation period of 10–14 days, followed by a septicaemic illness, *enteric fever*, quite unlike the diarrhoea and vomiting that are characteristic of food poisoning.

Other salmonellae adapted to particular animal hosts include Cholerae-suis (pigs), Dublin (cattle), Gallinarum-pullorum (poultry), Abortus-equi (horses) and Abortus-ovis (sheep). These are all responsible for considerable morbidity, mortality and economic loss among domestic animals. All can cause human illness, but only strains of Cholerae-suis and Dublin do so regularly. Strains of *S.* Typhimurium DT 104 isolated from human infection appear to have originated from bovine sources; but whether these strains can be considered as host-adapted to farm animals remains to be established. The rest of the 2000 or so serotypes of salmonellae show no apparent host preference. The extent to which they cause human infection appears to result from their prevalence in domestic food animals at any particular time and on the opportunity for contamination of food in which further multiplication can take place. In developed countries most human infections are caused by a relatively small number of locally prevalent serotypes.

## PATHOGENESIS

In common with many pathogenic enteric bacteria, strains of *S. enterica* require a range of pathogenic mechanisms to enable them to survive passage through the digestive tract, colonize a host and cause disease. The lack of a good animal model of *Salmonella* pathogenicity has impeded research into how these bacteria cause disease; however, it is anticipated that the availability of gene sequences will allow the mechanisms to be understood more fully. In general terms, infection is initiated by the ingestion of a sufficient number of organisms to survive the stomach acid barrier and the effects of digestive bile prior to colonization of the gut mucosa, and to express the mechanisms resulting in overt disease.

### Infective dose

For human infections, the number of bacteria that must be swallowed in order to cause infection is uncertain and varies with the serotype. The accepted dictum that large inocula of these bacteria are required for induction of human illness is based largely on volunteer studies. In most of these the median infective dose for most serotypes, including Typhi, has varied from $10^6$ to $10^9$ viable organisms. However, investigation of outbreaks suggests that in natural infection the infective dose might be fewer than 1000 viable organisms.

Many factors are thought to influence the infective dose. There appears to be considerable strain-to-strain variation in virulence even within a single serotype. Systematic variation in pathogenicity between serotypes is less easy to demonstrate outside the host-adapted strains. The vehicle of ingestion may also influence pathogenesis. Organisms ingested in water and other drinks may be carried through the stomach relatively rapidly, and evade the effect of gastric acid. Similarly, the administration of antacids, or the effects of gastric resection, reduces the infective dose. Bacteria within particles of food would also evade the action of stomach acids.

### Host factors

Host factors are also likely to be important, particularly the nutritional and immune status of the host. Host variables can, however, be confusing; for example, age-specific isolation rates for salmonellae, as for some other gut pathogens, are higher for children less than 1 year of age than for any other age group, but this reflects the fact that a higher proportion of infections are investigated in this age group.

### Initiation of infection

Once salmonellae enter the lumen of the intestine they need to be able to tolerate the action of digestive bile and compete with the prevailing gut flora for adhesion sites on the gut mucosa. Certain serotypes, such as *S.* Typhimurium, express type-1 fimbriae, which enable them to adhere to α-mannose-containing molecules on the microvilli of the ileal mucosa; however, surprisingly little is known about the range of fimbriae expressed. Strains of *S.* Enteritidis are thought to express at least three different fimbrial structures (Fig. 24.2).

*Salmonella* serotypes such as Typhimurium and Enteritidis also express an adhesion mechanism that does not involve fimbriae. Certain strains of enteric

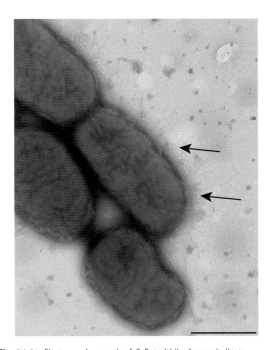

**Fig. 24.2** Electron micrograph of *S.* Enteritidis. Arrows indicate fimbriae. Bar = 0.5 μm. (From Zuckerman AJ 2004 *Principles and practice of clinical virology*, 5th edn. John Wiley & Sons Ltd, Chichester.)

bacteria carry deoxyribonucleic acid (DNA) sequences that encode several pathogenic mechanisms, termed *pathogenicity islands*. In common with strains of Verocytotoxin-producing *Escherichia coli* belonging to serogroup O157 (see Ch. 26), strains of *S.* Typhimurium and *S.* Enteritidis have pathogenicity islands that encode an adhesion mechanism comprising both a bacterial adhesin and the adhesin receptor, which is translocated into the host intestine. This process enables these bacteria to insert their own binding site into the gut, unlike fimbriae, which require host-derived binding sites located in the intestinal wall.

Attachment to the host mucosa is followed by degeneration of the microvilli to form breaches in the cell membrane through which the salmonellae enter the intestinal epithelial cells. For certain strains, further multiplication in these cells and in macrophages of the Peyer's patches follows. Some bacteria penetrate into the submucosa and pass to the local mesenteric lymph nodes. All of the clinical manifestations of infection with salmonella, including diarrhoea, begin after ileal penetration where inflammation of the ileal mucosa results in the efflux of water and electrolytes resulting in diarrhoea. For strains of *S.* Typhi, infection involves invasion of the bloodstream and various organs.

## CLINICAL SYNDROMES

Although salmonellae can cause a wide spectrum of clinical illness there are four major syndromes, each with its own diagnostic and therapeutic problems:

- enteric fever
- gastroenteritis
- bacteraemia with or without metastatic infection
- the asymptomatic carrier state.

Although uncommon, infection with *Salmonella* can result in sequelae, including reactive arthritis (*Reiter's syndrome*).

### Enteric fever

Enteric fever is caused by strains of *S.* Typhi or *S.* Paratyphi A, B or C; although *S.* Paratyphi B, which gene sequence analysis suggests is a variant of *S.* Java, is more likely to cause non-typhoidal diarrhoea. The clinical features tend to be more severe with *S.* Typhi (*typhoid fever*). After penetration of the ileal mucosa the organisms pass via the lymphatics to the mesenteric lymph nodes, whence after a period of multiplication they invade the bloodstream via the thoracic duct. The liver, gall bladder, spleen, kidney and bone

marrow become infected during this primary bacteraemic phase in the first 7–10 days of the incubation period. After multiplication in these organs, bacilli pass into the blood, causing a second and heavier bacteraemia, the onset of which approximately coincides with that of fever and other signs of clinical illness. From the gall bladder, a further invasion of the intestine results. Peyer's patches and other gut lymphoid tissues become involved in an inflammatory reaction, and infiltration with mononuclear cells, followed by necrosis, sloughing and the formation of characteristic typhoid ulcers occurs.

### Onset

The interval between ingestion of the organisms and the onset of illness varies with the size of the infecting dose. It can be as short as 3 days or as long as 50 days, but is usually about 2 weeks. The onset is usually insidious. Early symptoms are often vague: a dry cough and epistaxis associated with anorexia, a dull continuous headache, abdominal tenderness and discomfort are among the most common symptoms. Diarrhoea is uncommon and early in the illness many patients complain of constipation.

### Progression

In the untreated case the temperature shows a stepladder rise over the first week of the illness, remains high for 7–10 days and then falls during the third or fourth week. Physical signs include a relative bradycardia at the height of the fever, hepatomegaly, splenomegaly and often a rash of *rose spots*. These are slightly raised, discrete, irregular, blanching, pink macules, 2–4 mm in diameter, most often found on the front of the chest. They appear in crops of up to a dozen at a time and fade after 3–4 days, leaving no scar. They are characteristic of, but not specific for, enteric fever.

### Relapse

Apparent recovery can be followed by relapse in 5–10% of untreated cases. Relapse is usually shorter and of milder character than the initial illness, but can be severe and may be fatal. Severe intestinal haemorrhage and intestinal perforation are serious complications that can occur at any stage of the illness.

### Morbidity and mortality

Classical typhoid fever is a serious infection that, when untreated, has a mortality rate approaching 20%. It is notoriously unpredictable in its presentation and course. Mild and asymptomatic infections are not uncommon. In endemic areas, and particularly where it co-exists with schistosomiasis, chronic infection can present with fever of many months' duration, accompanied by chronic bacteraemia. Occasionally, diarrhoea may dominate the picture from the outset, particularly in paratyphoid infections, which sometimes present as typical gastroenteritis no different from that caused by most *S. enterica* serotypes.

## Gastroenteritis and food poisoning

Acute gastroenteritis is characterized by vomiting, abdominal pain, fever and diarrhoea. It can be caused by ingestion of a wide variety of bacteria or their products, several viruses, and a number of vegetable toxins and inorganic chemicals. The term *bacterial food poisoning* is conveniently restricted to cases and epidemics of acute gastroenteritis that are caused by the ingestion of food contaminated by bacteria or their toxins. In bacterial food poisoning, the bacteria need the opportunity to multiply in the food to reach an infective concentration before being eaten. Infections such as hepatitis A or bacillary dysentery, in which food may be an incidental vector, are not usually considered to be examples of food poisoning. Strains of *S. enterica* commonly cause food poisoning worldwide.

### Clinical features

The most common clinical manifestation of infection with non-invasive salmonella serotypes is diarrhoea, often accompanied by headache, malaise and nausea. The incubation period is usually 8–48 h, the onset abrupt, and the clinical course short and self-limiting. Symptoms vary from the passage of two or three loose stools, which may be disregarded by the sufferer, to a severe and prostrating illness with the frequent passage of watery, green, offensive stools, fever, shivering, abdominal pain and, in the most severe cases, dehydration leading to hypotension, cramps and renal failure. Vomiting is rarely a prominent feature of the illness.

Severe infections occur most often in the very young and the elderly, although mild subclinical infections also occur in these age groups. Infections with certain serotypes in those already ill or debilitated from other causes are likely to be more severe and life-threatening. In most cases the acute stage is over within 2–3 days, although it may be more prolonged. Persistent or high fever suggests bacteraemia, possibly with metastatic infection.

## Bacteraemia and metastatic disease

Bacteraemia is a constant feature of enteric fever caused by strains of *S.* Typhi and Paratyphi A and C. Rarely, complications of infection with other salmonellae can occur. Transient bacteraemia occurs in up to 4% of cases of acute gastroenteritis, but in most cases the organisms are cleared from the bloodstream without ill effect.

Occasionally, dissemination of the bacilli throughout the body results in the establishment of one or more localized foci of persisting infection, especially where pre-existing abnormality makes a tissue or organ vulnerable. Atherosclerotic plaques within large arteries, damaged heart valves, joint prostheses and other implants are all susceptible to metastatic infection.

Osteomyelitis is most often found in long bones, costochondral junctions and the spine. Multiple bony sites may be affected, and sickle cell anaemia is an important predisposing factor. Suppurative arthritis can occur either as an extension of contiguous osteomyelitis or as a primary infection.

Meningitis is a particularly serious complication of infection in neonates and very young children. Abscess formation can occur in almost any organ or tissue. Even in the absence of obvious tissue damage, the ability of salmonellae to enter and survive within macrophages and other cells, particularly in the liver and biliary tree, but also in bone marrow and the kidney, leads occasionally to persistent infection and the chronic carrier state.

## The prolonged carrier state

Most people infected with salmonella continue to excrete the organism in their stools for days or weeks after complete clinical recovery, but eventual clearance of the bacteria from the body is usual. A few patients continue to excrete the salmonellae for prolonged periods. The term *chronic carrier* is reserved for those who excrete salmonellae for a year or more. Chronic carriage can follow symptomatic illness or may be the only manifestation of infection. It can occur with any serotype, but is a particularly important feature of enteric fever: up to 5% of convalescents from typhoid and a smaller number of those who have recovered from paratyphoid fever become chronic carriers, many for a lifetime. The bacilli are most commonly present in the gall bladder, less often in the urinary tract, and are shed in faeces and sometimes in urine. The long duration of the carrier state enables the enteric fever bacilli to survive in the community in non-epidemic times and to persist in small and relatively isolated communities.

Age and sex are important determinants of the frequency of carriage, at least of *S.* Typhi. After enteric fever, fewer than 1% of patients under 20 years old become carriers, but this proportion rises to more than 10% in patients over 50 years of age. At all ages women become carriers twice as often as men.

The duration of excretion following infection with other salmonellae is less well documented, but more than 50% of patients stop excreting the organisms within 5 weeks of infection, and 90% of adults are culture negative at 9 weeks. The duration of excretion is significantly greater in children aged under 5 years, but virtually all permanent carriers are adults.

## LABORATORY DIAGNOSIS

Selective media, such as desoxycholate–citrate agar or xylose–lysine desoxycholate agar, are used for the isolation of salmonella bacteria from faeces. Fluid enrichment media, such as tetrathionate or selenite broth, are also useful to detect small numbers of salmonellae in faeces, foods or environmental samples. Suspicious colonies from the culture plates are tested directly for the presence of *Salmonella* somatic (O) antigens by slide agglutination and subcultured to peptone water for the determination of flagellar (H) antigen structure and further biochemical analysis. A presumptive diagnosis of salmonellosis can often be made within 24 h of the receipt of a specimen, although confirmation may take another day, and formal identification of the serotype takes several more days. A negative report must await the result of enrichment cultures – at least 48 h.

Several commercial PCR assays are available. In common with all PCR assays involving clinical, environmental and food samples, the numbers of bacteria and amounts of DNA can be below the levels required for successful amplification.

### Enteric fever

#### Blood culture

Bone-marrow culture is the most reliable method for the diagnosis of enteric fever. The organisms may also be recovered from the bloodstream at any stage of the illness, but are most commonly found during the first 7–10 days and during relapses. The organisms can also be recovered from the blood clot from a sample taken for serological tests. The clot is digested with streptokinase or minced, and incubated in broth.

#### Stool and urine culture

Specimens of faeces and urine should be submitted for examination, although the isolation of salmonella from these specimens may indicate merely that the patient is a carrier. In typhoid fever, patients' stools may contain salmonella from the second week and urine cultures from the third week of the infection. In paratyphoid B infections the clinical course may be much shorter than in typhoid; diarrhoea may occur early and stool cultures are often positive in the first week of the illness.

### Serological tests

Infections with both invasive and non-invasive serotypes may induce specific serum antibodies to *Salmonella* surface antigens, although serological tests have been applied extensively only in the routine diagnosis of infection with *S.* Typhi and *S.* Paratyphi A, B and C. The Widal agglutination test, formerly used for the detection of specific O, H and Vi antigens, has been largely replaced by sensitive and specific methods such as enzyme-linked immunosorbent assay (ELISA) and immunoblotting. In interpreting the results of serology, account must be taken of antibodies acquired by previous infection or vaccination.

Cross-reacting antibodies from previous exposure to other salmonellae may confuse the results of serodiagnosis. For example, the O antigens of *S.* Typhi are expressed by other serotypes such as Enteritidis (see Table 24.1). Antibodies specific for group 'd' flagellar antigens can be used to differentiate infections caused by *S.* Typhi from other serotypes that share O antigens.

Use of serology in the search for typhoid carriers, for example in the routine examination of food handlers and waterworks employees, is of doubtful value.

### Food poisoning

The laboratory diagnosis of bacterial food poisoning depends on isolation of the causal organism from samples of faeces or suspected foodstuffs. The more common food-poisoning serotypes, such as Enteritidis or Typhimurium, may be characterized more fully by phage typing and antibiotic resistance typing (see above). Strains can be differentiated further by plasmid and pulsed-field gel electrophoresis typing so that the isolates from patients may be matched with those from the infected food and from a suspected animal source.

## TREATMENT

### Enteric fever

The introduction of chloramphenicol in 1948 transformed a life-threatening illness of several weeks' duration associated with a mortality rate of more than 20% into a short-lasting febrile illness with a mortality rate of less than 2%. Many patients can be treated adequately with oral chloramphenicol from the outset. Initial intravenous therapy with the drug may be necessary for the more severely ill patient, who may have anorexia, abdominal distension and, perhaps, vomiting. The intramuscular route gives inadequate blood levels. Treatment should be maintained for 14 days because relapse is more frequent with a shorter course.

The problem of bone marrow toxicity and the emergence of plasmid-mediated chloramphenicol resistance in many parts of the world prompted the search for alternative agents. Amoxicillin and co-trimoxazole are as effective as chloramphenicol, and are used widely. However, simultaneous resistance to these drugs has become increasingly common in strains of *S.* Typhi in several endemic areas, and imported multiresistant typhoid is being encountered worldwide. Fluoroquinolones such as ciprofloxacin and cephalosporins such as ceftriaxone and cefixime have emerged as the drugs of choice for the treatment of typhoid.

### Gastroenteritis

Management of salmonella gastroenteritis includes replacement of fluids and electrolytes, and control of nausea, vomiting and pain. Drugs to control the hypermotility of the gut are contra-indicated; they may give symptomatic relief for a while, but it is easy to transform a trivial gastroenteritis into a life-threatening bacteraemia by paralysing the bowel.

Antibiotics have no part to play in the management in most cases. Randomized, placebo-controlled, double-blind studies have failed to show any benefit from any antibiotic on the duration and severity of the diarrhoea or the duration of fever; some antibiotics seemed to prolong the carrier state. If a patient is clearly at increased risk of bacteraemia and generalized invasion, an antibiotic may protect against this serious complication. Such patients include infants under 3 months of age, patients with a malignancy, haemoglobinopathy or chronic gastrointestinal disease such as ulcerative colitis (especially when treated with steroids), and patients who are immunosuppressed for other reasons. Treatment with an

appropriate agent (see above) should continue until the gastroenteritis has resolved completely.

### Salmonella bacteraemia

Established salmonella bacteraemia requires aggressive antimicrobial treatment with ciprofloxacin, chloramphenicol, co-trimoxazole or high-dose ampicillin. Uncomplicated bacteraemia should be treated for 10–14 days. A careful search for focal metastatic disease should be undertaken, especially when relapse follows cessation of treatment. Surgical drainage of metastatic abscesses may be required, with surgical intervention if heart valves or large vessels are affected.

In salmonella meningitis in infancy, treatment with chloramphenicol or ampicillin may be unsuccessful in up to a third of cases caused by sensitive strains. As cefotaxime and ceftriaxone penetrate into the cerebrospinal fluid reasonably well and are highly active against most salmonellae, they offer an effective alternative.

Resistance to any of the drugs used to treat invasive infection may occur, so treatment should be supported by susceptibility testing whenever possible.

### Chronic asymptomatic carriers

The chronic carrier state presents a particularly difficult therapeutic challenge. The principal site of carriage is the biliary tract, and the presence of gall stones can influence the carriage of *S.* Typhi and *S.* Paratyphi A; concomitant biliary disease also has significant implications for therapy. When the patient has chronic cholecystitis or gallstones, antibiotics alone are most unlikely to eradicate the infection. Cholecystectomy together with appropriate antibiotic treatment results in cure in about 90% of cases, but has significant risk, not least from metastatic infection from dissemination of the organisms during surgery.

In the absence of biliary disease, prolonged courses of ampicillin, amoxicillin, co-trimoxazole or ciprofloxacin may cure up to 80% of carriers. However, it is difficult to justify even moderately heroic efforts to cure a condition that has little if any ill effect on the individual and not much direct public health importance. The chronic human carrier is the principal reservoir of enteric fever salmonellae, but even in the developing world direct person-to-person spread by asymptomatic carriers is uncommon. 'Typhoid Mary', who is reputed to have caused many infections by her cooking, was an exception and must have had peculiar personal habits. Normal personal hygiene, adequate sanitation and a reliable supply of potable water are the real safeguards against enteric fever. Prolonged carriage of other *S. enterica* serotypes is of even less public health importance, and rarely if ever justifies exclusion from any employment, or intrusive efforts to eradicate the infection.

Typhoid carriers may develop high levels of serum IgG-class antibodies to the Vi capsular polysaccharides; detection of such antibodies warrants faecal screening for *S.* Typhi and Paratyphi.

## EPIDEMIOLOGY AND CONTROL

The typhoid and paratyphoid bacilli are essentially human parasites. Human beings are the reservoir host and most infections can be traced to a human source, or at least to a source of human sewage. All other salmonellae have animal hosts.

### Enteric fever

#### Incidence

Historically, strains of *S.* Typhi have been the major cause of typhoidal illness; however, in certain parts of the world, such as Asia, the predominant cause of enteric fever is *S.* Paratyphi A. In 2000, an estimated 21.7 million cases of typhoid fever occurred with 217 000 deaths. In parts of sub-Saharan Africa, strains of *S.* Enteritidis and *S.* Typhimurium are major causes of bloodstream infections. In England and Wales, *S.* Typhi and *S.* Paratyphi account for most systemic infections (Fig. 24.3).

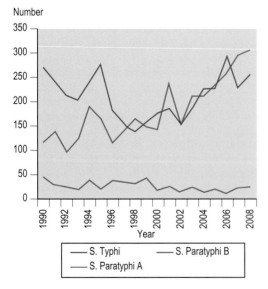

**Fig. 24.3** Human cases of *S.* Typhi and *S.* Paratyphi identified in England and Wales during 1990–2008. (Health Protection Agency data.)

### Sanitation

The control of enteric fever is in theory straightforward. Cases occur from the ingestion of food or water contaminated with human sewage carrying typhoid or paratyphoid bacilli. Outbreaks occur when numbers of people are infected from a primary source. This may be a single meal or a briefly contaminated water supply, or may be a water supply or source of food contaminated and available for ingestion over a longer period. Secondary transmission from patients infected by the primary source is rare.

Enteric fever is a public health problem only where the wide public availability of wholesome drinking water and the provision of adequate means for the proper disposal of human excreta do not exist. In these circumstances the organisms can be spread widely from carriers and from convalescent and sick persons, possibly helped by cultural factors such as food habits, occupation and personal behaviour. In such communities the selection of control measures may be difficult, and provision of adequate sanitation and pure water may need to be supplemented by prophylactic immunization.

### Vaccination

Heat-killed, phenol-preserved whole-cell vaccines containing a mixture of cultures of Typhi, Paratyphi A and Paratyphi B (TAB) have been used for many years in countries with a high endemic level of typhoid fever. Such preparations confer considerable, although not absolute, protection against typhoid for about 3 years. There has always been doubt about the value of the paratyphoid components and monovalent typhoid vaccines are now preferred. Capsular (Vi) polysaccharide vaccines have largely replaced whole-cell vaccines. Alternatively, an oral live-attenuated typhoid vaccine is used.

Travellers to endemic areas in which there are high carriage rates and poor standards of hygiene should be offered immunization, especially if they intend to visit rural areas or to live 'rough'. However, the risk to the air traveller with full board at a reputable hotel is so small that typhoid immunization may be unnecessary.

### Salmonella food poisoning

No other zoonosis is as complex in its epidemiology and control as salmonellosis. The biology of different *S. enterica* serotypes varies widely and epidemiological patterns differ greatly between geographical areas, depending on climate, population density, land use, farming practices, food-processing technologies and consumer habits.

## Sources

The carcasses or products (cooked meats, eggs, milk) of naturally infected domestic animals are the most common sources of food poisoning. Flesh may be infected when an ill, septicaemic animal is slaughtered, but in most cases the salmonellae important in human infection cause only mild or inapparent infection in their animal hosts, and abattoir and shop cross-contamination with intestinal contents from a carrier animal is a more important hazard. Poultry (particularly hens), ducks and turkeys are the most significant reservoirs of food poisoning salmonellae in the UK. Pigs share the honours with poultry in much of northern Europe, whereas beef cattle are important sources in the USA. Duck eggs have always been a problem, as they can be infected in the oviduct before the egg is shelled. Hen eggs acquire their shells higher in the oviduct and are less commonly infected in this way, although they can be contaminated on the outside if laid on soil contaminated by infected hen faeces.

## Food contamination

Rats and mice are commonly infected with food-poisoning salmonellae and may contaminate human food with their faeces. Food poisoning may occasionally be caused by food contaminated by a human case or carrier. Thus, even if the foodstuff is initially free from salmonellae, the chance of contamination 'from the hoof to the home' is high, and the more sophisticated the manipulation of the food, the greater the chance of contamination. For example, one egg containing salmonellae, if eaten by an individual, probably will not give rise to an infection. On the other hand, if such an egg is pooled with others free from salmonellae, as in preparing a mayonnaise or a Hollandaise sauce for communal consumption, and if conditions of temperature and time allow multiplication of the salmonellae, there will be the potential for an outbreak of infection among those who eat the contaminated food.

A clean carcass can be contaminated at the abattoir by instruments or by hanging in contact with an infected carcass in the chilling hall or during transportation to the wholesale and retail butchers' premises. The aggregation of calves or pigs in holding pens greatly increases the occurrence of cross-infection before slaughter. Infection in pigs is most often due to the feeding of swill containing infected animal matter, a practice that is difficult to prevent.

There is a close correspondence between the types of salmonellae prevalent in animals, especially pigs and poultry, and the types causing human infection. Strains of S. Typhimurium, which is a primary pathogen in a wide variety of animals, are common, and S. Enteritidis has become prevalent in the UK in poultry flocks. Strains belonging to serotypes such as Heidelberg, Brandenburg, Panama and Virchow are rarely found in animals and yet may be responsible for widespread human infections. More needs to be learned about the epidemiology of such infections. Since 1998 there has been a steady decline in the numbers of salmonellas causing intestinal infection in England and Wales, largely due to vaccination of broiler flocks and restrictions of the importation of eggs from abroad.

## Food preparation

Infection of food with salmonellae is not in itself sufficient to cause food poisoning. It is necessary for the infected food to be moist and to be held long enough under conditions that will allow the bacteria to grow, for instance overnight in a warm kitchen or several days in a cool larder. If the food is then eaten without further cooking, infection may follow. Although cooking of liquid foods will render them safe, cooking of solid foods often fails to do so because of the relatively poor rate of heat penetration into the food. A cold or chilled joint of meat, a poultry carcass or a large meat pie may be heated in an oven until the surface is well cooked, while the central part is still insufficiently heated to destroy vegetative bacteria.

## Outbreaks

Food-poisoning incidents occur most dramatically as explosive outbreaks among members of a community sharing communal meals, as in factories, hospitals or schools or at a celebratory feast, although sporadic incidents affecting a single family or a single person are much more common and much more difficult to track to a source. In the UK, salmonellae account for about 75% of the incidents of food poisoning in which a causal agent is identified. However, this may only reflect the fact that salmonellosis is relatively easy to confirm bacteriologically and is therefore more readily recognized.

## Surveillance

Efficient surveillance of diseases caused by *Salmonella* has been facilitated by accurate strain discrimination achieved with serotyping, phage typing, antimicrobial resistance typing and pulsed-field gel electrophoresis. Several online networks have been established to enable the rapid exchange of information relating to strains, outbreaks of disease, etc.

## Prevention

The principles of the prevention of salmonella food poisoning are:

- raising of animals free from infection
- elimination of contamination by rodents at all levels of food production
- prevention of contamination by human handlers at the wholesale, retail and hotel levels.

The barriers of economic husbandry, out-of-date premises and, perhaps the most important of all, the need for continuing education of food handlers at all levels of production make implementation of these principles difficult. To reduce the incidence of food poisoning, whether due to salmonellae or to other bacteria, two basic precepts must be observed:

1. Raw foodstuffs of animal origin, which are always potentially contaminated, must never have direct or indirect contact with cooked foods.

2. Foodstuff thought to be contaminated should be treated or held under temperature conditions that prevent the organisms from growing.

Cooked foods should be served and eaten immediately after cooking and while still hot, or cooled rapidly and held at refrigerator temperature until eaten, so that at least the inoculum eaten by any individual is small. It is often found that the food incriminated in an outbreak had been cooked several hours or even a day or two before and then left at room temperature before being reheated immediately before serving. This procedure ensures that salmonellae that survived the initial cooking or gained access to the food from contaminated kitchen surfaces or implements had excellent opportunities to multiply in the interval before being warmed up for consumption.

As in most other endeavours to control the spread of infection, the human element is the weakest link in the chain, so that health education, particularly of food handlers, is a most important and continuing requirement.

## RECOMMENDED READING

Chart H, Cheasty T, de Pinna E, et al: Serodiagnosis of *Salmonella enterica* serovar Typhi and *S. enterica* serovars Paratyphi A, B and C human infections. *Journal of Medical Microbiology* 56:1161–1166, 2007.

Crawford RW, Rosales-Reyes R, Ramírez-Aguilar Mde L, et al: Gallstones play a significant role in *Salmonella* spp. gallbladder colonization and carriage. *Proceedings of the National Academy of Sciences USA* 107:4353–4358, 2010.

Crump JA, Mintz ED: Global trends in typhoid and paratyphoid Fever. *Clinical Infectious Diseases* 50:241–246, 2010.

House D, Bishop A, Parry C, et al: Typhoid fever: pathogenesis and disease. *Current Opinion in Infectious Diseases* 14:573–578, 2001.

Morpeth SC, Ramadhani HO, Crump JA: Invasive non-Typhi *Salmonella* disease in Africa. *Clinical Infectious Diseases* 49:606–611, 2009.

Raffatellu M, Wilson RP, Winter SE, Bäumler AJ: Clinical pathogenesis of typhoid fever. *Journal of Infection in Developing Countries* 30:260–266, 2008.

Threlfall EJ: Antimicrobial drug resistance in *Salmonella*: problems and perspectives in food- and water-borne infections. *FEMS Microbiology Reviews* 26:141–148, 2002.

Wain J, House D, Parkhill J, et al: Unlocking the genome of the human typhoid bacillus. *Lancet Infectious Diseases* 2:163–170, 2002.

Zhang S, Kingsley RA, Santos RL, et al: Molecular pathogenesis of *Salmonella* enterica serotype typhimurium-induced diarrhea. *Infection and Immunity* 71:1–12, 2003.

### Websites

Centers for Disease Control and Prevention. Salmonella Infection (Salmonellosis). http://www.cdc.gov/ncidod/diseases/submenus/sub_salmonella.htm

Enter-Net. http://www.hpa.org.uk/AboutTheHPA/WhatTheHealthProtectionAgencyDoes/InternationalWork/EnterNet/

Health Protection Agency. Salmonella. http://www.hpa.org.uk/infections/topics_az/salmonella/menu.htm

PulseNet. http://www.pulsenetinternational.org

PulseNet Europe. http://www.pulsenetinternational.org/networks/Pages/europe.aspx

Sanger Institute. http://www.sanger.ac.uk/resources/downloads/bacteria/salmonella.html

# 25 Shigella

## Bacillary dysentery

*H. Chart*

## KEY POINTS

- *Shigella* species cause bacillary dysentery.
- The infective dose is very small.
- *Sh. dysenteriae* type 1 produces a toxin that resembles the Verocytotoxin of certain strains of *E. coli* and is responsible for the most serious forms of shigellosis.
- *Sh. flexneri, Sh. boydii* and *Sh. sonnei* cause enteric disease of varying severity.
- Sonnei dysentery is the most prevalent form of shigellosis in developed countries.
- Most cases of shigellosis do not require antibiotics. Treatment with ciprofloxacin is indicated in severe cases. Ampicillin, tetracyclines and trimethoprim are suitable alternatives, but resistance is common.

Dysentery, the bloody flux of biblical times, is a clinical entity characterized by the frequent passage of bloodstained mucopurulent stools. Aetiologically it is divisible into two main categories, amoebic and bacillary. Both forms are endemic in most countries with a warm climate. Bacillary dysentery, caused by members of the genus *Shigella*, is also prevalent in many countries with temperate climates.

## DESCRIPTION

The genus *Shigella* is subdivided on biochemical and serological grounds into four species:

- *Sh. dysenteriae* – serogroup A
- *Sh. flexneri* – serogroup B
- *Sh. boydii* – serogroup C
- *Sh. sonnei* – serogroup D.

Strains of *Shigella* spp. are typical members of the Enterobacteriaceae and are closely related to the genus *Escherichia*. Studies focusing on the ancestral lineage of these bacteria suggest that *Sh. boydii* is related only distantly to other members of the genus *Shigella*, which are more closely related to enteroinvasive serotypes of *E. coli* (see p. 285).

Microscopically and culturally shigellae are indistinguishable from other enteric Gram-negative bacilli. They are non-motile, non-capsulate and appear not to express fimbriae. Strains of *Shigella* spp. share lipopolysaccharide (LPS) antigens with strains of *E. coli* but the LPS structures are distinct and merely share common epitopes.

The distinction between strains of *Shigella* spp. and *E. coli* depends on a limited number of diagnostic tests including motility, production of lysine decarboxylase and the utilization of citrate. *Sh. dysenteriae* type 1 produces Shiga toxin and this differentiates it from other members of the genus.

All strains express LPS somatic antigens which form the basis for the *Shigella* serotyping scheme. There are 13 serotypes of *Sh. dysenteriae* of which type-1 is much the most important as a cause of severe bacillary dysentery. *Sh. boydii* can be subdivided into 18 specific serotypes. The six serotypes of *Sh. flexneri* can each be further subdivided into subtypes. Strains of *Sh. sonnei* are serologically homogeneous, and a variety of other markers such as the ability to produce specific colicines, the carriage of drug resistance or other plasmids, or lysogeny by a panel of bacteriophages are used to discriminate between strains for epidemiological purposes.

## CLINICAL FEATURES

The incubation period is usually between 2 and 3 days, but may be as long as 8 days. The onset of symptoms is usually sudden, and frequently the initial symptom is abdominal colic. This is followed by the onset of watery diarrhoea, and in all but the mildest cases this is accompanied by fever, headache, malaise and anorexia. Many episodes resolve at this point, but others progress to abdominal cramps, tenesmus and the frequent passage of small volumes of stool, predominantly consisting of bloody mucus. The symptoms typically last about 4 days, but may continue for 14 days or more. Infection may affect the nervous system resulting in seizures and encephalitis. Shigellosis is occasionally associated with the development of Reiter's syndrome (reactive arthritis).

The severity of the clinical illness is to some extent associated with the species involved. Infection with *Sh. dysenteriae* 1 is usually associated with a severe illness in which prostration is marked and, in young children, may be accompanied by febrile convulsions. Members of the *Sh. flexneri* and *Sh. boydii* groups may also cause severe illness. In contrast, dysentery associated with *Sh. sonnei (Sonnei dysentery)* in an otherwise healthy person may be confined to the passage of a few loose stools with vague abdominal discomfort, and the patient often continues at school or work.

Strains of *Sh. dysenteriae* 1 have been responsible for many cases of the haemolytic uraemic syndrome that accompanies outbreaks of dysentery in several countries. The condition, with its triad of haemolytic anaemia, thrombocytopenia and acute renal failure, can be caused by many pathogens (in particular, *E. coli* O157; see p. 286). It is associated with complement activation and disseminated intravascular coagulation, and in some parts of the world is one of the most common forms of acute renal failure in children.

Death from bacillary dysentery is uncommon in the developed world; it occurs mostly at the extremes of life or in individuals who are suffering from some other disease or debilitating condition.

## PATHOGENESIS

*Shigella* spp. are pathogens of man and other primates, and the pathogenesis of infection with these bacteria and enteroinvasive *E. coli* (EIEC; see p. 285) is very similar. The infective dose is small: bacillary dysentery may follow the ingestion of as few as ten viable bacteria. The site of infection is the M cells in the Peyer's patches of the large intestine. Strains of *Shigella* spp. are non-motile and it is not known how the bacteria reach and adhere to M cells.

Association with the intestinal mucosa initiates mucosal inflammation leading to apoptosis, which is thought to facilitate the invasion of the M cells, after

which the bacteria are phagocytosed. The shigellae multiply within the epithelial cells and spread laterally into adjacent cells and deep into the lamina propria. The infected epithelial cells are killed, and the lamina propria and submucosa develop an inflammatory reaction with capillary thrombosis. Patches of necrotic epithelium are sloughed and ulcers form. The cellular response is mainly by polymorphonuclear leucocytes, which can be seen readily on microscopic examination of the stool, together with red cells and sloughed epithelium.

Dysentery bacilli rarely invade other tissues. Transient bacteraemia can occur but septicaemia with metastatic infection is rare.

## Pathogenic mechanisms

In common with most bacteria, shigellae require a range of pathogenic mechanisms to cause disease. They are tolerant to the conditions of low pH encountered in the human stomach and the action of bile.

Pathogenic strains of shigellae, like entero-invasive *E. coli*, carry a plasmid of 100–140 MDa, which encodes the pathogenic mechanisms involved with eukaryotic cell invasion. Expression of the mechanisms encoded on the virulence plasmid are thermoregulated such that strains become invasive when growing at 37°C but not at 30°C, and regulation is by both plasmid and chromosomally located elements. Plasmid-encoded proteins are required for bacteria to break free from cellular endosomes and for the migration between epithelial cells.

Long-chain lipopolysaccharide plays a role in virulence by preventing the effects of serum complement. The lipid A component has been implicated in causing localized cytokine release, and the resultant inflammatory response and cellular disruption enable these bacteria to enter intestinal cells. *Sh. flexneri* and *Sh. sonnei* express an aerobactin-mediated high-affinity iron uptake system; however, as *Sh. dysenteriae* 1 does not express this siderophore, the role of aerobactin in the pathogenesis of the disease is unclear.

## Shiga toxin

*Sh. dysenteriae* 1 produces a potent protein toxin (*Shiga toxin*) very similar to Verocytotoxin (VT)-1 expressed by strains of Verocytotoxigenic *E. coli* (VTEC; see p. 286); however, in contrast to VTEC, the genes encoding Shiga toxin are located on the chromosome. Expression of Shiga toxin has been shown to be iron regulated, with toxin production increasing under conditions of iron restriction.

Shiga toxin is a subunit toxin comprising an A portion and five B subunits. The A subunit possesses the biological activities of the toxin, and the B subunits mediate specific binding and receptor-mediated uptake. In common with the Verocytotoxins of *E. coli*, Shiga toxin binds to globotriosylceramide ($Gb_3$) molecules present on the surface of certain eukaryotic cells. During pathogenesis, release of the inflammatory mediators tumour necrosis factor and interleukin-1 increases the number of $Gb_3$ receptors on the surface of eukaryotic cells, enhancing the binding of toxin to these cells.

Like Verocytotoxin, Shiga toxin becomes internalized by host cells and remains active within endosomes, eventually reaching the Golgi apparatus. Within the host cell the A subunit divides to form portions $A_1$ and $A_2$; the $A_1$ portion of the toxin prevents protein synthesis and causes cell death. Haemolytic uraemic syndrome is thought to be caused by the action of Shiga toxin on kidney tissues; however, Shiga toxin has also been shown to have neurotoxic properties and the role of this toxin in the pathogenesis of bacillary dysentery remains to be elucidated fully.

## LABORATORY DIAGNOSIS

A specimen of faeces is always preferable to a rectal swab. Rectal swabs do not allow adequate macroscopic and microscopic examination of the stool, and unless taken properly and bearing obvious faecal material may be no more than a swab of peri-anal skin. Moreover, because of drying of the swab, pathogenic species die quite rapidly, and may not survive transport to the laboratory.

The faeces are inoculated on desoxycholate citrate agar or MacConkey agar. Mucus, if present in the specimen, may be used as the inoculum. After overnight incubation, pale non-lactose-fermenting colonies are tested by standard biochemical and sugar utilization tests to differentiate them from other enterobacteria. Identity is confirmed by agglutination tests with serotype-specific rabbit antisera, unless the strain is *Sh. sonnei*. A DNA-array-based assay has been developed to detect the recognized serotypes of *Shigella* spp.

Strains of *Shigella* spp. can be detected with polymerase chain reaction (PCR) tests targeting the genes encoding the invasion plasmid antigen H (*ipa*H) although this assay will also detect certain strains of invasive *E. coli*. The genes for *Shigella* enterotoxin 2 can be detected with the ShET-2 PCR and strains with the genes encoding an aerobactin-mediated iron uptake system can be identified with a PCR using primers targeting the *iuc* gene complex. Plasmid pattern analysis and colicine typing can also be used to characterize strains of *Sh. sonnei*.

Expression of Shiga toxin can be detected by Vero and HeLa cell tests (see p. 286) and immunoassays designed for the Verocytotoxin produced by certain *E. coli* strains.

Patients infected with *Sh. dysenteriae* 1 produce serum and salivary antibodies to the lipopolysaccharide antigens, but tests for the antibodies are not available routinely.

## TREATMENT

Most cases of shigella dysentery, especially those due to *Sh. sonnei*, are mild and do not require antibiotic therapy. Maintaining good nutrition is essential. Symptomatic treatment with the maintenance of hydration by use of oral rehydration salt solution (see Table 30.1, p. 318) is all that is required. As with salmonella infections, drugs that impair gut motility should be avoided.

Treatment with a suitable antibiotic is necessary in the very young, the aged or the debilitated, and in those with severe infections. The World Health Organization recommends the use of ciprofloxacin, ceftriaxone and pivmecillinam for the treatment of dysentery in children. There is no evidence that antibiotics reduce the period of excretion of the organisms, and they should not be used in the asymptomatic person, either prophylactically or in attempts to hasten clearance after recovery.

## EPIDEMIOLOGY

During the twentieth century, infections due to *Sh. dysenteriae* 1 and *Sh. boydii* declined and strains of *Sh. sonnei* became dominant in the UK and other European countries. In England and Wales more than 16 000 cases of Sonnei dysentery were recorded in 1992. The incidence then declined steadily to an annual average of fewer than 1000 notified cases between 1998 and 2004 (Fig. 25.1). Infections caused by *Sh. flexneri* have also steadily declined to around 250 cases/year, but are still more common than those caused by *Sh. boydii* (50–100 cases/year) or *Sh. dysenteriae* (40–50 cases/year), most of which are contracted abroad. Globally, shigellosis remains a major problem particularly in tropical areas of the developing world, where shigellosis is endemic. It has been estimated that some 5 million cases require hospital

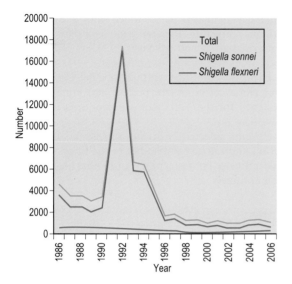

**Fig. 25.1** Faecal isolates of shigellae (total), *Sh. sonnei* and *Sh. flexneri*, in England and Wales 1986–2004. (Health Protection Agency data.)

children at school undoubtedly plays a part. The disease can be endemic among adults living in residential institutions where high standards of hygiene are difficult to maintain, and has in the past been a scourge in gaols and in armies in the field. The seasonal distribution of bacillary dysentery in the UK is bimodal, with the highest incidence in spring and a second peak in October and November. The incidence is at its lowest in summer, when school children are on holiday. As this is the period when flying insects are most abundant, this suggests that in the UK insects play little, if any, part in transmission. In certain settings, where disposal of human faeces is inadequate, flies may also serve as vectors for the spread of *Shigella* bacteria.

Occasional epidemics of bacillary dysentery have been traced to water supplies when chlorination of the supply has not been instituted or has been defective. Such water-borne epidemics are usually spectacular in the large numbers of people simultaneously infected and in the speed with which they can be terminated when the water supply is adequately treated. Epidemic infection may also follow the contamination of milk or ice cream.

treatment and about 600 000 die every year. Young children are particularly vulnerable.

### Sources and spread

Bacillary dysentery is highly contagious and is usually spread by the faecal–oral route. The case or carrier, after contaminating his or her hands while cleansing at toilet, may contaminate the lavatory flush-handle, door knobs, washbasin taps, hand towels and other objects that, when handled by another individual, allow transfer of the dysentery bacteria to the recipient's hands and to the mouth. The carrier may also infect bedding and, in the case of young children, may contaminate toys. Dysentery bacilli are also liberated into the air in an aerosol when an infected loose stool is flushed from the toilet and, after settling on the surfaces of toilet seats, furniture and surroundings, may survive for some days in a moist atmosphere. Infection can also occur among those who indulge in sexual practices involving anal–oral contact. Contamination of foods, particularly those that are to be consumed raw, are a major source of infection.

An important feature of the epidemiology of bacillary dysentery in the UK and other countries with good environmental sanitation is that the main patient group involved is school-aged children, particularly primary school children. Neglect of toilet hygiene by

### CONTROL

The mild and often fleeting nature of the clinical illness associated with *Sh. sonnei* infection means that frequently the patient with bacillary dysentery remains ambulant and follows his or her daily labour and leisure pursuits, remaining in circulation as a disperser of the causal organism. The pressure on toilet facilities, particularly in schools, allows hand-to-mouth spread of the bacilli. The provision of washbasins in the same compartment as the toilet pedestal would allow some reduction in spread, especially if flushing mechanisms and washbasin taps could be operated by foot instead of by hand.

During diarrhoea, faecal soiling of the fingers can be heavy, and hand washing, although very important, will at best only reduce the numbers of bacteria present. The normal disinfecting effect of the skin fatty acids and competing skin organisms may take up to half an hour to destroy the rest. People with dysentery should stay off work and, as far as possible, out of circulation until the symptoms have subsided, especially when their work involves the preparation of food or direct contact with other people. Asymptomatic carriers are far less important in the spread of this disease and seldom, if ever, need to be excluded from any employment.

## Control of an outbreak

Outbreaks of dysentery in schools and other institutions are notoriously difficult to control. In nursery school outbreaks, infection is usually widespread before the first cases have been notified, with considerable environmental contamination. Some children will be incubating the infection; others will have recovered from the diarrhoea but still be excreting the organisms. In this situation the acute case is far more important in the spread of infection than the symptomless excreter. There is little to be gained by trying to ascertain bacteriologically who is infected and who is not once the cause of the outbreak has been established, as there is little reason to exclude an asymptomatic carrier and it is pointless to seek confirmation of a clearly symptomatic case. The practical course is usually to keep children away from school.

Having determined the exclusion policy it is important to try to stop hand-to-hand spread among those who remain at school. Supervision of children using the lavatory, supervised hand washing before meals, frequent disinfection of toilets, including seats, lavatory chain and door handles, and the general use of paper towels all play a part.

Similar principles can be applied to outbreaks in residential institutions or a hospital ward. The most important single factor in all these situations is the need for adequate communication. Teachers, nurses, parents and all who are involved in trying to control the outbreak need to have explained to them exactly how the infection spreads, and the reasons for the measures taken or not taken. Finally, the temptation to use antibiotics prophylactically in an attempt to limit the spread must be resisted.

## Vaccination

Infection with a given species of *Shigella* spp. results in high levels of mucosal IgA-class antibodies which confer protection against subsequent infection with the same species; however, there is only limited protection against infection with a heterologous species. Research has focused on two prototype *Shigella* vaccines, a live attenuated oral vaccine and the other a parenteral vaccine comprising *Shigella* LPS conjugated to a carrier protein. Achieving a useful vaccine, capable of proving broad protection, has been hampered by the large number of different epidemiologically significant serotypes of *Shigella*.

### RECOMMENDED READING

Ashkenasi S: Shigella infections in children: new insights. *Seminars in Pediatric Infectious Diseases* 15:246–252, 2004.

Kingcombe CI, Cerqueira-Compos ML, Farber JM: Molecular strategies for the detection, identification and differentiation between enteroinvasive *Escherichia coli* and *Shigella* spp. *Journal of Food Protection* 68:239–245, 2005.

Levine MM, Kotloff KL, Barry EM, et al: Clinical trials of Shigella vaccines: two steps forward and one step back on a long, hard road. *National Revues in Microbiology* 5:540–553, 2007.

Li Y, Cao B, Liu B, et al: Molecular detection of all 34 distinct O-antigen forms of Shigella. *Journal of Medical Microbiology* 58:69–81, 2009.

Lopez EL, Prado-Jimenez V, O'Ryan-Gallardo M, Contrini MM: Shigella and Shiga toxin-producing *Escherichia coli* causing bloody diarrhea in Latin America. *Infectious Disease Clinics of North America* 14:41–65, 2000.

Nhieu GT, Sansonetti PJ: Mechanism of Shigella entry into epithelial cells. *Current Opinion in Microbiology* 2:51–55, 1999.

Niyogi SK: Shigellosis. *Journal of Microbiology* 43:133–143, 2005.

Sansonetti PJ: Molecular and cellular mechanisms of invasion of the intestinal barrier by enteric pathogens: the paradigm of *Shigella*. *Folia Microbiologica* 43:239–246, 1998.

Sasakawa C: Molecular basis of pathogenicity of *Shigella*. *Reviews in Medical Microbiology* 6:257–266, 1995.

Vu DT, Sethabutr O, Von Seidlein L, et al: Detection of *Shigella* by a PCR assay targeting the ipaH gene suggests increased prevalence of shigellosis in Nha Trang, Vietnam. *Journal of Clinical Microbiology* 42:2031–2035, 2004.

Yang YG, Song MK, Park SJ, Kim SW: Direct detection of *Shigella flexneri* and *Salmonella typhimurium* in human feces by real-time PCR. *Journal of Microbiology and Biotechnology* 17:1616–1621, 2007.

### Websites

Centers for Disease Control and Prevention: *Shigellosis.* http://www.cdc.gov/nczved/divisions/dfbmd/diseases/shigellosis/

Health Protection Agency: http://www.hpa.org.uk/Topics/InfectiousDiseases/InfectionsAZ/Shigella/

International Centre for Diarrhoeal Disease Research: http://www.icddrb.org/

World Health Organization: Shigella. http://www.who.int/topics/shigella/en/

# Escherichia

Urinary tract infection; travellers' diarrhoea; haemorrhagic colitis; haemolytic uraemic syndrome

*H. Chart*

Strains of *Escherichia coli* and related Gram-negative bacteria predominate among the aerobic commensal flora in the gut of human beings and animals. These bacteria are present wherever there is faecal contamination, a phenomenon that is exploited by public health microbiologists as an indicator of faecal pollution of water sources, drinking water and food. The species encompasses a variety of strains, which may be purely commensal or possess combinations of pathogenic mechanisms that enable them to cause disease in man and other animals.

## DESCRIPTION

Strains of *E. coli* are usually motile and may express fimbriae (Fig. 26.1). Some, especially those from extra-intestinal infections, may produce a polysaccharide capsule. They grow well on non-selective media and usually (with the exception of certain Verocytotoxin-producing strains) ferment lactose, producing large red colonies on MacConkey agar. They grow over a wide range of temperature (15–45°C); some strains are more heat-resistant than other members of the Enterobacteriaceae and may survive 60°C for 15 min or 55°C for 60 min. Certain strains are haemolytic when grown on media containing suitable erythrocytes.

*E. coli* can be differentiated from other enteric Gram-negative bacteria by the ability to utilize certain sugars and by a range of other biochemical reactions. Many characteristic reactions, such as indole production and the formation of acid and gas from lactose and other carbohydrates, take place at 44°C as well as at 37°C.

DNA–DNA recombination studies show that *E. coli* and *Shigella* spp. form a single genetic group, and it is therefore to be expected that intermediate strains will occur. Certain atypical types of *E. coli* are non-motile and anaerogenic, and often ferment lactose late or not at all.

### Antigenic structure

Serotyping is based on the somatic lipopolysaccharide (LPS) (O), flagellar (H) and capsular (K) antigens, as detected in agglutination assays with specific rabbit antibodies. More than 200 different O-antigens have been described and others continue to emerge. Serotyping detects cross-reactions as a result of shared

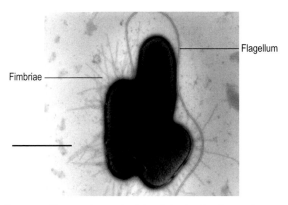

Fimbriae

Flagellum

**Fig. 26.1** Electron micrograph of *E. coli* showing flagellum and fimbriae (arrowed). Bar = 0.5 μm.

**Table 26.1** K antigens of *E. Coli*

| Property | Group I | Group II |
| --- | --- | --- |
| Molecular weight (Da) | >100 000 | <50 000 |
| Acidic component | Hexuronic acid, pyruvate | Glucuronic acid, phosphate, KDO, NeuNAc |
| Heat stability (100°C, pH 6) | All stable | Mostly labile |
| O groups | 08, 09 | Many |
| Chromosome site | *His* | *SerA* |
| Expressed at 17–20°C | Yes | No |
| Electrophoretic mobility | Low | High |

KDO, ketodeoxyoctonate; NeuNAc, *N*-acetylneuraminic acid.

epitopes on the LPS expressed by strains of *E. coli*, and may occur with organisms belonging to the genera *Brucella, Citrobacter, Providencia, Salmonella, Shigella* and *Yersinia*.

More than 50 H antigens have been identified. Most are monophasic, but rare diphasic strains have been reported. There are only a few significant cross-reactions between them and with the H antigens of other members of the Enterobacteriaceae. Because certain strains of *E. coli* cease to express flagella during growth in vitro, strains may need to be grown in semi-solid agar (Craigie tubes) to induce flagella expression. Obtaining a motile phenotype can take several days and sequence-typing of the *fliC* gene has been considered as a rapid alternative to serotyping.

The term 'K antigen' was formerly used collectively for surface or capsular antigens (designated L, A and B) that prevent flagella-specific antibodies from binding to the somatic antigens. In modern usage, 'K antigen' refers to the acidic polysaccharide capsular antigens, and those of *E. coli* may be divided into two groups (groups I and II; Table 26.1) that largely correspond to the former A and L antigens. Due to the complexity of available tests, strains of *E. coli* are not routinely K-typed.

### Fimbrial antigens

Strains of *E. coli* may express both sex pili and more than one type of fimbrial structure (see p. 159). Within a given culture, there may exist individual cells with fimbriae and others with none, and there is reversible variation between the fimbriate and the non-fimbriate phase.

Type-1 fimbriae can mediate adhesion to a wide range of human and animal cells that contain the sugar mannose. Such adhesion might be involved in

pathogenicity and there are some examples of this. Filamentous protein structures resembling fimbriae cause mannose-resistant haemagglutination, and probably play an important part in the pathogenesis of diarrhoeal disease and urinary tract infection. They include the K88 antigen found in strains causing enteritis of pigs, the K99 antigen found in strains causing enteritis of calves and lambs, and the colonization factor antigens (CFAs) or coli surface (CS) antigens expressed by enterotoxigenic *E. coli* (ETEC) that cause human diarrhoeal disease.

Fimbriae that are of importance in urinary tract infection and cause mannose-resistant haemagglutination are distinguished according to their receptor specificities. These include the P fimbriae that bind specifically to receptors present on the P blood group antigens of human erythrocytes and uroepithelial cells.

## PATHOGENESIS

Strains of *E. coli* possess a range of different pathogenic mechanisms. The polysaccharides of the O and K antigens protect the organism from the bactericidal effect of complement and phagocytes in the absence of specific antibodies. However, in the presence of antibody to K antigens alone, or to both O and K antigens, opsonization may occur.

Many strains express haemolysin(s), and in general strains of *E. coli* isolated from human extra-intestinal infections are more likely to be haemolytic than strains isolated from the faeces of healthy human beings. Haemolysin production is an important pathogenic mechanism for releasing essential ferric ions bound to haemoglobin, and the expression of certain haemolysins has been shown to be regulated by iron.

Strains of *E. coli* can express siderophores, such as enterobactin, which remove ferric ions from mammalian iron transport proteins like transferrin and lactoferrin (see Ch. 13). Some strains also express the siderophore, aerobactin; this may be plasmid-mediated. The ability of strains of *E. coli* to acquire ferric ions is a recognized pathogenic mechanism. Expression of the aerobactin-mediated iron-uptake system is a common feature of strains isolated from patients with septicaemia, pyelonephritis and lower urinary tract infection. Some strains may also utilize siderophores produced by certain species of fungi (e.g. ferrichrome, coprogen, rhodoturulic acid) to acquire iron from environmental sources.

## CLINICAL SYNDROMES

### Urinary tract and septic infections

*E. coli* is the most common cause of acute, uncomplicated urinary tract infection outside hospitals, as well as causing hospital-associated urinary tract sepsis. These bacteria may also cause neonatal meningitis and septicaemia, sepsis in operation wounds and abscesses in a variety of organs.

As many as 80% of *E. coli* strains that cause neonatal meningitis and 40% of those isolated from infants with septicaemia but without meningitis express a K1 antigen. Strains possessing the K1 or the K5 antigen may be more virulent than those with other K antigens, as they share structural identity with host components.

Strains that cause urinary tract infection often originate from the gut of the patient, with infection occurring in an ascending manner. The ability of *E. coli* to infect the urinary tract may be associated with fimbriae that specifically mediate adherence to uroepithelial cells.

### Epidemiology

Urinary tract infection occurs more frequently in women than in men because the shorter, wider, female urethra appears to be less effective in preventing access of the bacteria to the bladder. Sexual intercourse may be a predisposing factor. The high incidence in pregnant women can be attributed to impairment of urine flow due partly to hormonal changes and partly to pressure on the urinary tract. Other causes of urinary stagnation that may predispose to urinary tract infection include urethral obstruction, urinary stones, congenital malformations and neurological disorders, all of which occur in both sexes. In men, prostatic enlargement is the most common predisposing factor. Catheterization and cystoscopy may introduce bacteria into the bladder and therefore carry a risk of infection.

Most urinary tract infections are thought to be caused by organisms originating from the patient's own faecal flora. However, the prevalence of various serotypes of *E. coli* in urinary tract infections varies with geographical location, suggesting that *E. coli* causing such infections are specific pathogens for the urinary tract. Pathogenic strains, possibly transmitted in contaminated foods, are able to colonize the bowel, and in individuals with predisposing factors may cause a urinary tract infection. The prevalence of infections due to a particular strain may therefore increase for a time in a locality.

### Laboratory diagnosis

Clinical specimens may be stained by Gram's method for microscopical examination, and are cultured on MacConkey agar or other suitable media. In the case of suspected urinary tract infection, culture is semi-quantitative; in acute *E. coli* infections the organism is generally present in pure culture at a count of $10^5$ or more per millilitre of urine. For more serious infections, strains should be referred to a reference laboratory for serotyping.

### Treatment and control

In the absence of acquired resistance, *E. coli* is susceptible to many antibacterial agents, including ampicillin, cephalosporins, tetracyclines, quinolones, aminoglycosides, trimethoprim and sulphonamides. Many strains, however, have acquired plasmids conferring resistance to one or more of these drugs, and antimicrobial therapy should be guided by laboratory tests of sensitivity if possible.

Uncomplicated cystitis usually responds to minimal treatment with oral agents such as trimethoprim or nitrofurantoin, but more serious infections require specific antimicrobial therapy based on laboratory results. In particular, bacterial meningitis is a medical emergency and vigorous early treatment with cefotaxime and gentamicin is required.

Urinary catheterization and cystoscopy require rigorous aseptic technique to minimize the introduction of bacteria into the bladder. Bladder irrigation and systemic treatment with antimicrobial agents has been used in catheter-associated infections, but such treatment is seldom more than palliative and encourages infections with resistant organisms.

## Diarrhoea

Although *E. coli* is normally carried in the gut as a harmless commensal, it may cause gastrointestinal disease ranging in severity from mild, self-limiting diarrhoea to haemorrhagic colitis and the associated, potentially life-threatening, *haemolytic uraemic syndrome*. Such strains fall into at least five groups, each associated with specific serotypes (Table 26.2) and with different pathogenic mechanisms:

1. *Enteropathogenic E. coli* (EPEC), which cause infantile enteritis, especially in tropical countries.
2. *Enterotoxigenic E. coli* (ETEC), which are responsible for community-acquired diarrhoeal disease in areas of poor sanitation and are the most common cause of travellers' diarrhoea.
3. *Enteroinvasive E. coli* (EIEC), which cause an illness resembling shigella dysentery in patients of all ages.
4. *Verocytotoxin-producing E. coli* (VTEC), which cause symptoms ranging from mild, watery diarrhoea to haemorrhagic colitis and haemolytic uraemic syndrome.
5. *Enteroaggregative E. coli* (EAggEC), which cause chronic diarrhoeal disease in certain developing countries.

### Enteropathogenic E. coli *(EPEC)*

**Pathogenesis.** EPEC strains belonging to characteristic serogroups (Table 26.2) were originally identified epidemiologically as a cause of diarrhoeal disease in infants. Some such strains, notably serogroup O26, have acquired the genes for expression of

**Table 26.2** The major groups of diarrhoea-causing *E. coli*

| Pathogenic group | Common serogroups |
|---|---|
| Enteropathogenic *E. coli* (EPEC) | O26, O55, O86, O111, O114, O119, O125, O126, O127, O128, O142, O158 |
| Enterotoxigenic *E. coli* (ETEC) | O6, O8, O15, O25, O27, O63, O119, O125, O126, O127, O128, O142 |
| Enteroinvasive *E. coli* (EIEC) | O78, O115, O148, O153, O159, O167 |
| Verocytotoxin-producing *E. coli* (VTEC) | O26, O111, O112ac, O124, O136, O143, O144, O152, O157[a], O164 |
| Enteroaggregative *E. coli* (EAggEC) | More than 50 'O' serogroups |

[a]Other serogroups are far less common than O157 in human disease.

Verocytotoxin and are classified as VTEC (see below). EPEC may adhere to HEp-2 tissue culture cells in small discrete 'localized adhesion' clusters, a phenotype encoded by the adherence factor plasmid (pEAF); strains which carry the pEAF are termed 'typical' EPEC (tEPEC) while those without this plasmid are termed 'atypical' EPEC (aEPEC).

Colonization of the upper part of the small intestine occurs in infantile enteritis associated with EPEC. Electron microscopy of intestinal biopsy specimens shows that the bacteria become intimately associated with the mucosal surface and are partially surrounded by cup-like projections ('pedestals') of the enterocyte surface. In areas of EPEC attachment the brush border microvilli are lost. Adhesion to the gut wall and the subsequent mucosal damage has been termed an 'attaching and effacing' lesion. The genes responsible are located on a pathogenicity island located on the *E. coli* chromosome. EPEC use a novel mechanism of adhesion in which the receptor for the adhesin is synthesized by the bacteria and inserted in the host gut wall to provide a binding site. One of the proteins involved, intimin, is expressed on the bacterial cell surface as an adhesin; the other key protein, the translocated intimin receptor (Tir) is synthesised by the EPEC and inserted into the host cell membrane to allow intimin attachment. EPEC-associated toxins have not been detected.

**Laboratory diagnosis.** Stool specimens are plated on media such as MacConkey agar. Bacteria fermenting lactose are identified as *E. coli* and serotyped based on somatic and flagellar antigens. Strains belonging to EPEC-associated serogroups may be putative EPEC but detecting the *eae* genes by PCR can provide an accurate identification.

**Epidemiology.** Since 1971 few epidemics of EPEC enteritis have been reported in the UK or the USA, although a satisfactory explanation for the decline has not been put forward. Strains responsible for sporadic cases that continue to occur in the UK, especially in the summer months, possess the same pathogenic mechanisms as those that caused earlier outbreaks.

EPEC enteritis is common in communities with poor hygiene where sporadic cases and frequent outbreaks occur in the general community as well as in institutions. The importance of EPEC as a cause of enteritis in adults is difficult to evaluate because few laboratories perform the relevant tests.

### Enterotoxigenic E. coli *(ETEC)*

**Pathogenesis.** ETEC produce a heat-stable enterotoxin or a heat-labile enterotoxin, or both. In addition, they usually express fimbriae that are specific for

| Table 26.3 | Differential properties of heat-labile toxins (LT) of *E. coli* | |
|---|---|---|
| | LT-I | LT-II |
| Tissue culture changes[a] | ± | ± |
| Molecular weight (kDa) | | |
|    A subunit | 26 | 28 |
|    B subunit | 11.5 | 11.8 |
| Isoelectric point | 8.5 | 6.8[b], 5.4[c] |
| Genetic location | Plasmid | Chromosome |
| Action | Binds to gangliosides | Activates cAMP |

[a]Chinese hamster ovary, Y1 cells or Vero cells.
[b]LT-IIa.
[c]LT-IIb.
cAMP, cyclic adenosine monophosphate.

| Table 26.4 | Differential properties of heat-stable toxins (ST) of *E. coli* | |
|---|---|---|
| | ST-I (ST$_a$) | ST-II (ST$_b$) |
| Molecular weight (kDa) | 2 | 5 |
| Infant mouse test | + | − |
| Methanol | Soluble | Insoluble |
| Pig intestinal loop | + | + |
| Rabbit ileal loop | + | − |
| Rat gut loop | + | − |
| Action | Activates cGMP | Unknown (cyclic nucleotides) |

cGMP, cyclic guanosine monophosphate.

the host animal species and that enable the organisms to adhere to the epithelium of the small intestine. Infection is usually of brief duration, often beginning with the rapid onset of loose stools and accompanied by variable symptoms, including nausea, vomiting and abdominal cramps.

Heat-labile enterotoxin (LT) is closely related to the toxin produced by strains of *Vibrio cholerae*. There are two main forms, termed LT-I and LT-II (Table 26.3). Different forms of LT-I associated with human, porcine and chicken infection have been described; similarly, two forms of LT-II (LT-IIa and LT-IIb) have been detected. Although these toxins have a degree of structural variation, they are all subunit protein toxins comprising one A subunit and five B subunits with molecular weights of 26 000–28 000 Da and 11 500–11 800 Da, respectively. The mechanism by which diarrhoea is caused is identical to that of cholera toxin (see p. 315).

In contrast to LTs, the heat-stable enterotoxins (STs) of *E. coli* (Table 26.4) have a low molecular weight which confers heat stability and poor antigenicity. There are two major classes, designated ST-I (ST$_a$) and ST-II (ST$_b$). Variants of ST-I have been associated with porcine and human infections. ST-I is detected by immunoassay or by molecular genetic methods. This toxin activates guanylate cyclase activity, resulting in an increase in the level of cyclic guanosine monophosphate (cGMP). The activity of ST-I is rapid, whereas LTs act after a lag period. The mechanism of secretion caused by ST-I, via cGMP, is not fully understood but calcium appears to play a role. ST-I is plasmid encoded, and these plasmids may also encode the genes for LT, adhesive factors and antibiotic resistance.

ST-II is distinguished from ST-I by its biological activity and its insolubility in methanol. The mechanism of action is not known but it appears not to act via cyclic adenosine monophosphate (cAMP) or cGMP. Molecular methods have superseded animal models for detecting these organisms.

Enterotoxin alone is not sufficient to enable *E. coli* to cause diarrhoea. The organism must first bind to specific receptors on the mucosal surface of the epithelial cells of the small intestine This adhesion is usually mediated by fimbriae expressing *colonization factor antigens* (CFAs) or *coli surface* (CS) antigens. Plasmids that simultaneously carry genes for both CFAs and enterotoxin production have been described.

The first colonization factor to be recognized in *E. coli* was a fimbrial antigen, K88, controlled by a transferable plasmid. Several more have subsequently been found in human strains of ETEC and, no doubt, others remain to be discovered. The properties of some important colonization factors are shown in Table 26.5.

### Laboratory diagnosis

Tissue culture assays formerly used for detecting LT have been replaced by immunological techniques. Most laboratories now screen for LT-producing strains of *E. coli* by a rapid PCR test. Other tests include an enzyme-linked immunoabsorbent assay (ELISA) in which LT present in culture supernates is captured with gangliogide GM$_1$ and detected with toxin-specific rabbit antibodies; a precipitin test (the *Biken* test) on bacterial colonies growing on an agar medium containing rabbit antibodies specific for LT and commercial latex particle agglutination tests.

**Table 26.5** Properties of some important human colonization factors

| Colonization factor | Components | Mannose-resistant haemagglutinin | | | Fimbrial type | Associated toxin | Associated serogroups |
| | | Human | Bovine | Guinea-pig | | | |
| --- | --- | --- | --- | --- | --- | --- | --- |
| CFA-I | | + | + | – | Rod-like | ST or ST/LT | O4, O7, O15, O20, O25, O63, O78, O90, O104, O110, O126, O128, O136, O153, O159 |
| CFA-II | CS1 | (+) | + | – | Rod-like | ST/LT | O6, O139 |
| | CS2 | – | + | – | Rod-like | ST/LT | O6 |
| | CS3 | – | + | – | Fibrillar | ST/LT | O8, O78, O80, O85, O115, O128, O139, O168 |
| CFA-III | | – | – | – | Rod-like | LT | O25 |
| CFA-IV | CS4 | + | + | – | Rod-like | ST/LT | O25 |
| | CS5 | + | + | + | Helical | ST | O6, O29, O92, O114 |
| | CS6 | – | – | – | None | ST or LT | O115, O167, O25, O27, O79, O89, O92, O148, O153, O159, O169 |

(+), weak reaction; CS, coli surface antigen; LT heat-labile toxin; ST, heat-stable toxin.

ST toxin is usually detected by ELISA tests with specific monoclonal antibody.

*Epidemiology.* In developing countries ETEC is a major cause of death in children under the age of 5 years. These strains also commonly cause diarrhoea in travellers visiting countries where ETEC are endemic.

The sources and modes of spread of ETEC infection in countries with a warm climate are not well understood, but it seems likely that water contaminated by human or animal sewage plays an important part in the spread of infection.

## Enteroinvasive E. coli (EIEC)

*Pathogenesis.* EIEC, like *Shigella dysenteriae*-1 (see Ch. 25), cause disease by invading intestinal epithelium. Infection is by ingestion; only a small number of bacteria need to be swallowed as they are relatively resistant to gastric acid and bile, and pass readily into the large intestine where they multiply in the gut lumen. The bacteria pass through the overlying mucous layer, attach to the intestinal epithelial cells and are carried into the cell by endocytosis into an endocytic vacuole, which then lyses. The ability to cause the vacuole to lyse is an important virulence attribute, as organisms unable to do this cannot spread to neighbouring cells. After lysis of the vacuole the bacteria multiply within the epithelial cell and kill it. Spread to neighbouring cells leads to tissue destruction and consequent inflammation, which is the underlying cause of the symptoms of bacillary dysentery.

Pathogenicity depends on both chromosomal and plasmid genes. A large plasmid carries genes for the expression of outer membrane proteins that are required for invasion as well as genes necessary for the insertion of these proteins into the cell membrane. Plasmid genes are also required for the ability to escape from the endocytic vacuole and to invade contiguous host cells. Chromosomal genes encoding pathogenic mechanisms include those required for the expression of long-chain LPS and those encoding an aerobactin-mediated iron-sequestering system.

*Laboratory diagnosis.* The controversial Serény test, in which the bacteria are tested for the ability to cause conjunctivitis in guinea-pigs, and former tissue culture methods have been superseded by molecular techniques to detect the genes encoding the invasion plasmid antigen (*ipaH*) and aerobactin expression (*iuc*).

*Epidemiology.* The epidemiology and ecology of EIEC have been poorly studied, but there appears to be no evidence of an animal or environmental reservoir. Surveys suggest that they cause about 5% of all diarrhoeas in areas of poor hygiene. In the UK and USA, outbreaks are occasionally described, especially in schools and hospitals for the mentally handicapped. Infections are usually food-borne but there is also evidence of cross-infection. The most common serogroup is O124.

## Verocytotoxigenic E. coli (VTEC)

Strains of *E. coli* expressing a protein cytotoxic for Vero cells were discovered in 1977. Once epidemiologists were aware of VTEC, the importance of these bacteria in human disease became apparent and a link was established with two diseases of previously unknown aetiology: *haemorrhagic colitis* and *haemolytic uraemic syndrome*. Outbreaks were first recognized in the USA in 1982, and strains of VTEC belonging to serogroup O157 emerged as the major cause. Since then, outbreaks and sporadic cases have been reported in several other countries and VTEC belonging to many other serotypes have been described. Well publicized major episodes in the USA, Canada, Japan and Scotland have heightened general awareness of the importance of this disease.

**Pathogenesis.** Human VTEC infection is associated with a range of clinical symptoms from mild, non-bloody diarrhoea to the severe manifestations of haemolytic uraemic syndrome; a wide spectrum of illness can occur even within a single outbreak.

Haemorrhagic colitis is a grossly bloody diarrhoea, usually in the absence of pyrexia. It is usually preceded by abdominal pain and watery diarrhoea. Haemolytic uraemic syndrome is characterized by acute renal failure, micro-angiopathic haemolytic anaemia and thrombocytopenia. It occurs in all age groups, but is more common in infants and young children, and is a major cause of renal failure in childhood. The syndrome is usually associated with a prodromal bloody diarrhoea, but an 'atypical' form occurs without a diarrhoeal phase. It may be accompanied by thrombotic thrombocytopenic purpura in which the clinical features are further complicated by neurological involvement and fever.

VTEC have also been implicated as a cause of disease in animals, particularly calves and pigs.

The biological properties, physical characteristics and antigenicity of Verocytotoxin (VT) are very similar to those of Shiga toxin, produced by strains of *Sh. dysenteriae* type 1 (see p. 276), but the genes encoding VT in *E. coli* are carried on a lambda-like bacteriophage whereas those encoding Shiga toxin in *Sh. dysenteriae* type 1 are located on the chromosome. There are two antigenically distinct forms: VT1 and VT2. Antibodies prepared to VT1 neutralize Shiga toxin, whereas antibodies specific for VT2 do not. Variant forms of VT2 have been described in strains of human and porcine origin. The genes controlling production of these variant toxins are not phage encoded, and the toxin receptor also differs from that used by VT1 and VT2 (Table 26.6).

**Table 26.6** Differential properties of verocytotoxins expressed by *E. coli*

|  | VT1 | VT2 | VT2v[a] |
|---|---|---|---|
| Synonym | SLT1 | SLT2 | SLT2v |
| Cytotoxicity |  |  |  |
| Vero cells | + | + | + |
| HeLa cells | + | + | − |
| Molecular weight (kDa) |  |  |  |
| A subunit | 32 | 35 | 33 |
| B subunit | 7.7 | 10.7 | 7.5 |
| Genes phage-encoded | + | + | − |

[a]Human and porcine variants.

Like Shiga toxin, VT1 and VT2 comprise A and B subunits. For both toxins the A subunit possesses the biological activities of the toxin and the B subunits mediate specific binding and receptor-mediated uptake of the toxin. VT1 and VT2 bind to globotriosylceramide ($Gb_3$) molecules present on the surface of certain eukaryotic cells. In contrast VT2 variant toxins bind to globotetraosylceramide ($Gb_4$). During infection with VTEC the inflammatory mediators, tumour necrosis factor and interleukin-1, in combination with LPS, increase the number of ceramide receptors on the surface of eukaryotic cells, enhancing the binding of VT to these cells. Infection also results in expression of VT molecules that bind to $Gb_3$ receptors located in the kidneys, leading to haemolytic uraemic syndrome. Molecules of $Gb_3$ have been detected on mammalian erythrocytes that have $P^k$ antigens. About 75% of the human population carries this antigen, and such people may have protection from developing haemolytic uraemic syndrome.

VT1 and VT2, like Shiga toxin, are cytotoxic for Vero and HeLa cells, although certain VT2 variant toxins do not bind to HeLa cells, which do not express $Gb_3$ receptors.

VT causes a direct, dose-dependent, cytotoxic effect on human umbilical cord endothelial cells in culture; actively dividing cells are the most sensitive. Micro-angiopathy of the capillaries is a characteristic renal lesion in haemolytic uraemic syndrome, supporting the hypothesis that vascular endothelial cells are primary targets for VT.

Once bound to the eukaryotic cell surface, the holotoxin becomes internalized by host cells and remains active within endosomes. The toxin eventually reaches the Golgi apparatus by mechanisms as yet unknown. At some point within the host cell, the A subunit becomes enzymically 'nicked' to form portions $A_1$

(28 kDa) and A$_2$ (4 kDa); the A$_1$ portion of the toxin prevents protein synthesis and results in cell death.

Strains of O157 VTEC express an 'attaching and effacing' phenotype and, in common with strains of EPEC, the genes involved are located on a pathogenicity island located on the *E. coli* chromosome (see p. 283). Although the mechanisms of bacterial adhesion expressed by O157 VTEC are similar to those of EPEC, antigenic variation in, for example, the respective intimin and Tir proteins, has been detected. Owing to the similarity in structure between Verocytotoxin and Shiga-toxin expressed by *Shigella dysenteriae*-1, VTEC have been termed Shiga-toxin-producing *E. coli* or STEC; however this can be misleading since VT2 is quite distinct from VT1 and Shiga toxin. Similarly, strains of VTEC have been termed 'enterohaemorrhagic' owing to the symptoms of disease they cause, but since few strains of VTEC cause this form of disease the term must be used with caution.

***Laboratory diagnosis.*** The proportion of VTEC in the faecal flora may be low, often less than 1%, so that testing of individual colonies from culture plates may not always detect the pathogen. In foods or faecal extracts VTEC can be concentrated with immunomagnetic beads, small magnetic spheres coated with O157-specific rabbit antibodies which 'capture' the VTEC O157 and can be harvested with a magnet. The *vtx* genes encoding VT1 and VT2 can be detected with DNA probes and PCR. Electrophoretic and gene sequence analysis techniques provide strain discrimination and characterization in outbreaks of infection.

Although 95% of *E. coli* ferment sorbitol, O157 VTEC do so only slowly. This property is exploited by replacing the lactose present in MacConkey agar with sorbitol. Most strains of O157 VTEC produce colourless colonies after overnight incubation and these can be tested with an O157 LPS-specific antiserum in a simple agglutination assay. An O157-specific PCR assay has also been developed but putative strains of *E. coli* O157 should be confirmed by routine bacteriological examination and serotyping. Toxigenicity is confirmed by gene probes, by PCR, by testing strains for a cytotoxic effect on Vero cells or by a VT-specific ELISA.

Infection with VTEC O157 results in high levels of serum antibodies to the O157 LPS antigens but not to the flagellar proteins. These antibodies may be detected for several months after infection, providing valuable retrospective evidence of exposure or recovery from acute infection. Polyacrylamide gel electrophoresis and immunoblotting remain the most sensitive means of detecting antibodies to *E. coli* O157

**Fig. 26.2** Isolations of *E. coli* O157 in England and Wales. (Health Protection Agency Data.)

LPS, techniques which can also be used to detect salivary antibodies.

***Epidemiology.*** In England and Wales numbers of isolates of VTEC O157 have ranged from 361 cases in 1991 to a peak of 1087 cases in 1997 (Fig. 26.2). Outbreaks have occurred in the community, in nursing homes for the elderly, in day care centres for young children and following visits to petting farms. The most severe clinical manifestations are usually seen in the young and the elderly.

Food is an important source and outbreaks of disease due to VTEC O157 have been associated with hamburger meat, cooked meat products, unpasteurized apple juice, unpasteurized milk and radish sprouts. VTEC have also been isolated from healthy heifers on farms associated with milk-borne incidents, and it is now generally accepted that cattle are a major reservoir.

### Enteroaggregative E. coli (EAggEC)

EAggEC are characterized by their ability to adhere to tissue culture cells, such as HEp-2, in an aggregative or 'stacked brick' pattern, a property usually encoded on a 60-MDa plasmid. Such strains were first reported in 1987 as a cause of chronic diarrhoea in malnourished children in Chile, and were reported subsequently in many other countries. Occasional outbreaks have occurred in Europe, including the UK, and travellers to endemic regions may become infected. EAggEC may be present in the faeces of apparently healthy members of the population, but EAggEC diarrhoea is comparatively rare in industrialized countries.

***Pathogenesis.*** How EAggEC causes diarrhoea is poorly understood. Volunteer studies have failed to identify the infective dose, and the site of adhesion within the human host is not known. The characteristic pattern of adhesion to HEp-2 cells may be a putative pathogenic mechanism. Strains of EAggEC may express fimbriae, but adhesion to HEp-2 cells can also occur in the absence of these structures and for certain strains adhesion involves cell surface charge. Some, but not all, strains produce an ST-like toxin. Similarly, some isolates express haemolysins, an aerobactin-mediated high-affinity iron uptake system and a range of haemagglutinins; however, apart from the ability to adhere to HEp-2 cells in the stacked-brick formation, these strains are generally quite distinct.

***Epidemiology.*** Strains of EAggEC belong to very diverse combinations of O and H type, and even within an outbreak of diarrhoeal disease strains with several different serotypes may be isolated. The diversity of serotypes and pathogenic mechanisms observed suggests that the genes encoding the aggregative phenotype may be accepted readily by strains of commensal and potentially pathogenic strains of *E. coli*.

***Laboratory diagnosis.*** The pattern of adhesion to HEp-2 cells on a glass slide has been considered as the 'gold standard' for detecting EAggEC; however, since the bacteria also stick to the glass non-specifically, the significance of the adhesion assay has come into question. Aggregative adhesion gene probes and PCRs based on the *aat* genes, encoding the anti-aggregation protein transporter, have proved useful as rapid screening methods.

## Treatment and control of *E. coli* enteritis

### General measures

As with most diarrhoeal disease, the early administration of fluid and electrolytes is the most important single factor in preventing the death of the patient in severe infections. Antimicrobial drugs play a minor role. Despite the potentially serious consequences of VTEC infection, the use of antibiotics in this condition is controversial; certain antimicrobial drugs have been shown to increase expression of Verocytotoxin, so that administration of antibiotics may be counterproductive.

The most effective means of preventing infection is to avoid exposure to the infecting agent. Contaminated food and water are probably the most important vehicles of ETEC infection in developing countries. The provision of safe supplies of water together with education in hygienic practice in the handling and production of food particularly that given to young children, are essential. Travellers to countries with poor hygiene, especially in the tropics, should select eating places with care and, if possible, should consume only hot food and drinks, or bottled water. Self-peeled fruits are probably safe, but salads should be avoided. Unheated milk should always be considered unsafe.

The spread of infantile enteritis in hospitals and nurseries is mainly from patient to patient, generally on the hands of attendants, or from contaminated infant feeds. It can be prevented only by very strict hygiene. Infected patients, and recently admitted patients suspected of being infected, must be isolated by barrier nursing techniques to prevent faecal spread. In some cases outbreaks can be terminated only by closing the ward or nursery and cleaning thoroughly before reopening.

VTEC infections are acquired most frequently from meat, unpasteurized milk and direct contact with animals. Food-borne infections should be avoided by normal food hygiene with particular attention to processing and handling cooked meat products separately from raw meat, and the thorough cooking of raw meats, especially if minced.

### Vaccination

The most extensive studies of the use of vaccines have so far been in the veterinary field. Trials of a potential vaccine for human use, prepared by cross-linking a synthetically produced ST with the non-toxic B subunit of LT, were inconclusive.

### Inhibition of enterotoxin activity

Activated charcoal, bismuth subsalicylate and non-steroidal anti-inflammatory drugs inhibit or reverse the secretory effects of enterotoxins in experimental animals and may be of value in the prevention or treatment of diarrhoea.

An experimental silica-based compound designed to bind VT synthesized by bacteria in the intestine, preventing toxin from entering the patient's tissues has been advocated for infection with VTEC. However, as symptoms follow the effects of toxin, such treatment may have only limited value.

### Antimicrobial prophylaxis

Several antimicrobial drugs, including doxycycline, trimethoprim and fluoroquinolones reduce the incidence of diarrhoea in travellers to tropical areas. However, the widespread use of antibiotic prophylaxis has been criticized on the grounds of drug toxicity and because of the rick of encouraging the development and spread of drug resistance.

## OTHER *ESCHERICHIA* SPECIES

*E. blattae* was first described among bacteria isolated from the gut of the cockroach. It differs from *E. coli* in several ways and would probably be better placed in another genus. It has not been reported from human clinical specimens. *E. fergusonii, E. hermanii* and *E. vulneris* have been recovered from various clinical specimens, especially faeces and wounds, but their clinical significance is usually unclear.

RECOMMENDED READING

Chart H: Clinical significance of Verocytotoxin-producing *Escherichia coli* O157, *World Journal of Microbiology and Biochemistry* 16:719–724, 2001.

Chart H, Cheasty T: Human infections with Verocytotoxin-producing *Escherichia coli* O157 – 10 years of *E. coli* O157 serodiagnosis, *Journal of Medical Microbiology* 57:1389–1393, 2008.

Croxen MA, Finlay BB: Molecular Mechanisms of *Escherichia coli* pathogenicity, *Nature Reviews Microbiology* 8:26–38, 2010.

Deisingh AK, Thompson M: Strategies for the detection of *Escherichia coli* O157:H7, *Journal of Applied Microbiology* 96:419–429, 2004.

Gunn GJ, McKendrick IJ, Ternent HE, et al: An investigation of factors associated with the prevalence of verocytotoxin producing *Escherichia coli* O157 shedding in Scottish beef cattle, *The Veterinary Journal* 174:554–564, 2007.

Huang DB, Okhuysen PC, Jiang Z-D, DuPont HL: Enteroaggregative *Escherichia coli*: an emerging enteric pathogen, *American Journal of Gastroenterology* 99:383–389, 2004.

Jenkins C, Chart H, Willshaw GA, et al: Association of putative pathogenicity genes with adherence characteristics and fimbrial genotypes in typical enteroaggregative *Escherichia coli* from patients with and without diarrhoea in the United Kingdom, *European Journal of Clinical Microbiology and Infectious Disease* 26:901–906, 2007.

Jenkins C, Tembo M, Chart H, et al: Detection of enteroaggregative *Escherichia coli* in faecal samples from patients in the community with diarrhoea, *Journal of Medical Microbiology* 55:1493–1497, 2006.

Kaper JB, Nataro JP, Mobley HLT: Pathogenic *Escherichia coli*, *Nature Reviews: Microbiology* 2:123–140, 2004.

Lynn RM, O'Brien SJ, Taylor CM, et al: Childhood hemolytic uremic syndrome, United Kingdom and Ireland, *Emerging Infectious Diseases* 11:590–596, 2005.

Matthews L, McKendrick IJ, Ternent H, et al: Super-shedding cattle and the transmission dynamics of *Escherichia coli* O157, *Epidemiology and Infection* 134:131–142, 2006.

Sanchez J, Holmgren J: Virulence factors, pathogenesis and vaccine protection in cholera and ETEC diarrhea, *Current Opinions in Immunology* 17:1–11, 2005.

## Websites

Centers for Disease Control and Prevention: *Escherichia coli* infection. http://www.cdc.gov/ecoli/.

Health Protection Agency: Escherichia coli. http://www.hpa.org.uk/Topics/InfectiousDiseases/InfectionsAZ/EscherichiaColi/.

Health Protection Agency: *Escherichia coli* O157. http://www.hpa.org.uk/Topics/InfectiousDiseases/InfectionsAZ/EscherichiaColiO157/.

# Klebsiella, enterobacter, proteus and other enterobacteria

Pneumonia; urinary tract infection; opportunist infection

*H. Chart*

The genera described in this chapter conform to the general definition of the Enterobacteriaceae in that they are aerobic or facultatively anaerobic, ferment glucose and produce catalase but not oxidase. Together with organisms of the genera *Salmonella* (see Ch. 24), *Shigella* (see Ch. 25), *Escherichia* (see Ch. 26) and *Yersinia* (see Ch. 35), they are commonly referred to as enterobacteria. Species of clinical interest are listed alphabetically in Table 27.1, along with common synonyms.

## KLEBSIELLA

### CLASSIFICATION

The name *Klebsiella aerogenes* was originally used for the non-motile, capsulate, gas-producing strains commonly found in human faeces and in water; certain biochemically atypical *Klebsiella* strains isolated from the respiratory tract of man and animals were designated *K. pneumoniae*. The name *K. pneumoniae* is now used for the species as a whole, and the former *K. aerogenes* is referred to as *K. pneumoniae* subspecies *aerogenes*. The atypical respiratory strains are included in the subspecies *ozaenae, pneumoniae* and *rhinoscleromatis* (Table 27.1). A further species, *K. oxytoca*, is encountered occasionally in clinical specimens.

### DESCRIPTION

Klebsiellae are non-motile, capsulate Gram-negative rods about 1–2 μm long. They are facultative anaerobes, but growth under strictly anaerobic conditions is poor. They may survive drying for months and remain viable for many weeks at room temperature. Species can be differentiated by simple biochemical tests. Capsular material is produced in greater amounts on media rich in carbohydrate. In these conditions the growth on agar is luxuriant, greyish white and extremely mucoid (Fig. 27.1). The polysaccharides of the different capsular types are complex acid polysaccharides, and resemble the K antigens of *Escherichia coli* (see p. 280–1).

**Table 27.1** Principal genera and species of Enterobacteriaceae of clinical interest

| Genus | Species | Synonyms |
|-------|---------|----------|
| Citrobacter | Cit. amalonaticus | Levinea amalonatica |
| | Cit. freundii | |
| | Cit. koseri | C. diversus, L. amalonatica |
| Cronobacter | C. sakazakii | |
| Edwardsiella | E. tarda | E. anguillimortifera |
| Enterobacter | Ent. aerogenes | K. mobilis |
| | Ent. cloacae | |
| | Ent. agglomerans | Erwinia herbicola |
| Escherichia[a] | | |
| Hafnia | H. alvei | Ent. alvei, Ent. hafniae |
| Klebsiella | K. oxytoca | |
| | K. pneumoniae | |
| | ssp. aerogenes | K. aerogenes |
| | ssp. ozaenae | K. ozaenae |
| | ssp. pneumoniae | K. pneumoniae |
| | ssp. rhinoscleromatis | K. rhinoscleromatis |
| Morganella | M. morganii | Pr. morganii |
| Proteus | Pr. mirabilis | |
| | Pr. vulgaris | |
| Providencia | Prov. alcalifaciens | |
| | Prov. rettgeri | Pr. rettgeri |
| | Prov. stuartii | |
| Salmonella[a] | | |
| Serratia | S. liquefaciens | Ent. liquefaciens |
| | S. marcescens | |
| | S. odorifera | |
| Shigella[a] | | |
| Yersinia[a] | | |

[a]See appropriate chapter.

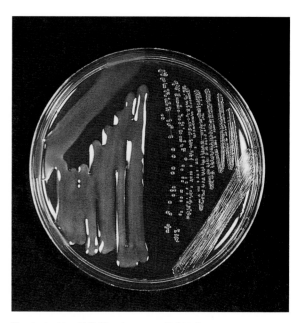

**Fig. 27.1** Mucoid (left) and non-mucoid (right) variants of *Klebsiella* species on carbohydrate-rich medium. (Courtesy of George Sharp and Richard Edwards, Queen's Medical Centre, Nottingham.)

## Antigenic structure

About 80 capsular (K) antigens are presently recognized. Types K1, K2, K3, K5 and K21 are of particular significance in human disease, and the prevalence of these types limits the usefulness of capsular serotyping as an epidemiological tool.

Strains express long-chain lipopolysaccharide (somatic or O antigens) and 12 O-types are recognized, although somatic antigen typing can be hampered by capsular polysaccharide layers. Certain O-antigens are identical to or related to *E. coli* O-antigens. It is therefore possible to divide *Klebsiella* strains into a small number of groups which may be further subdivided into capsular types, but this is of little practical value in classification.

There is some association between antigenic structure, biochemical activities and habitat. Members of capsular types 1–6 occur most frequently in the human respiratory tract. Considerable overlap occurs with capsular antigens of unrelated organisms; capsular type 2, for example, is immunologically similar to the type 2 pneumococcus.

## Typing methods

Many *Klebsiella* strains produce bacteriocins which are distinct from colicins of *E. coli*. They have a narrow range of activity on other klebsiellae and epidemiological analysis may be improved by the use of bacteriocins as an adjunct to capsular serotyping. Phage typing has also been used, and biotyping has been recommended instead of serotyping for use in less well-equipped laboratories.

Molecular typing methods include the polymerase chain reaction (PCR) with 16S-23S rDNA. Capsular antigens can be detected by means of the capsular 'swelling' reaction (p. 34), but various other techniques are used, including counter-current immunoelectrophoresis and enzyme-linked immunosorbent assay (ELISA).

## PATHOGENESIS

*Klebsiella* spp. are primarily a cause of infections involving the urinary tract but may also cause soft-tissue infections, endocarditis, central nervous system

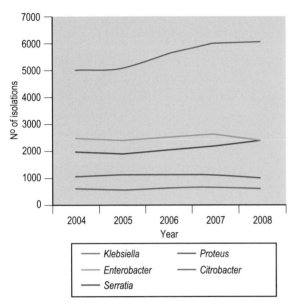

**Fig. 27.2** Isolations selected from Gram-negative bacilli bacteraemia. Laboratory reports for England, Wales and Northern Ireland 2004 to 2008. (Health Protection Agency data.)

infections, and cases of severe bronchopneumonia, sometimes with chronic destructive lesions and multiple abscess formation in the lungs (*Friedländer's pneumonia*). In many cases there is also bacteraemia (Fig. 27.2), and the mortality rate is high. This condition is usually but not always associated with capsular types 1–5, which are often biochemically atypical. Strains of *K. pneumoniae* expressing the K1 capsular antigens have emerged as a cause of pyogenic liver abscesses.

Colonization of the respiratory tract is very common in hospital patients receiving antibiotics, but its clinical significance is often difficult to assess. Some debilitated patients develop bronchopneumonia in which a *Klebsiella* spp. appears to be the primary infecting agent. Klebsiellae are naturally resistant to many antibiotics and readily acquire resistance to most others. The emergence of the species as an important cause of infection in hospitals is undoubtedly related to the use of antibiotics.

The *ozaenae* and *rhinoscleromatis* subspecies of *K. pneumoniae* take their names from the diseases with which they are associated. Rhinoscleroma is a chronic upper respiratory tract disease that occurs in many parts of the world, where it is associated with prolonged exposure to crowded and unhygienic conditions. The lesions occur in the nose, larynx, throat and, to a lesser extent, the trachea, and consist of granulomatous infiltrations of the submucosa. Ozaena

(atrophic rhinitis) is an uncommon, chronic disease of the nasal mucosa, in which *K. pneumoniae* ssp. *ozaenae* is of disputed significance.

## Pathogenic mechanisms

Expression of a polysaccharide capsule is a major pathogenic mechanism providing strains with protection against opsonization and the action of serum complement. Adhesion to host tissues has been attributed to the expression of a range of fimbrial and non-fimbrial adhesins. In common with other members of the Enterobacteriaceae, klebsiellae express type 1 fimbriae that exhibit mannose-sensitive haemagglutination and probably play a role in adhesion to the human host. Strains may also express type 3 fimbriae, which may be used to adhere to material in the environment. Additional fimbrial structures (type 6 and KPF-28) and non-fimbrial adhesins have been described. Adhesins CF29K and CS31A are plasmid-encoded and enable strains to adhere to cultured human intestinal cell lines. Such strains may also be invasive, a process which involves an outer membrane protein, OmpX.

In common with many enteric bacteria, klebsiellae express an enterobactin-mediated iron-sequestering system which uses ferric siderophore receptors antigenically related to those expressed by strains of *E. coli*. Less frequently strains of *Klebsiella* may also express an aerobactin-mediated high-affinity iron-uptake system, encoded on a plasmid. The importance of iron in infections with klebsiellae can be illustrated by the fact that strains are particularly virulent in patients with iron-overload conditions such as thalassaemia. Heat-labile and heat-stable toxins have been described in strains isolated from burns patients; however, the role played by these toxins in the pathogenesis of disease remains to be determined.

## TREATMENT

Clinical isolates of *Klebsiella* characteristically produce a β-lactamase that renders them resistant to ampicillin and amoxicillin, but combinations of these drugs with β-lactamase inhibitors such as clavulanic acid are usually effective. Klebsiellae are normally susceptible to cephalosporins, especially β-lactamase-stable derivatives such as cefuroxime and cefotaxime, and to fluoroquinolones. Resistance to chloramphenicol and tetracyclines varies from strain to strain; they are often sensitive to gentamicin and other aminoglycosides, but transferable enzymic resistance to aminoglycosides is common in some hospitals.

Multi-resistant strains of *Klebsiella* species sometimes cause serious hospital infection problems.

Klebsiella infection of the urine often responds to trimethoprim, nitrofurantoin, co-amoxiclav or oral cephalosporins. Pneumonia and other serious infections require vigorous treatment with an aminoglycoside or a cephalosporin such as cefotaxime.

Attempts to produce protective vaccines have so far proved fruitless.

## ENTEROBACTER

### DESCRIPTION

*Enterobacter* species have many features in common with those of the genus *Klebsiella*, but are readily distinguished by their motility, although non-motile variants occur occasionally. *Ent. cloacae* is clinically the most important species. *Ent. agglomerans*, an anaerogenic, yellow-pigmented organism, formerly known as *Erwinia herbicola*, is also encountered occasionally. Strains of *Ent. amnigenus* and *Ent. asburiae* have also been isolated from human infections.

The colonies of *Enterobacter* strains may be slightly mucoid. In general, their fermentative activity is more limited than that of typical klebsiellae. Serotyping and phage typing schemes have been developed to characterize strains of *Ent. cloacae,* with numerous O- and H-types currently recognized. Outbreak strains have been characterized using pulsed-field gel electrophoresis.

### PATHOGENESIS

The normal habitat of *Enterobacter* spp. is probably soil and water, but the organisms are occasionally found in human faeces and the respiratory tract. Infection of hospital patients, notably of the urinary tract, occurs. *Enterobacter* spp. are also an important cause of bacteraemia, but much less so than *Klebsiella* spp (Fig. 27.2).

The pathogenic mechanisms are poorly understood. In common with certain strains of *Klebsiella*, they express type 1 and type 3 fimbriae. Most strains also express an aerobactin-mediated iron-uptake system, which is generally associated with extra-intestinal human bacterial pathogens. Strains may produce a haemolysin resembling the α-haemolysin produced by strains of *E. coli*. Very rarely strains hybridize with gene probes for Verocytotoxin 1 (see p. 286).

An outer membrane protein, termed OmpX, may be a pathogenic factor for strains of *Ent. cloacae*. This protein appears to reduce production of porins, leading to decreased sensitivity to β-lactam antibiotics, and might play a role in host cell invasion.

### TREATMENT

*Enterobacter* strains produce a chromosomal β-lactamase with cephalosporinase activity and are nearly always highly resistant to penicillins and many cephalosporins. Many are also resistant to tetracyclines, chloramphenicol and streptomycin, although most are sensitive to other aminoglycosides, including gentamicin. Most strains are susceptible to fluoroquinolones, co-trimoxazole and carbapenems. *Enterobacter* strains differ from *Serratia* strains in being sensitive to the polymyxins.

## CRONOBACTER

### DESCRIPTION

*Chronobacter sakazakii* is one of several related species and subspecies of *Cronobacter* formerly included with the genus *Enterobacter*. Strains can be detected by 16S-23S rRNA gene sequencing.

### PATHOGENESIS

*C. sakazakii* is an emerging pathogen associated with powdered milk, causing necrotizing enterocolitis, sepsis and meningitis in infants. In England, Wales and Northern Ireland, 72 cases of bacteraemia were identified in 2004, declining to 30 in 2008. The mechanisms by which disease is caused appear to include adhesion to the host tissues, multiplication within host tissues and possibly toxins.

### TREATMENT AND CONTROL

Disease usually responds to treatment with ampicillin and gentamicin. Infections associated with powdered milk can be prevented by sterilization of the milk products during production by irradiation or other means. Avoidance of consumption of dried milk by breastfeeding obviates the risk.

## HAFNIA

### DESCRIPTION

*Hafnia alvei* was also formerly placed in the genus *Enterobacter*. At present the genus contains only one species.

Strains of *H. alvei* are motile, non-capsulate, Gram-negative rods that grow well on general laboratory media at 30–37°C and can be differentiated by biotyping. There is an antigenic scheme for *H. alvei* that includes many serotypes and strains can be characterized further by phage-typing.

### PATHOGENESIS

Strains are found in the faeces of man and other animals, and also in sewage, soil, water and dairy products. *H. alvei* is encountered in blood, urine or wounds of hospital patients as an opportunist pathogen. Strains express mannose-resistant and mannose-sensitive haemagglutination indicating expression of type-1 fimbriae. A siderophore-mediated high-affinity iron uptake mechanism has been described and the bacteria can utilize siderophores expressed by strains of *E. coli*. Some strains can cause 'attaching and effacing' lesions of intestinal cells, as described for strains of enteropathogenic *E. coli* (EPEC; see p. 283).

### TREATMENT

Strains are usually sensitive to carbapenems, chloramophenicol, quinolones, aminoglycosides and trimethoprim, but resistant to penicillins.

## SERRATIA

### DESCRIPTION

Although numerous *Serratia* species have been described, *S. marcescens* is the one most commonly encountered in clinical specimens. Several others, including *S. liquefaciens* (formerly known as *Ent. liquefaciens*) and *S. odorifera*, are sometimes isolated.

*Serratia* spp. are motile Gram-negative rods that grow well on laboratory media at 30–37°C and utilize most carbohydrates with the production of acid and gas. They vary considerably in size, ranging from small coccobacilli to rods indistinguishable from other enterobacteria. Capsules are not normally formed, except on a well aerated medium poor in nitrogen and phosphate. Certain strains of *S. marcescens* produce red-pigmented colonies on agar. The pigment, prodigiosin, is formed only in the presence of oxygen and at a suitable temperature, which is not necessarily the same as that for optimal growth. Certain organisms unrelated to *S. marcescens*, including an actinomycete and certain Gram-negative rods isolated from seawater, also form prodigiosin.

### Typing methods

Several typing methods have been developed, including bacteriocin and phage typing. Strains may also be differentiated by electrophoretic and molecular methods, such as PCR, ribotyping and pulsed-field gel electrophoresis. Plasmid typing has been used, but not all strains carry plasmids.

### PATHOGENESIS

*S. marcescens* and other *Serratia* species are widely distributed in nature, but faecal carriage is uncommon in the general human population. Pigmented strains may cause concern by giving rise to red colours in food or by simulating the appearance of blood in the sputum or faeces. Pigmented and non-pigmented strains are found occasionally in the human respiratory tract and in faeces. Most infections occur in hospital patients; they include infections of the urinary and respiratory tracts, meningitis, wound infections, septicaemia (Fig. 27.2) and endocarditis. Some strains become established endemically in hospitals and may cause outbreaks of infection. *Serratia* spp. can multiply at ambient temperatures in fluids containing minimal nutrients, and outbreaks have followed the introduction of the organisms directly into the bloodstream in contaminated transfusion fluids. Only a small proportion of the strains responsible for infection are pigmented.

### Pathogenic mechanisms

*Serratia* spp. may express a range of fimbriae including those exhibiting mannose-sensitive and mannose-resistant haemagglutination, although the tissue specificity of these adhesins is unknown. Some strains express cell surface components causing them to be highly hydrophobic, and this may be involved in adhesion to eukaryotic cell surfaces. The expression of long-chain LPS has been described as a pathogenic mechanism for *S. marcescens*. A 56-kDa protease, which may be involved in host tissue damage, has been detected in virulent strains of *S. marcescens*. An iron-regulated haemolysin has been described, but a role for this toxin in the pathogenesis of disease has not been demonstrated. *Serratia* spp. also expresses an enterobactin-mediated high-affinity iron-uptake system and some may acquire ferric ions mediated by aerobactin. Toxins resembling *E. coli* verocytotoxin and heat-labile toxin have been described.

## TREATMENT

*Serratia* strains are commonly resistant to cephalosporins. Resistance to ampicillin and gentamicin is variable, but many strains destroy these antibiotics enzymically. An aminoglycoside, such as gentamicin, is usually the most reliable first-line choice. Fluoroquinolones or carbapenems may be useful in recalcitrant cases.

**Fig. 27.3** Swarming growth of *Pr. mirabilis* inoculated centrally on to a blood agar plate and incubated overnight at 37°C. (Courtesy of George Sharp and Richard Edwards, Queen's Medical Centre, Nottingham.)

## *PROTEUS* AND RELATED GENERA

## CLASSIFICATION

The history of the genera *Proteus, Providencia* and *Morganella* is inextricably linked, and they are best considered together.

There has been much debate over the taxonomy of this group, with successive proposals to combine and separate the genera *Proteus* and *Providencia*. The organisms once known as biotypes A and B of *Proteus inconstans* are now regarded as separate species of the genus *Providencia: Providencia alcalifaciens* and *Prov. stuartii*. Similarly, *Proteus rettgeri* is now known as *Prov. rettgeri*, even though it resembles *Proteus* spp. rather than other organisms of the genus *Providencia* in producing urease. The former *Pr. morganii* has been allocated to a new genus, *Morganella*, and is known as *Morganella morganii*. This leaves only *Pr. vulgaris* and *Pr. mirabilis* in the genus *Proteus*.

much like that of other coliform bacteria. Strains of *Proteus* spp. can be differentiated from *Morganella* spp. and *Providentia* spp. by their ability to swarm on suitable agar media; the swarming characteristically takes place in a discontinuous manner, with each period of outward progress followed by a stationary period (Fig. 27.3). Various methods have been devised to inhibit swarming, mainly to avoid interference with the isolation of clinically more important organisms.

The various species are differentiated by standard biochemical tests.

Phage-typing, bacteriocin-typing and serotyping schemes are used for strain descrimination. Swarming *Proteus* strains exhibit the Dienes phenomenon (the mutual inhibition of swarming), and this forms the basis for a precise method of differentiation among such strains. Test organisms are inoculated on to the surface of an agar plate, and those that show no line of demarcation in areas where the swarming growths meet are regarded as identical.

## DESCRIPTION

There is considerable morphological variation, but in agar-grown cultures the microscopical appearance is

## PATHOGENESIS

*Pr. mirabilis* is a prominent cause of urinary tract infection in children and of bacteraemia (Fig. 27.2).

Other strains of *Proteus* and *Providencia* are usually isolated from hospital patients, especially in elderly men following surgery or instrumentation. Septicaemia generally occurs only in patients with serious underlying conditions or as a complication of urinary tract surgery, but outbreaks of septicaemia, often with meningitis, may occur among the newborn in hospitals. A variety of other infections, usually of surgical wounds or bedsores, occur in hospitals and are usually considered to originate from the gut flora.

*M. morganii* is uncommon in human disease but occasionally causes infections in hospital patients.

## Pathogenic mechanisms

These bacteria are characteristically highly motile and chemotaxis may play a part in pathogenesis. Strains of *Proteus* spp. express mannose-resistant haemagglutination and may also produce calcium-dependent and calcium-independent haemolysins in addition to a range of proteases such as an IgAase. *M. morganii* exhibits mannose-sensitive haemagglutination and expresses phenolate and hydroxamate siderophores for high-affinity iron uptake.

*Proteus* spp. and other urease-producing organisms create alkaline conditions in the urine and may provoke the formation of calculi (stones) in the urinary tract.

## TREATMENT

Most strains of *Pr. mirabilis* do not produce β-lactamase; they are consequently moderately sensitive to benzylpenicillin and fully sensitive to ampicillin and most other β-lactam antibiotics. *Pr. vulgaris* strains are usually resistant to penicillins and many cephalosporins, although they may be sensitive to β-lactamase-stable derivatives such as cefotaxime. All strains are resistant to polymyxins and tetracyclines. *Proteus* and *Providencia* strains are inherently sensitive to aminoglycosides, but enzymic or non-enzymic resistance mechanisms are now common.

*Pr. mirabilis* urinary tract infections usually respond to ampicillin or trimethoprim but nitrofurantoin is not effective. Treatment of infection associated with renal stones is often unsuccessful. Serious infection with other *Proteus, Providencia* or *Morganella* strains can often be treated with an aminoglycoside or a cephalosporin such as cefotaxime. However, susceptibility is unpredictable and treatment should be guided by laboratory findings.

## CITROBACTER

## DESCRIPTION

The genus *Citrobacter* was first proposed for a group of lactose-negative or late lactose-fermenting Gram-negative bacilli that share certain somatic antigens with salmonellae and were also known as the Ballerup-Bethesda group. These organisms are now known as *Citrobacter freundii*. Other species included in the genus are *Cit. koseri* (formerly known as *Cit. diversus*) and *Cit. amalonaticus*. They grow well on ordinary media and are unpigmented. Mucoid forms sometimes occur.

Serotyping schemes based on the LPS antigens have been developed for *Cit. freundii* and *Cit. koseri*. Antigen–antibody cross-reactions between strains of *Citrobacter* spp. and strains of *Salmonella* and *E. coli* have been described. For example, certain strains of *Cit. freundii* share LPS epitopes with *E. coli* expressing O157 antigens.

## PATHOGENESIS

*Citrobacter* spp. are often found in human faeces and may be isolated from a variety of clinical specimens. They do not often give rise to serious infections but may cause bacteraemia (Fig. 27.2).

*Cit. koseri* occasionally causes neonatal meningitis; in this condition there is a high mortality rate and the formation of cerebral abscesses is common.

Pathogenic mechanisms expressed by strains of *Citrobacter* spp. are poorly understood. Strains of *Cit. koseri* express type 1 (mannose-sensitive) fimbriae and occasional strains produce a form of *E. coli*, Verocytotoxin type 2.

## TREATMENT

*Cit. freundii* is usually sensitive to aminoglycosides, fluoroquinolones and chloramphenicol; sensitivity to ampicillin, tetracycline and cephalosporins varies. Resistance to aminoglycosides occurs frequently among *Cit. koseri* strains. Choice of treatment should be based on laboratory tests of susceptibility.

## EDWARDSIELLA

*Edwardsiella tarda, E. hoshinae* and *E. ictaluri* belong to a group of enterobacteria with distinctive properties, originally described as the 'Asakusa group'. Members of the genus are small, motile, facultatively anaerobic Gram-negative rods. They are facultative anaerobes and grow optimally at 37°C. Strains are biochemically inactive compared with other members of the Enterobacteriaceae but will utilize glucose. They grow well on ordinary media but produce only small colonies 0.5–1 mm in diameter after 24 h.

*Edwardsiella* spp. are principally associated with freshwater environments and can be isolated from healthy amphibia, reptiles and fish. *E. tarda* is most frequently associated with human disease. Two biotypes of *E. tarda* exist in nature with most human infections caused by biotype 2. Wound infection is most common, but meningitis and septicaemia have been reported. This bacterium is rarely found in the faeces of healthy people, but a higher isolation rate has been found in patients with diarrhoea. Some strains produce a heat-stable toxin causing fluid accumulation in the infant mouse test developed for detecting *E. coli* heat-stable toxin I.

## OTHER GENERA

Various other Gram-negative bacilli, more or less related to those described in this chapter, surface occasionally in clinical specimens, usually from seriously ill, immunologically vulnerable patients. Identification is best left to specialist reference laboratories. Where a pathogenic role is suspected, priority should be given to the often unpredictable antimicrobial susceptibility pattern of the isolate so that appropriate treatment can be started quickly.

RECOMMENDED READING

Baumgartner A, Grand M, Liniger M, Iversen C: Detection and frequency of *Cronobacter* spp. (*Enterobacter sakazakii*) in different categories of ready-to-eat foods other than infant formula, *International Journal of Food Microbiology* 136:189–192, 2009.

Janda JM, Abbott SL: The genus *Hafnia*: from soup to nuts, *Clinical Microbiology Reviews* 19:12–18, 2006.

Kurz CL, Chauvet S, Andrès E, et al: Virulence factors of the human opportunistic pathogen *Serratia marcescens* identified by *in vivo* screening, *European Molecular Biology Organization Journal* 22:1451–1460, 2003.

Lund BM, Sussman M, Jones D, Stringer MR, editors: *Enterobacteriaceae in the Environment and as Pathogens*, Society of Applied Bacteriology Symposium Series, No. 17, Oxford, 1988, Blackwell Scientific (published as a supplement to *Journal of Applied Bacteriology* 65).

O'Hara CM, Brenner FW, Miller JM: Classification, identification and clinical significance of *Proteus, Providencia*, and *Morganella, Clinical Microbiology Reviews* 13:534–546, 2000.

Podschun R, Ullmann U: *Klebsiella* spp. as nosocomial pathogens: epidemiology, taxonomy, typing methods, and pathogenicity factors, *Clinical Microbiology Reviews* 11:589–603, 1998.

Williams P, Tomas JM: The pathogenicity of *Klebsiella pneumoniae*, *Reviews in Medical Microbiology* 1:196–204, 1990.

### Websites

Health Protection Agency: *Bacteraemia*. http://www.hpa.org.uk/infections/topics_az/bacteraemia/menu.htm.

MicrobeWiki: Enterobacter. http://microbewiki.kenyon.edu/index.php/Enterobacter.

Virtual museum of bacteria: Klebsiella pneumoniae. http://www.bacteriamuseum.org/species/Kpneumoniae.shtml.

# 28 Pseudomonads and non-fermenters

Opportunist infection; cystic fibrosis; melioidosis

*J. R. W. Govan*

## KEY POINTS

- Pseudomonads are aerobic, saprophytic and innately resistant bacteria causing opportunist infections in man, animals, plants and insects. The most important pseudomonad species responsible for human infections are *Pseudomonas aeruginosa*, *Burkholderia pseudomallei* and members of the *Burkholderia cepacia* complex.
- *Pseudomonas aeruginosa* is an important cause of hospital-acquired infections, especially in intensive care units and in neutropenic patients. Infections range from topical to systemic and may be trivial or life-threatening.
- Mucoid forms of *Ps. aeruginosa* are a major cause of chronic debilitating and life-threatening respiratory infections in individuals with cystic fibrosis.
- *Burkholderia pseudomallei* is the causative agent of melioidosis, a serious tropical infection of man and animals endemic in South-East Asia and Northern Australia.
- The *Burkholderia cepacia* complex causes life-threatening pulmonary infections in individuals with cystic fibrosis or chronic granulomatous disease.
- The term 'glucose non-fermenters' includes *Acinetobacter* spp. and describes a group of saprophytes that are distinct from the oxidative pseudomonads. They cause hospital-acquired opportunist infections, particularly in intensive care units.

*In wine there is truth, in beer there is strength, in water there are pseudomonads!*

(adaptation of German proverb)

The term *pseudomonads* describes a large diverse group of aerobic, non-fermentative, Gram-negative bacilli, originally contained within the genus *Pseudomonas*. Presently, the group comprises more than 100 species. Most are saprophytes found widely in aquatic environments, including rivers and ponds, in the rhizosphere of plants, and in a variety of other moist environments. The group includes important pathogens for man, animals, plants and insects.

Historically, the genus *Pseudomonas* has been used as a taxonomic dumping ground for novel species, often with diverse phenotypic characteristics. However, comprehensive analyses of the group have led to revised classifications, and many pseudomonads of clinical interest have been allocated to new genera including *Burkholderia, Brevundimonas, Delftia, Ralstonia, Pandoraea* and *Stenotrophomonas* (Table 28.1).

*Pseudomonas aeruginosa* is the species most commonly associated with human disease but *Burkholderia pseudomallei* has long been recognized as an important pathogen in tropical countries. Members of the *Burkholderia cepacia* complex are important pathogens in immunocompromised patients, particularly in individuals with cystic fibrosis or chronic granulomatous disease. *Stenotrophomonas maltophilia* also infects immunocompromised patients, with a mortality rate reaching 60% in patients with haematological malignancies. Several other pseudomonads are occasionally isolated from clinical specimens as true opportunistic pathogens; these include *Ps. fluorescens, Ps. putida, Ps. stutzeri* and various 'glucose non-fermenters'. In immunocompromised patients, it is important to distinguish whether culture of these bacteria reflects invasive infection rather than transitory colonization.

There are several reasons for the pre-eminence of *Ps. aeruginosa* as an opportunistic human pathogen:

- its adaptability
- its innate resistance to many antibiotics and disinfectants
- its armoury of putative virulence factors
- an increasing supply of patients compromised by age, underlying disease or immunosuppressive therapy.

**Fig. 28.1** Genome size of *Burkholderia cepacia* compared with that of *Haemophilus influenzae* and *Escherichia coli*.

**Table 28.1** The principal genera and species of pseudomonads of clinical interest

| Genus | Species |
|---|---|
| Pseudomonas | Ps. aeruginosa |
| | Ps. fluorescens |
| | Ps. putida |
| | Ps. stutzeri |
| | Ps. mendocina |
| Burkholderia | B. pseudomallei |
| | B. mallei |
| | B. cepacia complex[a] |
| | B. gladioli |
| Delftia | D. acidovorans |
| Comamonas | C. testosteroni |
| Stenotrophomonas | Sten. maltophilia |
| Ralstonia | R. pickettii |
| Brevundimonas | Brev. diminuta |
| Pandoraea | P. apista |

[a]See text pp. 303–4.

The *Ps. aeruginosa* genome is unusually large (6.3 Mb); *Burkholderia pseudomallei* (7.2 Mb) and *B. cepacia* (7.7 Mb) have even bigger, multi-replicon genomes, equalling those of protozoa (Fig. 28.1). Genomic and proteomic studies are providing valuable insights into the versatility, virulence and resistance of these important pathogens; e.g., analysis of hypervirulent *Ps. aeruginosa* has led to the identification of novel and sometimes chimeric 'pathogenicity islands'.

## PSEUDOMONAS AERUGINOSA

### DESCRIPTION

*Ps. aeruginosa* is a non-sporing, non-capsulate, non-fastidious Gram-negative bacillus; it is usually motile by virtue of one or two polar flagella. It is a strict aerobe but can grow anaerobically if nitrate is available as a terminal electron acceptor. The organism grows readily on a wide variety of culture media, over a wide temperature range, and emits a sweet grape-like odour that is easily recognized. Most strains produce diffusible pigments; typically, the colony and surrounding medium is greenish-blue due to production of a soluble blue phenazine pigment, *pyocyanin*, and the yellow–green fluorescent pigment *pyoverdin*; additional pigments include *pyorubrin* (red) and *melanin* (brown). Some isolates (10–15%) produce pigment only when grown on pigment-enhancing media. Individual colonies vary from dwarf to large mucoid types; most commonly, they are relatively large and flat with an irregular surface, a translucent edge and an oblong shape with the long axis parallel to the line of inoculum.

*Ps. aeruginosa* differs from members of the Enterobacteriaceae by deriving energy from carbohydrates by an oxidative rather than a fermentative metabolism. The species is inactive in carbohydrate fermentation tests, and only glucose is utilized. However, all strains give a rapid positive oxidase reaction (within 30 s) and this is a useful preliminary test for non-pigmented isolates.

Typing of *Ps. aeruginosa* isolates for epidemiological purposes originally relied on serotyping, susceptibility to phages and bacteriocin production. These techniques have been superseded by molecular typing methods, including DNA fingerprinting by pulsed-field gel electrophoresis of *Xba*1 or *Spe*1 restriction endonuclease digests (currently the 'gold standard') and multilocus sequence typing (see Ch. 3).

## PATHOGENESIS

*Ps. aeruginosa* is pathogenic for a wide range of animal, plant and insect hosts. In man, it can infect almost any anatomical surface or organ causing an expanding spectrum of infections with variable morbidity and mortality. Community infections are uncommon and usually mild, but in hospital and other healthcare settings, *Ps. aeruginosa* infections are more common, more varied and more severe.

### Community infections

Infections such as otitis externa and varicose ulcers are often chronic, but not disabling. In contrast, corneal infections, in particular keratitis resulting from contaminated contact lenses or other sources, are extremely painful and can be rapidly destructive. Recreational and occupational factors associated with

*Ps. aeruginosa* infections include the relatively mild whirlpool or Jacuzzi® rash (an acute self-limiting folliculitis) and serious industrial eye injuries, which may lead to panophthalmitis.

## Hospital infections

Infections in hospital or other healthcare settings can be localized, as in catheter-related urinary tract infection, infected ulcers, bedsores, burns and eye infections. However, in vulnerable patients compromised by age or diseases such as leukaemia, acquired immune deficiency syndrome (AIDS), and chemotherapy-induced neutropenia, pseudomonas infections often become bacteraemic and the organism may be cultured from various organs post mortem. *Ps. aeruginosa* septicaemia or necrotizing pneumonia, though uncommon, is associated with a high mortality rate in neutropenic patients. Patients in critical care units are at particular risk; *Ps. aeruginosa* is the second most common cause of ventilator-associated pneumonia. Septicaemic infections are uniquely characterized by the black necrotic skin lesions known as *ecthyma gangrenosum*.

## Cystic fibrosis

The lungs of individuals with cystic fibrosis are particularly susceptible to life-threatening infections caused by *Ps. aeruginosa* and members of the *Burkholderia cepacia* complex. Initial pulmonary infection with typical non-mucoid forms of *Ps. aeruginosa* occurs in early childhood and is often asymptomatic. This is followed by the emergence of mucoid alginate-producing variants, which grow within protective bacterial biofilms or microcolonies, and are associated with a damaging inflammatory response (Fig. 28.2). Subsequent repeated and debilitating episodes of pulmonary exacerbation are the main cause of morbidity and mortality. Once transition to the mucoid phenotype has occurred, eradication of *Ps. aeruginosa* is seldom if ever achieved. Although not so well recognized, a similar transition to mucoidy occurs in patients with chronic bronchiectasis caused by *Ps. aeruginosa*.

## Virulence factors

Most isolates of *Ps. aeruginosa* exhibit an armoury of cell-associated and extracellular virulence factors that can initiate or maintain infection. These include exotoxin A and exoenzyme S, and various cytotoxic proteases, phospholipases and rhamnolipids, as well as hydrogen cyanide and the toxic pigment pyocyanin.

**Fig. 28.2**  Gram-stained sputum from patient harbouring mucoid *Ps. aeruginosa*. Note spawn-like microcolony and adjacent phagocytes. (Original magnification ×400.)

The intracellular action of exotoxin A is similar to that of diphtheria toxin fragment A (see Ch. 17). Fluorescein provides *Ps. aeruginosa* with a potent bacterial siderophore to compete with mammalian iron-binding proteins such as transferrin. In association with pyocyanin, this also explains the characteristic blue–green pus of pseudomonas-infected wounds.

*Ps aeruginosa* exhibits highly evolved sensory systems, including quorum sensing, that allow regulation and coordinate expression of multiple virulence factors; also various export systems, most importantly a type III secretion system that allows injection of toxin or damaging effector proteins directly into the cytoplasm of host cells. The alginate-like exopolysaccharide, composed of D-mannuronic acid and L-guluronic acid, which is responsible for the mucoid colonial phenotype (Fig. 28.3), acts as a further virulence determinant.

The individual importance of these virulence factors depends upon the site and nature of infection:

- The direct action of proteases and the indirect activation of an excessive inflammatory response through bacterial flagella and lipopolysaccharide play important roles in corneal ulceration.
- Exotoxin and proteases (in particular elastase) are important in burn infections and septicaemia.
- Alginate and quorum sensing molecules are associated with the formation and architecture of biofilms within airways that are associated with debilitating chronic pulmonary infection in patients with cystic fibrosis or bronchiectasis.
- Pyochelin and pyoverdin act as important siderophores.

**Fig. 28.3** Alcohol extraction of alginate from mucoid *Ps. aeruginosa*.

## LABORATORY DIAGNOSIS

Material should be cultured on a selective medium that enhances the production of pyocyanin to aid detection. A selective medium containing acetamide as the sole carbon and nitrogen source may be used for enrichment from water or soil. About 10–15% of isolates do not produce detectable pigment even on suitable media; in such cases, a positive oxidase test provides rapid presumptive evidence of the identity. Presumptive identification of isolates exhibiting atypical phenotypic features can be made with an appropriate commercial multitest system.

Various reliable polymerase chain reaction (PCR) assays are also available. Tests for serum antibodies against pseudomonas antigens have no place in diagnosis except in patients with cystic fibrosis or chronic obstructive pulmonary disease, where detection of increasing precipitating antibodies correlates directly with immune-mediated lung damage.

## TREATMENT

Treatment of *Ps aeruginosa* infection remains challenging. Most isolates are intrinsically resistant to commonly used antimicrobial agents, and this problem is exacerbated by strains exhibiting acquired and mutational resistance to agents with antipseudomonal activity. Multidrug resistant strains are increasingly common.

Aminoglycosides (gentamicin, amikacin and tobramycin) and β-lactam compounds (piperacillin, ticarcillin, ceftazidime and carbapenems) are often used, alone or in combination. Combinations provide the potential for antibacterial synergy and reduced antibiotic resistance, but there is little evidence of clinical superiority. Fluoroquinolones such as ciprofloxacin exhibit good activity against *Ps. aeruginosa* and penetrate well into most tissues, but resistance may develop. Unlike most antipseudomonal agents, ciprofloxacin can be given orally. Monotherapy with broad-spectrum β-lactam agents such as ceftazidime and imipenem is possible but resistance occurs rapidly; thus monotherapy should be avoided in the treatment of chronic infections. In patients presenting with acute febrile neutropenia, empiric antimicrobial therapy should include at least one antipseudomonal antibiotic.

Polymyxins, though nephrotoxic, show good activity against *Ps. aeruginosa* and resistance is unusual. Interest in these agents has been revived as a 'treatment of last resort' for multiresistant *Ps. aeruginosa*. Aerosolized delivery of colistin (polymyxin E) or tobramycin directly into the lungs has proved safe and clinically effective in the management of *Ps. aeruginosa* lung infection in individuals with cystic fibrosis. New formulations of tobramycin, colistin, ciprofloxacin, and amikacin that are suitable for aerosol delivery may provide improved treatment options in cystic fibrosis and other lung infections.

The results of trials of multicomponent pseudomonas conjugate vaccines in the management of cystic fibrosis lung disease have been disappointing.

## EPIDEMIOLOGY

The ability of *Ps. aeruginosa* to persist and multiply in moist environments and equipment including sinks, drains, flower vases, hydrotherapy pools, ponds, rivers, humidifiers, washing machines and even in distilled water, is of particular importance in infection control. Consumption of salad vegetables contaminated with pseudomonas is a potential risk for immunocompromised patients in intensive care units. The organism is resistant to, and may multiply in, many disinfectants and antiseptics commonly used in hospitals. It can be a troublesome contaminant in pharmaceutical preparations and may cause ophthalmitis following the faulty chemical 'sterilization' of contact lenses.

*Ps. aeruginosa* has relatively low intrinsic virulence but accounts for approximately 10% of all hospital-acquired infections. Such infections usually originate from exogenous sources but some patients suffer endogenous infection, particularly of the urinary tract. Healthy carriers usually harbour strains in the gastrointestinal tract, but in the open community the carriage rate seldom exceeds 10–15%. In contrast, acquisition of *Ps. aeruginosa* in a hospital is rapid, and

**Fig. 28.4** Jacuzzi® or whirlpool rash caused by *Pseudomonas aeruginosa.*

up to 30% of patients may excrete the organisms within a few days of admission.

Burned patients are especially at risk; the presence of the organism in ward air, dust and in eschar shed from the burns suggests that infection can be airborne. However, contact spread is probably more important than the airborne route. Transmission may occur directly via the hands of medical staff, or indirectly via contaminated apparatus. Severely burned patients and those with chest injuries who require artificial ventilation are highly susceptible to *Ps. aeruginosa*; pulmonary infection frequently precedes septicaemia, which is often fatal. Intensive care equipment can be difficult to clean and infection can undoubtedly be spread by this source.

Severe eye infections caused by *Ps. aeruginosa*, in particular keratitis, may result from contaminated contact lenses, industrial eye injuries or the introduction of contaminated medicament during ophthalmic procedures. Extremely painful ear infections acquired under the hyperbaric conditions of deep-sea diving operations have been reported

The warm, moist and aerated conditions under which *Ps. aeruginosa* thrives are ideally met in poorly maintained recreational hot tubs or whirlpools. Ear infections and an irritating folliculitis (Fig. 28.4) may be acquired from such sources.

Epidemics of gastrointestinal infection can occur in newborn and young infants in maternity units and paediatric wards, and may result from contaminated milk feeds. Other important *Ps. aeruginosa* infections in infants include septicaemia and meningitis.

## CONTROL

Prevention is easier than cure; once *Ps. aeruginosa* has gained access to a niche in the hospital environ-

ment, particularly in hospital water supplies, or has established infection, it is notoriously difficult to eradicate. Three guidelines to control infection are offered in the knowledge that it is not always easy to put them into practice:

1. Patients at a high risk of acquiring infection with *Ps. aeruginosa* (e.g. a patient being evaluated for organ transplantation) should not be admitted to a ward where cases of pseudomonas infection are present.
2. Antimicrobial and other therapeutic substances and solutions must be free from *Ps. aeruginosa*. Particular danger exists when multidose ointments, creams or eye drops are used to treat several individuals over a period. Contamination of a sterile preparation can easily occur between uses, and *Ps. aeruginosa* readily multiplies at a range of temperatures in many medicaments. Contamination of medicinal products is also a hazard with other pseudomonads, including the *Burkholderia cepacia* complex and *Ps. fluorescens*.
3. In hospital units, episodes of cross-infection due to a single strain may occur as sporadic infections in individual patients over a period of months or years. For this reason, it is advantageous to identify highly transmissible epidemic strains by 'fingerprinting' all clinically relevant isolates with a suitable typing system.

## BURKHOLDERIA

Although most of the presently 30 known *Burkholderia* species are saprophytes, *B. pseudomallei*, *B. mallei* and the *B. cepacia* complex are important human or animal pathogens.

## BURKHOLDERIA PSEUDOMALLEI

The environmental saprophyte *B. pseudomallei* causes melioidosis, a life-threatening tropical infection of man and animals in Southeast Asia and Northern Australia. In endemic areas the organism is found in soil and surface water, particularly rice paddy fields and monsoon drains. Isolation rates are highest during the rainy season and in still rather than flowing water.

The incidence of melioidosis is increasing; it has emerged in South America and the acquisition of *B. pseudomallei* in individuals with cystic fibrosis has been reported after recreational visits to Southeast Asia. As laboratory facilities can be limited in the rural tropics published cases may represent only the 'tip of the iceberg'. In northeastern Thailand, *B. pseudomallei* is responsible for up to 20% of community-acquired bacteraemias and the species is the most common cause of fatal community acquired pneumonia in Northern Australia.

A closely related species, *B. mallei*, causes *glanders*, a potentially fatal infectious disease of horses, mules and donkeys. Laboratory-acquired infection with either organism is a serious risk (hazard category 3) and both are regarded as potential bioterrorism agents.

## MELIOIDOSIS

Human infection is acquired mainly percutaneously through skin abrasions or by inhalation of contaminated particles, especially during monsoon rains. Melioidosis commonly presents as pyrexia. The clinical manifestations are protean and range from dormant subclinical infection, diagnosed by the presence of specific antibodies, to acute pneumonia or chronic pulmonary infection that may resemble tuberculosis and other conditions, leading to a fulminating septicaemia with a mortality rate of 80–90%. The organism can survive intracellularly within the reticulo-endothelial system, and this may account for latency and the emergence of symptoms resembling other infections many years after exposure. Suppurative parotitis is a characteristic presentation of melioidosis in children.

### Laboratory diagnosis

*B. pseudomallei* can be difficult to identify in laboratories with little experience of the organism. The organism may be seen, usually in very small numbers, as small, bipolar-stained Gram-negative bacilli in exudates, and can be cultured on appropriate media from sputum, urine, pus or blood, producing wrinkled or mucoid colonies after several days of growth. Fresh cultures emit a characteristic pungent odour of putrefaction. The organism is oxidase positive and motile but does not produce diffusible pigments. Formal identification by gas liquid chromatography and 16S rDNA sequencing should be confirmed by a reference laboratory.

Enzyme-linked immunosorbent assay (ELISA) for a conserved *B. pseudomallei* lipopolysaccharide antigen allows identification of specific antibodies in the evaluation of pyrexia of unknown origin. However, where melioidosis is endemic a high rate of seropositivity due to childhood exposure to *B. pseudomallei* or

subclinical exposure to the less virulent *B. thailandensis* limits this form of diagnosis. In some cases serologic diagnosis may require the use of the patient's own isolate as the reference strain.

### Treatment

Accurate and early diagnosis, including culture of *B. pseudomallei*, and appropriate antibiotic therapy are key to successful management. The optimum treatment of severe melioidosis is unclear. Intravenous ceftazidime, followed by a combination of co-trimoxazole and doxycycline, is emerging as the treatment of choice. Imipenem or meropenem have sometimes been effective when treatment with ceftazidime has proved unsuccessful. Prolonged treatment is necessary to avoid relapse.

## BURKHOLDERIA CEPACIA COMPLEX

*B. cepacia*, the cause of soft rot of onions, is also an important human pathogen causing life-threatening respiratory infection in immunocompromised patients, particularly those treated in intensive care or with chronic granulomatous disease. In cystic fibrosis, anxiety over *B. cepacia* is based on the innate multiresistance of the organism to antibiotics, its transmissibility by social contact, and the risk of *cepacia syndrome*, an acute, fatal necrotizing pneumonia, sometimes accompanied by bacteraemia, which occurs in 20–30% of infected patients.

The *B. cepacia* complex comprises 17 phenotypically similar but genetically distinct species (genomovars). With few exceptions, all have been isolated from cystic fibrosis patients: The species with the most medical relevance are *B. cenocepacia*, *B. multivorans*, *B. dolosa,* and *B. gladioli*. Around 90% of human infections are caused by *B. multivorans* and *B. cenocepacia*.

In cystic fibrosis accurate identification is vital for the implementation of optimal treatment regimens and infection control procedures to reduce patient-to-patient spread, and in the management of patients selected for lung transplantation. Laboratory identification from clinical specimens and from environmental sites is challenging, as most commercially available multitest kits may misidentify *Ps. aeruginosa*, *Achromobacter xylosoxidans, Stenotrophomonas maltophilia, Acinetobacter baumanni* and various other species as *B. cepacia* complex. Use of selective media is essential and presumptive phenotypic identification should be confirmed by RecA sequencing and PCR assays.

*B. cepacia* complex isolates produce several putative virulence determinants, including proteases, catalases, haemolysin, exopolysaccharide, cable pili and other adhesins. In vitro the lipid A of these bacteria stimulates pro-inflammatory cytokines tenfold more than *Ps. aeruginosa* lipid A.

The organisms are intrinsically resistant to most antibiotics, including polymyxins. Some are susceptible to ceftazidime, trimethoprim, tetracycline and chloramphenicol. The carbapenem, meropenem, appears the most active agent. Unfortunately, human infections are usually intractable to therapy unless combinations of three or four antibiotics are used. Strict infection control measures, including segregation, are necessary to limit the spread of highly transmissible strains.

## GLUCOSE NON-FERMENTERS

The heterogeneous group of aerobic Gram-negative bacilli commonly referred to as *glucose non-fermenters* is taxonomically distinct from the carbohydrate-fermenting Enterobacteriaceae and the oxidative pseudomonads. Their clinical relevance is based on their role as opportunistic pathogens in hospital-acquired infections and their intrinsic resistance to many antimicrobial agents. They grow easily on common culture media, but unequivocal identification may be difficult as most species are relatively inert in the biochemical tests used in identification of Gram-negative bacteria. Susceptibility to antibiotics is very variable and treatment should be based on the results of laboratory tests.

- *Acinetobacter* species are saprophytes found in soil, water and sewage, and occasionally as commensals of moist areas of human skin. The organisms survive well in the hospital environment, and now account for around 10% of nosocomial infections in intensive care units in Europe. Serious infections, including meningitis, osteomyelitis, wound infections (including war wounds), pneumonia and septicaemia, are most commonly associated with *A. baumannii*. Patients in intensive care units are at particular risk. Isolates are often inherently resistant to many antimicrobial agents, including β-lactam agents (other than carbapenems), aminoglycosides and quinolones.
- *Alcaligenes* and *Achromobacter* species are saprophytes found in moist environments, including those in hospital wards, and are associated with a range of hospital-acquired opportunistic infections, including septicaemia and ear discharges.
- *Eikenella corrodens* is a commensal of mucosal surfaces. It may cause a range of infections, in particular endocarditis, meningitis, pneumonia, and infections of wounds and various soft tissues.
- *Chryseobacterium* (formerly *Flavobacterium*) *meningosepticum* is a saprophyte whose natural habitat is soil and moist environments, including nebulizers; it may cause opportunistic nosocomial infections, particularly in infants. As the name suggests, this species is associated with meningitis, and has been responsible for high mortality in epidemic outbreaks.

RECOMMENDED READING

Bergogne-Bérézin E, Towner KJ: *Acinetobacter* spp. as nosocomial pathogens: microbiological, clinical and epidemiological features, *Clinical Microbiology Reviews* 9:148–165, 1996.

Estes DM, Dow SW, Schweizer HP, Torres AG: Present and future therapeutic strategies for melioidodosis and glanders, *Expert Reviews of Antiinfective Therapy* 8:325–338, 2010.

Govan JRW: *Burkholderia cepacia* complex and *Stenotrophomonas maltophilia*. In Bush A, Alton E, Davies J, et al, editors: Cystic Fibrosis in the 21st Century. Progress in Respiratory Research, vol 34, Basel, 2006, Karger, pp 145–152.

Hodgson K, Engler C, Govan B, et al: Comparision of routine bench and molecular diagnostic methods in identification of *Burkholderia pseudomallei*, *Journal of Clinical Microbiology* 47:1578–1580, 2009.

Kerr KG, Snelling AM: *Pseudomonas aeruginosa*: a formidable and ever-present adversary, *Journal of Hospital Infection* 73:338–344, 2009.

Mahenthiralingam E, Urban TA, Goldberg JB: The multifarious, multireplicon *Burkholderia cepacia* complex, *Nature Reviews* 3:1–14, 2005.

Peix A, Ramirez-Bahena M-H, Velazquez E: Historical evolution and current status of the taxonomy of genus *Pseudomonas*, *Infection, Genetics and Evolution* 9:1132–1147, 2009.

Willcox MDP: *Pseudomonas aeruginosa* infection and inflammation during contact lens wear: A review, *Optometry and Vision Science* 84:273–278, 2007.

### Websites

Health Protection Agency. Pseudomonas. http://www.hpa.org.uk/Topics/InfectiousDiseases/InfectionsAZ/PseudomonasAeruginosa/

Health Protection Agency. Melioidosis. http://www.hpa.org.uk/Topics/InfectiousDiseases/InfectionsAZ/Melioidosis/

International *Burkholderia cepacia* Working Group: http://www.go.to/cepacia

Pseudomonas Genome Database: http://www.pseudomonas.com

UK Cystic Fibrosis Microbiology Consortium: http://www.cfmicrobiology.org.uk

# 29 Campylobacter and helicobacter

## Enteritis; polyneuropathy; gastritis; peptic ulcer disease; gastric cancer

*J. M. Ketley and A. H. M. van Vliet*

## KEY POINTS

- *Campylobacter jejuni*, a food-borne pathogen generally associated with faecal contamination of food or water, is a common cause of bacterial enteritis.
- This flagellate, spiral and toxigenic micro-aerobe is capable of invading host cells.
- The generally self-limiting clinical presentation includes acute abdominal pain followed by diarrhoea with blood and leucocytes; antibiotic treatment is required only in severe cases.
- *Helicobacter pylori* is a flagellated spiral micro-aerobe causing peptic ulcer and gastritis. Infection is a risk factor for gastric cancer.
- It produces a cell-damaging toxin and a system that alters host cell signal transduction pathways.
- The transmission route is unclear. Colonization and disease rates are falling in industrialized countries.
- Treatment is by eradication of *H. pylori* using a combination of antibiotics and proton pump inhibitors.

*Campylobacter* and *Helicobacter* are phylogenetically related, spirally shaped, flagellate bacteria. They are adapted to colonizing mucous membranes and penetrate mucus with particular facility. In most industrialized countries *Campylobacter jejuni* is the most frequently identified cause of acute infective diarrhoea, causing much morbidity and economic loss. Lifelong colonization of the stomach with *Helicobacter pylori* is essentially the cause of 'idiopathic' peptic ulceration, and a notable risk factor for the development of gastric cancer.

## CAMPYLOBACTER

Campylobacters were first isolated in 1906 from aborting sheep in the UK. Originally thought to be vibrios, they were later placed in their own genus with *C. fetus* as the type species. The discovery that *C. jejuni* and *C. coli* commonly cause acute enteritis in man was not made until the late 1970s.

Several other species, such as *C. upsaliensis, C. lari* and the closely related bacterium *Arcobacter butzleri*, are occasionally associated with diarrhoea, mainly in children in developing countries. *C. fetus* is a major cause of abortion in sheep and cattle worldwide. It is a rare cause of human fetal infection and abortion, and infrequently causes bacteraemia in patients with immune deficiency. Several other species of *Campylobacter*, notably *C. concisus* and *C. rectus*, are associated with periodontal disease.

## CAMPYLOBACTER JEJUNI AND C. COLI

### Description

*C. jejuni* and *C. coli* are small, spiral, Gram-negative rods with a single flagellum at one or both poles (Fig. 29.1); this endows the bacteria with rapid darting motility. They are sensitive to oxygen and superoxides, yet oxygen is essential for growth, so micro-aerobic and capnophilic conditions must be provided for their cultivation. They are often called 'thermophilic campylobacters' because they grow best at 37–42°C. Campylobacters are inactive in many conventional biochemical tests, including metabolism of sugars, but they are strongly oxidase- and catalase-positive. Under laboratory conditions they are easily destroyed by heat and other physical and chemical agents. Campylobacters undergo coccal transformation under adverse conditions, a change controversially associated with a viable, non-culturable state.

**Fig. 29.1** Electron micrograph of *C. jejuni* showing single unsheathed bipolar flagella (original magnification ×11 500). (Photomicrograph courtesy of Dr AL Curry and DM Jones, Manchester Public Health Laboratory.)

Campylobacters readily take up from their surroundings naked DNA, which can be incorporated into the genome making them genetically diverse. *C. jejuni* and *C. coli* are closely related and phenotypically similar, but they can be differentiated by polymerase chain reaction (PCR) tests.

A capsular polysaccharide forms the major antigen for the Penner serotyping system. Bacteriophages able to infect campylobacters are also used in strain typing. Genetic 'fingerprinting' methods, such as multi-locus sequence typing (see p. 37) are available alternatives to more classical methods for epidemiological studies.

## Pathogenesis

*C. jejuni* accounts for 80–85% of human campylobacter infections in most parts of the world. As few as 500 to 800 organisms can initiate infection, presumably protected from stomach acid within the bolus of ingested food. The jejunum and ileum are the first sites to become colonized, and the infection extends distally to affect the terminal ileum and, usually, the colon and rectum. The organisms can translocate across the epithelial cell layer and are able to invade host cells. Symptoms are usually evident within 7 days. In well-developed infections, mesenteric lymph nodes are enlarged, fleshy and inflamed, and there may be transient bacteraemia. Histological examination of the mucosa shows an acute neutrophil response, oedema and, sometimes, superficial ulceration. These mucosal changes are indistinguishable from those seen in salmonella, shigella or yersinia infections.

Understanding of the mechanisms by which campylobacters cause enteric disease is limited. Colonization of the intestine requires factors such as chemotactic motility, iron-uptake systems and several potential adhesins. Diarrhoea is likely to result from disruption of the intestinal mucosa due to cell invasion and the production of toxin(s) (Fig. 29.2). Both *C. jejuni* and *C. coli* produce at least one toxin, cytolethal distending toxin, which blocks the cell cycle of host cells, but its precise role in virulence is unclear. Infection is influenced by the extent of the associated cellular immune response

Analysis of the complete genome sequence of several *C. jejuni* strains has revealed the existence of many genes responsible for the production of various glycans, as well as the presence of short hypervariable sequences. These so-called 'homopolymeric tracts' can act as a genetic switch and many are present in genes responsible for glycan biosynthesis. The amount of the genome invested in glycan biosynthesis indicates an important role for glycans in campylobacters. The genes responsible for glycosylation of the lipo-oligosaccharide, capsule and flagellum are highly variable, suggesting a role in avoidance of host immune responses or adaptation to other environmental changes. In contrast, genes involved in general protein glycosylation are highly conserved. Disruption of glycosylation pathways in *C. jejuni* affects host cell invasion and intestinal colonization. Extensive glycosylation may reflect molecular mimicry of host epitopes as part of a strategy to avoid host immune responses.

### Immune response

Specific humoral antibodies appear within 10 days of onset, peak in 2–4 weeks, and then decline rapidly. Most of the antibody is in the form of immunoglobulin (Ig) G, but healthy persons exposed to repeated infection show a progressive increase in IgA, which provides substantial immunity. Mild clinical symptoms, such as mild watery diarrhoea or even asymptomatic colonization, may reflect increased levels of immunity and/or development of tolerance from repeated infections.

### Clinical features

The typical features of campylobacter enteritis are shown in Figure 29.3. The average incubation period is 3 days, with a range of 1–7 days. The illness may start with abdominal pain and diarrhoea, or there may be an influenza-like prodrome of fever and generalized aching, sometimes with rigors and sweating. Abdominal pain and diarrhoea are the main symptoms. Nausea is common, but vomiting is less pronounced. Severe watery diarrhoea may lead to prostration. Leucocytes are almost always present in

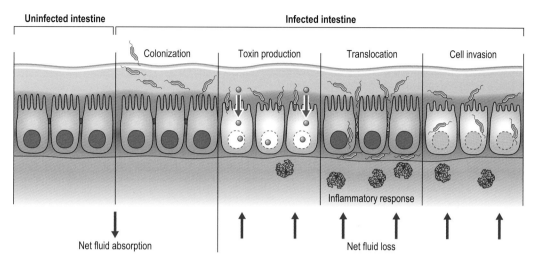

**Fig. 29.2** The pathogenesis of *Campylobacter jejuni* and *C. coli*. Net fluid absorption occurs across the undamaged ileal and colonic epithelium. On infection of the host intestine, campylobacters use chemotactic motility to reach the mucous layer and colonize the epithelial surface. Campylobacters translocate directly across the cell layer, invade host cells and produce a cytotoxin. Cell damage disrupts the integrity of the mucosal cell layer and stimulates an inflammatory response. Disruption of the absorptive function of the epithelium and, possibly, stimulation of secretion leads to diarrhoeal disease.

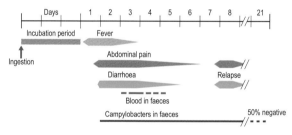

**Fig. 29.3** Typical course of untreated campylobacter enteritis of average severity. There is considerable variation among individual patients.

the faeces, and frank blood may be apparent. Symptoms usually resolve within a few days, but excretion of bacteria may continue for several weeks. Prolonged carriage occurs only in patients with immunodeficiency. Campylobacter enteritis cannot be distinguished clinically from salmonella or shigella infection, but abdominal pain tends to be more severe in campylobacter infection. Indeed, a common reason for patients with campylobacter enteritis to be admitted to hospital is suspected acute appendicitis. Occasionally, illness starts with symptoms of colitis without preceding ileitis, which can make it difficult to distinguish from acute ulcerative colitis. In developing countries infection often presents as milder diarrhoea and asymptomatic colonization is common. Clinical differences are mostly due to host immune status, the development of tolerance, or variation in strain virulence.

## Complications

Two conditions may arise 1–2 weeks after the onset of illness:

1. Reactive (aseptic) arthritis, typically affecting the ankles, knees and wrists, affects 1–2% of patients. It may be incapacitating, but is ultimately self-limiting.
2. Guillain–Barré syndrome, a form of peripheral polyneuropathy, affects around 1 in 1000 infected individuals per year; it may cause serious and potentially fatal paralysis lasting for several months. It is thought that antibodies to lipo-oligosaccharide epitopes, present in some strains, cross-react with the myelin in nerve sheaths, causing demyelination.

## Laboratory diagnosis

Faecal specimens should be refrigerated pending delivery to the laboratory. Specimens sent by post should be placed in an appropriate transport medium.

### Microscopy

The motility and morphology of campylobacters are sufficiently characteristic for a rapid presumptive diagnosis to be made by direct microscopy of fresh faeces, in either wet preparations or stained smears. This is occasionally useful, but is not done routinely.

## Culture

Isolation of campylobacters from faeces requires some form of selective culture to inhibit competing faecal flora. Charcoal-based blood-free agar containing bile acids, cefoperazone or other selective antimicrobial agents is widely used. Plates are incubated in closed jars or specialized incubators with the oxygen tension lowered to 5–15% and carbon dioxide raised to 5–10%. Incubation at 42–43°C gives added selectivity against other faecal flora and more rapid growth of *C. jejuni* and *C. coli*, but may exclude other *Campylobacter* species. Plates are incubated for 48 h. Colonies are typically flat with a tendency to spread on moist agar. *Campylobacter* species sensitive to antimicrobial agents in selective media can be isolated by inoculating a membrane (pore size 0.45–0.65 μm) laid on non-selective media. Campylobacters are small enough to swim through the membrane, which is removed before incubation.

## Serology

Serology can be useful in patients presenting with aseptic arthritis or Guillain–Barré syndrome occurring after diarrhoea that was not investigated. Group-specific complement fixation tests and enzyme-linked immunosorbent assay (ELISA) can detect recent infection with *C. jejuni* or *C. coli*.

## Epidemiology

### Incidence

Campylobacter enteritis is the most common form of acute infective diarrhoea in most developed countries. In the UK, laboratory reports indicate an annual incidence of about 1 per 1000 population, but the true figure is probably much higher. The disease occurs among all age groups (especially young adults), shows a pronounced summer peak and is often associated with travel.

In developing countries, infection is hyperendemic, and children are repeatedly exposed to infection from an early age. By the time they are 2–3 years old, children have developed substantial immunity that lasts into adulthood. The maintenance of immunity probably depends on continuous exposure to infection.

### Sources and transmission

*C. jejuni* and *C. coli* are found in a wide variety of animal hosts, notably birds, an adaptation that is reflected in their high optimum growth temperature which mimics the avian body temperature. Figure 29.4 summarizes the principal sources and routes of transmission to human beings. There is a constant shedding of the bacteria from wild birds and other animals into the surface water of lakes, rivers and streams, in which campylobacters can survive for many weeks at low temperatures. Farm animals are often infected from such sources and flies have also been implicated in spread. Cattle are commonly infected, and raw milk often becomes contaminated. The distribution of raw or inadequately pasteurized milk and untreated water has caused major outbreaks of campylobacter enteritis, some affecting several thousand people. Direct contact with infected animals or their products can also give rise to infection.

At least 60% of chickens sold in shops are contaminated with campylobacters, and contaminated broiler chickens are thought to account for about 50% of human infections in industrialized countries. Red meats are less often contaminated.

Properly cooked poultry and meats do not pose a risk, but cross-contamination to other foods, such as bread and salads, probably accounts for many infections. Unlike salmonellae, campylobacters do not multiply in food, so explosive food-poisoning outbreaks are rare. Most infections are sporadic or confined to one household; the spread of infection between individuals is of minor importance.

## Treatment

Campylobacteriosis is usually self-limiting and patients seldom require more than fluid and electrolyte replacement. Antimicrobial treatment should be reserved for patients with severe or complicated infections. Erythromycin is effective if given early in the disease. Ciprofloxacin and other fluoroquinolones are also effective, but resistance rates are rising.

## Control

The wide distribution of campylobacters in nature precludes any possibility of reducing the reservoir of infection. Efforts are mostly directed to interrupting transmission and reducing numbers of *Campylobacter* in poultry. The purification of water and the heat treatment of milk are obvious and basic measures. The control of colonization in broiler chickens merits high priority, but the means to achieve this are beset with difficulty. Terminal γ-irradiation or chemical washes of carcasses can eliminate campylobacters and other pathogens, but public acceptability is a problem.

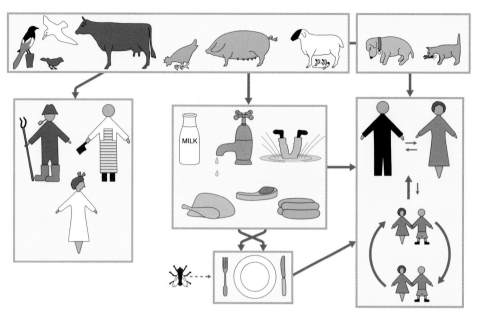

**Fig. 29.4** Sources and transmission of *C. jejuni* and *C. coli*. Top boxes: animal reservoirs and sources of infection (the sheep has just given birth to a dead campylobacter-infected lamb). Left-hand box: transmission by direct occupational contact (farmer, butcher, poultry processor). Right-hand boxes: transmission by direct domestic contact (puppy or kitten with campylobacter diarrhoea; intra-familial spread, mainly from children). Central box: indirect transmission through consumption of untreated water, raw milk, raw or undercooked meat and poultry, food cross-contaminated from raw meats and poultry; possible transmission from flies. (From document VPH/CDD/FOS/84.1 by permission of the World Health Organization, which retains the copyright.)

## HELICOBACTER

Remarkably, *H. pylori*, which colonizes roughly half of the world's population, remained undiscovered until 1982 when Warren and Marshall in Western Australia overturned the dogma that bacteria could not colonize the stomach. The discovery revolutionized the treatment of duodenal and gastric ulcers and earned them a Nobel Prize in 2005.

Over 20 species of *Helicobacter* are now officially recognized, with more awaiting formal recognition. One group, the gastric helicobacters, colonizes the stomachs of animals; the monkey, cat, dog, ferret and cheetah each harbour their own species. The entero-hepatic group colonizes the intestines and liver of a wide range of animals, mostly rodents, and enteric *Helicobacter* spp. have been linked to the development of inflammatory bowel disease in man. *H. cinaedi* and *H. fennelliae* are associated with proctitis in homosexual men.

Less common helicobacters, originally named '*H. heilmannii*', are found in the human stomach and are associated with gastritis, ulcers and malignancy. Molecular studies suggest transmission from an animal source. The bacteria are more tightly spiralled than *H. pylori*, with up to 12 sheathed polar flagella.

They belong to two groups: one closely related to a pathogenic gastric helicobacter of pigs, and the other to canine and feline helicobacters.

## *HELICOBACTER PYLORI*

### Description

*H. pylori* is a Gram-negative, spirally shaped bacterium. It is strictly micro-aerophilic, requires carbon dioxide and a rich growth media, but it has a tuft of sheathed unipolar flagella, unlike the unsheathed flagella of campylobacters (Fig. 29.5; cf. Fig. 29.1). It is biochemically inactive in most conventional tests, but produces an exceptionally powerful urease, almost 100 times more active than that of *Proteus vulgaris*, which is vital to its survival in the stomach. When exposed to adverse conditions *H. pylori* undergoes coccal transformation more rapidly than *C. jejuni* and is more fragile, a point of importance when referring samples to a laboratory.

### Antigens and strain typing

Although various antigens are expressed by *H. pylori*, serotyping is of limited practical value. However, its

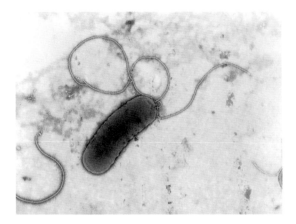

**Fig. 29.5** *H. pylori* showing multiple sheathed unipolar flagella (original magnification ×11 500). (Photomicrograph courtesy of Dr AL Curry and DM Jones, Manchester Public Health Laboratory.)

**Fig. 29.6** Section of gastric mucosa showing colonization with *H. pylori* (Warthin–Starry silver stain; original magnification ×1400). (Photomicrograph courtesy of Mr GH Green, Worcester Royal Infirmary.)

genetic diversity can be exploited by molecular typing based on DNA analysis. Like campylobacters, *H. pylori* exhibits considerable genetic diversity arising from natural competence, a high mutation rate and frequent recombination events. In consequence a host can be colonized by a population of closely related variants analogous to the 'quasi-species' observed with certain viruses.

## Pathogenesis

### Site of infection

*H. pylori* is highly adapted and lives only on gastric mucosa. Colonization ceases abruptly where gastric mucosa ends, for example in areas of intestinal metaplasia in the stomach. Conversely, areas of gastric

metaplasia elsewhere in the gut, notably the duodenum, may become colonized with *H. pylori*, thus setting the scene for ulceration.

The gastric antrum is the most favoured site, but other parts of the stomach may be colonized, especially in patients taking an acid-lowering drug such as an $H_2$ antagonist or proton pump inhibitor, or in subjects with a natural lower acid output. The bacteria are non-invasive, being present in the mucus overlying the mucosa. Although gastric acid is potentially destructive to *H. pylori*, protection is provided by its powerful urease, which acts on the urea passing through the gastric mucosa to generate ammonia, and this may neutralize acid around the bacteria. Colonization often extends into gastric glands (Fig. 29.6). Where they are numerous, the underlying mucosa usually shows a superficial gastritis of the type known as chronic active or type B gastritis (not to be confused with type A atrophic auto-immune gastritis of pernicious anaemia). This is characterized by infiltration with chronic inflammatory cells and polymorphonuclear leucocytes. Mucus-secreting foveolar cells often show damage where the bacteria are numerous.

### The course of infection

After an incubation period of a few days, patients suffer a mild attack of acute achlorhydric gastritis with symptoms of abdominal pain, nausea, flatulence and bad breath. Colonization results in the formation of mucosa-associated lymphoid tissue (MALT) and infiltration of polymorphonuclear leucocytes, together producing the active gastritis. Symptoms last for about 2 weeks, but hypochlorhydria may persist for up to a year. Despite a substantial humoral antibody response, infection and chronic active gastritis persist, but after several decades there may be a progression to atrophic gastritis and intestinal metaplasia. Conditions are then inhospitable for *H. pylori*, which disappears or is much reduced in number.

### Associated disease

The outcome of infection by *H. pylori* reflects an interaction between strain virulence, pro-inflammatory host genotypes, and environmental factors. Despite the presence of chronic active gastritis, most infections are symptomless, and endoscopic appearances of the stomach are normal. However, in some infected persons the chronic active gastritis forms a launch pad for more serious clinical outcomes, such as gastric and duodenal ulcers, non-ulcer dyspepsia and gastric malignancies.

*Peptic ulceration.* *H. pylori* is actively involved in the pathogenesis of peptic ulceration unrelated to non-steroidal anti-inflammatory agents or the Zollinger–Ellison syndrome. Infection is virtually a prerequisite for ulceration, and elimination of *H. pylori* allows healing of ulcers without recurrence. Recurrent ulceration is almost always associated with recrudescence of infection.

The topographical pattern of gastritis is a predictor of clinical outcome. In antral predominant gastritis, hyperacidity induced by *H. pylori* via increased gastrin production promotes duodenal gastric metaplasia and this leads to colonization of the duodenum, inflammation and finally ulceration. With corpus-predominant gastritis or pangastritis, host interactions lead to the suppression of acid production and destruction of parietal cells. Consequently duodenal ulceration is not evident, although hypoacidity can lead to epithelial changes and gastric gland atrophy that increase the risk of gastric ulceration.

*Non-ulcer dyspepsia.* Some cases of non-ulcer dyspepsia are associated with *H. pylori* as eradication has a small but significant effect on dyspepsia and prevents the development of peptic ulcers in some patients. Although there is currently no way of identifying such patients, a 'test and treat' strategy is justified on economic grounds.

*Gastric cancer.* Atrophic gastritis resulting from longstanding infection with *H. pylori* is associated with an increased risk of developing gastric cancer. In addition, gastric MALT lymphoma is strongly associated with *H. pylori* infection, and in most cases complete regression has been observed after eradication of the infection.

*Other disease.* *H. pylori* infection has been associated statistically with several conditions outside the digestive tract, including coronary heart disease, iron deficiency anaemia and cot death. Although these are of great potential importance, the links remain unproven because of possible confounding factors. Epidemiological data link eradication of *H. pylori* infection with increased rates of oesophageal cancer, allergy and asthma.

### Virulence factors

Some strains of *H. pylori* produce a vacuolating toxin (VacA) and a cytotoxin (CagA). As well as providing acid protection, urease may also promote colonization in other ways. In addition, host factors strongly influence the outcome of infection.

The *cagA* gene is a marker for strains that confer an increased risk of both peptic ulceration and gastric malignancy, although other factors play a role as strains lacking the toxin can still cause gastritis. The gene forms part of a pathogenicity island, which also encodes a secretion system capable of injecting bacterial macromolecules, including CagA and peptidoglycan, into host cells. The injected CagA protein is phosphorylated by a host kinase and subsequently interacts with various signal transduction pathways to affect epithelial cell morphology and behaviour. Peptidoglycan binds to the intracellular NOD1 receptor and contributes to the initiation or continuation of a proinflammatory immune response. An anti-apoptotic effect may aid bacterial persistence on the gastric epithelium.

The vacuolating toxin has been associated with pore formation in host cell membranes, the loosening of the tight junctions between epithelial cells (thus affecting mucosal barrier permeability), and specific immune suppression. The *vacA* gene, present in all *H. pylori* strains, exhibits a high degree of polymorphism. Each allele encodes different VacA types associated with an increased risk of certain patterns of gastroduodenal disease.

In addition to VacA and CagA, *H. pylori* expresses adhesin proteins that allow reversible adhesion to host receptors mostly present in inflamed tissue, including sialyl-Lewis X and the ABO-bloodgroup antigens.

## Laboratory diagnosis

Non-invasive tests are used for initial screening. Definitive tests of infection depend on finding *H. pylori* in specimens of gastric mucosa obtained by biopsy.

### Non-invasive tests

*Serology.* Serological tests, mostly based on ELISA or latex agglutination, detect antibodies to *H. pylori* or its products and are used to screen patients with dyspepsia. They are less useful for screening children and are unreliable for excluding infection in elderly patients, or as a test for cure in patients who have received treatment (owing to variable persistence of antibody). The accuracy of rapid bedside tests of whole blood is poor.

*Urea breath test.* This test detects bacterial urease activity in the stomach by measuring the output of carbon dioxide resulting from the splitting of carbon-13 or carbon-14 labelled urea into carbon dioxide and ammonia; infected patients give high readings. The test has excellent sensitivity and specificity, but carbon-14 is weakly radioactive, so it is not used in children. A mass spectrometer is needed to assay non-radioactive carbon-13. The urea breath test cannot be used during or directly after antibiotic therapy.

***Faecal antigen test.*** Stool antigen tests that detect *H. pylori* antigens in faeces are available. Tests based on the use of monoclonal antibodies are more accurate than polyclonal antibody tests and have the potential to supplant serology for routine screening.

***Polymerase chain reaction (PCR).*** DNA probes for the direct detection of *H. pylori* in gastric juice, faeces, dental plaque and water supplies have been developed. Some can also detect genes expressing antibiotic resistance and presence of the *cagA* pathogenicity island. Newer versions can detect *H. pylori* within a few hours. Present methods are unsuitable for general use because clinical samples may contain compounds that inhibit the reaction.

### Invasive tests

***Collection of specimens.*** Ideally, patients for endoscopy should not have received antibiotics or proton pump inhibitors for 1 month before the test. Mucosal biopsy specimens are taken from the gastric antrum within 5 cm of the pylorus, and preferably also from the body of the stomach. For maximum sensitivity, duplicate specimens are taken: one for histopathology (placed in fixative); the other for culture (placed in the neck of a sterile bottle made humid by adding a tiny amount of normal saline). Specimens for culture must be processed as soon as possible, certainly on the same day, or placed in transport medium.

***Biopsy urease test.*** This is a simple and cheap test that can be performed at the bedside. A biopsy specimen is placed into a small quantity of urea solution with a dye such as phenol red, which detects alkalinity resulting from the formation of ammonia. Most infected patients (70%) give a positive result within 2 h; 90% after 24 h. Newer tests have faster reaction times and a test with monoclonal antibody promises higher sensitivity and specificity.

***Histopathology and microscopy.*** Histopathology provides a permanent record of the nature and grading of a patient's gastritis as well as detecting *H. pylori*. Organisms can be seen in sections stained with haematoxylin and eosin, but more specific stains make the task easier (see Fig. 29.6). The bacteria can also be seen in smears of biopsy material stained with Gram's stain. Fluorescein-based molecular probes under development are potentially able to detect *H. pylori* and its virulence factors.

***Culture.*** Culture is no more sensitive than skilled microscopy of histological sections, but has several advantages: isolates can be tested for antimicrobial resistance and typed for epidemiological studies; information about the presence of virulence factors can inform clinical outcome.

Rich growth media (commonly including lysed or whole animal blood or complement-inactivated serum), selective agars and incubation conditions similar to those used for campylobacters are used for primary isolation (see p. 308). Sensitivity is increased if a non-selective medium is used in parallel. High humidity is essential. Plates are left undisturbed for 3 days and incubated for a week before being discarded as negative. *H. pylori* forms discrete domed colonies, unlike the effuse colonies of *C. jejuni* and *C. coli*.

### Epidemiology

Man appears to be the sole reservoir and source of *H. pylori*. Infection is presumed to be by the oral–oral or, possibly, faecal–oral route, and has been suggested to be mostly intrafamilial. Volunteer studies indicate that the adult infectious dose is relatively high, but infections resulting from lower doses may resolve quickly whereas higher doses lead to persistent infection.

Infection rates are strongly related to poor living conditions and overcrowding during childhood. There is a steady rise in seropositivity with increasing age (about 50% infected by the age of 60 years in industrialized countries). In developed nations progressively fewer children are becoming colonized, but most children in developing countries are infected by the time they reach puberty. High rates of infection correlate broadly with high rates of gastric cancer. The so-called 'African enigma', in which high seropositivity is associated with low gastric cancer risk, may be due to intestinal helminth infection driving the local immune response towards a protective T helper cell 2 (Th2), rather than the deleterious Th1 response.

Inmates of psychiatric units and orphanages and professional staff carrying out endoscopy examinations show higher than average infection rates. Nosocomial infection from inadequately disinfected endoscopes has also occurred.

### Treatment

Elimination of *H. pylori* infection is not always necessary and is associated with an increase in prevalence of other inflammatory diseases and oesophageal cancer. Two unequivocal indications for treatment are:

- peptic ulcer disease
- gastric MALT lymphoma.

Possible indications are:

- patients with non-ulcer dyspepsia refractory to conventional treatment
- patients with a family history of gastric carcinoma.

In vitro, *H. pylori* is sensitive to most β-lactam antibiotics, macrolides, tetracyclines and nitroimidazoles, but resistant to trimethoprim. In practice, the choice of antibiotic is dependent on stability in acid, activity against very slow growing organisms and diffusion into the gastric mucus layer, and this limits treatment to four main antibiotics: amoxicillin, clarithromycin, tetracycline and metronidazole. It is also sensitive to bismuth subcitrate or subsalicylate and partially sensitive to the acid-lowering proton pump inhibitors omeprazole and lansoprazole.

To eradicate *H. pylori* infection, at least two antimicrobial agents must be given in combination with an acid-lowering agent (triple therapy), as monotherapy rapidly leads to antibiotic resistance. A popular regimen is a 1-week course of the macrolide clarithromycin, plus amoxicillin and omeprazole (or lansoprazole). These regimens eliminate *H. pylori* in about 90% of patients. Alternative therapies usually contain tetracycline; use of metronidazole is now avoided due to its mutagenic properties and the prevalence of resistance. Similar regimens are used with children but eradication rates are generally lower than those in adults.

Recrudescence of infection demands a repeat biopsy with culture and sensitivity testing of the infecting strain. Treatment failure may result from poor compliance or antibiotic resistance, which is common for metronidazole and clarithromycin, but still rare for tetracycline and amoxicillin. Some fluoroquinolones are active against *H. pylori* and changes in treatment regimen may improve compliance and eradication rates.

## Control

Social deprivation is the dominant factor governing the prevalence of *H. pylori* infection. In western society, social advancement has brought about a reduction of infection, and peptic ulcer disease is on the decline. However, this is far from the case in developing countries, where a cheap and effective vaccine would be valuable, particularly for the prevention of gastric cancer.

RECOMMENDED READING

Blaser MJ, Atherton JC: *Helicobacter pylori*: biology and disease, *Journal of Clinical Investigation* 113:321–333, 2004.
Gerrits MM, van Vliet AH, Kuipers EJ, Kusters JG: *Helicobacter pylori* and antimicrobial resistance: molecular mechanisms and clinical implications, *Lancet Infectious Diseases* 6:699–709, 2006.
Gilbreath JJ, Cody WL, Merrell DS, Hendrixson DR: Change is good: variations in common biological mechanisms in the epsilonproteobacterial genera *Campylobacter* and *Helicobacter*, *Microbiology and Molecular Biology Reviews* 75:84–132, 2011.
Janssen R, Krogfelt KA, Cawthraw SA, et al: Host-pathogen interactions in *Campylobacter* infections: the host perspective, *Clinical Microbiology Reviews* 21:505–558, 2008.
Ketley JM, Konkel ME, editors: *Campylobacter: Molecular and Cellular Biology*, Norwich, 2005, Horizon Bioscience.
Kusters JG, van Vliet AH, Kuipers EJ: Pathogenesis of *Helicobacter pylori* infection, *Clinical Microbiology Reviews* 19:449–490, 2006.
Nachamkin I, Szymanski CM, Blaser MJ: *Campylobacter*, ed 3, Washington, 2008, ASM Press.
Young KT, Davis LM, Dirita VJ: *Campylobacter jejuni*, *Nature Reviews, Microbiology* 5:665–679, 2007.

## Websites

Centers for Disease Control and Prevention: Campylobacter. http://www.cdc.gov/nczved/divisions/dfbmd/diseases/campylobacter/
Centers for Disease Control and Prevention: *Helicobacter pylori* and Peptic Ulcer Disease. (Archived site.) http://www.cdc.gov/ulcer/keytocure.htm
Health Protection Agency: Campylobacter. http://www.hpa.org.uk/infections/topics_az/campy/menu.htm
Health Protection Agency: Helicobacter pylori. http://www.hpa.org.uk/infections/topics_az/helicobacter/menu.htm
Helicobacter Foundation: http://www.helico.com/
Nobel Foundation: The Nobel Prize in Physiology or Medicine, 2005. http://nobelprize.org/nobel_prizes/medicine/laureates/2005/press.html
World Health Organization: Campylobacter. http://www.who.int/topics/campylobacter/en/

# 30 Vibrio, mobiluncus, gardnerella and spirillum

Cholera; vaginosis; rat bite fever

*H. Chart*

## KEY POINTS

- *Vibrio cholerae* belonging to serogroup O1 is the causative agent of epidemic cholera.
- *V. cholerae* O139 is emerging as a cause of epidemic cholera.
- Cholera toxin is the key pathogenic mechanism, causing extensive loss of water and electrolytes in the form of rice-water stools; death from cholera can be prevented with rehydration therapy.
- *V. parahaemolyticus* is a major cause of diarrhoea in Japan and South-East Asia; infection is associated with the consumption of seafood.
- Infection with *V. vulnificus* may result in rapid-onset and fatal septicaemia, particularly in people with conditions of iron overload, and is associated with the consumption of seafood.
- *Mobiluncus* spp. and *Gardnerella vaginalis* are a major cause of bacterial vaginosis; changes in the normal vaginal flora appear to permit these organisms to cause disease.
- *Spirillum minus* causes rat bite fever.

## VIBRIO

The *Vibrio* genus includes more than 30 species commonly found in aquatic environments. Some cause disease in human beings as well as in marine vertebrates and invertebrates. The most important pathogens of man are *Vibrio cholerae, V. parahaemolyticus* and *V. vulnificus*, but various other species are occasionally implicated as opportunist pathogens. Historically, vibrios have been associated almost exclusively with epidemic and pandemic cholera caused by a particular antigenic form of *V. cholerae*.

## DESCRIPTION

Vibrios are short Gram-negative rods, which are often curved and actively motile by a single polar flagellum (Fig. 30.1). Nearly all produce the enzyme oxidase and give a positive indole reaction. The genus can be divided into non-halophilic vibrios, including *V. cholerae* and other species that are able to grow in media without added salt, and halophilic species such as *V. parahaemolyticus* and *V. vulnificus* that require salt for growth. Vibrios grow readily on ordinary media provided that their requirements for electrolytes are met, and grow best when abundant oxygen is present. Most grow at 30°C but some of the halophilic species grow poorly at 37°C, whereas *V. cholerae, V. parahaemolyticus* and *V. alginolyticus* grow at 42°C.

Vibrios have a low tolerance to acid and prefer alkaline conditions (growth range pH 6.8–10.2, optimum pH 7.4–9.6).

## VIBRIO CHOLERAE

### Description

Strains of *V. cholerae* can be differentiated by their lipopolysaccharide O-antigens into some 130 different serogroups. The classical cause of epidemic cholera possesses the O1 antigen, and is known as *V. cholerae* O1. Other serogroups are collectively known as 'non-O1 *V. cholerae*' and correspond to strains formerly known as *non-agglutinable vibrios* or *non-cholera vibrios*. Some of these strains can cause diarrhoea in man. All strains of *V. cholerae* share the same flagellar (H) antigen.

Strains of *V. cholerae* O1 may be further subdivided on the basis of their O antigens into the subtypes

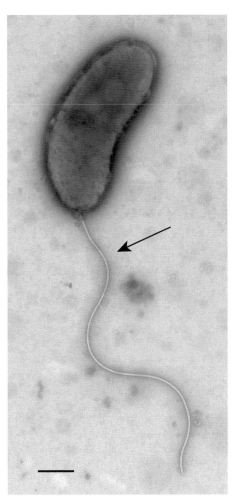

**Fig. 30.1** Electron micrograph of *Vibrio cholerae* showing typical short rod morphology with a single polar flagellum. Bar = 2 μm.

*Inaba* and *Ogawa*; some strains possess determinants of both of these subtypes and are known as subtype *Hikojima*.

There are two biotypes of *V. cholerae* O1: the *classical* and *El Tor* biotypes. The El Tor variant is distinguished from the classical biotype by the ability to express a haemolysin on sheep erythrocytes, resistance to polymyxin B, agglutination of chicken erythrocytes and a positive Voges–Proskauer test. The two biotypes can also be recognized by their differential susceptibility to specific phages IV and V.

*V. cholerae* O139, which has emerged as a new epidemic strain (see below), may have evolved from *V. cholerae* O1, but with a modified lipopolysaccharide structure.

## Pathogenesis

### Clinical manifestations

Cholera is characterized by the sudden onset of effortless vomiting and profuse watery diarrhoea. Although vomiting is a common feature, the rapid dehydration and hypovolaemic shock, which may cause death in 12–24 h, are related mainly to the profuse, watery, colourless stools with flecks of mucus and a distinctive fishy odour – *rice water stools* – which contain little protein and are very different from the mucopurulent blood-stained stools of bacillary dysentery. Anuria develops, muscle cramps occur, and the patient quickly becomes weak and lethargic with loss of skin turgor, low blood pressure and an absent or thready pulse. There are, however, all grades of severity, and milder cases cannot be distinguished clinically from other secretory diarrhoeas. Symptomless infections are common.

### Pathogenic mechanisms

*V. cholerae* requires two major pathogenic mechanisms to cause disease:

1. the ability to produce cholera toxin
2. expression of toxin-co-regulated pili.

The sequence of events leading to cholera is confined to the gut. The cholera vibrios are ingested in drink or food and, in natural infections, the dose must often be small. After passing the acid barrier of the stomach the organisms begin to multiply in the alkaline environment of the small intestine, where they migrate towards epithelial cells, facilitated by active motility and the production of mucinase and other proteolytic enzymes. Once the organism has penetrated the mucous layer it adheres to the enterocyte surface. In addition to toxin, co-regulated pili, haemagglutinins and lipopolysaccharide have also been implicated in adhesion.

Once adherent, the bacteria produce a potent enterotoxin known as *cholera toxin*. The toxin consists of five B subunits (molecular weight 11 600 Da) and a single A subunit (molecular weight 27 200 Da), and has structural, functional and antigenic similarity to heat-labile toxin expressed by strains of enterotoxigenic *Escherichia coli* (ETEC; see p. 283–4). The A subunit is made up of two peptides ($A_1$ and $A_2$) linked by a single disulphide bridge. The B subunit binds to sugar residues of ganglioside $GM_1$ on the cells lining the villi and crypts of the small intestine. It is thought that insertion of the B subunit into the host cell membrane forms a hydrophilic transmembrane channel through which the toxic A subunit can pass into the cytoplasm. Reduction of the disulphide bond releases the $A_1$ portion of the molecule, which has enterotoxic activity. The cholera enterotoxin causes the transfer of adenosine diphosphoribose (ADP ribose) from nicotinamide adenine dinucleotide (NAD) to a regulatory protein, which is part of the adenylate cyclase enzyme responsible for the generation of intracellular cyclic adenosine monophosphate (cAMP). The result is irreversible activation of adenylate cyclase and overproduction of cAMP. This in turn causes inhibition of uptake of $Na^+$ and $Cl^-$ ions by cells lining the villi, together with hypersecretion of $Cl^-$ and $HCO_3^-$ ions. This blocks the uptake of water, which normally accompanies $Na^+$ and $Cl^-$ absorption, and there is a passive net outflow of water across mucosal cells, leading to serious loss of water and electrolytes.

*V. cholerae* may express one or more of four haemolysins: thermo-stable direct haemolysin, El Tor haemolysin, thermo-labile haemolysin and thermostable haemolysin. The latter three are found in pathogenic strains of *V. cholerae*, and all are thought to contribute to virulence.

Some strains of *V. cholerae* O1 that cause diarrhoea produce a toxin that differs in antigenic nature, receptor site, mode of action and genetic homology from cholera toxin.

## Non-O1 V. cholerae

Non-O1 strains of *V. cholerae* cause mild, sometimes bloody, diarrhoea, often accompanied by abdominal cramps. Symptoms may occasionally be severe, in which case the disease resembles cholera. Wound infections may occur in patients exposed to aquatic environments, and bacteraemia and meningitis have been reported.

These strains may elaborate a wide range of virulence factors, including enterotoxins, cytotoxins, haemolysins and colonizing factors. A few produce cholera toxin.

## Laboratory diagnosis

Stool specimens are inoculated into alkaline peptone water, in which vibrios grow rapidly and accumulate on the surface. After incubation for 3–6 h a loopful from the surface is inoculated on to a suitable solid medium such as thiosulphate–citrate–bile salts–sucrose (TCBS) agar. On this medium *V. cholerae* forms yellow sucrose-fermenting colonies, which are tested for the enzyme oxidase and for agglutination with rabbit antibodies specific for the O1 lipopolysaccharide antigens before biochemical confirmation. A

fluorogenic test based on the production of lysyl aminopeptidase by *Vibrio* spp. has been developed.

Cholera toxin can be detected by the same techniques described for *E. coli* heat-labile toxin (see p. 284), but these assays have largely been replaced by antibody-based commercial kits or by rapid molecular methods. The haemolysins expressed by *V. cholerae* can be detected in polymerase chain reaction (PCR) assays with primers for the *tcpA* genes and cholera toxin can be characterized by targeting the *ctxB* genes: *ctxB*1 has been associated with the classical biotypes; *ctxB*2 has been linked with El Tor strains isolated in Australia; and *ctxB*3 has been associated with strains from South America.

## Epidemiology

### V. cholerae O1

A series of six pandemics of cholera, originating in the Bengal basin, ravaged the world in the nineteenth and twentieth centuries. Subsequently, cholera was contained within the endemic foci and surrounding areas of India and Bangladesh until 1961, when a seventh pandemic due to the El Tor biotype of *V. cholerae* O1, originally isolated from pilgrims at the quarantine station known as El Tor, began to supplant the classical biotype in India. By 1973 the El Tor biotype had entirely displaced the classical biotype in Bangladesh and spread to Indonesia, the Far East and Africa. In 1991 it reached South America, where the first epidemic in that subcontinent of the twentieth century occurred in Peru. By December 1993 more than 820 000 cases of cholera, with almost 7000 deaths, had occurred, and the epidemic had involved all Latin American countries except Uruguay (Fig. 30.2). Since 1993, the number of cases in the western hemisphere has continued to fall. The vast majority of cases of cholera now occur in Africa and Asia.

Infection is generally spread by contaminated water or foods such as uncooked seafood or vegetables. The source of the contamination is usually the faeces of carriers or patients with cholera, but contamination can probably sometimes occur from natural aquatic reservoirs. Cholera is characteristically an infection of crowded communities with poor standards of hygiene and shared communal water supplies such as tanks, ponds, canals or rivers used for bathing, washing and household use. Outbreaks occur either as explosive epidemics, usually in non-endemic areas, or as protracted epidemic waves in endemic areas. The seasonal incidence is fairly consistent in different endemic regions, although the climatic conditions during epidemic waves may be distinctive for each region. For

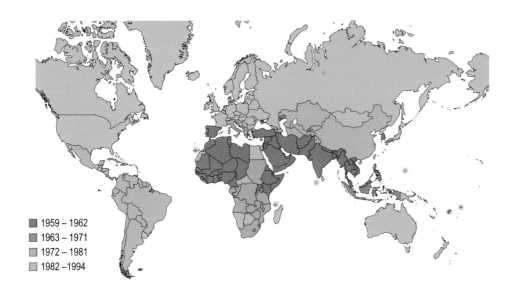

1959 – 1962
1963 – 1971
1972 – 1981
1982 –1994

**Fig. 30.2**   Areas reporting indigenous cholera to the World Health Organization 1959–1994. (Redrawn from data in: Public Health Laboratory Service 1991 *Communicable Disease Report Review* 1: R48–R50 and WHO 1995 *Weekly Epidemiological Record* 70: 201–208.)

example, in Bangladesh the cholera season (November to February) follows the monsoon rains and ends with the onset of the hot dry months. In Calcutta the main epidemic wave (May to July) rises to its peak in the hot dry season and ends with the onset of the monsoon, but extends inland to neighbouring states during the rainy season.

Spread of infection is facilitated by the high ratio of symptomless carriers to clinical cases, which varies from 10:1 to 100:1 depending on living conditions and biotype. Symptomless carriers occur much more frequently in El Tor than in classical infections.

## V. cholerae *O139*

In the 1990s cases of cholera indistinguishable from disease caused by *V. cholerae* O1 were reported in India and Bangladesh.

The new strain did not agglutinate with antisera to any of the O serogroups and was assigned to a new serogroup, O139 Bengal. However, it closely resembles *V. cholerae* O1 El Tor biochemically and physiologically, and may eventually attain the status of a subtype (*Bengal*) of that organism alongside the subtypes *Inaba* and *Ogawa*.

*V. cholerae* O139 is associated with free-living aquatic amoebae and other members of the zooplanktonic flora, which may act as a reservoir for the organism. In Spring 2000, an estimated 30 000 cases occurred in Dhaka, Bangladesh.

## Other non-*O1* V. cholerae *serogroups*

Strains belonging to serogroups other than O1 and O139 occur widely in aquatic environments, and many infections are associated with exposure to saline environments or consumption of seafood. They appear to survive and multiply in a wide range of foods, and it is likely that food-borne outbreaks occur as with other enteric pathogens.

## Treatment

In cholera absolute priority must be given to the life-saving replacement of fluid and electrolytes. Oral rehydration therapy is often sufficient, but severe cases may require intravenous rehydration. The World Health Organization (WHO) promotes the use of oral rehydration therapy in all cases of severe diarrhoea, including that due to *V. cholerae*. The recommended formula is shown in Table 30.1.

Tetracyclines, chloramphenicol and co-trimoxazole reduce the period of excretion of *V. cholerae* in the stools of patients with cholera. Tetracycline is often given to reduce environmental contamination and the risk of cross-infection. Tetracycline-resistant strains of *V. cholerae* O1 El Tor began to appear in the 1970s and were soon followed by the appearance of strains resistant to a wide range of antimicrobial agents, including penicillins, streptomycin, chloramphenicol, sulphonamides and trimethoprim.

**Table 30.1** Formulation of oral rehydration solution recommended by the World Health Organization

| Constituent | Amount (g)<sup>a</sup> |
|---|---|
| Sodium chloride | 2.6 |
| Potassium chloride | 1.5 |
| Trisodium citrate | 2.9 |
| Glucose (anhydrous) | 13.5 |

*a*To be dissolved in 1 L of clean drinking water.

## Control

Public health measures used in the control of any disease spread by faecal contamination are of value in the control of cholera. Most important are the provision of safe drinking water supplies and the proper disposal of human faeces.

Although cholera can be life threatening it is easily prevented and treated. Cholera among travellers is rare and few infections are reported from industrialized countries.

### Vaccines

The immune response to cholera is directed against the bacterium rather than the toxin. It is specific for a given serotype. Infection with the classical biotype is followed by almost complete immunity for several years, but infection with the El Tor biotype confers little or no immunity. It is not surprising, therefore, that the development of effective vaccines has proved difficult.

Traditional whole-cell vaccines are not very effective and are no longer recommended for travellers. Oral vaccines that combine purified B subunit and killed whole cells are now widely available and appear to be safe and protective.

## VIBRIO PARAHAEMOLYTICUS

## Description

*V. parahaemolyticus* is a halophilic vibrio and does not grow in the absence of sodium chloride. This property is conveniently demonstrated by inoculating the organism on to cystine–lactose–electrolyte-deficient (CLED) agar, which supports the growth of non-halophilic vibrios but not halophilic species. Strains of *V. parahaemolyticus* from clinical specimens generally form green, non-sucrose-fermenting colonies on TCBS agar, but sucrose-fermenting strains are found in estuarine and coastal waters.

Strains associated with gastroenteritis usually express a thermostable haemolysin which causes β-haemolysis of human red cells in Wagatsuma's agar, a special medium containing mannitol. This haemolysis is known as the *Kanagawa phenomenon.*

## Pathogenesis

*V. parahaemolyticus* can cause explosive diarrhoea, but symptoms usually abate after 3 days. Other symptoms include abdominal pain, nausea and vomiting, and there may be blood in the stools. A few extra-intestinal infections have been reported, particularly from wounds.

Kanagawa-positive strains cause diarrhoea in volunteers. In contrast, volunteers have ingested $10^{10}$ cells of Kanagawa-negative strains without ill effects. Kanagawa-positive strains also adhere to human intestinal cells, whereas Kanagawa-negative strains do not. The heat-stable haemolysin disrupts the cytoskeleton of cell membranes, and causes fluid accumulation in the rabbit ileal-loop toxin test. *V. parahaemolyticus* also produces a thermo-labile haemolysin that causes morphological changes in tissue culture cells resembling those caused by cholera toxin and the heat-labile enterotoxin of *E. coli*.

Most strains from seafood and the environment are Kanagawa negative, although positive colonies can usually be found if a sufficient number are tested. It is likely that a few Kanagawa-positive strains multiply selectively in the human intestine as infection develops and predominate in the stools of patients with diarrhoea.

## Laboratory diagnosis

The faeces of patients with a history of recent consumption of seafood may be examined by the methods used for *V. cholerae*. In the examination of seafood and sea or estuarine waters for halophilic species, including *V. parahaemolyticus*, enrichment culture in alkaline peptone water containing 1% sodium chloride is used. Around 13 O-types (somatic antigens) and 71 K-types (capsular antigens) are recognized; serotype O3:K6 has been detected widely in India, Asia, Africa and Latin America.

## Epidemiology

*V. parahaemolyticus* is a common cause of diarrhoea in Japan and South-East Asia. It also causes illness associated with seafood in many other countries, including the USA and the UK. The organisms are common in fish and shellfish and in the waters from which they are harvested. Infections occur more frequently in the warmer months when the organisms are most prevalent in the aquatic environment. There is a particular risk associated with the consumption of raw seafood prepared and eaten in Japanese-style restaurants.

Extra-intestinal infections are always associated with exposure to the aquatic environment or handling of contaminated seafood.

## Treatment and control

Patients with diarrhoea generally require only fluid replacement therapy. Infection can be avoided by normal food hygiene procedures and by refrigeration of seafood to reduce the possibility of bacterial multiplication. For wound infections and septicaemia, the most effective antimicrobial agents include tetracyclines, ciprofloxacin, ceftazidime and gentamicin.

## VIBRIO VULNIFICUS

This halophilic species differs from other vibrios by utilizing lactose. There are three biotypes of *V. vulnificus* based on physiological, biochemical and serological properties. Biotype 1 is the predominant human pathogen. Biotype 2 infects eels and biotype 3 causes human wound infections.

## Pathogenesis

There are three distinct clinical syndromes:

1. Rapid onset of fulminating septicaemia followed by the appearance of cutaneous lesions. More than 50% of those with primary septicaemia die. The condition is invariably associated with the consumption of raw shellfish. It is thought that the organisms enter the bloodstream by way of the portal vein or the intestinal lymph system. Elderly males with liver function defects due to alcohol abuse and people with iron-overload conditions are particularly susceptible, but any deficiency in the immune system may be a contributing factor.
2. A rapidly progressing cellulitis following contamination of a wound sustained during exposure to salt water. Infections of this kind occur in otherwise healthy persons as well as in the debilitated, and are characterized by wound oedema, erythema and necrosis, which progresses to septicaemia only occasionally. The infection can be rapidly fatal.

3. Acute diarrhoea following the consumption of shellfish. This is less common; victims generally have mildly debilitating underlying conditions. Death is rare.

### Pathogenic mechanisms

Strains of *V. vulnificus* are acid tolerant, surviving in stomach acid by breaking down amino acids to produce amines and $CO_2$. A capsular polysaccharide and long-chain lipopolysaccharide enable pathogenic strains to resist phagocytosis and the killing effects of human serum complement. Two siderophores, a catechol (vulnibactin) and a hyroxamate, have been reported indicating the presence of high-affinity iron-uptake systems; however, many strains are unable to obtain ferric ions bound to human transferrin. Patients with iron overload disorders such as haemochromatosis are highly susceptible; high levels of free serum iron are thought to facilitate the rapid septicaemia observed in patients infected with this organism.

Several toxins may contribute to tissue damage. They include a metalloprotease, a collagenase, a mucinase and a cytotoxin. A vascular permeability factor has also been described. Strains of *V. vulnificus* express El Tor haemolysin and thermo-labile haemolysin, but a role in pathogenesis has not been demonstrated.

### Epidemiology

Infections occur most frequently in areas where the water temperature remains high throughout the year, such as the mid-Atlantic and Gulf coast states of the USA. They are much more common during the warmer months of the year when *V. vulnificus* is most abundant. Wound infections are associated with injuries sustained in the aquatic environment, whereas septicaemic infections are associated with the consumption of raw shellfish.

### Treatment

*V. vulnificus* wound infections and primary septicemia require early antimicrobial treatment to reduce morbidity and mortality from the illness and to prevent complications. The most effective antimicrobial agents include: tetracyclines; fluoroquinolones such as ciprofloxacin; ceftazidime; and gentamicin. Because of the high case-fatality rates, it is particularly important for clinicians to suspect *V. vulnificus* wound or bloodstream infections in persons with shellfish or warm seawater exposure and a history of chronic liver disease or conditions of iron overload.

## *VIBRIO ALGINOLYTICUS*

### Description

*Vibrio alginolyticus* is a halophilic organism formerly regarded as biotype 2 of *V. parahaemolyticus*. It fails to grow on CLED agar but grows in the presence of 10% sodium chloride. It forms large, yellow (sucrose-fermenting) colonies on TCBS. There is pronounced swarming on non-selective solid media.

### Pathogenesis

*V. alginolyticus* causes wound and ear infections. Clinical features include mild cellulitis and a seropurulent exudate. The pathogenic mechanisms are not fully understood although genetic homology between *V. alginolyticus*, *V. cholerae* and *V. parahaemolyticus* has been shown.

### Epidemiology

This organism is widely distributed in seawater and seafood and is probably the most common vibrio found in these sources in the UK. It occurs in large numbers throughout the year. Infections are invariably associated with exposure to sea water. Strains appear to be sensitive to ciprofloxacin.

## OTHER VIBRIOS

- *Photobacterium damsela* is a halophilic marine vibrio found in tropical and semitropical aquatic environments. It is associated with severe infections of wounds acquired in warm coastal areas.
- *Vibrio fluvialis* is easily confused with *Aeromonas hydrophila*, but can be differentiated by growth on media containing 6% sodium chloride. Patients experience diarrhoea, abdominal pain, fever and dehydration. Low numbers of *V. fluvialis* can be isolated from fish and shellfish, and from warm seawater. It seems likely that infection is from contaminated seafood. Strains of *V. fluvialis* express El Tor haemolysin, and a vacuolating toxin acting on HeLa cells, but the role of these in pathogenesis has not been demonstrated.
- *Vibrio hollisae* is associated with bacteraemia and diarrhoea, especially in warm coastal areas, such as the Gulf of Mexico. Infections are strongly associated with the consumption of raw seafood. The organism is difficult to isolate because it grows poorly on TCBS agar. Strains of *V. hollisae* exhibit gene sequences homologous with those encoding the thermo-stable haemolysin of *V. parahaemolyticus*.
- *Vibrio mimicus* is a non-halophilic vibrio named for its similarity to *V. cholerae* and occurrence in similar environments. Most isolates are from the stools of patients who develop gastroenteritis after consumption of raw oysters, although a few cases of otitis media have also been reported. In vitro, strains of *V. mimicus* express thermo-stable direct haemolysin, El Tor haemolysin and thermo-labile haemolysin.
- *Vibrio furnissii* is most commonly isolated from stool samples. It has occasionally been implicated in gastroenteritis.

Other aquatic organisms that are probably related to vibrios include *Aeromonas* spp. and *Plesiomonas shigelloides*. *Aeromonas* spp., notably *A. hydrophila*, have been implicated in diarrhoea and occasionally cause more serious infection in compromised individuals. *A. salmonicida* is an economically important pathogen of fish. *P. shigelloides* is an organism of uncertain taxonomic status that sometimes causes water-borne outbreaks of diarrhoea in warm countries.

## *MOBILUNCUS*

The name *Mobiluncus* was first proposed for a group of curved, motile, Gram-variable, anaerobic bacteria isolated from the vagina of women with bacterial vaginosis. Its taxonomic position is uncertain. Studies of 16S RNA suggest that the genus is most closely related to *Actinomyces*.

## DESCRIPTION

There are two subspecies: *M. curtisii* and *M. mulieris*; *M. curtisii* can be divided further into two subspecies *M. curtisii* ssp. *curtisii* and *M. curtisii* ssp. *holmesii*. *M. curtisii* is short rod (mean length 1.5 μm) and Gram-variable, whereas *M. mulieris* is longer (mean length 3.0 μm) and Gram-negative. Both have multiple flagella originating from the concave aspect of the cells. Cell wall studies have revealed no outer membrane, but both species are thought to be Gram-negative.

## PATHOGENESIS

### Bacterial vaginosis

*Mobiluncus* spp. are isolated from 97% of women with bacterial vaginosis (non-specific vaginitis) and is rarely found in the vagina of healthy women. Bacterial vaginosis appears to be a polymicrobial infection, with certain organisms playing a key role, especially when they overgrow the lactobacilli of the normal flora, raising the vaginal pH above 4.5. The condition is characterized by the presence of a thin, homogeneous vaginal discharge with a characteristic 'rotten fish' smell. This becomes more pronounced on alkalization, and can be evoked by placing a drop of potassium hydroxide solution on the fresh exudate on a slide or the speculum used for the vaginal examination. The characteristic smell is ascribed to amines produced by one or more of the bacterial species that form the complex microbial flora of the vagina.

*Mobiluncus* are frequently found in association with *Gardnerella vaginalis* (see below) and with other organisms that may also be of aetiological importance. It appears that both the combination of species and their relative numbers are of importance in the development of the syndrome. The organisms may be isolated from the urethra of male consorts of infected women but do not persist in men once condom use is implemented.

*Mobiluncus* spp. are occasionally isolated from extragenital sites, especially from breast abscesses. A fatal case of bacteraemia caused by *M. curtisii* has been reported.

### Pathogenic mechanisms

The mechanisms that allow *Mobiluncus* spp. to cause disease are poorly understood. They express pili and are able to obtain iron from lactoferrin, but the role of these in the pathogenesis of disease is speculative. Strains of *Mobiluncus* spp. express a relatively thermostable toxin that is cytotoxic for Vero (African green monkey) cells, but a role in pathogenesis has not been demonstrated. Primates can be infected experimentally and animal studies may help to elucidate the pathogenesis of vaginitis.

## LABORATORY DIAGNOSIS

Microscopy of fresh unstained vaginal exudate reveals epithelial cells covered with adherent bacteria (*clue cells*). *Mobiluncus* spp. can be grown in Columbia blood broth and peptone–starch–dextrose broth containing 10% horse serum. The organisms are essentially anaerobic but grow slowly in 5% oxygen in nitrogen. They do not produce oxidase or catalase but ferment sugars.

A multiplex PCR comprising primers for both *Mobiluncus* spp. and *G. vaginalis* has been applied to cases of bacterial vaginosis.

## TREATMENT

Treatment of bacterial vaginosis aims to restore the normal vaginal flora by eliminating *Mobiluncus* and other organisms that may be involved. Oral or intravaginal metronidazole and clindamycin have been successfully used. Although *M. mulieris* is more susceptible than *M. curtisii* to metronidazole, treatment with this drug appears to eliminate all *Mobiluncus* species in patients with vaginosis.

## GARDNERELLA

*Gardnerella vaginalis* (formerly *Corynebacterium vaginale* or *Haemophilus vaginalis*) is commonly isolated together with *Mobiluncus* spp. in bacterial vaginosis. It has been implicated in cases of cervical cancer and infections of the urinary tract, but because the organism is frequently present in the vagina of asymptomatic patients its role in disease is equivocal.

## DESCRIPTION

*G. vaginalis* is a non-motile, non-sporing, microaerophilic coccobaccilus. It is Gram-variable, but because the cell wall contains lipopolysaccharide it appears to be Gram-negative.

## LABORATORY DIAGNOSIS

*G. vaginalis* grows on various media, such as Columbia agar containing colistin and nalidixic acid as selective agents. Plates are incubated at 35–37°C in 5–10% carbon dioxide for 2–3 days. On media containing human erythrocytes, the organism produces zones of β-haemolysis. *G. vaginalis* does not produce oxidase or catalase, but ferments starch and hydrolyses hippurate, and these properties provide a means of presumptive identification. Genes encoding the 60 kDa heat-shock protein chaperonin *Cpn* 60 can be used to detect *G. vaginalis* by PCR.

## PATHOGENESIS

Whether *G. vaginalis* can cause disease in isolation is unclear. The organisms may simply flourish in the vaginal environment provided by other bacteria. Infections with *G. vaginalis* are associated with proteolysis yielding nitrous products such as cadavarines and putrescines which contribute to the characteristic odour resulting from these infections. The ability to lyse human red cells offers a mechanism for acquiring metabolic iron and may aid multiplication. Similarly, *G. vaginalis* can acquire ferric ions from human lactoferrin. Strains produce various mucinases such as sialidase and proline dipeptidase, which are thought to damage the vaginal mucosa as part of the pathogenic process. Patients infected with *G. vaginalis* produce IgA antibodies to the haemolysin, but whether these can be used for serodiagnosis is not known.

## TREATMENT

For the treatment of bacterial vaginosis, see *Mobiluncus* (above).

## SPIRILLUM MINUS

The organism commonly known as *Spirillum minus* is of uncertain taxonomic position since a type-strain for this taxon has not been identified. Along with *Streptobacillus moniliformis* (see p. 348) it is one of the causes of rat bite fever in humans.

## DESCRIPTION

*S. minus* is a spiral Gram-negative organism about 2–5 μm in length and 0.2 μm in diameter. Longer forms of up to 10 μm may be observed. The regular short coils have a wavelength of 0.8–1.0 μm. The organisms are very actively motile, showing darting movements like those of a vibrio. The movement is due to polar flagella, which vary in number from one to seven at each pole. The organisms can be demonstrated in fresh specimens by dark-ground illumination or by staining with Giemsa or Leishman stains. The organism has not been reliably cultivated on artificial media and many of its properties are unknown. It can be cultured in vivo by intraperitoneal injection into guinea-pigs or mice.

## LABORATORY DIAGNOSIS

In rat bite fever, *S. minus* may be demonstrated in the local lesion, in the regional lymph glands or in the blood by direct microscopy or by animal inoculation. In theory, *S. minus* DNA may be amplified by broad range bacterial 16S rRNA gene primers.

## PATHOGENESIS

*S. minus* is transmitted to humans by animal bite; human-to-human transmission has not been recorded. The clinical syndrome of rat bite fever begins with an acute onset of fever and chills 1–4 weeks after the bite, although infection without fever may occur. The bite usually heals before the onset of symptoms but it often re-ulcerates. Local lymphadenopathy and lymphangitis develop with the onset of fever and systemic disease. A generalized rash with large brown to purple macules is usually observed, but some patients present with urticarial lesions. A roseolar rash may spread from the area of the original bite. Fever usually declines within 1 week before returning again after a few days; the fever may then recur in an episodic fashion for months or even years.

Endocarditis, meningitis, hepatitis, nephritis and myocarditis are rare complications. In most untreated cases, symptoms resolve within 2 months, after 6–8 episodes of fever, and fewer than 6.5% of untreated cases are fatal.

## EPIDEMIOLOGY

*S. minus* occurs naturally in wild rats and other rodents, causing bacteraemia. Human rat bite fever occurs mainly in Africa, Japan (where it is known as *sodoku*) and the Far East. There have been a few reports from Europe and the USA. The disease is prevalent in laboratory workers who handle rats, and in children who live in rat-infested homes.

## TREATMENT

Infections respond to treatment with penicillin, erythromycin and tetracyclines. In the rare case of endocarditis the addition of an aminoglycoside may be of value.

# RECOMMENDED READING

Chiang S-R, Chuang Y-C: *Vibrio vulnificus*: clinical manifestations, pathogenesis and antimicrobial therapy, *Journal of Microbiology, Immunology, and Infection* 36:81–88, 2003.

Chou TN, Lee YT, Lai YY, et al: Prognostic factors for primary septicemia and wound infection caused by *Vibrio vulnificus*, *American Journal of Emergency Medicine* 28:424–431, 2010.

Forsum U, Holst E, Larsson PG, et al: Bacterial vaginosis – a microbiological and immunological enigma, *Acta Pathologica, Microbiologica et Immunologica Scandinavica* 113:81–90, 2005.

Jenkins SG: Rat-bite fever, *Clinical Microbiology Newsletter* 10:57–59, 1988.

Jones MK, Oliver JD: *Vibrio vulnificus*: disease and pathogenesis, *Infection and Immunity* 77:1723–1733, 2009.

Sack DA, Sack RB, Nair GB, Siddique AK: Cholera, *Lancet* 363:223–233, 2004.

Safa A, Nair GB, Kong RY: Evolution of new variants of *Vibrio cholerae* O1, *Trends in Microbiology* 18:46–54, 2010.

Sanchez J, Holmgren J: Virulence factors, pathogenesis and vaccine protection in cholera and ETEC diarrhea, *Current Opinion in Immunology* 17:1–11, 2005.

Spiegal CA: Bacterial vaginosis, *Reviews in Medical Microbiology* 13:43–51, 2002.

## Websites

Centers for Disease Control and Prevention: Vibrio vulnificus. http://www.cdc.gov/nczved/divisions/dfbmd/diseases/vibriov/

Centers for Disease Control and Prevention: Vibrio parahaemolyticus. http://www.cdc.gov/nczved/divisions/dfbmd/diseases/vibriop/

Health Protection Agency: *Cholera.* http://www.hpa.org.uk/infections/topics_az/cholera/menu.htm

Todar's Online Textbook of Bacteriology: Vibrio cholerae *and Asiatic Cholera.* http://textbookofbacteriology.net/cholera.html

# 31 Haemophilus

## Respiratory infections; meningitis; chancroid

*M. P. E. Slack*

## KEY POINTS

- Most strains of *Haemophilus influenzae* are non-capsulate but some strains possess a polysaccharide capsule (types a–f).
- *H. influenzae* type b (Hib) is a major human pathogen that causes invasive infections, including meningitis and epiglottitis.
- Non-capsulate strains cause 90% of non-invasive respiratory infections, including otitis media and acute exacerbations of chronic obstructive airway disease.
- Following the introduction of Hib conjugate vaccine, the number of invasive *H. influenzae* infections declined dramatically; most invasive infections are now caused by non-typable strains.
- 15–20% of *H. influenzae* strains are ampicillin resistant ($\beta$-lactamase-mediated); ceftriaxone is the treatment of choice for invasive disease.
- Conjugate Hib vaccine is routinely offered to infants at 2, 3, 4 and 12 months in the UK.
- *H. ducreyi* causes chancroid, sexually transmitted genital ulcers that are common in Africa and South-East Asia but rare in the UK. Single-dose therapy with azithromycin or ceftriaxone is effective.
- Chancroid lesions may facilitate the transmission of HIV.

*Haemophilus influenzae* is associated with a variety of invasive infections such as meningitis, epiglottitis, pneumonia and septic arthritis, and localized disease of the respiratory tract including bronchitis and otitis media. Other haemophili of medical importance include *H. ducreyi*, the causative organism of chancroid, and *H. parainfluenzae*. Two related organisms, *H. aphrophilus* and *H. paraphrophilus*, are now combined as a single species within the genus *Aggregatibacter* as *A. aphrophilus*; like *H. parainfluenzae* they are occasionally encountered in patients with infective endocarditis and other miscellaneous conditions.

During the influenza pandemic of 1889–1892, Pfeiffer noted the constant presence of large numbers of small bacilli in the sputum of patients affected with the disease and suggested that the bacillus was the causative agent. Although the true aetiological agent of influenza was shown in 1933 to be a virus, it remains possible that secondary infection with *H. influenzae* contributed to the high mortality rate seen in the 1889–92 and 1918–19 pandemics.

## DESCRIPTION

Haemophili are small, pleomorphic, Gram-negative rods or coccobacilli with occasional longer, filamentous forms (Fig. 31.1). Some strains of *H. influenzae* produce a polysaccharide capsule, which is demonstrable by capsule stains and a *Quellung reaction* (swelling of the capsule) with type-specific antisera. There are six capsular types, designated a–f, which can be identified by a polymerase chain reaction (PCR) method. The most important is type b, a polymer of ribosyl ribitol phosphate.

All species of *Haemophilus* are catalase and oxidase positive; they reduce nitrate to nitrite and ferment glucose. Patterns of acid production from other carbohydrates are used to differentiate the species. *H. influenzae* can be divided into eight biotypes on the basis of indole production, urease activity and ornithine decarboxylase reactions. Biotypes I–III are the most common, and most invasive (type b) organisms are biotype I.

**Fig. 31.1** Gram stain of cerebrospinal fluid showing *Haemophilus influenzae*: Gram-negative pleomorphic coccobacilli.

**Table 31.1** Clinical spectrum of *Haemophilus influenzae* infections

| Type of infection | Age group | Strains |
|---|---|---|
| Invasive | 90% children <4 years[a] | 90% *H. influenzae* type b[a] 10% non-capsulate strains 1% types e and f |
| Neonatal and maternal | Neonates; pregnant and parturient women | >90% non-capsulate strains |
| Non-invasive respiratory | Children and adults | >90% non-capsulate strains |

[a]Percentages observed before the introduction of Hib conjugate vaccine; since the introduction of routine vaccination, the epidemiology has changed (see text).

## Growth requirements

Growth depends on a requirement for two factors, termed X and V:

- X factor (haemin) is required for the synthesis of cytochrome *c* and other iron-containing respiratory enzymes.
- V factor is nicotinamide adenine dinucleotide (NAD), NAD phosphate or certain unidentified precursor compounds. It is essential for oxidation-reduction processes in cell metabolism.

Different species of *Haemophilus* require either or both of these factors, and growth factor dependence forms an important step in identification.

Ordinary blood agar contains X and V factors, but growth of *H. influenzae*, which requires both factors, is poor. Growth is enhanced if the medium is supplemented with NAD. Streaking an organism that excretes this substance (e.g. *Staphylococcus aureus*) across the surface of the agar stimulates growth in its vicinity (satellitism). Heating blood agar for a few minutes at 70–80°C until it turns brown (chocolate agar) much improves the growth of *H. influenzae*. This process removes serum NADase, which limits the amount of V factor, and also liberates extra X and V factors from the red cells into the medium. X factor is heat stable, but heating of media at 120°C for several minutes destroys V factor.

Anaerobic growth considerably reduces the haemin requirement of X-dependent species. *A. aphrophilus* has a requirement for carbon dioxide, but this character may be lost on subculture. *H. influenzae* does not require a carbon dioxide-enriched atmosphere, but often grows better in such conditions.

## *HAEMOPHILUS INFLUENZAE*

### Pathogenesis

*H. influenzae* is an obligate parasite of human mucous membranes; it is not found in any other animal species. It colonizes the throat and nasopharynx, and to a lesser extent the conjunctivae and genital tract. The species is associated with two types of infection which are quite distinct in their epidemiological profiles: invasive infections and non-invasive infections (Table 31.1).

#### Invasive infections

Most invasive infections are caused by *H. influenzae* type b (Hib). Meningitis is the most common manifestation, but *H. influenzae* also causes epiglottitis, septic arthritis, osteomyelitis, pneumonia and cellulitis. In some cases the patient develops a bacteraemia without a clearly defined focus of infection.

These infections are unusual in the first 2 months of life, but are otherwise seen mainly in early childhood. Most cases occur in children under 2 years of age, but acute epiglottitis has a peak incidence between 2 and 4 years of age. The incidence of invasive disease in children has been reduced dramatically in countries where a conjugate Hib vaccine has been introduced, and consequently the epidemiology is changing (see below).

The polysaccharide capsule is the major virulence factor for Hib. When the organism invades the bloodstream, the capsule enables the organisms to evade phagocytosis and complement-mediated lysis in the non-immune host. The rarity of infections in the first 2 months of life correlates with the presence of

**Fig. 31.2** Incidence of *H. influenzae* meningitis during the first 5 years of life and the corresponding mean level of anti-*H. influenzae* type b (Hib) capsular polysaccharide antibodies. (From Peltola H, Käyhty H, Sivonen A, Mäkelä H 1977 *Haemophilus influenzae* type b capsular polysaccharide vaccine in children: a double blind field study of 100 000 vaccinees 3 months to 5 years of age in Finland. *Pediatrics* 60: 730–737. ©1977 by the American Academy of Pediatrics.)

maternal capsular antibodies, and the occurrence of infection in early infancy with the absence of such antibodies. As the prevalence and mean level of capsular antibodies in the population rise, *H. influenzae* type b infections become less common (Fig. 31.2).

What determines whether acquisition of type b organisms in a susceptible host will lead to asymptomatic carriage and the stimulation of protective antibodies, or to the induction of invasive disease, is unclear. However, animal experiments suggest that when invasion occurs the organism penetrates the submucosa of the nasopharynx and establishes systemic infection through the bloodstream.

The type b capsular polysaccharide facilitates all phases of the invasion process. Other virulence factors that may be involved include:

- fimbriae, which assist attachment to epithelial cells
- immunoglobulin A (Ig A) proteases, which are also involved in colonization
- outer membrane proteins and lipopolysaccharide, which may contribute to invasion at several stages.

Initiation of invasive infection may be potentiated by intercurrent viral infection. Host genetic factors and immunosuppression may also play a role. It is unclear whether it is exposure to *H. influenzae* type b, or some other organism (e.g. *Escherichia coli* K100) possessing cross-reacting antigens, that usually stimulates natural protective antibody production.

Since the introduction of routine infant immunization with conjugate Hib vaccine, invasive disease caused by non-capsulate (non-typable) strains has become more common than that caused by Hib in the

UK. Meningitis and bacteraemia due to non-capsulate *H. influenzae* is sometimes seen in the neonate. Infections with non-capsulate strains may also occur in children and adults. Pneumonia and bacteraemia are the most common manifestations, often in patients with an underlying disease, notably chronic lung disease or malignancy. The highest rates occur in patients aged over 60 years, and the case fatality rate is high.

Invasive infections due to *H. influenzae* of serotypes other than b (principally types a, e and f) are uncommon. The spectrum of disease is similar to that seen with type b.

### Non-invasive disease

*H. influenzae* produces a variety of local infections, which are often associated with some underlying physiological or anatomical abnormality. Most are caused by non-capsulate strains. The most common are:

- otitis media
- sinusitis
- conjunctivitis
- acute exacerbations of chronic obstructive airway disease
- pneumonia.

Acute sinusitis and otitis media are usually initiated by viral infections, which predispose to secondary infection with potentially pathogenic components of the resident microbial flora. The mechanisms may involve:

- obstruction to the outflow of respiratory secretions
- decreased clearance of micro-organisms via the normal mucociliary mechanism
- depression of local immunity.

Acute exacerbations of chronic obstructive airway disease are similarly initiated by acute viral infections. Respiratory viruses compromise an already impaired mucociliary clearance mechanism in patients with chronic lung disease and allow bacterial colonization of the lower respiratory tract. In this situation *H. influenzae* can establish purulent infection and further damages pulmonary function by a direct toxic effect on cilia.

### Laboratory diagnosis

Gram-stained smears of cerebrospinal fluid, pus, sputum or aspirates from joints, middle ears or sinuses can provide a rapid presumptive identification. Haemophili tend to stain poorly, and dilute carbol fuchsin is a better counterstain than neutral red or safranin.

The viability of *H. influenzae* in clinical specimens declines with time, particularly at 4°C. Specimens should therefore be transported to the laboratory and cultured without delay. Chocolate agar is a good, general purpose, culture medium and can be used without further supplementation for specimens obtained from sites that would normally be expected to be sterile. Plates should be incubated in an aerobic atmosphere enriched with 5–10% carbon dioxide.

Specimens of expectorated sputum inevitably become contaminated by upper respiratory flora, commonly including *H. influenzae*, and the finding of the organism in such specimens does not necessarily signify involvement in disease. Support for the significance of *H. influenzae* is provided if, in a purulent sample, the organism is present as the predominant isolate, or in a viable count of over $10^6$ colony-forming units per mL. Addition of bacitracin (10 international units/mL) facilitates the selective isolation of *H. influenzae* from mixed cultures of respiratory organisms. Obtaining bronchial secretions by broncho-alveolar lavage reduces the problem of contamination with commensal organisms.

The temptation to obtain throat swabs in patients with suspected acute epiglottitis should be resisted, as attempts to obtain the sample may precipitate complete airway obstruction. Blood culture is indicated for patients with suspected invasive disease and is usually positive in those with acute epiglottitis.

## Identification

*H. influenzae* grows poorly on blood agar. On chocolate agar the colonies are smooth, grey or colourless (Fig. 31.3), with a characteristic seminal odour.

Confirmation of the identity depends on demonstrating a requirement for one or both of the growth factors, X and V:

- *H. influenzae* requires both X and V factors.
- *H. parainfluenzae* requires V factor alone.
- *A. aphrophilus* (*H. aphrophilus*) and *H. ducreyi* require X factor alone.

The culture is plated on nutrient agar that is deficient in both X and V factor, and paper discs containing X factor, V factor and X + V factor are placed on the surface of the agar. After overnight incubation, growth is observed around the discs supplying the necessary growth factors (Fig. 31.4).

PCR techniques are used to identify *Haemophilus* species in clinical specimens and as confirmatory tests on isolates. The capsular type of *H. influenzae* isolates is determined by slide agglutination with type-specific antisera, or a PCR-based method.

## Antigen detection

The detection of type b polysaccharide antigen in body fluids or pus is useful, particularly in patients who received antibiotics before specimens were obtained. A rapid latex agglutination test with rabbit antibody to type b antigen is used most commonly.

In the absence of confirmatory cultures, the results should be regarded with caution as some serotypes of *Streptococcus pneumoniae* and *E. coli* may share similar antigens.

**Fig. 31.3**  Culture of *H. influenzae* on chocolate agar.

**Fig. 31.4**  Determination of the growth factor requirement of *H. influenzae*. Growth around the disc containing both X and V factors (right-hand disc), but not round discs of the individual factors (left-hand discs), indicates that the organism is *H. influenzae* (see text).

## Antibiotic sensitivity tests

Accurate determination of the antibiotic susceptibility of *H. influenzae* requires careful standardization of the methodology. Disc tests are less reliable for detecting enzyme-mediated ampicillin (β-lactamase) and chloramphenicol (chloramphenicol acetyltransferase) resistance than microbiological or biochemical techniques that demonstrate antibiotic inactivation.

## Treatment

*H. influenzae* is usually susceptible to ampicillin (or amoxicillin), chloramphenicol and tetracyclines. Among cephalosporins, compounds such as cefuroxime, cefotaxime and ceftriaxone are highly active. Other antibiotics active against *H. influenzae* include co-amoxiclav, ciprofloxacin, azithromycin and clarithromycin.

Ceftriaxone (or a related cephalosporin such as cefotaxime) is the antibiotic of first choice for the treatment of meningitis and acute epiglottitis. It is bactericidal for *H. influenzae*, achieves good concentrations in the meninges and cerebral tissues, and is highly effective.

β-Lactamase mediated resistance to ampicillin is now encountered in up to 15% of type b strains and about 20% of invasive non-capsulate isolates in the UK. Occasional strains are resistant to ampicillin through alterations in penicillin binding protein 3 (β-lactamase-negative ampicillin resistance–BLNAR) and a few strains demonstrate both mechanisms of resistance. For these reasons ampicillin should not be used as a single agent in meningitis when *H. influenzae* is a possibility and the results of sensitivity tests are not available. Resistance to chloramphenicol may also be encountered, but in most parts of the world this remains uncommon.

Antibiotic therapy is only one component of the clinical management of patients with haemophilus meningitis and full supportive care is required to achieve the most favourable outcome. Skilled medical and nursing care is also vital in the management of acute epiglottitis, where maintenance of a patent airway is crucial.

For the treatment of less serious respiratory infections, such as otitis media, sinusitis and acute exacerbations of chronic bronchitis, oral antibiotics such as amoxicillin, co-amoxiclav and clarithromycin are all effective.

## Epidemiology of invasive disease

Non-capsulate *H. influenzae* are present in the nasopharynx or throat of 25–80% of healthy people; capsulate strains (about half of which are capsular type b) are present in 5–10%. *H. influenzae* type b is an important cause of serious systemic infection in children throughout the world. Meningitis is more common in winter months, in families of low socioeconomic status and in household contacts of a case. The disease is usually seen in the youngest member of a family and uncommonly in children who have no siblings. Household contacts of patients with invasive disease have an increased risk of acquiring infection if they are less than 5 years of age. The risk for children under 2 years of age is 600–800-fold higher than the age-adjusted risk for the general population.

Outbreaks of infection have been described in close communities, such as nursery schools. Contact with a case in a day care centre or nursery has also been associated with increased attack rates in children under 2 years of age, although the calculated risk is lower than that seen in household contacts.

Very high incidence rates have been reported in certain populations of Australian Aborigines, American Indians and Inuits. In these racial groups the peak incidence of infection occurs at a younger age. By contrast, very low rates have been reported in Hong Kong Chinese. It is possible that socio-economic considerations are important in determining such racial differences, but host genetic factors may also play a role. Immunosuppression, whether iatrogenic or associated with malignancies (especially Hodgkin's disease), asplenia or agammaglobulinaemia, also predispose to invasive disease. There is seasonal variation, with most cases occurring during the winter months.

The mortality rate associated with *H. influenzae* meningitis is around 5%. Neurological sequelae, including intellectual impairment, seizures and profound or severe hearing loss, may be present in 10–20% of survivors.

## *H. influenzae* type b disease in the UK

Before the introduction of conjugate Hib vaccine into the infant immunization schedule in 1992, approximately 1500 cases of invasive Hib disease, including 900 cases of meningitis, occurred in the UK every year, with 60 deaths. Immunization rates have remained high (about 93%), and between 1992 and 1999 *H. influenzae* type b disease in children less than 5 years old fell by 95% (Fig. 31.5). In 1998 only 21 cases of invasive Hib disease in children under 5 years were reported in England and Wales. From 1999 there was a small but gradual increase in the number of

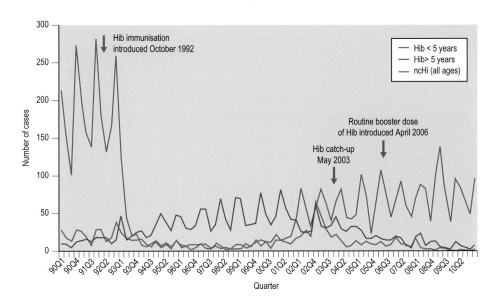

**Fig. 31.5** Quarterly incidence of invasive *H. influenzae* type b (Hib) and non-capsulate *H. influenzae* (ncHi) infections in England and Wales, January 1990 to December 2010. (Data from Health Protection Agency Centre for Infections.)

cases, most notably in fully immunized children born in 2000 and 2001, but also in older children and adults. In 2003 children over 6 months and under 4 years of age were offered a booster dose of Hib vaccine and in 2006 a routine booster dose of Hib vaccine, given in combination with meningococcus group C conjugate vaccine, was incorporated into the UK infant immunization schedule. These campaigns have had a marked effect on the incidence of invasive Hib disease, most dramatically in 1–4-year-olds, but also in older children and adults.

## Control

### Active immunization

Early haemophilus vaccines consisting of purified type b capsular polysaccharide were poorly immunogenic in children less than 2 years old and in patients with immune deficiency. Conjugate vaccines in which the polysaccharide is covalently coupled to proteins such as tetanus toxoid, a non-toxic variant of diphtheria toxin, *Neisseria meningitidis* outer membrane protein or diphtheria toxoid produce a lasting anamnestic response, which is not age-related and may be effective in high-risk patients who respond poorly to polysaccharide vaccine alone. In the UK, *H. influenzae* type b vaccine is offered routinely to infants at 2, 3 and 4 months of age as part of a pentavalent diphtheria, tetanus, pertussis, polio, Hib vaccine (see Ch. 70). A Hib booster dose (in combination with meningococcus C vaccine), given at 12 months of age, was introduced in 2006. Immunization of infants significantly reduces pharyngeal carriage of Hib, but has no effect on the carriage of other capsular types or non-capsulate strains.

Conjugate Hib vaccine is recommended for children and adults with splenic dysfunction, because they are at increased risk of invasive Hib infection.

### Prophylaxis

Rifampicin (20 mg/kg (maximum 600 mg) for children >3 months and adults; 10 mg/kg for infants <3 months) given orally once daily for 4 days eradicates carriage of *H. influenzae* and prevents secondary infection in household and nursery contacts.

Unvaccinated or partially vaccinated (including those who were immunized only in infancy) siblings of the index case who are younger than 10 years old should be appropriately immunized with the Hib conjugate vaccine. The index case should also be given a dose of Hib vaccine before discharge from hospital to ensure high levels of antibodies and long-term protection against Hib. Household contacts and the index case should be given rifampicin chemoprophylaxis to eradicate carriage if there is a vulnerable individual in the household (an immunosuppressed or asplenic person of any age, or any child younger then ten years – this may be the index case).

When two or more cases of Hib disease occur in a nursery or playgroup within 120 days, chemoprophylaxis should be offered to all room contacts – carers and children. Any unvaccinated or partially vaccinated children under 10 years of age should be appropriately immunized against Hib.

The widespread use of conjugate vaccine may soon render chemoprophylaxis unnecessary.

## OTHER HAEMOPHILI

### *H. influenzae* biogroup aegyptius

This organism, formerly known as the *Koch–Weeks bacillus* and *H. aegyptius*, is now classified as a subgroup of *H. influenzae*. It is indistinguishable from *H. influenzae* biotype III in routine tests, but can be identified by a PCR method. It causes a purulent conjunctivitis and *Brazilian purpuric fever*, a clinical syndrome first recognized in Brazil in 1984, in which conjunctivitis proceeds to an overwhelming septicaemia resembling fulminating meningococcal infection. This virulent clone has not been reported since the early 1990s. Ampicillin in combination with chloramphenicol has been successful when treatment has been started sufficiently early.

### *H. ducreyi*

*H. ducreyi* is responsible for a sexually transmitted infection, chancroid, which is most prevalent in tropical regions, particularly Africa and South-East Asia. Patients present with painful penile ulcers (soft sore or soft chancre) and inguinal lymphadenitis. Typical small Gram-negative bacilli can be seen in material from the ulcers or in pus from lymph node aspirates. It is likely that the lesions of chancroid have facilitated the transmission of human immunodeficiency virus (HIV) in some tropical countries.

*H. ducreyi* is an extremely fastidious organism requiring specialized culture media. A multiplex PCR has been developed for the simultaneous amplification of DNA targets from *H. ducreyi*, *Treponema pallidum* and herpes simplex virus types 1 and 2.

Susceptibility to antimicrobial agents varies geographically. Many strains are β-lactamase producers and resistance to tetracycline and co-trimoxazole is common. Chancroid is best treated with azithromycin, ceftriaxone, ciprofloxacin or erythromycin. Azithromycin and ceftriaxone have the advantage of single-dose therapy. Strains with intermediate resistance to ciprofloxacin or erythromycin have been reported. Treatment failures are much more likely in patients with concurrent HIV infection. The use of condoms dramatically reduces the transmission of *H. ducreyi*. All sexual partners should be identified by contact tracing and treated.

An unrelated Gram-negative rod, *Calymmatobacterium granulomatis*, causes a somewhat similar sexually transmitted disease, granuloma inguinale or donovanosis, in parts of the tropics. Intracellular organisms, known as Donovan bodies (not to be confused with the Leishman–Donovan bodies of leishmaniasis), can be demonstrated in the stained smears from the lesions. Tetracyclines are usually used in treatment.

### Related organisms

*H. parainfluenzae*, *A. aphrophilus* (formerly *H. aphrophilus* and *H. paraphrophilus*; see p. 324) and *A. actinomycetemcomitans* (formerly *Actinobacillus actinomycetemcomitans*) are occasionally implicated in human disease, notably infective endocarditis, but also dental infections, lung abscess and brain abscess. Endocarditis is usually treated successfully with a combination of ampicillin and gentamicin.

## RECOMMENDED READING

Alfa M: The laboratory diagnosis of *Haemophilus ducreyi*, *Canadian Journal of Infectious Diseases and Medical Microbiology* 16:31–34, 2005.

Coker TR, Chan LS, Newberry SJ, et al: Diagnosis, microbial epidemiology and antibiotic treatment of acute otitis media in children, *Journal of the American Medical Association* 304:2161–2169, 2010.

Harrison LH, Simonson V, Waldman EA: Emergence and disappearance of a virulent clone of *Haemophilus influenzae* biogroup aegyptius, cause of Brazilian Purpuric Fever, *Clinical Microbiology Reviews* 21:594–605, 2008.

Kelly DF, Moxon ER, Pollard AJ: *Haemophilus influenzae* type b conjugate vaccines, *Immunology* 113:163–174, 2004.

Ladhani S, Neely F, Heath PT, et al: Recommendations for the prevention of secondary *Haemophilus influenzae* type b (Hib) disease, *Journal of Infection* 58:3–14, 2009.

Ladhani S, Slack MPE, Heath PT, et al: Invasive *Haemophilus influenzae* disease, Europe, 1996–2006, *Emerging Infectious Diseases* 16:455–462, 2010.

Peltola H: Worldwide *Haemophilus influenzae* type b disease at the beginning of the 21st century: global analysis of the disease burden 25 years after the use of the polysaccharide vaccine and a decade after the advent of conjugates, *Clinical Microbiology Reviews* 13:302–317, 2000.

Tristram S, Jacobs MR, Appelbaum PC: Antimicrobial resistance in *Haemophilus influenzae*, *Clinical Microbiology Reviews* 20:368–389, 2007.

Ulanova M, Tsang RSW: Invasive *Haemophilus influenzae* disease: changing epidemiology and host-parasite interactions in the 21st century *Infection, Genetics and Evolution* 9:594–605, 2009.

Watt JP, Wolfson LJ, O'Brien KL, et al: Burden of disease caused by *Haemophilus influenzae* type b in children younger than 5 years: global estimates, *Lancet* 374: 903–911, 2009.

### Websites

Clinical Effectiveness Group (British Association for Sexual Health and HIV, BASSH): 2007 National Guideline for the Management of Chancroid. http://www.bashh.org/documents/85/85.pdf

UK Department of Health. *Haemophilus influenzae* type b (Hib) Immunization. http://www.dh.gov.uk/prod_consum_dh/groups/dh_digitalassets/@dh/@en/documents/digitalasset/dh_125943.pdf

# 32 Bordetella

## Whooping cough

*N. W. Preston*

## KEY POINTS

- Whooping cough is caused by *Bordetella pertussis,* and occasionally by *B. parapertussis.*
- Paroxysmal cough, typically with vomit and whoop, lasts for several weeks or even months.
- Pertussis is a human disease (most severe in children) and has no animal or environmental reservoir.
- Clinical diagnosis is unreliable in mild cases.
- Bacterial culture is the optimal method of laboratory confirmation.
- Therapy for established cases is unsatisfactory.
- Immunity to *B. pertussis* infection is serotype-specific.
- Vaccine containing the three serotype antigens is safe, and is effective if the vaccination schedule is optimal.
- Eradication of whooping cough by childhood vaccination is an achievable goal.

The genus *Bordetella* constitutes one of the groups of very thin ovoid or rod-shaped Gram-negative bacilli, often described as parvobacteria. The genus contains two notable human pathogens, *Bordetella pertussis* and *B. parapertussis*, which cause one of the most frequent and serious bacterial respiratory infections of childhood in communities not protected effectively by vaccination.

## DESCRIPTION

Bordetellae used to be classified in the genus *Haemophilus*. However, growth is not dependent on either of the nutritional factors X and V (see p. 325), and *B. parapertussis* and *B. bronchiseptica* do not require blood for their growth. The three species resemble one another in being small Gram-negative bacilli, in causing infection of the respiratory tract, and in sharing some surface antigens.

### *Bordetella pertussis*

This is the most fastidious of the bordetellae. It produces toxic products that must be absorbed by a culture medium containing charcoal, or starch, or a high concentration of blood as in the original Bordet–Gengou medium. Because agglutination forms an important part of identification, a smooth growth is essential, and this is best provided by charcoal–blood agar. *B. pertussis* is a strict aerobe, with an optimal growth temperature of 35–36°C. Even under these conditions it usually takes 3 days for colonies to be visible to the naked eye.

Typical colonies are shiny, greyish white, convex, and with a butyrous consistency. By slide agglutination, they react strongly with homologous (pertussis) antiserum, and weakly or not at all with parapertussis antiserum, depending on the specificity of the reagent. Subculture reveals no growth on nutrient agar.

The organism produces three major agglutinogens (1, 2 and 3) which can be detected by the use of absorbed single-agglutinin sera. Factor 1 is common to all strains; the three serotypes pathogenic to man (type 1,2, type 1,3 and type 1,2,3) also possess factor 2 or factor 3 or both factors, and these type-specific agglutinogens have a vital role in immunity to infection.

### *Bordetella parapertussis*

This organism is readily distinguished from *B. pertussis* by its ability to grow on nutrient agar, with the production of a brown diffusible pigment after 2 days (Table 32.1). It also grows more rapidly than *B. pertussis* on charcoal–blood agar, and is agglutinated more strongly by parapertussis than by pertussis antiserum.

*B. parapertussis* usually causes less severe illness than *B. pertussis*, and is uncommon in most countries,

**Table 32.1** Differential properties of *B. pertussis* and *B. parapertussis*

| Property | *B. pertussis* | *B. parapertussis* |
|---|---|---|
| Duration of incubation to yield visible colonies | 3 days | 2 days |
| Growth on nutrient agar | None | Good |
| Pigment diffusing in medium | None | Brown |
| Slide agglutination with: | | |
|     Pertussis antiserum | Strong | Weak |
|     Parapertussis antiserum | Weak | Strong |

although occasionally it has been responsible for outbreaks of whooping cough.

### Bordetella bronchiseptica

Colonies of this species are visible on nutrient agar after overnight incubation; it differs from the other species by also being motile and by producing an obvious alkaline reaction in the Hugh and Leifson medium that is used to differentiate oxidative from fermentative action on sugars. It is therefore placed by some taxonomists in the genus *Alcaligenes*; however, it is readily distinguished from the intestinal commensal *Alcaligenes faecalis* by its rapid hydrolysis of urea.

Although rarely encountered in human infections, *B. bronchiseptica* is a common respiratory pathogen of animals, especially laboratory stocks of rodents. Because it shares antigens with other bordetellae, animals must be checked for freedom from bordetella antibody before they are used in the preparation of specific antisera. For this reason, sheep or donkeys have sometimes been used in preference to rodents.

## PATHOGENESIS

Whooping cough is a non-invasive infection of the respiratory mucosa, with man as the only natural host. In a typical case, an incubation period of 1–2 weeks is followed by a 'catarrhal' phase with a simple cough but no distinctive features. Within about a week, this leads into the 'paroxysmal' phase, with increasing severity and frequency of paroxysmal cough, which may last for many weeks and be followed by an equally prolonged 'convalescent' phase.

In the initial preventable stage of the infection there is colonization of the ciliated epithelium of the bronchi and trachea with vast numbers of bacteria whose agglutinogens play a vital and type-specific role in attachment. *B. pertussis* produces a tracheal cytotoxin that paralyses the cilia and leads to paroxysms of coughing as an alternative means of removing the increased mucus. Another bacterial product, called pertussis toxin, is responsible for the characteristic lymphocytosis in uncomplicated whooping cough. A subsequent increase in the number of neutrophils, together with fever, suggests bronchopneumonia or other secondary infection, maybe with pyogenic cocci. Blockage of airways may cause areas of lung collapse, and anoxia may lead to convulsions, although with modern intensive care the disease is rarely fatal.

## Clinical features

Pertussis (severe cough) has been recognized as a clinical entity for several centuries. Typically, the child suffers many bouts of paroxysmal coughing each day; during these, with no pause for air intake, the tongue is protruded fully, fluids stream from the eyes, nose and mouth, and the face becomes cyanotic; when death seems imminent, a final cough clears the secretions and, with a massive inspiratory effort, air is sucked through the narrowed glottis, producing a long high-pitched whoop – hence the term *whooping cough*. Such attacks often terminate with vomiting. Between them the patient does not usually appear ill.

If a characteristic attack is witnessed, a diagnosis of pertussis is usually made on clinical grounds alone. However, the illness is often mild and atypical, especially in:

- older children and adults
- younger children who have been incompletely immunized
- very young infants partially protected by maternal antibody.

In these cases, the laboratory has a vital role in diagnosis, because similar coughing may be caused by a variety of viruses and such illness is generally mild and of short duration. Here, the term *pseudo-whooping cough* has been aptly applied. False diagnosis may create a popular impression of pertussis as a trivial disease; and it is recommended that, in the absence of positive bacterial culture, whooping cough should not be diagnosed for paroxysmal coughing lasting less than 3 weeks. With genuine pertussis, the illness is likely to persist for months rather than weeks. Furthermore, because pertussis vaccine cannot be expected to protect against viral infection, estimates of vaccine efficacy require an accurate diagnosis. Thus, a study in the UK found an efficacy of 93% against pertussis confirmed by bacterial culture, compared with only 82% for cases diagnosed solely on clinical criteria.

In developing countries, whooping cough is still a major cause of death; however, in developed countries, concern is focused on a very prolonged and frightening illness with possible respiratory and neurological sequelae, on the anxiety and exhaustion of parents, and on the heavy use of hospital and community medical resources.

## Experimental infection in animals

Some, though not all, of the features of human disease have been produced in animals. Thus, marmosets and rabbits develop catarrh during prolonged colonization of the respiratory tract; they produce a similar range of agglutinin response to vaccination, and this immunity shows evidence of serotype specificity.

However, the mouse, which has long been used in the evaluation of pertussis vaccine potency, does not show these features. It can be infected and even killed by degraded organisms of serotype 1, which have lost the type-specific agglutinogens (2 and 3) that are necessary for human infection. It also reveals additional properties of pertussis toxin that are not seen in human beings: histamine sensitization, and islets activation (including hyperinsulinaemia and hypoglycaemia). Furthermore, pertussis toxin and other components of the organism – filamentous haemagglutinin and pertactin – are virulence factors in the mouse; but their role in human infection is uncertain. It is therefore necessary to interpret with caution experimental evidence from mice or other small rodents.

## LABORATORY DIAGNOSIS

### Bacterial culture

Because atypical clinical cases occur frequently, laboratory confirmation of the diagnosis is often essential. Bacterial culture has the highest specificity of the tests available. In the absence of really effective therapy, accuracy in the diagnosis is more important than speed. Bacterial culture has the additional advantage that the isolate can be serotyped and genotyped, and thus provide valuable epidemiological information.

So rarely has a positive culture been obtained from a healthy person, other than one incubating the disease, that a false-positive result can be discounted. Moreover, with good technique of swabbing and culture, the organism can be recovered up to 3 months from the onset of illness when coughing persists. This casts doubt on the widespread belief that the bacterium is eliminated in a few weeks, and has implications for the transmission of infection.

Although the disease is mainly in the lower respiratory tract, the organism can be recovered readily from the nasopharynx. 'Cough plates' and postnasal swabs are unsatisfactory because of overgrowth by commensal bacteria. A pernasal swab acquires fewer commensals, and these can be suppressed by penicillin (0.25 unit/mL = 0.15 mg/L) or cefalexin (30 mg/L) in the charcoal–blood agar plate; higher concentrations may suppress bordetellae. Pernasal swabs on flexible wire are available commercially; the tip is directed downwards and towards the midline, passing gently along the floor of the nose for about 5 cm (depending on the patient's age) until stopped by the posterior wall of the nasopharynx. Practice in swabbing is necessary – initially with a co-operative adult! If old enough, patients should be warned to expect a tickling sensation but no pain; and a child's head should be held steady. Ideally, a segment of the culture plate should be inoculated immediately after withdrawal of the swab. The use of transport medium reduces the isolation rate. A single swab may yield a negative culture, but isolation rates of up to 80% may be achieved by taking specimens on several successive days.

In the laboratory, the inoculum is spread to give separate colonies, and the plate is incubated for at least 7 days before being discarded as negative. Because of the prolonged incubation, the medium should have a depth of 6–7 mm (40 mL in a 9-cm dish) and a bowl of water may be placed in the incubator to reduce drying of the culture. Cefalexin tends to give 'rough' growth, which may have to be subcultured on cefalexin-free medium for reliable serological identification.

### Detection of bacterial antigens or DNA

Bordetella antigens may be detected in serum and urine in tests with specific antiserum. Alternatively, bacteria in nasopharyngeal secretions are labelled with fluorescein-conjugated antiserum and examined by ultraviolet microscopy. This method has the theoretical advantage, compared with culture, of detecting dead bordetellae. However, false-negative results are likely unless the patient's own antibody is removed from the bacteria by enzyme before application of the fluorescent reagent. Moreover, false-positive results may occur because of serological cross-reactions with organisms such as staphylococci, yeasts, haemophili and moraxellae, some of which resemble bordetellae microscopically. Bordetella antiserum should be absorbed with these organisms, but appropriate reagents are not readily available. Reports on the high specificity of this test lack conviction in the absence of reliable evidence on the true diagnosis.

There have been numerous studies of the polymerase chain reaction (PCR) in the detection of bordetella DNA in nasopharyngeal specimens, by the use of various primers. However, the method is relatively expensive and technically demanding compared with culture; and as yet there is a lack of consensus on its diagnostic reliability, with the need to detect both *B. pertussis* and *B. parapertussis*, and then to distinguish between them. Moreover, to be of epidemiological value, these methods would need modification to enable them to identify the serotype of the infecting strain of *B. pertussis*.

Furthermore, a test with very high sensitivity may merely detect the transient presence of a small number of bacteria attempting to colonize the mucosa before being eliminated from an immune host; such scanty bacteria would constitute a minimal risk of transmission to contacts.

### Detection of bordetella antibody

Sera and nasopharyngeal secretions can usefully be examined for antibody. However, a negative result does not exclude pertussis because the serological response is often slow and weak, especially in very young children. More importantly, a positive result needs careful interpretation because antigens are shared with other organisms (see above). Even with insensitive tests, such as agglutination, pertussis antibodies are readily detected in the sera of healthy persons. More sensitive techniques, such as enzyme-linked immunosorbent assay (ELISA), are liable to increase the number of false-positive results and thereby give spurious respectability to a diagnosis that should rightly be 'pseudo-whooping cough'. The need at present in serological diagnosis is not for greater sensitivity but for greater specificity. Even then, the detected antibody may be an 'anamnestic' response to previous pertussis infection or vaccination, provoked non-specifically by a current, antigenically unrelated, illness.

The ready detection of antibody in adolescents and adults, resulting from past infection or vaccination, has led some to believe that these people are an important reservoir of pertussis infection, despite the rarity of a positive culture on pernasal swabbing.

Nevertheless, bacterial agglutination may be a useful guide in the serodiagnosis of pertussis, provided that sera are absorbed with type 1 organisms and titrated for the more specific agglutinins 2 and 3, and that paired sera are taken about 3 weeks apart to detect a greater than fourfold rise in titre. This requires a serum sample of at least 0.5 mL on each occasion.

### Differential blood count

Although lymphocytosis is a characteristic response to pertussis infection, many cases of true pertussis do not develop a significant increase in circulating lymphocytes; conversely, there are so many other causes of lymphocytosis that a positive result lacks diagnostic specificity.

## TREATMENT

### Antimicrobial drugs

Most antibiotics have little or no clinical effect when the infection is well established, even though the organism may be sensitive in vitro.

The drug of choice is a macrolide such as azithromycin, clarithromycin or erythromycin, which may reduce the severity of the illness if given before the paroxysmal stage. If given for at least 14 days, erythromycin has sometimes eliminated the organism and so reduced the exposure of contacts. However, positive cultures are frequently obtained after short periods of erythromycin therapy.

A macrolide may also be given to protect non-vaccinated infants, although it seems unrealistic to expect this treatment to be maintained throughout the several months that the older sibling (or adult) may remain infectious.

Appropriate antibiotics should, of course, be administered to patients who show signs of secondary bacterial infection.

### Other measures

Cough suppressants and corticosteroids may control the paroxysms, but may be harmful by encouraging retention of secretions. Cyanosis and anoxia can be reduced by avoiding sudden noises, excitement or excessive medical examination, which tend to precipitate paroxysms. Mucus and vomit should be removed to prevent their inhalation.

Treatment with pertussis immunoglobulin has been tried, but with limited success, probably because such materials have never been checked for the presence of all three agglutinins.

Because of the dearth of effective therapy for whooping cough, the widespread use of pertussis vaccine is of supreme importance (see below).

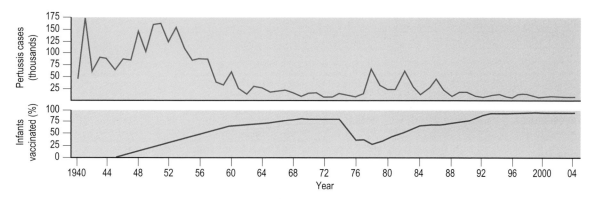

**Fig. 32.1** Whooping cough in England and Wales 1940–2004.

## EPIDEMIOLOGY

### Source and transmission of infection

Most new cases arise from patients (usually children, occasionally adults) with typical symptoms, presumably because the paroxysmal cough provides an efficient means of droplet dissemination. Atypical cases have only a minor role in transmission; long-term asymptomatic carriage is unknown. The degree of contact is important: 80–90% of non-immune siblings exposed in the household become infected, compared with less than 50% of non-immune child contacts at school. Antibiotic therapy may reduce transmission, but is not completely effective.

### Incidence and mortality

Pertussis infection occurs worldwide, affects all ages, and is a major cause of death in malnourished populations. In developed countries the mortality rate has gradually declined with a combination of improved socio-economic conditions, availability of intensive care in hospitals, and antibiotic therapy to combat secondary infection. However, the latter constitute an unnecessary use of medical resources for a disease that is eminently preventable by vaccination.

The disease is most severe and the morbidity rate highest in the first 2 years of life; most fatal cases are in infants less than 1 year old. Even very young babies are not immune: maternal antibody does pass to the fetus, but it rarely contains all three agglutinins and protection is incomplete.

Although one attack usually confers long-lasting immunity, infection with a different serotype of the organism can occur subsequently.

The disease occurs in epidemic waves at about 4-year intervals – the time needed to build up a new susceptible population after the 'herd' immunity produced by an epidemic. Figure 32.1 illustrates the pattern for England and Wales up to 2004, since when the situation has remained unchanged. The maintenance of a 4-year cycle presumably results from the interaction of various factors, such as the degree of artificial immunity produced by high vaccination rates, and the levels of natural immunity that follow either large epidemics or a high background incidence of endemic pertussis in inter-epidemic intervals.

Figure 32.1 also illustrates how variations in the rates of uptake of pertussis vaccine have affected the incidence of whooping cough more than the steady improvement in the general health of the population that continued throughout the period. After the gradual introduction of pertussis vaccination during the 1950s, there was a steady reduction in the size of epidemics until the 1970s. Unfounded fear of brain damage caused a loss of faith in the vaccine, and three large epidemics occurred before the slow restoration of confidence in the vaccine began to take effect.

### Prevalence of serotypes

The three serotypes of *B. pertussis* pathogenic for man are liable to spontaneous reversible variation, in vitro and in vivo, between types 1,2 and 1,3 via 1,2,3. Fimbriae are readily demonstrable on strains possessing agglutinogen 2, aiding colonization of the respiratory mucosa; serotypes 1,2 and 1,2,3 predominate among the strains isolated from patients in non-vaccinated communities.

Table 32.2 shows the occurrence of serotypes of *B. pertussis* in different communities. In the 1960s, many countries used type 1,2 vaccine, and these two serotypes were suppressed. However, type 1,3 organisms, which have a weak agglutinogen 1 component, became predominant in these countries, and caused infection

**Table 32.2**    Occurrence of serotypes of *B. pertussis* in different communities

| Community | Antibody in serum | | | Prevalence of serotypes of *B. pertussis* in cases of whooping cough[a] | |
|---|---|---|---|---|---|
| | 1 | 2 | 3 | 1,2[b] | [1],3[c] |
| Non-vaccinated | Little if any | | | High | Low |
| Vaccinated with: | | | | | |
|    type 1,2 | +++ | +++ | − | Low | High[d] |
|    type [1],3[c] | + | − | +++ | High[d] | Low |
|    type 1 (degraded) | + | − | − | High[d] | Low |
|    type 1,2,3 (before final elimination) | +++ | +++ | ++[e] | Lower | Higher |

[a]Spontaneous reversible variation occurs, in vitro and in vivo, between types 1,2 and 1,3 via 1,2,3.
[b]Type 1,2 is fimbriate, with colonizing advantage.
[c]The square brackets [1] indicate a weak agglutinogen 1 component, so that type 1,3 vaccine does not protect against type 1,2 infection, and vice versa.
[d]Infection occurs even in vaccinated children.
[e]The immune response to agglutinogen 3 is weaker than for agglutinogens 1 and 2.

even in vaccinated children before the vaccine was modified in the late 1960s by addition of agglutinogen 3. Similarly, countries that used a vaccine deficient in agglutinogen 2, or in both agglutinogens 2 and 3, saw a predominance of type 1,2 infection, even in vaccinated children.

To be effective, it seems, a vaccine must contain all three agglutinogens, as recommended by the World Health Organization. However, because the agglutinin 3 response is usually the weakest (when type 1,2,3 vaccine is used), type 1,3 organisms are the last to be eliminated from a community with an effective vaccination programme.

## Genotypes

It is not possible to trace the spread of infection by serotyping isolates because there are only three serotypes and they undergo spontaneous variation. In contrast, more than 40 genotypes have been demonstrated in macro-restriction profiles by pulsed-field gel electrophoresis of DNA digests. Isolates within a household have been shown to belong to the same genotype, but the technique is probably too expensive and time-consuming for routine use.

## CONTROL

### Treatment and quarantine

Antibiotics and immunoglobulins currently available are not very effective for the treatment of patients or the protection of contacts. Because patients typically

**Table 32.3**    Plain and adsorbed pertussis vaccine

| Vaccine | Immune response | Adverse reactions |
|---|---|---|
| Plain | Weaker | More |
| Adsorbed (onto adjuvant) | Stronger | Fewer |

disseminate the organism for many weeks or months, and because children are infectious even before the most characteristic symptoms develop, control of the disease by quarantine is unrealistic.

### Vaccination

Vaccination is safe and more than 90% effective and is strongly recommended. The vaccines still in widespread use are suspensions of whole bacterial cells, killed by heat or chemicals, and are administered by deep intramuscular injection. Adsorption of the bacteria on to an adjuvant, such as aluminium hydroxide, enhances the immune response (particularly important with agglutinogen 3) and also causes fewer adverse reactions (Table 32.3).

Three conditions are essential for good protection:

1. Presence of all three agglutinogens in the vaccine
2. Use of adsorbed vaccine (i.e. with adjuvant)
3. A minimum of three doses, at monthly intervals.

Since there is little passive protection from the mother and effective active immunity cannot be achieved until after the third injection of vaccine, the first dose is given as soon as a good response can be obtained. In many countries, therefore, the first injection is recommended at 3 months of age. In the UK and some other countries, concern for the vulnerability of the young infant prompted a start at 2 months, although the immune response is somewhat weaker and there have been doubts about the effectiveness of this early start. An upsurge of invasive infection with *Haemophilus influenzae* type b followed in the Netherlands when the policy of giving the first dose at 3 months was changed to 2 months. For these and other aspects of vaccination, see also Chapter 70.

## Safety of pertussis vaccine

Minor adverse reactions occur in about one-half of vaccinated children, and can be considered as part of the normal immune response. Parents should therefore be warned to expect possible erythema and local swelling, slight feverishness, and crying. Of much more concern are possible neurological sequelae, but the National Childhood Encephalopathy Study in the UK and several other studies have shown that pertussis vaccination merely triggers the manifestation of neurological disorders that would occur in any case, and there is no firm evidence that the vaccine causes serious long-term adverse side-effects.

## Contra-indications to pertussis vaccination

Severe adverse reaction to a previous dose has been considered the only firm contra-indication. A current feverish illness (not merely snuffles) is cause for postponement until the child is well. Parental concern over a possible neurological contra-indication is due reason for consultation with a paediatrician. Allergy is not a contra-indication; neither is age – children who missed vaccination in infancy may receive the normal three-dose course. Vaccination is also sometimes advised for adults, such as nurses and doctors in appropriate hospitals.

## Acellular pertussis vaccine

Although doubts about the efficacy and safety of whole-cell pertussis vaccine have passed, the urge to identify the essential protective components persists. Trials in different countries (including one with type 1,2 prevalence and another with type 1,3 prevalence), and with vaccines containing various components, may reveal a correlation between the protection of children and the response to individual pertussis antigens and type-specific agglutinogens.

A large-scale trial with good diagnostic criteria in Sweden showed that antibodies to pertussis toxin and filamentous haemagglutinin do not confer protection in the child, although these antigens have been incorporated in nearly all acellular vaccines because they provide mouse-protection (see above). This trial did indicate a correlation between agglutinin titres and protection of children, and it showed that whole-cell vaccine had a higher efficacy than any of the acellular vaccines used. Moreover, the whole-cell vaccine has an additional adjuvant effect on other antigens given simultaneously; in the UK an increase in *Haemophilus influenzae* type b infections followed the replacement of whole-cell pertussis vaccine with an acellular product owing to a reduced antibody response.

Acellular vaccines are now used in various countries, but without any assurance that they produce an adequate response to both agglutinogens 2 and 3. Moreover, they are very expensive, putting a questionable burden on limited national health resources, especially in developing countries where the need is greatest.

## Eradication

Vaccination aims at a herd immunity, which breaks the cycle of transmission because the organism dies before finding a new susceptible host (see Ch. 70).

In several countries, good whole-cell vaccine is available. Eradication is possible, but even if high levels of vaccination of infants are maintained it will be some years before adequate herd immunity is achieved within the child population.

RECOMMENDED READING

Editorial: Pertussis: adults, infants, and herds, *Lancet* 339:526–527, 1992.
Health Protection Agency: Laboratory confirmed cases of pertussis in 2009; and Quarterly vaccination coverage in the UK, *Health Protection Report* 4:No.25, 2010.

Jenkinson D: Natural course of 500 consecutive cases of whooping cough: a general practice population study, *British Medical Journal* 310:299–302, 1995.
Khattak MN, Matthews RC: Genetic relatedness of *Bordetella* species as determined by macrorestriction digests resolved by pulsed-field gel

electrophoresis, *International Journal of Systematic Bacteriology* 43:659–664, 1993.

Lang F, editor: *Encyclopedia of Molecular Mechanisms of Disease*, ed 2, Heidelberg, 2008, Springer.

Preston NW: Pertussis (whooping-cough): the road to eradication is well sign-posted but erratically trodden, *Infectious Diseases Review* 2:5–11, 2000.

Preston NW: Why the rise in *Haemophilus influenzae* type b infections? *Lancet* 362:330–331, 2003.

Preston NW: Diagnosis and prevention of pertussis, *Lancet* 368:1769, 2006.

Preston NW, Matthews RC: Immunological and bacteriological distinction between parapertussis and pertussis, *Lancet* 345:463–464, 1995.

Preston NW, Matthews RC: Acellular pertussis vaccines: progress but déjà vu, *Lancet* 351:1811–1812, 1998.

Salmaso S and the Eurosurveillance editorial team: Pertussis vaccine schedules across Europe, *Eurosurveillance* 9:70–71, 2004.

# 33 Legionella

Legionnaires' disease; Pontiac fever

*J. Hood and G. F. S. Edwards*

## KEY POINTS

- *Legionella* species are water-borne bacilli and include *L. pneumophila*, which is responsible for a form of pneumonia known as legionnaires' disease, and a less serious influenza-like illness called Pontiac fever.
- Many serogroups of *L. pneumophila* are recognized, but human infection is almost always caused by serogroup 1.
- Legionnaires' disease is diagnosed by demonstrating the organism in sputum or soluble antigen in urine.
- High-dose macrolide, e.g. erythromycin, with or without rifampicin, is used for treatment.
- Suppression of the organism in air-conditioning systems and water supplies in public buildings (common immediate sources) is central to control of the disease.

The Legionellaceae are Gram-negative rods whose natural habitat is water. There are more than 50 genetically defined species, of which much the most important is *Legionella pneumophila*. This species can be subdivided on the basis of deoxyribonucleic acid (DNA) relationships into three subspecies:

- *L. pneumophila* ssp. *pneumophila* and *L. pneumophila* ssp. *fraseri*, which have been described in human disease
- *L. pneumophila* ssp. *pascullei*, which has so far been isolated only from the environment.

Eighteen *Legionella* species have been associated with human disease (Table 33.1), but most infections are caused by just one of the many serogroups of *L. pneumophila*: serogroup 1. Other serogroups and species, such as *L. micdadei, L. bozemanii* and *L. longbeachae*, account for a few cases; other species rarely cause infection. *L. longbeachae* infections make up more

than a quarter of diagnosed infections in Australia and New Zealand and may be increasing in Europe. Infection is usually acquired accidentally and the disease is not transmissible from person to person.

Legionellae give rise to two main clinical syndromes:

1. *Legionnaires' disease*, a pneumonia that may progress rapidly unless treated with appropriate antibiotics. In previously healthy subjects the mortality rate is about 10%, but in those with nosocomial infection the rate may be much higher.
2. *Pontiac fever*, a brief febrile influenza-like illness that may be slow to resolve fully, but does not cause death.

Legionellae have rarely been associated with other infections such as prosthetic valve endocarditis or wound infection, but these are usually nosocomial infections.

## DESCRIPTION

In biological material (e.g. sputum or lung) or in water deposits legionellae are short rods or coccobacilli, but in culture they become longer and are sometimes filamentous. Although they are weakly Gram-negative, they stain poorly with Gram's stain, but may be stained by a silver impregnation method. Specific fluorescent antibody stains are used diagnostically. The organisms may be numerous, particularly in patients who are infected in hospital or who are immunosuppressed, but are often present only in very small numbers in the scanty sputum that is characteristic of legionnaires' disease. They have not been demonstrated in patients with Pontiac fever.

Legionellae are exacting in their growth requirements and grow best on buffered charcoal yeast-extract agar (BCYE), which contains iron plus cysteine

**Table 33.1** *Legionella* species associated with human disease

| Species | Number of serogroups | Autofluorescence under ultraviolet light |
|---|---|---|
| L. anisa | 1 | + |
| L. birminghamensis | 1 | − |
| L. bozemanii | 2 | − |
| L. cincinnatiensis | 1 | − |
| L. dumoffii | 1 | + |
| L. feeleii | 2 | − |
| L. gormanii | 1 | + |
| L. hackeliae | 2 | − |
| L. Jordanis | 1 | − |
| L. lansingensis | 1 | − |
| L. longbeachae | 2 | − |
| L. maceachernii | 1 | − |
| L. micdadei | 1 | − |
| L. parisiensis | 1 | + |
| L. pneumophila | 16 | − |
| L. sainthelensi | 2 | − |
| L. tucsonensis | 1 | + |
| L. wadsworthii | 1 | − |

+, Blue–white fluorescence; −, no autofluorescence.

as an essential growth factor. Some legionellae grow better in the presence of 2.5–5% carbon dioxide at 35–36°C. Colonies usually appear after incubation for 48 h to 5 days, but species other than *L. pneumophila* may take up to 10 days. Colonies have a 'cut glass' appearance on examination under the plate microscope. Colonies of some *Legionella* species show blue–white (or red – not yet seen in species isolated from man) autofluorescence on illumination with long-wave ultraviolet light (see Table 33.1).

Species and serogroups within species are characterized by specific heat-stable lipopolysaccharide antigens. Serogroups may be differentiated further on the basis of serology into serotypes, but this presently applies almost entirely to *L. pneumophila* serogroup 1. Subtyping is usually by the use of monoclonal antibodies in an immunofluorescence test. Similarities or differences between strains of the same serogroup may be revealed by genetic studies, and this may be useful in the investigation of possible outbreaks. Molecular methods, including gene sequencing, are being used increasingly for speciation and typing.

## PATHOGENESIS

### Legionnaires' disease

Infection is almost always due to *L. pneumophila* serogroup 1. The illness is characterized by:

- an incubation period of 2–10 days
- high fever
- respiratory distress
- confusion, hallucinations and, occasionally, focal neurological signs.

Once infection is established the patient develops pneumonic consolidation with an outpouring of proteinaceous fibrinous exudate, containing macrophages and polymorphs, into the alveoli. Despite the outpouring of cells, patients usually produce little sputum. Infection may extend to involve two or more lobes of the lung and renal impairment leading to renal failure may occur. The severity of the disease may range from a rapidly progressing fatal pneumonia to a relatively mild pneumonic illness. The mechanism of the distant toxic effects of the infection on the nervous system is unknown.

Patients who are debilitated, for example by immunosuppression or surgery, are more prone to infections, and their infections are usually more severe than those encountered as sporadic community cases. Smoking is a predisposing factor. The deterioration in body defences associated with ageing is also important: the disease is most common in those over the age of 40 years, with a peak in the 60–70-year age group. The only generally accepted mode of infection is inhalation of an aerosol of fine water droplets containing the organism, but some believe that aspiration of water containing legionellae can also lead to infection; evidence for a route of infection is often missing in sporadic cases, even when an environmental source of the organism has been identified. There is presently no convincing evidence that ingestion plays a part in pathogenesis, although the demonstration of *L. pneumophila* in bowel contents raises this as a possibility.

Animal models provide some insight into the train of events in the lungs. Guinea-pigs infected by inhalation of an aerosol containing legionellae develop a lobular pneumonia that rapidly becomes confluent. Instillation of a protease produced by *L. pneumophila* into the lungs of guinea-pigs produces a pneumonia that appears to be the same as that caused by inhalation of intact bacteria.

At the cellular level, legionellae are engulfed by monocytes and can survive therein as intracellular parasites. The duration of intracellular parasitization is unknown but the persistent excretion of group-specific legionella antigen in the urine of some patients, as opposed to its more transient appearance in most cases of legionella pneumonia, suggests that in some patients intracellular parasitism may be prolonged. There is, however, no evidence of a chronic carrier state or chronic infection.

## Pontiac fever

The pathogenesis of this non-pneumonic, non-fatal form of legionella infection is not understood. Living legionellae have been isolated from sources of infection associated with outbreaks of Pontiac fever, and legionella antigen has been demonstrated in the urine of some cases, indicating that appreciable quantities of legionellae have been involved in the infection.

## LABORATORY DIAGNOSIS

The tests used are listed in Table 33.2. Respiratory secretions (sputum, bronchial aspirate or washings), as well as pleural fluid, lung biopsy or autopsy material, should be examined by microscopy and culture. Gram-stained films are of little value except to demonstrate the presence of other pathogens and organisms that may interfere with the isolation of legionellae. Blood culture is an unrewarding procedure. Cultures are made on BCYE medium with and without antibiotics added to suppress other respiratory tract flora. Potentially contaminated material such as sputum or post-mortem material may also be heated at 50°C for 30 min in order to diminish growth by less heat-stable respiratory tract organisms that may inhibit growth of legionellae in culture. In heavy infections, growth on BCYE medium (but not on standard media) may appear after incubation for 48 h at 36°C in air, preferably enriched with 2.5% carbon dioxide. Some less common species may take longer to grow and cultures should be incubated for 10–14 days. Colonies having a 'cut glass' appearance by plate microscopy, and those fluorescing blue–white under ultraviolet light, are Gram stained, and subcultured on to blood agar or cysteine-deficient medium to show that they will *not* grow on these media. Cultures are identified by use of specific antisera in an immunofluorescence test or by gene sequencing.

The polymerase chain reaction (PCR) is also used to detect and type legionellae in clinical material; it is quicker than culture and sometimes allows typing of organisms when culture is unsuccessful. Immunofluorescent staining with monoclonal or polyclonal antisera is specific, but legionellae are usually hard to find in the scanty sputum produced by patients.

## Antigen tests

The examination of urine for legionella antigen by enzyme-linked immunosorbent assay (ELISA) is a rapid and specific method of identifying *L. pneumophila* as the likely cause of a pneumonia. Most legionella infections are now diagnosed by urine antigen tests, but failure to detect urinary antigen does not exclude infection with legionellae other than *L. pneumophila* serogroup 1.

## Serology

Although antibodies take at least 8 days to develop after the onset of infection, some patients may not reach hospital until this period has elapsed, so it is worthwhile examining serum for antibodies to *L. pneumophila* on admission to hospital. Further sera should be taken at intervals to show the development of antibodies or a rise in antibody titre. Antibodies usually develop after 8–10 days of illness and then increase in titre, but some patients may not produce antibody for some weeks or, rarely, for several months.

- A four-fold or greater rise in antibody titre in a typical clinical case indicates infection with legionella.
- A single titre of 256 or more is presumptive of infection.

In some cases proven by culture, lower titres may be found, especially when death occurs early in the illness. Antibody may persist for months or years and can be a source of confusion, as may cross-reacting antibody produced by some patients with *Campylobacter* infection. At present the only fully validated antibody test is that for infection by *L. pneumophila* serogroup 1, although patients proven by bacterial culture to be infected by other legionellae produce antibodies to the infecting strain.

## TREATMENT

An intravenous macrolide (often azithromycin) is the standard therapy in legionella pneumonia. In severe cases a fluoroquinolone (usually ciprofloxacin) or

**Table 33.2** Diagnostic tests for legionella infection

| Nature of test | Test | Appropriate specimen |
|---|---|---|
| Detection of whole organism | Culture | Sputum or other clinical material |
| Detection of specific DNA | PCR | |
| Detection of soluble antigen | ELISA | Urine |
| Detection of antibody | FAT | Serum |
| | ELISA | |

ELISA, enzyme-linked immunosorbent assay; FAT, fluorescent antibody test; PCR, polymerase chain reaction.

rifampicin is usually added. Aminoglycoside and β-lactam antibiotics are not effective.

Susceptibility testing of clinical isolates is rarely justified. It is technically demanding and, as person-to-person transmission of infection does not occur, antibiotic use is unlikely to contribute to the development of resistance in other patients.

## EPIDEMIOLOGY

In 1976 an outbreak of 182 cases of pneumonia, mainly affecting members of the American Legion, occurred at a convention in Philadelphia. This form of pneumonia became known as *legionnaires' disease*, and the bacterium associated with it as *L. pneumophila*. Since that time, legionella pneumonia has been recognized as the only acute *bacterial* pneumonia that may occur in outbreak form. This is due to the dissemination of the bacteria in aerosols, which may travel as much as 1–2 km from the source.

Infected aerosols are usually generated from warm water sources, typically:

• the ponds in cooling towers of refrigeration plants in air-conditioning systems
• domestic hot water systems in hotels and hospitals
• warm water in nebulizers and oxygen line humidifiers
• whirlpool spa baths and showers.

Legionellae are engulfed by, and survive within, free-living amoebae, and the bacteria may be protected from drying and disinfectants when present in amoebic cysts. Community outbreaks may occur on a fairly large scale and the source of infection in such outbreaks is invariably a cooling tower in which the bacteria are harboured in the water of the pond associated with the apparatus. Smaller outbreaks have been associated with domestic water supplies in hospitals, spas and hotels, and also with whirlpool spas. So-called sporadic cases may, on careful epidemiological examination, prove to be associated with cooling towers. About a third of patients with legionnaires' disease in the UK acquire their infection abroad, usually from domestic water supplies in hotels; apparently sporadic cases account for many others. There is a convincing association between *L.*

*longbeachae* infection and gardening; this and several other legionellae have been isolated from compost.

Legionnaires' disease is more prevalent in late summer and autumn. This may be due to an increase in bacterial numbers in water from natural sources and in cooling towers.

The route and source of infection of Pontiac fever are the same as in legionnaires' disease. Pontiac fever may affect all age groups, including children. The attack rate is high, with almost all of those exposed to the infection source being affected, whereas in legionnaires' disease the attack rate is low.

## CONTROL

There is no vaccine. Nevertheless, unlike most forms of bacterial pneumonia, the disease may be prevented by the eradication of *Legionella* species in the various kinds of water source that may give rise to aerosol production. It is therefore important that any outbreak, or even one case occurring in hospital, is investigated to try to identify possible sources of an infectious aerosol so that it can be eradicated. Information about cases must be notified to epidemiological centres so that any association between cases may be established; once the source has been identified, legionellae can be eradicated from water in several ways:

• heat
• disinfection with chlorine or other biocides, including chlorine dioxide
• copper–silver ionization.

Water systems in hotels and hospitals should be managed so that hot water is heated to above 60°C before distribution and does not lie stagnant and cooling in the pipes. As legionellae do not multiply in cold water, cold water supplies should be kept below 20°C; water should not be allowed to stagnate, as it may warm up and allow the multiplication of legionellae. It may be necessary in some infected water systems to dose continuously with a suitable biocide (see above). Cooling towers should be disinfected with chlorine or other biocides in a way that ensures that the growth of legionellae and possible supporting organisms, such as algae or amoebae, is suppressed.

RECOMMENDED READING

Amsden GW: Treatment of legionnaires' disease, *Drugs* 65:605–614, 2005.
Diederen BM: *Legionella* spp. and legionnaires' disease, *Journal of Infection* 56:1–12, 2008.
Fields BS, Benson RF, Besser RE: Legionella and legionnaires' disease: 25 years of investigation, *Clinical Microbiology Reviews* 15:506–526, 2002.
Newton HJ, Ang DK, van Driel IR, Hartland EL: Molecular pathogenesis of infections caused by *Legionella pneumophila*, *Clinical Microbiology Reviews* 23:274–298, 2010.
Stout JE, Yu VL: Legionellosis, *New England Journal of Medicine* 337:682–687, 1997.

# 34 Brucella, bartonella and streptobacillus

Brucellosis; Oroya fever; trench fever; cat scratch disease; bacillary angiomatosis; rat bite fever

*M. J. Corbel*

## KEY POINTS

- Brucellae are highly infectious coccobacilli that cause a septicaemic illness, undulant fever. Most human disease is caused by *Brucella melitensis*, *B. abortus* or *B. suis*.
- The disease is a typical zoonosis most commonly acquired from infected animals, or from infected meat or dairy products.
- Brucellosis is diagnosed by isolation of the organism from blood; alternatively serology or polymerase chain reaction tests can be used.
- Brucellosis is treated with a tetracycline, usually in combination with an aminoglycoside or rifampicin.
- *Bartonella bacilliformis* is a highly infectious agent causing the sandfly-disseminated diseases, Oroya fever (Carrion's disease) and verruga peruana in parts of South America.
- The organism infects blood cells and can be diagnosed in stained blood or tissue aspirates. Alternatively, PCR methods are used.
- Other bartonellae cause trench fever and cat scratch disease. Endocarditis can complicate these infections.
- Chloramphenicol, macrolides, aminoglycosides, fluoroquinolones and tetracyclines are used in the treatment of bartonella infections.
- *Streptobacillus moniliformis* is one of the causes of a septicaemic illness, rat bite fever. Treatment with penicillin or a tetracycline is usually effective.

## BRUCELLA

The genus *Brucella* comprises a group of Gram-negative coccobacilli that can infect a wide range of mammals ranging from rodents to killer whales. They are of particular zoonotic and economic importance as a cause of highly transmissible disease in cattle, sheep, goats and pigs. Infection in pregnant animals often leads to abortion, and involvement of the mammary glands may cause the organisms to be excreted in milk for months or even years. Human infections arise through direct contact with infected animals, including handling of infected carcasses; indirectly from a contaminated environment; or through consumption of infected dairy produce or meat.

Brucellosis is a typical zoonosis, and person-to-person infection does not play a significant role in transmission. Infection may remain latent or subclinical, or it may give rise to symptoms of varying intensity and duration. Brucellosis can present as an acute or subacute pyrexial illness that may persist for months or develop into a focal infection that can involve almost any organ system. The characteristic intermittent waves of increased temperature that gave the name *undulant fever* to the human disease are now usually seen only in long-standing untreated cases.

## DESCRIPTION

### Classification

The *Brucella* genus comprises a group of closely related bacteria that probably represent variants of a single species. For convenience these have been classified into nomen species that differ from one another in their preferred animal host, genetic arrangement, phage sensitivity pattern, and oxidation of certain amino acids and carbohydrates. The main human pathogens are *Brucella abortus*, *B. melitensis*, *B. suis* and *B. canis*. The first three may be further subdivided into biovars associated with various animal hosts. *B. abortus* has a preference for cattle and other Bovidae, *B. melitensis* for sheep and goats. The first three biovars of *B. suis* preferentially infect pigs, whereas the fourth and fifth biovars have reindeer or caribou and rodents, respectively, as natural hosts. The biovars differ in their sensitivity to dyes, in production of hydrogen sulphide and in agglutination by sera monospecific for A and M epitopes. Various molecular typing methods are also used to differentiate subtypes down to the level of individual strains.

*B. cetaceae* and *B. pinnipediae*, isolated from dolphins, porpoises, killer whales and seals, appear to be pathogenic for man. Newly designated species include *B. microti* from voles and *B. inopinata* isolated from a breast implant recipient with a brucellosis-like syndrome.

## Morphology

Brucellae are Gram-negative coccobacilli or short bacilli, occurring singly, in groups or short chains. They are non-motile, non-capsulate and non-sporing.

## Culture characteristics

*Brucella* spp. are aerobic. However, *B. ovis* and many strains of *B. abortus*, when first cultured, are unable to grow without the addition of 5–10% carbon dioxide. All strains grow best at 37°C in a medium enriched with animal serum and glucose.

On clear solid medium, smooth, transparent and glistening ('honey droplet') colonies appear after several days. However, the organisms can mutate, especially in liquid media, forming 'rough' colonies on subculture. There is a corresponding loss in virulence and an antigenic change, so that they are no longer readily agglutinated by homologous antisera prepared against normal smooth strains. Identification can be made by the polymerase chain reaction (PCR) with appropriate primers or by a combination of biochemical, cultural, phage typing and serological tests. Rapid gallery tests may misidentify *Brucella* spp. and this has resulted in laboratory-acquired infections; they are not recommended.

## Sensitivity and survival

Brucellae may be killed at a temperature of 60°C for 10 min, but dense suspensions, such as laboratory cultures, can require more drastic heat treatment to ensure their inactivation. Infected milk is rendered safe by efficient pasteurization. Brucellae are very sensitive to direct sunlight and moderately sensitive to acid, so that they tend to die out in sour milk and in cheese that has undergone lactic acid fermentation. The organisms can survive in soil, manure and dust for weeks or months, and remain viable in dead fetal material for even longer. They have been isolated from butter, cheese and ice cream prepared from infected milk. They may survive in carcass meat, pork and ham for several weeks under refrigeration. Pickling and smoking reduce survival. They are susceptible to common disinfectants if used at appropriate concentration and temperature. They are sensitive in vitro to a wide range of antibiotics, only a few of which are effective therapeutically.

## Antigenic structure

In all smooth strains the dominant surface antigen is a lipopolysaccharide (LPS) O chain, which, depending on the three-dimensional structure of the polysaccharide portion, forms A, M or C epitopes. These are common to all smooth species, but the distribution of A and M depends on biovar. Rough strains do not produce the O chain but have a common R epitope. The LPS has endotoxin activity of relatively low pyrogenicity and elicits limited antibody-mediated protection. The organisms behave as 'stealth pathogens' and evade innate immune responses; effective immunity is dependent on specific cell-mediated and cytotoxic responses elicited by a variety of protein antigens.

## PATHOGENESIS

The incubation period is usually about 10–30 days, although infection may persist for several months before causing any symptoms. *B. melitensis* and *B. suis* tend to cause more severe disease than *B. abortus* or *B. canis*. Infection by any species may give rise to a variety of non-specific symptoms and, without the fluctuating temperature to act as a guide, diagnosis may be difficult. Pointers to the diagnosis are a history of occupational exposure or recent travel to endemic areas with consumption of milk products.

Brucellae can enter the body through skin abrasions, through mucosal surfaces of the alimentary or respiratory tracts, and sometimes through the conjunctivae, to reach the bloodstream by way of regional lymphatics. The organisms are facultative intracellular parasites and subsequently localize in various parts of the reticulo-endothelial system with the formation of abscesses or granulomatous lesions, resulting in complications that may involve any part of the body. Brucellae surviving within cells may cause relapses of acute disease, or a chronic syndrome may develop that is associated with continued illness and vague symptoms of malaise, low-grade fever, lassitude, insomnia, irritability and joint pain. Such 'chronic brucellosis' may follow an acute attack or develop

**Table 34.1** Results of serological tests used in the diagnosis of brucellosis

| Type of brucellosis | Agglutination test | Mercaptoethanol test | Complement fixation test | ELISA |
|---|---|---|---|---|
| Acute | + | ± | + | + |
| Chronic | (±) | + | + | + |
| Past infection | (−) | − | − | (−) |

(−), weak or negative; ELISA, enzyme-linked immunosorbent assay.

insidiously over several years without previous acute manifestations. It rarely responds to antibiotic therapy and is probably a post-infectious response similar to the 'myalgic encephalomyelitis syndrome'.

# LABORATORY DIAGNOSIS

Brucellosis is confirmed in man by isolating the organisms from blood or other tissue samples and by serological and other tests. In animals, culture may be attempted from abortion material, placenta, milk, semen or samples of lymphoid tissue, mammary gland, uterus or testis collected post mortem.

Brucellae are easily transmitted by aerosols, ingestion and percutaneous inoculation. Samples suspected to contain brucellae must be treated as high risk. Cultures must be handled under containment conditions appropriate to hazard group 3 pathogens.

## Blood culture

When brucellosis is suspected, blood culture should be attempted repeatedly, not only during the febrile phase. Because the organisms may be scanty, at least 10 mL of blood should be withdrawn on each occasion, 5 mL being added to each of two blood culture bottles containing glucose–serum broth. One of these bottles should be incubated in an atmosphere containing 10% carbon dioxide. Preliminary lysis and centrifugation of the blood improves the isolation rate. Other materials such as bone marrow, solid tissue samples or exudates are also suitable for culture.

Subculture should be made on to serum–dextrose agar every few days; alternatively, a two-phase Castaneda culture system, in which the broth is periodically allowed to flow over agar contained within the blood culture bottle, may be used. Blood cultures should be retained for 6–8 weeks before being discarded as negative. Automated blood culture systems may also be used.

*B. melitensis* and *B. suis* are more frequently isolated from blood than are *B. abortus* or *B. canis*.

## Serological tests

In the absence of positive cultures, the diagnosis of brucellosis usually depends on serological tests, the results of which tend to vary with the stage of the infection (Table 34.1).

In some rural communities the sera from a proportion of the normal population are reactive in low dilutions in serological tests because of previous subclinical infection.

### Serum agglutination test

This test usually becomes positive 7–10 days after onset of symptoms. During the acute stage of the disease, levels of agglutinins associated with both immunoglobulin (Ig) M and IgG continue to rise. As high-titre sera may not cause agglutination in low dilution (the *prozone* effect), a range of serum dilutions from 1 in 10 to greater than 1 in 1000 should be made.

As the disease progresses from the acute to the chronic phase and the organisms become localized intracellularly in various parts of the body, the IgM antibodies decrease; the agglutination titre falls and may become undetectable even while the patient is still ill. The absence of agglutination therefore does not rule out the possibility of infection. Persisting antibodies that are no longer capable of agglutinating may be detected by complement fixation, antiglobulin or enzyme-linked immunosorbent assay (ELISA) tests. In latent or chronic infection, the complement fixation test is likely to be positive, whereas in cases of past infection it is negative.

### Mercaptoethanol test

Low-titre agglutinins due to residual IgM may persist for months or even years after the infection has cleared. Testing in the presence of mercaptoethanol, which destroys the agglutinating ability of IgM, was formerly used to indicate the continuing presence of IgG and the likelihood of persisting infection, but is no longer considered reliable.

## Enzyme-linked immunosorbent assay

The ELISA for IgG and IgA antibodies shows a good correlation with active disease, especially in long-standing infection. It has largely replaced the anti-human globulin (Coombs') test, formerly used for detecting non-agglutinating (IgG) antibodies.

The O chain of smooth *Brucella* LPS is structurally related to the LPS antigens of various other Gram-negative bacteria. False-positive cross-reactions in agglutination, complement fixation and ELISA tests are produced by antibodies to *Yersinia enterocolitica* O9, *Salmonella* O30, *Escherichia coli* O157, *Francisella tularensis*, *Stenotrophomonas maltophilia* and *Vibrio cholerae*. Tests using protein antigens are more specific but may cross react with *Ochrobactrum* spp. – environmental bacteria closely related to *Brucella* that are occasionally implicated in opportunistic infections.

## Other diagnostic tests

PCR methods can detect *Brucella* specifically and also give an indication of species and biovar. Promising results have been obtained in clinical studies, but no standard procedure is yet available.

The Rose Bengal plate test, a rapid slide agglutination test with a buffered stained antigen, is widely used as a screening test in farm animals, but also gives good results in human brucellosis. It is not affected by prozones or immunoglobulin switching. Positive results should be confirmed by a quantitative method.

The brucellin skin test, similar to the tuberculin test (see p. 216), does not differentiate active from past or subclinical infection and is no longer recommended.

## TREATMENT

Brucella infections respond to a combination of streptomycin or gentamicin with tetracycline, or to rifampicin and doxycycline. Tetracycline alone is often adequate in mild cases. Fluoroquinolones may be used in combination with rifampicin or tetracyclines but are not recommended for monotherapy. Treatment should be continued for at least 6 weeks. Co-trimoxazole and rifampicin can be used in children. In patients with endocarditis and neurobrucellosis, a combination of a tetracycline, aminoglycoside and rifampicin is recommended.

Serum antibody titres usually decline sharply after effective treatment. The chronic post-infectious form without localizing lesions responds poorly to treatment.

## EPIDEMIOLOGY

*B. abortus* has been eradicated from cattle in most developed countries, although there has been a resurgence in some parts of Europe. It was formerly common in dairy farmers, veterinarians and abattoir workers, but is now rare. Nearly all human cases in the UK are now acquired abroad; most are caused by *B. melitensis*, which is still prevalent in Mediterranean countries, the Middle East, central and southern Asia, and parts of Africa and South America.

Human brucellosis due to *B. suis* is largely an occupational disease arising from contact with infected pigs or pig meat. It was once common in the USA, chiefly among those who handled raw meat shortly after slaughter. It occurs in feral pigs in Australia and the USA, and is a hazard to hunters. It is widespread in domesticated pigs in various African, Asian and South American countries; biovar 4 is found only in the Arctic regions of North America and Russia.

Brucellae have potential as agents of biological warfare or bioterrorism and this possibility should be borne in mind in the event of unexplained outbreaks.

## CONTROL

The live-attenuated *B. abortus* strain S19 vaccine has been used to protect cattle from abortion and so reduce spread of the disease. It can interfere with subsequent diagnostic serology and has been widely replaced by the rough strain *B. abortus* RB51, which may give comparable protection, but does not induce interfering antibodies and is less hazardous to man, though not innocuous.

The live-attenuated smooth strain *B. melitensis* Rev I is used to protect sheep and goats from *B. melitensis* infection. Vaccination of pigs is not widely practised, although the attenuated *B. suis* strain 2 has been used in China.

Effective and non-reactogenic vaccines are not currently available for human vaccination. Pasteurization eliminates the risk of brucellosis from the consumption of infected milk or milk products. However, there remains the possibility of infection due to contact with infected animals or their tissues. Veterinary surgeons, farmers and laboratory workers are particularly at risk.

Eradication depends on elimination of the infection from domestic animals by a policy of compulsory testing of the animals and slaughtering of positive reactors.

## BARTONELLA

The genus *Bartonella*, which is distantly related to *Brucella*, comprises at least 20 species of very small Gram-negative bacilli, most of which have been implicated in various febrile and localizing diseases in man.

- *Bartonella bacilliformis* is the cause of Oroya fever or Carrion's disease and verruga peruana. It is spread by sandflies.
- *Bart. quintana* is the cause of *louse-borne trench fever*.
- *Bart. henselae* and *Bart. clarridgeiae* are the most common causes of *cat scratch disease* and can be transmitted by fleas and possibly ticks.

Other *Bartonella* species have been identified as pathogens of dogs and other mammals. Some, including *Bart. vinsoni* (and its various subspecies), *Bart. elisabethae*, *Bart. alsatica*, *Bart. koehlerae* and *Bart. mayotimonensis* occasionally cause a range of syndromes involving many organ systems in man including bacteraemia and endocarditis. *Bart. grahami* has been implicated in ocular disease.

## BARTONELLA BACILLIFORMIS

*Bart. bacilliformis* is responsible for outbreaks of a severe and often fatal disease of man in the mountainous regions of Peru, Colombia and Ecuador. The name Oroya fever was given after an epidemic of the disease in 1870 during the building of a railway between Lima and Oroya, when 7000 labourers died within a few weeks. The infection is spread by sandflies, usually *Lutzomyia verrucarum* and *L. peruensis*.

After recovery from Oroya fever the patient may develop a skin eruption known as verruga peruana. Individuals may remain bacteraemic and act as reservoirs of infection long after recovery from the illness, or after asymptomatic infection, which probably occurs in more than 50% of those exposed. *Bart. bacilliformis* is pathogenic only to man.

### Description

*Bart. bacilliformis* is a small, strictly aerobic, Gram-negative coccobacillus. The organisms occur singly, in pairs, chains or clumps. In older cultures they tend to be extremely pleomorphic. They are motile through a cluster of about ten flagella situated at one end of the cell. The organism grows best at 25–28°C and at pH 7.8.

### Pathogenicity

After an incubation period of about 20 days, Oroya fever presents as a high fever followed by progressively severe anaemia due to blood cell destruction. There may be enlargement of the spleen and liver, and haemorrhages into the lymph nodes.

The case fatality rate in untreated cases of Oroya fever may be over 40%, although the overall fatality rate for all forms of the infection is probably only 0.1%. Verruga peruana is a form of bacillary angiomatosis; it may occur without the initial attack of Oroya fever or may develop several weeks after recovery. A pleomorphic skin eruption of reddish, round, elevated, hard nodules may become secondarily infected, producing ulcers and haemorrhagic lesions. The rash usually appears mainly on the legs, arms and face, although all parts of the body may be affected. The condition may persist for as long as a year, but is rarely fatal.

### Laboratory diagnosis

In both Oroya fever and verruga peruana, bartonellosis is confirmed by demonstrating the organisms in smears of blood or tissue aspirates stained by Giemsa or immunofluorescent stain. They are seen packing the cytoplasm of the cells and adhering to the cell surfaces.

*Bartonella* spp. are dangerous pathogens and should be handled under class 3 containment conditions. *Bart. bacilliformis* is readily cultured in semi-solid nutrient agar supplemented with rabbit serum and haemoglobin, similar to that used for the culture of leptospires (p. 376). Visible growth may take up to 10 days. PCR or serology is used for identification.

Blood culture should be carried out at all stages of infection. It may be difficult to isolate the organisms from the blood when the verruga stage has developed, and culture from the skin lesions is rarely productive.

PCR tests offer a rapid and reliable diagnosis, but are usually available only from reference laboratories. *Bart. bacilliformis* antibodies can be detected by various serological tests, but they are common in inhabitants of endemic areas and not necessarily diagnostic of active disease.

### Treatment

Chloramphenicol can drastically reduce the mortality rate in Oroya fever and the frequently associated salmonella infections. Penicillin, streptomycin, tetracyclines, rifampicin, fluoroquinolones and clarithromycin may also be effective in uncomplicated cases. A combination of two antimicrobials is recommended in severe cases. Blood transfusion may be necessary in severe cases of anaemia.

## Control

No vaccine is available. Insecticides are used to eliminate the sandfly vector in likely breeding sites inside and outside houses and surrounding areas. As the insects bite only at night, individuals may protect themselves by withdrawing from affected areas at nightfall.

## BARTONELLA QUINTANA

This organism was formerly classified among the rickettsiae as *Rochalimaea quintana*. However, unlike the rickettsiae, these organisms can grow in cell-free media and they tend to be epicellular rather than strictly intracellular parasites of man. Unlike *Bart. bacilliformis* the organism does not possess flagella, although it may exhibit a twitching movement owing to fimbriae.

*Bart. quintana* was first identified as the cause of the febrile illness known as *trench fever* among the troops in the First World War. It is transmitted by the body louse, *Pediculus humanus*, under unhygienic living conditions and is not uncommon among homeless people in some countries. Trench fever is a bacteraemic condition typically associated with periodic febrile episodes lasting for about 5 days. *Bart. quintana* has also been implicated in cases of angiomatosis and endocarditis. The organism may be isolated from the blood of patients by culture on blood agar. *Bart. vinsoni* and its subspecies are similar and can cause an identical syndrome.

## BARTONELLA HENSELAE

*Bart. henselae* has been isolated from the blood and lymph nodes of patients suffering from *cat scratch disease*, a severe condition of regional lymphadenopathy and fever resulting from the scratch or bite of an infected cat. Cat fleas and ticks may be responsible for transmission. *Bart. clarridgeiae*, which can be differentiated from *Bart. henselae* by its flagella, can cause an identical syndrome.

An organism known as *Afipia felis* has also been implicated in a small proportion of cases of cat scratch disease. It is morphologically similar to *Bart. henselae*, but differs biochemically, genetically and in being culturally less fastidious.

*Bart. henselae* and, less frequently, *Bart. quintana* and other species have been identified in the blood and tissues of individuals suffering from two severe clinical syndromes associated with human immunodeficiency virus (HIV) or other immunosuppressant conditions:

1. *Bacillary angiomatosis*, which produces proliferative vascular lesions in the skin, regional lymph nodes and various internal organs.
2. *Bacillary peliosis*, which affects the liver and spleen.

## Diagnosis

*Bart. henselae* may be cultured from the pus or lymph node samples of patients with cat scratch disease, and from blood, lymphoid tissue, liver and spleen of patients with bacillary angiomatosis or peliosis. In tissue sections the organisms are best demonstrated by silver stain or an immunospecific stain. ELISA, with various protein antigens, is the most useful serological test.

Conventional blood culture often fails to detect endocarditis. Most *Bartonella* species can be detected and differentiated by PCR methods.

## Treatment

Tetracyclines, aminoglycosides, chloramphenicol, clarithromycin and fluoroquinolones are all effective against bartonella infections. In cases of endocarditis a combination of gentamicin and doxycycline is recommended. Treatment may need to be prolonged for at least 6 weeks.

## STREPTOBACILLUS MONILIFORMIS

*Streptobacillus moniliformis* is one of the causes of *rat bite fever* in man, the other being *Spirillum minus* (see p. 322). It is a common commensal of the nasopharynx of rodents, and sometimes causes epizootic disease in mice and rats, resulting in otitis media, multiple arthritis and swelling of the feet and legs. Laboratory workers who handle rodents are most at risk. Rarely, outbreaks of infection occur as a result of the ingestion of milk or other food contaminated by rats.

## DESCRIPTION

*S. moniliformis* is Gram-negative, non-motile, non-capsulate and highly pleomorphic. The organisms appear as short bacilli, forming chains interspersed with long filaments that may show oval or spherical lateral swellings.

It is a facultative anaerobe that benefits from added carbon dioxide and a moist atmosphere. It grows best at 37°C and pH 7.6. Culture media must contain blood, serum or ascitic fluid. Loeffler's serum medium is satisfactory. Media may be made selective by addition of colistin and nalidixic acid. After incubation for 2 days, discrete, granular, greyish yellow colonies 1–5 mm in diameter are visible on the surface, and minute 'fried egg' colonies appear in the depth of the medium. The latter are L-phase variants (see pp. 20–1) that have little or no virulence for laboratory animals. They develop spontaneously and are thought to have a defective mechanism for cell wall formation. Cultural and biochemical variants occur and have been used to define biotypes.

*S. moniliformis* is killed in 30 min by a temperature of 55°C. In culture it survives for only a few days, although it may remain viable for up to a 1 week in serum broth at 37°C. With the exception of the L-forms, *S. moniliformis* is susceptible to penicillin, and both forms are sensitive to streptomycin and tetracycline.

## PATHOGENICITY

In man the organism usually enters the body through wounds caused by rodent bites. It multiplies and invades the lymphatics and bloodstream, causing a feverish illness with severe toxic symptoms and sometimes complications such as arthritis, endocarditis and pneumonia.

Infection acquired by ingestion of contaminated water, milk or food is known as *Haverhill fever*, a condition characterized by fever, sore throat, rash, polyarthritis and erythema. The duration of the illness varies from a few days to several weeks. Endocarditis, hepatitis and amnionitis may develop as complications. In the pre-antibiotic era a case fatality rate of about 10% was reported; the rate is much lower nowadays with effective treatment.

## LABORATORY DIAGNOSIS

An acute febrile illness associated with asymmetric arthropathy, a maculopapular rash involving the extremities and a history of contact with rodents may point to the diagnosis.

*S. moniliformis* can be isolated in culture from the patient's blood during the acute phase of the illness and from the synovial fluid of those who develop arthritis. Growth occurs in serum broth as a characteristic granular sediment, appearing like 'cotton wool balls' that do not disintegrate on shaking.

Mice are highly susceptible to intraperitoneal inoculation of infected blood or joint fluid, as a result of which they develop either a rapidly fatal generalized condition or a more chronic disease with swelling of the feet and legs.

ELISA is the method of choice for detecting antibodies. A PCR test may also be used for detection of human and rat infections. Specific agglutinins may be detected in the patient's serum as early as 10 days or as late as several weeks after the rat bite, but is no longer recommended. A false-positive reaction in the VDRL test (Venereal Disease Research Laboratory slide test; see p. 370) is seen in about 25% of patients.

## TREATMENT

Penicillin, clarithromycin or oral tetracycline is usually effective.

RECOMMENDED READING

Andre JM, Freydiere AM, Benito Y, et al: Rat bite fever caused by *Streptobacillus moniliformis* in a child: human infection and rat carriage diagnosed by PCR, *Journal of Clinical Pathology* 58: 1215–1216, 2005.

Boot R, Oosterhuis A, Thuis HC: PCR for the detection of *Streptobacillus moniliformis*, *Laboratory Animals* 36:200–208, 2002.

Corbel MJ, Beeching NJ: Brucellosis. In Kasper DL, Braunwald E, Fauci A, editors: *Harrison's Principles of Internal Medicine*, ed 17, New York, 2008, McGraw Hill, pp 973–976.

Graves MH, Janda JM: Rat bite fever (*Streptobacillus moniliformis*): a potential emerging disease, *International Journal of Infectious Diseases* 5:151–155, 2001.

Jensen WA, Fall MZ, Rooney J, et al: Rapid identification and differentiation of *Bartonella* species using a single step PCR assay, *Journal of Clinical Microbiology* 38:1717–1722, 2000.

Lopez-Goni I, Moriyon I, editors: *Brucella. Molecular and Cellular Biology*, Wymondham, 2004, Horizon Bioscience.

Madkour MM: *Madkour's Brucellosis*, Berlin, 2001, Springer.

Murray PR, Corbel MJ: Brucella. In Borriello SP, Murray PR, Funke G, editors: *Topley and Wilson's Microbiology and Microbial Infections*, ed 10, Vol. 2, London, 2005, Hodder Arnold, pp 1719–1751.

Rolain JM, Brouqui P, Koehler JE, et al: Recommendations for the treatment of human infections caused by Bartonella species, *Antimicrobial Agents and Chemotherapy* 48:1921–1933, 2004.

Wullenweber M: *Streptobacillus moniliformis* – a zoonotic pathogen. Taxonomic considerations, host species, diagnosis, therapy, geographical distribution, *Laboratory Animals* 29:1–15, 1995.

# 35 Yersinia, pasteurella and francisella

Plague; pseudotuberculosis; mesenteric adenitis; pasteurellosis; tularaemia

M. J. Corbel

## KEY POINTS

- *Yersinia pestis* is the cause of human plague, transmitted to humans from rats and other rodents by their fleas. Pneumonic plague is transmitted from person to person by droplet infection.
- There are three main types of disease: bubonic, pneumonic and septicaemic plague. All are highly fatal without prompt treatment.
- The organism is readily cultured, but a polymerase chain reaction method is preferred for diagnosis as the organism is hazardous to handle.
- Aminoglycosides and chloramphenicol are commonly used in the treatment of plague.
- *Y. pseudotuberculosis* is an animal pathogen that occasionally causes human infection, which may be subclinical or severe.
- *Y. enterocolitica* causes a usually mild enteritis, but can give rise to a septicaemia, which may be fatal if untreated.
- *Pasteurella multocida* sometimes infects man, usually through animal bites.
- Pasteurella infection usually responds to penicillin or other antibiotics.
- *Francisella tularensis* is the cause of tularaemia, a febrile illness that can be severe and life-threatening. It is usually acquired from infected animals.
- Streptomycin or gentamicin is the antibiotic of choice.

The organisms within these three genera are animal pathogens that, under certain conditions, are transmissible to man, either directly, or indirectly through food and water or via insect vectors. They are Gram-negative coccobacilli, formerly contained within one genus, *Pasteurella*. Molecular genetics has indicated a completely separate identity for the three genera,

each with its own disease manifestations in man and animals:

1. *Yersinia* belongs to the Enterobacteriaceae and includes many non-pathogenic environmental species and three closely related pathogenic species.
2. *Pasteurella* is closely related to the *Actinobacillus–Haemophilus* group.
3. *Francisella* is distantly related to *Legionella*.

## YERSINIA

### YERSINIA PESTIS

*Yersinia pestis*, the *plague bacillus*, is essentially a parasite of rodents. In certain parts of the world, burrowing animals such as ground squirrels, gerbils and voles act as reservoirs of infection that may be transmitted by fleas to susceptible animals such as bandicoots, marmots, squirrels and rats. The animals suffer from outbreaks of plague, and their fleas may transmit the infection to man, giving rise to sporadic disease referred to as *wild* or *sylvatic plague*. Farmers or trappers who come into contact with infected animals are at risk.

More serious for man is *urban plague*, resulting from the spread of infection among rats, especially the black rat, *Rattus rattus*, which used to flourish around human habitation. Outbreaks of human plague, following epidemics in rats, have in the past sometimes developed into pandemics.

### Description

*Y. pestis* is a Gram-negative, non-sporing, non-motile, short coccobacillus. It occurs singly, in pairs or, when in liquid culture, in chains. Pleomorphism is marked, especially in old cultures in which pear-shaped or globular cells, suggestive of yeast cells (*involution forms*; see p. 20), may be seen. In smears from exudates and in cultures grown at 37°C they are frequently capsulate. In smears from tissues stained by methylene blue or Giemsa stain they show characteristic bipolar staining ('*safety pin*' appearance).

*Y. pestis* grows aerobically or anaerobically at 0–37°C (optimum 27°C), although small inocula may not grow aerobically in ordinary culture media. Small, slightly viscid, translucent, non-haemolytic colonies develop on blood agar within 24 h. Growth occurs on MacConkey's medium but tends to autolyse after 2–3 days.

It is killed at 55°C in 5 min and by 0.5% phenol in 15 min. It is sensitive to drying but may remain viable in moist culture for many months, especially at low temperatures.

## Pathogenesis

The heat-stable somatic antigen complex of *Y. pestis* comprises a rough-type lipopolysaccharide (LPS), which has endotoxin activity and is believed to contribute to the terminal toxaemia of plague. The heat-labile Fraction 1 (F1) protein capsular antigen helps the organism to resist phagocytosis and is a protective immunogen. This, and many other proteins associated with pathogenicity, is encoded by three plasmids. The largest, which is very similar to the virulence plasmids of *Y. enterocolitica* and *Y. pseudotuberculosis*, contains genes activated at low calcium concentration that express various outer membrane and secreted proteins with a variety of functions, such as inhibition of phagocytosis and intracellular killing. The V antigen, part of the type III secretion system, helps to suppress the innate immune response and facilitate infection and is an important protective antigen. *Y. pestis* also produces a plasminogen activator and fibrinolysin, which may play a critical role in the initial stages of infection. A pathogenicity island encodes other proteins associated with virulence including cell surface adhesion and iron acquisition factors, some common to *Y. pseudotuberculosis* and *Y. enterocolitica*.

Three severe forms of human plague are described: bubonic, pneumonic and septicaemic plague. All may occur at different stages in the same patient. The disease may also present as pharyngitis or meningitis.

### Bubonic plague

The transfer of *Y. pestis* from rats to man through the bites of infected fleas may occasionally result in a localized infection, known as *pestis minor*, with mild constitutional symptoms. More often the lymph nodes draining the area of the flea bite become affected, and the resulting adenitis produces intensely painful swellings or *buboes* in the inguinal, axillary or cervical regions, depending on the position of the bite. From these primary buboes the plague bacilli may spread to all parts of the body. Complications such as bronchopneumonia, septicaemia or meningitis may follow. In the absence of adequate antibiotic therapy administered early in the course of the disease, the case fatality rate may exceed 50%.

### Pneumonic plague

This can develop in patients presenting with bubonic or septicaemic plague. It may also be acquired as a primary infection by inhalation of droplets infected with *Y. pestis*, usually from an individual with pneumonic disease or as a result of exposure to aerosols generated from cultures. A severe bronchopneumonia develops. As disease progresses, the sputum becomes thin and blood stained; numerous plague bacilli are demonstrable in stained films or on culture of the sputum. This type of plague is highly contagious and is almost invariably fatal unless treated very early.

### Septicaemic plague

This may occur as a primary infection or as a complication of bubonic or pneumonic plague. The bacilli spread rapidly throughout the body and the outcome is almost invariably fatal, even in treated cases. Purpura may develop in the skin ('*Black Death*'), and disseminated intravascular coagulation is usually present. It should be noted that bacteraemia can occur in bubonic or pneumonic plague but is usually intermittent in the early stages.

Pointers to the disease include a sudden onset of high fever accompanied by prostration in individuals recently returned from an endemic area, or with a history of occupational exposure.

## Laboratory diagnosis

Pneumonic plague is easily acquired in the laboratory by inhalation of aerosols generated from *Y. pestis* cultures. These and clinical specimens suspected of containing the organism should be handled only under containment conditions appropriate for hazard group 3 pathogens. Animals used for diagnostic tests must be housed under insect-free containment conditions and handled with strict precautions.

Plague is confirmed by demonstrating the bacilli in fluid from buboes or local skin lesions in the case of bubonic plague, in the sputum in pneumonic plague, and in blood films and by blood culture when septicaemic plague is suspected. Blood culture may be intermittently positive in all forms of the disease. Post mortem, the bacilli can usually be isolated from a wide range of tissues, especially spleen, lung and lymph nodes.

Smears of exudate or sputum are stained with methylene blue, Wayson stain (a mixture of basic fuchsin, methylene blue and phenol), Giemsa stain or with an immunospecific stain. Characteristic bipolar-stained coccobacilli are confirmed as *Y. pestis* by culturing samples on blood agar and incubating at 27°C. If exudate is inoculated subcutaneously into guinea-pigs or white rats, or on to their nasal mucosa, infection follows and the animals die within 2–5 days. The bacilli may then be isolated from the blood or from smears of spleen tissue taken post mortem.

Characteristic colonies growing on blood agar plates are identified presumptively by various cultural and biological tests, by demonstrating chain formation in broth culture, and by 'stalactite' growth from drops of oil layered on the surface of fluid medium. Demonstration of the F1 capsular antigen by immunospecific staining confirms the presence of *Y. pestis* except in the case of rare non-capsulate strains.

Serology is most likely to be useful in the convalescent stage. The complement fixation and a haemagglutination tests formerly used have now been largely superseded by an enzyme-linked immunosorbent assay (ELISA) with F1 antigen.

A polymerase chain reaction (PCR), with primers based on F1 gene sequences, offers a rapid and less hazardous means of diagnosis than culture.

## Treatment

*Y. pestis* is sensitive to many antibiotics, including aminoglycosides, fluoroquinolones, chloramphenicol, co-trimoxazole and tetracyclines, but not penicillin.

When plague is suspected, patients should be isolated and respiratory precautions observed for at least the first 48 h of treatment. Antibiotic therapy should be started without waiting for confirmation of the diagnosis.

Intramuscular streptomycin or intravenous gentamicin is highly effective. Chloramphenicol (given intravenously for the first 4 days) is recommended in patients with meningitic symptoms. Tetracycline may be adequate in uncomplicated bubonic plague if given in large doses within 48 h of onset, and continued for 10 days. Experience with other antibiotics is limited, but there are indications that ciprofloxacin is effective.

Although monotherapy is usually adequate, strains carrying antibiotic resistance plasmids have been reported, and combined therapy may be advisable until the sensitivity of the strain is known.

Plague is a toxigenic infection and antibiotics will not prevent death once the bacteraemia has exceeded a certain threshold. Most patients treated within 18 h of onset can be expected to survive.

## Epidemiology

Plague was introduced into Europe from Asia in the thirteenth century and led to the great pandemic known as the Black Death, when about a quarter of the population of Europe succumbed to the disease.

Plague largely disappeared from Europe in the seventeenth century, perhaps because the black rat was displaced by the spread of the brown (sewer) rat, *Rattus norvegicus*, which is susceptible to plague but does not commonly frequent human dwellings. Improvements in housing may also have played an important part in the elimination of plague from Europe.

The bacilli are transmitted between animals and from animals to man by fleas, notably, but not exclusively, *Xenopsylla cheopsis*, an ectoparasite of rats. In cool humid weather fleas multiply and plague spreads readily among susceptible rats. In hot dry weather, on the other hand, the fleas die out, limiting the spread of infection. The persistence of endemic plague requires a fine balance between maintenance hosts with a relatively high resistance to lethal infection and transmission to more susceptible hosts such as rats. These conditions occur in a limited number of locations.

When a flea feeds on the blood of a sick animal, plague bacilli are sucked into the insect's midgut, where they multiply to produce a biofilm that may block the proventriculus, a process promoted by secreted bacterial proteins. When the host animal dies, the flea seeks an alternative host, which may be another rodent or human being. Because the 'blocked' flea is unable to suck readily, some of the infected midgut content is regurgitated and injected into the bite wound of the new victim.

When the epizootic among rats has reached a stage at which the number of susceptible animals has greatly decreased through death or immunity, it tends to die out, as does any human epidemic associated with it.

Domestic cats may become infected through contact with rodents. The animals may develop atypical disease and then transmit the infection to their owners or to veterinarians by the percutaneous or respiratory routes.

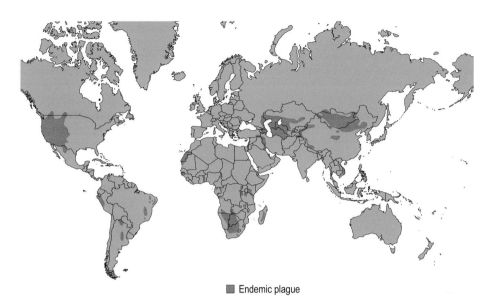

Endemic plague

**Fig. 35.1**  Areas where endemic plague is known to have persisted.

The sputum of persons suffering from pneumonic plague contains large numbers of plague bacilli, and under favourable conditions the disease spreads rapidly through the community by droplet infection, independently of rodents or fleas. Close contact is required and epidemics are most likely to occur when overcrowding in insanitary accommodation allows the infected droplets to spread readily from person to person. Cool, humid conditions favour transmission.

Endemic foci of wild rodent plague persist in many rural parts of the world, including North and South America, Africa and many parts of Asia (Fig. 35.1). Constant surveillance must be maintained to prevent its spread to urban populations, especially in areas where living conditions are below standard.

*Y. pestis* has been used as a biological warfare agent. Its potential application in bio-terrorism is of major concern.

## Control

### Bubonic plague

Periodic surveys are advocated in endemic areas to determine the prevalence of rodents and fleas so that control measures can be taken. Rats may be destroyed by rat poison and fleas by the liberal application of insecticide to rat runs.

Other control measures include the construction of rat-proof dwelling houses and buildings such as warehouses in dockland areas. The fumigation of ships and measures to prevent rats gaining access to ships and aircraft help to prevent the spread of plague from one country to another.

### Pneumonic plague

Patients suffering from pneumonic plague should be isolated, with full respiratory precautions. Overcrowding of houses and other accommodation should be avoided. Co-trimoxazole, ciprofloxacin or tetracyclines administered to immediate contacts may afford some degree of protection.

### Vaccination

Killed vaccines confer significant protection against bubonic but not pneumonic plague, but are no longer widely available. Live vaccines prepared from avirulent strains such as *Y. pestis* EV76 are used in some countries, but can cause severe reactions. Neither type reliably confer long-term immunity, and revaccination is necessary at 6-month intervals if exposure to infection continues. Candidate vaccines based on recombinant F1 and V antigens or fusion proteins have been submitted for licensing but are not yet commercially available.

## YERSINIA PSEUDOTUBERCULOSIS

*Y. pseudotuberculosis* can cause disease in many species of wild and domesticated animals and birds. Although presentation can vary widely, it typically causes a fatal septicaemia, often accompanied by formation of small whitish nodules in the viscera ('*pseudotuberculosis*'). The infection is indirectly transferable to man, usually through contaminated food or water.

## Description

*Y. pseudotuberculosis* is a small, ovoid, Gram-negative bacillus, with a tendency to bipolar staining. Genetically it is very similar to *Y. pestis*, which is probably a rough variant that has acquired additional plasmids encoding virulence factors. Initial growth may be best under anaerobic conditions. Isolation can be improved by 'cold enrichment' in buffered saline incubated at 4°C with periodic subculture for up to 6 weeks.

The organisms may be differentiated from *Y. pestis* by:

- motility when grown at 22°C
- ability to produce urease
- lack of the F1 antigen as shown by immunospecific staining or PCR.

There are eight major O serotypes, several of which can be separated into subtypes based on thermostable LPS somatic antigens. Unlike *Y. pestis* LPS, these are of smooth type and their specificity is determined by the O chain structure. The core regions are common to all serotypes and to *Y. pestis*. Thermolabile flagellar antigens are present in cultures grown at 18–26°C. Many other protein antigens are shared with *Y. pestis* and *Y. enterocolitica*.

## Pathogenesis

Like other yersiniae, *Y. pseudotuberculosis* carries a plasmid encoding factors essential for pathogenicity including a type III secretion system. At least one enterotoxin is also produced, as well as *invasin* and iron-regulated proteins encoded by a chromosomal pathogenicity island.

Clinical disease ranges in severity from subclinical to severe. Gastrointestinal manifestations are common; acute ileitis and mesenteric lymphadenitis are the most characteristic usually accompanied by fever, diarrhoea and pain simulating acute or subacute appendicitis. Infection occasionally results in a severe typhoid-like illness with fever, purpura and enlargement of the liver and spleen, which is usually fatal.

All age groups may be attacked but young males aged 5–15 years seem to be more frequently affected. Recovery is usually uneventful, although immunological sequelae such as erythema nodosum or reactive arthritis develop in some patients.

## Laboratory diagnosis

Infection in man is confirmed by isolation of the organism in culture from blood, local lesions or mesenteric nodes, particularly the ileocaecal nodes. PCR has been used experimentally.

Specific serum antibodies are detected and measured by tube or micro-agglutination tests performed during the acute phase of the illness with smooth suspensions of strains of serotypes I–VI grown at 22°C. ELISA or haemagglutination of red cells sensitized with LPS can also be used. The antibodies decline rapidly and reach low levels within 3–5 months.

## Treatment

Unlike *Y. pestis*, *Y. pseudotuberculosis* is usually sensitive in vitro to penicillins; it is also usually sensitive to aminoglycosides, chloramphenicol, tetracyclines, co-trimoxazole and fluoroquinolones.

Ileitis and mesenteric adenitis are usually self-limiting. Septicaemia demands parenteral treatment with ampicillin, chloramphenicol, gentamicin or tetracycline.

## Epidemiology

Many animal species suffer from the infection, but there is little proof of direct transmission to man. Most human infections probably result from the ingestion of contaminated water, vegetables or other food.

About 90% of all human cases in Australia, Europe and North America are attributed to strains of serotype I, followed by serotypes II and III, whereas in Japan serotypes IV and V predominate.

## YERSINIA ENTEROCOLITICA

By far the most common manifestation of *Y. enterocolitica* infection is acute enteritis, which may simulate acute appendicitis. Like many environmental species of *Yersinia*, it may also occasionally cause opportunist infection in compromised patients, and rarely may present as a plague-like syndrome with fulminant septicaemia.

## Description

Morphologically and culturally, *Y. enterocolitica* resembles *Y. pestis* and *Y. pseudotuberculosis* but grows more readily; it differs from them antigenically, biochemically and genetically.

At least 54 different O antigens and 19 H factors have been identified, so that a large number of serotypes are recognized. Serotypes O:3, O:5,27, O:8 and O:9 account for most human infections; other serotypes are probably non-pathogenic in immunocompetent individuals.

## Pathogenesis

*Y. enterocolitica* infects primarily the lymphoid tissue of the small intestine and ileocaecal junction. It carries a low calcium response plasmid and pathogenicity island encoding factors similar to those of *Y. pseudotuberculosis*. It causes mild and occasionally severe enteritis, mesenteric lymphadenitis and terminal ileitis. Septicaemia, which is often fatal, is most common in the elderly or in patients with predisposing conditions such as cirrhosis, iron overload or immunosuppression. Pneumonia and meningitis are rare presentations. Post-infectious complications include erythema nodosum, polyarthritis, Reiter's syndrome and thyroiditis. In young children the infection may produce fever, diarrhoea, abdominal pain and vomiting. The symptoms may last for several weeks.

## Laboratory diagnosis

The organism is isolated from blood, lymph nodes or other tissues on blood agar or MacConkey's agar. Isolation from contaminated sources such as faeces is best done by cold enrichment in buffered saline incubated at 4°C for up to 6 weeks, followed by plating on a selective medium. Identity is confirmed by biochemical tests and motility.

The serotype may be determined by slide agglutination with specific rabbit antisera. Serum antibodies are measured by agglutination tests against appropriate O antigens. A significant rise in the titre to 160 or more over a 10-day period indicates acute infection. ELISA may also be used. Cross-reactions occur between serotype O9 and smooth *Brucella* strains. These are very difficult to differentiate. PCR may be of value but is difficult to apply to highly contaminated materials such as faeces.

## Treatment

*Y. enterocolitica* is sensitive to many antibiotics, including aminoglycosides, chloramphenicol, co-trimoxazole, fluoroquinolones and tetracyclines, but is resistant to penicillin. Sensitivity to other β-lactam antibiotics is variable.

Uncomplicated gastrointestinal infection is usually self-limiting and treatment is indicated only in severe cases. Tetracycline is probably the drug of choice. Invasive infections such as septicaemia require intensive parenteral antibiotic treatment. Limited data are available on the optimum treatment but fluoroquinolones appear effective.

## Epidemiology

*Y. enterocolitica* has been isolated from caseous abscesses resembling those of pseudotuberculosis, from blood and infected wounds, and from the intestinal contents of apparently healthy animals of many species throughout the world. Pigs carry pathogenic serotypes quite frequently, cattle, sheep and goats less so.

Human disease usually results from ingestion of contaminated food or from contact with the environment. Raw pork, milk and drinking water have been implicated as sources. Person-to-person transmission also occurs.

Blood transfusion is a significant hazard as the organism can grow in refrigerated blood from donors with 'silent' bacteraemia. Flies are believed to play a role in transmission by contaminating food, and infection has been demonstrated in fleas and lice. However, enteric infection is the usual route of transmission and preventive measures are those appropriate for foodborne disease.

## PASTEURELLA

### PASTEURELLA MULTOCIDA

*Pasteurella multocida* (formerly *P. septica*) is a commensal or opportunist pathogen of many species of domestic and wild animals and birds. Human beings occasionally become infected, especially following animal bites. It is subdivided into three subspecies.

## Description

*P. multocida* organisms are aerobic and facultatively anaerobic coccobacilli, which are appreciably smaller than those of *Yersinia* species, although they are often pleomorphic in culture. They are Gram-negative, non-motile, non-sporing and capsulate in culture at the optimal growth temperature of 37°C. In smears of blood or tissue stained with methylene blue they show bipolar staining. *P. multocida* does not grow on MacConkey's medium.

Five capsular antigens A, B, D, E and F (C is not valid) and at least 11 somatic LPS antigens have been identified. The expression of the capsule is affected by cultural conditions and is lost in rough strains, which also fail to express smooth type O antigens.

The organisms are killed in a few minutes at 55°C and by 0.5% phenol in 15 min. They may survive and remain virulent in dried blood for about 3 weeks, and in culture or infected tissues for many months if kept frozen.

## Pathogenesis

*P. multocida* can be extremely virulent to many species of animals and birds, causing *fowl cholera* and haemorrhagic septicaemia, which are usually fatal. It also causes respiratory infections and contributes to the pathogenesis of atrophic rhinitis in pigs. Carriage of the organism is usually asymptomatic but stress may provoke fatal systemic infection.

The capsule is essential for full virulence, at least in mice and rabbits, and is the major protective antigen. Iridescent smooth strains show the greatest pathogenicity; mucoid strains are of reduced virulence and rough strains are avirulent. A dermonecrotic protein toxin, a cytotoxin and a neuraminidase probably account for many of the local manifestations of infection, but the bacteria also contain LPS with endotoxin activity.

Human infections usually present as a local abscess at the site of a cat or dog bite, with cellulitis, adenitis and, sometimes, osteomyelitis. *P. multocida* is also implicated in infections of the respiratory system such as pleurisy, pneumonia, empyema, bronchitis, bronchiectasis and nasal sinusitis.

Rare manifestations of disease include meningitis or cerebral abscess (usually following head injury), endocarditis, pericarditis or septicaemia, and infections of the eye, liver, kidney, intestine and genital tract.

A history of a recent animal bite or of occupational exposure are indicators for suspecting a *Pasteurella* infection. The organisms may also be carried commensally in the respiratory tract and can cause infection after surgical operation or cranial fracture.

## Laboratory diagnosis

Material from bite wounds, blood cultures, cerebrospinal fluid (in cases of meningitis) or respiratory secretions (in suppurative chest infections) are cultured on blood agar. The organisms are identified by various cultural and biochemical tests. Serology is unhelpful. PCR is potentially useful but rarely available.

## Treatment

Infections usually respond to penicillin but β-lactamase positive strains occur. Tetracycline, erythromycin or co-trimoxazole are suitable alternatives. In cases of osteomyelitis following dog or cat bites, antibiotic therapy must be continued for at least 8 weeks.

## Epidemiology

*P. multocida* is carried in the nasopharyngeal region of many species of wild and domestic animals. In human infections following animal bites, the organism passes directly to the person in the animal's saliva. Cat bites are particularly hazardous. Human beings may also become infected through breathing droplets generated by the coughing of animals suffering from respiratory infection. Pig farmers may be particularly at risk.

The disease in farm animals can be prevented by vaccination with preparations derived from killed capsulate bacteria. This is not practicable for human infections because of their rarity.

## OTHER *PASTEURELLA* SPECIES

*Pasteurella* spp. other than *P. multocida* and closely related bacteria formerly classified as *Pasteurella*, including *Avibacterium*, *Bibersteinia*, *Mannheimia*, *Gallibacterium* and *Phocoenobacter* spp., are rarely implicated as human pathogens.

- *P. caballi* causes respiratory and genital infections in horses and has caused bite wound infections in man.
- *P. dagmatis* has been associated with bite wounds and endocarditis.
- *P. (Mannheimia) haemolytica* causes pneumonia and haemorrhagic septicaemia in sheep, buffalo and cattle, and various diseases in poultry and other domesticated animals. It has been isolated from human cases of endocarditis, septicaemia and wound infection. It differs from *P. multocida* in forming haemolytic colonies on blood agar and by its ability to grow on MacConkey's medium.
- *P. (Actinobacillus) pneumotropica* is frequently isolated from the respiratory tract of laboratory animals. It has occasionally been isolated from human cases of septicaemia, upper respiratory tract infections and from animal bite wounds.
- *P. stomatis* has been isolated from cat bite wounds.
- *P. volantium* has been isolated from the human oropharynx.

## FRANCISELLA

### FRANCISELLA TULARENSIS

*Francisella tularensis* produces *tularaemia* in man and certain small mammals, notably rabbits, hares, beavers and various rodent species. It occasionally causes large epizootics in lemmings and other small rodents. It can be transmitted by direct contact, by biting flies, mosquitoes and ticks, by contaminated water or meat, or by aerosols.

### Description

When first isolated from infected tissue, *F. tularensis* is a very small, non-motile, non-sporing, capsulate, Gram-negative coccobacillus. In culture larger, pleomorphic, even filamentous, forms are present. It stains poorly with methylene blue but carbol fuchsin (10%) produces characteristic bipolar staining. Four biovars are recognized:

- Type A (formerly *F. tularensis tularensis* or *F. tularensis nearctica*) is found only in North America, is often transmitted by ticks and is highly pathogenic.
- Type B (formerly *F. tularensis palaearctica* or *F. tularensis holarctica*) occurs in Europe, Asia and North America, is transmitted by mosquitoes and is much less virulent.

*F. novicida* and *F. philomiragia* are now regarded as biovars of *F.tularensis* and have been reported from North America as rare causes of human disease.

*F. tularensis* is strictly aerobic. It will not grow on ordinary nutrient media, but grows well on blood agar containing 2.5% glucose and 0.1% cysteine hydrochloride. The *novicida* and *philomiragia* biovars are less fastidious.

*F. tularensis* is killed by moist heat at 55°C in 10 min, but may remain viable for many years in cultures maintained at 10°C, and for many days in moist soil and in water polluted by infected animals.

### Pathogenesis

Little is known about mechanisms of pathogenicity. A carbohydrate capsule is essential for virulence. A smooth type LPS is also present in the outer membrane, but apparently has low endotoxin activity. Certain outer membrane proteins elicit protective immunity and presumably contribute to pathogenesis.

In animals suffering from tularaemia the bacteria are present in large numbers within the cells of the liver and spleen, including macrophages.

Most human cases are sporadic, although occasional large outbreaks have been reported. After an acute onset with fever, rigors and headache, the disease develops manifestations that vary according to the route of entry of infection.

Following cutaneous inoculation through direct contact with infected animals or a fly or tick bite, a small punched-out skin ulcer develops at the point of entry, accompanied by enlargement of the draining lymph nodes even to the extent of bubo formation (*ulceroglandular form*). If entry is via the conjunctiva a similar syndrome will develop involving the eye and pre-auricular nodes (*oculoglandular form*). A glandular form without ulceration also occurs. Inhalation of infected dust or droplets, or ingestion of contaminated meat or water, is more likely to lead to pulmonary or typhoidal disease, respectively. Either can be preceded or accompanied by painful pharyngitis.

Type A strains cause severe and, in the pre-antibiotic era, often fatal disease. Disease caused by type B strains is much less severe and associated with very low mortality rates, but can cause prolonged disability.

### Laboratory diagnosis

*F. tularensis* is extremely dangerous to handle in the laboratory and hazard group 3 containment is required for all manipulations and animal work. All suspect samples should be labelled 'High risk'.

Human infections are usually diagnosed by inoculating tissue samples or the discharge from local lesions on to glucose–cystine blood agar or cystine heart agar, and identifying any characteristic small mucoid colonies. Alternatively, the exudate may be inoculated into guinea-pigs or mice and the liver and spleen of the infected animals cultured post mortem. PCR methods targeting outer membrane protein genes are now preferred to culture. Ribosomal sequence typing can aid identification.

Serology is most likely to be positive after 3 weeks. Rising *F. tularensis* antibody titres or individual agglutinin titres of 160 are diagnostic. ELISA with confirmatory western blotting is now replacing agglutination as the preferred method. Serum from cases of brucellosis may cross-react with *F. tularensis* and vice versa, usually to relatively low titre. Western blotting permits differentiation of cross-reactions.

## Treatment

*F. tularensis* is sensitive to aminoglycosides, chloramphenicol, fluoroquinolones and tetracyclines, but resistant to most β-lactam antibiotics. Streptomycin and gentamicin are the antibiotics of choice in tularaemia and are usually curative. Treatment should be continued for at least 10 days (14 days if ciprofloxacin is used). Tetracyclines or chloramphenicol in high dosage are also effective, but relapse may occur with these bacteriostatic agents unless treatment is prolonged.

## Epidemiology

Tularaemia has a worldwide distribution, but occurs mainly in the northern hemisphere. Cases have been reported from North America, from several European countries, including Scandinavia, and from Asia. It has not so far been identified in the UK.

It is a typical zoonosis, spread mainly by insects or ticks among lagomorphs and rodents. It is transmitted to humans through:

- handling of infected animals, such as rabbits or hares
- tick, mosquito or fly bites
- inhalation of contaminated dust (e.g. during harvesting or mowing)
- ingestion of contaminated water (as a result of pollution with the carcasses or excreta of infected rodents) or meat.

The organism is highly infectious, with a minimum infectious dose of about ten viable bacteria for the most virulent strains. Laboratory workers are especially at risk through handling infected laboratory animals or cultures of the organism. Person-to-person transmission of infection apparently does not occur. *F. tularensis* has been developed as a biological warfare agent and has potential application in bio-terrorism. A vaccine based on the live-attenuated LVS strain confers some protection. Immunity is dependent on cell mediated responses to outer membrane proteins. Antibodies although diagnostically useful, are not protective.

RECOMMENDED READING

Abdel-Haq NM, Asmar BI, Abrahamson WM, Brown WJ: *Yersinia enterocolitica* infection in children, *The Pediatric Infectious Disease Journal* 19:954–958, 2000.

Agger WA: Tularemia, lawn mowers and rabbits' nests, *Journal of Clinical Microbiology* 43:4304–4305, 2005.

Bottone EJ: *Yersinia enterocolitica*; overview and epidemiologic correlates, *Microbes and Infection* 1:323–333, 1999.

Butler T: Plague. In Ledingham JEG, Warrell DA, editors: *Concise Oxford Textbook of Medicine*, Oxford, 2000, Oxford University Press, pp 1625–1628.

Dennis DT, Campbell GL: Plague and other yersinia infections. In Kasper DL, Braunwald E, Fauci AS, et al, editors: *Harrison's Principles of Internal Medicine*, ed 16, New York, 2005, McGraw-Hill, pp 921–929.

Feodorova VA, Corbel MJ, Prospects for new plague vaccines, *Expert Review of Vaccines* 8:1721–1738, 2009.

Janda WM, Mutters R: *Pasteurella, Mannheimia, Actinobacillus, Eikenella, Kingella, Capnocytophaga* and other miscellaneous Gram-negative rods. In Borriello SP, Murray PR, Funke G, editors: Topley and Wilson's Microbiology and Microbial Infections, ed 10, Vol 2, London, 2005, Hodder Arnold, pp 1648–1691.

Schmitt P, Splettstosser W, Porsch-Ozcurumez M, et al: A novel ELISA and a confirmatory western blot useful for diagnosis and epidemiological studies of tularaemia, *Epidemiology and Infection* 133:759–766, 2005.

Wanger A: Yersinia. In Borriello SP, Murray PR, Funke G, editors: Topley and Wilson's Microbiology and Microbial Infections, ed 6, Vol 2, London, 2005, Hodder Arnold, pp 1458–1473.

Wilson WJ, Erler AM, Nasarabadi SL, et al: A multiplexed PCR-coupled liquid bead array for the simultaneous detection of four biothreat agents, *Molecular Cell Probes* 19:137–142, 2005.

# 36 Non-sporing anaerobes

## Wound infection; periodontal disease; abscess; normal flora

*R. P. Allaker*

## KEY POINTS

- Non-sporing anaerobes are found as part of normal flora in health.
- Most infections with anaerobes are of endogenous origin and are often polymicrobial. They act as opportunistic pathogens at damaged and necrotic tissue sites.
- Production of putrid odour is a common feature of infection.
- *Fusobacterium nucleatum* is often recovered from head and neck infections.
- Anaerobic Gram-negative rods, especially *Bacteroides fragilis* and anaerobic Gram-positive cocci, are the most common cause of non-clostridial anaerobic infections.
- Black-pigmented *Porphyromonas* and *Prevotella* species occur in abscesses and soft tissue infections in various parts of the body.
- Penicillins and nitroimidazoles, especially metronidazole, are the main agents used for treatment.

The significance of obligate anaerobes in general and of non-sporing anaerobes in particular is now well recognized. This heightened awareness of the important role that such organisms play, both as part of the normal microbial flora of the body and in a wide variety of infections, has come about largely through the application of greatly improved laboratory techniques for the isolation and cultivation of anaerobic bacteria, and the pioneering efforts of 'anaerobe enthusiasts' in various parts of the world.

A bewildering range of anaerobes is found in the mouth and oropharynx, gastrointestinal tract and female genital tract of healthy individuals as part of the commensal flora. These include Gram-positive and Gram-negative cocci, rods and filaments, as well as a number of spiral forms (Table 36.1). Most infections with these organisms are of endogenous origin, except in the case of animal and human bite wounds, where the infecting organisms, usually mixed, are derived from the mouth of the aggressor.

The flora of the lower intestinal tract, in particular, harbours vast numbers of anaerobes; quantitative studies on the bacterial flora of human faeces (Table 36.2) reveal a total content of over $10^{10}$ anaerobes per gram of faeces.

Many of the bacteria isolated from anaerobic infections are opportunist pathogens. Such organisms are particularly likely to set up infections in damaged and necrotic tissue, when they are translocated to sites other than their normal habitat, or in a host that is compromised or debilitated in a way that leads to impairment of immunological or other defence mechanisms. Anaerobic infections of the head, neck and respiratory tract are often associated with organisms found in the mouth, whereas infections in the abdominal and pelvic regions are more commonly associated with gut bacteria.

## FEATURES OF ANAEROBIC INFECTIONS

### Clinical signs

A common, but not invariable, feature is the production of a foul or putrid odour. Foul-smelling pus or discharge should always alert the clinician to the likelihood that anaerobes are present, as no other organisms produce this effect, but the absence of this sign does not necessarily exclude the involvement of anaerobic bacteria. Other clues to the clinical diagnosis are listed in Box 36.1.

### Polymicrobial flora

Infections involving non-clostridial anaerobes are often polymicrobial. The composition of these mixed infections varies according to the site affected. The

359

**Table 36.1** Anaerobic bacteria found as part of normal flora in man[a]

| | Skin | Mouth | Gastrointestinal tract | Genitourinary tract |
|---|---|---|---|---|
| **Gram-positive bacilli** | | | | |
| Actinomyces | − | + | + | + |
| Bifidobacterium | − | + | + | + |
| Clostridium | − | − | + | + |
| Eubacterium | − | + | + | + |
| Lactobacillus | − | + | + | + |
| Propionibacterium | + | + | + | + |
| **Gram-positive cocci** | | | | |
| Coprococcus | − | − | + | − |
| Gemmiger | − | − | + | − |
| Peptococcus | − | + | + | + |
| Peptostreptococcus | + | + | + | + |
| Ruminococcus | − | − | + | − |
| Sarcina | − | − | + | − |
| Streptococcus | + | + | + | + |
| **Gram-negative bacilli** | | | | |
| Anaerobiospirillum | − | + | + | (?) |
| Anaerorhabdus | − | − | + | (?) |
| Bacteroides | − | + | + | + |
| Bilophila | − | − | + | + |
| Butyrivibrio | − | − | + | − |
| Centipeda | − | + | + | (?) |
| Desulfomonas | − | − | + | − |
| Fusobacterium | − | + | + | + |
| Leptotrichia | − | + | + | − |
| Mitsuokella | − | + | + | (?) |
| Porphyromonas | − | + | + | + |
| Prevotella | − | + | + | + |
| Selenomonas | − | + | + | − |
| Succinimonas | − | − | + | − |
| Succinivibrio | − | − | + | − |
| Wolinella | − | + | + | − |
| **Gram-negative cocci** | | | | |
| Acidaminococcus | − | − | + | + |
| Megasphaera | − | − | + | − |
| Veillonella | − | + | + | + |
| **Spirochaetes** | | | | |
| Treponema | − | + | + | + |
| Other spiral forms | − | + | + | + |

−, Not usually found; +, commonly present; (?), presence uncertain (further data required).
[a]Data from various sources.

complexity may vary from two or three species up to a dozen or more, and may include strict anaerobes, facultatively anaerobic and micro-aerophilic organisms. Such combinations frequently comprise mixtures of Gram-negative rods (such as *Bacteroides*, *Prevotella* and *Fusobacterium* species) and Gram-positive cocci (such as streptococci). In most cases, with the occasional exception of actinomycosis, it is not possible to accurately predict which organisms are present from the clinical presentation, although the detection of red fluorescing pus under ultraviolet light usually indicates the involvement of one of the black-pigmented *Porphyromonas* species.

## LABORATORY DIAGNOSIS

When anaerobic infection is suspected, it is important that adequate clinical specimens are collected and transported as soon as possible to the bacteriology

**Table 36.2** The bacterial flora of faeces of English subjects

| Bacterial group | Mean bacterial count[a] |
|---|---|
| Gram-negative anaerobic rods | 9.8 |
| *Bifidobacterium* spp. | 9.8 |
| *Clostridium* spp. | 5.0 |
| *Veillonella* spp. | 4.2 |
| *Lactobacillus* spp. | 6.5 |
| *Bacillus* spp. | 3.7 |
| Enterobacteria | 7.9 |
| *Streptococcus* spp. | 7.1 |
| *Enterococcus* spp. | 5.8 |
| Total anaerobes | 10.1 |
| Total aerobes | 8.0 |

[a]$Log_{10}$ viable organisms per gram of faeces.
From Hill M J, Drasar B S, Hawksworth G et al 1971 Bacteria and aetiology of cancer of large bowel. *Lancet* 1: 95–100.

**Box 36.1** Some clinical signs and indicators of non-clostridial anaerobic infections

- Presence of foul-smelling pus, discharge or lesion
- Production of a large amount of pus (abscess formation)
- Proximity of lesion to mucosal surface or portal of entry
- Failure to isolate organisms from pus ('sterile' pus)
- Infection associated with necrotic tissue
- Deep abscesses
- Gas formation in tissues (crepitus)
- Failure to respond to conventional antimicrobial therapy
- Pus that shows red fluorescence under ultraviolet light (*Porphyromonas* spp.)
- Detection of 'sulphur granules' in pus (actinomycosis)
- Infection of human or animal bite wound
- Gram-negative bacteraemia
- Septic thrombophlebitis

Adapted from Finegold and George (1989).

laboratory, preferably under reducing conditions. After direct microscopical examination of the material, appropriate culture media should be inoculated for incubation in an anaerobic cabinet or in anaerobic jars. As many anaerobes are relatively slow growing, it is essential that cultures are incubated for several days before being discarded. In mixed infections, fast-growing aerobic or facultatively anaerobic organisms are often detected within 24 h, whereas some anaerobes may require incubation for 7–10 days before their colonies can be recognized.

In some laboratories, gas–liquid chromatography is carried out directly on pus and other clinical specimens in order to detect metabolic products, such as butyric and propionic acids, that are characteristic of certain anaerobes. Molecular based techniques are also increasingly used for the rapid identification of anaerobes.

## GRAM–NEGATIVE BACILLI

### *Fusobacterium* spp.

Fusobacteria colonize the mucous membranes of human beings and animals, and are generally regarded as commensals of the upper respiratory and gastrointestinal tracts. They tend to form long filamentous rods, often with pointed ends, sometimes described as *fusiform* or spindle shaped. Species such as *F. nucleatum*, *F. periodonticum* and *F. naviforme* are generally isolated from the oral cavity and are often associated with infections of this and related sites. *F. nucleatum*, the most studied species, is frequently recovered from mixed infections of the head and neck region, including dental abscesses and the central nervous system, and is also quite commonly isolated from transtracheal aspirates and pleural fluid. Five subspecies are recognized; *animalis*, *fusiforme*, *nucleatum*, *polymorphum* and *vincentii*. *F. nucleatum* subspecies *nucleatum* is an important periodontal pathogen, particularly during the period when quiescent periodontitis becomes active.

*F. necrophorum* is an important animal pathogen. It is associated with human necrobacillosis and occasionally infections similar to those caused by *F. nucleatum*.

*F. mortiferum*, *F. necrogenes*, *F. gonidiaformans* and *F. varium* are generally isolated from the gastrointestinal and urogenital tracts of man and animals. These species, together with *F. nucleatum*, are often associated with mixed intra-abdominal infections, perirectal abscesses, osteomyelitis, decubitus, and other ulcers and various soft tissue infections. *F. ulcerans* is associated with tropical ulcers but may be found in other sites.

### *Leptotrichia buccalis*

This species shares a number of properties with the fusobacteria. It is normally considered to be an oral species, but also occurs outside the oral cavity. It has been reported in acute necrotizing ulcerative gingivitis (*Vincent's gingivitis*), together with *Treponema*, *Porphyromonas* and *Fusobacterium* species. Some isolates described as *L. buccalis* probably represent separate species within the genus.

### *Bacteroides, Porphyromonas* and *Prevotella* species

Bacteria once thought of as typical members of the genus *Bacteroides*, especially those isolated from human beings, form three broad groups according to

**Table 36.3**  Current taxonomic status of *Bacteroides*, *Porphyromonas* and *Prevotella* species

| Group | Species |
|---|---|
| Saccharolytic (*B. fragilis* and related species) | *B. fragilis*, *B. caccae*, *B. eggerthii*, *B. ovatus*, *B. stercoris*, *B. thetaiotaomicron*, *B. uniformis*, *B. vulgatus*, *Parabacteroides distasonis*, *Para. merdae* |
| Moderately saccharolytic (*Prevotella* spp.) | *Prev. melaninogenica*, *Prev. bivia*, *Prev. buccae*, *Prev. buccalis*, *Prev. corporis*, *Prev. denticola*, *Prev. disiens*, *Prev. enoeca*, *Prev. heparinolytica*, *Prev. intermedia*, *Prev. loescheii*, *Prev. nigrescens*, *Prev. pollens*, *Prev. oralis*, *Prev. oris*, *Prev. oulorum*, *Prev. tannerae*, *Prev. veroralis*, *Prev. zoogleoformans*, *Prev. salivae*, *Prev. shahii*, *Prev. multiformis*, *Prev. marshii*, *Prev. baroniae* |
| Asaccharolytic (*Porphyromonas* spp.) | *P. asaccharolytica*, *P. catoniae*, *P. gingivalis*, *P. endodontalis*, *P. uenonis* |
| Other (uncertain taxonomic status) | *B. splanchnicus* |

whether they are asaccharolytic, moderately saccharolytic or strongly saccharolytic (Table 36.3):

1. The asaccharolytic, pigmented species are classified in the genus *Porphyromonas*, which includes the important periodontal pathogen *P. gingivalis*.
2. The moderately saccharolytic species that are inhibited by 20% bile and are largely indigenous to the oral cavity are assigned to the genus *Prevotella*.
3. The genus *Bacteroides* is now restricted to *B. fragilis* and related species that are saccharolytic and grow in 20% bile.

To add to the taxonomic complexity, many other former *Bacteroides* species that are usually isolated from nonhuman sources have undergone reclassification. *B. gracilis* and *B. ureolyticus* now belong to the genus *Campylobacter*, and the former *B. ochraceus* now belongs to the genus *Capnocytophaga*.

### Infections with *Bacteroides*, *Porphyromonas* and *Prevotella* species

*Bacteroides* species and related Gram-negative rods are, together with anaerobic cocci, the most common cause of non-clostridial anaerobic infections in man. Organisms of the *B. fragilis* group are particularly significant, as they are the most commonly isolated and tend to be more resistant to antimicrobial agents than most anaerobes.

*B. fragilis* itself is substantially outnumbered by other *Bacteroides* species in the normal bowel microflora, but is often associated with intra-abdominal and soft tissue infections below the waist. *B. fragilis* is also the most common anaerobe found in bacteraemia, and has even occasionally been reported from head and neck infections, despite its apparent absence from the normal flora of the mouth. Species of the *B. fragilis* group account for about a quarter of all anaerobes isolated from clinical specimens.

Black-pigmented species, including those from the genera *Porphyromonas* and *Prevotella*, occur in abscesses and soft tissue infections in various parts of the body. They are rarely isolated in pure culture. *P. gingivalis* is associated with chronic adult periodontitis and *P. endodontalis* with dental root canal (endodontic) infections.

## GRAM-POSITIVE ANAEROBIC COCCI

Gram-positive anaerobic cocci comprise part of the normal microbial flora of the mouth, gastrointestinal tract, genitourinary tract and skin (see Table 36.1). Most are found as part of the flora of the bowel and are not usually considered to be significant in infections.

However, several genera of clinically significant strictly anaerobic Gram-positive cocci, formerly regarded as belonging to the genus *Peptostreptococcus*, are now recognized (Box 36.2). They are not easy to identify precisely, and are often described simply as 'anaerobic cocci'.

### Infections with anaerobic cocci

Anaerobic cocci are isolated from infections in various parts of the body, particularly from abscesses (Box 36.3). They are often found in association with other anaerobic, facultatively anaerobic or aerobic organisms. As with all mixed infections, it is difficult to assess the contribution of each individual organism to the pathogenic process. However, there is sufficient evidence from both clinical and experimental studies to confirm their pathogenic potential.

## GRAM-NEGATIVE ANAEROBIC COCCI

Among genera recorded as part of the normal flora of the gastrointestinal tract (see Table 36.1), only *Veillonella* is found regularly at other sites. In the mouth,

**Box 36.2**  Currently recognized species (human) of Gram-positive anaerobic cocci

- *Peptococcus niger*
- *Peptostreptococcus anaerobius*
- *Peptoniphilus asaccharolyticus*
- *Peptoniphilus harei*
- *Peptoniphilus ivorii*
- *Peptoniphilus lacrimalis*
- *Finegoldia magna*
- *Parvimonas micra*
- *Anaerococcus hydrogenalis*
- *Anaerococcus lactolyticus*
- *Anaerococcus octavius*
- *Anaerococcus prevotii*
- *Anaerococcus tetradius*
- *Anaeroccus vaginalis*

**Table 36.4**  Some characteristics of anaerobic non-sporing Gram-positive rods

| Genus | Common sites | Acid end-products |
|---|---|---|
| *Propionibacterium* | Skin, mouth, gut, vagina | Propionic acid |
| *Bifidobacterium* | Gut, mouth, vagina | Acetic and lactic acids |
| *Lactobacillus* | Mouth, gut, vagina | Lactic acid (major end-product) |
| *Actinomyces* | Mouth, gut, vagina | Succinic, lactic and acetic acids |
| *Eubacterium*[a] | Mouth, gut, vagina | Butyric and other acids |

[a]Taxonomy currently undergoing revision; includes several different genera.

**Box 36.3**  Types of infection and clinical specimens from which anaerobic Gram-positive cocci are isolated

- Blood cultures
- Central nervous system (including brain abscesses)
- Head and neck infections (including ear)
- Dental abscesses and infected root canals
- Periodontal diseases and infected oral implants
- Human and animal bites
- Pleural infections
- Abdominal infections
- Genitourinary tract infections
- Decubitus ulcers
- Foot ulcers
- Osteomyelitis

although they are present in significant numbers in the normal flora of the mouth, skin, gastrointestinal and female genitourinary tracts, and are isolated from a variety of types of infection. The main genera and some of their characteristics are listed in Table 36.4.

## Infections with Gram-positive rods

Any of these bacteria can occur as components of mixed anaerobic infections, and *Actinomyces* species can undoubtedly adopt a pathogenic role. Most cases of actinomycosis are caused by *Actinomyces israelii* and are cervicofacial, although the disease can also occur in the thorax, abdomen and female genital tract (see Ch. 20). *Actinomyces* species are not themselves strict anaerobes, but *A. israelii* requires good anaerobic conditions for primary isolation, and plates should be incubated for 7–10 days.

*Propionibacterium propionicum* is morphologically and biochemically very similar to *A. israelii*. It is particularly associated with infection of the tear duct in the condition called *lachrymal canaliculitis*. The significance of other genera in infections is not clear. Some species are found in acne; they are also isolated occasionally in infective endocarditis and in infections associated with implanted prostheses. *Eubacterium* species are a large group (possibly mistaken for *Actinomyces* species in some reports), many of which are being reclassified into new genera, including *Slackia* and *Eggerthella*. These bacteria may play a role in infections around intra-uterine devices; others, for example *Slackia exigua*, may be involved in human periodontal disease. There is only limited evidence for the pathogenicity of *Bifidobacterium* species, although *Bif. dentium* has been isolated occasionally

for example, this genus is a regular component of supragingival dental plaque and the tongue microflora. Veillonellae are able to use some of the lactic acid produced by bacteria such as streptococci and lactobacilli that potentially induce dental caries.

The role of *Veillonella* species and other anaerobic Gram-negative cocci in disease, if any, has not been clearly established, although they may be isolated from a variety of clinical conditions. In general, they are regarded as a minor component of mixed anaerobic infections, and antimicrobial chemotherapy is not generally directed specifically against them.

## NON-SPORING GRAM-POSITIVE RODS

The spore-forming genus *Clostridium* is well known for its involvement in serious infections (see Ch. 22). The role of anaerobic non-sporing Gram-positive rods, on the other hand, is less well understood, from pulmonary infections; bifidobacteria can also be isolated from dental caries lesions by use of appropriate cultural methods.

## SPIRAL-SHAPED MOTILE ORGANISMS

Several *Treponema* species are found in the mouth and elsewhere in the body (see Table 36.1). They are thought to be an important component of the mixed anaerobic infection associated with acute necrotizing ulcerative gingivitis along with fusobacteria and *Prev. intermedia*, and may also contribute to other forms of periodontal disease. The proportion of motile spiral organisms seen by dark-ground microscopy in samples from the gingival pocket increases markedly when there is evidence of periodontal destruction.

Motile, spiral-shaped, Gram-negative anaerobes of the genus *Anaerobiospirillum* have been isolated from patients with diarrhoea and from bacteraemia. Although comparatively rarely isolated from man, they can cause serious infections. The distribution and normal habitat of this and other morphologically similar organisms are not well understood. In some cases the source of infection may be domestic animals and pets.

## TREATMENT

In many infections caused by anaerobes the most important aspect of treatment is surgical. This often involves drainage of pus from abscesses, but may also include debridement, curettage and removal of necrotic tissue. For minor infections surgical drainage alone may be sufficient, but in many cases antimicrobial chemotherapy is also indicated. The main groups of agents used are the penicillins and the nitroimidazoles, particularly metronidazole. Other agents with good anti-anaerobe activity include chloramphenicol, clindamycin and cefoxitin, but resistant strains occur.

Metronidazole is effective against virtually all obligate anaerobes, including *Bacteroides*, *Porphyromonas*, *Prevotella* and *Fusobacterium* species, but not against facultatively anaerobic or micro-aerophilic bacteria such as actinomyces and streptococci. Resistance to metronidazole is still relatively uncommon.

Most anaerobic species are sensitive to benzylpenicillin, but members of the *B. fragilis* group are usually resistant. Such resistance is associated with β-lactamase production and these organisms are usually susceptible to combinations of penicillins with β-lactamase inhibitors (e.g. co-amoxiclav) and to carbapenems such as imipenem.

### RECOMMENDED READING

Allaker RP, Young KA, Langlois T, et al: Dental plaque flora of the dog with reference to fastidious and anaerobic bacteria associated with bites, *Journal of Veterinary Dentistry* 14:127–130, 1997.

Borriello SP, Murray PR, Funke G, editors: *Topley and Wilson's Microbiology and Microbial Infections*, Vol. 2 *Bacteriology*, Oxford, 2005, Wiley-Blackwell.

Duerden BI, Drasar BS, editors: *Anaerobes in Human Disease*, London, 1991, Edward Arnold.

Finegold SM, George WL, editors: *Anaerobic Infections in Humans*, San Diego, 1989, Academic Press.

Fuller R, Perdigon G, editors: *Gut Flora, Nutrition, Immunity, and Health*, Oxford, 2003, Blackwell Publishing.

Marsh P, Martin MV: *Oral Microbiology*, Edinburgh, 2009, Churchill Livingstone.

Wilson M: *Bacteriology of Humans*, Oxford, 2008, Blackwell Publishing.

### Website

List of Prokaryotic Names with Standing in Nomenclature. http://www.bacterio.cict.fr/

# 37 Treponema and borrelia

## Syphilis; yaws; relapsing fever; Lyme disease

### A. Cockayne

---

## KEY POINTS

- The genus *Treponema* includes the agents of syphilis (*T. pallidum*), yaws (*T. pertenue*), bejel (*T. endemicum*) and pinta (*T. carateum*). All are essentially morphologically and antigenically identical spirochaetes, which cannot be cultivated in vitro.
- These diseases, if untreated, characteristically progress to chronic disease through distinct early and late stages and pathologies whose appearance is separated by latent periods of variable length.
- Diagnosis of syphilis, which is primarily sexually transmitted, is made by clinical observation and confirmed serologically.
- All of these organisms are sensitive to benzylpenicillin, which can be used to treat the early stages of disease.
- The genus *Borrelia* includes agents of Lyme disease (*B. burgdorferi* sensu lato) and relapsing fevers (*B. recurrentis* and others), all of which are transmitted to man by ticks or lice.
- Lyme disease, if untreated, may progress through distinct clinical phases (stages 1–3), resulting in later pathology (e.g. arthritis, neurological damage) in some individuals.
- Relapsing fevers are characterized by recurring periods of fever and remission associated with antigenic variation of the borreliae. Infection may be fatal.
- Lyme disease is diagnosed clinically and confirmed serologically. Doxycycline may be used to treat the early stages.

Members of the genera *Treponema* and *Borrelia* are spirochaetes. Human diseases caused by these bacteria (Table 37.1) include syphilis, which has been known for thousands of years, and infections such as Lyme disease, the true prevalence and geographical distribution of which are still being evaluated.

Treponemal infections may be spread from person to person by intimate physical contact, by contact with infectious body fluids or, in some instances, by fomites. The treponemes that infect man are obligate human parasites, and no other natural hosts are known. In contrast, borreliae are transmitted to man by infected ticks or lice. The borreliae that cause Lyme disease and endemic relapsing fever also infect many other animal species, which act as reservoirs of infection; man is an unfortunate incidental host in the natural history of these pathogens.

Characteristically, treponemal and borrelial infections occur in several distinct clinical stages. These may be separated by periods of remission, and each stage may have a particular associated pathology. Commonly the causative organism is detectable in early lesions but is much more difficult to identify in later disease. The pathogen spreads from the initial site of infection to many organs via the bloodstream and, despite a vigorous immune response, in some untreated cases these infections may be progressive, destructive and, in some instances (e.g. tertiary syphilis), fatal. In other cases only the early symptoms are apparent and the later pathology is not seen.

Antigenic variation contributes to bacterial virulence for the relapsing fever borreliae but in general the pathogenic mechanisms employed by spirochaetes are poorly understood. No extracellular toxins have yet been identified, and the mechanisms that enable these organisms to persist in tissues despite vigorous immune responses remain unclear. *Borrelia burgdorferi* and other borreliae can vary their surface lipoproteins to avoid the immune system. The paucity of exposed antigenic proteins on the surface of *Treponema pallidum* may contribute to immune evasion. It is also likely that the later manifestations of the treponemal and some borrelial infections involve auto-immune phenomena.

In addition to the pathogenic species, many other spirochaetes form part of the normal bacterial flora

**Table 37.1** Principal human diseases caused by spirochaetes

| Organism | Disease | Distribution | Primary mode of transmission | Animal reservoirs |
|---|---|---|---|---|
| *T. pallidum* | Syphilis | Worldwide | Sexual-congenital | None |
| *T. pertenue* | Yaws | Tropics and subtropics | Direct contact | None |
| *T. endemicum* | Bejel | Arid, subtropical or temperate areas | Mouth-to-mouth via utensils | None |
| *T. carateum* | Pinta | Arid, tropical Americas | Skin-to-skin contact | None |
| *B. recurrentis* | Epidemic relapsing fever | Central, East Africa; South American Andes | Louse bites | None |
| *Borrelia* spp. | Endemic relapsing fever | Worldwide[a] | Tick bites | Yes |
| *B. burgdorferi* sensu lato | Lyme disease | Worldwide[a] | Tick bites | Yes |

[a]Distribution governed by presence of tick vectors.

of the mouth, gut and genital tract. Morphological and antigenic similarities between pathogenic and commensal spirochaetes may cause problems in the clinical and serological diagnosis.

## DESCRIPTION

Spirochaetes are slender unicellular helical or spiral rods (Fig. 37.1) with a number of distinctive ultrastructural features used in the differentiation of the genera (Fig. 37.2). The cytoplasm is surrounded by a cytoplasmic membrane, and a peptidoglycan layer contributes to cell rigidity and shape. In *Treponema* species, fine cytoplasmic filaments are visible in the bacterial cytoplasm (Fig. 37.3), but these are absent in *Borrelia* species. Members of both genera are actively motile; several flagella are attached at each pole of the cell and wrap around the bacterial cell body. In contrast to other motile bacteria, these flagella do not protrude into the surrounding medium but are enclosed within the bacterial outer membrane. Treponemal flagella are complex, comprising a sheath and core (Fig. 37.4), whereas those of *Borrelia* species are simpler and similar to the flagella of other bacteria. The spirochaetal outer membrane is unusually lipid rich and, at least in some treponemes, appears to be protein deficient and to lack lipopolysaccharide. This may account for the susceptibility of these organisms to killing by detergents and desiccation.

Although the treponemes are distantly related to Gram-negative bacteria, they do not stain by Gram's method, and modified staining procedures are used. Moreover, the pathogenic treponemes cannot be cultivated in laboratory media and are maintained by subculture in susceptible animals. In contrast, borreliae stain Gram-negative, and many pathogenic species can be cultured in vitro in enriched, serum-containing, media.

**Fig. 37.1** Electron micrograph of *T. pallidum*. The flagella (arrowheads) are inserted at the tip and follow the helical contour of the bacterial cell enclosed within the outer membrane. Bar = 0.1 μm. (Photograph courtesy of Professor CW Penn.)

## *TREPONEMA*

*Treponema* species pathogenic for man include the causative agents of venereal *syphilis* and the non-venereal treponematoses, *yaws*, *bejel* and *pinta*.

The spirochaetes causing these different infections are micro-aerobic and morphologically identical:

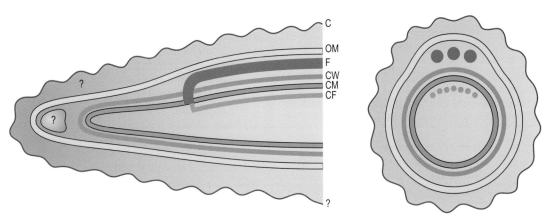

**Fig. 37.2** Schematic representation of the structure of *T. pallidum* in longitudinal and cross-section: C, postulated capsular layer; OM, outer membrane; F, flagellum; CW, cell wall peptidoglycan; CM, cytoplasmic membrane; CF, cytoplasmic filaments (absent in borreliae). Areas of uncertainty (indicated by question marks) include the existence and form of the capsule, the continuity or otherwise of the outer membrane over the tip of the organism, the nature and form of the tip structure, and the exact juxtaposition of the ends of the cytoplasmic filaments with the bacterial flagellar basal bodies. (After Strugnell R, Cockayne A, Penn CW 1990 Molecular and antigenic analysis of treponemes. *Critical Reviews in Microbiology* 17: 231–250.)

**Fig. 37.3** Electron micrograph of a detergent- and protease-treated *T. pallidum* cell showing cytoplasmic filaments (arrowheads) in the bacterial cytoplasm. Bar = 0.1 μm.

**Fig. 37.4** Electron micrograph of a detergent-treated *T. pallidum* cell showing the complex structure of the treponemal flagellum. Both sheathed (S) flagella and the thinner flagellar cores (C) are visible. Bar = 0.1 μm.

tightly coiled helical rods, 5–15 μm long and 0.1–0.5 μm diameter. They show only subtle antigenic differences and are characterized primarily by the clinical syndromes they cause and minor differences in the pathology induced in experimental animals.

## TREPONEMA PALLIDUM SSP. PALLIDUM (T. PALLIDUM)

*T. pallidum*, the causative agent of syphilis, was first isolated from syphilitic lesions in 1905. Infection

is usually acquired by sexual contact with infected individuals and is most common in the most sexually active age group of 15–30-year-olds. *Congenital syphilis* usually occurs following vertical transmission of *T. pallidum* from the infected mother to the fetus in utero, but neonates may also be infected during passage through the infected birth canal at delivery. Infection in utero may have serious consequences for the fetus. Rarely, syphilis has been acquired by transfusion of infected fresh human blood.

## Pathogenesis

Untreated syphilis may be a progressive disease with *primary*, *secondary*, *latent* and *tertiary* stages. *T. pallidum* enters tissues by penetration of intact mucosae or through abraded skin.

The bacteria rapidly enter the lymphatics, are widely disseminated via the bloodstream and may lodge in any organ. The exact infectious dose for man is not known, but in experimental animals fewer than ten organisms are sufficient to initiate infection. The bacteria multiply at the initial entry site forming a *chancre*, a lesion characteristic of primary syphilis, after an average incubation period of 3 weeks. The chancre is painless and most frequently on the external genitalia, but it may occur on the cervix, peri-anal area, in the mouth or anal canal. Chancres usually occur singly, but in immunocompromised individuals, such as those infected with the human immunodeficiency virus (HIV), multiple or persistent chancres may develop. The chancre usually heals spontaneously within 3–6 weeks, and 2–12 weeks later the symptoms of secondary syphilis develop. These are highly variable and widespread but most commonly involve the skin where macular or pustular lesions develop, particularly on the trunk and extremities. The lesions of secondary syphilis are highly infectious.

These lesions gradually resolve and a period of latent infection is entered, in which no clinical manifestations are evident, but serological evidence of infection persists. Relapse of the lesions of secondary syphilis is common, and latent syphilis is classified as early (high likelihood of relapse) or late (recurrence unlikely). Individuals with late latent syphilis are not generally considered infectious, but may still transmit infection to the fetus during pregnancy and their blood may remain infectious.

Late or tertiary syphilis may develop decades after the primary infection. It is a slowly progressive, destructive, inflammatory disease that may affect any organ. The three most common forms are *neurosyphilis*, *cardiovascular syphilis* and *gummatous syphilis* – a rare granulomatous lesion of the skeleton, skin or mucocutaneous tissues. Isolation of *T. pallidum* from patients with late syphilis is usually impossible, and much of the observed pathology may be due to autoimmune phenomena.

## TREPONEMA PALLIDUM SSP. PERTENUE (T. PERTENUE)

*T. pertenue* is the causative agent of *yaws*, a disease that is endemic among rural populations in tropical and subtropical countries such as Africa, South America, South-East Asia and Oceania. Eradication programmes sponsored by the World Health Organization reduced the number of cases to fewer than 2 million in the 1970s, but termination of the programmes led to a resurgence of pockets of disease, particularly in West Africa.

Infection with *T. pertenue* occurs non-venereally following contact of traumatized skin with exudate from early yaws lesions. Infection is usually acquired before puberty. The incubation period is 3–5 weeks, and the initial lesions usually occur on the legs. The papular lesions enlarge, erode and usually heal spontaneously within 6 months. Eruption of similar lesions occurs weeks to months later, and relapse is common. Secondary lesions may involve bones, particularly the fingers, long bones and the jaw. Late yaws is characterized by cutaneous plaques and ulcers, and thickening of the skin on the palms and soles of the feet. Gummatous lesions may also develop. In contrast to syphilis, neurological and cardiovascular damage does not occur. As affected individuals acquire infection early in life, they are essentially non-infectious at childbearing age, and congenital yaws is unknown.

## TREPONEMA PALLIDUM SSP. ENDEMICUM (T. ENDEMICUM)

This organism causes a non-venereal, syphilis-like disease called *endemic syphilis* or *bejel*. Bejel is endemic in Africa, western Asia and Australia, and affects mainly children in rural populations where living conditions and personal hygiene are poor. Transmission is by direct person-to-person contact and by sharing of contaminated eating or drinking utensils.

The initial lesion is usually oral and may not be detected. Secondary lesions include oropharyngeal mucous patches, condyloma lata and periostitis. Late lesions involve gummata in the skin, nasopharynx and bones. As in yaws, the cardiovascular and central nervous systems are not involved, and congenital infection is rare because of the early age of infection.

## TREPONEMA CARATEUM

Unlike the other treponematoses, the manifestations of *pinta*, caused by *T. carateum*, are confined to the skin. Although these lesions are non-destructive, they cause disfigurement with associated social problems for infected individuals. Pinta is probably the oldest human treponemal infection, with distribution now restricted to arid rural inland regions of Mexico, Central America and Colombia.

Spread of infection is by direct contact with infectious lesions. After a 7–21-day incubation period, small erythematous pruritic primary lesions develop, most commonly on the extremities, face, neck, chest or abdomen. The primary lesions enlarge and coalesce, and once healed may leave areas of hypopigmentation. Disseminated secondary lesions appear 3–12 months later and may become dyschromic. Recurrence of lesions is common for up to 10 years after the initial infection. The depigmented lesions are characteristic of the later stages of pinta but do not cause any serious harm.

## OTHER TREPONEMA SPECIES

Treponemes are implicated in several other human infections. The microbial flora associated with these conditions is complex, and the exact role of the spirochaetes in the aetiology of infection remains to be determined. Moreover, the taxonomic status of some of these organisms is uncertain.

### Oral infections

*T. denticola*, *T. socranskii* and *T. pectinovorum* form part of the normal flora, and the numbers of these organisms increase in acute necrotizing ulcerative gingivitis and chronic adult periodontal disease. *T. vincentii* (or Vincent's spirillum) is similarly associated with ulceromembranous gingivitis or pharyngitis, *Vincent's angina*. Several spirochaetes appear to be involved in the aetiology of a similar condition called *trench mouth*.

### Gastrointestinal infections

Several as yet unidentified weakly haemolytic spirochaetes have been implicated in the aetiology of persistent diarrhoea and rectal bleeding in certain human populations. A morphologically similar but genetically distinct organism, *Brachyspira* (formerly *Serpulina*) *hyodysenteriae*, is the cause of swine dysentery.

### Skin lesions

*Tropical ulcer* is a chronic skin condition in which spirochaetes of unknown identity have been implicated, usually in association with fusiform bacteria (see p. 361) and other organisms.

## LABORATORY DIAGNOSIS

The inability to grow most pathogenic treponemes in vitro, coupled with the transitory nature of many of the lesions, makes diagnosis of treponemal infection impossible by routine bacteriological methods. Although spirochaetes are detectable by microscopy in primary and secondary lesions, diagnosis is based primarily on clinical observations and confirmed by serological tests. For practical purposes, the serological responses to all these pathogens are identical, and only their use in the serodiagnosis of syphilis is considered here.

### Direct microscopy

Treponemes can be visualized directly in freshly collected exudate from primary or secondary lesions by dark-ground or phase-contrast microscopy. Although this method allows a rapid definitive diagnosis to be made, it is rather insensitive because primary lesions may contain relatively few bacteria. In addition, care must be taken to differentiate between pathogenic and commensal spirochaetes, which may occasionally contaminate such material. More sensitive and specific results may be obtained using fixed material in an immunofluorescence assay with an anti-treponemal antibody.

### Serological tests

Infection with *T. pallidum* results in the rapid production of two types of antibody:

1. Specific antibodies directed primarily at polypeptide antigens of the bacterium
2. Non-specific antibodies (reagin antibodies) that react with a non-treponemal antigen called *cardiolipin*.

The mechanism of induction of non-specific antibodies remains unclear. Cardiolipin is a phospholipid extracted from beef heart, and it is possible that a similar substance, present in the treponemal cell or released from host cells damaged by the bacterium, may stimulate antibody production.

Historically, assays for non-specific antibody were used as routine screening tests for evidence of syphilis because of their low cost and technical simplicity. Enzyme immunosorbent assays that detect specific treponemal antibodies are increasingly replacing the older tests for screening purposes.

## Non-specific serological tests for syphilis

The *rapid plasma reagin* (RPR) test, which has now largely superseded the earlier *Venereal Disease Research Laboratory* (VDRL) test, is a non-specific serological test for syphilis that uses cardiolipin as antigen. Immunoglobulin (Ig) M or IgG antibody present in positive sera causes a suspension of this lipoidal antigen to flocculate, and the result can be read rapidly by eye. Both of these assays may be used as screening tests, and are positive in approximately 70% of primary and 99% of secondary syphilitics, but are negative in individuals with late syphilis. These tests can be used quantitatively, and increases in antibody titres with time may be used to confirm a diagnosis of congenital syphilis. The RPR assay is not suitable for use with cerebrospinal fluid.

As a positive result in these tests usually indicates active infection, they can also be used to monitor the efficacy of antibacterial therapy.

## Tests for specific antibody

***Fluorescent treponemal antibody absorption (FTA-Abs) test.*** This is an indirect immunofluorescence assay in which *T. pallidum* is used as an antigen. Acetone-fixed treponemes are incubated with heat-treated sera, and bound antibody is detected with a fluorescein-labelled conjugate and ultraviolet microscopy. The serum is first absorbed with a suspension of a non-pathogenic treponeme, which removes non-specific cross-reactive antibodies that may be directed against commensal spirochaetes. The FTA-Abs test is positive in approximately 80, 100 and 95% of primary, secondary and late syphilitics, respectively, and, unlike the RPR and VDRL tests, remains positive following successful therapy.

***T. pallidum haemagglutination assay (TPHA).*** In this test, *T. pallidum* antigen is coated on to the surface of red blood cells, and specific antibody in test sera causes haemagglutination. As in the FTA-Abs assay, sera are pre-absorbed with a non-pathogenic treponeme to remove antibody against commensal spirochaetes. The TPHA test is less sensitive than the FTA-Abs test in primary syphilis (positive in 65%), but both give similar results for secondary and late syphilis; the TPHA also remains positive for life following infection. This assay can be used to detect localized production of anti-treponemal antibodies in cerebrospinal fluid, a marker of neurosyphilis. The *T. pallidum particle agglutination (TPPA)* test works on the same principle as the TPHA, but treponemal antigen is coated on to coloured gelatin particles rather than red blood cells.

***Enzyme immunoassay.*** In these tests monoclonal anti-*T. pallidum* antibodies are used to detect antibody responses to individual treponemal antigens. This allows rapid screening of large numbers of samples with potentially enhanced specificity. Assays that detect either IgM or IgG are available. Positive results should be confirmed by a second specific test such as the TPHA.

## Problems in the serological diagnosis of syphilis

Occasionally, both the non-specific and specific tests produce false-positive results. The RPR and VDRL assays may give a transient positive result following any strong immunological stimulus such as acute bacterial or viral infection or after immunization. More persistent false-positive results occur in individuals with autoimmune or connective tissue disease, in drug abusers and in individuals with hypergamma-globulinaemia. False-positive results usually become apparent when negative results are found in specific serological tests, but in some cases FTA-Abs results may also be positive or borderline.

Rarely, the FTA-Abs test may be positive and the nonspecific VDRL test negative. Lyme disease (see below) induces antibodies that react in the FTA-Abs but not in the VDRL assay. Other spirochaetal diseases such as relapsing fever, yaws, pinta and leptospirosis may give positive results in both specific and non-specific tests. Of particular difficulty is the differential diagnosis of syphilis and yaws in immigrants from areas in which yaws is endemic.

Some of the newer enzyme immunoassays are less sensitive in cases of primary syphilis.

Direct detection of spirochaetal deoxyribonucleic acid (DNA) in clinical material by molecular methods, such as the polymerase chain reaction (PCR), may have a future role in confirming a diagnosis of syphilis in difficult or atypical cases.

## TREATMENT

All the pathogenic treponemes are sensitive to benzylpenicillin, and prolonged high-dose therapy with procaine penicillin has been the traditional method of treatment for primary and secondary syphilis. So far there have been no reports of penicillin resistance. If penicillin allergy is a problem, erythromycin, tetracycline or chloramphenicol may be used. There are reports of treatment failure with erythromycin, and an erythromycin-resistant variant of *T. pallidum* has been isolated. In late syphilis, aqueous benzylpenicillin is used, as this penetrates better into the central nervous system. In neurosyphilis, successful eradication of the organism may not result in a clinical cure. More aggressive and prolonged antibiotic therapy may be required in HIV-positive patients with syphilis owing to impaired immune function.

Antibiotic therapy of syphilitics, particularly with penicillin, characteristically induces a systemic response called the *Jarisch–Herxheimer reaction*. This is characterized by the rapid onset (within 2 h) of fever, chills, myalgia, tachycardia, hyperventilation, vasodilatation and hypotension. The response is thought to be due to release of an endogenous pyrogen from the spirochaetes.

## EPIDEMIOLOGY AND CONTROL

### Syphilis

The widespread introduction of antibiotic therapy shortly after the Second World War produced a dramatic decrease in the incidence of syphilis, but the disease remained endemic within the general population. Geographically localized outbreaks of syphilis, associated with specific recreational activities and lifestyles, now occur in countries such as the UK.

In the mid-1980s most cases of syphilis in developed countries occurred in male homosexuals. The advent of HIV and the acquired immune deficiency syndrome (AIDS) in the 1980s reduced the incidence among this group owing to changes in sexual practices. The early 1990s saw a resurgence of syphilis among the heterosexual population in the USA, resulting in an increased incidence among women and in the number of cases of congenital syphilis. Subsequent changes in sexual practices among homosexual men have reversed this trend: significantly more cases of primary and secondary syphilis now occur in men than women and, among males, over 60% of cases occur in men who have sex with men. The incidence of congenital syphilis has fallen from 2435 cases in 1994 to 427 in 2009. Total reported numbers of cases of syphilis in the USA were 46 291 in 2008 and 44 828 in 2009.

In the UK ongoing outbreaks of syphilis in various regions have seen the number of cases rise consistently from 2000, peaking at around 3700 cases of infectious syphilis in 2007. Most cases of infectious syphilis (>70%) currently occur among men who have sex with men but significant numbers of cases are still detected in heterosexual men and women. Syphilis therefore continues to pose major public health issues. The potential for congenital infection and the acquisition of syphilis by blood transfusion mean that screening programmes of all pregnant women and blood donations are still required.

Control of syphilis is achieved by treating index cases and any known contacts. Treatment of contacts is important as some may be incubating the infection even if they have no overt signs of disease.

Control of the disease may have additional benefits: primary syphilis increases the risk of HIV infection two- to five-fold, presumably by permitting easier access of the virus through damaged skin or mucosal membranes.

### Other treponematoses

The incidence of the other treponematoses is influenced primarily by socio-economic factors. Prevention and control involve treatment of individuals with active or latent disease and contacts, and improvement of living conditions and personal hygiene.

## BORRELIA

The two principal human diseases associated with borreliae are *relapsing fever*, caused by *Borrelia recurrentis* and several other *Borrelia* species, and *Lyme disease* or *Lyme borreliosis*, a multi-system infection caused by *B. burgdorferi* sensu lato. The bacteria causing these infections are morphologically similar helical rods, 8–30 μm long and 0.2–0.5 μm in diameter, with three to ten loose spirals. Antigenic and genetic differences are used to differentiate the species.

## RELAPSING FEVERS

Relapsing fevers are characterized clinically by recurrent periods of fever and spirochaetaemia.

*Endemic* or *tick-borne relapsing fever* is a zoonosis caused by several *Borrelia* species, including *B. duttoni*, *B. hermsii*, *B. parkeri* and *B. turicatae*, and is transmitted to man by soft-bodied *Ornithodoros* ticks. The natural hosts for these organisms include rodents and other small mammals on which the ticks normally feed. The disease occurs worldwide, reflecting the distribution of the tick vector.

*Epidemic* or *louse-borne relapsing fever* is caused by *B. recurrentis*, an obligate human pathogen transmitted from person to person by the body louse, *Pediculus humanus*. The incidence is influenced by socio-economic factors such as lack of personal hygiene, and, historically, increases during periods of war, famine and other social upheaval. The disease still occurs in central and eastern Africa and in the South American Andes.

The spirochaetes causing the two forms of relapsing fever differ in their mode of growth in the arthropod vector, and this influences the way in which human infection is initiated. *B. recurrentis* grows in the haemolymph of the louse but does not invade tissues. As a result the louse faeces are not infectious and the bacterium is not transferred through eggs to the progeny. Human infection occurs when bacteria released from crushed lice gain entry to tissues through damaged or intact skin, or mucous membranes. Spirochaetes causing tickborne relapsing fever invade all the tissues of the tick, including the salivary glands, genitalia and excretory system. Infection occurs when saliva or excrement is released during feeding. Transovarial transmission to the tick progeny maintains the spirochaete in the tick population.

## Pathogenesis

In both forms of relapsing fever, acute symptoms, including high fever, rigors, headache, myalgia, arthralgia, photophobia and cough, develop about 1 week after infection. A skin rash may occur, and there is central nervous system involvement in up to 30% of cases. During the acute phase there may be up to $10^5$ spirochaetes per cubic millimetre of blood. The primary illness resolves within 3–6 days, and terminates abruptly with hypotension and shock, which may be fatal. Relapse of fever occurs 7–10 days later, and several relapses may take place.

Each episode of spirochaetaemia is terminated by the development of specific anti-spirochaete antibody. Subsequent febrile episodes are caused by borreliae that differ antigenically, particularly in outer membrane protein composition, from those causing earlier attacks. As the cycle of fever and relapse continues, the borreliae tend to revert back to the antigenic types that caused the original spirochaetaemia, and ultimate clearance of the infection appears to be due to antibody-mediated killing.

In general, louse-borne relapsing fever has longer febrile and afebrile periods than tick-borne infection, but fewer relapses. The case fatality rate varies from 4–40% for louse-borne infection and from 2–5% for tick-borne relapsing fever, with myocarditis, cerebral haemorrhage and liver failure the most common causes of death.

## Laboratory diagnosis

Definitive diagnosis of relapsing fevers is made by detection of borreliae in peripheral blood samples. Thick or thin blood smears are stained with Giemsa or other stains such as acridine orange.

Although antibodies to the borreliae are produced during infection, serological tests are complicated by antigenic variation and the tendency to relapse. Serological tests for syphilis are positive in 5–10% of cases.

## Treatment

Tetracycline, chloramphenicol, penicillin and erythromycin have been used successfully. As in the treatment of syphilis, antibiotics may elicit a Jarisch–Herxheimer reaction.

Prevention of infection involves avoidance or eradication of the insect vector. Insecticides can be used to eradicate ticks from human dwellings, but elimination from the environment is not feasible. Prevention of louse-borne infection involves maintenance of good personal hygiene, and delousing if necessary.

## LYME DISEASE

Lyme disease, originally called *Lyme arthritis*, was recognized as an infectious condition in 1975 following an epidemiological investigation of a cluster of cases of suspected juvenile rheumatoid arthritis that occurred in Lyme, Connecticut, USA. A common factor in these cases was a previous history of insect bite, and the infectious agent, *B. burgdorferi*, was subsequently isolated from an *Ixodes* tick. Retrospective serological data suggest that Lyme disease was endemic in the USA as early as 1962, and the clinical manifestations of this infection have been known in Europe, including the UK, since the early 1900s. Lyme disease has also been reported in Scandinavia, eastern Europe, China, Japan and Australia.

The natural hosts for *B. burgdorferi* are wild and domesticated animals, including mice and other rodents, deer, sheep, cattle, horses and dogs. The larger animal hosts such as deer are probably more important in maintaining the size of tick populations rather than acting as a major source of *B. burgdorferi*. Infection in these animals may be inapparent, although clinical infection has been observed in cattle, horses and dogs.

*B. burgdorferi* is transmitted to man by ixodid ticks that become infected while feeding on infected animals. The principal vectors in the USA are *Ixodes dammini* and *I. pacificus*, and in Europe, *I. ricinus*. The life cycle of these ticks involves larval, nymph and adult stages, all of which are capable of transmitting infection, although the nymphal stage is most commonly implicated. In areas endemic for Lyme disease, 2–50% of ticks may carry *B. burgdorferi*. The bacterium grows primarily in the midgut of the tick, and transmission to man occurs during regurgitation of the gut contents during the blood meal. Transmission efficiency appears to be relatively low, but increases with the duration of feeding.

Although there is general similarity, clinical manifestations may differ in the USA and Europe. This variation is due in part to significant differences in the bacterial strains causing infection in the two continents, and has resulted in the division of *B. burgdorferi* into three distinct genospecies:

- *B. burgdorferi* sensu stricto is the sole cause of Lyme disease in the USA where Lyme arthritis is a common complication of infection.
- *B. afzeli* and *B. garinii* are responsible for most Lyme disease in Europe, and are associated with chronic skin and neurological symptoms, respectively.

Several other genetically distinct isolates of *B. burgdorferi* have been identified in ticks, but their importance in human infection has yet to be established.

Lyme disease may be a progressive illness, and is divided into three stages:

- *Stage 1* is characterized by a spreading annular rash, *erythema chronicum migrans* (ECM), which occurs at the site of the tick bite 3–22 days after infection. Lesions may contain very small numbers of bacteria, and the disproportionate intensity of the pathology seen may be due to stimulation of cytokines such as tumour necrosis factor-$\alpha$ and secondary mediators. The bacterium also spreads to various other organs. In the USA, secondary lesions similar to those of ECM are common. Malaise, fatigue, headache, rigors and neck stiffness may also be apparent. The rash and secondary lesions fade within 3–4 weeks.
- *Stage 2* develops in some patients after several weeks or months. These patients exhibit cardiac or neurological abnormalities, musculoskeletal symptoms or intermittent arthritis.
- *Stage 3* may ensue months to years later, when patients present with chronic skin, nervous system or joint abnormalities.

Congenital infection may occur with serious, potentially fatal, consequences for the fetus.

## Laboratory diagnosis

Once a clinical diagnosis has been made, culture of the spirochaete from suitable biopsy material provides a definitive diagnosis, but this is a lengthy, specialized technique that is not widely available. As the organism is also difficult to detect in histological sections,

serological tests are used routinely for the confirmation of Lyme disease, although PCR techniques are used in some laboratories.

Specific IgM antibodies develop within 3–6 weeks of infection. The earliest response appears to be against the bacterial flagellum and later against outer surface proteins. Subsequently, IgG antibodies are produced, and the highest titre is detectable months or years after infection.

An indirect immunofluorescence test is available, but enzyme-linked immunosorbent assay (ELISA) is now widely used. Immunoblotting with a panel of carefully selected recombinant antigens is used to confirm serological results. Serological diagnosis of early Lyme disease may still pose problems, as antibodies to the bacterium are slow to develop in some individuals and the formation of immune complexes may affect the test results. Antibodies that cross-react with *B. burgdorferi* may be produced after infection with other spirochaetes, and sera from patients with Lyme disease may give a positive FTA-Abs test, although the VDRL test is negative.

Serological evidence of infection may be detectable in the apparent absence of overt disease. The significance of these findings is unclear but it is possible that such individuals may develop late complications of Lyme disease.

## Treatment

Penicillins, macrolides, cephalosporins and tetracyclines have all been used successfully. Reports suggest that treatment with tetracyclines (doxycycline) produces fewer late complications than penicillin therapy. About 15% of patients experience a Jarisch–Herxheimer reaction after antibiotic therapy. Despite antibiotic treatment, some patients suffer from minor late complications of the disease, which may be mediated immunologically and may require supplementary immunosuppresive therapy, or may indicate low-level persistence of the organisms.

Antibiotic therapy may reduce or abolish the antibody response, and this may interfere with the serological confirmation of infection.

## Epidemiology and control

The geographical distribution of Lyme disease is governed by that of the tick vector and its associated animal hosts. Forestry workers and farmers are particularly at risk, but infection is also increasingly associated with recreational activities. In the UK, Lyme disease occurs in areas that support large populations of wild or domesticated animals on which ixodid ticks feed. Infection may also be acquired after travel to countries where Lyme disease is endemic. It is difficult to accurately assess the true incidence of Lyme disease, because infection may be mild or asymptomatic and consequently not detected. In 2008, there were 813 laboratory-confirmed cases in the UK but estimated case numbers range from 1000–3000 per year. By comparison, approximately 30 000 confirmed cases were reported in the USA in 2009.

Prevention of infection involves avoidance of endemic areas and education of the public regarding the possible risks of infection in these localities. Eradication of the tick vectors or mammalian hosts from such areas is not feasible. A vaccine to protect residents and visitors in areas in which Lyme disease is endemic would be useful, but attempts to develop effective and safe recombinant vaccines against *B. burgdorferi* have so far been unsuccessful.

## RECOMMENDED READING

Andersson LC, Bergstrom S: Current issues in relapsing fever, *Current Opinion in Infectious Disease* 22:443–449, 2009.

Antal GM, Lukehart SA, Meheus AZ: The endemic treponematoses, *Microbes and Infection* 4:83–94, 2002.

Cullen PA, Haake DA, Adler B: Outer membrane proteins of pathogenic spirochetes, *FEMS Microbiology Reviews* 28:291–318, 2004.

Edwards AM, Dymock D, Jenkinson HF: From tooth to hoof: treponemes in tissue-destructive diseases, *Journal of Applied Microbiology* 94:767–780, 2003.

Egglestone SI, Turner AJ: Serological diagnosis of syphilis: PHLS Syphilis Serology Working Group, *Communicable Disease and Public Health* 3:158–162, 2000.

Herremans T, Kortbeek L, Notermans DW: A review of diagnostic tests for congenital syphilis in newborns, *European Journal of Clinical Microbiology and Infectious Disease* 29:495–501, 2010.

Lee V, Kinghorn G: Syphilis: an update, *Clinical Medicine* 8:330–333, 2008.

Marques AR Lyme disease: a review, *Current Allergy and Asthma Reports* 10:13–20, 2010.

### Websites

Centers for Disease Control and Prevention: Syphilis. http://www.cdc.gov/std/syphilis/

Health Protection Agency. Diagnosis and treatment of Lyme borreliosis. http://www.hpa.org.uk/web/HPAweb&HPAwebStandard/HPAweb_C/1204031510081

# 38 Leptospira

## Leptospirosis; Weil's disease

*M. Picardeau*

## KEY POINTS

- The term leptospirosis is used to describe all infections in man and animals, regardless of the clinical presentation or strain of *Leptospira* involved.
- The incidence rate is low in Europe (fewer than 1 case/100 000 inhabitants) and associated predominantly with occupational or recreational exposure.
- Antibiotics offer some benefit if started within 4 days of the onset of illness, and preferably within 24–48 h.
- Animals that acquire infection may not develop discernible disease, but become long-term carriers, so-called *maintenance hosts*.
- More than 200 pathogenic serovars are known and each is able to infect a range of animals that may become long-term carriers capable of infecting others. The organisms can also survive for long periods in the environment. Together, these features make control of leptospirosis a substantial challenge.

The recognition of human leptospirosis as a distinct clinical entity is usually attributed to Adolf Weil of the University of Heidelberg in 1886, although the disease had been described in animals since the mid 19th century. The term *Weil's disease* acknowledges Weil's observations in differentiating what was later proven to be a leptospiral infection from other forms of infective jaundice.

In 1914, Ryokichi Inada and his colleagues in Kyushu, Japan, observed spiral organisms in the livers of guinea-pigs inoculated with blood taken from Japanese miners with infectious jaundice, presumed to be Weil's disease. They named the organisms *Spirochaeta icterohaemorrhagiae*, reflecting their spiral shape and the fact that human infections were associated with jaundice (icterus) and haemorrhage. In Europe, similar organisms were demonstrated in some cases of jaundice in German soldiers involved in the First World War. In 1917, another Japanese scientist, Hideyo Noguchi, recognized that the organisms associated with Weil's disease differed from other known spirochaetes and proposed the genus name *Leptospira*, meaning a 'slender coil'. Today, more than 300 serovars have then been isolated from the environment, animals and man.

Leptospirosis is a zoonosis and has one of the widest geographical distributions of any zoonotic disease. The highest incidence is found in tropical and subtropical parts of the world. Probably every mammal has the potential to become a carrier of some serovar of *Leptospira*. These carriers harbour leptospires in their kidneys and excrete the bacteria into the environment when they urinate. This enables spread among their own kind and to other species, including human beings, who may directly or indirectly come into contact with their urine.

In man, the disease varies in severity from a mild self-limiting illness to the fulminating and potentially fatal disease described by Weil. Fortunately, full recovery without long-term morbidity is the most frequent outcome.

## DESCRIPTION

### Classification

The family Leptospiraceae belongs to the order Spirochaetales and can be subdivided into three genera: *Leptospira*, *Leptonema* and *Turneriella*. Only *Leptospira* spp. are considered to be pathogenic for animals and man.

The genus *Leptospira* was originally divided into two groups:

- *Leptospira interrogans* sensu lato (pathogenic strains)
- *L. biflexa* sensu lato (saprophytic strains).

These two groups differ in their nutritional requirements and other phenotypic properties. For example, the growth of pathogenic strains is inhibited by the purine analogue 8-azaguanine, whereas saprophytic strains grow normally in the presence of this compound. Similarly, unlike *L interrogans*, *L. biflexa* can grow at low ambient temperature (11–13°C).

More recently, genotypic classification has defined 20 species of Leptospira:

- 9 pathogenic species (*L. interrogans, L. kirschneri, L. borgpetersenii, L. santarosai, L. noguchii, L. weilii, L. alexanderi, L. alstoni,* and *L. kmetyi*)
- 6 saprophytic species (*L. biflexa, L. wolbachii, L. meyeri, L. vanthielii, L. terpstrae* and *L. yanagawae*)
- 5 'intermediate' species (*L. inadai, L. broomii, L. fainei, L. wolffii* and *L. licerasiae*), which are of unclear pathogenicity.

*Leptospires* are serologically classified in serovars, defined on the basis of structural heterogeneity in the carbohydrate component of the lipopolysaccharide (LPS). More than 200 different pathogenic serovars are currently recognized.

The genetic classification of *Leptospira* does not correlate with the phenotypic classification because serovars of the same serogroup may be distributed between different species. However, the serological classification is still widely used as it provides useful information for clinical or epidemiological investigations. The accepted nomenclature is generic name, followed by species name, followed by serovar, followed by strain (if appropriate). For example:

- *Leptospira* (generic name) *interrogans* (species name) serovar Icterohaemorrhagiae
- *Leptospira* (generic name) *interrogans* (species name) serovar Hardjo strain Hardjoprajitno.

The complete DNA sequence of strains belonging to two pathogenic species, *L. interrogans* and *L. borgpetersenii*, and one saprophytic species, *L. biflexa*, have been determined and this should provide insight into the molecular mechanisms of the survival and persistence of *Leptospira* in host and environment.

## The organism

Leptospires range between about 6 and 20 μm in length, but are only about 0.1 μm in diameter, which allows them to pass through filters that retain most other bacteria. They are Gram-negative, but take up conventional stains poorly. They can be visualized by Giemsa staining, silver deposition,

fluorescent antibody methods or electron microscopy. These bacteria are so thin that they are best viewed by dark-field microscopy. They have a helical-cell shape with one or both ends appearing hooked and they rotate rapidly around their long axis (Fig. 38.1).

*Leptospira* spp. possess a double-membrane structure composed of a cytoplasmic membrane, the periplasm and the outer membrane that contains the LPS and many membrane-associated lipoproteins which are the main targets for the host immune response. Two endoflagella with their free ends towards the middle of the bacteria lie in the periplasmic space between the cell wall and the outer envelope, and are wrapped around the cell wall. Each flagellum is attached to a basal body located at either end of the cell. The flagella are similar in structure to those of other bacteria and are responsible for motility, but the mechanism involved in their rapid movement is incompletely understood.

Leptospires are killed rapidly by desiccation, extremes of pH (e.g. gastric acid) and antibacterial substances that occur naturally in human and bovine milks. They are susceptible to low concentrations of chlorine and are killed by temperatures above 40°C (after about 10 min at 50°C and within 10 s at 60°C).

## Metabolism

Leptospires require aerobic or micro-aerophilic conditions for growth. Adequate sources of nitrogen, phosphate, calcium, magnesium and iron (as a haem compound or ferric ions) are essential. They can use fatty acids as their major energy source, but are unable to synthesize long-chain fatty acids with 15 or more carbon atoms. Pathogenic species require the presence of unsaturated fatty acids to utilize saturated fatty acids. Vitamins $B_1$ (thiamin) and $B_{12}$ (cyanocobalamin) are also essential and the addition of biotin is needed for the growth of some strains. These components are provided in Ellinghausen–McCullough–Johnson–Harris (EMJH) medium.

Optimal growth of pathogenic species in culture takes place at 28–30°C at pH 7.2–7.6. They are slow growing with a generation time of about 20 h: colonies are visible after 3–4 weeks on solid medium, whereas saprophytes grow more rapidly (colonies are visible after 1 week). Culture media do not generally contain selective agents as leptospires may be sensitive to them, so great care must be taken to avoid bacterial or fungal contamination at the time of inoculation and during the prolonged incubation period.

**Fig. 38.1**  Appearance of living leptospires as seen by dark-field microscopy. Note the very fine coils and characteristic hooked ends. (From an original painting by Dr Cranston Low. In Low RC, Dodds TC 1947 *Atlas of Bacteriology.* Livingstone, Edinburgh.)

## PATHOGENESIS

The pathogenesis of leptospirosis is incompletely understood, but a vasculitis resulting in damage to the endothelial cells of small blood vessels is probably the main underlying pathology.

Infection is acquired by direct or indirect contact with infected urine, tissues or secretions. Ingestion or inhalation of leptospires is not thought to pose a risk and human-to-human spread is very rare. Leptospires generally gain entry through small areas of damage on the skin or via mucous membranes. It is possible that they may also pass through waterlogged skin, although this is probably not a major route of infection.

The term 'leptospirosis' is used to describe all infections in both man and animals, regardless of the clinical presentation or strain of *Leptospira* involved. There are no serovar-specific disease patterns, although some serovars tend to cause more severe disease than others. In the past many names (epidemic pulmonary haemorrhagic fever, cane cutter's disease, Fort Bragg fever, Weil's disease, autumnal fever, etc.) were used to describe the particular clinical presentation or to reflect occupational, geographical, seasonal or other epidemiological features of leptospiral disease. Because of this, the full range of disease presentations was not appreciated and, even now, leptospiral infection may not be suspected unless the patient has the classically severe disease involving the liver and kidneys described originally by Weil. Some reports suggest that human infection with some serovars can, in rare cases, cause abortion.

## Clinical features

Typically, acute symptoms develop 5–14 days after infection, although rarely the incubation period can be as short as 2–3 days or as long as 30 days. The infection presents with an influenza-like illness characterized by the sudden onset of headache, muscular pain, especially in the muscles of the lower back and calf, fever and occasionally rigors. Conjunctival suffusion and a skin rash may be seen in some cases.

During a bacteraemic phase lasting 7–8 days after the onset of symptoms, the leptospires spread via the blood to many tissues, including the brain. In severe cases the illness often follows a biphasic course: the bacteraemic phase is followed by an 'immune' phase, with the appearance of antibody and the disappearance of recoverable leptospires from the blood. In this phase patients may show signs of recovery for a couple of days before the fever, rigors, severe headaches and meningism return. Bleeding may occur, together with signs and symptoms of jaundice and renal impairment. Typically, bilirubin concentrations are markedly raised, but other liver function test results may be only moderately increased.

In some cases of leptospirosis, pulmonary manifestations of infection are predominant. Patients can present with cough, shortness of breath or haemoptysis. In severe cases, adult respiratory distress syndrome and pulmonary haemorrhage can supervene and lead to death.

In severe fulminating disease the patient may die within the first few days of illness, but with appropriate treatment the prognosis is usually good. Many deaths throughout the world are due to the failure to provide adequate supportive management, especially in relation to the maintenance of renal function. Generally, patients are well within 2–6 weeks but some require up to 3 months to recover fully. In a few patients, symptoms persist for many months, but neither long-term carriage of leptospires nor chronic disease has been conclusively demonstrated in man.

After infection, immunity develops against the infecting strain, but may not fully protect against infection with unrelated strains.

## LABORATORY DIAGNOSIS

The initial diagnosis must rely on the medical history and clinical findings backed up with details of possible occupational or recreational exposure.

### Serology

Antibodies can usually be demonstrated by the sixth day after symptoms have developed (Fig. 38.2), although their detection may be delayed if antibiotics were administered early in the course of the illness.

The microscopic agglutination test (MAT), which can indicate the likely infecting serogroup or serovar, is generally accepted as the 'gold standard'. Doubling dilutions of patient's serum are titrated against pools of reference serovars representing the most common serogroups. After incubation, tests are read by dark-field microscopy; 50% agglutination of the leptospires by the patient's or control serum represents a positive result. Sera collected soon after the onset of symptoms often show cross-reactivity to different serogroups in the microscopic agglutination test. In contrast, sera obtained during the convalescent phase of the illness generally show a significantly higher titre to the infecting serogroup or serovar.

Most other tests give no indication of the infecting serovar. Several enzyme-linked immunosorbent assay (ELISA) kits offer ease of use together with relatively good sensitivity and specificity. Most detect IgM antibodies, which, are detectable in the acute phase of the illness and may remain for several months after infection (Fig. 38.2).

### Examination of blood and urine

The detection of leptospires in blood offers the earliest confirmation of infection. In theory, leptospirosis can be diagnosed by dark-field microscopy of blood taken during the first week of illness or, much less reliably, in urine during the second week. Dark-field microscopy of blood is technically demanding as Brownian movement of collagen fibrils, red blood cell membranes and other artefacts can resemble viable leptospires. Examination of urine is seldom worthwhile as a method of early diagnosis of infection in man.

Culture of blood may be useful in severe fulminating disease. Identification of infecting serovars requires specialized techniques that are available only in national reference laboratories. In recent years, PCR-based methods have been described and these assays are now used in many diagnostic and reference laboratories for the detection of leptospires in biological fluids of patients. Molecular diagnostic techniques offer the potential for more rapid diagnosis of leptospirosis than the currently available serological methods. This is of particular value in the critically ill patient. Reference laboratories can advise on the examination of cerebrospinal fluid or other tissue, including those taken at post mortem.

## TREATMENT

Antibiotics offer some benefit if started within 4 days of the onset of illness, and preferably within 24–48 h. In severe illness, intravenous benzylpenicillin is the drug of choice. For milder infections a 7–10-day course of oral amoxicillin is appropriate. Patients allergic to penicillins can be treated with erythromycin.

The value of antibiotic treatment is probably overestimated and few trials have been conducted. However, supportive management to maintain tissue and organ function, such as the temporary maintenance of renal function by dialysis, may be life-saving.

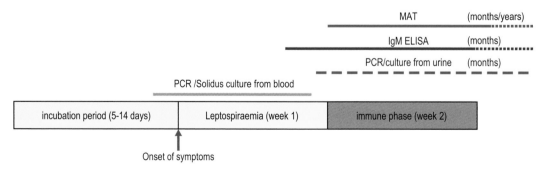

**Fig. 38.2** Disease kinetics of leptospirosis. Infection produces leptospiraemia in the first few days after exposure. Leptospires are then cleared from the bloodstream as the titres of serum agglutinating antibodies increase (immune phase). Leptospires are also transiently shed in urine for long periods. ELISA, enzyme-linked immunosorbent assay; MAT, microscopic agglutination test; PCR, polymerase chain reaction.

## EPIDEMIOLOGY

Animals that acquire infection may not develop discernible disease, but become long-term carriers – so-called *maintenance hosts*. Many rodents fall into this category. For example, rats acquiring inapparent infection with pathogenic strains may carry the bacteria in the convoluted tubules of the kidney (possibly life-long), resulting in chronic excretion of viable leptospires in their urine. Similarly, cattle may become a maintenance host for serovar Hardjo, dogs for serovar Canicola, and pigs for serovar Pomona or Bratislava. The reasons for this tolerance are unclear, as infection with other serovars may cause illness of varying severity followed by the transient shedding of the leptospires in the urine for only a few weeks. Moreover, an animal may become a long-term maintenance host for one serovar and yet develop disease and transient carriage after infection with another.

Changes in industrial, agricultural and social practices may result in the rapid change of both the density and type of animal populations in an area, with subsequent change in the predominant serovars of *Leptospira* causing disease in people and animals.

Viable leptospires are present in the semen of infected animals; in rodents a significant increase in the carriage of leptospires is seen once sexual maturity has been reached. Spread across the placenta occurs in several animal species, leading to infection and possibly death of the fetus.

Outside the animal host, leptospiral survival is favoured by warm, moist conditions at neutral or slightly alkaline pH. This no doubt contributes to the seasonal pattern of human infections, which peak in the summer months in both hemispheres. Even small reductions below pH 7.0 markedly reduce the survival of leptospires. The anaerobic conditions and low pH of raw sewage explains their short survival time compared with that in aerated sewage. Salt water is also relatively toxic to leptospires. They do not survive well in undiluted cow's milk and therefore drinking unpasteurized milk poses minimal risk. However, they will survive in water at pH 7.0 or in damp soil for up to 1 month. If the soil is saturated with urine they may survive for up to 6 months, indicating the potential for long-term exposure to an infection risk even if the reservoir host has been removed for some time.

Leptospirosis in man is an emerging disease with more 500 000 severe cases occurring annually; case fatality rates exceed 10%. The disease is expected to become more important due to predicted global climate changes and rapid urbanization in developing countries where slum settlements have produced the conditions for epidemic rat-borne transmission of the disease.

Exposure to virulent leptospires may be direct, through contact with the urine or tissues of infected animals. Direct exposure is generally associated with particular occupations that bring human beings into contact with animals (e.g. butchers, veterinary surgeons, animal breeders, hunters or pet owners). Indirect exposure, through contact with freshwater or humid environment contaminated with the urine of an infected animal, is more common. Such indirect exposure is associated with particular occupations (e.g. sewer workers, rice-field workers) or situations (e.g. triathlon participants, military manoeuvres). In slum communities in developing countries, indirect exposure from rats is thought to be the main source of infection.

Infections related to exposure to surface waters have shown a significant rise in industrialized countries. The increase is almost certainly due to the greater recreational use of surface waters for activities such as canoeing, rafting, fishing, and the use of rivers for the swimming section of triathlon competitions. There has also been an increase in cases of leptospirosis acquired abroad, particularly among travellers on adventure holidays with water contact. In England and Wales between 1990 and 2004, leptospirosis was acquired by 111 travellers, 60 of whom had been to South-East Asia, compared with 194 indigenous cases.

Morbidity and mortality from leptospirosis have declined markedly because of improved hygiene levels in industrialized countries. In countries with limited facilities for medical care death may occur in 25% or more cases.

## CONTROL

With more than 200 known pathogenic serovars, each able to infect a wide range of animals that may become long-term carriers capable of infecting others, together with the organisms' ability to survive for long periods in the environment, the complete prevention or eradication of leptospirosis is impossible.

Mass immunization of domestic livestock will prevent clinical disease in the animals and reduce the risk of human acquisition of infection.

To be fully effective, a vaccine should not only protect against disease in the animal but also prevent the establishment of the carrier state and the shedding of viable leptospires in the urine. It is also important that the vaccine contains antigens representing circulating serovars, as protection will be optimal only against the vaccine components. Current vaccines protect for only 1–2 years and the economics of farming may influence a farmer's decision as to whether or not to immunize cattle. Cuba and China have used vaccines for mass prevention campaigns in human populations and France has used a human vaccine containing only serovar Icterohaemorrhagiae since 1981.

Awareness of leptospirosis through the education of doctors, employers and the general public has helped to develop safer practices or procedures in the workplace and during recreational pursuits. This awareness should include consideration of leptospirosis in the differential diagnosis of fever in the returning

tourist. Measures to reduce rodent populations in the vicinity of human activity, such as removing rubbish, especially waste food, and prevention of the access of rats into buildings is most important. Simple measures to reduce the risks of acquiring infection also include covering cuts and abrasions with waterproof plasters and wearing protective footwear before exposure to surface waters.

In parts of the world where the prevalence of human infection in certain groups is high, selective human immunization schemes may be of benefit if a suitable vaccine is available. Antimicrobial prophylaxis with doxycycline may be of value in high-risk exposure situations in which prompt medical help is unavailable.

## RECOMMENDED READING

Faine S, Adler B, Bolin C, Perolat P: *Leptospira and Leptospirosis*, ed 2, Melbourne, 1999, MediSci.

Kmety E, Dikken H: *Classification of the Species* Leptospira interrogans *and History of its Serovars*, Groningen, 1993, University Press.

Ko AI, Goarant C, Picardeau M: Leptospira: the dawn of the molecular genetics era for an emerging zoonotic pathogen, *Nature Reviews Microbiology* 7: 736–747, 2009.

Levett PN: Leptospirosis, *Clinical Microbiology Reviews* 14:296–326, 2001.

### Websites

eMedicine: Leptospirosis in humans. http://www.emedicine.medscape.com/article/220563-overview

Centers for Disease Control and Prevention. Leptospirosis. http://www.cdc.gov/ncidod/dbmd/diseaseinfo/leptospirosis_g.htm

International Leptospirosis Society (ILS): http://www.med.monash.edu.au/microbiology/staff/adler/ils.html

# 39 Chlamydia

## Genital and ocular infections; infertility; atypical pneumonia

*D. Mabey and R. W. Peeling*

### KEY POINTS

- Chlamydiae are obligate intracellular bacterial pathogens with a unique growth cycle.
- *C. trachomatis* is the most common bacterial sexually transmitted infection, and the leading infectious cause of blindness.
- *C. pneumoniae* is an important cause of community acquired pneumonia.
- Chlamydial infections are frequently asymptomatic.
- Serious sequelae of chlamydial infection (blindness, pelvic inflammatory disease, infertility) are caused by immune response-driven scarring and fibrosis.
- Diagnosis requires laboratory tests, preferably nucleic acid amplification tests.
- Treatment is with doxycycline, erythromycin or azithromycin.
- It is important to treat sexual partners of patients with chlamydial genital tract infection.
- Prevention depends on interrupting the transmission chain: there are no effective vaccines.

Chlamydiae are obligate intracellular bacterial pathogens of eukaryotic cells with a characteristic dimorphic growth cycle quite distinct from that of other bacteria, involving alternation between a metabolically inert, infectious, spore-like elementary body, which can survive in the extracellular environment, and a metabolically active, replicating reticulate body, which cannot. They are widely distributed in nature and are responsible for a variety of human infections affecting the eye, and the genitourinary and respiratory tracts.

*Chlamydiae* were first described in 1907 by Halberstaedter and von Prowazek, who observed cytoplasmic inclusions in conjunctival scrapings taken from children with trachoma and from monkeys inoculated with ocular material from these children. They named them *Chlamydozoa*, from the Greek words χλαμυς (cloak) and ζοον (animal), because of the way in which the inclusions were draped around the nucleus. Similar inclusions were soon observed in conjunctival scrapings taken from neonates with conjunctivitis, and from the cervix of their mothers. Most human infections are caused by *Chlamydia trachomatis*, which was first grown, in mouse brain and subsequently in eggs, from a patient with lymphogranuloma venereum (LGV) in the 1930s. The more fastidious trachoma biovar was not isolated until 1957. It was first grown in tissue culture in 1965, making it possible for the first time to study the epidemiology and clinical features of *C. trachomatis* infection on a large scale.

## DESCRIPTION

### Classification

The *Chlamydia* genus (order Chlamydiales; family Chlamydiaceae) comprises nine species of which two are primarily human pathogens: *C. trachomatis*, causing ocular and genital infections; and *C. pneumoniae*, causing mainly respiratory disease. The other species infect animals: *C. psittaci* (chiefly birds); *C. abortus* (sheep); *C. felis* (cats); *C. pecorum* (cattle); *C. suis* (pigs); *C. muridarum* (mice) and *C. caviae* (guinea pigs). *C. psittaci, C. abortus* and *C. felis* are occasionally transmitted to man. A taxonomic reclassification, based on ribosomal DNA sequence data, assigned *C. pneumoniae, C. psittaci* and *C. abortus* to a new genus, *Chlamydophila*. However, this new taxonomy has not been universally accepted and is not used here.

The species *C. trachomatis* contains two biovars: the more invasive LGV biovar (serovars L1–L3) replicates in macrophages, invades lymph nodes and causes a systemic infection; the more common trachoma biovar is largely confined to squamo-columnar epithelial cells of the eye (serovars A–C) and genital tract (serovars D–K) (Table 39.1). Serovars are defined by the presence of specific epitopes on the major outer membrane protein. Serovars A–C differ

**Table 39.1**  Human infections caused by chlamydiae

| Site of infection | Disease | Sequelae | Organism (serovars) |
|---|---|---|---|
| Eye | Trachoma | Conjunctival scarring, trichiasis, blindness | *C. trachomatis* (A, B, Ba, C) |
| | Inclusion conjunctivitis | | *C. trachomatis* (D–K) |
| | Ophthalmia neonatorum | | *C. trachomatis* (D–K) |
| Genital tract | | | |
| Male | Non-specific urethritis, proctitis, epididymitis | ? Urethral stricture | *C. trachomatis* (D–K) |
| Female | Cervicitis, urethritis, endometritis, salpingitis, PID, perihepatitis | Tubal infertility, ectopic pregnancy | *C. trachomatis* (D–K) |
| | Abortion, premature birth | | *C. trachomatis* (D–K) |
| Male and female | Lymphogranuloma venereum | Scarring, lymphoedema, rectal stricture | *C. trachomatis* (L1–L3) |
| Respiratory tract | Neonatal pneumonia | | *C. trachomatis* (D–K) |
| | Pharyngitis, bronchitis, pneumonia | | *C. pneumoniae* |
| | Psittacosis, ornithosis | | *C. psittaci* |

PID, pelvic inflammatory disease.

from serovars D–K in that they are unable to synthesize tryptophan, owing to disruption of the *trpA* gene.

Chlamydiae have one of the smallest bacterial genomes, containing around 1 million base pairs. Virtually all strains of *C. trachomatis* also contain a 4.4-MDa plasmid of unknown function. Genomes of several *C. trachomatis* serovars have been sequenced, and show a high level of conservation of gene order and content (>99%). A high degree of genetic conservation is also seen across *Chlamydia* species, with *C. trachomatis* and *C. muridarum,* for example, being >95% identical. The fact that chlamydiae replicate within an intracellular vacuole probably explains the high degree of conservation, since it does not allow them to exchange genetic material with other bacteria.

## Biology

Chlamydiae probably evolved from host-independent, Gram-negative ancestors. They are 'energy parasites' relying on the host cell for synthesis of ATP. The chlamydial envelope possesses bacteria-like inner and outer membranes. The infectious elementary body is electron dense, DNA rich and approximately 300 nm in diameter. The cell wall does not contain peptidoglycan, and its rigidity is maintained by extensive disulphide linking of the major outer membrane protein, which makes up some 60% of the outer membrane. The elementary body binds to the host cell and enters by 'parasite-specified' endocytosis. Fusion of the chlamydia-containing endocytic vesicle with lysosomes is inhibited and the elementary body begins its unique developmental cycle within the eukaryotic cell.

The major outer membrane protein is reduced to a monomeric form and acts as a porin, allowing nutrients to enter the organism from the host cell. After about 8 h the elementary body differentiates into the larger (800–1000 nm), non-infectious, metabolically active *reticulate body*, which divides by binary fission. By 20 h post-infection, a proportion of reticulate bodies has begun to reorganize into a new generation of elementary bodies (Fig. 39.1). These reach maturity up to 30 h after entry into the cell and rapidly accumulate within the endocytic vacuole, which may contain more than 1000 organisms. They are released by lysis of the host cell 30–48 h after the start of the cycle.

## PATHOGENESIS

After an incubation period of 5–10 days, *C. trachomatis* elicits an acute inflammatory response with a purulent exudate. A period of chronic inflammation ensues, with the development of sub-epithelial follicles, and this leads eventually, in some cases, to fibrosis and scarring. This scarring process is responsible for much of the morbidity associated with *C. trachomatis*, in both the genital tract and the eye. It is particularly likely to be seen after repeated infections.

Study of virulence determinants of *C. trachomatis* is difficult, since it has not so far proved possible to manipulate chlamydiae genetically. However, the availability of the complete genome of several *C. trachomatis* strains has provided some insights. The serovar D genome contains genes homologous with those coding for virulence factors in other bacteria, including a cytotoxin gene, and genes encoding a type

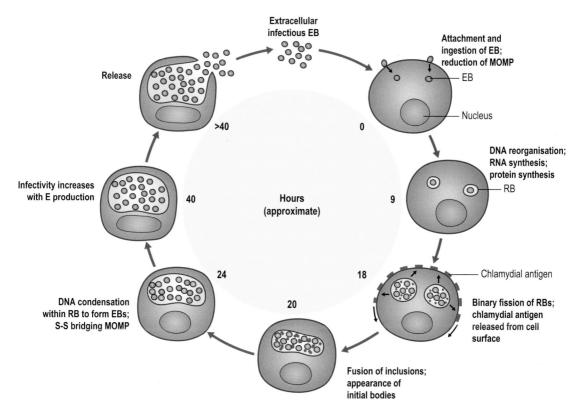

**Fig. 39.1** The growth cycle of chlamydiae. EB, elementary body; MOMP, major outer membrane protein; RB, reticulate body.

III secretion pathway (see p. 17). A conserved chlamydial protease, proteasome-like activity factor, is secreted into the host cell cytoplasm, where it interferes with the assembly and surface expression of HLA (human leucocyte antigen) molecules and inhibits apoptosis. In a non-human primate model genetic variations in six C. trachomatis genes that appear to be associated with increased virulence have been identified.

The epidemiology of C. trachomatis infection suggests that a degree of protective immunity follows natural infection. The prevalence and bacterial load of ocular infection is lower in adults than in children in trachoma endemic communities, and the duration of infection is shorter. Similarly, genital C. trachomatis infection is most prevalent in the youngest sexually active age groups, and the chlamydial isolation rate for men with non-gonococcal urethritis is lower in those who have had previous episodes. Killed whole organism vaccines provide some degree of protection against ocular C. trachomatis infection in man and non-human primates. Serovar-specific monoclonal antibodies to the major outer membrane protein neutralize C. trachomatis in vitro, but there are few data to suggest that either IgG or IgA antibody is protective. The intracellular development of C. trachomatis is inhibited by interferon-γ, and evidence from animal models and studies of human ocular infection suggest that cell-mediated immune responses, mediated by CD4+ lymphocytes are important for the clearance of infection.

Vaccine studies in primates suggest that vaccination could provoke more severe disease on subsequent challenge, implying that much of the damage caused by C. trachomatis infection may be immunopathological in origin. This would be in keeping with the histopathology of C. trachomatis infection, in which the lymphoid follicle is the hallmark. Follicles contain typical germinal centres, consisting predominantly of B lymphocytes, with T cells, mostly CD8+, in the parafollicular region. The inflammatory infiltrate between follicles comprises plasma cells, dendritic cells, macrophages, and polymorphonuclear leucocytes, with T and B lymphocytes. Fibrosis is seen at a late stage, typically in trachoma and pelvic inflammatory disease. T lymphocytes are also present and outnumber B cells and macrophages.

A chlamydial heat-shock protein (hsp 60), homologous with the GroEL protein of *Escherichia coli*, elicits antibody responses that are associated with the damaging sequelae of *C. trachomatis* infections in both the eye and genital tract. In-vitro interferon-γ interferes with the chlamydial development cycle, leading to persistent infection with continuing release of hsp 60. It is not known whether the immune response to hsp 60 is itself the cause of immunopathological damage, or merely a marker of more severe or prolonged infection. Studies of gene expression at the site of ocular infection have shown the importance of innate immune pathways and NK (natural killer) cell activation, and suggest that matrix metalloproteinases 7 and 9 play an important role in the scarring process. Polymorphisms in immune response genes encoding tumour necrosis factor-α, interferon-γ and interleukin-10 are associated with the development of severe scarring following ocular *C. trachomatis* infection.

## CLINICAL FEATURES

### Chlamydia trachomatis

### Genital infection

The clinical manifestations of genital *C. trachomatis* infection are similar to those of gonorrhoea, but are usually less severe, as *C. trachomatis* infection elicits a less intense acute inflammatory response than *Neisseria gonorrhoeae*. Many chlamydial infections are asymptomatic. Long term sequelae such as infertility and ectopic pregnancy are generally caused by fibrosis and scarring of the fallopian tubes following prolonged or repeated infections, and may develop even in those with few or no symptoms.

*Infection in men.* *C. trachomatis* is detectable in the urethra of up to 50% of men with symptomatic non-gonococcal urethritis. The incubation period is 7–21 days, compared to 2–5 days for gonorrhoea. Patients present with a history of dysuria, usually accompanied by a mild to moderate mucopurulent urethral discharge. *C. trachomatis* is responsible for a proportion of cases of chronic (persistent or recurrent) non-gonococcal urethritis. Since mixed infections are common, treatment of gonococcal urethritis with an antibiotic ineffective against *C. trachomatis* may result in post-gonococcal urethritis.

*C. trachomatis* is responsible for up to 70% of cases of acute epididymitis in young men (35 years of age or less) in developed countries. Patients present with unilateral scrotal pain, swelling and tenderness, often accompanied by fever. Most give a history of current or recent urethral discharge. In older patients, epididymitis and epididymo-orchitis tend to be caused by urinary-tract pathogens. There is no good evidence that chlamydial infection leads to male infertility or to acute or chronic prostatitis.

Both LGV and non-LGV strains of *C. trachomatis* can cause proctitis in those who practise receptive anal intercourse. Non-LGV strains cause a milder disease, which may be asymptomatic or give rise to rectal pain, bleeding and muco-purulent anal discharge.

*Infection in women.* *C. trachomatis* typically infects the columnar epithelial cells of the endocervix. It does not affect the squamous epithelium of the vagina. Infection is associated with a mucopurulent discharge from the cervix visible on speculum examination, and with hypertrophic cervical ectopy that tends to bleed on contact. Most infected women have no symptoms. The prevalence of cervical infection is no higher among women who complain of vaginal discharge than among those who do not, suggesting that it is not a cause of symptomatic vaginal discharge.

*C. trachomatis* has been implicated as a cause of the urethral syndrome, characterized by dysuria, frequency and sterile pyuria. Clinical signs of urethritis, such as urethral discharge or meatal redness, are not usually found.

Infection may spread from the endocervix to the endometrium and fallopian tubes, causing *pelvic inflammatory disease*. This is more likely to occur after trauma to the cervix due, for example, to termination of pregnancy, insertion of an intra-uterine contraceptive device, or delivery. Histologic evidence of endometritis can be found in up to 50% of women with mucopurulent cervicitis due to *C. trachomatis,* and is more common in those with a history of abnormal vaginal bleeding. Classic signs of pelvic inflammatory disease may be present (fever, lower abdominal pain and tenderness, and cervical motion tenderness), but chlamydial pelvic inflammatory disease may be subclinical. Spread to the peritoneum may result in perihepatitis (the *Curtis–Fitz-Hugh syndrome*), which may be confused with acute cholecystitis in young women. *C. trachomatis* infection has also been associated with post-partum endometritis.

*C. trachomatis* is the major cause of pelvic inflammatory disease in developed countries. Infertility may be the first indication of asymptomatic tubal disease. It occurs in about 10% of women following a single upper genital tract infection and in up to 50% after two or three episodes. Infertility may result from endometritis, from blocked or damaged fallopian tubes, or from abnormalities of ovum transportation caused by damage to the ciliated epithelial surface. Other consequences of salpingitis are chronic pelvic pain and ectopic pregnancy. Following chlamydial pelvic inflammatory disease, the risk of ectopic pregnancy increases 7–10-fold.

Some studies have shown *C. trachomatis* infection to be associated with low birth weight and pre-term delivery, but others have failed to confirm this. In general, infection was diagnosed and treated at a later stage of gestation in those studies which found a correlation between infection and adverse birth outcome than in those that did not.

Infection has been weakly associated with bartholinitis and should be considered in the absence of other known pathogens. A significant association between cervical chlamydial infection and cervical squamous cell carcinoma, but not adenocarcinoma, has been established, and it has been suggested that chlamydial infection may enhance the effect of oncogenic papillomaviruses.

### Adult paratrachoma (inclusion conjunctivitis) and otitis media

Adult chlamydial ophthalmia commonly results from the accidental transfer of infected genital discharge to the eye. It usually presents as a unilateral follicular conjunctivitis, acute or subacute in onset. The features are swollen lids, mucopurulent discharge, papillary hyperplasia and later, follicular hypertrophy, and occasionally punctate keratitis. About one-third of patients have otitis media, and complain of blocked ears and hearing loss. The disease is generally benign and self-limiting. Patients and their sexual contacts should be investigated for genital chlamydial infection and managed appropriately.

### Reactive arthritis

Arthritis occurring with or soon after non-gonococcal urethritis is termed '*sexually acquired reactive arthritis*'. Conjunctivitis and other features characteristic of Reiter's syndrome are seen in about one-third of patients. *C. trachomatis* has also been associated with 'seronegative' arthritis in women. Viable chlamydiae have not been detected in the joints of patients with this condition, which is probably the result of immunopathology. Despite this, early tetracycline therapy has been advocated by some investigators.

### Neonatal infections

Conjunctivitis appears in 20–50% of infants exposed to *C. trachomatis* infecting the cervix at birth. A mucopurulent discharge and occasionally pseudomembrane formation occur 1–3 weeks later. It usually resolves without visual impairment.

About half of the infants who have conjunctivitis also develop pneumonia, although a history of recent conjunctivitis and bulging eardrums are found in only half of the cases. Chlamydial pneumonia usually begins between the fourth and eleventh week of life, preceded by upper respiratory symptoms. There is tachypnoea, a prominent, staccato cough but usually no fever, and the illness is protracted. Radiographs show hyperinflation of the lungs with bilateral diffuse, symmetrical, interstitial infiltration and scattered areas of atelectasis. Children infected during infancy are at increased risk of obstructive lung disease and asthma.

### Lymphogranuloma venereum

The clinical course of LGV can be divided into three stages. The primary stage at the site of inoculation; the secondary stage in the regional lymph nodes, and/or the anorectum; and the tertiary stage of late sequelae affecting the genitalia and/or rectum.

***Primary stage.*** After an incubation period of 3–30 days, a small, painless papule, which may ulcerate, occurs at the site of inoculation. The primary lesion is self-limiting and may pass unnoticed by the patient. Among patients with LGV presenting with buboes in Thailand, more than half had not been aware of an ulcer.

***Secondary stage.*** This occurs some weeks after the primary lesion. It may involve the inguinal lymph nodes, or the anus and rectum. The inguinal form is more common in men than women, since the lymphatic drainage of the upper vagina and cervix is to the retro-peritoneal rather than the inguinal lymph nodes. LGV proctitis occurs in those who practise receptive anal intercourse, probably due to direct inoculation.

The cardinal feature of the inguinal form of LGV is painful, usually unilateral, inguinal and/or femoral lymphadenopathy (bubo). Enlarged lymph nodes are usually firm and often accompanied by fever, chills, arthralgia and headache. Biopsy reveals small discrete areas of necrosis surrounded by proliferating epithelioid and endothelial cells, which may enlarge to form stellate abscesses that may coalesce and break down to form discharging sinuses. In women, signs include a hypertrophic suppurative cervicitis, backache and adnexal tenderness.

Clinical features of anorectal disease include a purulent anal discharge, pain and bleeding due to an acute haemorrhagic proctitis or proctocolitis, often with fever, chills and weight loss. Proctoscopy reveals a granular or ulcerative proctitis. Computed tomography or magnetic resonance imaging scans may show pronounced thickening of the rectal wall, with enlargement of iliac lymph nodes. Enlarged inguinal nodes may also be palpable.

Cervical adenopathy due to LGV has been reported after oral sex. A follicular conjunctivitis has also been described following direct inoculation of the eye, which may be accompanied by pre-auricular lymphadenopathy. Other rare manifestations of the secondary stage include acute meningoencephalitis, synovitis and cardiac involvement.

*Tertiary stage.* This appears after a latent period of several years, but is rare. Chronic untreated LGV leads to fibrosis, which may cause lymphatic obstruction and elephantiasis of the genitalia in either sex, or rectal strictures and fistulae. Rarely, it can give rise to the syndrome of esthiomene (Greek: 'eating away') with widespread destruction of the external genitalia.

## Trachoma

The clinical signs of trachoma are best seen in the conjunctival surface of the everted upper eyelid. Active or inflammatory trachoma, which is usually seen in children in endemic communities, is a follicular keratoconjunctivitis. Subjects in whom five or more follicles of >0.5 mm diameter are seen in the central subtarsal conjunctiva are defined by the World Health organization (WHO) as having *follicular trachoma*. In some cases the inflammation is severe enough to obscure the conjunctival blood vessels. If more than half the blood vessels are obscured, this is defined as intense inflammatory trachoma. Blood vessels may be seen growing into the cornea, usually at its superior margin; this is known as *pannus*. *C. trachomatis* can be detected in a proportion of cases of follicular trachoma, but not in all cases, since the follicles can persist for weeks or months after the infection has resolved. Repeated episodes of inflammatory trachoma lead eventually to conjunctival scarring. As the scars contract they cause the lid margin to turn inwards (*entropion*), and the lashes to abrade the cornea (*trichiasis*). This causes extreme discomfort, damages the cornea, and leads eventually to blindness due to corneal opacity.

## C. pneumoniae

*C. pneumoniae* causes pneumonia, pharyngitis, bronchitis, otitis and sinusitis with an incubation period of about 21 days. It may be a significant cause of acute exacerbations of asthma, and is one of the most common causes of community-acquired pneumonia, but is seldom identified as the causal agent because laboratory tests for its diagnosis are not widely used. It is a chronic, often insidious, respiratory pathogen to which there appears to be little immunity. Seroepidemiological studies indicate that some 60–80% of people worldwide become infected with *C. pneumoniae* during their life.

## C. psittaci

*C. psittaci* is an important cause of infections in a wide range of birds and is shed in nasal secretions and droppings. Nasal secretions contaminate the feathers, where they dry and produce a highly infectious dust in which the organism can survive for months. This may give rise to severe pneumonia in man, called *ornithosis* or *psittacosis* depending on the bird species from which the infection was derived. The agricultural economy is also affected, as large outbreaks of ornithosis have been reported in turkeys, geese and ducks. There are import controls in many countries to restrict the movement of birds, which are rendered more infectious by travel-induced stress.

The incubation period is about 10 days, and the illness ranges from an 'influenza-like' syndrome, with general malaise, fever, anorexia, rigors, sore throat, headache and photophobia, to a severe illness with delirium and pneumonia. The illness may resemble bronchopneumonia, but the bronchioles are involved as a secondary event and sputum is scanty. The organism disseminates through the body, and there may be meningoencephalitis, arthritis, pericarditis or myocarditis, or a predominantly typhoidal state with enlarged liver and spleen. Endocarditis has been described.

## LABORATORY DIAGNOSIS

The laboratory diagnosis of chlamydial infection depends on detection of the organisms or their antigens or nucleic acid and, to a much lesser extent, on serology (Table 39.2). In urogenital infection the highest bacterial load of *C. trachomatis* is found in the endocervix in women and in the urethra in men. An endocervical swab is therefore needed for the diagnosis of infection by culture or antigen detection assay. However, the greater sensitivity of nucleic acid amplification tests for *C. trachomatis* means that self-administered vaginal swabs and 'first-catch' urine specimens give equivalent results to endocervical swabs when using these assays. Samples to be tested can be transported to the laboratory at room temperature, making home-based screening for *C. trachomatis* possible.

## Culture

Centrifugation of specimens onto cycloheximide-treated McCoy or HeLa cell monolayers, followed

**Table 39.2** Advantages and disadvantages of diagnostic tests for *C. trachomatis*

| Factor considered | Culture | Direct fluorescent antibody | Enzyme immunoassay | Nucleic acid amplification |
|---|---|---|---|---|
| Sensitivity | <70% | 70–100% | <50–70% | Up to 100% |
| Specificity | 100% | Up to 98% (reader dependent) | 95–98% | Up to 99% |
| Appropriate specimens | Cervical/urethral/ocular swabs | Cervical/urethral/ocular swabs | Cervical/urethral/ ocular swabs | Cervical/urethral/ocular swabs, urine (men), vaginal swabs |
| Speed/temperature for transport of specimen | Rapid or at low temperature | Room temperature | Room temperature if specimen in buffer | Room temperature if <48 h, 4°C if >48 h |
| Storage requirements | 4°C if overnight, −70°C or liquid nitrogen if long term | 4°C if short term | 4°C if 3–5 days, freezing if longer | 4°C if not processed in 7 days; −70°C if long term |
| Evaluation of adequacy of specimen | Not possible | Host cells seen under microscope | Not possible | Determine whether host DNA present |
| Special equipment or procedure | Centrifuge, biological safety cabinet, $CO_2$ incubator, microscope | Fluorescence microscope | ELISA reader | Dedicated equipment for nucleic acid amplification and detection |
| Processing of specimen | Laborious | Simple | Relatively simple, amenable to batching | Requires precautions against false positive results due to laboratory contamination |
| Reading of test | Subjective and moderately tedious | Subjective and tedious | Objective and simple | Objective and simple |
| Time to result | 48–72 h | 30 min | 3 h | 2–4 h |
| Cost | High | Moderate | Low | Very high |

by incubation and then staining with a fluorescent monoclonal antibody or with a vital dye, to detect inclusions, has been widely used for the diagnosis of *C. trachomatis* infection. One blind passage may increase sensitivity. However, cell-culture techniques are no more than 70% sensitive compared to nucleic acid amplification tests and are slow and labour intensive. Because culture is essentially 100% specific, it still has a role in medico-legal cases. *C. pneumoniae* is even more difficult to grow than C. *trachomatis*. *C. psittaci* is a hazard group 3 pathogen and few laboratories attempt to grow it.

## Direct immunofluorescence

Microscopic detection of elementary bodies with species-specific fluorescent monoclonal antibodies is rapid and, for *C. trachomatis* oculogenital infections, highly sensitive and specific in the hands of skilled observers. However, the test is laborious and interpretation is subjective. It is best used in settings where few specimens are tested, or for confirming positive results obtained with other tests.

## Nucleic acid amplification tests

By enabling amplification of a nucleic acid sequence specific to the chlamydial species, the polymerase chain reaction assay, the strand displacement assay and the transcription mediated amplification technique have overcome problems of poor sensitivity.

Commercial assays for *C. trachomatis* based on each of these three amplification methods are available and widely used. The first two assays amplify nucleotide sequences of the cryptic plasmid, which is present in multiple copies in each chlamydial elementary body. However, a rare variant of *C. trachomatis* has been described which lacks the plasmid, giving rise to false negative results with these assays. The transcription mediated amplification reaction is directed against rRNA, which is also present in multiple copies. These sensitive assays have replaced culture as the 'gold standard' for the diagnosis of *C. trachomatis* infection. Nucleic acid amplification tests for *C. pneumoniae* and *C. psittaci* are not commercially available.

## Enzyme immunoassays

Enzyme immunoassays that detect chlamydial antigens, usually the genus specific lipopolysaccharide, have largely been replaced by the more sensitive nucleic acid amplification test.

## Point of care tests

Over 20 rapid strip tests based on the immunochromatographic detection of chlamydial lipopolysaccharide are commercially available. They can give a result within 15–20 min of sample collection, but most lack sensitivity compared to nucleic acid amplification methods.

## Serological tests

Serological tests are of no value in uncomplicated genital *C. trachomatis* infection. In pelvic inflammatory disease, in LGV and in the Curtis–Fitz-Hugh syndrome, serology may be useful if a rising titre can be demonstrated. *C. trachomatis* IgM antibody is the 'gold standard' for the diagnosis of chlamydial pneumonia in babies. Pneumonia due to *C. pneumoniae* and *C. psittaci* is usually diagnosed serologically, but depends on the demonstration of IgM antibodies or an IgG titre >512 by microimmunofluorescence, or a rise in antibody titre in a convalescent sample. Immunofluorescence and enzyme immuno-assays are commercially available, but have not been rigorously evaluated.

## TREATMENT

Chlamydiae are intracellular and hence insensitive to aminoglycosides and other antibiotics that do not penetrate cells efficiently. Tetracyclines and macrolides are the mainstay of treatment. Treatment is often started before a microbiological diagnosis can be established, so additional broad-spectrum antibiotics are needed to cover gonococcal and, in the case of pelvic inflammatory disease, anaerobic infections. Treatment of sexual partners is essential to prevent reinfection.

Uncomplicated *C. trachomatis* infections are treated with a single dose of azithromycin 1 g, or with doxycycline 100 mg twice daily for 7 days. Chlamydial pelvic inflammatory disease is treated with a 14-day course of doxycycline 100 mg twice daily. Clinically significant resistance to these antibiotics has not been reported. Doxycycline is contra-indicated in pregnancy. Azithromycin 1 g as a single dose, and amoxicillin 500 mg three times daily for 7 days, are safe and effective in pregnant women. Ofloxacin is active against *C. trachomatis* at a dose of 300 mg twice daily for 7 days, but is not widely used. Ophthalmia neonatorum and neonatal pneumonia due to *C. trachomatis* should be treated with erythromycin syrup by mouth, 50 mg/kg daily divided into four doses, for 14 days.

There has been no adequate study comparing antibiotic regimens for LGV, *C. pneumoniae* or *C. psittaci* infection. Recommended treatment for LGV is doxycycline 100 mg twice daily, or erythromycin 500 mg four times daily, for 21 days. Azithromycin has been used successfully in some cases, although a 1 g single dose is unlikely to be sufficient. Large collections of pus should be aspirated, using a lateral approach through normal skin. Macrolides or tetracyclines are recommended for the treatment of infection with *C. pneumoniae* and *C. psittaci*. Prolonged courses may be required in patients with pneumonia.

Ocular infection can be effectively treated with a single oral dose of azithromycin (20 mg/kg, maximum 1 g) but, in trachoma endemic communities, reinfection rapidly occurs and mass treatment of entire communities is therefore recommended.

## EPIDEMIOLOGY

*C. trachomatis* is the most common bacterial sexually transmitted infection, and the most common infectious cause of blindness. Genital infection is common in all sexually active populations, and prevalence is usually highest in the young. In the UK, the number of reported chlamydial infections trebled between 1996 and 2005. Similar increases were seen in other Western countries over this period, including Sweden and Canada, despite active screening programmes. It is not clear to what extent this is due to an increased incidence, or to an increase in the number of people tested with the sensitive nucleic acid amplification tests that have been widely used since the late 1990s. The overall incidence of reported chlamydial infection in the UK in 2005 was 223 per 100000 total population, with the highest rate (1300 per 100000) in women aged 16–19. The WHO has estimated that, in 2005, there were 101 million new cases of genital chlamydial infection.

LGV is rare in industrialized countries, but is endemic in parts of Africa, Asia, South America and the Caribbean. Its epidemiology is poorly defined, because LGV is often indistinguishable clinically from chancroid and other causes of genital ulceration with bubo formation, and it has been difficult to obtain laboratory confirmation. Among patients presenting with buboes to a sexually transmitted disease clinic in Bangkok 10% were found to have LGV, and an epidemic of LGV has been reported among crack cocaine users in the Bahamas. In 2003, an outbreak of LGV proctitis due to the L2 serovar was reported among homosexual men in the Netherlands, and since then over one thousand cases have been reported in homosexual men in Europe and North America; most affected men were HIV-positive.

Trachoma, caused by *C. trachomatis* transmitted from eye to eye, disappeared from Europe and North America in the 20th century as living standards improved, but remains endemic in poor rural populations in Africa and Asia. WHO estimates that at least 40 million people have trachoma, and that 8 million are blind or visually impaired as a result.

## Molecular epidemiology

Typing isolates of *C. trachomatis* is potentially of great value. It could help to map sexual networks, and to distinguish between treatment failure and reinfection in clinical trials. If associations could be found between particular strains and particular clinical findings, it could help to identify virulence determinants of *C. trachomatis* and increase understanding of the pathogenesis of infection.

The first typing method for *C. trachomatis*, the micro-immunofluoresence test, was based on the ability of monoclonal antibodies to distinguish 13 (later increased to 17) serotypes of *C. trachomatis*. More recently genital and ocular strains of *C. trachomatis* have been genotyped following amplification of the *ompA* gene which encodes the major outer membrane protein, either by sequencing, or by restriction fragment length polymorphism analysis of the amplified product; but *ompA* genotyping is not sufficiently discriminatory to distinguish between persistent infection and reinfection with a common genotype.

A multi-locus sequence typing method, targeting six variable genes identified through genome sequencing projects, has been used to investigate a variant of *C. trachomatis* lacking the plasmid detected by commonly used nucleic acid amplification tests.

## CONTROL AND PREVENTION

Health education and condom promotion, especially for the youngest sexually active age groups, may help to reduce the incidence of genital *C. trachomatis* infection. Syndromic management of symptomatic infections, and partner notification, may also play a role, but since a high proportion of chlamydial infections is asymptomatic in both sexes, these measures are unlikely to be successful on their own. A screening programme for *C. trachomatis* at primary health care level in the USA has been shown to reduce the incidence of upper genital tract infection and its complications in women. Screening programmes have been introduced in some European countries, in which young people presenting to health services for any reason are offered a test for *C. trachomatis*; but the public health impact of such opportunistic screening programmes remains to be demonstrated. Where reinfection rates are high retesting of positive cases 6 months after treatment has been recommended.

No vaccine is presently available. Recent research has focused on the development of a subunit vaccine against *C. trachomatis*, which provides protection without eliciting immunopathology. Purified preparations of major outer membrane protein were protective in murine models, provided the native trimeric structure of the protein was maintained. In non-human primates, a similar preparation of major outer membrane protein reduced peak shedding from the ocular surface, but had no effect on the duration of infection or on ocular disease.

The strategy for trachoma control recommended by WHO is based on the acronym SAFE: Surgery for trichiasis; mass treatment with Antibiotics; Facial cleanliness; and Environmental improvement to reduce the transmission of *C. trachomatis* from eye to eye.

RECOMMENDED READING

Brunham RC, Rey-Ladino J: Immunology of chlamydia infection: implications for a *Chlamydia trachomatis* vaccine, *Nature Reviews Immunology* 5:149–161, 2005.
Kuo CC, Jackson LA, Campbell LA, Grayston JT: *Chlamydia pneumoniae* (TWAR), *Clin Microbiol Rev* 8:451–461, 1995.
Low N, Bender N, Nartey L, et al: Effectiveness of chlamydia screening: systematic review, *Int J Epidemiol* 38:435–448, 2009.
Mabey D, Solomon A, Foster A: Trachoma, *Lancet* 362:223–229, 2003.
Stephens RS, Kalman S, Lammel C, et al: Genome sequence of an obligate intracellular pathogen of humans: *Chlamydia trachomatis*, *Science* 282:754–759, 1998.
Van der Bij AK, Spaargaren J, Morré SA, et al: Diagnostic and clinical implications of anorectal lymphogranuloma venereum in men who have sex with men: a retrospective case-control study, *Clinical Infectious Diseases* 42:186–194, 2006.

# 40 Rickettsia, orientia, ehrlichia, anaplasma and coxiella

Typhus; spotted fevers; scrub typhus; ehrlichioses; Q fever

*D. H. Walker and Xue-Jie Yu*

## KEY POINTS

- Rickettsiae are small obligately intracellular bacteria that are associated with insects or ticks during at least part of their transmission cycle.
- *Rickettsia* and *Orientia* cause spotted fevers, typhus fevers and scrub typhus by infecting and damaging endothelial cells, resulting in increased vascular permeability, oedema, adult respiratory distress syndrome, meningoencephalitis and rash.
- *Ehrlichia* and *Anaplasma* reside in persistently infected vertebrate hosts such as deer, dogs or rodents, and are transmitted by feeding ticks.
- *Ehrlichia and Anaplasma* target human monocytes or granulocytes, where they grow to microcolonies in cytoplasmic vacuoles.
- The frequent absence of antibodies to rickettsiae, orientiae and ehrlichiae early in the course of illness hinders laboratory diagnosis, making clinico-epidemiologic suspicion of the diagnosis and empirical treatment, preferably with doxycycline, essential.
- *Coxiella burnetii* thrives in the acidic phagolysosome of macrophages, has a stable extracellular form and infects human beings who inhale aerosols from birth fluids or the placenta of infected animals.

Few diseases have had a greater impact on the course of human history than epidemic typhus. Hans Zinsser's classic book *Rats, Lice and History* provides a graphic account of how *Rickettsia prowazekii*, the aetiological agent of this louse-borne disease, has caused millions of deaths and much human suffering in conditions of famine, poverty and war. Epidemic typhus now occurs mainly in poor populations in developing countries as world conditions have improved, but various other rickettsial diseases are still widely distributed.

The rickettsiae (*Rickettsia* and *Orientia* species) and anaplasmas (*Anaplasma, Ehrlichia* and *Neorickettsia* species) of medical importance are obligately intracellular bacteria mostly transmitted by arthropod vectors. Molecular studies reveal that *Rickettsia* species, *Orientia tsutsugamushi*, *Ehrlichia* species and *Anaplasma* species evolved from a common ancestor.

*Coxiella burnetii*, an intracellular bacterium found in ticks, is more closely related to *Legionella pneumophila*, but is conveniently considered here alongside the rickettsia group.

## RICKETTSIA AND ORIENTIA

## DESCRIPTION

The genera *Rickettsia* and *Orientia* include organisms responsible for numerous diseases in many parts of the world (Table 40.1). The pioneering research of Ricketts and others in the early twentieth century demonstrated the rickettsial aetiology of Rocky Mountain spotted fever and epidemic louse-borne typhus. Several other diseases, including murine typhus and Mediterranean spotted fever, were later shown to be rickettsial infections. Previously unrecognized spotted fevers caused by *R. japonica, R. africae* and *R. honei* were discovered in the 1980s and 1990s in Japan, Africa and Australia, indicating that much remains to be learned about these organisms. Other rickettsiae, poorly understood and presumed to be non-pathogenic, have been isolated, primarily from arthropods, including herbivorous insects.

Rickettsiae are small ($0.3–0.5 \times 0.8–1.0$ μm) Gram-negative bacilli. They reside in the cytosol of host cells (Fig. 40.1). All pathogens are associated with a flea, louse, mite or tick vector. Species pathogenic for man parasitize endothelial cells almost exclusively. Rickettsiae have a small genome (approximately 1

**Table 40.1** Human diseases caused by *Rickettsia* and *Orientia* species

| Species | Disease | Geographical distribution | Mode of transmission | Primary vectors | Main vertebrate hosts |
|---------|---------|--------------------------|---------------------|-----------------|----------------------|
| **Typhus group** | | | | | |
| *R. prowazekii* | Epidemic typhus | Extant foci in Africa, North and South America | Louse faeces | *Pediculus humanus corporis* | Man, flying squirrels |
| *R. typhi* | Murine typhus | Primarily tropics and subtropics | Flea faeces | *Xenopsylla cheopis* and other fleas | Rodents and other small mammals |
| **Spotted fever group** | | | | | |
| *R. akari* | Rickettsialpox | USA, Ukraine, Croatia, Korea, Turkey, Mexico | Bite of mouse mite | *Liponyssoides sanguineus* | House mice; possibly other rodents |
| *R. australis* | Queensland tick typhus | Australia | Bite of tick | *Ixodes holocyclus* | Unknown |
| *R. conorii* | Boutonneuse fever | Europe, Africa, Middle East, India | Bite of tick | *Rhipicephalus sanguineus* | Unknown |
| *R. japonica* | Japanese spotted fever | Japan and north-eastern Asia | Bite of tick | *Dermacentor, Haemaphysalis, Ixodes* spp. | Unknown |
| *R. rickettsii* | Rocky Mountain spotted fever | North and South America | Bite of tick | *Dermacentor* spp., *Rh. sanguineus, Amblyomma cajennense* | Rodents, opossums, dogs and other small mammals |
| *R. africae* | African tick bite fever | Africa and West Indies | Bite of tick | *A. hebraeum, A. variegatum* | Unknown |
| *R. parkeri* | American tick bite fever | North and South America | Bite of tick | *A. maculatum, A. americanum, A. triste* | Unknown |
| *R. sibirica* | North Asian tick typhus | Northern Asia | Bite of tick | *Dermacentor, Haemaphysalis* spp., etc. | Rodents and other small mammals |
| *R. honei* | Flinders Island spotted fever | Australia and South-East Asia | Bite of tick | *Bothriocroton hydrosauri* | Unknown |
| *R. slovaca* | Tick-borne lymphadenopathy | Eurasia | Bite of tick | *Dermacentor marginatum, D. reticularis* | Unknown |
| *R. felis* | Flea-borne spotted fever | Worldwide | Flea; undetermined mechanism | *Ctenocephalides felis* | Opossums |
| **Scrub typhus group** | | | | | |
| *Orientia tsutsugamushi* | Scrub typhus | Asia, Australia, islands of south-west Pacific and Indian oceans | Bite of larval mite | *Leptotrombidium* spp. | Rodents (especially rats) |

Mb) and lack genes encoding many essential enzymes. Thus they depend on the host for nutrition and building blocks, and are yet to be cultivated outside eukaryotic cells. Like the chlamydiae (see Ch. 39), rickettsiae have a typical Gram-negative bacterial cell wall, including a bilayered outer membrane that contains lipopolysaccharide, and are energy parasites that transport adenosine triphosphate (ATP) with a unique translocase.

The genus *Rickettsia* is divided into two antigenically distinct groups based on their lipopolysaccharide: the typhus group and the spotted fever group. The immunodominant rickettsial outer membrane protein A (OmpA) exists only in the spotted fever group rickettsiae. Another major outer membrane protein, OmpB, exists in all *Rickettsia* species. OmpA and OmpB both contain cross-reactive and species-specific epitopes.

The scrub typhus rickettsiae are antigenically distinct and appear to be fundamentally different. They have been classified into a related but distinct genus as *Orientia tsutsugamushi* (see Table 40.1). The cell wall lacks lipopolysaccharide, peptidoglycan and a slime layer, and appears to derive its structural integrity from proteins linked by disulphide bonds. *O. tsutsugamushi* exhibits multiple major antigenic proteins with both strain-specific and cross-reactive epitopes.

**Fig. 40.1** Electron micrograph of a cell infected with *R. rickettsii*, showing the dilatation of the endoplasmic reticulum of host cells that occurs as a result of injury associated with infection by spotted fever group rickettsiae.

**Fig. 40.2** Electron micrograph of a cell infected with *R. prowazekii*. The rickettsiae continue to multiply within the cell until it is completely packed with organisms and bursts. In contrast to cells infected with spotted fever group rickettsiae, the ultrastructural appearance of cells infected with typhus group rickettsiae remains normal until the cell lyses. The region of the cell containing rickettsiae is indicated by the arrowhead.

## PATHOGENESIS

### Invasion and destruction of target cells

Rickettsiae normally enter the body through the bite or faeces of an infected arthropod vector. They are disseminated through the bloodstream, attach to endothelial cells by OmpA, OmpB and other autotransporter surface proteins, enter endothelial cells by induced phagocytosis, escape from the phagosome, multiply intracellularly and eventually destroy their host cells. Cell culture studies suggest that spotted fever and typhus group rickettsiae destroy the host cell by different mechanisms. After infection with *R. prowazekii* or *R. typhi*, the rickettsiae continue to multiply until the cell is packed with organisms (Fig. 40.2) and then bursts, possibly as a result of membranolytic activity; before lysis, host cells appear ultrastructurally normal.

Spotted fever group rickettsiae seldom accumulate in large numbers and do not burst the host cells, but stimulate polymerization of F-actin tails which propel them through the cytoplasm and into filopodia, from which they escape the cell or spread into an adjacent cell (Fig. 40.3). Two proteins, RickA and Sca2, act as critical regulators of actin-based movement in spotted fever group, but not in typhus rickettsiae. Infected cells exhibit signs of membrane damage associated with an influx of water, which is sequestered within cisternae of dilated rough endoplasmic reticulum (see Fig. 40.1). Rickettsiae damage host cell membranes at least in part by stimulating production of free oxygen radicals by endothelial cells.

**Fig. 40.3** Electron micrograph of *R. conorii* escaping from a host cell. Note the location of the rickettsiae within host cell filopodia.

Scrub typhus rickettsiae also escape from the phagosome, reside free in the cytosol, and are released from host cells soon after infecting them, but little is known about the mechanism(s) by which these organisms damage cells.

### Pathological lesions

All members of the genera *Rickettsia* and *Orientia* cause widespread microvascular injury leading to the destruction and dysfunction of infected endothelial cells. The pathological manifestations result more from direct rickettsial injury than from immuno-pathological mechanisms mediated via cytokines and cytotoxic T lymphocytes, inflammation, intra-vascular coagulation or endotoxin. Interference with normal circulation and increased vascular per-meability following damage of blood vessels can cause life-threatening encephalitis and non-cardiogenic pulmonary oedema.

## CLINICAL ASPECTS OF RICKETTSIAL DISEASES

### Epidemic typhus

Headache and fever develop 6–15 days after infection with *R. prowazekii*. A macular rash, often noted 4–7 days after the patient becomes ill, first appears on the trunk and axillary folds and then spreads to the extremities. In mild cases the rash may begin to fade after 1–2 days, but in more severe cases it may last much longer and become haemorrhagic. Severe cases may also develop pronounced hypotension and renal dysfunction. The mental state of the patient may progress from dullness to stupor and even coma. Although the prognosis is grave for comatose patients, prompt appropriate treatment may be life-saving.

Individuals who survive a primary infection of louse-borne typhus may develop a relatively milder reactivation of latent infection many years later. This is referred to as recrudescent typhus or *Brill–Zinsser disease*. Such individuals are nevertheless immune to a second louse-borne infection.

### Flea-borne fevers

Patients infected with *R. typhi* develop symptoms similar to those of epidemic typhus. Fatal cases are uncommon but occasionally occur, particularly in the elderly. Although murine typhus is much milder than epidemic typhus, it is still severe enough to require several months of convalescence. *R. felis* is maintained transovarially in cat fleas and causes a similar illness.

### Tick-borne spotted fever

There are many clinical similarities among the tick-borne rickettsioses of the spotted fever group. The most severe is Rocky Mountain spotted fever, for which the average annual case-fatality rate for 1981–1998 was 3.3%. Risk factors for fatal infection include older age, glucose-6-phosphate dehydrogenase defi-ciency and delayed tetracycline treatment.

Patients become ill within 2 weeks of infection. Early symptoms include fever, severe headache and myalgia, often accompanied by anorexia, vomiting, abdominal pain, diarrhoea, photophobia and cough. An eschar ('*tache noire*') frequently occurs at the site of the tick bite in all spotted fever group infections except Rocky Mountain spotted fever. A maculopapular rash usually develops within 3–5 days. The rash of spotted fever usually develops first on the extremi-ties rather than on the trunk. Absence of a rash does not exclude rickettsial infection, because a dispropor-tionate number of fatal cases of Rocky Mountain spotted fever are of the 'spotless' variety. Spotted fever group rickettsiae are found within the endothe-lial cells and less often macrophages of vertebrate hosts, but *R. rickettsii* can also invade vascular smooth muscle.

Vascular damage in severe cases may result in haemorrhagic rash, hypovolaemia, hypotensive shock, non-cardiogenic pulmonary oedema and impairment of central nervous system function. A ful-minant form of Rocky Mountain spotted fever some-times kills the patient within 5 days of the onset of symptoms; this form of the disease is more common in black males who are deficient in glucose-6-phos-phate dehydrogenase, and may be related to haemoly-sis in these patients. Infection confers long-lasting immunity.

### Rickettsialpox

The clinical course of rickettsialpox is similar to that of other spotted fever group infections and includes development of fever, headache and an eschar at the site where the infected mite fed. The rash is initially maculopapular but often becomes vesicular. Fever lasts for about a week, and patients usually recover uneventfully.

### Scrub typhus

Scrub typhus may be mild or fatal, depending on host factors and presumably the virulence of the infecting strain. Symptoms develop 6–18 days after being fed upon by infected mite larvae (chiggers). The disease is characterized by sudden onset of fever, headache, and myalgia. A maculopapular rash often develops 2–3 days after onset of the illness. An eschar is often apparent at the site of the bite with enlargement of local lymph nodes. Progression of the disease may be accompanied by interstitial pneumonitis, general-ized lymphadenopathy and splenomegaly. Death may result from encephalitis, respiratory failure and circu-latory failure. Patients who survive generally become afebrile after 2–3 weeks, or sooner if treated appropriately. Scrub typhus confers only transient immunity, and re-infection may occur with heterologous or homologous strains.

## LABORATORY DIAGNOSIS

Timely and accurate diagnosis of rickettsial disease followed by administration of an appropriate antibiotic may mean the difference between death of the patient and uneventful recovery. The lack of widely available, reliable diagnostic tests that can detect the disease in its early stages remains a problem, particularly as symptoms are often non-specific. The rash may appear at a late stage in the infection or not at all, and may resemble exanthemata of many other diseases. The presence or significance of an eschar, if present, is also commonly overlooked.

### Serological methods

Rickettsial diseases are usually acute and short-lasting. Antibodies appear in the second week of illness, when the patient is usually on the way to recovery. Death may occur before detectable levels of antibody are present. Serology is therefore not suitable for early diagnosis of rickettsial infections and is used mainly to confirm the diagnosis for epidemiologic investigations.

The traditional *Weil–Felix test*, which relies on agglutination of the somatic antigens of non-motile *Proteus* species, is no longer recommended because of unacceptably poor sensitivity and specificity. More reliable diagnostic tests including immunofluorescence and enzyme immunoassay are now commercially available.

### Isolation of rickettsiae

Isolation of the organism provides conclusive proof of rickettsial infection. However, it is seldom attempted because of lack of facilities or expertise and because of the presumed danger to laboratory personnel. Such dangers have been overemphasized in this era of antibiotics, but use of containment facilities is appropriate.

Rickettsiae can be isolated in cell culture, in laboratory animals such as mice or guinea-pigs, or in embryonated chicken eggs. Cell culture yields timely results and is widely used for isolation of rickettsiae from clinical samples. Rickettsiae can be detected in cell culture 48–72 h after inoculation by the shell vial assay.

### Detection of rickettsiae in tissue

Skin biopsies from the centre of petechial lesions can be examined by immunohistochemistry. This approach is virtually 100% specific and has a sensitivity of 70%. Rickettsiae can be visualized for up to 48 h after the administration of appropriate drugs, allowing diagnosis of infection post mortem. A method has been developed for capturing detached, circulating endothelial cells by antibody-coated magnetic beads and immunocytological detection of intracellular rickettsiae.

### Polymerase chain reaction (PCR)

Detection of rickettsial DNA by PCR is more rapid than isolation and allows specific identification, but the test is not generally available. It is also insensitive, particularly early in the course of the infection when therapeutic decisions should be made. Peripheral blood mononuclear cells, skin biopsy and tache noire specimens from the site of the bite can be used.

PCR amplification of highly conserved rickettsial genes can also be used. A single primer pair that amplifies all or most rickettsiae can be designed from the genes encoding 16S ribosomal ribonucleic acid (*rrs*), a 17-kDa protein (*htr*), citrate synthase (*gltA*) or *ompB*. A suitable approach is to use a conserved genus-specific primer pair to amplify a rickettsial gene and then to identify the species by restriction fragment length polymorphism analysis or DNA sequencing. Scrub typhus can be diagnosed by PCR amplification of the 56-kDa protein gene of *O. tsutsugamushi*.

## TREATMENT

The drug of choice for treating rickettsial infections of all types and in all age groups is doxycycline. Chloramphenicol is an alternative, but is less effective and carries a higher risk of death. Both drugs are rickettsiostatic and allow the patient's immune system time to respond and control the infection. Sulphonamides should not be administered as they exacerbate rickettsial infections; β-lactam and aminoglycoside antibiotics are ineffective. Some new quinolones and macrolides have antirickettsial effects in vitro, but clinical experience in severe rickettsioses is lacking. Short courses of doxycycline do not cause significant dental staining in young children.

Owing to the difficulties of accurate diagnosis and the risks involved in misdiagnosis, empirical tetracycline therapy is appropriate for patients who have had a fever for 3 days or more and a history consistent with the epidemiological and clinical features of rickettsial disease. The case fatality rate is increased significantly if treatment is delayed for more than 5 days.

Intensive nursing care, management of fluids and electrolytes, and administration of red blood cells to patients who develop anaemia may be needed. Surgery may also be necessary to remove digits and extremities that develop ischaemic necrosis.

## EPIDEMIOLOGY

### Typhus group infections

#### Epidemic typhus

*R. prowazekii* is transmitted from person to person by the body louse, *Pediculus humanus corporis*; the organisms are present in the faeces of infected lice and enter through the bite wound or skin abrasions. *R. prowazekii* causes a fatal infection of the louse, which is therefore incapable of long-term maintenance of the rickettsiae, and human beings appear to be reservoirs of epidemic typhus. Patients who suffer a bout of recrudescent typhus (Brill–Zinsser disease) circulate sufficient rickettsiae in their blood to infect approximately 1–5% of lice that feed on them – enough to initiate new epidemics of the disease. *R. prowazekii* is maintained in an enzootic cycle in North America involving flying squirrels and their fleas and lice.

#### Murine typhus

Murine typhus is distributed worldwide, particularly in tropical and subtropical coastal regions where the disease is an occupational hazard of working in rat-infested areas such as markets or ports. This disease is maintained in an enzootic cycle involving rats and their fleas, which remain infected for life. Even the inefficient rate of transovarial transmission in fleas may play an important role in maintaining the rickettsiae in nature. Man is infected by the contamination of abraded skin, respiratory tract or conjunctiva with infective flea faeces, in which the rickettsiae can survive for as long as 100 days under optimal conditions of temperature and humidity.

### Spotted fever group infections

#### Tick-borne infections

Tick-borne rickettsiae of the spotted fever group are maintained in enzootic cycles involving ticks and their wild animal hosts. Ticks are the primary reservoirs of the rickettsiae, and maintain the organisms by both trans-stadial transmission (during moulting of larva to nymph and thence to adult tick) and transovarial or vertical transmission. Some horizontal transmission (tick to rodent to tick) is likely to be essential to the survival of virulent rickettsiae in nature because these rickettsiae are somewhat pathogenic to ticks.

Man becomes infected following the bite of infected ticks or through contamination of abraded skin or mucous membranes. People place themselves at risk when they enter areas infested with infected ticks. Infection may also occur through bites of ticks of domestic dogs or if partially fed ticks rupture during manual deticking of dogs. Rocky Mountain spotted fever is endemic in the Americas, especially in the southeastern and south-central USA. In 2007, 2221 cases were reported. A nonfatal illness, African tick bite fever, is often observed in travellers returning from safari in southern Africa.

#### Rickettsialpox

*R. akari* is maintained in an enzootic cycle that involves house mice (*Mus musculus*) and their mites. The arthropod vector is also the primary reservoir and can maintain the organism by trans-stadial and transovarial transmission. Other rodents and their ectoparasites may be able to maintain the rickettsiae in rural areas, but their importance remains unknown. Rickettsialpox is primarily an urban disease associated with mice-infested buildings.

### Scrub typhus

The nymphal and adult stages of the mites transmitting *O. tsutsugamushi* are free living and do not feed on animals. The parasitic larvae (chiggers) occur in habitats that have been disturbed by the loss or removal of the natural vegetation. The area becomes covered with scrub vegetation, which is the preferred habitat for chiggers and their mammalian hosts, and gives the disease its name. The disease is often localized because of the restricted habitat of the chiggers. Persons entering infected areas are at risk.

## CONTROL

It is virtually impossible to eradicate rickettsial infections because of their enzootic nature. Measures aimed at reducing rodent or ectoparasite populations may help to reduce the risk of infection. In addition to delousing infested persons, their clothing and bedding should be decontaminated.

**Table 40.2** Human diseases caused by *Ehrlichia, Anaplasma* and *Neorickettsia* species

| Species | Disease | Geographical distribution | Means of transmission | Primary vectors |
|---|---|---|---|---|
| *E. chaffeensis* | Monocytic ehrlichiosis | North and South America, Africa, Asia | Tick bite | *Amblyomma americanum* |
| *A. phagocytophilum* | Granulocytic anaplasmosis | USA, Eurasia | Tick bite | *Ixodes spp.* |
| *E. ewingii* | Ehrlichiosis ewingii | USA | Tick bite | *A. americanum* |
| *N. sennetsu* | Sennetsu ehrlichiosis | Japan, Southeastern Asia | ? Fluke-infested fish | |

Persons entering areas endemic for spotted fever group infections should wear protective clothing treated with tick repellent. Individuals should also examine themselves carefully for ticks as soon as possible after returning from tick-infested areas. The probability of infection is decreased if the tick is removed soon after it attaches. Transmission may require up to 24 h of feeding, perhaps because starved ticks require a partial blood meal if they are to reactivate the virulence of the rickettsiae as well as inject organisms into the feeding site in their saliva.

There is no safe, effective vaccine for any of the rickettsial diseases. The attenuated E strain of *R. prowazekii* induces protective immunity, but is unsuitable for general use because it causes a mild form of typhus in 10–15% of those inoculated and reverts to a virulent state after animal passage. Inactivated Rocky Mountain spotted fever vaccines afford incomplete protection and are no longer available. A recombinant or attenuated vaccine that contains cross-protective antigens stimulating cellular immunity could protect against both typhus and spotted fever rickettsioses. Scrub typhus vaccines derived from killed rickettsiae do not prevent infection, and experimental recombinant subunit vaccines are ineffective in animals.

Antimicrobial prophylaxis is not recommended for infections with *Rickettsia* species, as they are only rickettsiostatic and disease develops as soon as the antibiotic is discontinued. Prolonged prophylaxis with weekly doses of doxycycline is effective against scrub typhus, but is probably inappropriate except under exceptional circumstances, for instance during military operations.

## EHRLICHIA AND ANAPLASMA

## DESCRIPTION

The first human ehrlichial disease was recognized in 1954 when *Neorickettsia* (formerly *Ehrlichia*) *sennetsu* was identified as the cause of an illness

**Fig. 40.4** Electron micrograph of *E. chaffeensis* within a cytoplasmic vacuole. (Micrograph by courtesy of Dr Vsevolod L Popov.)

resembling glandular fever in Japan. *Ehrlichia chaffeensis, Anaplasma phagocytophilum* and *E. ewingii* later emerged as the causes of tick-borne diseases in the USA. *Ehrlichia* and *Anaplasma* species are transmitted through the bite of ticks. *N. sennetsu* is suspected to infect a fluke and to cause infection when ingested with parasitized raw fish (Table 40.2).

These organisms are small Gram-negative bacteria. They multiply within membrane-bound cytoplasmic vacuoles, usually in various phagocytes, and form characteristic microcolonies resembling mulberries, termed morulae (Latin: *morum*, mulberry) (Fig. 40.4). Electron microscopy reveals two distinct morphological forms, larger reticulate and smaller dense-core cells, which are the replicating and infectious forms, respectively, in a developmental cycle.

## PATHOGENESIS

*Anaplasma* and *Ehrlichia* species can establish prolonged, even persistent, infections in vivo, and some species, including *E. chaffeensis*, kill heavily infected cells in vitro. Cytokine-associated immunopathological mechanisms are probably important. *A. phagocytophilum* and *E. chaffeensis* evade the host immune system by antigenic variation and by modulating the host defences, respectively.

The tropism for phagocytes indicates that these organisms have evolved strategies for evading the microbicidal activities of the macrophage or granulocyte. Within phagocytes *A. phagocytophilum* and *E. chaffeensis* block the fusion of phagosome-containing bacteria with lysosomes to prevent killing by lysosomal enzymes. *A. phagocytophilum* prevents killing mediated by reactive oxygen species by lowering reduced nicotinamide adenine dinucleotide phosphate (NADPH) oxidase activity in neutrophils. To accommodate a slow generation time (about 8 h), *Anaplasma* and *Ehrlichia* prolong their host cells' lifespan by inhibiting apoptosis.

Antibody to ehrlichiae confers passive protection, and cellular immunity is crucial to recovery. Suppression of neutrophil function by *A. phagocytophilum* may predispose to opportunistic infection.

## Clinical aspects of infection

### Human monocytic ehrlichiosis

The disease begins 1–2 weeks after a bite of an infected tick. Clinical features frequently include fever, headache, myalgias, nausea, arthralgias and malaise. Other manifestations include cough, pharyngitis, lymphadenopathy, diarrhoea, vomiting, abdominal pain and changes in mental status. A fleeting or transient rash involving the extremities, trunk, face or, rarely, the palms and soles appears in 30–40% of patients about 5 days after onset. The rash may be petechial, macular, maculopapular or diffusely erythematous.

Cytopenia early in the course of the illness may provide presumptive clues to the diagnosis. Mild to moderate leucopenia is observed in approximately 60–70% of patients during the first week of illness, with the largest decreases occurring in the total neutrophil count. Thrombocytopenia occurs in 70–90% of patients. Mildly or moderately raised hepatic transaminase levels are noted in most patients at some point during their illness.

About 50% of patients need admission to hospital. Those with severe disease may develop acute renal failure, metabolic acidosis, respiratory failure, profound hypotension, disseminated intravascular coagulopathy, myocardial dysfunction and meningoencephalitis; about 3% die. Death is more common in elderly men and immunocompromised individuals, including those infected with human immunodeficiency virus (HIV).

### Human granulocytic anaplasmosis

The incubation period is 7–10 days after a bite by an infected tick. Clinical signs and symptoms are similar to those of human monocytic ehrlichiosis, but the disease is less severe and the mortality rate is less than 1%. Rash and central nervous system involvement are rare.

Human granulocytic ehrlichiosis caused by *E. ewingii* elicits similar signs and symptoms. The infection has been observed mainly in immunocompromised patients with no fatalities.

## LABORATORY DIAGNOSIS

*Ehrlichia* and *Anaplasma* species grow intracellularly, and isolation is difficult. Human infections are diagnosed mainly by demonstrating the development of specific antibodies during convalescence. Indirect immunofluorescence methods use cell culture-propagated organisms. *E. chaffeensis, A. phagocytophilum* and *E. ewingii* are detected diagnostically by PCR with specific primers to amplify the ehrlichial DNA. Human granulocytic anaplasmosis can often be diagnosed by identification of characteristic morulae in Giemsa-stained peripheral blood neutrophils; *E. chaffeensis* is seldom detected in monocytes in blood smears.

## TREATMENT

Doxycycline shortens the course of infection and reduces mortality. The use of chloramphenicol is not recommended.

## EPIDEMIOLOGY

Deer and ticks are involved in the ecology of human monocytic and granulocytic ehrlichioses and of granulocytic anaplasmosis. Deer, canines, rodents and domestic ruminants are important reservoirs. Immature ticks obtain ehrlichiae from the blood of infected animals; the organisms are maintained trans-stadially but not transovarially, and are transmitted during a subsequent blood meal. Human infections are strongly associated with the season of tick activity, history of tick bite and distribution of the vectors. Most cases of human monocytic ehrlichiosis are reported between March and November in the south-central and southeastern USA, where *Amblyomma americanum* is prevalent. Human granulocytic anaplasmosis occurs from March to December in the northern states.

## COXIELLA

### DESCRIPTION

Query or Q fever, first identified as a distinct clinical entity in 1935 after an outbreak of typhoid-like illness among abattoir workers in Australia, is a widespread disease with an almost global distribution. The aetiological agent, *C. burnetii*, is a fastidious intracellular prokaryote, genetically related to *Legionella* species.

*C. burnetii* is a pleomorphic coccobacillary bacterium with a Gram-negative type of cell wall. The organisms typically grow within the phagolysosome of macrophages of the vertebrate host (Fig. 40.5). Structurally distinct large and small cell variants have been described, suggesting that the organism has a developmental cycle. In acidic conditions, similar to those found within a phagolysosome, it actively metabolizes a variety of substrates and can accomplish significant levels of macromolecular synthesis. Prolonged cultivation in vitro results in phase variation due to deletion of genes involved in the synthesis of lipopolysaccharides analogous to the smooth to rough transitions observed in other bacteria. Phase I organisms are representative of strains in nature, whereas phase II organisms appear in laboratory cultures and are avirulent for laboratory animals.

### PATHOGENESIS

Human infection usually follows inhalation of aerosols containing *C. burnetii*. Entry into the lungs results in infection of the alveolar macrophages and a brief

**Fig. 40.5** Immunoperoxidase staining of *C. burnetii* in alveolar macrophages in a patient with Q fever. (Micrograph by courtesy of Dr J Stephen Dumler.)

rickettsaemia. Most infections are subclinical, and only 2% of persons infected with *C. burnetii* are admitted to hospital. The incubation period for the acute form of the disease is usually about 2 weeks but can be longer.

Typical acute Q fever is a self-limiting flu-like syndrome with high fever (40°C), fatigue, headache and myalgia. The patient may also suffer pneumonitis, hepatic and bone marrow granulomata, and meningoencephalitis. Chronic infections can develop, with the organism persisting in cardiac valves and possibly other foci. Endocarditis is rare, but potentially fatal, and may be accompanied by glomerulonephritis, osteomyelitis or central nervous system involvement.

Reactivation of latent infection may occur during pregnancy, and the organism is shed with the placenta or abortus.

### LABORATORY DIAGNOSIS

Diagnosis relies on the demonstration of specific antibodies in an indirect immunofluorescence assay or enzyme immunoassay. Immunofluorescence assay titres peak at 4–8 weeks. PCR amplification has been used to detect *C. burnetii* DNA in clinical samples from acute and chronic Q fever patients.

Isolation of *C. burnetii* from patient specimens is a specialized procedure and is not generally recommended because of the extremely infectious nature of the organism.

### TREATMENT

Most infections resolve without antibiotic treatment, but administration of doxycycline reduces the duration of fever in the acute infection and is definitely recommended in cases of chronic infection. In Q-fever endocarditis, long-term administration of a combination of two drugs among doxycycline, ciprofloxacin and rifampicin has been suggested.

*C. burnetii* may be recovered from some patients after months or even years of continuous treatment. In addition to antibiotic therapy, the haemodynamic status should be monitored. Valve replacement may be necessary in some cases of Q-fever endocarditis.

### EPIDEMIOLOGY

Q fever has been found on all continents except Antarctica, but most cases are reported from the UK and France. Elsewhere, the disease often goes unreported, is misdiagnosed, or causes such a mild infection that treatment is not sought. The main reservoirs of the disease are wild and domestic cattle, sheep and goats. Ticks can maintain *C. burnetii* by trans-stadial and transovarial transmission. Faeces of infected ticks contain very large numbers of *C. burnetii*, but arthropods are not an important source of infection.

*C. burnetii* may be the most infectious of all bacteria. Human infections generally follow inhalation of aerosols or direct contact with the organisms in the milk, urine, faeces or birth products of infected animals. The organism can survive on wool for 7–10 months, in skimmed milk for up to 40 months and in tick faeces for at least 1 year. Most individuals acquire the disease as an occupational hazard. Cases are common among abattoir workers and those associated with livestock rearing or dairy farming. Although Q fever normally occurs as isolated, sporadic cases, well-documented outbreaks have been reported.

## CONTROL

Elimination of infected reservoir hosts is probably impossible because of chronic infections among the animals and the ability of the organism to survive for long periods in the external environment. Exposure can be reduced by construction of separate facilities for animal parturition, destruction of suspect placental membranes, heat treatment of milk (74°C for 15 s) and efforts to reduce the tick population. Abattoir workers should take care while handling carcasses, especially in the removal and dissection of mammary glands and inner organs. Animal hides should be kept wet until the salting procedure begins. Appropriate containment procedures should be observed in laboratories working with this highly infectious organism.

Inactivated whole-cell vaccines derived from phase I organisms have been developed and generate a protective response.

## RECOMMENDED READING

Audy JR: *Red Mites and Typhus*, London, 1968, Athlone Press.

Carlyon JA, Fikrig E: Invasion and survival strategies of *Anaplasma phagocytophilum*, *Cellular Microbiology* 5:743–754, 2003.

Dalton MJ, Clarke MJ, Holman RC, et al: National surveillance for Rocky Mountain spotted fever, 1981–1992: epidemiologic summary and evaluation of risk factors for fatal outcome, *American Journal of Tropical Medicine and Hygiene* 52:405–413, 1995.

Dumler JS: Ehrlichioses and anaplasmosis. In Guerrant RL, Walker DH, Weller PF, editors: *Tropical Infectious Diseases. Principles, Pathogens, and Practice*, ed 3, Philadelphia, 2010, Elsevier Saunders, pp 339–341.

Hechemy KE, Avsic-Zupanc T, Childs JE, Raoult DA, editors: *Rickettsiology: Present and Future Directions*, New York, 2003, Academy of Sciences.

Kawamura A, Tanaka H, Tamura A: *Tsutsugamushi Disease*, Tokyo, 1995, University of Tokyo Press.

Maurin M, Raoult D: Q fever, *Clinical Microbiology Reviews* 12:518–553, 1999.

Paddock CD, Childs JE: *Ehrlichia chaffeensis*: a prototypical emerging pathogen, *Clinical Microbiology Reviews* 16:37–64, 2003.

Treadwell TA, Holman RC, Clarke MJ, et al: Rocky Mountain spotted fever in the United States, 1993–1996, *American Journal of Tropical Medicine and Hygiene* 63:21–26, 2000.

Walker DH: *Rickettsia rickettsii* and other spotted fever group rickettsiae (Rocky Mountain spotted fever and other spotted fevers). In Mandell GL, Bennett JC, Dolin R, editors: *Principles and Practice of Infectious Diseases*, ed 7, Vol. 2, Philadelphia, 2009, Elsevier Churchill Livingstone, pp 2499–2507.

Walker DH, Raoult D: *Rickettsia prowazekii* (epidemic or louse-borne typhus). In Mandell GL, Bennett JC, Dolin R, editors: *Principles and Practice of Infectious Diseases*, ed 7, Vol. 2, Philadelphia 2009, Elsevier Churchill Livingstone, pp 2521–2524.

Kim I–S, Walker DH: Scrub typhus. In Guerrant RL, Walker DH, Weller PF, editors: *Tropical Infectious Diseases. Principles, Pathogens, and Practice*, ed 3, Philadelphia, 2010, Elsevier Saunders, pp 334–338.

Zhang JZ, Sinha M, Luxon BA, Yu X-J: Survival strategy of obligately intracellular *Ehrlichia*: novel modulation of immune response and host cell cycles, *Infection and Immunity* 72:498–507, 2004.

# 41 Mycoplasmas

## Respiratory and genital tract infections

*D. Taylor-Robinson*

## KEY POINTS

- Mycoplasmas pathogenic for man include the genera *Mycoplasma* and *Ureaplasma*. They are found in the respiratory and genital tracts of man and many animal species, and sometimes invade the bloodstream to gain access to joints and other organs.
- Mycoplasmas are the smallest organisms that grow in cell-free bacteriological media. They lack a rigid cell wall containing peptidoglycan; hence they are not susceptible to β-lactam or glycopeptide antibiotics. Infections are treated principally with macrolides, tetracyclines or fluoroquinolones.
- *M. pneumoniae* is a pathogen for the human respiratory tract, sometimes resulting in pneumonia, especially in children.
- *M. genitalium* and *U. urealyticum* cause acute non-gonococcal urethritis in men and are also implicated in chronic disease; *M. genitalium* also causes balanoposthitis.
- Various mycoplasmas and ureaplasmas are associated with genital infections in women, including bacterial vaginosis, post-partum fever, cervicitis, endometritis and salpingitis.
- Mycoplasmas, most often ureaplasmas, are responsible for about two-fifths of the cases of suppurative arthritis occuring in patients with hypogammaglobulinaemia. *M. fermentans* has been detected in the joints of patients with chronic arthritides.

Mycoplasmas are the smallest prokaryotic organisms that can grow in cell-free culture medium. They are found in man, animals, plants, insects, soil and sewage. The first to be recognized, *Mycoplasma mycoides* ssp. *mycoides*, was isolated in 1898 from cattle with pleuropneumonia. As other pathogenic and saprophytic isolates accumulated from veterinary and human sources they became known as pleuropneumonia-like organisms (PPLO), a term long superseded by 'mycoplasmas'. Mycoplasma (Greek: *mykes*, fungus; *plasma*, something moulded) refers to the filamentous (fungus-like) nature of the organisms of some species and to the plasticity of the outer membrane resulting in pleomorphism.

The term mycoplasma(s) is often used, as here, in a trivial fashion to refer to any member of the class Mollicutes ('soft skins'), which embraces 5 families, 8 genera and over 200 species. The family Mycoplasmataceae contains the mycoplasmas that are of importance in human medicine. It is subdivided into two genera:

- *Mycoplasma*, of which there are at least 120 named species, 14 of which are of human origin.
- *Ureaplasma*, urea-hydrolysing organisms (trivially termed ureaplasmas), of which there are seven species, two of which are of human origin.

Organisms in the genus *Spiroplasma* cause disease in plants and insects, and those in genus *Acholeplasma* are ubiquitous in nature. Several species of *Haemobartonella* and *Eperythrozoon* are also placed within the genus *Mycoplasma* on the basis of their 16S ribosomal RNA (rRNA) sequence similarities.

Mycoplasmas are distributed widely in nature, and various species cause economically important infections in domestic animals, other mammals, birds and reptiles as well as man. In addition, mycoplasmas are of concern to those who use cell cultures because mycoplasmal contamination may severely affect the cells.

Ureaplasmas were known originally as T strains or T mycoplasmas – 'T' for 'tiny' to indicate the small size of the colonies in comparison with those produced by other mycoplasmas. Many animals are infected by ureaplasmas. Those of avian, bovine, canine and feline origin are antigenically distinct from the human strains and have been placed in separate species. Ureaplasmas of human origin, formerly classified as *Ureaplasma urealyticum*, comprise at least 14 serovars and fall into two groups differentiated in several ways, most importantly by genome size. Strains of small genome size include the serovars 1, 3, 6 and 14 within the species *U. parvum*, whereas those of larger genome size include the other ten serovars and these remain within *U. urealyticum*.

## DESCRIPTION

### Reproduction

Mycoplasmas, like conventional bacteria, multiply by binary fission. However, cytoplasmic division may not always be synchronous with genome replication, resulting in the formation of multinucleate filaments and other shapes. Subsequent division of the cytoplasm by constriction of the membrane at sites between the genomes leads to chains of beads that later fragment to give single cells. Budding occurs when the cytoplasm is not divided equally between the daughter cells. The minimal reproductive unit of mycoplasmas is a roughly spherical or bottle-shaped cell about 200–250 nm in diameter. Organisms of this order initiate growth in cell-free medium and make up, with larger forms (0.5–1.0 μm diameter), the substance of the characteristic agar-embedded colonies.

### Morphology

Cell morphology varies with the species, environmental conditions and the stage of the growth cycle. Light microscopy reveals pleomorphic organisms, which may range from spherical through coccoid, coccobacillary, ring and dumb-bell forms, to short and long branching (Fig. 41.1), beaded or segmented filaments.

Several mycoplasmas, including *M. pneumoniae*, *M. genitalium* (Fig. 41.2) and *M. penetrans* of human origin, have specialized structures at one or both ends by which they attach to respiratory or genital tract mucosal surfaces. Sections of the terminal structures of the two former mycoplasmas may exhibit a dense rod-like core when viewed by electron microscopy.

Mycoplasmas, unlike conventional bacteria, do not have a rigid cell wall containing peptidoglycan. This also differentiates them from bacterial L-forms for which the absence of the cell wall is a temporary environmental change. The mycoplasma cell is limited by a membrane, 7.5–10 nm wide, in which two electron-dense layers are separated by a translucent one (Fig. 41.3). Some species have an extramembranous layer, which, in the case of *M. mycoides* ssp. *mycoides*, for example, comprises galactan and has a dense capsular appearance. Some others, including *M. genitalium*

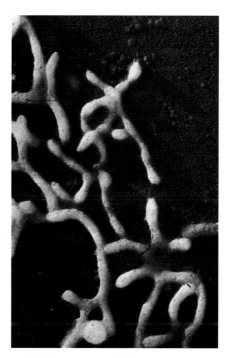

**Fig. 41.1** Electron micrograph of *M. mycoides* ssp. *mycoides* (bovine origin), gold shadowed, to show branching filaments (original magnification ×28 000). (From Rodwell AW, Abbot A 1961 The function of glycerol, cholesterol and long-chain fatty acids in the nutrition of *Mycoplasma mycoides*. *Journal of General Microbiology* 25: 201–214.)

and *M. pneumoniae*, have surface spikes (sometimes described as a 'nap'), somewhat coarser than those seen on myxoviruses, which may contribute, through adhesin proteins, to attachment of the organisms to eukaryotic cells. *M. gallisepticum* (avian), *M. genitalium* and *M. pneumoniae* attach to neuraminic acid receptors. Close adherence enables the mycoplasma to insert nucleases and other enzymes into the cell and to take from it the products of enzyme activity, such as nucleotides. Adherence to erythrocytes (*haemadsorption*), tissue culture cells, spermatozoa and other eukaryotic cells may be demonstrated with certain mycoplasmas, including *M. pneumoniae*, *M. genitalium* and *M. agalactiae* (shown in Fig. 41.4). Some mycoplasmas, including *M. pneumoniae*, *M. genitalium* and *M. hominis*, invade eukaryotic cells.

The electron-lucent part of the membrane comprises lipids with the long chains of the fatty acids arranged inwards and polar groups to the external and internal parts of the organisms; the electron-dense layers consist of protein and carbohydrate. The mycoplasma membrane is the site of many metabolic reactions involving membrane-bound enzymes and transport mechanisms. Cholesterol, or carotenoid/

**Fig. 41.2** Electron micrograph of *M. genitalium* (human origin), negatively stained, to show flask-shaped appearance and terminal specialized structure covered by extracellular 'nap' (original magnification ×120 000). (From Tully JG, Taylor-Robinson D, Rose DL et al 1983 *Mycoplasma genitalium*, a new species from the human urogenital tract. *International Journal of Systematic Bacteriology* 33: 387–396.)

**Fig. 41.3** Electron micrograph of *M. pulmonis* (of murine origin); thin section illustrating trilaminar membrane (arrow) (original magnification ×75 000).

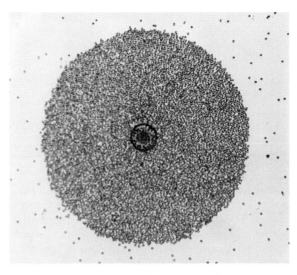

**Fig. 41.4** Colony of *M. agalactiae* (of caprine origin) showing adherent guinea-pig erythrocytes (phenomenon of haemadsorption).

carotenol, is interspersed between the phospholipid molecules and plays an important part in maintaining membrane integrity in the face of varying external osmotic pressures and in the absence of the rigid cell wall found in other bacteria. However, the presence of cholesterol renders the cell membrane susceptible to damage with agents such as saponin, digitonin and some polyene antibiotics (e.g. amphotericin B) that complex with sterols. As expected, mycoplasmas are completely resistant to β-lactam and other antibiotics that influence bacterial cell wall synthesis and also to lysozyme.

Mycoplasmas are prokaryotes (p. 10) and the cytoplasm does not contain endoplasmic reticulum, but is packed with ribosomes. Ribosomal protein synthesis is inhibited by antibiotics such as tetracyclines, aminoglycosides and macrolides.

The genome of *M. genitalium* is the smallest known so far (580 kb). It is not much larger than that of a large poxvirus, an indication of the small amount of genetic information needed for a free-living existence and the reason why mycoplasmas have a paucity of biochemical activity and are nutritionally fastidious.

### Viruses and plasmids

Fourteen viruses have been identified: six in *Acholeplasma*, four in *Mycoplasma* and four in *Spiroplasma* species. They are rod-shaped (Fig. 41.5) or enveloped spheres that bud from the mycoplasma membrane surface, or are polyhedral with a tail. Those that have been examined in detail contain single- or

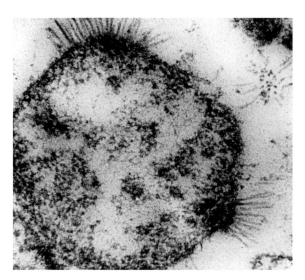

**Fig. 41.5** Rod-shaped virus particles (75 × 7.5 nm) radiating from the surface of an *A. laidlawii* cell (original magnification ×100 000).

double-stranded DNA in circular or linear form. There is evidence for integration of the viral genome into the mycoplasmal chromosome, especially in spiroplasmas, and this may provide a mechanism for the promotion of genetic diversity. There is no evidence, however, that the viruses influence mycoplasmal pathogenicity. Viral release is continuous and is not accompanied by cell lysis. Plasmids, so far regarded as cryptic, have been detected in *Acholeplasma, Mycoplasma* and, most frequently, *Spiroplasma* species.

## Cultivation

Mycoplasmas have limited biosynthetic abilities, so that they need a rich growth medium containing natural animal protein (usually blood serum) and, in most cases, a sterol component. Serum supplies not only cholesterol but also saturated and unsaturated fatty acids for membrane synthesis, components that the organisms cannot synthesize. A medium that has been widely used for isolation contains bovine heart infusion (PPLO broth) with fresh yeast extract and horse serum. However, these components vary in their ability to support growth and success may depend on use of different batches of the components, sera from other animal species or the addition of various supplements.

Cultivation of spiroplasmas is more difficult. A medium designated SP-4 has been helpful in their isolation and also in the isolation of fastidious mycoplasmas, such as *M. pneumoniae*, *M. fermentans* and *M. genitalium,* which is notoriously difficult to isolate.

Although various specific formulations have been described for the isolation of ureaplasmas, most mycoplasmal media containing urea may be suitable. The sterol-independent organisms also grow readily on these media, but serum, which often promotes growth, is not usually essential.

A strategy using Vero (African green monkey) cell cultures has been described for isolating *M. genitalium*. The inoculated cell cultures are monitored for mycoplasmal growth by polymerase chain reaction (PCR) technology followed, when there are signs of growth, by subculture to mycoplasmal medium. However, investigators should be aware of the dangers inherent in the widespread use of cell cultures which may become contaminated by mycoplasmas.

Most mycoplasmas are facultatively anaerobic but, because organisms from primary tissue specimens often grow only under anaerobic conditions, an atmosphere of 95% nitrogen and 5% carbon dioxide is preferred for primary isolation. The optimal temperature for growth of most mycoplasmas and ureaplasmas from man or animals is 36–38°C, but is lower for acholeplasmas and spiroplasmas.

### Colonial morphology

On agar, mycoplasmas often produce colonies that have a 'fried egg' appearance, with an opaque central zone of growth within the agar and a translucent peripheral zone on the surface (Fig. 41.6). However, some, such as *M. pneumoniae* on primary isolation, have a mulberry appearance without the peripheral zone. The size of the colonies varies widely: colonies of some bovine mycoplasmas and most acholeplasmas may exceed 2 mm in diameter, and are visible to the naked eye. Nevertheless, most require low-power microscopic magnification. Colonies of ureaplasmas are characteristically small (15–60 μm in diameter), mainly because they usually lack the peripheral zone of growth. However, the size and appearance of all mycoplasmal colonies depend on the constituents and degree of hydration of the medium, the agar concentration, atmospheric condition and age of the culture.

### Biochemical reactions

Most mycoplasmas use glucose (or other carbohydrates) or arginine as a major source of energy; a few use both or do not metabolize either substrate. In most mycoplasmas the respiratory pathways are flavin-terminated so that the haem compounds, cytochromes and catalase are absent. The unique and distinctive biochemical feature of ureaplasmas is the conversion of urea to ammonia by urease.

**Fig. 41.6** Colonies of *M. hominis* (of human origin) (up to 110 μm in diameter) with typical 'fried egg' appearance (oblique illumination; original magnification ×150).

*Mycoplasma, Ureaplasma* and certain other species depend on sterol. Thus, they fail to grow in serum-free media and are inhibited by digitonin, distinguishing them from the species that do not require sterol. In addition, most *Mycoplasma* species and ureaplasmas produce hydrogen peroxide, which causes some lysis of guinea-pig or other erythrocytes when these are suspended in agar over developing colonies. *M. pneumoniae* produces clear zones of β-haemolysis. About one-third of all *Mycoplasma* species display the phenomenon of haemadsorption (Fig. 41.4).

## Antigenic properties

DNA analysis and sequencing has made a fundamental contribution to the taxonomy of mycoplasmas. Amplification of part of the 16S rRNA gene by PCR plays an important role in the rapid identification of some mycoplasmas and ureaplasmas, and simplifies species classification. Nevertheless, identification and speciation are often accomplished by the use of specific antisera containing antibodies that reflect their different antigenic compositions. The western blot technique is useful in assessing the importance of particular antigens, but gel diffusion and immuno-electrophoresis techniques are important for studying the antigenic structure and the relationships between them. For sero-epidemiological studies and for serological diagnosis, more sensitive tests, such as indirect haemagglutination, the enzyme-linked immunosorbent assay (ELISA) and micro-immunofluorescence, are used.

The way in which different antigens function is exemplified by considering *M. pneumoniae*. The glucose- and galactose-containing membrane glycolipids of the organism are haptens, which are antigenic only when bound to membrane protein. They induce antibodies that react in complement-fixation, metabolism-inhibition and growth-inhibition tests. Glycolipids of the mycoplasma have a structure fortuitously similar to that in the human brain. The cross-reactivity of the brain glycolipids with antibodies to *M. pneumoniae* could feasibly account for the neurological manifestations of *M. pneumoniae* infection (vide infra). Furthermore, the ability of the organisms to alter the I antigen on erythrocytes sufficiently to stimulate anti-I antibodies (cold agglutinins) leads to an autoimmune response and damage to erythrocytes.

*M. pneumoniae* has two major surface proteins, including the P1 protein involved in attachment, that are recognized by the host; antibody to them is detected in convalescent sera and respiratory secretions. Variation in the P1 protein has led to the recognition of two subtypes of strains, which may vary epidemiologically and in pathogenicity.

Variable membrane lipoproteins of several mycoplasmas form an antigenic variation system that provides a means of escaping from the host immune response; the variations are restricted to a small number of protein antigens and do not appear to alter the total cell protein profiles of the organisms.

## PATHOGENESIS

The *Mycoplasma* and *Ureaplasma* species that have been isolated from man, either from the respiratory tract (mostly the oropharynx) or from the urogenital tract, are shown Table 41.1. *M. pneumoniae, M. genitalium, M. hominis, M. fermentans* and *U. urealyticum* unequivocally cause disease or are strongly associated with disease. *M. amphoriforme* was recovered from the respiratory tract of patients with antibody deficiency and chronic bronchitis, but its relation to this disease or, indeed, others is not clear.

The mechanisms whereby mycoplasmas and ureaplasmas cause disease are multifactorial and include the following:

- Adherence of mycoplasma organisms to host cells, the adhesins of *M. pneumoniae* and *M. genitalium* being proteins P1 and MgPa, respectively.

**Table 41.1** Mycoplasmas/ureaplasmas of human origin: anatomical site of detection and some properties

| Mycoplasma | Frequency of detection | | Metabolism of | Preferred pH | Haemadsorption[a] |
|---|---|---|---|---|---|
| | Respiratory tract | Urogenital tract | | | |
| M. amphoriforme | ? Rare | Not reported | Glucose | 7.5 | ? |
| M. buccale | Rare | Not reported | Arginine | 7.0 | − |
| M. faucium | Rare | Not reported | Arginine | 7.0 | + |
| M. fermentans[d] | Common | Quite common | Glucose and arginine | 7.5 | − |
| M. genitalium[d] | Very rare | Rare[b] | Glucose | 7.5 | + |
| M. hominis[d,e] | Rare | Common | Arginine | 7.0 | − |
| M. lipophilum | Rare | Not reported | Arginine | 7.0 | − |
| M. orale | Common | Not reported | Arginine | 7.0 | + |
| U. parvum[e] | Rare | Common | Urea | 6.0 or less | +[c] |
| M. penetrans[d] | Not reported | Rare | Glucose and arginine | 7.5 | + |
| M. pirum[d] | Not reported | ? | Glucose and arginine | 7.5 | ? |
| M. pneumoniae | Rare[b] | Very rare | Glucose | 7.5 | + |
| M. primatum | Not reported | Rare | Arginine | 7.0 | − |
| M. salivarium | Common | Rare | Arginine | 7.0 | − |
| M. spermatophilum | Not reported | Rare | Arginine | 7.0 | − |
| U. urealyticum[e] | Rare | Common | Urea | 6.0 or less | − |

[a]Chick red blood cells.
[b]Rare, except in disease.
[c]Serovar 3 only.
[d]Reported in rectum of homosexual men.
[e]Reported in the anal canal of women attending a genitourinary medicine clinic.

- The ability of some mycoplasmas to invade host cells.
- The production of toxins by *M. pneumoniae* and some other mycoplasmas.
- The stimulation of pro-inflammatory cytokines.
- Antigenic variation which enables the mycoplasma to evade the protective immune systems of the host.
- Immunological responses of the host, for example, autoimmune ones causing disease, and an exaggerated response to a repeat infection leading to worse disease.
- The ability of mycoplasmas to develop antibiotic resistance culminating sometimes in chronic disease.

## Respiratory infections

### Mycoplasmal pneumonia

Pneumonias not attributable to any of the common bacterial causes were labelled historically as *primary atypical pneumonias*. In one variety associated with the development of cold agglutinins, a filterable micro-organism, first called the *Eaton agent*, was isolated in embryonated eggs. Inhibition by chlortetracycline and gold salts, and cultivation on cell-free medium eventually clinched its mycoplasmal nature.

The organism was named *M. pneumoniae*, and its importance as a cause of respiratory disease was confirmed in numerous studies.

*Epidemiology.* *M. pneumoniae* infection occurs world wide. Although endemic in most areas, there is a preponderance of infection in late summer and early autumn in temperate climates; in some countries, such as the UK, epidemic peaks have been observed about every 4 years. Spread is fostered by close contact, for example in a family. Overall, *M. pneumoniae* may cause only about one-sixth of all cases of pneumonia, but in certain confined populations, such as military recruits, it has been responsible for almost half of the cases of pneumonia. Children are infected more often than adults, and the consequence of infection is also influenced by age. Thus, in school-aged children and teenagers, about a quarter of infections culminate in pneumonia, whereas in young adults fewer than 10% do so. Thereafter, pneumonia is even less frequent, although the severity tends to increase with the age of the patient.

*Clinical features.* *M. pneumoniae* infections often have an insidious onset, with malaise, myalgia, sore throat or headache overshadowing and preceding chest symptoms by 1–5 days. Cough, which starts around the third day, is characteristically dry, troublesome and sometimes paroxysmal, and becomes a prominent feature. Physical signs such as râles become apparent, frequently after radiographic evidence of pneumonia. Most often this amounts to patchy opacities, usually of one of the lower or middle lobes. About 20% of patients suffer bilateral pneumonia, but pleurisy and pleural effusions are unusual. The course of the disease is variable; cough, abnormal chest signs and radiographic changes may extend over several weeks and relapse is a feature. A prolonged paroxysmal cough simulating the features of whooping cough may occur in children. Despite these signs and symptoms, most patients are not seriously ill and few warrant admission to hospital. However, very severe infections have been reported in adults, usually in those with immunodeficiency or sickle cell anaemia, although death is rare. Apart from being involved in some exacerbations of chronic bronchitis, there is an unproven suggestion that *M. pneumoniae* might not only exacerbate asthma, but sometimes be a primary cause of asthma in children.

Disease is limited usually to the respiratory tract. Extra-pulmonary manifestations include:

- Stevens–Johnson syndrome and other rashes
- arthralgia
- meningitis or encephalitis (and other neurological sequelae including, rarely, Bell's palsy)
- haemolytic anaemia
- myocarditis
- pericarditis.

Haemolytic anaemia with crisis is an auto-immune phenomenon brought about by cold agglutinins (anti-I antibodies). Some of the other complications, such as the neurological ones, may arise in a similar indirect way, although *M. pneumoniae* has been isolated from cerebrospinal fluid.

### Other respiratory infections

*M. hominis* and ureaplasmas, in particular, have been associated with respiratory disease in the newborn, as described below.

*M. hominis* has produced sore throats when given orally to adult volunteers; however, it does not seem to cause naturally occurring sore throats in children or adults possibly because the dose encountered is smaller.

*M. fermentans* has been associated with adult respiratory distress syndrome with or without systemic disease, and with pneumonia in a few children with community-acquired disease. *M. genitalium* has been isolated, together with *M. pneumoniae*, from the respiratory secretions of a few adults but its role, if any, in respiratory disease seems small.

### Urogenital infections

As listed in Table 41.1, various mycoplasmas and ureaplasmas, most frequently *M. hominis* and *U. urealyticum,* have been isolated most frequently from the urogenital tract. Use of the PCR technique has enabled some mycoplasmas, for example *M. fermentans* and especially *M. genitalium*, to be detected far more often than would otherwise be the case.

### Urogenital infections in men

Although *M. hominis* may be isolated from about 20% of men with acute non-gonococcal urethritis (NGU), it has not been incriminated as a cause. There is increasing evidence to implicate *U. urealyticum*, but not *U. parvum*, in this acute condition; *U. urealyticum* is the most likely species involved in some chronic cases.

*M. genitalium* has been strongly implicated worldwide as a cause of about 25% of cases of acute NGU; it also causes chronic NGU, usually in those who have been treated inadequately. In addition, there is preliminary evidence that *M. genitalium* causes balanoposthitis and it might be involved in some cases of acute epididymitis. However, there is no evidence that this or other mycoplasmas cause acute or chronic prostatitis.

There is evidence that ureaplasmas may occasionally cause acute epididymitis, but it is very doubtful that they have any role in male infertility. The idea that *M. genitalium* could have a role in infertility is based on the possibility that it might be involved in causing epididymitis and its known ability to adhere to spermatozoa.

### Reproductive tract disease in women

*M. hominis* and, to a lesser extent, ureaplasmas are found in the vagina of women who have bacterial vaginosis in much larger numbers, up to 10 000-fold in the case of *M. hominis*, than in healthy women. Thus, it is possible that, with various other bacteria, they may contribute to the development of the condition. However, it seems very unlikely that *M. hominis* causes disease if present in small numbers. *M. genitalium* has been associated strongly with cervicitis, despite the criteria used to define the condition being variable.

*M. hominis* has been isolated from the endometrium and fallopian tubes of about 10% of women with laparoscopically confirmed pelvic inflammatory disease (PID), together with a specific antibody response. This suggests a causal role, but the significance of *M. hominis* is difficult to judge with confidence as several other micro-organisms, including *Chlamydia trachomatis* (Ch. 39), may be found at the same time. Ureaplasmas have also been isolated directly from affected fallopian tubes, but the absence of antibody responses and failure to produce salpingitis in subhuman primates make them an even less likely cause of disease at this site.

The pathogenic potential of *M. genitalium* in PID seems greater; it has been associated significantly with endometritis, and antibody responses to the mycoplasma in some patients with the disease and produces endometritis, parametritis and salpingitis in subhuman primates. However, reports of detection of *M. genitalium* in laparoscopically derived fallopian tube specimens by PCR technology are few and this decisive approach needs to be taken whenever the opportunity arises.

The part that *M. hominis* is likely to play in infertility in women as a result of tubal damage is small. In contrast, serology has shown a strong association between *M. genitalium* and tubal factor infertility.

### Disease associated with pregnancy and the newborn

*M. hominis* and ureaplasmas have been isolated from the amniotic fluid of women with severe chorioamnionitis who had pre-term labour. Similarly, ureaplasmas have been isolated from spontaneously aborted fetuses and stillborn or premature infants more frequently than from induced abortions or normal full-term infants.

Isolation of ureaplasmas from the internal organs of aborted fetuses, together with some serological responses and an apparently diminished occurrence following antibiotic therapy, suggest that these organisms may have a role in abortion. However, bacterial vaginosis is strongly associated with pre-term labour and late miscarriage and, as *M. hominis* and ureaplasmas are part of the extensive microbial flora of bacterial vaginosis, they may act with a multitude of other micro-organisms and not independently. There is, so far, inadequate evidence to associate *M. genitalium* with pre-term outcome of pregnancy.

The same considerations relate to the role of other genital mycoplasmas, particularly ureaplasmas, in causing low birth-weight in otherwise normal full-term infants. Bacterial vaginosis has been largely ignored in defining this association. A study in which women given erythromycin in the third trimester delivered larger babies than those given a placebo has not been confirmed in later trials. However, in infants

of less than 1000 g with a ureaplasmal respiratory tract infection acquired in utero or at the time of delivery, congenital pneumonia and the likelihood of death or chronic lung disease is about double that in uninfected infants of similar or greater birthweight. Inflammatory cytokines have been found in tracheal aspirates from these very low birthweight infants with respiratory ureaplasmal infection. There is considerable support for this scenario but no evidence of a reduction in the incidence of chronic disease has yet been found when preterm infants have been treated with erythromycin. Although there is uncertainty surrounding this particular issue, premature infants are prone to meningitis, with or without further neurological damage, as a result of *M. hominis* or ureaplasmas gaining access to the cerebrospinal fluid within the first few days of life.

After an abortion or even a normal delivery, *M. hominis* has been isolated, apparently in pure culture, from the blood of about 10% of febrile women, about half of them developing an antibody response, but not from afebrile women who aborted or from healthy pregnant women. Observations of this kind have also been made for ureaplasmas and it seems that both micro-organisms induce fever, possibly by causing endometritis.

### Urinary infection and calculi

*M. hominis* has been isolated from the upper urinary tract of patients with acute pyelonephritis and may cause a small proportion (possibly about 5%) of such cases. Ureaplasmas do not seem to be involved in pyelonephritis. However, the fact that they produce urease, induce crystallization of struvite and calcium phosphates in urine in vitro, and calculi experimentally in animal models, raises the question of whether they cause calculi in the human urinary tract. In support of this, ureaplasmas are more often found in the urine and calculi of patients with infective-type stones than in those with metabolic stones.

### Joint infections

Evidence that ureaplasmas are involved in the aetiology of sexually acquired reactive arthritis is based on synovial fluid mononuclear cell proliferation in response to specific ureaplasmal antigens. Ureaplasmas also have a role in suppurative arthritis in hypogammaglobulinaemic patients (vide infra). *M. genitalium* has been reported in the joints of patients with Reiter's disease or rheumatoid arthritis, but the significance of this remains unclear. *M. fermentans* has been found by a PCR assay in the joints of about

20% of patients with rheumatoid arthritis and in those of patients with other chronic inflammatory rheumatic disorders, but not in the joints of patients with non-inflammatory arthritides. However, whether this mycoplasma is simply attracted to an inflammatory site and is behaving as an innocent bystander remains to be determined.

## Infections in immunocompromised patients

*M. pneumoniae* pneumonia in immunodeficient patients may be severe and the organisms may persist for many months in the respiratory tract of hypogammaglobulinaemic patients, despite apparently adequate antibiotic treatment. A few hypogammaglobulinaemic patients develop suppurative arthritis and mycoplasmas are responsible for at least two-fifths of the cases. The mycoplasmas mainly involved are *M. pneumoniae, M. salivarium* (usually regarded as non-pathogenic), *M. hominis* and, particularly, ureaplasmas. In some cases involving ureaplasmas, the arthritis has been associated with subcutaneous abscesses, persistent urethritis and chronic cystitis. Although sometimes responding to antibiotic treatment, these organisms and disease may persist for many months despite concomitant use of anti-inflammatory and γ-globulin replacement therapy.

Haematogenous spread of *M. hominis* leading to septic arthritis, surgical wound infections and peritonitis seems to occur more often after organ transplantation and in other patients on immunosuppressive therapy. Particularly common are sternal wound infections in heart and lung transplant patients.

The suggestion that *M. fermentans* infection of the peripheral blood monocytes of human immunodeficiency virus (HIV)-positive subjects may lead to a more rapid development of AIDS now seems highly unlikely. Similarly, nothing has emerged to support the notion that *M. penetrans* is associated with HIV positivity or with Kaposi's sarcoma.

## LABORATORY DIAGNOSIS

### Respiratory infections

Because the clinical manifestations of *M. pneumoniae*-induced disease are often insufficiently distinct for definitive diagnosis, laboratory help is required. Isolation is not often attempted because of insensitivity and the time required. In the past reliance was often placed on serology, notably the complement fixation test. However, specificity is relative since cross-reactivity with *M. genitalium* is sometimes seen.

A four-fold or greater rise in antibody titre, with a peak at about 3–4 weeks, is indicative of a recent *M. pneumoniae* infection, but because paired sera are not always available or because of the delay in acquiring a second serum, a single antibody titre of 64–128 has been used to institute therapy in a suggestive clinical setting.

Serology and culture have largely been superseded by PCR technology, which is specific, sensitive and rapid. If an *M. pneumoniae* isolate is required, a sensible approach is to test specimens by both the PCR assay and culture, and to continue the culture procedure only for those specimens that prove to be PCR positive.

The cold agglutinin test is non-specific and unreliable. Of a gamut of other tests, the enzyme immunoassay is sensitive and specific, and there are formats for testing paired sera or a single serum. The Immuno-Card® test (Meridian Diagnostics) for IgM is simple and rapid and has proved reliable, especially in children. The Remel enzyme immunoassay detects IgM and IgG simultaneously and is sensitive and specific.

Attempted isolation of *M. pneumoniae* (and *M. fermentans*) requires the use of mycoplasmal SP4 broth medium supplemented with penicillin and glucose, and phenol red as a pH indicator. After inoculation with sputum, throat washing, pharyngeal swab or other specimen, the medium is incubated at 37°C, and a colour change (red to yellow), which may take up to 3 weeks or longer, indicates fermentation of glucose by multiplying organisms. The broth is then subcultured on agar medium to await the development of colonies, which are identified specifically by immunofluorescence with a specific antiserum or by other serological methods.

Diagnostic procedures for other mycoplasmas that might be found in the respiratory tract are considered below.

### Urogenital infections

Culture still has a place in the detection of some genital mycoplasmas and ureaplasmas. Material from urethral, cervical or vaginal swabs, or a centrifuged deposit from urine, is added to separate vials of liquid mycoplasmal medium containing phenol red and 0.1% glucose, arginine or urea. *M. genitalium* metabolizes glucose and changes the colour of the medium from red to yellow. *M. fermentans* also metabolizes glucose but also converts arginine to ammonia, as do *M. hominis* and *M. primatum*. Ammonia is also produced when ureaplasmal urease breaks down urea and the colour changes from yellow to red.

*M. hominis* multiplies in most routine blood culture media if gelatin (1% w/v) is added to overcome the inhibitory effect of sodium polyanethol sulphonate, included as an anticoagulant.

Kits designed to isolate and identify *M. hominis* and ureaplasmas, and to provide antimicrobial susceptibility profiles, are available commercially. They are of particular value if the need to detect these micro-organisms arises infrequently. Phylogeny-based rapid identification of urogenital mycoplasmas and ureaplasmas, based on the amplification of a part of the 16S rRNA gene by PCR, has also been described.

DNA primers specific for practically all *Mycoplasma* and *Ureaplasma* species, including *M. fermentans*, *M. genitalium*, *U. urealyticum* and *U. parvum*, have been developed and used for amplification by PCR. This technique is much more sensitive than culture for detecting the two former mycoplasmas and is the only reliable way of determining their presence in clinical specimens.

Genital mycoplasmal infections stimulate antibody responses, but the various techniques to detect them are rarely used diagnostically.

## TREATMENT

The in-vitro sensitivity of several mycoplasmas and ureaplasmas to various antibiotics used in treatment is shown in Table 41.2. These micro-organisms are completely resistant to β-lactam or glycopeptide antibiotics.

### Mycoplasmal pneumonia

*M. pneumoniae* is sensitive to erythromycin and moderately sensitive to the tetracyclines in vitro and these antibiotics have been used widely in clinical practice. Though they have sometimes proved less effective for treating pneumonia than in planned trials, it is still worthwhile administering a macrolide or a tetracycline to adults, and erythromycin to children and pregnant women.

Newer macrolides, such as clarithromycin and azithromycin, and the newer fluoroquinolones, are highly active in vitro and certainly have a place in treatment, although macrolide resistance may sometimes be an issue. The fluoroquinolones seem to have a cidal effect, an important attribute which may be useful as tetracyclines and macrolides only inhibit growth. Failure to kill the organisms, together with the fact that they may become intracellular, probably explains persistence in the respiratory tract long after clinical recovery, as well as clinical relapse in some patients. Furthermore, a functioning immune system has been shown to be important in eradication, some hypogammaglobulinaemic patients, for example, experiencing persistence of the organisms for months or years. A veterinary pleuromutilin antibiotic (Econor®) has been used with some success to treat mycoplasmal respiratory infections in immunocompromised subjects.

Antibiotic treatment of *M. pneumoniae* or other mycoplasma-induced infection should start as soon as possible, based on clinical suspicion, and a course of at least two weeks is justified. The wait for laboratory confirmation is now less pressing in view of the rapidity of PCR technology.

### Urogenital infections

Treatment must take into account the fact that several different micro-organisms may be involved and that a precise microbiological diagnosis may not be attainable. Thus, patients with NGU should receive an antibiotic that is active against *C. trachomatis*, ureaplasmas and *M. genitalium*. Azithromycin, which is used increasingly for chlamydial infections, is also active

**Table 41.2** Susceptibility of some mycoplasmas and ureaplasmas to various antibiotics

| Antibiotic | *M. pneumoniae* | *M. hominis* | *M. genitalium* | *Ureaplasma* spp. |
|---|---|---|---|---|
| Tetracycline | + | + | +++ | ++ |
| Doxycycline | ++ | + | +++ | ++ |
| Erythromycin | +++ | − | +++ | ++ |
| Clarithromycin | +++ | − | +++ | +++ |
| Azithromycin | +++ | − | +++ | − |
| Clindamycin | +++ | +++ | + | + |
| Ciprofloxacin | ± | + | − | + |
| Sparfloxacin | +++ | +++ | ++ | +++ |
| Moxifloxacin | ++ | ++ | +++ | + |

+++, extremely sensitive; ++, very sensitive; +, moderately sensitive; ±, weakly sensitive; −, insensitive.

against a wide range of mycoplasmas, including *M. genitalium* and, to a lesser extent, ureaplasmas. This may be preferable to a tetracycline, because *M. genitalium* is less sensitive to tetracyclines and at least 10% of ureaplasmas are resistant. Some *M. genitalium* strains are, or have become, resistant to azithromycin and in this circumstance moxifloxacin has been used successfully.

A broad-spectrum antibiotic should also be included for the treatment of PID to cover *C. trachomatis, M. genitalium* and *M. hominis* as well as various anaerobic bacteria. As about 20% of *M. hominis* strains are resistant to tetracyclines, other antibiotics such as clindamycin or fluoroquinolones may need to be considered.

Fever following abortion or childbirth often settles within a few days, but if it does not therapy with a broad-spectrum antibiotic should be started, keeping the above comments in mind.

## MYCOPLASMAS AND CELL CULTURES

It is rare for primary cell cultures to become infected with mycoplasmas, but continuous cell lines do so frequently. Various species may be responsible. The effects of contamination include those caused by mycoplasmal enzymes and toxins, and those resulting from metabolism of cell culture media components or from changes in pH. Despite the presence of up to $10^8$ organisms per millilitre of culture fluid, there may be little effect on viral propagation, although it may decrease the yield. Occasionally, the yield may be increased as, for example, with vaccinia virus in *M. hominis*-infected cells.

Mycoplasmal culture methods and an indicator cell system with staining (e.g. Hoechst DNA dye) are used conventionally to detect contamination, but PCR methods have much greater sensitivity. Numerous procedures have been described to eliminate mycoplasmas from cell cultures, but none is consistently successful. Whenever possible it is easier to discard the cultures, replace them with mycoplasma-free cells and adhere to simple guidelines to prevent contamination. If it is imperative to save cells, treatment with an antibiotic that is likely to have mycoplasmacidal activity, such as a fluoroquinolone, identification of the contaminant and use of a specific antiserum, or a combination of these methods, is most likely to be successful in eradication.

### RECOMMENDED READING

Blanchard A, Browning G, editors: *Mycoplasmas: Molecular Biology, Pathogenicity and Strategies for Control*, Wymondham, UK, 2005, Horizon Scientific Press.

Furr PM, Taylor-Robinson D, Webster ADB: Mycoplasmas and ureaplasmas in patients with hypogammaglobulinaemia and their role in arthritis: microbiological observations over 20 years, *Annals of the Rheumatic Diseases* 53:183–187, 1994.

Maniloff J, McElhaney RN, Finch LR, Baseman JB, editors: *Mycoplasmas. Molecular Biology and Pathogenesis*, Washington, DC, 1992, American Society for Microbiology.

Taylor-Robinson D: Mycoplasmas and their role in human respiratory tract disease. In Myint S, Taylor-Robinson D, editors: *Viral and Other Infections of the Human Respiratory Tract*, London, 1996, Chapman and Hall, pp 319–339.

Taylor-Robinson D: *Mycoplasma genitalium* – an update, *International Journal of STD & AIDS* 13:145–151, 2002.

Taylor-Robinson D, Bebear C: Antibiotic susceptibilities of mycoplasmas and treatment of mycoplasmal infections, *Journal of Antimicrobial Chemotherapy* 40:622–630, 1997.

Taylor-Robinson D, Gilroy CB, Jensen JS: The biology of *Mycoplasma genitalium*, *Venereology* 13:119–127, 2000.

Taylor-Robinson D, Jensen JS: Genital mycoplasmas. In Morse SA, Ballard RC, Holmes KK, Moreland AA, editors: *Atlas of Sexually Transmitted Diseases and AIDS*, ed 4, London, 2011, Mosby, pp 64–75.

Taylor-Robinson D, Jensen JS: *Mycoplasma genitalium*: from chrysalis to multicolored butterfly, *Clinical Microbiology Reviews* 24:498–514, 2011.

Totten PA, Taylor-Robinson D, Jensen JS: Genital mycoplasmas. In Holmes KK, Sparling PF, Stamm WE, et al, editors: *Sexually Transmitted Diseases*, ed 4, New York, 2008, McGraw Hill, pp 709–736.

Tully JG, Razin S, editors: *Molecular and Diagnostic Procedures in Mycoplasmology. Diagnostic Procedures*, Vol. 2, London, 1996, Academic Press.

Waites KB, Taylor-Robinson D: *Mycoplasma* and *Ureaplasma*. In Murray PR, Baron EJ, Jorgensen JH, et al, editors: *Manual of Clinical Microbiology*, ed 10, Vol. 1. Washington, DC, 2011, American Society for Microbiology, pp 970–985.

# PART 4
## VIRAL PATHOGENS AND ASSOCIATED DISEASES

# 42 Adenoviruses

## Respiratory disease; conjunctivitis; gut infections

*J. S. M. Peiris and C. R. Madeley*

**KEY POINTS**

- Adenoviruses, comprising 51 serotypes in six species (A–F), commonly infect man, and can persist in lymphoid tissue.
- They cause (mostly) mild respiratory infections, especially in children, but can cause serious disease outbreaks in military recruits and severe multi-organ disease in immunocompromised patients.
- Types 1, 2, 5 and 6 are mostly endemic; types 3, 4 and 7 may be associated with epidemic disease.
- Types 40 and 41 cause diarrhoea, but others are also found in faeces without associated disease.
- Type 8 (and also types 19 and 37) causes epidemic keratoconjunctivitis.
- Similar viruses infect both animals and birds but are not known to cross species boundaries.
- The use of adenoviruses as vectors for gene and cancer therapy, and for vaccines against other diseases, is being explored but is not yet suitable for clinical use.

Adenoviruses were named from their original source, *adenoid tissue*, removed at operation and cultured as explants in vitro. Cellular outgrowth occurred readily, but this often deteriorated rapidly a week or 10 days later. The cause of the deterioration was found to be *adenovirus(es)* present in the original tissue and which replicated enthusiastically in the new cells growing from the explant.

This discovery initiated much research, which established that there were a considerable number of serotypes, mostly associated with mild *upper respiratory tract infections*. In addition, there were occasional serious (and even fatal) childhood *pneumonias* and infrequent, but readily transmissible, *eye infections*. Some of these infections, mostly in children and not always symptomatic, could persist for weeks or months. The focus of adenovirus research then shifted away from clinical virology with the discovery that some species could cause malignancies in laboratory rodents. As a result, virologists have thoroughly investigated adenovirus structure, replicative mechanisms and oncogenicity during the past 40 years.

Clinical interest revived in the middle 1970s with the discovery of two new serotypes (subsequently numbered types 40 and 41) linked (with several other hitherto unknown viruses) to that previously elusive entity '*viral gastroenteritis*'. This revival of clinical interest has been extended by the discovery in rapid succession of six new serotypes (numbered 42–47), most of them in patients with acquired immune deficiency syndrome (AIDS) and others (types 48–51). Further types (52–55) have also been proposed but their novelty has yet to be confirmed (see below, under Classification). Adenoviruses can cause serious disease in immunocompromised patients (e.g. bone marrow transplant recipients), but they may also be present in the stools of congenitally immunodeficient children with little or no associated pathology. The apparently low pathogenic potential of adenoviruses has encouraged those pursuing gene-therapy to explore their possible use as vectors for gene or vaccine delivery, or tumour treatment. Human genes (up to 7 kb in size) have been inserted into replication-crippled adenoviruses and these new gene(s) carried into cells by adenovirus infection in the hope that their expression can correct defects caused by absent or defective genes. Alternatively, similarly modified adenoviruses have been used to target tumour cells (which are often of epithelial origin), either to carry lethal mutations into the cell or to induce the surface expression of target viral antigens, making the cell vulnerable to normal immune mechanisms.

Both of these approaches show promise, but formidable technical problems remain to be overcome before either gene therapy or oncolysis becomes routinely useful. These include difficulties in making the transferred genes persist and in overcoming pre-existing immunity in the patient to the serotype(s) of adenovirus used. Interest in using adenoviruses

**Fig. 42.1** Group of adenovirus particles from a stool extract showing typical adenovirus morphology although apical fibres are not visible. Individual capsomers can be seen as surface 'knobs'. These virus particles should be compared with the model seen in (C). Negative contrast, 3% potassium phosphotungstate, pH 7.0 (magnification ×160 000). (B) Single adenovirus particle showing some of the apical fibres. This is an unusual finding. Negative contrast, 3% potassium phosphotungstate, pH 7.0 (magnification ×280 000). (C,D) Photograph of a model with pentons (P), peripentons (PE) and hexons (H) indicated. Note that the fibres (F) are attached to the penton.

in these ways has sparked further detailed molecular investigations into adenovirus structure and taxonomy.

## DESCRIPTION

Adenovirus virions provide a very good example of an *icosahedron*. Figure 42.1A shows a group of typical adenovirus particles, whereas Figures 42.1B–D compare a single virus particle, as seen by electron microscopy, with a model. The particles seen in Figure 42.1A do not show the apical fibres (they are rarely seen in situ by the electron microscope), but otherwise the particles in Figures 42.1A & B resemble the model closely.

The virion is 70–75 nm in size, depending on whether it is measured across the 'flats' or the apices,

and there are probably minor variations between preparations and, possibly, serotypes. The surface has 252 visible surface 'knobs', the capsomers. Twelve apical capsomers, each surrounded by five others, are known as *pentons*; 60 peripentons surround the pentons and 180 other capsomers make up the major part of the faces (Fig. 42.1D). Except for the pentons, all of the other capsomers are surrounded by six others, and are therefore called *hexons*.

From each penton projects an apical *fibre*; these vary greatly in length, from 9–31 nm. Some avian types have double fibres, but human strains have only single ones.

Adenoviruses contain a single piece of double-stranded DNA, 33–45 kbp in size, which codes for a considerable number of structural and non-structural proteins with molecular weights of 7500–400 000 Da. The ten structural proteins include three polypeptides that make up each hexon, one that forms the penton base and a glycoprotein for the fibre. These lie on the surface of the particle, whereas the other five are internal.

The pentons and fibres bear antigenic determinants that are 'type' specific, and antibody binding to them neutralizes virus infectivity. There are type-specific antigenic determinants on the hexons, but they carry genus-specific antigens as well. The same genus-specific antigens are found on all mastadenoviruses (see below), the genus to which the medically important human adenoviruses belong. These genus-specific antigens provide a basis for tests to detect adenoviruses and antibodies to them (by immunofluorescence, enzyme immuno-assays, complement fixation, etc. – see under laboratory Diagnosis, below).

## Classification

The family Adenoviridae comprises two genera:

1. *Mastadenovirus*, whose members infect mammalian species, including humans.
2. *Aviadenovirus*, whose members infect avian species. They are not relevant to this chapter as they do not infect humans.

The classification of *Mastadenoviruses* remains in a state of flux. Hitherto, up to 51 serotypes, identified using prepared animal antisera, were defined by neutralisation tests in cell culture. They were subdivided into six species (A–F) by differences in DNA homology (>20%), with members of the same species having >50% homology. Preparation of type-specific antisera, usually in rabbits, was, and is, a laborious and expensive task and these antisera to known adenovirus types are then used to compare novel strains with

previously known serotypes. More recently, alternative approaches using molecular methods offered quicker, simpler and less laborious ways to identify possible new strains. Four new strains designated types (not serotypes) 52–55 have been reported. They have been found by molecular methods, but their separate identity has not been confirmed serologically and it seems likely that type 55, for instance, is a recombinant between types 14 and 11. It is likely that it would still serotype as 14 although this has not been confirmed. How widespread such recombinants are is unknown at present. As pathogens, their immunological identity will be more important than genetic differences when considering whether to make a vaccine against them.

Consequently, since there are many uncertainties about the higher-numbered human adenoviruses, this edition refers only to types up to 51. Table 42.1 shows current classification into species and serotypes.

## REPLICATION

The virus attaches to susceptible cells by the apical fibres and is then taken into the cell, losing both fibres and pentons in the process. It then passes to the nucleus, losing the peripentons at the nuclear membrane. Inside the nucleus the DNA is released and the process of replication is initiated (see Ch. 7). About 20 early proteins are made, most of which are not incorporated into new particles. The late proteins are produced in quantity in the cytoplasm, are mostly structural, and are later transported back to the nucleus where new virus particles are assembled, appearing as crystalline arrays. The shutting down of host cell metabolism and the accumulation of

| Species[b] | Serotypes | No. of *Smal* fragments[c] | Oncogenicity in newborn hamsters | Tissues most commonly infected |
|---|---|---|---|---|
| A | 12, 18, 31 | 4–5 | High | Gut (no symptoms) |
| B | 3, 7, 11, 14, 16, 21, 34, 35, 50 | 8–10 | Low | Respiratory tract, kidney |
| C | 1, 2, 5, 6 | 10–12 | None | Respiratory tract, lymphoid tissue (tonsils and adenoids) |
| D | 8–10, 13, 15, 17, 19, 20, 22–30, 32, 33, 36–39, 42–49, 51 | 14–18 | None | Conjunctiva, gut, respiratory tract(?) |
| E | 4 | 16–19 | None | Conjunctiva, respiratory tract |
| F | 40, 41 | 9–12 | None | Gut |

Table 42.1 Properties and classification of adenoviruses of species A–F[a]

[a]Putative types 52–55 are not included in this table.
[b]More than 50% DNA homology between members.
[c]Restriction endonuclease digestion. Some small fragments probably not included.
Adapted with permission from Wadell G 2000 In: Zuckerman AJ, Banatvala JE, Pattison JR (eds) *Principles and Practice of Clinical Virology*, 4th edn, pp 307–327. John Wiley, Chichester.

**Table 42.2** Disease associated with adenovirus serotypes

| Disease | Those at risk | Associated serotypes |
|---|---|---|
| Acute febrile pharyngitis: | | |
|     Endemic | Infants, young children | 1, 2, 5, 6 |
|     Epidemic | Infants, young children | 3, 4, 7 |
| Pharyngoconjunctival fever | Older school-aged children | 3, 7 |
| Acute respiratory disease | Military recruits | 4, 7, 14, 14a, 21 |
| Pneumonia | Infants | 1, 2, 3, 7 |
| Follicular conjunctivitis | Any age | 3, 4, 11 |
| Epidemic keratoconjunctivitis | Adults | 8, 19, 37 |
| Haemorrhagic cystitis | Infants, young children | 11, 21 |
| Diarrhoea and vomiting | Infants, young children | 40, 41 |
| Intussusception | Infants | 1, 2, 5 |
| Disseminated infection | Immunocompromised (e.g. AIDS, renal, bone marrow and heart–lung transplant recipients) | 5, 11, 34, 35, 43–51 |

Adapted with permission from Wadell G 2000 In: Zuckerman AJ, Banatvala JE, Pattison JR (eds) *Principles and Practice of Clinical Virology*, 4th edn, pp 307–327. John Wiley, Chichester.

thousands of new virions results in rupture (lysis) and death of the infected cell with dissemination of the particles.

In cell cultures, this process causes the cells to round up, swell and aggregate into clumps resembling bunches of grapes. The cells then disintegrate as they lyse.

## CLINICAL FEATURES

Table 42.2 lists the more common associations of serotypes with disease. The great majority of infections with adenoviruses are not confirmed virologically and the full extent of adenovirus disease burden is under-reported. In addition, virus infection and replication are not invariably associated with disease. For example, a variety of serotypes are isolated from faeces without any evidence of gut pathology, and prolonged tonsillar carriage in children is common. However, some well recognized disease syndromes are caused by adenovirus infections.

### Respiratory diseases

These are usually mild upper respiratory tract infections with fever, runny nose and cough. Most are due to types 1–7, although higher serotypes may be involved sporadically. Types 1, 2, 5 and 6 are more commonly associated with endemic infections, whereas types 3, 4 and 7 are more epidemic. In children the associated clinical diagnoses include 'upper respiratory tract infection', wheezing and 'failure to thrive'. Adenovirus infections can mimic whooping cough in some patients.

These respiratory infections are rarely serious but, occasionally and unpredictably, may progress to a pneumonia that is both extensive and frequently fatal. The majority of these pneumonias occur in young children. Unlike other viral respiratory infections, adenoviruses may be associated with a raised white cell count and enhanced levels of C-reactive protein, and therefore may be confused with a bacterial infection.

In older children and young adults, some of these infections will be labelled 'colds', although epidemics of adenoviral infection with respiratory symptoms and fever occur in, for example, US military recruits, where strenuous exercise and close proximity combine both to make the victims more vulnerable and to facilitate spread. These outbreaks can be severe in both numbers and extent of disease – severe enough, in fact, to warrant the development of a trial vaccine. More recently, a variant adenovirus, type 14a, has emerged to cause an epidemic threat in the USA, especially in military encampments but also in the general population (see Gray & Chorazy 2009). Eye involvement is a common feature (see below), leading to such outbreaks being called pharyngoconjunctival fever. Types 3 and 7 are more often associated with these outbreaks, but other serotypes are found from time to time.

### Eye infections

Adenoviruses have been associated with several outbreaks of conjunctivitis in the UK, referred to as 'shipyard eye' because originally it was thought to be due to particles of steel swarf thrown up during welding and grinding. It was later shown that the real cause was an adenovirus transmitted through fluids, eyebaths and other instruments used to treat eye injuries in the shipyard First Aid Clinic, and which had become contaminated by virus from the index case. Use of properly sterilized instruments and single-dose preparations of eye ointment have now made this uncommon. Most such outbreaks have been due to adenovirus type 8 (although types 19 and 37 have also been involved). This is a difficult type to isolate, and sporadic cases may not be identified as readily as in outbreaks, which inevitably attract a more concentrated effort at diagnosis. Eye infections with type 8 do not usually cause systemic symptoms.

Conjunctivitis caused by other serotypes may occur in outbreaks of pharyngoconjunctival fever. This is a follicular conjunctivitis resembling that caused by *Chlamydia*, from which it should be differentiated, but the associated and usually marked adenovirus respiratory symptoms will provide a clue to the cause.

## Gut infections

The common respiratory serotypes (1–7) are frequently isolated from faeces; in young children, the same serotype may be recovered from both ends of the child. There is little evidence to link such isolates with disease in the gut. However, when faecal extracts from children with diarrhoea were examined by electron microscopy, typical adenoviruses were seen in some of the cases, often in very large numbers. Surprisingly, these morphologically typical viruses could not readily be isolated in cell culture and were later shown to be two hitherto unknown serotypes, 40 and 41. They cause a significant proportion of cases of endemic childhood diarrhoea (as opposed to outbreaks, often due to *noroviruses* – see Ch 56) and, in numbers of cases, are second only to rotaviruses. They may contribute up to one-third of those cases in which a virus is found. As with the other viruses found in diarrhoeal faeces, such adenoviruses may also be present in the faeces of apparently normal babies, although less frequently, but there is no doubt of their pathogenic potential for the gut. How they differ from the other non-pathogenic types found there is not known, nor whether they cause respiratory infections.

The role of adenovirus(es) in mesenteric adenitis and intussusception is unproven. Even when enlarged nodes are identified at laparotomy, it is not usual practice to excise one for diagnostic purposes, and direct evidence is lacking. Finding a coincidental adenovirus in faeces is not proof of involvement, nor is it clear how often adenitis precedes (and possibly initiates) intussusception. Where any such temporal association has been recorded it has involved the common serotypes 1, 2, 5 and 6.

Ten new serotypes (42–51) have been found, nine of them (43–51) in the faeces of patients with AIDS. Type 42 was isolated from the faeces of a normal child. Chronic diarrhoea is a feature of AIDS, although no causal role for these adenoviruses has been proven. Interestingly, these new serotypes were isolated and identified in cell culture (see below, under laboratory Diagnosis), suggesting that they are indeed 'new'. If so, both their origin and significance are unknown.

### Disease in transplant recipients

Adenoviruses may also be associated with hepatitis (in liver transplant patients) and pneumonitis, in immunocompromised patients. The serotypes involved are often uncommon ones (e.g. types 11, 34 and 35). Adenoviruses have been implicated as a major cause of systemic disease in bone marrow transplant recipients, rivaling cytomegalovirus as the main viral infectious threat in some transplant centres.

### Other diseases

There have been occasional reports of adenovirus (mostly types 11 and 21) recovered from the urine of children with haemorrhagic cystitis. The finding of virus provides a (possible) retrospective cause. In the newborn, adenoviruses may cause disseminated disease with a 'septic shock' form of presentation.

There are reports in the literature of recovery of adenoviruses from both the male and the female genital tracts. They may be transmitted sexually but are not recognized as the cause of a sexually transmitted disease.

There is no good evidence of adenoviruses being involved in initiating human tumours. Experimentally, adenoviruses may induce transformation of hamster cells in culture, and such transformed cells will induce tumours in laboratory animals. There is no evidence that this can occur in man, although it has been diligently sought. Under laboratory conditions adenoviruses can also form recombinants (i.e. hybrids) with simian virus 40 (SV40), a polyomavirus that contaminated early stocks of polio vaccine grown in monkey kidney cells. These recombinants, carrying part of the SV40 genome, are neither pathogenic nor oncogenic in man.

## PATHOGENESIS

Adenoviruses mostly infect mucosal surfaces (respiratory tract, gut and eye), although it is clear that not all such infection leads to overt disease. Different serotypes appear to prefer different regions of the body, perhaps due to the presence or absence of particular cellular receptors. Infection of an individual cell will cause its death, but several studies have documented prolonged respiratory and gut excretion in healthy children, lasting for weeks or months. Such respiratory 'carriage' is probably in lymphoid tissue (tonsils and adenoids), and gut carriage may be in the equivalent Peyer's patches, although this has not been documented.

Most infections with adenoviruses, whatever the primary site, probably spread to the gut as well. 'Respiratory' strains are frequently recovered from faeces and it seems improbable that this results solely from overflow from the upper respiratory tract. It is much more likely that faecal excretion follows a secondary gut infection, albeit asymptomatic in most cases. Types 40 & 41 are primary pathogens of the gut, infecting and damaging cells lining it. Death of the infected cells may lead to temporary malabsorption and diarrhoea in children, though not invariably.

The role of the nine recently discovered serotypes (43–51) in patients with AIDS is not known at present. All were recovered from faeces and had not been identified before. They extend the unanswered questions about adenoviruses: Where do new types come from? Do they arise by mutation and/or recombination? For further discussion of this topic, see de Jong et al 1999.

## LABORATORY DIAGNOSIS

### Direct demonstration of 'virus'

#### Detection of viral DNA

Conserved parts of the adenoviral genomic DNA can be detected by molecular detection methods (e.g. the very sensitive polymerase chain reaction) in a variety of clinical specimens. This may form part of a multiplex system to test, for example, for several respiratory viruses simultaneously, or in other conditions. This approach can be adapted to identify individual adenovirus serotypes, but is only available in reference laboratories.

#### Virus antigen

The presence of viral antigen in the nasopharynx may be identified by immunofluorescence with genus-specific antibodies (polyclonal or monoclonal) directly on aspirates (*not* swabs), provided that they contain respiratory cells. The presence of such infected cells usually indicates a significant infection, in contrast to asymptomatic carriage. Alternatively, viral antigen may be detected by enzyme immuno-assays, although these detect virus antigen alone without indicating where it was located. Hence, they cannot distinguish between a significant presence in respiratory cells (indicating invasion of the mucosal surface) and mostly silent (and clinically insignificant) carriage, probably in the tonsils and adenoids.

Viral antigen in the stools can also be detected by a variety of commercial genus-specific enzyme immuno-assays.

### Electron microscopy

Virus particles may be seen directly in stool extracts by electron microscopy, although this cannot identify serotypes. Nonetheless, where virus is seen, this is usually of type 40 or 41, particularly where large numbers are present (the level may reach more than $10^{10}$ particles per gram of faeces). The finding of virus in faeces by electron microscopy does not mean that virus is also present in the nasopharynx or eye(s).

### Culture

Adenovirus can be grown in cell culture from respiratory specimens (nasopharyngeal aspirates, and nose and throat swabs), eye swabs, faeces and, occasionally, urine. The speed of isolation is usually an indication of viral load in the specimen and can provide a pointer to the clinical significance of the finding. If isolation takes longer than 12 days it is less likely to be clinically significant, particularly with types 1, 2, 5 and 6.

Isolation of an adenovirus in cell culture from the faeces of patients with diarrhoea is by itself of little significance. As mentioned above, the diarrhoea-causing adenoviruses are not readily isolated in culture, and cultivable adenoviruses in the stool are not usually those associated with diarrhoea. Nevertheless, the diarrhoea-associated adenoviruses go through partial replication in 293 cells (an adenovirus-transformed human embryo kidney cell line), and the antigens induced in these cells are type-specific. They may be identified by immunofluorescence using type-specific antisera.

### Serology

A rise in antibody levels indicates recent infection (although not its site nor its nature), but absence does not exclude it, especially in babies. Complement fixation is the test most frequently used routinely; it provides only a genus-specific diagnosis. Genus- and type-specific enzyme immuno-assays have also been developed but are not used widely. Neutralization tests are both type-specific and more sensitive, but are not available as routine tests; neither is haemagglutination inhibition widely available. However, both tests may be used by reference laboratories or in research.

## TREATMENT

As most adenoviral infections are not life threatening in healthy individuals, there is little demand for specific treatment and no antiviral drugs are available that are unequivocally effective for adenoviral infections. Any treatment is therefore purely symptomatic. Ribavirin, ganciclovir, vidarabine and cidofovir have all been shown to have antiviral activity in vitro and there are anecdotal reports of their therapeutic use in immunocompromised patients, but with variable success.

## EPIDEMIOLOGY

Adenoviruses are endemic. Types 1–7 spread readily between individuals, presumably by droplets and direct or indirect contact with infected secretions. Faecal–oral transmission can also occur, and probably does, in areas with poverty, poor hygiene and overcrowding. However, it is probable that types 40 and 41, which are widespread causes of diarrhoea even in developed countries, are also spread via droplets.

Subtyping, which has shown, for example, eight subtypes of adenovirus type 7 (the prototype 7p and seven variants 7a–7g), also indicates geographical variation in distribution. Such detailed analysis is not routine, however, and no information on the subtype distribution of types 40 and 41 is available.

Only a minority of adenovirus infections are confirmed virologically.

## CONTROL

For the reasons discussed above under Treatment, there is little demand for a vaccine in the general population. Nevertheless, the problems with adenoviruses encountered by US armed forces in recruit camps led them to develop and use a live virus vaccine containing adenovirus types 4 and 7, administered orally in enteric capsules. This provided adequate protection from disease and was licensed for use but only in military personnel. This vaccine, which was phased out in 1999, is now being reintroduced for US armed forces. There is some evidence that immunity to adenovirus type 7 (contained in this vaccine) partially cross-protects against the newly emerged adenovirus 14a (see above). However vaccine use is not contemplated in the general population.

A careful and rigorous attention to aseptic technique and single-dose vials of materials for use in the eye is the best approach to preventing outbreaks of adenovirus eye infections. However, the component of conjunctivitis that is part of pharyngoconjunctival fever, which is primarily a respiratory infection, is not preventable by these means.

## ADENOVIRUS-ASSOCIATED VIRUSES

The adenovirus-associated viruses (adeno satellite viruses) are members of the Parvoviridae. They are about 22 nm in diameter, appear to be more hexagonal than circular in outline, and contain insufficient single-stranded DNA to replicate on their own. They form a genus, *dependoviruses*, indicating their dependence on a co-infection with an adenovirus (or herpes simplex virus) to provide the missing functions.

True adeno-associated virus has not been implicated in clinical disease. However, as with any other virus found in faeces, large numbers of parvovirus-like particles have been seen in extracts of diarrhoeal faeces, sometimes (but not invariably) combined with smaller numbers of adenoviruses. Neither virus grows in cell culture, leaving the significance of these observations obscure (see Ch. 47).

RECOMMENDED READING

Cody JJ, Douglas JT: Armed replicating adenoviruses for cancer virotherapy, *Cancer Gene Therapy* 16:473–488, 2009.

De Jong JC, Wermenbol AG, Verweij-Uijterwaal MW, et al: Adenoviruses from human immunodeficiency virus-infected individuals, including two strains that represent new candidate serotypes Ad50 and Ad51 of species B1 and D, respectively, *Journal of Clinical Microbiology* 37:3940–3945, 1999.

Echavarria M: Adenoviruses. In Zuckerman AJ, Banatvala JE, Griffiths PD, et al, editors: *Principles & Practice of Clinical Virology*, ed 6, Chichester, 2009, Wiley-Blackwell, pp 463–488.

Gray GC, Chorazy ML: Human adenovirus 14a: A new epidemic threat, *Journal of Inectious Diseases* 199:1413–1415, 2009.

Lenaerts L, De Clercq E, Naesens L: Clinical features and treatment of adenovirus infections, *Reviews in Medical Virology* 18:357–374, 2008.

Yamamoto M, Curiel DT: Current issues and future of oncolytic adenoviruses, *Molecular Therapy* 18:243–250, 2010.

# 43

# Herpesviruses

Herpes simplex; varicella and zoster; infectious mononucleosis;
B cell lymphomas; cytomegalovirus disease; exanthem subitum;
Kaposi's sarcoma; herpes B

*I. Johannessen and M. M. Ogilvie*

## KEY POINTS

- All herpesviruses persist for the lifetime of the host and establish a latent (non-replicating) state from which they may be reactivated under certain conditions.
- Cell-mediated immunity, especially the action of cytotoxic T lymphocytes, is essential in the control of herpesvirus infections.
- Acute necrotizing sporadic viral encephalitis caused by HSV is a medical emergency requiring urgent treatment with high-dose intravenous aciclovir that must be instigated empirically without delay and prior to laboratory confirmation.
- Genital herpes simplex may be due to HSV 1 or 2, and the individuals are often unaware that they have this recurring infection.
- A live-attenuated VZV vaccine can protect against chickenpox (varicella); it may boost immunity in older age groups with a reduction in the symptoms of zoster (shingles), which arises as a result of VZV reactivation.
- Glandular fever is a clinical presentation of primary EBV infection, mainly in the 15–25 years age group; most individuals have an asymptomatic infection in childhood.
- EBV is a recognized human tumour virus associated with certain epithelial and lymphoid tumours (e.g. B cell lymphoma post transplant).
- CMV is commonly acquired without symptoms; however, in the immunocompromised host, CMV disease is serious and merits prophylaxis or pre-emptive therapy.
- Less well known herpesviruses (HHV 6 and 7) cause a common childhood rash illness (exanthem subitum), whereas HHV 8 is associated with Kaposi's sarcoma.

Species-specific herpesviruses have been described for most animals and they share several features including their structure, mode of replication and the capacity to establish lifelong latent infections from which virus may be reactivated. Together, they form the herpesviridae family.

***Latent infection.*** Latency reflects persistent infection (as manifest by the presence of the viral genome) during which no infectious virus is produced, except during intermittent episodes of reactivation.

***Reactivation.*** Reactivation from the latent state may be restricted to asymptomatic virus shedding or manifest as clinical disease.

***Recurrence or recrudescence.*** These terms are used when reactivated virus produces clinically apparent disease.

The herpesviridae family is subdivided into 3 subfamilies: *alpha (α)-, beta (β)-* and *gamma (γ)-*herpesvirinae (see Table 43.1). The human α-herpesvirinae contain the genera *simplexvirus* (herpes simplex virus (HSV) 1 and 2) and *varicellovirus* (varicella zoster virus, VZV); the β-herpesvirinae consist of *cytomegalovirus* (cytomegalovirus, CMV) and *roseolovirus* (human herpes virus, HHV 6 and 7) genera; and the *γ-herpesvirinae* contain the *lymphocryptovirus* (Epstein–Barr virus, EBV) and *rhadinovirus* (Kaposi sarcoma-associated herpesvirus, KSHV) genera. Individual viruses are denoted by the taxonomic unit (family/subfamily) followed by an Arabic number (e.g. human herpesvirus (HHV) 4). However, vernacular and approved names are often used interchangeably (e.g. HHV 4 and EBV). At present, eight human herpesviruses (HHV 1–8) are recognized, and infection with each of HHV 1–7 has been shown to be common in all populations; studies with HHV 8 suggest it is an uncommon infection in developed countries. The herpes B virus of monkeys can be transmitted to man accidentally.

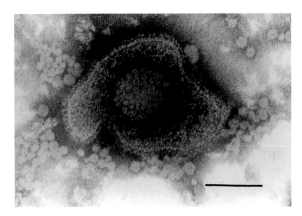

Fig. 43.1 Electron micrograph of HSV. Negative staining (2% phosphotungstic acid). Bar = 100 nm. (Prepared by Dr BW McBride.)

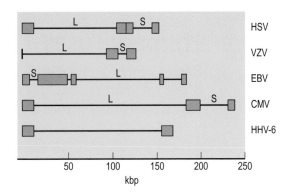

Fig. 43.2 Diagrammatic comparison of herpesvirus DNAs. Lines indicate long (L) and short (S) unique sequences, and repeated regions are boxed.

| Table 43.1 | Human herpesviruses (HHV) | | |
|---|---|---|---|
| Approved name | Vernacular name (see text) | Subfamily (-herpesvirinae) | Genus (-virus) |
| HHV 1 | HSV 1 | $\alpha_1$ | Simplex |
| HHV 2 | HSV 2 | $\alpha_1$ | Simplex |
| HHV 3 | VZV | $\alpha_2$ | Varicello |
| HHV 4 | EBV | $\gamma_1$ | Lymphocrypto |
| HHV 5 | CMV | $\beta_1$ | Cytomegalo |
| HHV 6 | – | $\beta_2$ | Roseolo |
| HHV 7 | – | $\beta_2$ | Roseolo |
| HHV 8 | KSHV | $\gamma_2$ | Rhadino |

## DESCRIPTION

Herpesviruses have a characteristic morphology (Fig. 43.1). The icosahedral protein capsid (average diameter 100 nm) consists of 162 hollow hexagonal and pentagonal capsomeres with an electron-dense core containing the DNA genome (together forming the *nucleocapsid*). Outside the capsid (in mature virus particles) is an amorphous proteinaceous layer, the *tegument*, surrounded by a lipid *envelope* derived from host cell membranes. Projecting from the trilaminar lipid host-derived envelope are *spikes* of viral glycoproteins. Cryo-electron micrographs indicate that the capsid is organized into at least three layers, with viral DNA inserted in the innermost layer. The average enveloped particle is approximately 200 nm in diameter.

The herpesvirus genome is linear double-stranded (ds) DNA that varies in length from 125–248 kbp with a base content ranging from 42–69 G+C mol% for the human herpesviruses. The presence of unique long and short ($U_L$, $U_S$) regions bounded by repeated and inverted short segments allows recombination

and isomeric forms in some cases (Fig. 43.2). Genes coding for viral glycoproteins, major capsid proteins, enzymes involved in DNA replication, and some transcripts associated with latency, have been identified. Conserved sequences appear in certain regions, and some genes show homology with regions of human chromosomes. Restriction endonuclease and genome sequence analysis permits epidemiological comparison of strains ('fingerprinting') within herpesvirus species.

Some herpesviruses are predominantly:

- neurotropic (HSV and VZV)
- lymphotropic (EBV, HHV 6 and 7).

## BIOLOGICAL CLASSIFICATION

Broad characteristics of the three herpes subfamilies include:

1. Alphaherpesvirinae (e.g. HSV, VZV and B virus): rapid growth in cultured cells, latency in sensory ganglia.
2. Betaherpesvirinae (e.g. CMV): slow growth in cultured cells, restricted host range.
3. Gammaherpesvirinae (e.g. EBV): growth in lymphoid cells.

The viruses are relatively thermo-labile and readily inactivated by lipid solvents such as alcohols and detergents.

## REPLICATION

After initial attachment of viral receptor-binding proteins to cell surface proteoglycans followed by specific binding to target cell receptors, the envelope of herpesviruses fuses with the cell membrane. The nucleocapsids cross the cytoplasm to the nuclear membrane; replication of viral DNA and assembly of capsids takes place within the nucleus. With HSV, it is known that the tegument proteins partake in transactivation of the first set of genes. Between 65 and 100 viral proteins are synthesized in an orderly sequence or cascade. Briefly, using HSV as an example, circularization of the herpesvirus genome in the cell nucleus results in the orderly transcription (by host RNA polymerase II) of a cascade of immediate early (IE; α), early (E; β) and late (L; γ) genes. IE proteins activate expression of E genes that include viral-derived enzymes (including DNA polymerase and thymidine kinase (TK)) involved in replication which is thought to proceed in a 'rolling circle' manner yielding a concatomer that is cut to genome-length DNA units. Induction by E gene products of L genes results in production of viral structural proteins that package around progeny DNA to give rise to new nucleocapsids.

The viral capsid proteins migrate from the cytoplasm to the nucleus where capsid assembly occurs, and new viral DNA is inserted and located in the inner shell. Viral glycoproteins are processed in the Golgi complex and incorporated into host cell membranes, from which the viral envelope is acquired, usually from the inner layer of the nuclear membrane as the virus buds out from the nucleus. It then passes by way of membranous vacuoles to reach the cell surface. Productively infected cells generally do not survive (*lytic infection*).

## HERPES SIMPLEX VIRUS

HSV is ubiquitous, infecting the majority of the world's population early in life and persisting in a latent form from which reactivation with shedding of infectious virus occurs, thus maintaining the transmission chain.

## DESCRIPTION

In contrast to other members of the group, HSV can be grown relatively easily in cells from a wide variety of animals so that far more extensive studies have been undertaken with this virus.

There are two distinct types of HSV: type 1 (HSV 1) and type 2 (HSV 2). These two types are generally (but not exclusively) associated with different sites of infection in patients (see below); type 1 strains are associated primarily with the mouth, eye and central nervous system (CNS), whereas type 2 strains are found most often in the genital tract.

### HSV glycoproteins

The envelope of HSV contains at least 11 glycoproteins. Three of the glycoproteins (g) are essential for production of infectious virus: gB and gD, which are involved in adsorption to and penetration into cells (alongside gC), and gH (together with gL), involved in fusion at entry and in the release of virus. Some of the glycoproteins have common antigenic determinants shared by HSV 1 and 2 (gB and gD) whereas others have specific determinants for one type only (gG).

## PATHOGENESIS

### Primary infection

The typical lesion produced by HSV is the *vesicle*, a ballooning degeneration of intra-epithelial cells, which contains infectious fluid. The basal epithelium is usually intact as vesicles penetrate the subepithelial layer only occasionally. The base of the vesicle contains multinucleate cells (*Tzanck cells*) and infected nuclei contain eosinophilic *inclusion bodies*. The roof of the vesicle breaks down and an ulcer forms. This happens rapidly on mucous membranes and non-keratinizing epithelia; on the skin, the ulcer crusts over, forming a scab, and then heals. A mononuclear cellular immune reaction is usual with the vesicle fluid becoming cloudy and cellular infiltration in the subepithelial tissue. After resorption, or loss, of the vesicle fluid, the damaged epithelium is regenerated. Natural killer (NK) cells play a significant role in early defence by recognizing and destroying HSV-infected cells. Herpesvirus glycoproteins synthesized during virus growth are inserted into host cell membranes, and some are secreted into extracellular fluid. The host's adaptive immune system responds to all these foreign antigens producing both cytotoxic (CD4$^+$ and CD8$^+$) and helper (CD4$^+$) T lymphocytes which activate primed B lymphocytes to produce specific antibodies, and are also involved in the induction of delayed hypersensitivity. The different glycoproteins have significant roles in generating these various cell responses; many induce neutralizing antibodies.

During the replication phase at the site of entry in the epithelium, virus particles enter the sensory nerve endings that penetrate to the parabasal layer of the epithelium and are transported, probably as nucleocapsids, along the axon to the nerve body (neurone) in the sensory (dorsal root) ganglion by retrograde axonal flow. Virus replication in a neurone ends in *lytic infection* and neuronal cell death; however, in some ganglion cells, a *latent infection* is established in which surviving neurones harbour the viral genome. Neurones other than those in sensory ganglia can be the site of herpesvirus latency. It is not clear whether true latency occurs at epithelial sites; there is some evidence of persistence of virus at peripheral sites, but this may be due to a reactivation with a low level of virus replication.

Antibody reduces the severity of infections although it does not prevent recurrences. Thus, neonates receiving maternal antibody transplacentally are protected against the worst effects of neonatal herpes. HSV 2 infection seems to protect against HSV 1, but previous HSV 1 infection only partly modifies HSV 2 disease.

## Latent infection

Latent infection of sensory neurones is a feature of the neurotropic herpesviruses, HSV and VZV; HSV 1 latency is the best understood. Only a small proportion (about 1%) of cells in the affected ganglion carry the viral genome as free circular episomes – estimated about 20 copies per infected cell. Very few virus genes are expressed in the latent state; in HSV, some viral RNA transcripts (latency-associated transcripts, LATs) are found in the nuclei, but no virus-encoded proteins have been demonstrated in the cells, so these infected neurones are not recognized by the immune system. Latent HSV genomes have been detected in post mortem studies on excised ganglia and other neuronal tissues. HSV 1 is regularly detected in:

- the trigeminal ganglion
- other sensory and autonomic ganglia (e.g. vagus)
- adrenal tissue and the brain.

HSV 2 latency in the sacral ganglia has been demonstrated. Either type may become latent in other ganglia.

## Reactivation and recrudescence

Reactivation processes are still not clearly understood. It is suggested that HSV DNA passes along the nerve axon back to the nerve ending where infection of epithelial cells may occur. Not all reactivation will result in a visible lesion; there may be asymptomatic shedding of virus only detectable by culture or DNA detection methods.

The factors influencing the development of recrudescent lesions are not yet clearly identified. An increase of CD8[+] T suppressor lymphocyte activity is common at the time of recurrences. Some mediators (e.g. prostaglandins), and a temporary decrease in immune effector cell function, particularly delayed hypersensitivity, may enhance spread of HSV. Certainly, the known triggers for recurrences are accompanied by a local increase in prostaglandin levels, and depression of cell-mediated immunity predisposes to herpes recurrence. The mechanism of reactivation is not known, but the event can be predicted accurately in those known to harbour latent virus. Thus, after bone marrow transplant, or high-dose chemotherapy, herpes simplex recurs in 80% of cases at a median interval of 18 days in the absence of prophylaxis.

In whatever way reactivation is achieved, it is a feature of HSV infection. It occurs naturally, and can be induced by a variety of stimuli such as:

- ultraviolet light (sunlight)
- fever
- trauma
- stress.

The interval between the stimulus and the appearance of a clinically obvious lesion is 2–5 days; this has been demonstrated regularly in patients undergoing neurological interference with their trigeminal ganglion, a common site of herpes latency.

## CLINICAL FEATURES

### Primary infection

Primary infection refers to the patient's initial acquisition of virus and, thus, occurs in those with no antibody against HSV (Table 43.2). It usually involves the mucous membranes of the mouth, but may include the lips, skin of the face, nose or any other site, including the eye and genital tract.

**Table 43.2** Types of herpes simplex virus (HSV) infection

| Type of infection | Antibody status of patient |
|---|---|
| *Primary*: first HSV infection (any type at any site) | Seronegative |
| *Latent*: no symptoms | Seropositive |
| *Recurrent*: recrudescence of the latent HSV type(s) | Seropositive |
| *Initial (non-primary)*: first episode of the heterologous HSV in a seropositive patient | Seronegative for infecting type; seropositive for latent type |
| *Re-infection (exogenous)*: with a strain that differs from the latent HSV type | Seropositive |

## Recurrence or recrudescence

Symptomatic recurrence is heralded by a prodrome in two-thirds of people, who experience pain or paresthesiae (tingling, warmth, itch) at the site followed by erythema and a papule, usually within 24 h. Progression to a vesicle and ulcer, with subsequent crusting, takes 8–12 days before natural healing occurs. Because of their association with febrile illness, the lesions are popularly known as *cold sores* or *fever blisters*. The most common sites are at the mucocutaneous junction of the lip (seldom inside the mouth), on the chin, or inside the nose. However, recurrent lesions can manifest at any site innervated by the affected neurone, determined by the site of initial infection.

Severe pain, extensive mucosal ulceration and delayed healing are features of recurrent herpes in severely immunocompromised patients. The ulcers provide entry for other infections. HSV viraemia after reactivation is uncommon, even in the immunocompromised individual, but can lead to disseminated infection in internal organs. Some sufferers experience *erythema multiforme* following their recurrent herpes, associated with reaction to certain herpes antigens; this may take the form of the Stevens–Johnson syndrome.

## Oral infection

Classically, primary HSV infection presents as an acute, febrile *gingivostomatitis* in pre-school children. Vesicular lesions ulcerate rapidly and are present in the front of the mouth and on the tongue (*stomatitis*). Gingivitis is usually present. Vesicles may also develop on the lips and skin around the mouth (*herpetic dermatitis*), and cervical lymphadenopathy can occur. The child is miserable for 7–10 days in an untreated case before the lesions heal. However, the majority of primary infections go unrecognized, the episode being attributed to teething or mistaken for 'thrush' (candida infection). In primary infection in older children and adults, there may also be an associated mononucleosis; pharyngitis is also notable. Viraemia with dissemination of HSV to internal organs is rare except in pregnancy (primary infection, with hepatitis), the neonate (see below), or the immunocompromised patient.

## Skin infection

### Herpetic whitlow

Hand infections with HSV are not uncommon, but other sites may be involved [e.g. as a result of sports such as *herpes gladiatorum* in wrestlers or rugby players (as a result of direct skin-to-skin contact)].

Three presentations of hand infections may be observed:

1. The classical primary lesion on the fingers or thumb of the toddler with herpetic stomatitis, due to autoinoculation.
2. Another classical and often primary infection is acquired by accidental inoculation in health-care workers (*traumatic herpes*). These infections may recur; the majority are HSV 1.
3. The most common hand lesions are recurrent, associated with HSV 2 and genital herpes, and are seen in young adults. Pain and swelling occur, and the vesicles become pustular, but, if in well keratinized areas, do not always ulcerate. Associated lymphangitis is common. Primary lesions take up to 21 days to heal, recurrent ones 10 days. Figure 43.3 shows recurrent lesions at an interval of 10 years.

### Eczema herpeticum

A severe form of cutaneous herpes may occur in children with atopic eczema – *eczema herpeticum* or *Kaposi's varicelliform eruption*. Vesicles resembling those of chickenpox may appear, mainly on already eczematous areas. Extensive ulceration results in protein loss and dehydration, and viraemia can lead to disseminated disease with severe, even fatal, consequences. A similar picture is seen occasionally in adults with pemphigus who develop herpes simplex. Patients with burns are also at risk. In each instance, early recognition and prompt antiviral therapy can be life-saving.

### Eye infection

HSV infection of the eye may be initiated during a childhood primary infection, or occur from transfer of virus from a cold sore. There may be periorbital *herpetic dermatitis* together with conjunctivitis, or keratoconjunctivitis associated with corneal ulceration. Typically, branching (dendritic) corneal ulcers are found. If these recur untreated, the result is corneal scarring and impairment of vision. More extensive ulceration occurs if steroids have been used, but deeper infiltrates are common in long-standing cases and benefit from combined steroid and antiviral therapy. The presence of typical herpes vesicles on eyelid margins is a useful clinical guide but is not always seen. The majority of eye infections are with HSV 1, and most patients with recurring eye disease are aged over 50 years. More than half of the corneal grafting performed in the UK is for HSV corneal

**Fig. 43.3** Herpetic whitlow on left index finger, photographed during recurrences in (A) 1984 and (B) 1994.

scarring, although the disease may recur in the graft. Acute retinal necrosis associated with HSV 1 or 2 is also recognized.

## Central nervous system infection

HSV may reach the brain in several ways. Viraemia has been detected during primary herpetic stomatitis, and infection may be carried within cells into the brain and meninges. Direct infection from the nasal mucosa along the olfactory tract is another possibility, but the most likely route is central spread from the trigeminal ganglia.

### HSV encephalitis

*Encephalitis* caused by HSV is a rare condition, but is the most common sporadic fatal encephalitis recognized in developed countries (1–2 cases per million population annually). The infection has a high mortality rate and significant morbidity in survivors of the acute necrotizing form. It presents:

- at any time of year
- at any age
- occasionally in the young, but more frequently in those aged 50–70 years.

Some 70% of cases are in people with serological evidence, and often a clinical history, of previous HSV infection. Recurrent lesions are seldom apparent at the same time as encephalitis. A prodrome of fever and malaise is followed by headache and behavioural change, sometimes associated with a sudden focal episode such as a seizure, or paralysis; coma usually precedes death. The temporal lobe is most frequently affected, and virus replication in neurones, followed by the oedema associated with the inflammatory response, accounts for the haemorrhagic necrosis and space-occupying nature of this form of the disease. More diffuse, milder disease has been recorded. Brainstem encephalitis is another serious manifestation.

Examination of cerebrospinal fluid (CSF) often demonstrates the presence of red cells and a lymphocytic response, but these findings are non-specific. Neuro-imaging can often suggest the diagnosis, the typical feature being the presence of focal lesions on CT or MRI (more sensitive) scans. Virus-specific diagnosis is considered below. Early clinical recognition, leading to prompt antiviral therapy, significantly reduces the 70% mortality rate and serious morbidity of untreated cases, but therapy must be started as soon as possible before confirmation of the diagnosis. HSV 1 is responsible for most cases of encephalitis where virus has been identified (outside the neonatal period; see below). HSV 2 encephalitis does occasionally occur in immunocompromised adults and may be seen more frequently in those infected with the human immunodeficiency virus (HIV).

### HSV meningitis

*Aseptic meningitis* caused by HSV is much less serious than encephalitis. HSV 2 is the usual cause and it reaches the CSF following radiculitis during genital herpes (see below). A lymphocytic reaction is seen in CSF, and there may be recurrent bouts of this meningitis (sometimes known as *Mollaret's meningitis*). HIV-infected patients may present with HSV meningitis.

## Genital tract infection

Both types of HSV can infect the genital tract. Although the more common association has been with type 2 virus, type 1 infection is not infrequent, particularly in young women, where it may account for more than half of genital infections. Genital infection may be acquired by autoinoculation from lesions elsewhere on the body, but most often results from intimate sexual contact, including oro-genital contact. The lesions are vesicular at first, but rapidly ulcerate.

- In the male, the glans and shaft of the penis are the most frequent sites of infection.
- In the female, the labia and vagina, or cervix, may be involved.
- In both sexes, lesions may spread to surrounding skin sites.

The incubation period is 2–20 days with an average of 7 days. A primary infection is usually the most severe, especially in women. Fever and malaise are accompanied by regional lymphadenopathy and urethritis, and vaginal discharge may be present. The whole episode lasts for 3–4 weeks, and high titres of virus are shed. In some cases, a lymphocytic meningitis develops, and urinary retention can also be a problem; these are manifestations of sacral radiculopathy. Where the infection is an initial genital herpes (but not a primary HSV) infection (see Table 43.2), the attack is generally less severe, but may still last for about 2 weeks.

## Recurrent genital herpes

This can be as frequent as six or more episodes a year. Although the attacks are milder and shorter than first

**Fig. 43.4** HSV 2 recurrence over the sacral region in an elderly patient.

episodes (around 7–10 days), the results are socially and psychologically distressing. Some patients experience prodromal symptoms in the distribution of the sacral nerves, but the patient is already infectious by this stage. Virus shedding from the genital tract is often asymptomatic. The patient or general practitioner may not recognize recurrent lesions as herpetic in origin, so that, in many instances, the risk of transmission to sexual partners is not appreciated. HSV 1 genital infection recurs less often than HSV 2, and, thus, carries a better prognosis. Either type is capable of transmission from mother to infant. Transplacental passage resulting in intra-uterine damage to the fetus has been recorded but is very rare, and probably limited to cases with substantial maternal viraemia. Ascending infection from the cervix may be more significant, especially when the membranes are ruptured for some time before delivery.

Genital herpes can be a significant problem in immunosuppressed patients, and may be seen as persistent, severe, peri-anal lesions (with or without proctitis) in many HIV-infected men that have sex with men (MSM). Genital herpetic ulcers are known to increase the risk of transmission of infection with HIV. Figure 43.4 shows recurrent HSV 2 over the sacrum in an elderly person; the latent virus in the sacral ganglion travels to the skin dermatome served as well as the internal mucosal site; the patient had been nursed on a rubber ring.

## Neonatal herpes

A rare (1.65 per 100 000 live births in the UK) but very serious infection, untreated neonatal herpes has a case fatality rate exceeding 60% with half of the survivors severely damaged. Virus, commonly HSV 2 (but this will vary according to a region's prevalence of HSV 1 infection of the genital tract), is acquired by passage through an infected genital tract. The greatest risk, with a 50% transmission rate (because there is more virus present and no transplacental antibody transfer has occurred), is when the mother has a primary HSV infection at the time of delivery. In contrast, with recurrent herpes at term, the transmission rate is only 5% or less.

Neonatal infection may present in 3 different ways:

1. *Skin, eye and mucous membrane (SEM) disease* at about 10–12 days post-partum. *Vesicular* lesions on the skin may be absent, or few in number, and are commonly located on the presenting part (e.g. the scalp; sites of trauma). Virus dissemination is the most serious complication and, without prompt antiviral treatment, disseminated disease (see below) will occur in 75% of cases with signs of general sepsis, including fever, poor feeding and irritability.
2. *Disseminated disease* presents during the first few days (often around day 6) of life with *pneumonitis* and *hepatitis* (manifest as hepatomegaly and jaundice) with or without signs of *aseptic* meningitis or encephalitis. Progressive liver failure with coagulopathy leads to death around day 16 in the most serious disseminated form.
3. *Encephalitis* (with or without dissemination to internal organs) manifests itself at around 2–3 weeks of age and, in the absence of prompt antiviral treatment, causes death or severe neurological morbidity.

Prompt high-dose antiviral therapy is the key to survival of the neonate with minimal morbidity, although local recurrent lesions can be expected, especially at skin sites, in the first year.

The prevention of neonatal herpes is difficult, the vast majority of infections occurring in babies born to women with no past history of genital herpes, and in whom the infection at term was either asymptomatic, or unrecognized clinically. Routine pre-term screening for virus shedding, particularly as applied to those with a past history, does not predict babies at risk. With the availability of type-specific antibody tests, susceptible women at risk of acquiring HSV 2 from partners can be identified. The discovery of lesions compatible with primary HSV infection during pregnancy necessitates consideration of antiviral therapy for the mother and (when occurring during the latter stages of pregnancy) caesarean section. If suspicious lesions are seen during labour, swabs (in virus transport medium, VTM) for virus culture and/or DNA amplification by PCR should be taken. Caesarean section may reduce the risk of infection if performed in the early stages of labour (before rupture of membranes, or shortly thereafter). However, if the mother is known to have moderate levels of antibody, the baby is unlikely to develop the disease.

Some cases of neonatal herpes are acquired just after birth from contact with sources of HSV other than the mother's genital tract. The clinical presentation is similar, although the virus is likely to be HSV 1 from oral or skin lesions of attendants or relatives.

In a case of suspected neonatal herpes, nasopharyngeal secretions, swabs (in VTM) from the skin, mouth and conjunctiva alongside CSF, urine and blood samples should be cultured and/or analysed by PCR.

## LABORATORY DIAGNOSIS

Virus detection (by culture and/or PCR) and serological studies both have their place in the diagnosis of infection with HSV. In all instances of acute infection, be it primary or recurrent, virus detection (e.g. using direct vesicle swabs sent in VTM) is the method of choice, as antibody responses are much less informative. Indeed, in recurrent episodes, the antibody titre may not vary. However, sensitive assays for immunoglobulin (Ig) G antibody, including type-specific antibody, have an important place in prospective testing.

### Herpesvirus detection

Direct diagnosis of HSV infection is available and should be sought in cases where there is any doubt as to the clinical diagnosis, or where rapid confirmation is required to guide the choice of therapy or other management.

Detection of viral DNA by PCR is the most sensitive and specific method of diagnosis. The two HSV types can be differentiated by using either type-specific primers in the PCR, or common primers followed by analysis with restriction enzymes or hybridization probes for each type.

Isolation of HSV is carried out in cultures of human diploid fibroblast cells. Growth is rapid, and within 24 h a *cytopathic effect* (CPE) may be visible, presenting as rounded, ballooned cells in foci that later expand and eventually involve the whole cell sheet. Virus is released from infected cells into the culture fluid – hence, the rapid spread of infection.

Herpesvirus particles may be demonstrated by electron microscope (EM) analysis of vesicle fluid or tissue preparations. Detection of viral antigens in cells by immunostaining (the use of labelled monoclonal antibodies directed against viral antigens) provides a rapid diagnosis on cells scraped from the base of lesions. In the most serious infections, easy access to the site of infection may not be possible.

## Antibody tests for HSV

Complement fixation tests (CFTs) are useful in the diagnosis of primary infections, when a significant change in antibody titre can be expected, but the assays are not widely available any longer in the UK. In the case of herpes encephalitis, a serological diagnosis depends on the demonstration of intrathecal synthesis of antibody to HSV. CFTs can be used, testing serum and CSF in parallel against HSV antigens and another unrelated antigen. In health, there is no antibody detectable by such tests in the CSF. If the serum antibody to CSF antibody ratio is diminished from the normal 200 : 1 to 40 : 1 (or less), and the blood–CSF barrier integrity is confirmed by other antibody (or albumin) being excluded from the CSF, intrathecal antibody synthesis is demonstrated. It is also helpful to check for the possible transfer of antibody from blood to CSF by means of an IgG index performed on the same serum and CSF samples. Tests on serum alone cannot confirm herpes encephalitis.

Enzyme immuno-assays (EIAs) are much more sensitive and specific than CFTs. When type-specific antigen preparations based on gG are used, type-specific antibody can be detected. Therapy often results in delayed appearance of these type-specific antibodies, and late convalescent samples (at 6 weeks) should be included.

## TREATMENT

Specific antiviral therapy has revolutionized the management of HSV infections over the past 30 years. Before the development of agents suitable for systemic use, topical application of the relatively non-selective idoxuridine was used successfully in the treatment of eye and skin infections. Aciclovir has a better therapeutic ratio and proven efficacy, when used early enough in appropriate dosage, for the whole range of acute HSV infections. Latency is not eradicated by this agent, which inhibits viral DNA synthesis. Aciclovir can also be used prophylactically to prevent reactivation in the immunocompromised individual, and long-term suppressive therapy has been particularly successful in the management of frequently recurring genital herpes and HSV-related erythema

multiforme. Patient-initiated early treatment can also abort or modify recurrences.

Aciclovir is the most widely used treatment for HSV, and the drug has an excellent safety record; it is available in preparations for topical, oral and intravenous use. It can be used in pregnancy as there is no evidence of adverse effects in infants of treated women although such use is not specifically licensed in the UK and, thus, requires careful risk assessment. Topical cream or ointment is suitable only for mild epithelial lesions, such as recurrent cold sores. Oral or intravenous therapy with aciclovir should be given for:

- any lesions that are not simply mild and superficial ones
- HSV-associated disease in the immunocompromised host
- CNS and systemic infection (intravenous therapy is required)
- any of the serious manifestations of HSV disease.

Dosage varies considerably, depending on the site of infection and whether the aim is suppression of recurrence, or therapy of established disease. Because the level of aciclovir achieved in the CSF is only half that in plasma, the dosage for the treatment of encephalitis has to be twice that for other systemic disease. Therapy must be maintained until clinical signs indicate a favourable response. In serious systemic disease, or in the severely immunocompromised host, therapy is continued for 2–3 weeks, or longer. In the neonate, 3 weeks' therapy at a higher (intravenous) dose should be followed by suppressive oral treatment for 6–12 months.

The poor bio-availability of oral aciclovir has led to the development of a pro-drug, valaciclovir, which is rapidly converted into aciclovir, producing significantly higher plasma levels after oral dosage. Another effective antiherpes agent, penciclovir, is given in the form of an oral pro-drug, famciclovir. Both of these agents are licensed for treatment of genital herpes, and may be administered less frequently than aciclovir.

Resistance to aciclovir can develop. The most common forms are HSV strains with deficient or altered virus-encoded thymidine kinase (TK); hence they cannot phosphorylate aciclovir to a monophosphate form which is key to further phosphorylation by cellular kinases into the triphospate active form. This has not been a significant clinical problem but it must be remembered, particularly in the severely immunocompromised host (e.g. acquired immune deficiency syndrome (AIDS), or following bone marrow transplant). A few resistant viruses with altered virus-encoded DNA polymerase have also been isolated and associated with clinical disease. With widespread use of aciclovir, more resistant strains may arise, and monitoring of the antiviral sensitivity of HSV isolates may be necessary. Strains resistant to aciclovir are generally also resistant to famciclovir, and foscarnet may be used as it does not require activation by viral TK.

## EPIDEMIOLOGY

HSV is probably transferred by direct contact with vesicular lesions and/or infectious fluid. Many children, especially in over-crowded conditions, acquire oral HSV 1 infections in the first years of life. Spread may not occur so readily in better social conditions with the result that primary infection is often delayed into young adulthood in developed countries. This is the usual time of exposure to genital herpes and, as a result, primary infections may be HSV 2 or HSV 1.

Sensitive EIAs, and type-specific assays, have shown that:

- some 60–90% of adults have had an HSV 1 infection
- many more adults have had HSV 2 infection than give a history of genital herpes.

Neonatal herpes is a rare complication in the UK. The rate of cases has increased in some populations as genital herpes has become more common.

## CONTROL

Transmission of herpes simplex can be reduced by:

- alleviating over-crowding
- simple hygiene measures (e.g. attention to adequate hand hygiene)
- education regarding the infectious stages
- the use of condoms.

Reference has already been made to the prevention of neonatal infection as has the use of prophylactic antiviral regimens to control predictable recurrence. Progress in understanding latency and reactivation will provide approaches to preventing reactivation. Protection from ultraviolet light, and the use of inhibitors of prostaglandin synthesis, may be useful in this context.

Experimental vaccines are under investigation, but none is licensed for use. Research into subunit vaccines based on the viral glycoproteins, or other significant viral proteins, may lead to an appropriate preparation to elicit the immune responses important in control of HSV. Recent trials have shown limited protection against genital tract disease. A vaccine that stimulates T cell immune responses may be required.

## VARICELLA–ZOSTER VIRUS (VZV)

Infection with VZV presents in two forms:

1. Primary infection: *varicella* (or chickenpox) is a generalized eruption.
2. Reactivated infection: *zoster* (or shingles) is localized to one (or a few) dermatomes.

## DESCRIPTION

The viruses isolated from varicella and zoster are identical. The virus has the morphology of all herpesviruses. Seventy genes code for 67 different proteins, including five families of glycoprotein genes. The glycoproteins gE, gB and gH are abundant in infected cells, and are present in the viral envelope (Fig. 43.5).

Following attachment (mediated primarily by gB) to cell surface glycosaminoglycans and fusion, the nucleocapsid enters the cell and viral DNA is released into the nucleus where virus replication takes place. Histological examination of infected epidermis reveals typical nuclear inclusions and multinucleate giant

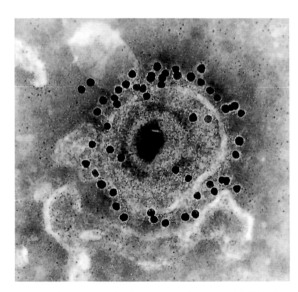

**Fig. 43.5** VZV showing the virus envelope glycoprotein I (gE) labelled with monoclonal antibody and goat anti-mouse IgG conjugated with 15 nm colloidal gold (original magnification ×150 000). (Micrograph taken by C. Graham, supplied by Dr E Dermott, Department of Microbiology and Immunobiology, Queen's University, Belfast, UK.)

cells identical to those of HSV. Human fibroblast cell cultures are most often used for isolation. Enveloped virus released from the nucleus remains closely attached to microvilli along the cell surface; studies of this 'cell-associated' characteristic, with infection being passed from cell to cell, have been limited compared with studies of the lytic HSV. The typical CPE appears in cell cultures in 3 days to 2–3 weeks.

Recently, the presence of geographically distinct VZV genotypes has been described, but little is known about the clinical significance of these findings. Antibodies to the three main glycoproteins all neutralize virus infectivity. One of these glycoproteins, gB, shares 49% amino acid identity with the gB of HSV, and this may account for the cross-reactive, anamnestic, antibody response that may be detected during infections with either virus.

## PATHOGENESIS

### Varicella

This is a disease predominantly of children characterized by a vesicular skin eruption (*chickenpox;* the origin of the term is unclear: from *chickpea* (the bean; refers to the look of the lesion) or the Old English term *gican* ('to itch')). Virus enters through the upper respiratory tract or conjunctivae, and may multiply in local lymph tissue for a few days before entering the blood and being distributed throughout the body. After replication in reticulo-endothelial sites, a second viraemic stage precedes the appearance of the skin and mucosal lesions. An alternative model has been proposed, based on studies in a humanised severe combined immunodeficient (hu-SCID) mouse model (bearing human skin xenografts). The work showed that activated human tonsillar T lymphocytes could be infected and, if given to the mice intravenously, homed rapidly to the skin grafts where VZV could be detected by 7 days (although the typical epidermal vesicular lesion did not appear for 10–21 days).

The VZV vesicles lie in the middle of the epidermis, and the fluid contains numerous free virus particles. Within 3 days, the fluid becomes cloudy with the influx of leukocytes; fibrin and interferon are also present. The pustules then dry up, scabs form, and they desquamate. Lesions in all stages are present at any one time while new ones are appearing. The clearance of virus-infected cells is dependent on functional T lymphocyte-mediated immune mechanisms and antibody-dependent cell cytotoxicity (ADCC). Persons deficient in these responses, and in interferon production, have prolonged vesicular phases and great difficulty in controlling the infection.

### Zoster

The pathogenesis of zoster (*shingles*) is not so well established as that of HSV recurrence. The latent virus is found in neurones and satellite cells in sensory ganglia, and more than one region of the genome is transcribed, although the state of the latent VZV is largely unknown. It seems likely that virus reaches the ganglion from the periphery by travelling up nerve axons, as HSV does, but there is also the possibility that, during viraemia, some virus enters ganglion cells. Another difference from HSV latency lies in the persistent VZV expression that has been detected in some mononuclear cells; this may have a role in VZV disease such as post-herpetic neuralgia (see below).

Reactivation of VZV as zoster can occur at any age in a person who has had a primary infection, which may or may not have been apparent clinically. The rate is greatest in persons aged ≥60 years and, as most primary infection takes place before the age of 20 years, there is usually a latent period of several decades. However, a much shorter latent period is seen in immunocompromised patients, and also in those who acquired primary infection in utero (see below) or in the first year of life. More than one episode of zoster is uncommon in any individual. The stimulus to reactivation is largely unknown, but virus travels from sensory ganglia to the peripheral site. Zoster is usually limited to one dermatome; in adults, this is most commonly in the thoracic or upper lumbar regions, or in the area supplied by the ophthalmic division of the trigeminal nerve. It is thought that this distribution is related to the density of the original varicella rash. There are associations with preceding trauma to the dermatome – injury or injections – with an interval of 2–3 weeks before the zoster appears. There is an associated suppression of specific T cell-mediated responses in acute zoster, but rapid secondary antibody responses are usually found. Reactivation occurs more commonly in T cell immunodeficiency states.

Viraemia may occur in the course of zoster but is unusual with pre-existing immunity normally being boosted rapidly. In the immunocompromised host, however, viraemia may lead to dissemination of zoster, either to internal organs or in a generalized manner reminiscent of varicella ('*disseminated zoster*').

## CLINICAL FEATURES

### Varicella

The incubation period averages 14–15 days but may range from 10 to 21 days. The patient is infectious for

2 days before, and for some days after, onset, while new vesicles are appearing and until all vesicles have crusted over.

The rash of varicella (*chickenpox*) is usually centripetal, being most dense on the trunk and head. Initially macular, the rash rapidly evolves through papules to the characteristic clear vesicles ('dew drops').

Presentations vary widely – from the clinically inapparent through to a severe febrile illness with a widespread itchy rash, especially in secondary cases in older members of a household. Usually a relatively mild infection in the young child, the complications of varicella, much more likely in adults, may cause significant morbidity and even mortality.

In the past, the main differential diagnosis was *smallpox* (Table 43.3). Another possibility is *monkeypox* if the travel or occupational history (or exotic pet handling) is suggestive of such exposure.

Secondary bacterial infection of skin lesions is the most common complication of varicella, mainly in the young child, and increases the amount of residual scarring. *Thrombocytopaenic* purpura occurs, especially in the immunocompromised host, and this may lead to *haemorrhagic chickenpox* which is life-threatening. A variety of organs may rarely be affected producing *arthritis,* myocarditis, *hepatitis*, glomerulonephritis and/or appendicitis. However, the two most frequent problems are related to the lungs and the CNS.

## Pneumonia

VZV pneumonitis is a serious complication, even in immunocompetent individuals. It is more likely to occur in adults, smokers, pregnant women, and immunocompromised hosts. Severity may vary from subclinical (evident only on radiography) to lifethreatening. Cough, dyspnoea, tachypnoea and chest pains begin a few days after the rash. Nodular infiltrates are seen in the lungs radiologically. Prompt antiviral therapy (see below) must be used in sufficient dosage and started at the first sign of pneumonia. Early investigations (imaging and gas exchange) are indicated in all smokers and immunocompromised patients with chickenpox.

## Central nervous system

Neurological complications include the common but benign cerebellar ataxia syndrome, and *aseptic meningitis.* Acute encephalitis is rare but more serious, and occurs mostly in the immunocompromised host. It may be confused with post-infectious *encephalopathy*, which, with other post-infectious manifestations such as transverse myelitis or Guillain–Barré syndrome, is immunologically mediated and not related to viral cytopathogenicity.

## Varicella in pregnancy

VZV can cross the placenta following maternal viraemia and infect the fetus. The infection may be more serious for the mother herself in pregnancy, with pneumonia being the major problem. Two types of intra-uterine infection are noted:

1. *Congenital varicella syndrome* (CVS) is a rare consequence of fetal infection in the first half of pregnancy (<1% of fetuses if maternal infection occurs during first 12 weeks of gestation; 2% if maternal infection occurs during 13–20 weeks of gestation). The characteristic features, usually unilateral, are scarring of the skin, damage to the musculoskeletal system (muscular atrophy, hypoplasia of the limbs, rudimentary or missing digits), as well as to the CNS (cortical atrophy, psychomotor retardation) and eyes (chorioretinitis, cataracts). Fetal infection is not inevitable. Silent intra-uterine infection can also occur: no damage is seen, but the baby is born with latent VZV infection, which may manifest as zoster in the first year of life.
2. *Neonatal varicella* is defined as varicella developing within the first 4 weeks of life, usually acquired from maternal varicella in late pregnancy (although, rarely, the exposure may occur post-natally, e.g. to an older sibling with chickenpox). The interval between maternal viraemia and delivery is important. If the maternal rash begins 7 days or more before delivery, her antibody response will have

**Table 43.3** Key differences between rashes of varicella and smallpox

| Feature | Varicella | Smallpox |
|---|---|---|
| Characteristic lesions | Blisters: domed small superficial single vesicles with clear fluid | Several layers of cells cover multifocal vesicles; early umbilication seen |
| Distribution | Centripetal: most on trunk, neck, face, proximal parts of limbs | Centrifugal: face, forearms and palms, soles of feet |
| Appearance at any one time | Pleomorphic: papules, vesicles and crusts may all be seen in one area | Lesions all at same stage in one affected area |

developed and been transferred across the placenta so that the baby does not develop disease. However, the infant is at serious risk if maternal varicella occurs 6 days or less before, or up to 2 days after, delivery; this allows viraemic spread across the placenta, before antibody is made and transferred to the baby. Because the usual respiratory entry route has been bypassed, the incubation period is reduced to (on average) 10 days. If infection arises, serious (and even fatal) disseminated disease may develop including pneumonitis and encephalitis. Such exposed neonates should be given passive immunization (see below) and consideration of prompt antiviral therapy, as should neonates of seronegative mothers exposed to any other source of VZV within the first 4 weeks of life.

## Zoster

This is the manifestation of reactivated VZV infection. *Zoster* takes the form of a localized eruption, is unilateral, and typically confined to one dermatome. Prodromal paresthesiae and pain in the area supplied by the affected sensory nerve are common before the skin lesions develop; these are identical to those of varicella except in their distribution. The evolution of the rash is similar, with some new vesicles appearing whilst the earliest ones are crusting; however, the whole episode in the majority of cases is confined to the affected dermatome and heals in 1–3 weeks. Acute pain is not always a feature, but its presence should alert to the possibility of zoster, and a search for early lesions, perhaps internal, is indicated. Occasionally there are no skin lesions – 'zoster sine herpete'.

*Disseminated* zoster is indicated by lesions appearing in the skin at distant sites (resembling the clinical picture of chickenpox) or, more seriously, by involvement of internal organs such as the lung and CNS (*meningitis, encephalitis* or *myelitis*). In the immunocompromised host, this results in severe disease with occasional fatalities. Patients with internal organ zoster may or may not present with a typical skin rash.

### Post-herpetic neuralgia

This is the most common complication of zoster, a risk in 50% of patients aged over 60 years, and results in significant morbidity in around 20% of cases. It is defined as intractable pain persisting for 1 month or more after the skin rash. Constant pain at the site, or stabbing pains or paraesthesiae, may continue for 1 year, or much longer in a number of individuals. This is an exhausting and disabling condition for which no satisfactory cure has been found; adequate early antiviral therapy may reduce the incidence.

### Ophthalmic zoster

Involvement of the ophthalmic division of the trigeminal nerve occurs in up to one-quarter of zoster episodes, with ocular complications in more than half of the patients. Corneal ulceration, stromal keratitis and *anterior* uveitis may result in permanent scarring, so this complication may threaten sight when the nasociliary branch is involved. Ocular complications are reduced in patients given oral aciclovir early in ophthalmic zoster. Occasionally, acute retinal necrosis is identified.

A contralateral hemiparesis due to granulomatous cerebral angiitis in the weeks following acute ophthalmic zoster is a recognized neurological complication. A more acute one, such as the *Ramsay–Hunt syndrome* (facial palsy with aural zoster vesicles), suggests that motor neurones can also be involved. Sympathetic ganglia may also be the site of latency, as indicated by cases in which the initial recrudescence has been in gastric mucosa with subsequent dissemination.

### Recurrent and chronic VZV

Immunocompromised individuals, most particularly those with CD4+ T cell lymphopenia due to HIV infection, may develop recurrent and chronic VZV infection. New lesions continue to appear, or re-appear after aciclovir therapy, often presenting an atypical hyperkeratotic appearance. Aciclovir-resistant VZV has been isolated in this situation.

## LABORATORY DIAGNOSIS

Typical presentations of varicella or zoster seldom need laboratory confirmation; however, atypical presentations merit investigation, especially in the immunocompromised host. Vesicular rashes due to enterovirus are sometimes confused with varicella and, in immunosuppressed individuals, various vesicular lesions may be mistaken for zoster. Localized vesicular lesions other than those on the face or genitalia are commonly misdiagnosed as due to zoster (see Fig. 43.4); many are due to recurrence of HSV, and this is readily shown by antigen detection and virus isolation, or by PCR. Thus, the approach to testing of vesicular lesions usually involves simultaneous HSV and VZV assessment by PCR.

## Virus detection

Early vesicular lesions provide the best diagnostic material. Vesicle fluid is collected in a capillary tube, aspirated with a fine needle and syringe, or lesions are swabbed directly (and sent in VTM). Direct examination by EM will reveal herpes particles; some of the fluid can be diluted in VTM and inoculated into tissue culture for virus isolation which takes between 5 days and 3 weeks. More rapid detection is possible with centrifugation-enhanced cultures ('shell vials'). If cells swabbed from the base of lesions are available, or biopsy tissue, virus antigens may be sought by immunostaining assays. VZV DNA amplification by PCR is used for the detection of VZV in CSF or aqueous humour, and routinely now for all types of samples. The latter two methods (immunostaining and PCR) are the ones most used for rapid diagnosis.

## Serological diagnosis

Antibody testing with VZV antigens can confirm a diagnosis of varicella by demonstration of seroconversion or rising titres of antibody between acute and convalescent serum samples; CFTs are still useful for this purpose but are not widely available any longer. CFTs are not sufficiently sensitive to determine past infection and, to assess immune status, assays need to be based on enzyme or radiolabelled methods, or immunostaining of infected cells. IgM to VZV is detectable by IgM capture systems in both varicella and zoster, appearing early in zoster. It is increasingly common to test for past infection (and therefore immunity) by measuring IgG antibody to VZV in those who are, or will become, immunocompromised, in women exposed antenatally to VZV, or in healthcare workers (or other adults) who are to be offered VZV immunization (see below).

## TREATMENT

VZV is not as sensitive to aciclovir as HSV, with 50% inhibitory dose ($ID_{50}$) values ranging from 4–17 μM aciclovir compared with 0.1–1.6 μM for HSV. This means that frequent high-dose oral or intravenous therapy is required against the virus. High-dose aciclovir given intravenously is effective in the treatment of varicella and zoster in the immunocompromised host. Oral aciclovir can be used to accelerate healing and reduce new lesion formation during zoster in immunocompetent patients if given early enough and may lower the rate of postherpetic neuralgia. Alternative preparations such as valaciclovir and famciclovir require less frequent dosing. Trials have shown that high-dose oral aciclovir shortens the course of varicella in immunocompetent children by 1 day if commenced within 24 h of the onset of the rash. The practical difficulties of achieving such an early start of treatment rule out routine use of aciclovir for all cases of varicella in immunocompetent children, but consideration should be given to treating all adults, and (where possible) adolescents and family contact cases who are known to develop more extensive disease. Treatment of VZV infection is given primarily to all 'high risk of complication' groups and should, thus, be considered for:

- neonates (within the first 4 weeks of life)
- immunocompromised patients
- those with ophthalmic zoster
- healthy individuals with varicella when there is an additional complicating factor such as pneumonia.

## EPIDEMIOLOGY

Varicella is partly seasonal, being spread mainly by the respiratory route in winter and early spring. Some cases result from contact with zoster and occur sporadically in any season. Varicella is highly infectious to susceptible close contacts (as a result of respiratory spread), as in a household; a past history of varicella is a good indicator of immunity since the clinical picture is quite distinct. The majority of children contract VZV between the ages of 4 and 10 years in western countries with around 8% of young adults remaining susceptible (Fig. 43.6). However, a much higher proportion of young adults remain susceptible in sub-tropical countries (for reasons that are not entirely clear). The rate of *pneumonitis* as a complication of varicella is surprisingly high in otherwise healthy adults (1 in 200; in children, the figure is 1 in 200 000), particularly pregnant women and smokers, who develop pneumonia in up to 10% of cases. Adult VZV pneumonitis may prove fatal without prompt antiviral therapy. Zoster is associated with decreased T cell function, and occurs with increased incidence in:

- old age
- the pre-AIDS phase of HIV infection
- organ transplant recipients
- patients receiving chemotherapy or radiotherapy for lymphoid malignancies.

In developed countries, the increasing survival of people beyond 65 years of age means that the incidence of zoster will increase. This may be exacerbated

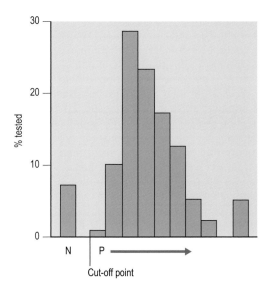

**Fig. 43.6** Distribution of antibody (IgG) to VZV in a young adult population (southern England). The proportion confirmed as negative (N) was 7.8%. P →, increasingly positive result.

by less natural boosting of immune responses as VZV decreases in countries offering childhood immunization for varicella.

## CONTROL

### Passive immunization

Passive immunity is partly protective for varicella as seen in infants with maternal antibody or patients given *varicella–zoster immunoglobulin* (VZIG) within 72 h of exposure. VZIG (in the UK), or another similar high-titre antibody preparation, is available for neonates, non-immune pregnant contacts, or immunocompromised contacts, of VZV. As most pregnant contacts will be immune, testing for VZV IgG antibody after exposure may prevent unnecessary use of costly VZIG. Current preparations seldom prevent infection, but do ameliorate disease. Importantly, VZIG reduces the rate of transmission to the fetus.

### Varicella vaccine

A live-attenuated varicella vaccine has been in use for some years in Japan and some European countries and was approved in the USA for routine childhood immunization in 1995. The vaccine strain (Oka), which can be distinguished from wild-type VZV by molecular analysis, is given by intramuscular injection. The vaccine is immunogenic in children with leukaemia in

remission and in healthy children and adults; vaccinees have resisted infection on close exposure to varicella. Some symptoms are noted around 10 days post-vaccination, and vesicles appear at the site of injection in up to 5% of individuals. Immunization does not prevent latency developing; however, the incidence of zoster in vaccinees compared with that in the naturally infected is not increased. In the USA, surveillance has confirmed a significant reduction in the incidence of varicella, especially in the 1–4 years age group, and a substantial fall in the mortality and complication rates. There have been reports of 'breakthrough' epidemics locally, even in well vaccinated cohorts, and a booster dose may be necessary. A large trial of vaccination in the elderly (over 60 years old) showed a 60% reduction in the incidence of zoster and post-herpetic neuralgia in those immunized with a high-titre preparation of Oka virus-based vaccine. Currently, in the UK, the VZV vaccine is not offered as part of the childhood immunization programme but, instead, to susceptible individuals who are in regular contact with those at risk of developing serious VZV illness. Thus, the vaccine is offered to non-immune health-care workers and healthy contacts of immunocompromised patients. The primary course consists of two vaccine doses administered 4–8 weeks apart.

## EPSTEIN–BARR VIRUS

In 1964, Epstein, Barr and Achong described herpesvirus particles in cells from a lymphoma in African children studied by Burkitt, who suspected an infectious aetiology of the tumour. The link between the new herpesvirus, denoted *Epstein–Barr virus* (EBV), and a variety of epithelial and lymphoid tumours is now clear. Primary infection with EBV

- is most often acquired in childhood when it is generally *asymptomatic*
- gives rise to infectious mononucleosis (also known as *glandular fever*) in up to a quarter of individuals when infection is delayed into adolescence.

Man is the only natural host, but EBV infection can be transmitted experimentally to some non-human (New World) primates (tamarin, marmoset; Old World primates are naturally immune as a result of infection with simian EBV homologues).

## DESCRIPTION

The characteristic morphology of EBV seen on EM is that of a herpesvirus. EBV cannot be grown in human fibroblast or epithelial cell lines and there is no completely productive or permissive system for culture of EBV. This lymphotropic virus is classified in the *gammaherpesvirinae* subfamily, genus *lymphocryptovirus*.

## REPLICATION

The full replication (productive, or lytic) cycle of EBV can take place in certain differentiated epithelial cells although it is not clear whether this is part of the natural life cycle of EBV infection in the human host. The B lymphocyte is the principal and essential cell infected through attachment of the major viral envelope glycoprotein gp350/220 to EBV receptors (primarily, the CD21 molecule) expressed on mature resting B lymphocytes. There are other receptors on cells of stratified squamous epithelium (e.g. in the oropharynx and ectocervix) and these epithelial cells can be infected through their basal aspect. Viral production is restricted to the differentiated cells of the granular layer and above, and virus is shed from the superficial cells. It is difficult to grow differentiating epithelia in culture, and most work on the lytic cycle of EBV has been done in B lymphoblastoid cell lines (BLCLs) in which a small proportion of the EBV-infected cells can be induced to produce virus.

The organization of the EBV genome differs from that of HSV, and some genes are present in one and not in the other. Approximately 80 proteins are encoded; many glycoproteins (gp) are known, including the major gp350/220, which mediates attachment to CD21, as well as gp25, gp42 and gp85, which bind a co-receptor (MHC class 2 molecules) on the target cell and are involved in membrane fusion. The latent (non-productive) state of EBV infection is established in a subset of resting memory B lymphocytes in which the EBV genome is maintained in the nucleus as multiple full-length covalently closed circular episomes. Specific EBV-encoded small RNA species (EBERs) are found in all cells infected with the virus. A variable number of EBV genes are expressed in the different forms of the latent state. These are principally genes coding for one or more of six EBV nuclear antigens (EBNA leader protein (LP), 1, 2, 3a-c) and two latent membrane proteins (LMP 1, 2). EBNA 1 maintains the EBV episome as the B cells divide, and is the only latent protein expressed in all types of EBV-associated tumours (see below). EBNA 2 and LMP 1 are both viral oncogenes that promote B cell proliferation. Latency involves different expression patterns of these latent viral proteins: all are expressed by BLCLs in culture as well as at the outset of primary EBV infection (*unrestricted latency*) which is followed by down-regulation of some, or all, of them (*restricted latency*) in the course of infection. Whilst all the lytic and latent proteins are involved in recognition by EBV-specific T cells that mediate immune control of the virus, such down-regulation of latent genes is one mechanism that facilitates persistent infection and immune evasion. An unrestricted latent virus expression profile is observed during infectious mononucleosis and in EBV-associated post-transplant lymphoproliferative disease whilst more restricted patterns are seen in other malignancies associated with this virus (see below). Interestingly, EBV encodes a homologue of interleukin (IL) 10 (viral IL 10, vIL10) that may play a role in immune modulation.

Although there are two types of EBV, type 1 and 2, their disease association is similar and no unique clinical significance has been attributed to either type.

The full lytic cycle of EBV replication is accompanied by the production of a large number of lytic proteins that include virus structural antigens resulting in the assembly of progeny virus. Although EBV does encode a viral TK, aciclovir is phosphorylated by cellular kinases in cells producing EBV. The viral DNA polymerase is sensitive to the active aciclovir triphosphate, and treatment with aciclovir reduces EBV production (at least *in vitro*) but has no effect on latency or the B cell proliferation induced by the virus.

## PATHOGENESIS

In primary infection, virus in saliva is thought to infect oropharyngeal B lymphocytes in tonsillar crypts, and the exact role of epithelial cells in the process is still unclear. This leads to activation of the infected cells, which progress to the local lymph nodes and on through the circulation with the potential to enter a productive (lytic) phase and release of progeny virus elsewhere in the body. Most shedding of virus takes place in the oral cavity (epithelial cells may have a role in this aspect of infection), and EBV can be detected regularly in the saliva of asymptomatic hosts, the amount increasing in immunosuppressed states.

Activated B lymphocytes secrete immunoglobulin, and EBV is a potent polyclonal activator of antibody production by B cells, independent of any accessory cells.

Recovery from primary EBV infection is associated with humoral and, primarily, cellular immune responses involving T cells; any delay in cellular control, or over-vigorous responses, will contribute to the severity of the infection. Thus, large initial infective doses may result in high numbers of circulating infected B lymphocytes followed by a marked T cell

**Fig. 43.7** Appearance and duration of diagnostic antibodies following primary EBV infection. EBNA, EBV nuclear antigen; VCA, viral capsid antigen.

response. The polyclonal B cell activation results in the transient appearance of a variety of antibodies (predominantly IgM), both autophile and heterophile. The cellular response is detected as a mononucleosis with large numbers of atypical *lymphocytes* in blood and infiltrating tissues that are EBV-specific T cells.

Antibody responses after EBV infection follow a characteristic pattern, with the initial IgM response to virus capsid antigens (VCA) persisting for some months. The latent EBNA complex elicits antibodies in late convalescence only, perhaps after release from B cells lysed by EBV-specific T cells (Fig. 43.7). Failure to produce antibody to the EBNAs is a feature of immunodeficiency states that may also be associated with increased levels of antibodies to EBV lytic cycle antigens [early antigen (EA) and VCA], reflecting a high virus replication rate. High IgA levels to VCA are found in those at risk of developing EBV-associated nasopharyngeal carcinoma (see below). Antibodies against the major viral envelope glycoprotein gp350/220 are neutralizing and may protect against re-infection.

## CLINICAL FEATURES

Primary infection with EBV is usually mild and unrecognized in the vast majority who acquire it in the first years of life.

### Infectious mononucleosis/glandular fever

*Infectious mononucleosis* (IM; or *glandular fever*, GF) is seen predominantly in the 15–25 years age group when primary EBV infection is delayed into adulthood. The incubation period is 30–50 days, and the onset is abrupt with a triad of sore throat, cervical lymphadenopathy and fever, often accompanied by malaise, headache, sweating (particularly at night) and gastrointestinal discomfort. A *mononucleosis* of atypical lymphocytes is observed in blood. Pharyngitis may be severe, accompanied by a greyish-white membrane and gross tonsillar enlargement. Lymphadenopathy becomes generalized, often with splenic enlargement and tenderness, mild hepatomegaly (and biochemical hepatitis) in some individuals and clinical jaundice in 5–10% of cases. Intermittent fevers with drenching sweats may occur daily over 2 weeks. A faint transient morbilliform rash may be seen; a maculopapular rash may follow ampicillin administration, due to immune complexes with antibody to ampicillin. The illness can last for several weeks, and prolonged and debilitating fatigue and lack of concentration are common in the aftermath.

### Complications of infectious mononucleosis/glandular fever

Complications are rare, but some can be serious:

- *acute* airway obstruction may occur as a result of the lymphoid enlargement and oedema; this merits emergency tracheostomy in some cases, but usually responds well to steroids
- *splenic* rupture (rare)
- *neurological* complications include *aseptic* meningitis, encephalitis and the Guillain–Barré syndrome.

### Other EBV-associated disease, tumours and immunosuppression

EBV is associated with an increasing number of diseases, including malignant tumours (Table 43.4). The role played by EBV in these conditions is not clear in all cases. Cellular immunodeficiency, associated with impaired T cell control of EBV-induced B cell proliferation, may result in EBV-driven B cell lymphoproliferations and lymphomas. This may be inherited (e.g. X-linked lymphoproliferative (or Duncan's) syndrome (X-LPS) due to a defective immunomodulatory SAP gene), acquired (e.g. in AIDS), or due to iatrogenic immunosuppression following transplantation surgery (post transplant lymphoproliferative disease, PTLD). In African Burkitt's lymphoma (BL), characterized by translocation of the cellular proto-oncogene *c-myc* gene into chromosomal locations driven by the highly active immunoglobulin promoters, EBV infection at an early age combines with chronic immunosuppression due to holoendemic malaria to promote further the development of

**Table 43.4** Diseases associated with EBV

| Disease | Cells infected | Link |
|---|---|---|
| Infectious mononucleosis ('glandular fever') | Naive B lymphocytes | Causal; acute primary infection |
| Oral hairy leukoplakia (seen in AIDS) | Differentiated epithelium along edge of tongue | Causal; productive recurrence in immunocompromised host |
| Nasopharyngeal carcinoma (especially in South-East Asia and China) | Anaplastic/undifferentiated nasopharyngeal epithelium (long latent period, >30 years) | All malignant cells contain EBV; co-factor(s) play a role and there is genetic risk |
| African (endemic) Burkitt's lymphoma | Monoclonal B cell tumour (short latent period, >5 years) | All malignant cells contain EBV; holoendemic malaria plays a role |
| Immunoblastic lymphoma (post-transplant/AIDS; X-linked lymphoproliferative syndrome) | Activated B lymphocytes | Over 90% of malignant cells contain EBV; immunodeficiency states, genetic defect |
| Hodgkin's lymphoma | Hodgkin-Reed-Sternberg cells (germinal-centre B lymphocytes) | 30–90% of malignant cells contain EBV (particular disease subsets) |
| Anaplastic gastric carcinoma | Epithelial cells | Malignant cells contain EBV (particular disease subsets) |
| T/NK cell lymphoma | T/NK lymphocytes | 30–100% of malignant cells contain EBV (particular disease subsets) |

highly aggressive BL tumours (endemic BL, eBL). Sporadic BL (sBL), that arises outwith equatorial Africa, is also associated with EBV in up to 50% of cases. *Hodgkin's lymphoma* (HL) is associated with EBV in approximately 50% of cases (particularly the *mixed cellularity* subset), and the anaplastic subset of nasopharyngeal carcinoma (NPC) is almost always associated with the virus.

## LABORATORY DIAGNOSIS

IM/GF is accompanied by the production of heterophile agglutinins that can be detected by a rapid slide agglutination test (the '*Paul–Bunnell test*'; related tests include the '*heterophile antibody test*' and the '*monospot test*'). Agglutination of horse or sheep red blood cells by serum absorbed to exclude a natural antibody is the basis of this test. Atypical lymphocytes, accounting for 20% of the lymphocytosis common in this condition, are seen in blood films. Definitive diagnosis requires the demonstration of IgM antibody to EBV VCA, or seroconversion of VCA IgG antibody. These tests, using indirect immunostaining (immunofluorescence) or, more commonly, EIAs, are generally available. Other serological tests may be applicable to aid serological diagnosis in special situations (e.g. EBNA and EA antibody tests by EIA).

Culture of EBV, from saliva or throat washings, is a research technique. Tissue sections can be immunostained for EBNA or other EBV proteins (Fig. 43.8), or probed for EBERs using *in-situ* hybridization techniques; these approaches, as well as PCR for EBV DNA in blood, are important in the diagnosis of disease in the immunocompromised host. The role of assessing levels of EBV DNA by PCR following transplantation to predict, diagnose or monitor treatment responses to PTLD is still being evaluated. Such measurements are not straight-forward in the solid organ transplant (SOT) setting although greater success has been achieved using EBV PCR to monitor high risk haematopoietic stem cell transplant (HSCT) recipients.

## TREATMENT

Aciclovir is of little value against EBV disease although it is sometimes included in regimes against PTLD. Whilst *reducing* immunosuppression in transplant recipients suffering PTLD is an option, this may put the grafted organ(s) at risk. *Adoptive humoral immunotherapy* using the agent rituximab, a humanized murine monoclonal antibody against the pan-B cell surface marker CD20, is effective against EBV-associated B cell tumours (including PTLD). Similarly, *adoptive cellular immunotherapy* employing autologous, or MHC-matched allogeneic, *EBV-specific T lymphocytes* has been shown to be effective in individuals that have not responded to any other treatment for PTLD.

## EPIDEMIOLOGY

EBV is transmitted by saliva, and a potential role for sexual transmission has also been proposed. Rarely, transmission has been reported following transfusion of blood products to seronegative recipients. Infection is widespread, with most of the population infected in

**Fig. 43.8** Liver needle biopsy of PTLD in a liver transplant recipient. (A) Portal area infiltrated with high-grade lymphoma showing slight spill-over into adjacent and relatively normal-looking liver tissue. (B) High-power view of the neoplastic infiltrate showing large, atypical, lymphoid blast cells. (C) EBV LMP immunohistochemistry decorates many of the neoplastic lymphoid cells. (D) EBNA 2 immunohistochemistry also highlights many tumour cell nuclei (brown is positive). (Courtesy of Dr COC Bellamy, Department of Laboratory Medicine, The Royal Infirmary of Edinburgh, UK.)

early life, even in developed countries. Increasing numbers of severely immunocompromised hosts are at risk of developing EBV-driven malignant lymphomas, including SOT and HSCT recipients. This can occur when donor virus is transmitted in grafted tissues or following reactivation of the recipient's own isolate. Primary EBV infection post transplant is a high-risk situation for PTLD development which explains why paediatric SOT recipients are at particular risk of the disease.

## CONTROL

Subunit vaccines based on the major membrane glycoprotein gp350/220 have been undergoing trials and shown to protect against tumour-inducing doses

of EBV in a cottontop tamarin model and against IM/GF in seronegative healthy human populations (although not through sterile immunity as EBV infection is not prevented). Screening for IgA antibodies to EBV VCA is used in populations at risk of NPC to detect pre-clinical cases although EBV PCR analysis is rapidly replacing such an approach.

## CYTOMEGALOVIRUS

Human cytomegalovirus (CMV) infects man, but there are other cytomegaloviruses that are specific for other animal species (e.g. murine CMV). The name derives from the CPE of CMV infection that results in a swollen state of infected cells (cytomegaly) in culture and in tissues. Nuclei of productively infected cells contain a large inclusion body, giving a typical 'owl's eye' appearance as can be seen by immunohistochemical staining under the light microscope. Whilst CMV is slowly proliferative in tissue culture, it replicates rapidly in the human body and can pose a serious threat to vulnerable individuals.

## DESCRIPTION

CMV has the same general structure as other herpesviruses but its target cell surface receptor(s) is not yet known for certain. Human fibroblast cells are required for isolation of the virus *in vitro*. In contrast, CMV replicates in *vivo* in epithelial cells in:

- salivary glands
- the kidney
- the respiratory tract
- other epithelial (or endothelial) sites.

CMV remains highly cell associated, and is sensitive to freezing and thawing. Virus shed in urine is stable at 4°C for many days.

## REPLICATION

The temporal regulation of viral protein synthesis in the growth cycle is more obvious in laboratory culture of the slower-growing CMV than with HSV. Non-structural IE protein (p72) appears in nuclei within 16 h of inoculation, whereas structural L proteins are produced after DNA synthesis; the typical CPE is often not recognizable for 5–21 days. Foci of swollen cells expand slowly as infection passes from cell to cell (Fig. 43.9). Passage and storage of virus are best achieved by trypsinization and passage as infected cells.

Human CMV does not produce a virus-specified TK; instead, the protein kinase product of CMV gene *UL97* carries out initial phosphorylation of ganciclovir in CMV-infected cells, and cellular kinases produce the active triphosphate form of the drug which inhibits the CMV DNA polymerase.

There are several families of glycoproteins in CMV, and these are important antigenic targets. Most neutralizing antibody is directed against gB.

## PATHOGENESIS

Primary infection with CMV may be acquired at any time, possibly from conception onwards and, similar to other herpesviruses, CMV persists in the host for

**Fig. 43.9** Focus of CMV infection (arrowed) in a tissue culture monolayer of human embryo fibroblasts.

life. Reactivation is common, and virus is shed in body secretions such as urine, saliva, semen, breast milk and cervical fluid. Mononuclear cells carry the latent virus genome and viral RNA transcripts of early genes have been detected in such cells. Bone marrow progenitor cells of the myeloid line may be the prime site of latency. Once their descendants have been activated to differentiate into tissue macrophages, the virus can enter the replication cycle. Recurrent infections may follow reactivation of latent (endogenous) virus, or re-infection with another (exogenous) strain. Isolates can be distinguished by restriction endonuclease analysis or PCR amplification followed by sequence analysis, and by variations in envelope glycoproteins (gB and gH). Endothelial giant cells (multinucleate cells) have been found in the circulation during disseminated CMV infection. These cells are fully permissive for CMV replication.

### Intra–uterine infection

Maternal viraemia may result in fetal infection in approximately 1 in 3 cases of primary CMV infection during pregnancy, and may lead to disease in the fetus. Infection may also be acquired in utero when the mother suffers CMV reactivation, but this rarely results in disease. Transplacental infection is probably carried by infected cells, and transmission is associated with a high viraemic load. CMV causes damage to target cells once they have formed rather than acting as a teratogenic agent.

## Perinatal infection

This is predominantly acquired from infected maternal genital tract secretions, or from breast-feeding (3–5% of pregnant women in Europe reactivate CMV). In the past, perinatal blood transfusion was rarely the source, but, as leukodepletion (removal of white blood cells) is now practised, this risk has been reduced.

## Postnatal infection

This can be acquired in many ways. Saliva containing CMV is spread among young children, and, at older ages, by kissing. Semen can contain high titres of virus, and may be a source of sexual transmission or artificial insemination-associated infection. Whole blood transfusion used to be (and donated organs remain) an important source of CMV. It is not known which donors are most likely to transmit infection, so all CMV IgG antibody-positive ('seropositive') cell and organ donors are considered as potentially infectious as the presence of antibody reflects the presence of persistent virus.

## Host responses

The host immune response to primary CMV includes humoral (IgM, IgG) and cellular (T lymphocyte) responses. Some of the T cell responses may contribute to immunopathology by reacting with MHC molecules induced by CMV. CMV early genes transactivate other viral and cellular genes, and there may be an important interaction with HIV, leading to the production of HIV from latently infected cells. Because CMV infects mononuclear cells, there is a degree of immunosuppression associated with the acute infection. Cell-mediated responses are crucial to the control of CMV as evident by the serious consequences of disseminated infection in the immunocompromised host. The incubation period for primary infection is 4–6 weeks; reactivation, after transplantation for instance, appears from 3 weeks onwards.

## CLINICAL FEATURES

### Congenital CMV infection

Congenital CMV infection is asymptomatic at birth in approximately 90% of infected babies, but approximately 10% of these may show sensorineural deafness and/or intellectual impairment in childhood as a result of progressive CMV infection. All congenitally infected infants excrete abundant virus in urine during the first year. Congenitally-infected babies that show symptoms at birth are said to have *cytomegalic inclusion disease* (*CID*) with:

- intrauterine growth retardation
- hepatosplenomegaly
- jaundice (*hepatitis*)
- thrombocytopenia
- CNS involvement – a significant problem with CMV: microcephaly, encephalitis and *chorioretinitis* are noted at birth (ultrasonography may detect such lesions in utero)
- other organ involvement including *myocarditis* and/or *pneumonitis*.

### Mononucleosis

Postnatal infection with CMV is seldom recognized clinically. *Respiratory tract infection* is common in infancy and a *mononucleosis syndrome* (reminiscent of symptomatic primary EBV infection) is seen occasionally, especially in young adults or when CMV is acquired from blood transfusion. Hepatitis, fever and atypical lymphocytosis are noted, but pharyngitis and lymphadenopathy are unusual and heterophile agglutinins are not found.

### Infection in the immunocompromised patient

Immunocompromised patients may develop symptoms as a result of primary, or recurrent, CMV infection. Dissemination of the virus in the blood, as indicated by a hectic fever, is a bad prognostic sign. The complications of CMV infection in cellular immunodeficiency include:

- pneumonitis: a high mortality rate in recipients of bone marrow allografts
- encephalitis: often fatal
- retinitis: may occur on its own (10–40% of patients with AIDS)
- oesophagitis/colitis: 5–10% of patients with AIDS
- hepatitis
- pancreatitis and/or adrenalitis.

CMV infection in transplant recipients is a significant cause of *direct* (caused by the virus) and *indirect* (caused by virus interactions with the immune system) morbidity that may culminate in loss of the grafted organ and even death. The mortality rate is high, particularly in allogeneic bone marrow recipients who develop an immunopathological pneumonitis associated with graft-versus-host disease. Transplant protocols all include *prophylaxis* or *pre-emptive therapy* for the prevention of CMV disease. The former approach entails routine administration of valganciclovir for a period of time post transplantation, and the latter involves regular measurements of CMV viral load in blood by PCR to detect virus with a view to instigating early treatment prior to symptomatic CMV disease.

Retinitis due to CMV recurrence is a feature of late-stage AIDS. Early recognition, antiviral treatment and maintenance therapy are important in slowing the progression towards blindness.

## LABORATORY DIAGNOSIS

Detection of CMV at the site of disease is the aim (if possible). Samples should include urine, saliva, broncho-alveolar lavage fluid, and/or biopsy tissue (if available), and peripheral blood collected in suitable (usually EDTA) anticoagulant.

### Virus detection

Rapid diagnostic methods can detect either viral DNA using hybridization or PCR assays, or CMV early antigen in cell cultures 24 h post-inoculation (Fig. 43.10). Conventional culture is used to isolate virus but this approach has been largely replaced by genome detection assays. High titres of CMV produce a CPE very quickly in tissue culture, but most cultures require 2–3 weeks. CMV must be demonstrated in a urine (or saliva) sample taken within the

**Fig. 43.10** CMV early antigen demonstrated in nuclei of human embryo fibroblasts by immunofluorescence after incubation for 24 h following centrifuge-assisted inoculation.

first 3 weeks of life to demonstrate congenital infection as later samples may reflect virus acquired in the postnatal period. Confirmation that CMV is related to a disease process comes from showing the presence of virus (by immunohistochemical or genome detection methods) in the affected tissues, or, in some cases, that a primary infection has occurred. The demonstration of CMV viraemia is a significant prognostic finding, by detection of leukocytes containing CMV late phosphoprotein antigen (pp65) or (nowadays) CMV DNA (by PCR); above certain levels, these approaches are predictive of clinical disease. The quantitative PCR assay has become important in detecting and monitoring CMV following transplantation.

### Serology for CMV

CFTs are adequate for showing sero-conversion after primary CMV infection in immunocompetent hosts but the assays are not widely available now. To screen for 'seropositive' status, a more sensitive assay, such as EIA for CMV IgG or total antibody (or latex agglutination assay), is appropriate. These tests can be done urgently for organ donor–recipient assessments. CMV IgM is found after primary or secondary infection, but it may not be possible to detect IgM in the neonate or immunocompromised patient.

## TREATMENT

Antiviral agents for CMV infections are available but serious side effects limit their use to life- or sight-threatening complications. Ganciclovir is the agent most often used, given intravenously. Marrow toxicity results in neutropenia, and there can be long-term loss of spermatogenesis. Clinically, treatment has been successful in CMV hepatitis, colitis and encephalitis, and progression of CMV retinitis in AIDS can be controlled with prolonged maintenance therapy. Ganciclovir-resistant virus has been found; usually a mutation in the protein kinase gene (*UL97*) is responsible but a DNA polymerase (product of the *UL54* gene) mutation may also occur. Foscarnet is an alternative agent that does not require phosphorylation but has serious side-effects (e.g. nephrotoxicity). Aciclovir is not effective therapy for CMV, but some benefit from high-dose prophylaxis against CMV in transplant recipients has been noted. Oral ganciclovir has been used for prophylaxis in transplant recipients for several years but has now been replaced by an oral pro-drug, valganciclovir, which provides systemic levels of ganciclovir equivalent to those achieved by intravenous therapy. Cidofovir is an alternative antiviral agent.

## EPIDEMIOLOGY

Primary CMV infection is acquired by 40–60% of persons by mid-adult life, and by more than 90% of those with multiple intimate exposures. Fewer than 5% of units of whole blood from seropositive donors result in transmission to seronegative recipients, whereas 80% of kidneys transmit infection from seropositive donors. The full extent of congenital CMV disease is not known, but this infection occurs in approximately 3 of 1000 live births in the UK and is the most common viral cause of congenital infection.

## CONTROL

Screening of organ donors (D) and recipients (R) is carried out prior to transplantation to prevent, where possible, a seronegative recipient (R–) receiving a solid organ from a seropositive donor (D+), in order to avoid the high risk D+/R– SOT situation. In the bone marrow transplant setting, a similar high risk situation involves D–/R+ HSCT procedures. Such tissue matching (when possible) reduces morbidity and mortality significantly for all forms of allogeneic transplant. Blood donor screening to select CMV-seronegative units for support of seronegative patients in transplant programmes, and for premature babies, is less important now with the use of leukodepletion. Antiviral prophylaxis (starting from time of transplant surgery), or pre-emptive treatment (starting from time of virus detection in blood), are routine procedures now in SOT and HSCT programmes for those at risk of CMV disease.

No CMV vaccine is licensed for use but trials continue. Experimental live-attenuated vaccines have been tried, but hopes rest on subunit vaccines, or on a combined approach.

## HUMAN HERPESVIRUSES 6 AND 7

## DESCRIPTION

The existence of further herpesviruses infecting man was not suspected until one was isolated in 1986 from the blood of patients with lymphoproliferative disorders, some of whom had AIDS. EM revealed a virus with characteristic herpesvirus features. DNA sequence studies showed this virus, now officially named human herpesvirus 6 (HHV 6), to be distinct from the then five known human herpesviruses, but closer to human CMV, with which it has some homology. Two variants have been identified on sequence analysis: HHV 6A and 6B. Although first isolated from B cells, HHV 6 was shown to infect CD4+ T cells preferentially. HHV 6B is the cause of a common disease of infancy called exanthem subitum or roseola infantum ('sixth disease') and may cause febrile convulsions in childhood, whereas variant 6A has much less clear disease association. Both variants do seem to play a role in disease (*bone marrow suppression, encephalitis*) in the immunosuppressed state following transplantation. The cell receptor for HHV 6 is CD46, a complement regulatory glycoprotein present on all nucleated cells. Bone marrow progenitor cells contain truly latent HHV 6; low-level persistent infection is found in salivary glands and brain cells.

In 1990, another new human herpesvirus was isolated in similar circumstances, and has been shown to be sufficiently distinct from other HHV to be denoted HHV 7. Primary infection with HHV 7 has been identified in some cases of *exanthem subitum* and *febrile convulsions* in childhood but its role post transplantation is unclear. A new genus, *roseolovirus,* has been established for HHV 6 and 7, which are members of the subfamily *betaherpesvirinae*, distantly related to human CMV, but with much smaller genomes.

## PATHOGENESIS AND CLINICAL FEATURES

Both HHV 6B and 7 are shed persistently in saliva, and both have been found in female genital secretions. Only HHV 7 is found in breast milk. It is known that HHV 6 may integrate into the human chromosome and can, thus, be inherited from either parent. Such congenital infection leads to a persistently high level of viral DNA within cells in blood. In most people, only low numbers of copies of HHV 6 or 7 are found in circulating cells.

### Exanthem subitum (Roseola infantum)

*Exanthem subitum* (ES) was long considered to be an infection caused by a virus, and transmission by blood was confirmed experimentally years before HHV 6 was isolated. The infection is extremely common in the first years of life, presenting between 6 months and 3 years of age with a sudden onset of fever (up to 39°C). The acute febrile illness due to these viruses accounts for 20% of all fevers of early childhood. The child is not usually ill, remaining alert and playful, with some throat congestion and cervical lymphadenopathy. Sometimes more pronounced respiratory symptoms occur with febrile convulsions. Fever usually persists for 3 days, when the temperature falls suddenly; a widespread *maculopapular* rash appears in around 10% of cases. HHV 6B has been isolated from peripheral blood in the acute febrile phase, in patients who subsequently produced a rash and in many who did not. Seroconversion is noted in convalescence, confirming a primary infection with HHV 6B. Some cases are associated with HHV 7 infection, but no other firm disease association has yet been found for HHV 7.

## Neurological disease

A British survey has confirmed the importance of roseoloviruses in neurological illness (*febrile convulsions* and encephalitis) in early childhood. Diagnosis is difficult as viral DNA is not always detected in CSF (and may then represent integrated HHV 6), but seroconversion to one of the viruses may confirm a primary infection. HHV 6 strains appear to remain thereafter in brain, and these viruses are now considered to be commensal in CNS. No clear association with demyelinating diseases, particularly multiple sclerosis, has been shown.

## Other associations

In the rare adult case, hepatitis and lymphadenopathy have been found, and sometimes a heterophile agglutinin-negative mononucleosis. Reactivation in immunocompromised hosts may be diagnosed by viral load or on the basis of serology, but this is difficult to interpret. HHV 6 and 7 reactivate in the first weeks after transplant and appear to make CMV disease worse, but the full extent of disease in the transplant recipient has still to be established. HHV 6 may cause *bone marrow suppression* and *encephalitis* following transplantation (HHV 6B is more often implicated than 6A).

Both HHV 6 and 7 infect T lymphocytes; indeed, HHV 7 uses the same receptor (CD4) as HIV. The potential significance of these interactions has still to be established.

## LABORATORY DIAGNOSIS

Isolation of HHV 6 or 7 involves co-cultivation of peripheral blood lymphocytes with mitogen-activated cord blood lymphocytes. Very large, refractile, multinucleate cells are produced in culture, and many intact enveloped virions are released into the culture medium. These viruses may be isolated from saliva, particularly HHV 7. Viral DNA detection (by PCR) is now the mainstay of routine diagnosis, with a multiplex assay capable of distinguishing HHV 6A from 6B and 7.

Confirmed laboratory diagnosis is currently available only from specialist laboratories. A particular source of confusion is the ability of HHV 6 to integrate (on occasion) into target cell chromosomes. Antibody tests are becoming more widely used, but results can be confusing. Antibody avidity tests can help to establish whether a primary infection has occurred, as the binding of recently acquired low-avidity IgG is easily disrupted by protein-denaturing agents. Both this method and PCR have proven useful in establishing the correct diagnosis of HHV 6- and 7-associated exanthem subitum in a substantial proportion of suspected cases of infant measles.

## TREATMENT

HHV 6 and 7 are sensitive to ganciclovir, but not to aciclovir. Foscarnet and cidofovir may also be used in serious cases, for example encephalitis in immunocompromised patients. However, treatment is seldom indicated clinically.

## EPIDEMIOLOGY

Antibody analysis to date has been based mainly on immunostaining studies with cells infected with either HHV 6 or 7 as antigens. High antibody titres to HHV 6 are found in young children in the first 4 years of life, reflecting recent primary infection in this age group. Primary infection, with viraemia and seroconversion, has also been detected in seronegative transplant recipients of liver or kidney grafts from seropositive donors. Possible transmission by blood transfusion has not been excluded. Infection with HHV 7 occurs, on average, slightly later in childhood. Older persons have lower levels of antibody, but more sensitive EIA tests reveal almost universal HHV 6B and 7 seropositivity. The full spectrum of disease associated with these viruses, and the extent of asymptomatic shedding, remain to be established.

## HUMAN HERPESVIRUS 8 (KAPOSI'S SARCOMA–ASSOCIATED HERPESVIRUS)

Sequences of DNA representing a completely new human herpesvirus were identified in 1994 in tissues from the epidemic form of Kaposi's sarcoma in patients with AIDS. The DNA fragments unique to the tumour tissue were found to have some homology with the gammaherpesvirus subfamily, including EBV. This virus, officially named HHV 8, but also referred to as *Kaposi's sarcoma-associated* herpesvirus (KSHV), is the latest human tumour virus.

HHV 8 is classified in the *rhadinovirus* genus of the *gammaherpesvirinae* along with known viruses of non-human primates. The genome is 165–170 kbp and encodes around 95 proteins, including a group that contains homologues of human proteins involved in cell growth regulation and cytokine production (IL 6; viral IL 6, vIL6). Like other herpesviruses, HHV 8 attaches to cells first via cell surface heparan sulphate and integrins through envelope glycoproteins gpK8.1 and gB. HHV 8 infects dividing B cells. It then proceeds to either a lytic replication cycle, releasing infectious virus, or enters latency, expressing only the latency-associated nuclear antigens (LANAs). LANA 1 maintains the HHV 8 episome whereas LANA 2 suppresses apoptosis via inhibition of p53-mediated transcription. Latency-associated membrane protein (LAMP) has functions reminiscent of EBV's LMP1 and 2 (see above).

## Kaposi's sarcoma

HHV 8 is strongly associated with all forms of Kaposi's sarcoma (KS). *Classic* KS was first described by the Austro-Hungarian dermatologist Moritz Kaposi in 1872 and affects elderly men of Mediterranean, Esatern European or Jewish backgrounds. The *endemic* form of KS was described in eastern Africa prior to the HIV epidemic, whereas *AIDS-associated* KS is an aggressive form of the disease that occurs in the context of HIV infection. Lastly, *iatrogenic* KS develops in immunosuppressed patients (e.g. organ transplant recipients) as a result of medical intervention. HHV 8 is not the sole driver of KS and other factors (e.g. immunosuppression) also play a role; however, KS only develops in individuals infected with HHV 8. The mucocutaneous neoplasm Kaposi described as 'a multifocal pigmented sarcoma' was the most common tumour in HIV-infected MSM before the advent of highly active antiretroviral therapy (HAART) and was one of the heralds of the AIDS pandemic in the early 1980s. A transmissible agent was long suspected in KS on epidemiological grounds, transmitted sexually but rarely by blood. Endothelial cells of vascular or lymphatic origin are involved; they have a characteristic spindle shape and are arranged in bundles. Although occurring at multiple sites in skin, lymph glands and the gastrointestinal tract, the tumour

itself does not lead to death. Local radiotherapy and systemic chemotherapy have been used in treatment. Lesions on exposed parts of the body are blue-reddish-brown plaques, sometimes raised, and are a cause of considerable concern for the affected individual.

## Body cavity–associated B lymphoma/primary effusion lymphoma/multicentric Castleman's disease

HHV 8 genomes have been found in lymphoma cells from AIDS-related B cell lymphomas termed *body cavity-associated B* lymphomas (BCBL) or *primary effusion lymphomas* (PEL). This condition presents as a malignant effusion in the pericardial, pleural or peritoneal spaces. Cell lines established from the tumours can be induced to produce viral proteins and particles, and have been used as a basis for diagnostic tests. A subset ('*plasma cell variant*') of another condition, multicentric Castleman's disease (MCD), is also strongly associated with HHV 8. MCD is a lymphoproliferative disorder that is often localized in the mediastinum, mesenterium or peripheral lymph nodes.

## LABORATORY DIAGNOSIS

DNA amplification by PCR is used to detect and monitor HHV 8 (viral load in blood). Lytic growth of HHV 8 can be induced in latently infected B cell lymphoma cell lines (many are co-infected with EBV) and, as a result, reagents for antibody testing can be produced – both infected cell lysates for immunoblots, and antigen-containing cells for immunostaining. Recombinant proteins have been synthesized and are useful for EIAs. Now that reagents free of EBV are available, the specific epidemiology of infection with this new herpesvirus is being studied.

## EPIDEMIOLOGY

Molecular sequence data have revealed five clades of HHV 8, termed A–E. Clade B predominates in Africa, whereas in Europe and North America clades A and C are more common. Serological surveys have shown that, unlike most of the human herpesviruses, HHV 8 infection is not common, at least in developed countries (fewer than 5% of blood donors in North America and northern Europe have anti-HHV 8 antibodies). Rates of seropositivity are higher in at-risk groups for KS, with up to 30% seropositivity rates in MSM. Confirmation of a high seropositivity rate (up to 60%) in adolescents and adults in most parts of sub-Saharan African countries, and studies on transmission, have shown a link between mothers and their children, and between siblings. Transmission from saliva is considered the most likely route, and the high rates in communities where over-crowding in childhood is seen support this. In Europe, there is increased seropositivity around the Mediterranean, and the presence of HHV 8 DNA in elderly Italians is highly predictive of the development of KS following organ transplantation or HIV infection.

## TREATMENT AND CONTROL

Ganciclovir has activity against HHV 8, and its use in CMV prophylaxis after organ transplantation may contribute to reducing the risk of reactivation and disease due to HHV 8 in seropositive recipients, or in seronegative recipients who have a seropositive donor. *Foscarnet* may be an alternative drug. Tumours associated with HHV 8 infection may regress if *reduction of immunosuppression* is possible (post-transplant) or following improvements in immunity with HAART (in patients with AIDS) – together with *local radiotherapy* and/or *chemotherapy*. *Rituximab* may also have some effect in patients with BCBL/PEL.

## CERCOPITHECINE HERPESVIRUS 1 (B VIRUS; HERPESVIRUS SIMIAE)

## DESCRIPTION

This virus, antigenically related to HSV, commonly infects Old World (Asiatic) macaque monkeys, causing a mild vesicular eruption on the tongue and buccal mucosa analogous to primary herpetic stomatitis in man. The infection rate in monkeys increases markedly if they are kept in crowded conditions and, although relatively benign in the monkey, this virus is potentially highly pathogenic for man.

Human infection with B virus is rare. It is usually acquired from a monkey bite or from handling infected animals without appropriate personal protective equipment (PPE). In one instance, the wife of an infected monkey handler became infected through contact with her husband's vesicles, and B virus has also been transmitted in the laboratory from infected monkey cell cultures. Within 5–20 days of exposure, local inflammation may appear at the site of entry, usually on the skin, accompanied by some itching, numbness and vesicular lesions. Ascending myelitis or

acute encephalomyelitis may follow, occasionally as long as 5 weeks after exposure, and may not always be recognized. Delay in specific therapy leads to a high mortality rate and serious neurological sequelae in survivors.

## DIAGNOSIS AND TREATMENT

Diagnosis by isolation of the virus from blood, vesicle fluid, conjunctival swabs or CSF is not always possible and such approaches pose significant problems for the laboratory as a result of safety concerns (ACDP Category 4 organism; see internet reference to ACDP). Herpesvirus particles may be detectable by EM of vesicle fluid. Definitive identification of the virus is available in specialist reference laboratories using immunostaining or DNA analysis by PCR. Demonstration of specific antibodies is complicated by cross-reacting HSV antibody, but new specific antigens based on recombinant glycoproteins offer improved serology. B virus is not as sensitive to aciclovir as HSV, requiring concentrations equivalent to those used for VZV. Treatment needs to be given promptly to be effective, and very high-dose intravenous aciclovir for 2 weeks or longer is recommended. Ganciclovir should be used when there is evidence of CNS involvement. Because of the small number of cases, the best therapeutic regimen is not well established.

## PREVENTION OF B VIRUS INFECTION

Guidelines have been issued for the protection of those handling monkeys or monkey tissues. These include:

- screening of macaque colonies when possible
- recommendations for training to prevent exposure
- safe handling and personal protective equipment (PPE) procedures
- immediate risk assessment and care of wounds
- information regarding the risks and nature of the infection.

Prophylaxis in the event of possible exposure involves prompt, rigorous wound washing and cleansing with 10% iodine in alcohol. A course of high-dose oral aciclovir, or valaciclovir, is reserved for prophylaxis of high-risk exposures, namely those on head, neck or torso, deep wounds, and where the source animal has lesions, recent stress or illness, or the material is of CNS or mucosal origin. After prophylaxis, a prolonged observation period is recommended as the onset of infection may be delayed.

## RECOMMENDED READING

Corey L, Wald A: Maternal and neonatal herpes simplex virus infections, *The New England Journal of Medicine* 361:1376–1385, 2009.

Fishman JA: Infection in solid organ transplant recipients, *The New England Journal of Medicine* 357:2601–2614, 2007.

Gershon AA, Gershon MD, Breuer J, et al: Advances in the understanding of the pathogenesis and epidemiology of herpes zoster, *Journal of Clinical Virology* 48: S2–S7, 2010.

Knipe DM, Howley PM, editors: Herpesviridae. In *Fields Virology*, ed 5, Philadelphia, 2007, Lippincott Williams & Wilkins, pp 2479–2904.

Mahy BWJ, Ter Meulen V, editors: Herpesviridae. In *Topley & Wilson's Microbiology & Microbial Infections: Virology*, ed 10, London, 2005, Hodder Arnold, pp 488–577.

Oxman MN: Zoster Vaccine: Current status and future prospects, *Clinical Infectious Diseases* 51: 197–213, 2010.

Parker A, Bowles K, Bradley JA, et al: Management of post-transplant lymphoproliferative disorder in adult solid organ transplant recipients – BCSH and BTS guidelines, *British Journal of Haematology* 149:693–705, 2010.

Zuckerman AJ, Banatvala JE, Schoub BD, et al: editors: Herpesviridae. In *Principles and Practice of Clinical Virology*, ed 6, Chichester, 2009, Wiley-Blackwell, pp 95–272.

## Websites

Advisory Committee on Dangerous Pathogens: Biological agents. The principles, design and operation of Containment Level 4 facilities. http://www.dh.gov.uk/prod_consum_dh/groups/dh_digitalassets/@dh/@en/documents/digitalasset/dh_4135259.pdf

British Transplantation Society: Active Standards and Guidelines. http://www.bts.org.uk/transplantation/standards-and-guidelines/

UK Department of Health: Varicella. http://www.dh.gov.uk/prod_consum_dh/groups/dh_digitalassets/@dh/@en/documents/digitalasset/dh_115138.pdf

# 44 Poxviruses

Smallpox; molluscum contagiosum; parapoxvirus infections

*T. H. Pennington*

## KEY POINTS

- Poxviruses are large cytoplasmic DNA viruses that infect a wide range of species.
- Smallpox is a generalized disease with a vesicular rash and associated with significant mortality.
- Live vaccine is used to eradicate disease, but is not risk free.
- Eradication was successful because only human beings are infected, the disease is easily recognized, transmitted to only a few contacts, and there is no carrier state. Bio-terrorism threatens the re-introduction of smallpox.
- Other human poxvirus infections are of minor significance and include molluscum contagiosum, monkeypox and orf.

The world's last naturally occurring case of smallpox was recorded in Merca, southern Somalia, in October 1977. This momentous event marked the end of a long campaign against smallpox, which in its 'modern' phase started with the introduction of vaccination by Edward Jenner at the end of the eighteenth century. With the eradication of smallpox, the importance of poxviruses in medical practice may appear to be much diminished, as the other naturally occurring viruses in this family that infect man nearly always cause only self-limiting and trivial skin lesions. Smallpox caused a generalized infection with a high mortality rate, and fell into that small group of viruses whose infections are commonly severe and frequently fatal. Notwithstanding their minor role today as human pathogens, poxviruses retain their importance, and their place in this book, for four reasons.

First, the successful smallpox eradication campaign is important in its own right as a major achievement. It is also important because it highlights the principles and problems associated with projects that aim to control infections by eradicating the pathogen. Smallpox was the first human disease to fall to this approach and remains the only successful example to date. (The announcement in June 2011 of the eradication of the cattle disease rinderpest (p. 551) marked the extinction of a second important pathogen; the end for polio (p. 484) and guinea worm (p. 660) is close.)

Second, work on the molecular biology of poxviruses has led to the identification of distinctive properties and to the development of techniques and approaches that have made it possible to move significantly towards constructing single-dose vaccines that protect simultaneously against a wide range of diseases. Genes coding for foreign non-poxvirus antigens have been inserted into the poxvirus genome so that the antigens are expressed during virus infection and induce immunity.

Third, no account of virus diseases in general and poxvirus infections in particular is complete without consideration being given to the events that followed the introduction of myxomatosis into Australia – by far the best studied example to date of the evolution of a new virus disease.

Finally, new poxviruses continue to be discovered – in 2009, a novel deer parapox virus was identified as the cause of disease in 2 deer hunters in the USA.

## DESCRIPTION

### Classification

A large number of different viruses belonging to the family Poxviridae have been described. They infect a wide range of vertebrate and invertebrate hosts. The subfamily Chordopoxvirinae contains all of the viruses that infect vertebrates; it is divided into six genera, each containing related viruses, which generally infect related hosts (Table 44.1). Thus, members of the genus *Leporipoxvirus* infect rabbits and squirrels, *Avipoxvirus* members infect birds, *Capripoxvirus* members infect goats and sheep, *Suipoxvirus* members infect swine, and *Parapoxvirus* members infect cattle and sheep. Some viruses, including that of molluscum contagiosum, which infects man, remain unclassified. By far the most intensively studied poxvirus is vaccinia virus, the Jennerian smallpox vaccine virus. This virus has been placed in the genus *Orthopoxvirus*, together with smallpox virus and some viruses that infect cattle and mice.

## The virion

Poxviruses are the largest animal viruses. Their virions are big enough to be seen as dots by light microscopy after special staining procedures. They are much more complex than those of any other viruses (Figs 44.1 and 44.2). They are also distinctive in that they do not show any discernible symmetry. The core contains the DNA genome and 15 or more enzymes that make up

a transcriptional system whose role is to synthesize biologically active polyadenylated, capped and methylated virus messenger RNA (mRNA) molecules early in infection. The core has a 9-nm thick membrane, with a regular subunit structure. Within the virion, the core assumes a dumbbell shape because of the large lateral bodies. The core and lateral bodies are enclosed in a protein shell about 12 nm thick (the outer membrane), the surface of which consists of irregularly arranged tubules, which in turn consist of a small globular

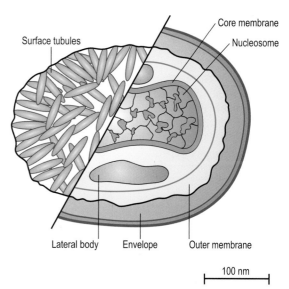

**Fig. 44.1** Structure of the vaccinia virion. Right-hand side, section of enveloped virion; left-hand side, surface structure of non-enveloped particle. (From Fenner F, Henderson DA, Arita I et al 1988 *Smallpox and its Eradication*. World Health Organization, Geneva.)

| Table 44.1 | Family: Poxviridae | |
|---|---|---|
| Subfamilies | Genera | Natural host |
| Chordopoxvirinae (contains all viruses that infect vertebrates) | *Leporipoxvirus* | Rabbits, squirrels |
| | *Avipoxvirus* | Birds |
| | *Capripoxvirus* | Goats and sheep |
| | *Suipoxvirus* | Swine |
| | *Parapoxvirus* | Cattle, sheep |
| | *Orthopoxvirus* | Man, cattle, mice |
| Entomopoxvirinae (viruses of insects) | | Insects |

**Fig. 44.2** Electron micrographs of poxviruses. (A) Molluscum contagiosum virus (MCV), ×15 000. (B) MCV showing internal structure, ×75 000 (prepared by N Atack). (C) Parapoxvirus: orf. Bar = 100 nm. (Courtesy of Dr DW Gregory.)

subunit. Virions released naturally from the cell are enclosed within an envelope that contains host cell lipids and several virus-specified polypeptides, including haemagglutinin; they are infectious. Most virions remain cell associated and are released by cellular disruption. These particles lack an envelope, so that the outer membrane constitutes their surface; they are also infectious. More than 100 different polypeptides have been identified in purified virions.

## The genome

Their DNA genomes range in mass from 85 MDa (para-poxviruses) to 185 MDa (avipoxviruses). The vaccinia virus genome has 186000 base pairs (123 MDa). The poxvirus genome is distinctive in that covalent links join the two DNA strands at both ends of the molecule, the genome thus being a single uninterrupted molecule that is folded to form a linear duplex structure. The occurrence of inverted terminal sequence repetitions is also a characteristic feature, identical sequences being present at each end of the genome.

## REPLICATION

Poxviruses are unique among human DNA viruses in that virus RNA and DNA synthesis takes place in the cytoplasm of the infected cell and they code for all the proteins needed for their replication. They have early and late phases of protein synthesis (see Ch. 7). Virion assembly takes place in the cytoplasm and proceeds in a series of steps which include the formation of spherical immature particles. The virus causes irreversible inhibition of host protein synthesis due to the functional inactivation and degradation of host cytoplasmic RNA molecules, leading to the death of infected cells.

## CLINICAL FEATURES

Smallpox virus had no animal reservoir and spread from person to person by the respiratory route. After infecting mucosal cells in the upper respiratory tract without producing symptoms, it spread to the regional lymph nodes and, after a transient viraemia, infected cells throughout the body. Multiplication of virus in these cells led to a second and more intense viraemia, which heralded the onset of clinical illness. During the first few days of fever the virus multiplied in skin epithelial cells, leading to the development of focal lesions and the characteristic rash. Macules

progressed to papules, vesicles and pustules, leaving permanent pockmarks, particularly on the face. Two kinds of smallpox were common in the first half of the twentieth century:

1. Variola major, or classical smallpox
2. Variola minor, or alastrim.

Variola major had case fatality rates varying from 10–50% in the unvaccinated. Variola minor caused a much milder disease and had case fatality rates of less than 1%. The viruses are very similar but can be distinguished in the laboratory by restriction enzyme fragment length polymorphisms of their genomes.

## CONTROL OF SMALLPOX

### Before vaccination

Before the introduction of vaccination, the control of smallpox relied on two approaches, variolation and isolation. Variolators aimed to induce immunity equivalent to that after natural infection. Susceptible individuals were deliberately infected with smallpox pus or scabs by scratching the skin or by nasal insufflation. Although the virus was not attenuated, infections had lower case fatality rates (estimated to be 0.5–2%) and were less likely to cause permanent pockmarks than those acquired naturally. Variolation was first recorded in China nearly 1000 years ago, and was practised in many parts of the world. In Afghanistan, Pakistan and Ethiopia the activities of variolators caused problems towards the end of the smallpox eradication programme in the 1970s because they spread virus in a way that evaded the measures erected to control natural virus transmission.

### Vaccination

Edward Jenner vaccinated James Phipps with cowpox virus on 14 May 1796 and challenged him by variolation some months later. He repeated this 'trial', as he called it, in other children, and the description of these events in his 'Inquiry' in 1798 led to the rapid worldwide acceptance of vaccination. Introduction of the vaccine virus into the epidermis led to the development of a local lesion and the induction of a strong immunity to infection with smallpox virus that lasted for several years. Although the essentials of *Jennerian vaccination* remained unchanged for the rest of its history, early vaccinators developed their own vaccine viruses, which became known as vaccinia. The origin of these viruses is obscure, and modern vaccinia viruses form a distinct species of orthopoxvirus,

**Table 44.2** Features of smallpox that facilitated its eradication

| Feature | Importance |
|---------|-----------|
| Disease severe | Ensured strong public and governmental support for eradication programme |
| Detection of cases easy because of characteristic rash and subsequent development of facial pockmarks | Facilitated containment of outbreaks and audit of success of programme |
| Slow spread and poor transmissibility | Facilitated containment of outbreaks by vaccination and isolation |
| Transmission by subclinical cases not important | Meant that control of spread by isolation of cases was an effective procedure |
| No carrier state in humans | Meant that control of spread by isolation of cases was an effective procedure |
| No animal reservoir | Meant that control of spread by isolation of cases was an effective procedure |
| Vaccine technically simple to produce in large amounts, in high quality and at low cost (in skin of ungulates) | Meant that vaccine availability was not an important constraint in the eradication programme |
| Vaccine delivery simple and optimized by use of re-usable, cheap, specially designed needles to deliver a standard amount of vaccine to scratches in skin | Meant that failure at the point of vaccination was not an important constraint in the eradication programme |
| Freeze-dried vaccine stocks were heat-stable with a very long shelf-life in the tropics | Meant that vaccine viability under adverse environmental conditions was not an important constraint in the eradication programme |

related to but very clearly distinct from the viruses of both cowpox and smallpox.

## The eradication campaign

Smallpox was brought under control by:

- routine vaccination of children – compulsory in some countries
- outbreak control by isolation and selective vaccination.

This was achieved gradually in Europe, the former USSR, North and Central America, and Japan, and the virus had been eradicated from all these areas by the mid-1950s. In 1959 this achievement prompted the World Health Organization (WHO) to adopt the global eradication of smallpox as a major goal. At this time 60% of the world's population lived in areas where smallpox was endemic. A slow reduction in disease was maintained for the next few years, but epidemics continued to be frequent. Consequently the WHO initiated its Intensified Smallpox Eradication Programme. This started on 1 January 1967 when the disease was reported in 31 countries. It had the goal of eradication within 10 years. The goal was achieved in 10 years, 9 months and 26 days.

From a starting point of 10–15 million cases annually, and against a background of civil strife, famine and floods, success came because of a major international collaborative effort – aided by some virus-specific factors (Table 44.2). At the beginning of 1976, smallpox occurred only in Ethiopia. Transmission was interrupted there in August of that year, although

an importation of virus into Somalia and adjacent countries had occurred by then. This was the last outbreak. The last case was recorded on 26 October 1977. There was a final, tragic death the following year after escape of the virus from a research laboratory; a reminder of the importance of biosecurity reinforced by the laboratory infections caused by the SARS virus in 2004 and the escape of foot and mouth virus from a reference laboratory in 2007. In the final years of the programme its emphasis moved from mass vaccination to a strategy of surveillance and containment. This strategy rapidly interrupted transmission because:

- cases were easy to detect owing to the characteristic rash
- patients usually transmitted disease to only a few people – and only to those in close face-to-face contact
- only persons with a rash transmitted infection.

The WHO Global Commission for the Eradication of Smallpox formally certified that smallpox had been eradicated from the world on 9 December 1979.

## Smallpox and bio-terrorism

After eradication, virus strains were kept in government laboratories in Atlanta and Novosibirsk Region, Russia. The possibility that virus could fall into unauthorized hands is small, but vaccine stocks have been ordered and contingency plans prepared. The experience from outbreaks in the past suggests that outbreaks could be controlled rapidly. There were

49 importations into Europe after 1949. The average number of cases was 14, justifying the characterization of the spread as slow and plodding. In some outbreaks, public pressure for protection led to unnecessary vaccinations, in turn leading to more deaths from vaccination (see below) than from smallpox. In spite of frequent misdiagnoses of early cases as chickenpox (see Ch. 43), the outbreaks were rapidly controlled. Fortunately smallpox spreads slowly.

## OTHER HUMAN POXVIRUS INFECTIONS

### Molluscum contagiosum

The lesions of this mild disease are small, copper-coloured, warty papules that occur on the trunk, buttocks, arms and face. It is spread by direct contact or by fomites. The lesion consists of a mass of hypertrophied epidermis that extends into the dermis and protrudes above the skin. In the epithelial cells very large hyaline acidophilic granular masses can be observed. They crowd the host cell nucleus to one side, eventually filling the whole cell. When material from the lesions is crushed, some of the inclusions burst open, liberating large numbers of virions. These have the size, internal structure and morphology of vaccinia virus. The infection has been transmitted experimentally to human subjects, but the virus has not been grown in cultured cells. The development of immunity is slow and uncertain. Lesions can persist for as long as 2 years, and re-infection is common.

### Monkeypox

This has been implicated occasionally in a smallpox-like condition in equatorial Africa. Its natural hosts are rodents. It may be fatal in unvaccinated humans, but is less transmissible from person to person than smallpox. Importation of infected Gambian pouched rats, that went on to infect captive prairie dogs, caused an outbreak of monkeypox in the USA in 2003.

### Parapoxvirus infections

The virions of parapoxviruses are characterized by a criss-cross pattern of tubes in the outer membrane (see Fig. 44.2C) and genomes that are considerably smaller (85 MDa) than those of other poxviruses. They infect ungulates and cause the human occupational diseases of *orf* and *milker's nodes*. The lesions of orf (which causes a disease in sheep known as contagious pustular dermatitis) are often large and granulomatous. Erythema multiforme is a relatively frequent complication. The lesions of milker's nodes are highly vascular, hemispherical papules and nodules. Both diseases are:

- self-limiting
- most common on the hands
- contracted by contact with infected sheep (orf) or cows (milker's nodes)
- occupational diseases, mainly seen in farm workers such as shepherds, slaughterhouse workers or butchers.

## VACCINIA

Vaccinia-like viruses infect cows and their milkers in Brazil. Whether they are remnants of the vaccination programme there, or naturally occurring viruses, is not clear.

### Vaccinia virus as a vaccine vector

The vaccinia virus genome can accommodate sizeable losses of DNA in certain regions, to the extent that as many as 25 000 base pairs can be lost without lethal effect. By replacing this non-essential DNA with foreign genes it has been possible to construct novel *recombinant virus strains*, which express the foreign genes when they infect cells. Recombinant vaccinia strains containing as many as four foreign genes, coding for combinations of bacterial, viral and protozoal antigens, have been constructed.

The advantages of this ingenious way of developing new vaccines are:

- they are applicable to many different antigens
- the possibility of constructing multivalent vaccines that could give protection against several diseases after a single 'shot'
- stimulates cell-mediated immunity
- the ease of administration
- cheapness of vaccinia as a vaccine.

A strain that expresses the rabies glycoprotein antigen is being used in Europe to protect foxes. Serious disadvantages remain for human diseases, however. These are primarily those associated with vaccinia virus itself, as its use was associated with a number of serious complications. The most important of these were:

- *progressive vaccinia*, a fatal infection that occurred in immunodeficient individuals
- *eczema vaccinatum*, a serious spreading infection that occurred in eczematous individuals

- *post-vaccinal encephalitis*, which, although rare, was severe and occurred in normal healthy individuals
- *myocarditis,* a recently described complication identified following large-scale vaccination of the US military in 2003.

These disadvantages preclude the use of vaccinia as a vector for foreign antigens in man, and work is being done on the modification of its virulence to circumvent these problems. So far, studies on virulence genes have shown that poxviruses code for an impressive array of factors that interfere with host defences. These include proteins that bind complement components, act as receptors for interleukin-1β, interferon and tumour necrosis factor, and synthesize steroids. These factors are all exported from infected cells. Factors that act inside cells include proteins that block the action of interferon, inhibit the post-translational modification of interleukin-1β, and prevent the synthesis of a neutrophil chemotactic factor. It is possible that abrogation of virulence factors such as these may lead to safer vaccines.

## MYXOMATOSIS: AN EVOLVING DISEASE

As a rule, virus infections are mild and self-limiting. Viruses are obligate parasites and it is not in their interests to cause the extinction or massive reductions in the size of host populations. It is reasonable to suppose that the type of disease caused by a virus reflects the outcome of a process in which host and virus have co-evolved to levels of resistance and virulence optimal for the maintenance of their respective population numbers. The high mortality rate of classical smallpox is considered by some to have been a major factor in the restriction of human population size, and this has been used to support the hypothesis that the association between smallpox and man has been established – in evolutionary terms – only in recent times, co-evolution of the relationship being a long way from equilibrium. It is impossible to test this hypothesis directly for variola, but the relationship between another poxvirus, myxoma virus, and the rabbit in Australia, has provided a dramatic example. This is the only example of co-evolution where changes in an animal host and virus and the evolution of a disease have been studied in real time.

Myxoma virus is South American. It causes a benign local fibroma in its natural host, the rabbit *Sylvilagus brasiliensis*, but causes *myxomatosis* in the European rabbit, *Oryctolagus cuniculus*. This is a generalized infection with a very high mortality rate. Field trials to test its efficacy as a measure for controlling the European rabbit were carried out in Australia in 1950. The virus escaped and caused enormous epidemics in the years that followed. The original virus caused infections with a case mortality rate greater than 99%, and rabbits survived for less than 13 days. Within 3 years virus isolates from epidemics had become much less virulent, causing infections with mortality rates of 70–95% and survival times of 17–28 days. Changes in the resistance of the rabbit also occurred, with mortality rates from infection falling (from 90% to 25% after challenge with strains of virus with modified virulence, for example) and symptomatology becoming less severe. In myxomatosis, natural selection favoured virus strains with intermediate virulence because such strains are transmitted more effectively than highly virulent strains, which kill their hosts too quickly, and non-virulent strains, which are poorly transmitted.

RECOMMENDED READING

Baxby D: *Jenner's Smallpox Vaccine*, London, 1981, Heinemann.
Damon IK: Poxviruses. In: Knipe DM, Howley PM, editors: *Field's Virology*, ed 5, Philadelphia, 2007, Lippincott Williams and Wilkins, pp 2947–2976.
Fenner F, Henderson DA, Arita I, et al: *Smallpox and its Eradication*, Geneva, 1988, World Health Organization.

Fenner F, Ratcliffe FN: *Myxomatosis*, Cambridge, 1965, Cambridge University Press.
Jenner E: *An Inquiry into the Causes and Effects of the Variolae Vaccinae*, London, 1798, Sampson Low.

# 45 Papillomaviruses and polyomaviruses

Warts: warts and cancers; polyomavirus associated nephropathy;
progressive multifocal leuco–encephalopathy

*H. A. Cubie, K. S. Cuschieri and C. Y. W. Tong*

## KEY POINTS

### Papillomaviruses

- Papillomaviruses are ubiquitous, found in most mammalian species as well as in birds and reptiles. More than 100 types of HPV are recognized.
- Some HPVs are associated with skin lesions such as common hand warts and plantar verrucas.
- More than 30 HPV types infect the genital mucosa and are associated with a variety of lesions ranging from benign genital warts to invasive cervical cancers.
- *E6* and *E7* are transforming genes of HPV whose protein products bind to cellular tumour suppressors p53 and Rb respectively.
- HPV types can be grouped into high-risk and low-risk types, dependent on their oncogenic potential.
- HPV-16 is the most common high-risk HPV worldwide, and is associated with more than 50% of cervical cancers.
- HPV vaccines based on L1 VLPs have been shown to be highly efficacious, over a period of at least 7 years, against infection and disease associated with the HPV types present in the vaccine.

### Polyomaviruses

- Merkel cell polyomavirus is the only human polyomavirus so far that is clearly associated with malignant tumours in humans.
- BKV and JCV are associated with diseases in immunosuppressed individuals.
- Polyomavirus-associated nephropathy (PVAN) caused by BKV is a significant cause of allograft dysfunction and graft loss after renal transplantation.
- Progressive multifocal leuco-encephalopathy (PML) caused by JCV is found mostly in patients with advanced HIV disease, but recently is also associated with the use of immune modulating therapeutic monoclonal antibodies.

Papillomaviruses and polyomaviruses are both characterized by having double-stranded DNA genomes, and were, for a long time, classified within the same virus family, the papovaviridae. While there are some notable homologies between Papillomaviruses and Polyoma viruses, more recent evidence showed significant dissimilar, genome level differences and in 2004, they were reclassified into 2 distinct virus families; the papillomaviridae and the polyomaviridae. For this reason, this chapter is divided into 2 distinct sections.

## GENERAL PROPERTIES

Papillomaviruses are very common, ancient viruses, thought to have existed when humans initially became a species. PVs are species-specific viruses that can infect an array of vertebrates, with the species name prefacing PV, e.g. bovine papillomavirus (BPV), canine papillomavirus (CPV) and human papillomavirus (HPV). Papillomaviruses are viruses that infect squamous epithelia and mucous membranes, and cause skin cells to proliferate. Infection with PVs can lead to benign or malignant consequences depending on a number of viral, host and environmental factors.

The malignant nature of PVs has been known for a long time. Eighty years ago, it was found that 25% of benign warts caused by cottontail rabbit PV underwent malignant change within a year, whereas in domestic rabbits up to 75% of lesions showed malignant change in the presence of tar which contains carcinogens. Similarly, cattle fed a diet containing bracken fern which contains the carcinogen quercetin, show malignant transformation of tumours of the alimentary canal (BPV type 4) and bladder (BPV type 2). Different types of HPV cause non-malignant warts and cancers seen in humans.

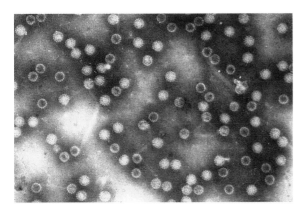

**Fig. 45.1** Electron micrograph of a wart virus from a plantar wart (phosphotungstic acid stain).

Papillomaviruses have:

- a diameter of 52–55 nm
- an icosahedral capsid composed of 72 capsomeres (Fig. 45.1)
- a supercoiled double-stranded DNA genome, with a single coding strand, a molecular weight of approximately $5 \times 10^6$ Da and consisting of about 7900 base pairs
- no envelope.

All papillomaviruses are dependent on the natural epithelial cell maturation or differentiation process of the cell for completion of their life cycle. Although viral DNA can be found in stem cells in the basal epithelial layer, whole virions are found only in terminally differentiated skin cells.

## HUMAN PAPILLOMAVIRUSES

### Genome organization

The HPV genome is divided into an early region with two large (E1 and E2) and several smaller (E4–E7) open reading frames and a late region with two large genes (L1 and L2). Separating the two is a non-coding region which contains regulatory elements. The E region largely encodes the proteins responsible for pathogenicity, while the L region encodes the structural proteins. The coding sequences are distributed in all three open reading frames with considerable overlap along a single strand of DNA. Cumulatively, HPV encodes 8 proteins. Unravelling the functions of these proteins has contributed significantly to our understanding of the pathogenicity of different HPV types and particularly to the transforming ability of some types.

## Life cycle

HPV requires breaks in the surface layers, sometimes referred to as micro wounds to infect basal epithelial cells. In most PVs, the L1 capsid protein binds to heparan sulphate proteoglycans on the basement membrane which facilitates a conformational change to the virus. This in turn exposes L2 which then facilitates transfer to a second, unknown epithelial receptor. The virus enters the cell in an endosome. Genome is uncoated and reaches the nucleus approximately 24h after initial attachment of virus. Recent evidence suggests this is through nuclear membrane pores following breakdown of the membrane during mitosis.

HPV does not encode its own polymerase, so in order to produce new virus particles, it must make use of the dynamic cellular resources available in a differentiating cell. Like other viruses, the productive life cycle for HPV has several stages. The first stages of uncoating and viral genome maintenance expression with a small a mount of genome amplification occur in the basal layer; high levels of genome amplification and particle assembly take place in the spinous and granular (suprabasal) layers while particle release is confined to the uppermost cornified layer. HPV completes these stages through a tightly regulated sequence of gene expression (Table 45.1) and maintains a stable extra-chromosomal state referred to as an episome throughout.

However HPV does not always complete a productive life cycle and where this organized pattern of events is lost, significant abnormal changes to the cell called transformation can occur. The usual life cycle is 'aborted'.

## Transformation

Transformation is an unlikely and unfortunate consequence of HPV infection. Transformation depends on several interlinking factors including HPV type, location and duration of infection, extent of immune response and environmental and constitutive risk factors. E6 and E7 are considered the primary transforming viral proteins (oncoproteins), although E5 plays a supporting role in enhancing the actions of both.

It is thought that integration of the viral genome into the host chromosome releases E6 and E7 from transcriptional control, leading to the de-regulated high-level protein production that is necessary for cell transformation. Most HPV-associated tumours therefore show integrated rather than episomal virus. E6 and E7 work cooperatively: E7 induces proliferation

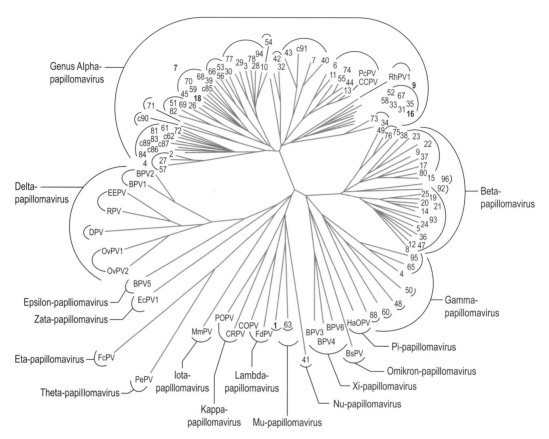

**Fig. 45.2** HPV phylogenetic tree. The majority of oncogenic HPVs are classified within the alpha genus; alpha species groups 9 and 7 contain types HPV 16 and 18 respectively (highlighted), which are responsible for the majority of cervical cancers. Adapted from de Villiers et al (2004) Virology 324:17–27.

of suprabasal cells which avoid apoptosis through the actions of E6. These oncoproteins target and disable pRb and p53, two key proteins involved in cell cycling that normally identify abnormal growth features and prevent proliferation. E6 and E7 can also act directly on centrosomes leading to genomic instability and abnormal mitosis which would normally trigger p53-mediated apoptosis. For these reasons p53 is often referred to as 'the guardian of the cell'. These viral–cellular interactions lead to unchecked growth of genetically unstable cells, vulnerable to secondary mutations and susceptible to malignant progression. The properties and affinities of E6 and E7 oncoproteins associated with high-risk HPV types are quite different to the properties of these proteins in low-risk HPV types.

## Classification of HPV

Due to their complex lifecycle, HPVs are difficult to culture in the laboratory so their characterisation has been performed through genome sequence analysis. The formal, systematic classification system defines an *HPV type* as a complete HPV genome whose L1 nucleotide sequence differs from that of any other genome by at least 10%, with HPV types distinguished by a number according to when they were discovered. Currently, well over 100 types of HPV are recognized and these are organized into separate *genera* (Fig. 45.2). Within the genera or 'major branches' of the phylogenetic tree, minor branches contain *HPV species* which unite types that are genomically distinct but similar in terms of their biological activity. Further subdivisions occur including HPV subtypes that differ by between 2–10% and HPV variants that differ by <2%.

Different HPVs have evolved to fill different biological niches and HPVs are frequently grouped according to the skin type and/or anatomical area with which they are associated. Consequently, the descriptive terms cutaneous HPVs, mucosal HPVs and genital HPVs are sometimes used, and these link

**Table 45.1**  Papillomavirus gene functions

| Gene | Function | Comments |
|------|----------|----------|
| E1 | Episomal maintenance | Frequently disrupted by integration |
| E2 | Regulation of transcription and replication. DNA-binding protein; very similar in BPV and HPV | Regulates transcription and viral replication in association with E1. Frequently disrupted by integration |
| E4 | Virion maturation, disrupts cytoskeleton | May facilitate release of virions from differentiated keratinocytes |
| E5 | Transforming function – alters signalling from growth factor receptors | Enhances transforming capabilities of E6 and E7 |
| E6 | Transforming function – binds to p53 and other pro-apoptotic proteins | Co-operates with E7 to stimulate cells into S phase, retard cell differentiation and increase efficiency of transformation |
| E7 | Major transforming gene – binds to members of pocket protein family such as Rb | Induces proliferation. Works cooperatively with E6 but is capable of transforming cells independently of E6 |
| L1 | Production of major capsid proteins, facilitates attachment and entry | Group- and type-specific determinants (for classification) |
| L2 | Production of minor capsid proteins, facilitates attachment and entry | Type-specific determinants (for classification) |
| URR (upstream regulatory region) | Regulation of gene function and initiator of viral replication | Non coding region. Contains both positive and negative transcriptional control elements. |

**Table 45.2**  Classification and clinical manifestations of HPV types

| Genus | Type | Clinical Associations |
|-------|------|----------------------|
| Alpha | HPV-2, -27, -57<br>HPV-6, -11<br>Species 9: HPV-16, -31, -33, -35, -51, -52, -56, -58, -59<br>Species 7: HPV-18, -45, -59 | Common skin warts and sometimes genital warts in children<br>Benign mucosal lesions – genital warts, laryngeal papillomas<br>Pre-invasive squamous and glandular lesions and cancers (high-risk types)<br>Pre-invasive squamous and glandular lesions and cancers (high-risk types) |
| Beta | HPV-5, -8 | Cutaneous benign and malignant lesions in immunosuppressed patients |
| Gamma | HPV-4, -65 | Cutaneous benign lesions |
| Mu | HPV-1, -63 | Cutaneous benign lesions, frequently on feet |

Adapted from Bernard SU 2005 The clinical importance of the nomenclature, evolution and taxonomy of human papillomaviruses. *Journal of Clinical Virology* 32S: S1–S6.

to different branches of the phylogenetic tree, e.g. cutaneous types form one clear branch and genital types with greatest malignant potential form a second branch.

Another way of stratifying HPV is as 'low-' or 'high-risk' (LR or HR) according to their potential association with cancer. Evidence for risk status comes from studies where the types detected in cancer cases are compared to the types detected in non-cancerous control tissue. A recent study of over 30 000 cervical cancers revealed the 13 most common

HR-HPV types to be -16, -18, -58, -33, -45, -31, -52, -35, -59, -39, -51 and -56, with HPV-16 and/or HPV-18 accounting for 70–76% of invasive cervical cancer in all world regions. Table 45.2 shows the clinical associations of HPV types.

## Transmission and epidemiology

HPV requires close skin to skin contact for transmission and most people will acquire an HPV infection at some point in their life. HPV is also a relatively stable virus and has been found in fomites such as damp surfaces and towels. Wet skin is more vulnerable to surface breaks hence the prevalence of plantar warts (verrucas; HPV-1) associated with swimming pool environments. Sexual contact/intimacy is the main route for transmission of HPV to the genital area, although transmission does not require penetrative sex. In males, HPV has been detected on several areas of the penis, the scrotum, the area surrounding the anus and the buttocks. Similarly in females, HPV can be found at all genital sites. Occasionally HPV can be transmitted to the genital areas by non-sexual routes; a mother with HPV can infect her child intrapartum and family studies have shown evidence of horizontal transmission between carer and child.

The mean duration of infection varies according to HPV type and age of the infected individual. Genital carriage of HPV decreases dramatically with age in females with highest prevalence around 40% in the 20–25 year group. Although there is less epidemiological data in males, recent evidence suggests infection levels are more consistent over the adult years. Most HPV infections clear within 1–2 years, depending on other influences including smoking, persistent oral contraceptive use, co-infection with other STIs and early age of first intercourse.

About 90% of genital warts are associated with the low-risk HPV-6 and HPV-11. HR-HPV such as HPV-16 and HPV-18 are more likely to be associated with subclinical or latent infections which can be detected by looking for HPV DNA. From many international studies, the median prevalence of high-risk HPV has been estimated to be 15% among women with normal cervical cytology. The peak prevalence is found in young women aged under 25 years, and declines with age. Persistent infection with HR-HPV carries a much greater risk of progression to cancer.

## Clinical features and pathogenesis of HPV infections

### Cutaneous warts

Cutaneous warts commonly infect the keratinized epithelium of the hands and feet, producing typical warts frequently seen in young children and adolescents (Fig. 45.3A). Typically, HPV-1 and HPV-4 are commonly found on the feet, whereas HPV-3 and HPV-10 are associated with flat warts and HPV types 2, 4 and 7 with common warts. HPV-7 can be particularly troublesome in butchers and fishmongers where frequent exposure to water causes maceration of the skin and facilitates virus entry and spread. Histologically, the lesions are benign with hypertrophy of all layers of the dermis and hyperkeratosis of the horny layer

(Fig. 45.4). They usually disappear spontaneously but occasionally may be resistant to treatment. Regrowth of the lesions after treatment is probably due to persistence of the virus in the skin surrounding the original wart.

Host factors contribute to the control and outcome of HPV infections. Both humoral and cell-mediated immune responses develop, with regression largely resulting from T helper ($T_H$) type 1-driven cytotoxic T cells and protection from subsequent infection with the same HPV type from $T_H2$ stimulation of B cells. Patients with primary or secondary cell mediated immunodeficiency have an increased risk of developing warts which can be extensive (Fig. 45.3B), persistent or recurrent. For example, in people suffering from the rare genetic skin disorder *epidermodysplasia verruciformis* (*EV*), in which there is a selective depletion of specific T cell clones, large plane warts associated with virus types such as HPV-5 and HPV-8 develop and persist for life. Similarly, up to 40% of renal allograft recipients develop cutaneous warts within a year of receiving the graft, rising to more than 90% in those with graft survival for longer than 15 years. EV-associated HPV types are found in a variety of lesions, including a high proportion of psoriatic skin lesions but also in normal skin and hair follicles in people with no immune defects, suggesting that the viruses are widespread and that development of visible lesions is well controlled by the immune system of healthy individuals.

### Anogenital warts

Genital HPV infections are very common in the general population and a huge increase in incidence has been reported in recent years. Anogenital warts (also known as *condylomata acuminata*; Fig. 45.3C) are found predominantly in sexually active adults and are the most common clinical manifestation.

In women, vulvar and vaginal warts are usually plainly visible, but on the cervix they may be indistinguishable from the normal mucosa without the aid of a colposcope to magnify the cervical epithelium. Subclinical lesions may proliferate and become clinically apparent if the immune response is disturbed, as in pregnancy. The application of 5% acetic acid causes whitening of epithelium in which there is a high concentration of nuclear material and reveals subclinical lesions as areas of densely white whorled epithelium known as flat or noncondylomatous warts (Fig. 45.3D). In men, the most common sites for lesions are the shaft of the penis, perianal skin and the anal canal. Subclinical infection on the penis can be detected using a colposcope and 5% acetic acid as in women.

**Fig. 45.3** Typical clinical presentations of HPV. (A) Common hand warts on child. (B) Extensive plantar warts in renal transplant patient. (C) Genital warts (condylomata acuminata). (D) Cervical flat wart after application of acetic acid. Courtesy of Dr MH Bunney and Dr EC Benton.

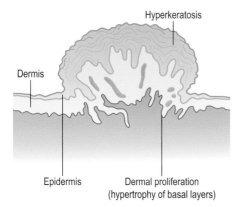

**Fig. 45.4** Diagrammatic representation of the histological appearance of a wart.

## Orolaryngeal lesions

***Recurrent respiratory papillomatosis (RRP).*** This is a rare condition characterized by the presence of benign squamous papillomata on the mucosa of the respiratory tract, most commonly on the larynx. It has a bimodal distribution with peaks of incidence in children under 5 and adults over 15 years of age, and is caused by infection with HPV types 6 and 11. Children acquire the disease by passage through an infected birth canal, whereas adults acquire the disease from orogenital contact with an infected sexual partner. The transmission rate is low. The disease presents with an abnormal cry in children and/or hoarseness of voice. As the lesions grow they may cause life-threatening upper airway obstruction that

**Fig. 45.5** HPV infection and pathogenesis of cervical cancer. CIN, cervical intra-epithelial neoplasia; HR, high risk.

requires emergency surgery. Recurrence after treatment is common. Malignant conversion of laryngeal papillomata has been described in the past, usually after radiotherapy to treat the initial lesion.

*Oral papillomatosis.* A variety of papillomata and benign lesions occur on the oral mucosa and tongue and are associated with a range of HPV types. The occurrence of multiple lesions on the buccal mucosa is known as oral florid papillomatosis. Subclinical lesions can be detected on the oral mucosa of normal adults after the application of acetic acid. The virus types here are those found more commonly in the genital tract, and infection is acquired during orogenital contact with an infected sexual partner.

## HPV and cancer

### Premalignant lesions of the genital tract

Malignant disease of the cervix is preceded by neoplastic change in the surface epithelium, a condition known as *cervical intra-epithelial neoplasia* (CIN). The initial transforming event takes place in the deepest layer of the epithelium, the germinal layer, and abnormal cells spread through the surface layers. This condition increases in severity from:

- CIN-I (low-grade squamous intra-epithelial lesions, LSIL in American classification) which can be associated with both low (including HPV-6 and HPV-11) and high-risk types and is very unlikely to progress

- CIN-II (high-grade or HSIL) in which abnormal cells including mitotic figures can be found up to the mid-epithelium with loss of stratification and differentiation. CIN-II often regresses spontaneously
- CIN-III (also called high-grade or HSIL, but with more extensive disturbance and mitotic figures including superficial layers of epithelium) which, if untreated, can progress to invasive cancer in a large proportion of affected individuals (Fig. 45.5).

Infection with multiple types is common but is not associated with an increased risk of progression. The development of intraepithelial neoplasia at other sites is similar (VIN for vulva; VAIN for vagina and AIN for anus) and HPV DNA can be detected in all grades of the premalignant lesions of the female and male genital tract.

### Invasive cancers

The association of HPV with invasive cancers of the skin and aero-digestive tract as well as the genital tract is well documented. Malignant conversion of skin warts occurs in about one-third of patients with EV at a relatively young age on skin exposed to sunlight, with HPV types 5 or 8 in more than 90% of squamous cancers. Malignant conversion of cutaneous warts also occurs in renal allograft recipients.

It is now recognized that a subset of oropharyngeal squamous cell cancers (OSCC), particularly those in the lingual and palatine tonsils, have an HR-HPV aetiology. The incidence of HPV-associated OSCC has risen in the last decade, particularly in individuals <50 years old who have been less exposed to the 'traditional' risk factors of drinking and smoking. Interestingly, HPV-associated OSCC has a better prognosis compared to HPV negative OSCC.

The most common association with invasive cancer, however, is with tumours of the anogenital tract. More than 99% of invasive cervical cancers contain HPV DNA. The proportion of cancers due to different HPV types varies around the world, and the incidence shows wide demographic, ethnic and socio-economic variation. Key facts include:

- Throughout the world, HPV-16 is by far the most common HR-HPV.
- HPV-16 is the cause of more than 50% of invasive cervical cancers worldwide.
- Cervical cancer is the second most common cancer of women worldwide with a mean incidence of 35 per 100 000.

HPV-18 and the related HPV-45 are found more frequently in the more aggressive adenocarcinomas. In-situ DNA hybridization of tumour biopsies has shown that HPV DNA is unevenly distributed throughout the tumour, suggesting that these cancers are polyclonal in origin.

In most animal cancers associated with papillomavirus there is a co-factor. In man the co-factors associated with genital tract malignancies are similar to those noted above for HPV infection with smoking, seminal fluid factors, immune status, long-term use of oral contraceptives and genetic background being most significant. In the development of HPV-related carcinomas at other sites, exposure to ultraviolet or ionizing radiation and chewing of betel-quid are additional risk factors. Thus:

- Women who smoke are at increased risk of CIN and cancer of the cervix.
- Women who are immunosuppressed, whether due to drug treatment (transplant recipients) or secondary to haematological malignancies (leukaemias) or to infection with human immunodeficiency virus (HIV), are also at increased risk of cervical cancer.

The incidence of anal cancer in men who have sex with men and in HIV-infected men is similar to that of cervical cancer. It is thought that the presence of a cellular transformation zone makes these sites more susceptible to the oncogenic effects of high-risk HPV infection. In contrast, vaginal, vulval and penile cancers are rare, and these areas lack a transformation zone.

## Laboratory diagnosis

### Morphological identification

HPV infection may be readily diagnosed when there are typical, visible clinical lesions. In cervical smears, HPV infection can be recognized morphologically by the presence of vacuolated cells with enlarged hyperchromatic nuclei described as *koilocytes*. However, koilocytes are not always present, are not sufficiently specific for HPV, and cannot differentiate between low- and high-risk HPV types. Histological examination of a biopsy taken from a lesion identified at colposcopy will show more specific features of HPV infection, including papillomatosis, hyperkeratinization of the surface layer, hypertrophy of the basal layers and disorganization of the epidermal structure (Fig. 45.4).

### Serology

The lack of native antigen hampered the development of serological assays for several years. However serological assays for HPV now exist using virus-like particles (VLPs) as a source of antigen. These assays are useful for natural history studies where past infection is assessed and also for monitoring vaccine induced immunity. However, as HPV has no viraemic phase, is non-lytic and creates little inflammation, natural infection induces a low-level antibody response with a <50% seroconversion rate. Consequently, serology tests lack sufficient sensitivity to be useful for clinical management.

### Molecular detection

Nucleic acid based detection of HPV DNA and RNA has been developed extensively for research, epidemiological and clinical use. Clinical applications often focus on the detection of DNA from a group of clinically relevant HR-HPV types and most are based on the detection of HPV-L1 DNA. Sensitivity is high but because infection is so common it is difficult to distinguish between clinically significant persistent infections and transient infections. RNA tests which detect transcription of E6 and E7 oncogenes have the potential to be more specific for disease. Work is also progressing on the detection of secondary markers known to be triggered by high level oncogenic expression including the cellular marker, p16INK4a. In research and surveillance, specialized genotype-specific assays are more relevant. These are often based on PCR amplification using consensus or degenerate primers followed by hybridization to type specific probes and colorimetric detection of the hybrids in nylon strips.

In cervical screening, HR-HPV DNA tests which give a presence/absence result are most frequently used and are extremely sensitive for the detection of high-grade cervical lesions (between 95–100%). Women who test negative are very unlikely to have significant disease. For effectiveness, cytology screening needs to be repeated regularly (every 3–5 years in the UK between ages 20–65) as it is only around 60% sensitive for the detection of significant lesions. Nevertheless, the lower specificity of HPV screening tests, particularly in young women (<30 years) who have high prevalence of infection means that tests should be performed only in appropriate contexts, where the result will be meaningful and help to inform patient management.

Cervical disease management systems incorporating HPV testing into the repertoire include:

### Triage of low-grade (cytological defined) abnormalities

While most low-grade abnormalities will clear, a proportion (15–20%) will harbour significant lesions. HPV testing is use to stratify risk, with HPV-negative women subjected to a less intensive clinical follow up than high-risk HPV-positive women.

### Post-treatment follow-up (test of cure)

After treatment of high-grade lesions, women are monitored to ensure their treatment has been successful. HPV testing can help to identify potential residual disease and reduce the intensity of follow-up in women who test HPV negative.

### HPV primary screening followed by cytology triage

Several European trials, together recruiting over 250 000 women, have shown the ability to detect high-grade disease more quickly with HPV screening than with cytology. New clinical testing algorithms based on HPV primary testing, followed by cytology of HPV-positive cases, are being introduced and will allow the screening interval to be increased to 5–6 years or longer in women over 30 years of age.

## Treatment and control

In most immunocompetent people, warts are a cosmetic nuisance and will eventually disappear spontaneously. Warts may be destroyed by cryotherapy with dry ice or liquid nitrogen, but simple topical treatment with salicylic acid at home is often successful. Genital warts are more problematic. They are the most common sexually transmitted infection and represent a significant burden to healthcare providers. In pregnant women, vaginal warts may occasionally grow to such a size that the birth canal is obstructed and surgical removal is required. Prevention of spread of wart viruses can be achieved by avoiding contact with affected individuals. Thus, the use of condoms will diminish the risk of spread of genital warts. Interferon, photodynamic therapy and indole-3-carbinol have been used for treatment of recurrent laryngeal warts after the reduction of tumour load by cautery or excision.

Many treatments can be used for genital warts including:

- antiproliferative agents such as podophyllin or 5-fluorouracil, although close monitoring is required
- destructive therapies such as trichloracetic acid, liquid nitrogen or surgical excision
- immunomodulators such as imiquimod, which activates monocytes/macrophages and causes direct release of interferon-α (self-applied topical treatment).

All of these treatments will remove the lesions but do not always eradicate the virus from surrounding normal epithelium. Incomplete treatment is the most common cause of recurrence of warts; all of a patient's warts must have disappeared with restoration of normal skin texture before a cure is considered. This is also true for treatment of CIN. Long-term follow-up to ensure clearance is a significant cost to health care and a significant anxiety for women.

## Vaccines

Vaccines are available which can prevent the development of papillomata and cancers in cattle and rabbits, consisting principally of virus-like particles of L1, or L1 with L2 proteins. The development and introduction of prophylactic vaccines for HPV based on genetically engineered virus-like particles has provided a unique opportunity to limit the spread of HPV infection and the global burden of HPV related cancers and its precursors. Two vaccines are currently licensed, one containing L1 of HPV-16 and HPV-18 (bivalent vaccine) and the other L1 of HPV-6, -11, -16 and -18 (quadrivalent vaccine). Both proved to be safe and highly efficacious in clinical trials, providing almost complete protection from high grade cervical disease associated with HPV-16 and HPV-18 (both vaccines) and from genital warts (quadrivalent vaccine). In 2008, the UK introduced

**Table 45.3**  History of human polyomavirus discoveries

| Abbreviation | Origin of name | Year of discovery | Diseases association |
|---|---|---|---|
| SV40 | Simian vacuolating agent | 1960 | Contamination of polio vaccines; association with human cancer controversial |
| BKV | Initials of patient | 1971 | Ureteric stenosis, haemorrhagic cystitis, polyomavirus associated nephropathy in transplant recipients |
| JCV | Initials of patient | 1971 | Progressive multifocal leuco-encephalopathy in immunosuppressed patients |
| KIV | Karolinska Institute | 2007 | Respiratory tract infection in young children, clinical significance unclear |
| WUV | Washington University | 2007 | Respiratory tract infection in young children, clinical significance unclear |
| MCV | Merkel cell polyomavirus | 2009 | Merkel cell carcinoma, a rare primary neuroendocrine malignant tumour of the skin |
| TSV | Trichodysplasia spinulosa associated polyomavirus | 2010 | Trichodysplasia spinulosa, a rare dermatological condition found only in immunosuppressed patients |

a national schoolgirl immunization programme for 12-13 year olds which has achieved record coverage of 80–90%. Vaccine is available in most countries, but is very expensive. For maximum effectiveness, population-based programmes with immunization before sexual debut should be implemented. While protection from infection is now possible, it will be many years before the ability of vaccine to prevent or halt cervical cancer development can be detected and even then only by implementing robust programmes of surveillance.

Therapeutic vaccines for the control of existing HPV-associated disease focus on HPV oncogenes and aim to generate potent E6 and E7-specific T cell-mediated immune responses. Modified DNA vaccines with improved immunogenicity provide a potentially promising approach and have reached the stage of clinical trials.

## POLYOMAVIRUSES

The term *polyomaviruses* literally stands for many (poly) tumour (oma) viruses, so called due to their ability to induce various tumours in experimental animals. So far, seven human polyomaviruses have been identified (Table 45.3). Initially, only murine and hamster polyomaviruses appeared to be oncogenic in their natural hosts. However, the more recently discovered Merkel cell polyomavirus has a clear association with Merkel cell carcinoma, a rare human neuro-endocrine cutaneous tumour found in the immunosuppressed or those exposed to sunlight. The older members BK virus and JC virus have no clear association with malignancies and both were named after the initials of the patients from whom they were first isolated.

The virions are 42–45 nm in size with a 72-capsomere icosahedral capsid. The genome consists of a double-stranded super-coiled loop of DNA, approximately 5100 bp in length, with both strands coding for virus proteins. Capsids contain three structural proteins, VP1, VP2 and VP3.

## Replication and transformation

There are three non-capsid regulatory proteins: large T (*T Ag*), small t and agnoprotein. Murine polyomaviruses have an additional middle *T Ag*. These are the first antigens to appear after infection; they accumulate in the nucleus, stimulate cellular growth and are important for replication. This is followed by a switch to transcription of the late region of the genome and production of the three structural capsid proteins. The growth cycle in culture is 36–44 h, and the release of mature virus particles follows lysis of the cell. The structural proteins determine host range and infectivity. BKV can be grown with difficulty in human embryonic kidney cells, whereas JCV, which is not only species but also tissue specific, replicates only in human embryo glial cell cultures. Recently, the 5-hydroxytryptamine 2A ($5HT_{2A}$) receptor for serotonin on the surface of glial cells was identified as the receptor protein for entry of JCV.

The early proteins are associated with immortalization and transformation of host cells. Large T antigen binds to both Rb and p53, and prevents the induction of cell death. Polyomaviruses do not have a viral DNA polymerase. Instead, they utilize the host DNA polymerase α/primase complex to which *T Ag* binds. *T Ag* also binds to double stranded (*ds*) DNA and has helicase activity to help to unwind the viral *ds*DNA for DNA replication.

## Clinical features and pathogenesis

Primary BKV and JCV infections are probably mostly asymptomatic. Rarely, upper respiratory tract symptoms, cystitis and encephalitis have been described. SV40 is primarily a simian virus. Its association with human infection is related to the inadvertent use of SV40 contaminated poliovirus vaccines in the 1950s and 1960s. The role, if any, of SV40 in human diseases is controversial. WUV and KIV are found in respiratory samples. Their role in human respiratory tract infection is at present unclear.

Reactivation of BKV and JCV is common, particularly in organ transplant patients, with up to 40% of renal allograft recipients and haematopoietic stem cell transplant (HSCT) patients excreting a polyomavirus in urine in the early months after transplantation. BKV reactivation is associated with haemorrhagic cystitis (HC) in HSCT patients and polyomavirus associated nephropathy (PVAN) in renal transplant patients. JCV is associated with progressive multifocal leuco-encephalopathy (PML), seen in immunosuppressed patients, most commonly patients with advanced HIV infection.

### Haemorrhagic cystitis (HC)

This is a common complication after HSCT. Early onset HC (<2 weeks) is probably not related to viral infection. However, late onset HC is often related to BK reactivation. BK virus excretors are 4 times more likely to develop HC than non-excretors and there is a strong temporal relationship between BK excretion and onset of HC. Pathogenesis may be related to immune reconstitution as its onset often coincides with engraftment.

### Polyomavirus-associated nephropathy (PVAN)

The association of BKV reactivation in the renal allografts of transplant recipients with graft dysfunction was made only in the last 10 years. Its discovery coincided with the introduction of newer more potent immunosuppressive agents such as tacrolimus and mycophenolate mofetil. So far, no specific immunsuppressive agents have been clearly associated with PVAN. Rather, the overall level of immunosuppression is thought to be responsible.

PVAN is mostly reported in patients receiving renal allografts and only rarely after other transplantations. Onset of PVAN occurs at a median time of about 6 months after transplantation and up to 1–5% of renal allografts are affected. Men are more likely to develop PVAN than females in most case series. The only presenting clinical feature is that of deterioration in graft function. Hence, the major differential diagnosis is allograft rejection. Renal biopsy is the gold standard for differentiation of these two conditions. However, non-invasive methods of diagnosis of PVAN are also available. Since the management of graft rejection is to increase immunosuppression whereas that of PVAN is to decrease it, an accurate diagnosis is necessary to inform management.

### Progressive multifocal leuco-encephalopathy (PML)

This condition, associated with the reactivation of JCV in the brain, was first described in 1958 in patients with *Hodgkin's lymphoma* and *chronic lymphocytic leukaemia*. Over the past 10 years, PML has been found almost exclusively in patients with acquired immune deficiency syndrome (AIDS). More recently, PML has also been described in patients receiving monoclonal antibody therapy such as rituximab and natalizumab.

Patients with PML have multiple foci of demyelination, usually affecting white matter in the cerebral hemispheres, but occasionally elsewhere in the central nervous system. Affected oligodendrocytes become swollen, with hyperchromatic nuclei and occasional basophilic inclusions pathognomonic of PML. Replication of the virus occurs in the nucleus, causing cell destruction and breakdown of the myelin sheath.

The clinical features depend on the areas affected. Symptoms include visual, mental and speech impairment, hemiplegia, loss of memory, personality change and dementia. Death usually occurs within 6 months of the first signs of the disease. Other causes of similar symptoms such as cerebral lymphoma, toxoplasmosis and tuberculosis need to be excluded.

## Laboratory diagnosis

In HC, polyomaviruses can be detected in large quantity in urine. The presence of BKV in the urine can be confirmed by BKV specific PCR. Patients with uncomplicated HC do not normally have significant BK viraemia (i.e. virus detectable in perpipheral blood).

The gold standard of PVAN diagnosis is histological examination of renal biopsy and identification of viral inclusion bodies in the renal tubular cells. The presence of polyomavirus can be confirmed by immunohistological staining using monoclonal antibodies against polyomavirus *T Ag*. Histology can also exclude or detect concomitant presence of graft rejection. Non-invasive methods such as urine cytology detection of polyomavirus infected uroepithelial cells (decoy cells) or detection of polyomavirus in urine by electron microscopy, though sensitive, are non-specific and have poor positive predictive values. The best non-invasive diagnostic method, with the highest positive predictive value, is quantitative plasma BK viral load. Serial plasma viral load can also be used to monitor the progress of the disease.

The 'gold standard' for diagnosis of PML depends on a combination of neuroimaging and biopsy. JCV DNA may not be detectable in the cerebrospinal fluid (CSF) even with the use of highly sensitive nested PCR. Intrathecal antibody detection may be useful if JCV DNA is negative in CSF.

Antibodies to polyomaviruses can be measured using haemagglutination inhibition (HAI) and enzyme-linked immunosorbent assay (ELISA). HAI uses whole virions and gives a species-specific result, whereas in ELISA disrupted virions or purified VP1 can be used to give a more sensitive and type-specific result. Rising titres and the presence of immunoglobulin M are diagnostic of recent infection. Failure to detect antibody to JCV nearly always excludes a diagnosis of PML.

## Transmission and epidemiology

Very little is known about the transmission of polyomaviruses. Both BKV and JCV are frequently detected in urine. Respiratory, sexual and fecal-oral routes of transmission are all possible. In human tissues, BKV DNA may be found in tonsils, lung, lymph nodes and spleen; and JCV DNA in lung, liver, spleen, lymph nodes and leucocytes.

Serological studies show that BKV infection is a common event in early childhood. By 3 years of age 50–60% of children have antibody, rising to almost 100% by the age of 10 years. JCV circulates independently of BKV in the community, and acquisition of antibodies is slower and increases steadily with age to about 60–70% in adulthood.

## Treatment

Cidofovir is active against polyomaviruses *in vitro*. As polyomaviruses do not carry viral DNA polymerase, the action of cidofovir is likely to be targeted against other proteins such as host polymerase or viral *T Ag*. Its clinical use in HC or PVAN has not been particularly successful. In addition, cidofovir is nephrotoxic and can only be used in very small doses in renal patients. Leflunomide is a mild immunosuppressive agent licensed for the treatment of rheumatoid arthritis. It also has anti-viral properties and has been used as a treatment for PVAN. It has significant haematological toxicity which can be restrictive and dose limiting. The main management of PVAN is pre-emptive reduction of immunosuppression. In order to achieve this, non-invasive surveillance methods for PVAN such as quantitative plasma viral load measurement need to be available.

There is no established treatment for PML. In HIV patients, the use of combination anti-retroviral therapy (cART) may prolong survival, but this could paradoxically also increase the damage through immune reconstitution inflammatory syndrome (IRIS). Several chemotherapeutic agents, including cytosine arabinoside (ARA-C, cytarabine), cidofovir and mefloquine, have been tried. With the recent discovery of JCV utilizing the serotonin receptor to enter into glial cells, there has been interest in investigating the use of 5HT2a antagonists.

## RECOMMENDED READING

Bosch FX: Prevention of Cervical Cancer: Progress and Challenges on HPV Vaccination and Screening, *Vaccine* 26:K1–K94, 2008

Dörries, K: The Human Polyomaviruses. In Zuckerman AJ, Banatvala JE, Schoub BD, et al, editors: *Principles and Practice of Clinical Virology*, ed 6, Chichester, UK, 2009, John Wiley & Sons Ltd.

Khalili K, Stoner GL, editors: *Human Polyomaviruses. Molecular and Clinical Perspectives*, New York, 2001, Wiley-Liss.

Li N, Franchesci S, Howell-Jones R, et al: HPV type distribution in 30,848 invasive cervical cancers worldwide: variation by geographical region, histological type and year of publication, *International Journal of Cancer* 128:927–935, 2011.

Marur S, D'Souza G, Westra WH, Forastiere AA: HPV-associated head and neck cancer: a virus-related cancer epidemic, *Lancet Oncology* 11:781–789, 2010.

McCance D: Papillomaviruses. In Zuckerman AJ, Banatvala J, Schoub BD, et al, editors: *Principles and Practice of Clinical Virology*, ed 6, Oxford, 2009, Wiley-Blackwell, pp 807–822.

Moody CA, Laimins LA: Human papillomavirus oncoproteins: pathways to transformation, *Nature Reviews in Cancer* 10:550–560, 2010.

# 46 Hepadnaviruses

## Hepatitis B virus infection; hepatitis delta virus infection

*C. Y. W. Tong*

## KEY POINTS

- Hepatitis B virus (HBV) causes acute hepatitis and chronic infection leading to chronic liver disease and hepatocellular carcinoma.
- HBV is a partially double-stranded DNA virus, carrying a reverse transcriptase-like enzyme to replicate viral DNA from an RNA intermediate.
- HBV is transmitted in blood, e.g. through intravenous drug use, by sexual intercourse and from mother to child during childbirth.
- There is considerable geographical variation in exposure; the highest rates are in the Far East, sub-Saharan Africa, Oceania and South America.
- An effective vaccine is available, given in three doses over 6 months. Universal vaccination of young children will reduce the chronic infection rate and long-term sequelae, including hepatocellular carcinoma.
- Treatment of chronic HBV infection includes a course of pegylated interferon or the use of long-term suppressive therapy with nucleos(t)ide analogues.

The hepadnaviridae are a family of hepatotropic DNA viruses with a unique life cycle involving an RNA intermediate and the use of a viral polymerase enzyme with reverse transcriptase activity. There are two recognized genera whose members are species-specific and cause acute and chronic infection of the liver. The genus *orthohepadnavirus* infects vertebral hosts including humans, great apes, woodchucks and ground squirrels, while the genus *avihepadnavirus* infects birds such as ducks, herons and storks. Hepatitis B virus (HBV) is the type species of *orthohepadnavirus*, a major cause of chronic liver disease and hepatocellular carcinoma (HCC) in humans. HBV infection also occurs in the wild in a number of non-human primate species, such as chimpanzees, orangutans and gibbons. Each of these species harbours variants of HBV distinct from those found in man.

## HEPATITIS B VIRUS

### Structure

The virion of HBV is a 42 nm double-shelled particle known as the Dane particle. The outer envelope of the virion is formed by hepatitis B surface antigen (HBsAg). The inner core, 27 nm in diameter, consists of hepatitis B core antigen (HBcAg) which encloses the viral genomic DNA and polymerase.

The outer envelope protein, HBsAg, is over-produced by HBV and excess HBsAg is found in abundance in the blood of chronically infected individuals as sub-viral particles. Two different forms of subviral HBsAg can be seen in the blood (Figs 46.1 and 46.2). The predominant form is a small, spherical particle with a diameter of 22 nm. A filamentous form is also present. Both types of particles are composed of lipid, protein and carbohydrate; they are not infectious and consist solely of surplus virion envelope. There may be as many as $10^{13}$ of the small particles and filaments per mL. The virions are present in much smaller numbers, usually by a factor of $10^3$ or more.

The viral DNA is about 3200 nucleotides long and is circular in configuration (Fig. 46.3). The long negative sense strand is complete, but there is a gap of variable length of about 1000 nucleotides in the complementary positive sense strand. This incomplete strand is closed by the viral polymerase when virus replication starts. There are four overlapping open reading frames on the circular viral DNA coding for the core, surface, polymerase and an X protein which is possibly an activator of transcription. An additional viral protein, the hepatitis B e antigen (HBeAg), is translated from the core open reading frame that encodes the HBcAg protein using an upstream

**Fig. 46.1** Electron micrograph of the particles in the blood of a patient infected with HBV (original magnification ×130 000). (Courtesy of Dr A Keen, University of Cape Town.)

**HBsAg**

22 nm diameter subviral particles

      Spheres    and    filaments

**Virion - Dane particle**

42 nm diameter, inner core 27nm diameter

- HBsAg
- HBV DNA
- HBcAg
- Polymerase

*HBeAg is a protein encoded in the core open reading frame and secreted into the blood stream, but it is not part of the virion

**HDV virion**

35 nm diameter

- HBsAg
- HDV RNA
- HDV antigen

**Fig. 46.2** Schematic diagram of particles and antigens of HBV and HDV.

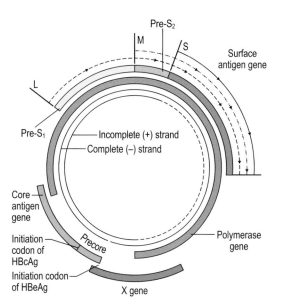

**Fig. 46.3** Gene organization of HBV DNA showing the four overlapping reading frames of core, polymerase, surface and X.

of the S reading frame known as pre-S$_2$. The protein from the L mRNA is the longest and comprises an additional pre-S$_1$ segment in addition to pre-S$_2$ and S. The L product is present only in the virions, whereas the M and S proteins are found in the virions as well as the subviral particles.

## Genetic variation

HBV can be classified into at least nine genotypes, A–I, based on a sequence divergence of >8% over the entire HBV genome. Some genotypes have a restricted geographical distribution, e.g. genotype E is found predominantly in sub-Saharan Africa, genotypes B and C in the Far East, and genotypes F and H in Central and South America. The HBsAg of all HBV genotypes contains a common 'a' determinant which is the main target of the protective antibody response. Immunity induced by infection or immunization with one HBV genotype cross-protects against infection with others.

## Stability

There is only limited success culturing HBV using primary hepatocyte cell culture and viral expression is often studied using cell lines with transfected HBV. It is therefore difficult to assess the stability of HBV. Indirect evidence has been obtained from the study of recipients of blood products treated in various ways and from chimpanzee inoculation experiments. Infectivity is lost after autoclaving at 121°C for 20 minutes

initiating codon. HBeAg is not found in the virion but is secreted from infected cells into the bloodstream, particularly during active viral replication. It is therefore frequently used as a marker indicating significant viral activity. The surface antigen gene is transcribed to produce three messenger RNAs (mRNAs): L, M and S. The S mRNA is the shortest but most abundantly produced. The product of the M mRNA is medium in length and consists of an additional portion or dry heat at 160°C for 1 h. HBV remains active after storage at 30–32°C for at least 6 months and when frozen at −15°C for 15 years. HBV in blood can withstand drying for at least 1 week. Effective chemical disinfectants include treatment with hypochlorite (10000 ppm available chlorine) for 10 min and 2% glutaraldehyde for 5 minutes. In clinical practice, chlorine based disinfectants are the ones most commonly used to disinfect environments contaminated with HBV. Glutaraldehyde was previously used to decontaminate endoscopes but was withdrawn due to toxicity. Effective substitutes include 0.2–0.35% peracetic acid, hypochlorous acid (superoxidised water) and chlorine dioxide.

## Replication

The exact cellular receptor and mechanism of entry of HBV into hepatocytes is still unknown. Once in the cytoplasm, the virus uncoats and the nucleocapsid is transported to the nucleus where replication of viral nucleic acid starts. The viral polymerase completes the positive sense strand to form a convalently closed circular (ccc) DNA. This cccDNA forms a minichromosome in association with host histone proteins and establishes the basis of the persistent infection. From the cccDNA, mRNAs are transcribed which are then translated to form the various viral proteins including HBsAg and HBcAg. A 3.5 kb mRNA that spans the entire length of the genome is packaged with the viral polymerase and a protein kinase into the core particles. The multi-function viral polymerase then reverse transcribes the packaged RNA into the negative strand genomic DNA. The same viral enzyme then creates the complementary positive strand DNA using the negative strand as template, but this process is left incomplete as the process stops when the nucleocapsid matures. The mature nucleocaspid is then transported to the cytoplasm to be associated with the envelope protein HBsAg in the endoplasmic reticulum to form progeny virions. Some nucleocaspids remain in the nucleus and contribute to the intra-nuclear pool of cccDNA, thus leading to amplification of infection. Integration of the viral DNA genome into a host chromosome can occur during the replication cycle. The position of integration appears to be random and may be important in the mechanism of carcinogenesis. However, unlike other viruses such as HIV, integration is not essential for the replication of HBV.

## ACUTE INFECTION

The incubation period of HBV infection ranges from 6 to 24 weeks, but is often about 2–3 months. Acute infection can be asymptomatic, particularly in children. Symptoms in the prodromal phase include malaise, anorexia, weakness, myalgia, nausea and vomiting. Presence of hepatitis is signalled by the appearance of jaundice and right upper quadrant abdominal pain, accompanied by pale stool and dark coloured urine. Paradoxically, the patient often feels physically better when the jaundice appears. Hepatocellular damage is detectable biochemically with elevated alanine transminase (ALT) levels before the onset of clinical jaundice, and persists after the jaundice has resolved. In some cases, immunological reactions due to circulating immune complexes may manifest as arthralgia, urticarial or maculopapular skin rash, polyarteritis nodosa or glomerulonephritis. Up to 1% of acute hepatitis B infections can become fulminant, resulting in acute liver failure.

## Pathology of acute infection

It is not possible to differentiate the various etiological agents of viral hepatitis at the histological level, as the changes are similar. In the acute stage there are signs of inflammation in the portal tracts; the infiltrate is mainly lymphocytic. In the liver parenchyma, infected hepatocytes show ballooning and form acidophilic (*Councilman*) bodies as they die.

HBV replicates in the hepatocytes, reflected in the detection of viral DNA and HBcAg in the nucleus and HBsAg in the cytoplasm and at the hepatocyte membrane. During the incubation period, high levels of virus are present before the host immune response develops to control the virus. During replication, HBcAg and HBeAg are also present at the cytoplasmic membrane. These antigens induce both B and T cell responses; damage to the hepatocyte can result from antibody-dependent, natural killer (NK) and cytotoxic T cell action. Expression of major histocompatibility complex (MHC) class I antigens is poor in hepatocytes but can be enhanced as interferons are produced in response to the infection. This in turn leads to increased antigen recognition and lysis of the infected hepatocytes. Thus, liver damage in HBV infection is mediated by an immunopathological mechanism.

## CHRONIC INFECTION

Most adults with acute HBV infection recover completely. Chronic infection occurs in 5–10% of adults, 20–50 % of children under the age of 6, and in over 90% of newborns who acquire the infection. Four stages of chronic infection are recognized (Fig. 46.4).

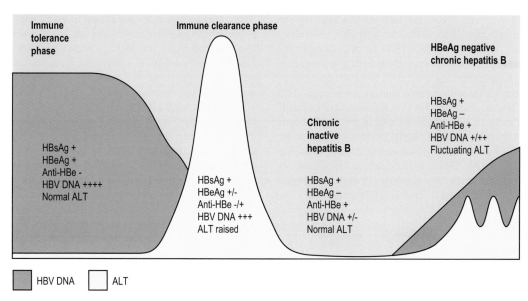

**Immune tolerance phase**

HBsAg +
HBeAg +
Anti-HBe -
HBV DNA ++++
Normal ALT

**Immune clearance phase**

HBsAg +
HBeAg +/-
Anti-HBe -/+
HBV DNA +++
ALT raised

**Chronic inactive hepatitis B**

HBsAg +
HBeAg –
Anti-HBe +
HBV DNA +/-
Normal ALT

**HBeAg negative chronic hepatitis B**

HBsAg +
HBeAg –
Anti-HBe +
HBV DNA +/++
Fluctuating ALT

■ HBV DNA    □ ALT

**Fig. 46.4**   Laboratory markers in different clinical phases of chronic hepatitis B.

1. Immune tolerance phase.
2. Immune clearance phase.
3. Inactive chronic infection phase.
4. HBeAg negative chronic hepatitis B – through emergence of hepatitis B variants.

The immune tolerance phase occurs mostly in children who acquired the infection at a young age, but is also seen in immunocompromised individuals. During this phase, the infected individual is immunologically tolerant to the presence of the virus, allowing the virus to replicate to very high levels without showing any symptoms. Serum HBV DNA levels are typically very high (>1 million IU/mL) and HBeAg is present with normal ALT levels. There is little evidence of necroinflammation or fibrosis on liver biopsy. Because of the high level of viraemia, these patients are highly infectious.

The immune clearance phase occurs when immune tolerance is lost. This typically occurs in early adulthood for those who were infected at a young age. This phase is characterized by HBeAg positivity, slightly lower level of HBV DNA (>200 000 IU/mL) compared to the immune tolerance phase, fluctuating levels of ALT and evidence of moderate to severe liver necroinflamamation and rapid progression of fibrosis. This phase may be confused with acute hepatitis due to similarity in symptoms and presence of low levels of IgM anti-HBc. The longer the duration of immune clearance, the more is the resultant liver damage.

For individuals who successfully clear active HBV infection, the phase of inactive chronic infection follows. Seroconversion from HBeAg to anti-HBe occurs and HBV DNA levels become very low (<2000 IU/mL) or undetectable, while ALT levels normalize. These individuals are asymptomatic but most remain HBsAg positive. As a result of successful immunological control of HBV, these patients tend to have a more favourable long-term outcome. Traditionally, these patients have been referred to as 'healthy hepatitis B carriers'. However, the use of such a term could result in a false sense of security, as between 10–20% may revert to active infection (reactivation) or change to the phase of HBeAg negative chronic hepatitis B through the emergence of viral variants. It is therefore necessary to have life long follow-up of patients with chronic inactive HBV infection.

In some patients, viral activity remains after seroconversion from HBeAg to anti-HBe. This is characterized by periodic fluctuating levels of HBV DNA and ALT. In these patients, a viral variant emerges (see section below) which is HBeAg negative but remains replication competent. The HBV DNA levels of these patients tend to be at a moderate level between 2000–200 000 IU/mL. Due to the fluctuating course, it is sometimes difficult to distinguish between patients in this phase with patients in the inactive phase. Nevertheless, a distinction is important as these patients have active disease and may progress to develop cirrhosis and HCC.

Approximately 0.5% per year of patients with inactive chronic hepatitis B will clear HBsAg. These individuals have resolved HBV infection and the presence of a past HBV infection is indicated by the presence of anti-HBc, with or without anti-HBs. However, in most cases, HBV is not completely cleared and reactivation can occur in the presence of immunosuppression such as after organ transplantation or treatment with immunosuppressive drugs. The risk for development of HCC is significantly reduced in these patients with resolved infection but not completely eliminated, particularly in older patients or those who have already developed cirrhosis. In some individuals, HBV DNA is persistently detectable in peripheral blood in the absence of HBsAg. These patients are said to have 'occult' HBV infection.

## Pathology and pathogenesis of chronic infection

In chronic hepatitis, damage extends out from the portal tracts, giving a piecemeal necrosis appearance. Some lobular inflammation is also seen. As the disease progresses, fibrosis and, eventually, cirrhosis develops. Chronic liver damage results from continuing, immune-mediated destruction of hepatocytes expressing viral antigens. In addition, autoimmune reactions may contribute to the damage as immune responses are induced to various liver-specific antigens.

Persistence of HBV is indicated by the continued presence of HBsAg and HBV DNA in the blood for more than 6 months. It is not yet clear what determines whether an individual will progress to the chronic state. There may be host genetic factors, but the absence, or relative inefficiency, of the immune response is important, as shown by the increased likelihood of chronic infection in the very young and the immunocompromised. In the neonate, infection occurs in the presence of maternal anti-HBc and HBeAg, which can cross the placenta. It is speculated that this results in tolerance through masking of HBcAg on hepatocyte membranes and thus prevention of its recognition by cytotoxic T cells and other immune mechanisms that could lead to clearance of the virus.

Other factors associated with increased risk of cirrhosis include older age or longer duration of infection, infection with HBV genotype C, high level of HBV DNA, heavy alcohol consumption and concurrent infection with hepatitis C virus (HCV), hepatitis D virus (HDV) or human immunodeficiency virus (HIV).

### Hepatocellular carcinoma (HCC)

There is considerable evidence that up to 80% of HCC worldwide is caused by chronic infection with HBV.

Thus, the highest rates are found in areas where HBV is endemic and where infection occurs at a very early age. Risk factors for HCC include male gender, a family history of HCC, older age, cirrhosis, infection with HBV genotype C, presence of core promoter variants (see section on variants below) and co-infection with HCV.

While only 5% of patients with cirrhosis develop HCC, between 60–90% of patients with HCC have underlying cirrhosis. Thus, a proportion of HCC occurs in the absence of cirrhosis. The prolonged presence (>40 years) of HBeAg and high levels of HBV DNA are independent risk factors of HCC. Integration of viral DNA is a possible mechanism of carcinogenesis as HBV DNA is often integrated in tumour cells but the site differs in different tumours. HCC can be prevented by vaccination. Experience from Taiwan, which has a high prevalence of both HBV infection and HCC, demonstrated that the introduction of universal childhood vaccination against HBV is effective in reducing the incidence of HCC in young adults.

### HBV variants

The frequency with which mutations appear in HBV is dependent on the high rate of replication of the virus and its dependence on replicating DNA via RNA and an RNA-dependent DNA polymerase. In highly viraemic individuals, as many as $10^{10}$ mutant genomes may arise each day. Most mutants are defective, but some may explain treatment failure or breakthrough infection.

### HBsAg variants

HBsAg variants arise as an escape mechanism during infection in the presence of anti-HBs. In babies given hyperimmune hepatitis B globulin (HBIG) and active immunization to reduce the risk of infection, but who are exposed to maternal virus during birth, the immune selection pressure from the HBIG and vaccine may result in the selection of HBsAg escape mutants. This is seen particularly in countries where universal childhood HBV vaccination has been practiced for many years, leading to breakthrough infection despite vaccination. Another scenario where immune selection pressure is intense is following liver transplantation for chronic hepatitis B. Immune selection pressure is exerted through the post-transplantation use of HBIG to protect the new liver from being re-infected with HBV.

HBsAg escape mutants mainly affect the 'a' determinant of HBsAg, the principal target of anti-HBs. The most common mutation observed is in position

145 of the HBsAg protein with an amino acid change from glycine to arginine (G145R). HBsAg escape mutants are transmissible and the widespread occurrence of HBsAg mutants would create considerable problems for the hepatitis B vaccination programme. In addition, many existing diagnostic assays for HBsAg use specific monoclonal antibodies that detect epitopes associated with the 'a' determinant. The presence of such mutations could lead to false negative diagnostic results when the monoclonal antibodies fail to bind to the mutated epitopes. Some cases of so-called 'occult HBV infection' are in fact due to false negative HBsAg, with detectable HBV DNA and no detectable antigenaemia.

### HBcAg variants

Mutations in the core promoter or pre-core coding regions of the core antigen open reading frame suppress the production of HBeAg, without affecting the synthesis of HBcAg and the assembly of complete virions. In the pre-core mutation variant, a stop codon is introduced between the initiation codons of HBeAg and HBcAg, so that full length HBeAg is no longer produced, but the production of HBcAg is unaffected. Individuals with these mutations are HBeAg negative but positive for HBV DNA. The absence of expression of HBeAg in such mutants is also believed to be an escape phenomenon enabling the virus to survive the cell mediated immune selection pressure from the host during the immune clearance phase. Core promoter mutations have been associated with the development of HCC in some studies.

### Polymerase variants

These are detected during therapy with nucleoside analogues and confer drug resistance. Their presence can affect the choice of drugs. The most well recognized mutation affecting the drug lamivudine is a change from methionine to valine or isoleucine at position 204 (M204V/I). This is often accompanied by another change at position 180 (L180M) which helps to maintain viral fitness and continuing replication. In HBV infected patients who receive a liver transplant, anti-viral prophylaxis is often given together with HBIG. Because the polymerase gene and the surface gene in HBV share the same region of the genome, although read in a different reading frame, mutations in the polymerase gene could force a mutation in the surface gene and vice versa. This could lead to complicated selections of mutants affecting both HBsAg and HBV polymerase.

## LABORATORY DIAGNOSIS

The laboratory can test for a wide range of HBV antigens and antibodies, using immnoassays based on enzyme reactivity (EIA) or chemiluminesence (CLIA). HBV DNA can be quantified in serum or plasma using real time polymerase chain reaction (PCR) assays. The standard screening test is for HBsAg, which, if present in the serum, indicates that the patient is currently infected with HBV.

### Acute infection

HBV DNA is the first detectable HBV marker in an acute infection followed shortly by HBsAg (Fig. 46.5) and both are present for some weeks before the onset of symptoms. In patients who have rapid viral clearance, antigenaemia is of short duration and may no longer be detectable at the onset of symptoms. If successive serum samples are examined, the development of anti-HBs will confirm recent primary infection, although there is considerable variation in the timing of the appearance of this antibody. HBV DNA may remain positive after disappearance of HBsAg. This creates a so-called 'window period' when an individual is HBsAg negative but remains infectious. In such cases, detection of IgM anti-HBc indicates that a primary infection has occurred recently.

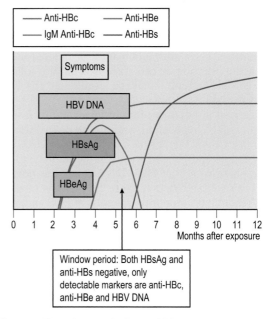

**Fig 46.5** HBV antigens, antibodies and DNA in a patient recovering from acute infection.

HBeAg is produced when virus is replicating and thus is usually found soon after HBsAg. IgM anti-HBc is a transient response and, if present in high titre, indicates a recent acute infection. Early disappearance of HBeAg and replacement with anti-HBe is a good prognostic sign for recovery. The presence of anti-HBs, occurring in about 90% of individuals after HBsAg clearance, indicates the development of immunity to further infection with HBV.

## Chronic infection

Chronic infection with HBV is defined by the presence of HBsAg for more than 6 months. During this time, IgM anti-HBc is replaced with IgG anti-HBc, although in some individuals with chronic active infection, IgM anti-HBc may persist at a low level. HBeAg remains detectable during the immune tolerance and immune clearance phases. It is replaced by anti-HBe either following successful immune clearance into the chronic inactive phase or the development of HBeAg negative mutants during chronic HBeAg negative hepatitis B. These two possible outcomes can be recognized by testing for HBV DNA levels. Chronic inactive HBV infection has a persistently low HBV DNA viral load (Fig. 46.6), whereas chronic HBeAg negative HBV infection often has fluctuating levels of HBV DNA at moderate to high levels.

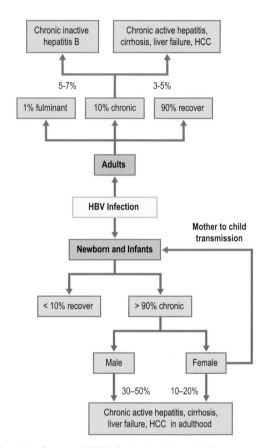

**Fig. 46.6** Outcome of HBV infection in adults and children.

## TREATMENT

The management of acute hepatitis B is usually supportive. Those with fulminant liver failure following acute infection or end stage liver failure following chronic infection may be candidates for liver transplantation.

The goal of treatment for chronic hepatitis B is to suppress HBV replication, prevent the progression of liver disease and thereby the development of cirrhosis, liver failure and HCC. Patients in the immune tolerance phase with high HBV DNA levels but normal ALT are not candidates for antiviral therapy. Instead, they should be monitored closely at 3–6 monthly intervals. Patients who have chronic inactive infection do not need antiviral treatment. For those who need treatment, the choice is between a course of interferon or long-term suppression with nucleoside or nucleotide analogues.

Interferon alpha ($\alpha$-IFN) is the first-line treatment option for patients without cirrhosis. Interferon has antiviral, anti-proliferative and immuno-modulatory effects. However, its efficacy is limited and only benefits a small proportion of patients. The current strategy is to use long acting pegylated interferon $\alpha$ for a finite duration of 24–48 weeks. In HBeAg positive individuals, a high pre-treatment ALT level, high histological activity score on liver biopsy, low HBV DNA levels and infection with genotype A or B, rather than C or D, are favourable prognostic indicators of treatment response. Seroconversion from HBeAg to anti-HBe occurs in approximately 30%, but <10% eventually clear HBsAg. Response to HBeAg negative disease is much less predictable and often requires a longer duration of therapy. Side effects are common and include influenza-like symptoms, neutropenia, thrombocytopenia, autoimmune thyroid disorders and psychiatric symptoms such as depression. An exacerbation of hepatitis is common, which is often a favourable indication of a subsequent response. However, in some patients, particularly those with existing cirrhosis, this can lead to hepatic decompensation.

Nucleoside or nucleotide analogues act as a false substrate after phosphorylation in infected hepatocytes and are incorporated into the growing DNA chains resulting in premature chain termination of HBV DNA synthesis. Lamivudine is a first generation nucleoside analogue in widespread use for some years. At a dose of 100 mg daily, lamivudine leads to a marked reduction or elimination of detectable HBV DNA in plasma in about 40% of HBeAg positive and 60–70% of HBeAg negative patients. Between 40–60% of patients have ALT normalization. Although toxicity is low, and in the long term the drug is generally tolerated well, prolonged administration is complicated by the emergence of antiviral resistance, manifested by the reappearance of HBV DNA in plasma and raised ALT levels after initial normalisation. Development of resistance associated mutations in the polymerase enzyme, particularly that of M204V/I, is common and can be detected in 14–32% after 1 year, and increases to 60–70% after 5 years of treatment. Development of resistance is more frequent in those who are immunosuppressed. Due to the rapid development of high-level resistance, lamivudine is now rarely used as a first line therapeutic agent. Instead, it is increasingly being used as a prophylactic agent to prevent HBV reactivation in the immunosuppressed.

Telbuvidine is a L-nucleoside analogue with potent anti-HBV activity. It is similar to lamivudine in mechanism of action and resistance profile but is more potent. However, its use is limited due to a high rate of resistance and cross-resistance with lamivudine. Emtricitabine is another L-nucleoside analogue with similar activity to that of lamivudine.

Adefovir is a nucleotide analogue of deoxyadenosine monophosphate that has demonstrated efficacy in suppressing HBV DNA (20–50%) and normalizing liver function (50–70%). Resistance to adefovir emerges less frequently than with lamivudine. Additionally, adefovir is effective against lamivudine-resistant mutants. Conversely, mutations that arise in response to adefovir therapy are sensitive to lamivudine. These observations led to the use of lamividune–adefovir combination therapy after failing lamivudine monotherapy. However, adefovir is not a very potent agent, and its use is now mostly superseded by newer antiviral agents such as entecavir and tenofovir.

Entecavir is a carbocyclic analogue of 2′ deoxyguanosine. It is a potent suppressor of HBV replication, resulting in loss of serum HBV DNA in 70–90%, and ALT normalization in 70–80% of patients. However, it is partially susceptible to the resistance associated mutations selected by lamivudine. Hence, a higher dose (1 mg instead of 0.5 mg) is required in the presence of lamivudine resistance. Development of full resistance to entecavir requires a two hit mechanism with initial selection of M204V/I followed by several entecavir specific mutations. As a result, treatment failure due to entecavir resistance is rare and is observed only in 3.6% of patients after 96 weeks of treatment. Entecavir resistant HBV is susceptible to adefovir or tenofovir.

Tenofovir is a nucleotide analogue initially approved for the treatment of HIV. It is often used in a co-formulation with emtricitabine. Tenofovir is structurally similar to adefovir, but because tenofovir is less nephrotoxic, a higher dose can be used, thus enhancing the antiviral activity significantly in comparison with adefovir. After 48 weeks of therapy with tenofovir, HBV DNA loss is achieved in 80–90% and ALT normalization in 70–80% of patients. So far, very little resistance against tenofovir has been described. The only limitation of its use is renal toxicity which requires monitoring of renal function and it is contra-indicated in patients with renal insufficiency. The combination of tenofovir with lamivudine or emtricitabine is often used in HIV/HBV co-infection in order to treat both viruses.

## EPIDEMIOLOGY

HBV is present in the blood as well as in body fluids such as semen, vaginal secretions and saliva. The presence of HBV in blood underlines the original association of infection with blood transfusion or the use of blood products and infections associated with needle-stick injuries. Sexual transmission is also recognized, as is that which occurs during close contact between family members, siblings, peers and residents in institutions. In these circumstances there will be frequent contact with blood and saliva; the virus gains entry through cuts and abrasions or across mucous membranes. Biting and scratching, sharing of household tools such as toothbrushes and razors could also be important factors. Vertical transmission from mother to child is one of the most important routes. Transmission occurs when maternal blood contaminates the mucous membranes of the baby during birth. Transplacental infection is thought to be quite rare unless maternal viral load is very high.

The World Health Organisation (WHO) has categorised three levels of HBV endemicity – high (≥8%), intermediate (2 to 7%) and low (<2%), based on the local prevalence of HBsAg. High-prevalence regions include sub-Saharan Africa, most of Asia and the Pacific islands. Intermediate-prevalence regions include the Amazon, southern parts of Eastern and Central Europe, the Middle East and the Indian sub-continent. Low-prevalence regions include most of

Western Europe and North America. Overall, it is estimated that one-third of the world's population has been infected with HBV and that 350 million individuals worldwide are chronically infected. Of these, between 15 and 40% will develop serious sequelae in their lifetime. In areas of low endemicity the risk of infection varies widely in different groups according to behaviour. Most cases occur in parenteral drug injectors sharing needles and syringes, and by sexual transmission, both homosexual and heterosexual. Screening of all blood donations using HBsAg and HBV DNA has virtually eliminated transmission by transfusion and blood products.

Healthcare personnel and laboratory workers are at risk of HBV infection through exposure to blood and body fluids of infected patients, although the degree of risk varies with the place and nature of their work, the care with which it is performed and their immune status. High-risk occupations include surgery, dental surgery, and obstetrics and gynaecology, which involve working with sharp instruments, often in restricted spaces. Operators may injure themselves and inoculate patients' blood. The spilling of a patient's blood will pose a threat only if there is contamination of unprotected abraded skin (intact skin is resistant to HBV penetration), or mucous membranes.

Patients are also at risk from infected staff, and episodes have been identified in which healthcare workers have transmitted HBV to their patients during invasive procedures, especially in difficult operations where the operator's hands are hidden and needles and instruments are guided by touch (exposure prone procedures).

## CONTROL

Broadly there are two approaches to the prevention of infection with HBV – modification of risk behaviour, and immunisation. Measures for the former include avoiding unprotected sexual contact by the use of condoms, and reducing needle sharing among injecting drug users through needle exchange schemes. Implementation of sensible infection control policies can reduce the risks considerably to healthcare workers and patients. It is essential that blood for transfusion and organ donors for transplantation are screened.

### Passive immunization

HBIG is prepared from donors with high titres of anti-HBs. Doses of 200–500 IU in 2–4 mL are given intramuscularly. The use of HBIG is indicated in the following situations:

- after accidental exposure if the victim is not vaccinated, or did not respond to the vaccine
- to babies born to infected mothers (in conjunction with active immunization)
- to prevent infection of a new liver transplanted into a recipient with chronic HBV infection.

HBIG must be given as soon as possible after exposure and preferably within 48 h; a second dose is given 4 weeks later to those who do not respond to current vaccines. Such a regimen does not give absolute protection, but an efficacy of 76% has been reported. In cases of needle-stick injuries, if the victim has not been vaccinated, HBIG should be used and a course of active immunization started, injecting the two materials into different body sites. To prevent mother to child transmission of HBV where the mother is highly infectious, e.g. the mother is HBeAg positive or HBV DNA viral load >1 million IU/mL, a combination of HBIG with active immunization given to the baby within 24 h of birth, is effective in as many as 90% of cases.

### Active immunization

Currently available vaccines are produced by cloning the surface antigen gene in yeast cells. The product is particulate and resembles the small particles seen in patients, although it is not glycosylated. The vaccine is administered with alum as adjuvant and injected intramuscularly; care should be taken to avoid injection into fat as this can reduce seroconversion rates. For this reason, injection into the deltoid muscle of the upper arm is recommended. The vaccine is free from major side effects; local swelling and reddening may occur in up to one in five recipients, with a slight fever in only a few cases.

Three doses of vaccine are given at 0, 1 and 6 months. Shorter schedules may be appropriate in some circumstances. The seroconversion rate is influenced by a number of factors, the most important of which are the age and sex of the vaccinee. Rates in excess of 95% are seen in young women, whereas the rate may drop to 80% in older men. Immunosuppressed patients show even lower rates, for example only 50–60% in patients on maintenance dialysis.

The duration of the response to vaccine is variable and dependent on the titre of anti-HBs achieved after completion of the course. A post-vaccination anti-HBs level >10 mIU/mL is considered as protective. However, to ensure a higher level of protection, a booster dose is often recommended if the anti-HBs level taken within 2–3 months after the third dose is <100 mIU/mL. If no response is detected (i.e. <10 mIU/mL), a course of three further doses should be given. A vaccine non-responder is defined as an individual who fails to develop immunity after two vaccine courses. Such individuals are not protected and must seek prophylaxis by passive immunization if they suffer accidental exposure. Those who are known to have responded can be given a booster if they are exposed to the virus. Some individuals show a drop in antibody level with time, but memory B cells will be activated on exposure to the virus and will provide sufficient protection against infection or at least to prevent the development of chronic infection.

## Who should be immunized?

Transmission from mother to child is an important route and requires intervention at birth (within 24 h) to protect the child. As most babies infected at birth will become chronically infected, it is essential to target this group. Dependent on the infectiousness of the mother, combined passive and active immunization or active immunization alone can be used. WHO has recommended universal childhood vaccination against HBV. Many countries have now incorporated this into their childhood vaccination programmes. Some countries, such as the UK, have adopted a selective infant vaccination strategy based on the result of antenatal HBV screening.

In the absence of a universal vaccination programme, the following groups should be targeted for HBV vaccination:

- Occupational risk groups – all healthcare workers who may have direct contact with patients' blood or body fluid, including doctors, nurses, cleaners, laboratory workers and paramedics. Other occupational risk groups such as police, fire and prison service staff, military personnel, morticians and embalmers.
- Babies of chronically infected mothers
- Injecting drug users
- Individuals who change sexual partners frequently
- Close family contacts and sexual partners of a case
- Families adopting children from endemic countries and foster carers
- Individuals with learning difficulties living in long-stay homes
- Patients needing frequent transfusions and/or blood products
- Patients with chronic renal failure
- Patients with chronic liver disease
- Inmates of custodial institutions
- Long stay travellers to endemic countries.

## THE DELTA AGENT (HEPATITIS D VIRUS, HDV)

The delta (δ) antigen was first identified in the late 1970s. Initially, it was thought to be an antigen of HBV, but it is part of another virus that cannot replicate without assistance from HBV. The specific helper function provided by HBV is its surface antigen, HBsAg, which also serves as the outer envelope of hepatitis D virus (HDV). HDV is a small (35–37 nm), enveloped particle containing a single, small, circular molecule of RNA of 1.7 kbp with an internal δ antigen enveloped by HBsAg (see Fig. 46.2). The origin of the virus is unknown and it has no homology with HBV. It has some resemblance with the satellite viruses of plants. However, it is also possible that the circular RNA of HDV is derived from an aberrant splicing event in human cells.

## CLINICAL FEATURES AND PATHOGENESIS

Hepatitis D virus (HDV) can only infect simultaneously with HBV (co-infection) or as a superinfection of an individual chronically infected with HBV. Co-infection has a better prognosis than superinfection, which often results in increase in severity of the chronic hepatitis with increased risk of developing cirrhosis, liver failure and HCC.

## DIAGNOSIS

Tests are available for HDV antigen, antibody and RNA. The sequence of appearance of the various markers in a patient co-infected with HBV and HDV is shown in Figure 46.7. The initial antibody response to HDV infection is IgM. In cases of superinfection, the test results are as illustrated in Figure 46.8. During the episode there may be a drop in the HBsAg titre, which, although usually still detectable, may disappear temporarily in a few cases. This can cause some diagnostic confusion. There may also be a reduction in HBV DNA levels which may result in a false assurance that the HBV infection is not active if HDV super-infection is not recognized.

**Fig. 46.7** Typical serological profile of simultaneous HBV and HDV co-infection.

**Fig. 46.8** Typical serological profile of chronic HBV with HDV super-infection.

## EPIDEMIOLOGY

There are an estimated 25 million HDV infected individuals in the world, but there is considerable geographical variation. Analysis of the RNA from different isolates has shown that there are at least eight different genotypes. Genotype 1 is of worldwide distribution; genotype 3 is found in the Amazon region; genotypes 2 and 4 in the Far East; and genotypes 5–8 in sub-Saharan Africa.

In the 1980s, it was thought that HDV was mainly associated with drug users and that controlling HBV through HBV vaccination or needle exchange schemes would be effective in eliminating HDV infection. There was an initial decrease in the prevalence of HDV in Europe, but it is increasingly recognized that HDV is not disappearing. Intravenous drug use is still an important factor; however it is no longer the sole driver of HDV spread. Immigrants from regions endemic for both HBV and HDV such as Eastern Europe and sub-Saharan Africa now constitute a higher proportion of infected cases in many cities. Despite having the highest prevalence of chronic HBV infection, the prevalence of HDV in South East Asia and China is very low.

## TREATMENT AND CONTROL

The only proven treatment of HDV infection is a prolonged course of pegylated interferon. However, this is not particularly successful as the sustained response rate after 48 weeks of treatment is less than 30%. There is no benefit in adding ribavirin or nucleos(t)ide analogues against HBV. The same general control measures as for HBV are also relevant for the control of HDV. HBV vaccine will prevent HDV co-infection, but there is no means of protecting against HDV superinfection.

RECOMMENDED READING

European Association for the Study of the Liver: EASL clinical practice guidelines: management of chronic hepatitis B, *Journal of Hepatology* 50:227–242, 2009.

Harrison TJ, Dusheiko GM, Zuckerman AJ: Hepatitis viruses. In Zuckerman AJ, Banatvala JE, Pattison JR, et al, editors: *2009 Principles and Practice of Clinical Virology*, ed 6, Chichester, 2009, Wiley, pp 273–320.

Lok ASF, McMahon BJ: Chronic Hepatitis B: AASLD Practice guidelines, *Hepatology* 50:1–36, 2009.

Seeger C, Zoulim F, Mason WS: Hepadnaviruses. In Knipe DM, Howley PM, editors: *Field's Virology*, ed 5, Philadelphia, 2007, Lippincott-Raven, pp 2977–3030.

Websites

Department of Health: Immunisation against infectious disease – 'The Green Book'. Chapter 18. Hepatitis B. http://www.dh.gov.uk/prod_consum_dh/groups/dh_digitalassets/@dh/@en/documents/digitalasset/dh_108820.pdf

Health Protection Agency: Hepatitis B. http://www.hpa.org.uk/infections/topics_az/hepatitis_b/menu.htm

# 47 Parvoviruses

## B19 infection; erythema infectiosum

*P. J. Molyneaux*

## KEY POINTS

- Parvoviruses, including B19, are the smallest viruses known to infect and cause human disease.
- B19 replicates in erythroid precursor cells, causing cell death.
- Spread is by respiratory, blood and transplacental routes.
- In healthy individuals, B19 causes immune-mediated rashes (fifth disease, slapped cheek syndrome) and arthropathy.
- In patients with underlying haematological disease, B19 may result in anaemia or a transient aplastic crisis.
- In immunocompromised patients, chronic anaemia or pure red cell aplasia may ensue.
- In pregnancy, maternal infection at 0–20 weeks' gestation may lead to fetal loss or non-immunological fetal hydrops.
- There is no specific antiviral therapy, and no available vaccine for B19.

Parvoviruses (*parvum* means small) have been isolated from a wide range of organisms, from arthropods to human beings. The family Parvoviridae is divided into two sub families: the Parvovirinae and the Densovirinae. The latter group infects only invertebrates. The Parvovirinae contain five genera: *Parvovirus, Dependovirus, Erythrovirus, Amdovirus* and *Bocavirus* (Table 47.1). They are differentiated by their replication:

- autonomous (*Parvovirus*)
- requirement for a helper virus (*Dependovirus*)
- replication in erythroid progenitor cells (*Erythrovirus*).

Only B19 within the genus *Erythrovirus* is known to be a human pathogen; erythroviruses distinct from B19 may yet be linked with human disease. Human bocavirus is a probable cause of lower respiratory tract infections and may have a role in gastroenteritis but neither is yet proven. Adeno-associated viruses (within the genus *Dependovirus*) and human parvovirus 4 (not yet classified) can be detected in human beings at various sites, but they have not been linked definitely with human disease (see p. 418).

## DESCRIPTION

The B19 virion (Fig. 47.1) is 20–25 nm in diameter, unenveloped, and contains a single strand of DNA (5.9 kilobase pairs). See Chapter 7 for details of replication. There are two capsid proteins, VP1 and VP2. B19 is genetically and antigenically stable with only one serotype, and is extremely resistant to lipid solvents, acid, alkali and high salt concentrations. It is relatively heat resistant as infectivity from high-titre virus can persist after 80°C for 72 h in clotting factor concentrates. The name B19 was given because it was first found in the blood of an asymptomatic blood donor (coded 19 in panel B) where it caused a false-positive result in an early test for hepatitis B surface antigen.

## PATHOGENESIS AND CLINICAL FEATURES

The clinical manifestations of B19 infection are due to either the direct effect of viral replication, which causes cell death, or the subsequent immune response. B19 attaches to cells through the blood group P antigen (globoside), and rare individuals who lack P antigen (p phenotype) are not susceptible to B19 infection. P antigen is present on mature erythrocytes, erythroid progenitors, megakaryocytes, vascular endothelium, placental cells, and fetal myocardial and liver cells. For B19 to replicate, it requires actively dividing cells; hence the cells most affected by B19 are the rapidly dividing red cell precursors in the bone

**Table 47.1** Taxonomic organization of Parvoviridae, their natural hosts and the diseases they cause

| Subfamily | Genus | Virus | Host | Disease |
|---|---|---|---|---|
| Densovirinae | Three genera | Densonucleosis viruses | Arthropods | Many fatal diseases |
| Parvovirinae | *Parvovirus* | Minute virus of mice | Mice | Subclinical |
| | | Feline panleucopenia virus | Cat | Enteritis, leucopenia, cerebellar ataxia |
| | | Canine parvovirus | Dog, fox | Enteritis, myocarditis |
| | | Porcine parvovirus | Pigs | Reproductive failure |
| | *Amdovirus* | Aleutian disease virus | Mink | Pneumonitis |
| | | Mink enteritis virus | Mink | Enteritis |
| | *Dependovirus* | Adeno-associated viruses | Man and others | Unknown |
| | *Erythrovirus* | Human parvovirus B19 | Man | Respiratory tract illness, aplastic crisis, erythema infectiosum/ fifth disease, fetal hydrops |
| | | Simian parvovirus | Monkey | Anaemia |
| | *Bocavirus* | Human bocavirus | Man | Unknown |
| | Unclassified | Human parvovirus 4 | Man | Unknown |

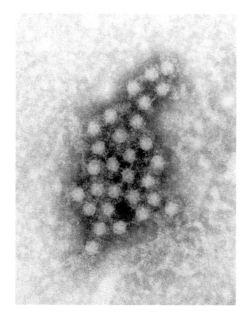

**Fig. 47.1** B19 particles in an immune electron microscopy preparation of serum from a child with a petechial rash and arthritis (original magnification ×200 000). (Courtesy of Dr Hazel Appleton, Health Protection Agency, London.)

**Fig. 47.2** Virological, haematological and clinical events during B19 virus infection of volunteers. (Reproduced with permission of John Wiley, Chichester).

marrow. The outcomes of infection depend on the immune competence and any red cell-related haematological dysfunction in the infected person. Development of antibody is needed to control B19 replication; capsid protein VP1 is the target for neutralizing antibody. After recovery, immunity is lifelong in normal individuals. Persistent and sometimes relapsing infection occurs in the immunocompromised as the little antibody they may produce in response to infection is not capable of neutralizing the virus and controlling the infection. Persistent infection can also develop in the fetus, the maternal viraemia giving ample

opportunity for infection of the placenta and fetus. Re-infection may occur, but is associated with illness only in the immunocompromised.

## Volunteer studies in humans

Experimental infection of healthy volunteers has revealed the steps in the pathogenesis of B19 infection (Fig. 47.2). The virus is infectious when given in nasal drops. One week later there is an intense viraemia with virus also present in respiratory secretions, but not in faeces or urine. At this time, a febrile influenza-like illness may occur, thought to be cytokine induced. The intense viraemia (up to $10^{11}$ particles per mL) lasts for only a few days before there is a brisk antibody response, initially of the immunoglobulin (Ig) M class, but followed rapidly by the appearance of IgG antibody. B19 viraemia can sometimes be detected for months after infection by polymerase chain reaction (PCR).

Haematological changes take place in the second week after inoculation. At 10 days after inoculation erythroid precursors are absent from the bone marrow and reticulocytes disappear from the peripheral blood; there is a small subclinical fall in the haemoglobin level. Lymphocyte, neutrophil and platelet counts sometimes fall transiently, but this is not due to lack of precursors in the bone marrow. Haematological changes are the direct result of virus-induced cell death of erythroid progenitor cells in bone marrow with interruption of erythrocyte production. No effect on the precursor cells of the myeloid series is observed.

The *rash* and *arthralgia* associated with B19 infection occur in infected volunteers during the third week after inoculation. As they follow the disappearance of the viraemia and occur when there is an easily detectable immune response, both are assumed to be immune mediated.

## Clinical disease caused by B19

There is a spectrum of clinical consequences of B19 infection (Table 47.2).

### Minor illness or subclinical infection

Asymptomatic or mild infection can occur at any age. In children this accounts for about half of all infections. A non-specific febrile respiratory tract illness is common at the viraemic phase; it is usually mild, but may mimic influenza.

### Rash illness

In healthy individuals, B19 can cause erythematous, macular or maculopapular or, less commonly, purpuric rashes. In its most distinct form the erythematous rash is called *erythema infectiosum* or *slapped cheek syndrome*, so called because of the intense erythema of the cheeks (Fig. 47.3). Rash illness is most common in children aged 4–11 years, and is sometimes called *fifth disease*, as it was the fifth of six erythematous rash illnesses of childhood in an old classification. Classically, it starts with facial erythema, followed by a maculopapular rash of the trunk and limbs. It lasts only a day or two, although transient recurrences may occur over 1–3 weeks. It may be exacerbated when the individual is hot, for example after exercise or a hot bath, and may be itchy. As it spreads out, there may be central clearing of the erythema which can give a lacy or reticular appearance (Fig. 47.4). There may be associated lymphadenopathy and joint symptoms.

Even during a community outbreak of slapped cheek syndrome, clinical diagnosis is not wholly reliable as the illness can be very similar to rubella (where arthropathy and lymphadenopathy may also occur). Cheek erythema is not always prominent, the rash may not appear lacy, and it may be on the palms and soles; rarely there are vesicles. A purpuric rash limited to the hands and feet in a gloves-and-socks distribution with pain, pruritus and oedema can also occur. In the absence of virology tests the most frequent clinical diagnoses made are rubella, allergy and 'viral illness'. Where the rash is purpuric, the platelet count is usually normal, but a transient thrombocytopenia may occur.

### Joint disease

Symptoms and signs of joint involvement may occur with or without rash illness, and B19 infection should

---

**Table 47.2** Spectrum of disease due to B19 related to host factors

| Disease | Host | Treatment |
| --- | --- | --- |
| Asymptomatic | Normal children and adults | |
| Respiratory tract illness | Normal children and adults | |
| Rash illness | Normal children and adults | |
| Erythema infectiosum, fifth disease, slapped cheek syndrome | Normal children | |
| Arthralgia | Normal adults | |
| Transient aplastic crisis | Patients with increased erythropoiesis | Blood transfusion |
| Persistent anaemia | Immunocompromised patients | Intravenous immunoglobulin |
| Congenital anaemia or hydrops | Fetus <20 weeks | Intra-uterine transfusion |

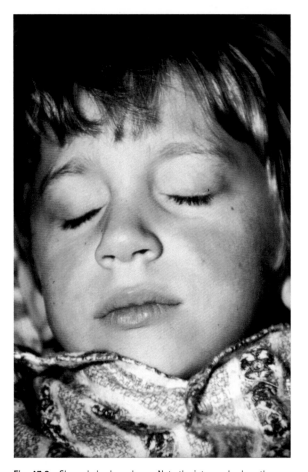

**Fig. 47.3** Slapped cheek syndrome. Note the intense cheek erythema and circumoral pallor. (Courtesy of Dr Ken Mutton, Medical Microbiology, Manchester Royal Infirmary.)

**Fig. 47.4** Late stage of B19 rash with central clearing showing lacy appearance.

be considered in the differential diagnosis of acute arthritis. This is more common in adults, especially women, of whom 80% have joint symptoms, compared with about 10% in childhood. Like the rash, the arthropathy is very similar to that seen with rubella, being a symmetrical arthralgia or arthritis involving mainly the small joints of the hands, although feet, wrists, knees, ankles and other joints may be affected. In children, the arthropathy may be less symmetrical. Arthropathy usually resolves within 2–3 weeks, but may occasionally persist or recur for months and very rarely for years. Some of these patients may be classified clinically as having early benign rheumatoid arthritis. However, B19 arthropathy is not destructive; if rheumatoid factor is detected it does not persist, and B19 virus infection is not causally linked to rheumatoid arthritis.

### Transient aplastic crisis

This is an acute transient event seen in those with various underlying haematological problems:

- decreased red cell survival (e.g. haemolytic disorders)
- where the bone marrow is 'stressed', for example because of haemorrhage or iron deficiency anaemia.

There is a virtual absence of red blood cell precursors in the bone marrow at the beginning of the crisis, followed by disappearance of reticulocytes from the peripheral blood and a subsequent fall in haemoglobin concentration. The cessation of erythropoiesis lasts for 5–7 days, and patients present with symptoms of acute anaemia, which can be life-threatening. Blood transfusion is required, but after a week or so specific antibody production controls viral replication, the bone marrow recovers rapidly, there is a reticulocytosis and the haemoglobin concentration returns to steady-state values.

Throughout the world, B19 infection is responsible for 90% of cases of transient aplastic crisis in those with underlying haemolytic disorders, most commonly in children with, for example, sickle cell anaemia, hereditary spherocytosis or thalassaemia.

### Persistent infection in the immunocompromised

The inability to mount an effective neutralizing antibody response to B19 results in persistent infection. This has been described in patients with:

- congenital immunodeficiency
- leukaemia
- acquired immune deficiency syndrome (AIDS)
- transplant recipients.

The bone marrow picture is typical of that seen in transient aplastic crisis with absent red cell precursors, but here results in *pure red cell aplasia*, ongoing viraemia and a non-specific febrile illness presenting with symptoms of chronic anaemia or a remitting and relapsing anaemia, without rash or joint disease.

**Fig. 47.5** Fetal hydrops due to B19. Note pallor of limbs. In-utero autolysis of fetus disguises pallor of body.

### B19 in pregnancy

Although B19 infection can cause fetal loss, most pregnancies result in the birth of a normal baby. There is no evidence of birth defects or developmental abnormalities in children exposed to B19 in utero.

Transplacental infection can occur during acute maternal infection, whether or not symptoms of B19 infection occur in the mother, before maternal antibody has developed and crossed the placenta to protect the fetus. Infection in the first 20 weeks can lead to intra-uterine death (increased risk 9%) and *non-immunological fetal hydrops* (risk 3%), of which about half die and are included in the 9%. This is in contrast to hydrops which occurs following Rhesus incompatibility and is immune mediated. The greatest risk of fetal loss is during the second trimester.

These effects are due to the immaturity of the fetal immune response and the shorter survival of fetal red cells. The large increase in red cell mass (in both the bone marrow and extramedullary sites of erythropoiesis) during the second trimester leads to the increased risk of developing anaemia at this time. The anaemia persists and becomes chronic because of ongoing viral replication. Infection of fetal myocardial cells can also occur, causing myocarditis. Both the anaemia and the myocarditis contribute to the development of cardiac failure, leading to the development of ascites and fetal hydrops (Fig. 47.5). Fetal loss is usually 4–6 weeks after maternal infection, but can be as long as 12 weeks later. Overall, B19 probably accounts for 10% of cases of fetal hydrops. A more effective fetal immune response reduces the risk of fetal loss in the third trimester; very rarely chronic anaemia in the newborn has followed intra-uterine infection.

### Other

In healthy people, case reports suggest that the manifestations of B19 may on occasion be very wide (e.g. meningitis, hepatitis, haemophagocytic syndrome or myocarditis). However, as both IgM and DNA may persist for months, some associations may be casual rather than causal.

## LABORATORY DIAGNOSIS OF B19 INFECTION

### Detection of virus

During pure red cell aplasia, and the acute illness of transient aplastic crisis, viraemia and throat virus excretion coincide with haematological changes, so detection of the viral genome in serum or bone marrow by DNA hybridization or PCR is the method of choice. Serum is the usual specimen examined; it contains high concentrations of virus and, if virus is not detected, it can serve as an acute-phase serum for antibody assays. While awaiting B19 detection results in those with anaemia, the reticulocyte count is a quick test that can be helpful as a low or absent count is consistent with current B19 infection, whereas a normal or raised count excludes the diagnosis. Hybridization or PCR are also used to investigate fetal samples. Virus culture is not appropriate as B19 does not grow in routine laboratory cell cultures.

### Antibody detection

In most cases B19-specific IgM is detectable within a day or two of the onset of the rash, although it may be up to 2 weeks before antibody is present in convincing amounts. Once B19-specific IgM has appeared in the serum, it rapidly reaches peak concentrations and is usually detectable for 2–3 months. High concentrations of IgG antibody are generally found by 1 month after infection, and IgG usually remains detectable for life. Diagnosis of recent infection can be made by demonstrating seroconversion or increasing amounts of IgG antibody.

### Investigations during pregnancy and infection in the fetus

At booking, all pregnant women should be advised to inform their general practitioner, midwife or obstetrician as soon as they develop a rash, unexplained arthropathy or are in contact with someone with a possible viral rash. Recommendations for investigating a pregnant woman who has had significant contact with possible B19 are summarized in Figure 47.6. Testing of a current sample for IgG and IgM should be initiated. Comparison to results in a stored blood (e.g. booking sample) taken prior to the contact may also be helpful. Where maternal infection is proven, whether or not symptoms have occurred, obstetric referral for investigations (e.g. fetal ultrasonography) should be arranged without delay as deterioration from early hydrops to intrauterine death can be rapid. Although fetal loss has been documented only with infection up to 20 weeks' gestation, investigation of rash or contact is recommended at any gestation and is also indicated for non-immune fetal hydrops.

The diagnosis of B19 infection in a fetus is complex. When fetal hydrops is found in an asymptomatic pregnant woman, maternal infection is likely to have occurred some weeks previously and B19 IgM may not be detectable in the mother or fetus. If available, a stored blood sample should be tested for IgG and IgM, looking for IgG seroconversion. Where fetal diagnosis is needed during pregnancy, testing of amniotic fluid or fetal blood for B19 DNA is appropriate. In placenta or fetal tissues taken at autopsy, diagnosis can be made by PCR or in-situ hybridization for B19 DNA on formalin-fixed, paraffin-embedded tissue sections (Fig. 47.7) or by demonstrating char-

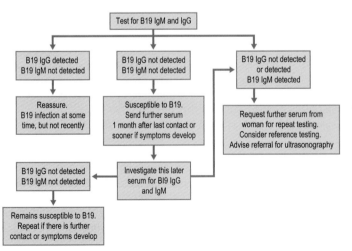

**Fig. 47.6** Investigation for B19 in a pregnant woman with significant exposure to rash illness. (Reproduced with modifications with permission of Health Protection Agency, London.)

**Fig. 47.7** In-situ hybridization using a pool of B19 oligonucleotide probes showing enlarged B19-infected erythroblasts in (A) fetal heart and (B) fetal liver from a fatal case of fetal hydrops. (Courtesy of Professor Heather Cubie, Specialist Virology Centre, Royal Infirmary, Edinburgh.)

**Fig. 47.8** Fetal liver (haematoxylin and eosin stain) from fetal hydrops showing characteristic B19-infected erythroblasts (arrows) with intranuclear inclusions and marginated chromatin. (Courtesy of Dr Elizabeth Gray, Pathology, Aberdeen Royal Infirmary.)

acteristic intranuclear inclusions in erythroid precursors (Fig. 47.8).

## EPIDEMIOLOGY

B19 infection is common and worldwide in distribution. Serological studies indicate that infection is most commonly acquired between 4 and 10 years of age, and by 15 years approximately 50% of children have antibody. Infection occurs throughout adulthood and up to 90% of elderly people are seropositive.

B19 virus infections are endemic throughout the year in temperate climates, with a seasonal increase in frequency in late winter, spring and early summer months. There are also longer-term cycles of infection with a periodicity of about 4–5 years. Most infections are transmitted by close contact by the respiratory route, with a seroconversion rate of 20–30% for day-care personnel in close contact with infected children. Asymptomatic blood donors with high-titre viraemia enable transmission by blood or blood products, and the stability and heat resistance of B19 enables transmission by heat-treated factor VIII and IX to haemophiliacs.

## MANAGEMENT

Most cases of B19 infection are mild and self-limiting, and specific treatment is not required other than symptomatic relief for joint disease. No antiviral drug is available. However, there are three situations (see Table 47.2) in which severe anaemia occurs as a consequence of B19 infection, and in each of these blood transfusion or intravenous immunoglobulin is indicated. In transient aplastic crisis, blood transfusion tides patients over the relatively short period of erythroid aplasia before the immune response rapidly clears the virus infection. In the immunocompromised there is a failure to produce neutralizing antibody, so management consists of blood transfusion plus a course of immunoglobulin over 5–10 days. This leads to disappearance of the viraemia, sometimes accompanied by the development of rash illness. If the viraemia recurs, further immunoglobulin is usually necessary. With infection during pregnancy, termination of pregnancy is not indicated as a fetus that survives B19 infection has a good prognosis. Although spontaneous resolution of hydrops due to B19 with the birth of a healthy baby has been documented, the overall fetal mortality rate is decreased with intra-uterine transfusion, which may need to be repeated.

Prevention of disease by isolating susceptible individuals is generally impractical as infections may be subclinical and symptomatic individuals are infectious before distinctive symptoms appear. In addition, as the rash and arthralgia of B19 infection are caused by immune reactions, not viraemia, those with rash or arthropathy are not infectious. However, susceptible pregnant healthcare workers should not care for those with transient aplastic crisis or pure red cell aplasia; those with these manifestations are likely to be infectious. Theoretically, susceptible individuals at risk of significant anaemia (e.g. immunocompromised children) could be protected temporarily by the administration of human immunoglobulin, but this has not been tried. Good hand hygiene should be encouraged.

There is as yet no licensed vaccine against B19 but, by analogy with the animal viruses where immunization against feline and canine parvoviruses is routine in veterinary practice, such a strategy would be expected to be very effective in man. Recombinant B19 virus-like particles can be produced that induce neutralizing antibodies and so are potentially suitable candidates for a human vaccine. At present, screening of at-risk groups is not recommended as vaccine and prophylaxis are not available.

## RECOMMENDED READING

Adler SP, Koch WC: Human parvovirus infections. In Remington JS, Klein JO, Wilson CB, Baker CJ, editors: *Infectious Diseases of the fetus and newborn infant*, ed 6, 2006, Elsevier Saunders, pp 867–893.

Berns K, Parrish CR: Parvoviruses. In Knipe DM, Howley PM, editors: *Virology*, ed 5, Philadelphia, 2007, Lippincott Williams & Wilkins, pp 2437–2477.

Brown KE: Human parvoviruses, including parvovirus B19 and human bocavirus. In Mandell GL, Bennett JE, Dolin R, editors: *Principles and Practice of Infectious Diseases*, ed 7, Philadelphia, 2010, Churchill Livingstone, pp 2087–2095.

Brown KE: The expanding range of parvoviruses which infect humans, *Reviews in Medical Virology* 20:231–244, 2010.

Faisst S: *Parvoviruses, from Molecular Biology to Pathology. Contributions to Microbiology*, Vol 4, Basel, 2000, Karger.

Jones MS, Kapoor A, Lukashov VL, et al: New DNA viruses identified in patients with acute viral infection syndrome, *Journal of Virology* 79: 8230–8236, 2005.

Lindner J, Karalar L, Schimanski S, et al: Clinical and epidemiological aspects of human bocavirus infection, *Journal of Clinical Virology* 43:391–395, 2008.

## Website

Health Protection Agency: Viral rashes in pregnancy. http://www.hpa.org.uk/infections/topics_az/pregnancy/rashes/default.htm

# 48 Picornaviruses

Meningitis; paralysis; rashes; intercostal myositis; myocarditis; infectious hepatitis; common cold

*I. Johannessen and S. M. Burns*

## KEY POINTS

- Picornaviruses pathogenic for man belong to the *enterovirus* (includes the former *rhinovirus* genus), *parechovirus* and *hepatovirus* genera.
- Enteroviruses cause a wide range of diseases including aseptic meningitis, poliomyelitis, encephalitis, maculopapular skin rashes, ulcerative exanthems, and myocarditis.
- Rhinoviruses are responsible for the most frequent of all human infections – the common cold.
- There are effective vaccines against polioviruses and hepatitis A virus.
- Enteroviruses are among the most stable viruses.
- Diagnosis of enterovirus infection now relies on nucleic acid detection.
- New enteroviruses regularly emerge and can cause major epidemics of disease.

The family picornaviridae comprises small (pico) RNA viruses with a diameter of 27–30 nm. It consists of 12 genera of which the *enterovirus* (incorporating the former *rhinovirus* genus)*, parechovirus* and *hepatovirus* genera are of considerable human importance, resulting in a variety of clinical manifestations including aseptic meningitis, encephalitis, myo- and pericarditis, respiratory tract infections, rashes, ulcerative exanthems, hepatitis, and the common cold. The *enterovirus* genus is divided according to genetic phylogeny into 10 species (Table 48.1), 7 of which (human enterovirus species A–D and human rhinovirus species A–C) contain (sero)types that infect humans. In the text that follows, the human enterovirus species A–D will be discussed together under the heading 'Enteroviruses' and the human rhinovirus species A–C (with emphasis on species A and B) together under the heading 'Rhinoviruses'.

## ENTEROVIRUSES

### DESCRIPTION

Viruses belonging to the human enterovirus species A–D of the genus *enterovirus* infect via the gut and are excreted in faeces, and include the echoviruses, coxsackieviruses and polioviruses. New enteroviruses continue to be isolated, but they are no longer subdivided into the three named groups. Instead they are called enterovirus and are numbered, for example, enterovirus 71. Hepatitis A, previously classified as enterovirus 72, has now been assigned its own genus, *hepatovirus*. The properties of entero- and rhinoviruses are compared in Table 48.2.

### Composition

The RNA genome is single-stranded and of positive sense (ss+ve RNA) and, therefore, can be translated directly by host ribosomes to generate viral proteins. It is surrounded by a capsid consisting of a protein shell arranged in icosahedral symmetry around the genomic RNA (together forming the *nucleocapsid*), the complete sequence of which is now known for several strains. Four major peptides are recognized in the shell: viral protein (VP) 1, VP2, VP3 and VP4, formed from a single precursor protein, VP0, by proteolytic cleavage. Specific neutralizing antibodies are considered to be the major mechanism of protection against infection. For example, four major antigenic sites on exposed surface loops of the VP1–3 proteins of polio type 3 have been identified. The virus is non-enveloped.

In addition to the properties listed in Table 48.2, all enteroviruses:

- attach to cells of the intestinal tract at specific receptor sites and replicate in the cytoplasm of the intestinal cells

- commonly cause asymptomatic immunizing infections which protect against future infections with the same virus
- occasionally cause infection of the central nervous system (CNS) and other target organs
- are commoner in children than in adults
- usually cause infections in late summer and early autumn (in temperate climates).

In recent years, over 30 additional enterovirus types have been described (type 73 onwards) as a result of nucleic acid sequence analysis.

## PROPERTIES OF ENTEROVIRUSES

In the presence of moist organic material, enteroviruses:

- survive at room temperature for weeks
- survive at 4°C for months
- are killed at 50–55°C.

They are stable in acid pH but rapidly inactivated by 0.3% formaldehyde and solutions giving a free residual chlorine concentration of 0.3–0.5 parts per million (ppm). However, chemical inactivation is ineffective when organic matter is present (e.g. in swimming baths).

### Polioviruses

There are three serotypes of poliovirus, identified by neutralization tests; their RNA molecules differ by 50% in hybridization studies. Two outstanding characteristics of the viruses are their affinity for nervous tissue and their narrow host range. Only human beings and non-human primates are susceptible – it was inoculation of samples from patients with paralytic poliomyelitis ('polio') into monkeys that led to the identification of the infectious nature of the disease in 1909. Cynomologus and rhesus monkeys can be infected by the oral route and develop paralysis; in chimpanzees, infection is often asymptomatic. Under the influence of steroids, monkeys become more susceptible to small parenteral doses of the viruses.

The prototype poliovirus strains are:

- type 1, the Brunhilde and Mahoney strains
- type 2, which includes the rodent-adapted strains, the Lansing and MEFI strains
- type 3, the Leon and Saukett strains.

The three types are antigenically distinct, but overlap occurs in neutralization tests. Type 1 is the common

| Table 48.1 Genetic phylogeny of the genus *enteroviruses* | |
|---|---|
| Enterovirus species | Serotypes |
| Human enterovirus A | Coxsackievirus A2–8, 10, 12, 14, 16 Enterovirus 71, 76, 89–91, 114 |
| Human enterovirus B | Coxsackievirus A9 Coxsackievirus B1–6 Echovirus 1–7, 9, 11–21, 24–27, 29–33 Enterovirus 69, 73–75, 77–88, 93, 97–98, 100–101, 106–107 |
| Human enterovirus C | Coxsackievirus A1, 11, 13, 17, 19–22, 24 Poliovirus 1–3 Enterovirus 95–96, 99, 102, 104–105, 109, 113, 116 |
| Human enterovirus D | Enterovirus 68, 70, 94, 111 |
| Human rhinovirus A | Rhinovirus 1–2, 7–13, 15–16, 18–25, 28–34, 36, 38–41, 43–47, 49–51, 53–68, 71, 73–78, 80–82, 85, 88–90, 94–96, 98, 100–101 |
| Human rhinovirus B | Rhinovirus 3–6, 14, 17, 26–27, 35, 37, 42, 48, 52, 69–70, 72, 79, 83–84, 86, 91–93, 97, 99 |
| Human rhinovirus C[a] | Rhinovirus C1–48[a] |
| Serotypes not yet assigned to species | Enterovirus 103, 108, 112, 115 |

[a]These are not serotypes but genetic types.

| Table 48.2 Some properties of picornaviruses | | |
|---|---|---|
| Property | Enteroviruses | Rhinoviruses |
| Size (nm) | 22–30 | 30 |
| Capsid | | |
|   Form | Icosahedral | Icosahedral |
|   Polypeptides | VP1, VP2, VP3, VP4 | VP1, VP2, VP3, VP4 |
|   RNA type | Single-stranded, positive-sense | Single-stranded, positive-sense |
|   RNA molecular weight (Da) | $2 \times 10^6$–$2.6 \times 10^6$ | $2.6 \times 10^6$ |
| Acid | Stable (pH 3–9) | Labile (pH 3–5) |
| Optimal temperature for growth (°C) | 37 | 33–34 |
| Density in caesium chloride (g/mL) | 1.34 | 1.39–1.42 |

epidemic type; type 2 is usually associated with endemic infections; type 3 has caused some epidemics. The size, chemical and physical properties of the three types are all identical, and so their antigenic properties provide one of the main methods of differentiating them.

## Echoviruses

Echoviruses were identified by cell culture of faeces of patients suffering from paralytic and non-paralytic illness. There are over 30 serotypes of these *Enteric Cytopathic Human Orphan* viruses and, true to their name, there is still no clear association of some types with specific disease. Echoviruses 22 and 23 have a very different RNA sequence and have been re-classified in a separate genus, *parechovirus* (see below). Most do not infect laboratory animals. Several types can agglutinate human group O red blood cells.

### Antigenic characters

Thirty-three distinct antigenic types have so far been distinguished by neutralization tests in cell cultures. Some cross-reactions occur. Antigenic variation is known to occur in types 4, 6 and 9, and may be a common occurrence under natural conditions.

## Coxsackieviruses

This group (of 30 serotypes) was named after the town of Coxsackie in New York State (USA) where the first member was isolated in 1948. This followed inoculation of faecal extracts from two patients with paralytic disease into newborn mice in which these viruses are pathogenic (as well as in hamsters). Two groups of viruses, A (1–24) and B (1–6), were recognized according to the histological nature and the types of lesions they produce in mice (Table 48.3).

**Table 48.3** Features of coxsackievirus infection in the laboratory

| | Types | Growth in MK cell culture | Effect in suckling mice |
|---|---|---|---|
| Coxsackie A virus | 1–24[a] | + | Paralysis |
| Coxsackie B virus | 1–6 | + | Spasticity |

MK, monkey kidney.
[a]Coxsackievirus A23 is now re-classified as echovirus 9.

### Growth in culture and mice

All group B coxsackieviruses, but only a few group A viruses, grow readily in monkey kidney cell cultures. The other type A viruses were isolated by inoculation of suckling mice. Type A7, which has caused paralytic disease, is identical to the Russian strain AbIV, thought at one time to be a fourth type of poliovirus. Mouse inoculation has not been used as a diagnostic test for years, having been replaced by RNA detection using reverse transcription–polymerase chain reaction (RT-PCR) analysis.

### Antigenic characters

Originally, 30 antigenic types were defined by cross-neutralization tests in mice or cell culture, and by cross-complement fixation tests (CFTs). Twenty-three have the features of group A (1–22, 24) and six have those of group B (1–6). Each of the six group B types is subject to antigenic variation, and sera from convalescent cases may show heterotypic responses. Coxsackievirus A23 has now been re-classified as echovirus 9.

## Other enteroviruses

Detailed examination of the characteristics of the viruses in cell culture and their ability to infect laboratory animals, which had been the basis of classification into polioviruses, coxsackieviruses or echoviruses, showed that these were not reliable features. Since 1970, new isolates are simply called enterovirus and given the next available consecutive number. Thus, enterovirus types 68, 69, 70 and 71 (and others) are now recognized as additions to the genus.

## REPLICATION

Knowledge of enterovirus replication is based on studies of poliovirus. Briefly, the ss+RNA genome acts as mRNA for translation of a single precursor polyprotein that is digested at specific sites by internal protease activity giving rise to viral proteins including a viral polymerase and individual proteases. As a pool of viral proteins accumulates, cytoplasmic RNA replication is favoured using the ss+RNA as a template for production of a ss-RNA copy giving rise to a double stranded RNA replicative intermediate that acts as a template for the production of further ss+RNA progeny genomes. The capsid coat is assembled as 12 pentamers of the structural VP1–4 proteins around the ss+RNA giving rise to infectious virus.

The end of replication is signalled by lysis of the host cell, with the release of new progeny virus particles.

## CLINICAL FEATURES AND PATHOGENESIS

The enteroviruses are associated with a wide variety of clinical presentations, although the majority of infections are asymptomatic. The main sites affected are:

- CNS (*aseptic* meningitis, *paralytic poliomyelitis, encephalitis*), particularly in children; persistent CNS infection (primarily *encephalitis*) may develop in immunocompromised patients
- skin and mucosa (*maculopapular* rashes, *ulcerative exanthem*)
- striated muscle (*intercostal myositis, myocarditis* accompanied by *pericarditis*)
- respiratory tract (*rhinitis, pharyngitis, bronchiolitis, pneumonia*)
- eyes (*conjunctivitis*)
- postnatal infection in neonates can be severe, extensive and occasionally fatal.

Maternal infection in pregnancy is not associated with congenital defects. There are additional controversial links between enterovirus infections and *chronic fatigue syndrome* (unlikely), and the onset of insulin-dependent (type 1) diabetes mellitus (possible), but further research is required to confirm this association.

### Polioviruses

There are three outcomes of poliovirus infection:

1. Asymptomatic infection, or a mild, transient 'influenza-like' illness; this is the most likely outcome with only 1% of infections resulting in recognizable clinical illness; the virus is excreted in faeces for a limited time, and an immunological response develops that protects against re-infection with the same strain.
2. *Aseptic meningitis*; infections with the same symptoms as above and evidence of CNS involvement with headache, photophobia, neck stiffness and back pain; rapid and complete recovery in less than 10 days is usual.
3. Paralytic poliomyelitis ('*polio*') in which the patient develops paralysis; this is the most dramatic form of the infection but is very uncommon, occurring in 1 in 1000 poliovirus infections in children, although 1 in 75 adults may be affected; the paralysis is usually flaccid

due to destruction of lower motor neurones, although invasion of the brainstem by the virus can lead to incoordination of muscle groups and painful spasms; paralysis occurs early in the illness but the extent is variable; often the paralysis is greatest initially; some function may return over the next 6 months; damage to nerve cells in the brainstem (bulbar paralysis) can lead to the inability to breathe and swallow.

The time between infection and the development of symptoms is usually 14 days but can range from 3–21 days. During this period several factors have an adverse effect on the outcome of infection:

- Increased muscular activity can lead to paralysis of the limbs used, possibly due to enhanced vascularity, either in the limb or the appropriate area of the spinal cord, allowing increased access of virus to nerve endings.
- Women in the third trimester of pregnancy can have severe disease, but there is no firm evidence of congenital defects in infants born to mothers with poliomyelitis; maternal infection acquired late in pregnancy may lead to perinatal infection and disease of the newborn.
- Injection of adjuvant-containing vaccines, and irritant substances such as heavy metals, can result in paralysis in the limb(s) that received the inoculation; paralysis develops (incidence 1 in 37 000 injections) when poliovirus is contracted within 1 month of receiving the inoculation.
- Patients who have had their tonsils removed have a higher chance of developing bulbar poliomyelitis which has been attributed to the reduction of secretory immunoglobulin (Ig) A in the pharynx and, thus, reduced neutralization of virus.

*Vaccine-associated paralysis* is a rare complication of oral live-attenuated polio vaccine, or following infection from contact with a vaccinee excreting virus. Non-polio enteroviruses have also been associated with CNS disease and paralysis (e.g. echovirus 4 and enterovirus 71); as with polio, paralysis is a rare manifestation of infection.

### Echoviruses

Most echovirus infections cause few, or no, clinical symptoms, but some have been associated with clinical syndromes including:

- aseptic meningitis
- paralysis
- maculopapular rash
- respiratory disease.

Less frequently, echoviruses may cause:

- myocarditis and pericarditis
- neonatal infection.

Infection can be widespread in a community, although only a few suffer from clinical illness. Symptoms occur following a short incubation period of 3–5 days (simple fever, upper respiratory symptoms or diarrhoea). Non-specific rashes of fleeting duration have been reported.

The onset of aseptic meningitis is abrupt, with severe headache and vomiting. Symptoms are self-limiting, and after a variable convalescent period a full recovery is made, although rare cases of paralysis do occur. Most of the echovirus types have been associated with sporadic cases of aseptic meningitis, or one of the other disease patterns already mentioned. A number of types have considerable epidemic potential, and the clinical features are very varied. For example, echovirus 9 epidemics have been common in Europe and North America as large outbreaks of a biphasic fever with a sore throat and a rash on the face, neck and chest and, less commonly, on the lower trunk and extremities. A minority of patients shows clinical signs of meningitis, but many without distinct clinical signs have a pleocytosis in the cerebrospinal fluid (CSF). In 2002, echovirus 13 was isolated from patients with aseptic meningitis in Korea.

Echovirus 16 epidemics have been called *Boston fever* after the city where the illness was first reported. Clinically, the infection starts with a sharp fever, abdominal pains and a mild sore throat. After 24–48 h, a pink discrete macular or maculopapular rash, mostly on the face, chest and back, appears in children. Echovirus 4, 6 and 30 epidemics have been associated particularly with aseptic meningitis in children and adults. Echoviruses 6, 9 and 11 have caused severe *neonatal* infections. The virus is probably transmitted during birth, or postnatally, from the mother or nursery attendants, who are asymptomatic. Circulatory collapse, hepatitis and meningoencephalitis develop and infection can spread rapidly to other infants in the nursery or special care baby unit. The type of virus circulating in the community at the time is usually implicated.

Echovirus 18 has been recovered from faeces of many infants in an outbreak of diarrhoea. The children had no rash and no severe CNS involvement or meningeal reaction. Several echoviruses have been isolated from cases of respiratory illnesses in children, in whom symptoms include upper respiratory tract illness, *bronchiolitis* and *pneumonitis* (*pneumonia*).

**Table 48.4** Features of human coxsackievirus infection

| Coxsackievirus group | Type | Clinical illness |
|---|---|---|
| A | 1–24[a] | Aseptic meningitis<br>Febrile illness<br>Herpangina<br>Hand, foot and mouth disease |
| B | 1–6 | Neonatal disease<br>Bornholm disease<br>Myocarditis, hepatitis<br>Aseptic meningitis |

[a]Coxsackievirus A23 is now re-classified as echovirus 9.

## Coxsackieviruses

### Group A viruses

These viruses give rise to a number of different illnesses (Table 48.4). Aseptic meningitis is caused by a number of types (e.g. 2, 4, 7, 9 and 23). Type A7 has given rise to epidemics of paralytic disease in Scotland, the former Soviet Union and elsewhere. Herpangina is an acute feverish disease with sore throat and pain on swallowing, usually in young children, characterized by lesions in the mouth consisting of papules on the anterior pillars of the fauces, soft palate, uvula, pharynx and tonsils; these papules become vesicles and finally shallow ulcers with a greyish base and punched-out edge. There are usually small numbers of lesions. A fine *maculopapular* rash ('*rubelliform*') is a feature of some Coxsackie infections. Outbreaks may be seen in nurseries and schools. Hand, foot and mouth disease presents as a mildly febrile ulcerative exanthem with painful stomatitis and a painful vesicular rash on the hands and/or feet (less frequently, on buttocks and external genitalia). Typically, it lasts about a week; most cases are seen in summer in children aged 1–10 years; cases can occur in clusters and in families. The viruses usually implicated are types 5 and 16.

Coxsackievirus A21 has caused epidemics of *rhinitis* and *pharyngitis* in camps of military recruits.

Coxsackievirus A24 caused a major outbreak of 6000 cases of *acute haemorrhagic conjunctivitis* in French Guyana in 2003. Molecular typing confirmed that this virus had been introduced from South-East Asia.

### Group B viruses

*Epidemic pleurodynia*, or *Bornholm disease*, first described on the Danish island of Bornholm, is characterized by fever and the sudden onset of agonizing stitch-like pains in the muscles of the chest, epigastrium or hypochondrium. Although the disease is most frequently recognized in its epidemic form, many sporadic cases occur. Pleurisy and pericarditis may complicate epidemic myalgia, although most cases recover within a week.

In newborn infants, severe and often fatal *myocarditis* has been reported, and the virus can be found in high concentrations in the myocardium at autopsy. Epidemics have occurred in nurseries when there is evidence of group B virus activity in a community. Myocarditis and pericarditis can occur in children and adults, and virus has been isolated from pericardial fluid.

Coxsackie B viruses are major causes of human myopericarditis, but this is a difficult diagnosis to confirm. Although severe in the neonate, it tends to follow a more benign course in the adult. The initial symptoms are often of an upper respiratory or 'influenza-like' illness followed 7–10 days later by clinical heart disease. Chest pain is a feature and electrocardiographic abnormalities such as tachycardia and arrhythmias have been found. On clinical examination, murmurs, rubs and, occasionally, pericardial effusions are detected.

Aseptic meningitis, sometimes with paralysis, is a common manifestation of infection due to group B viruses. Occasionally, a maculopapular rash is present.

## Enteroviruses 68–71 (Table 48.5)

### Enterovirus 68

This has been reported to cause pneumonia.

### Enterovirus 69

This virus has not yet been associated with significant clinical illness.

**Table 48.5** Illness associated with enteroviruses 68–72

| Enterovirus type | Clinical illness |
| --- | --- |
| 68 | Pneumonia and bronchiolitis |
| 69 | Isolated from an ill person in Mexico |
| 70 | Acute haemorrhagic conjunctivitis |
| 70, 71 | Paralysis, meningoencephalitis |
| 71 | Hand, foot and mouth disease |
| 72[a] | Hepatitis A |

[a]Reclassified as hepatovirus.

### Enterovirus 70

In 1969, outbreaks of *acute haemorrhagic conjunctivitis* spread throughout Africa and Asia; more recently the disease has occurred in Mexico. This condition is highly infectious and has a short incubation period of 24–48 h. Attack rates are very high where there is over-crowding and poor sanitation. Although subconjunctival haemorrhage is a complication, most patients recover within 7 days. Neurological complications can occur, including polio-like *paralysis*.

### Enterovirus 71

Like other enteroviruses, enterovirus 71 produces infections that are usually mild or inapparent. This virus was first recognized in 1969 in California when it was isolated from faeces of a 9-month old infant suffering from encephalitis. Since then it has been isolated from patients with a spectrum of illness. During an epidemic in Bulgaria in 1975, there was a high incidence of paralytic disease, mostly in children under 5 years of age. A large outbreak occurred in Malaysia in 1997 where 2140 children were affected and 27 cases of fatal myocarditis were reported. This was followed by a related large outbreak in Taiwan in 1998, which was characterized by hand, foot and mouth disease, and caused disability and even fatalities.

## PATHOGENESIS

All enterovirus infections follow a similar pattern, as illustrated in Figure 48.1 for poliovirus, with differences in the target organs (e.g. CNS, skin, heart or muscle). Due to the potential severity of infection and the availability of an animal model, most is known about poliomyelitis.

Virus is ingested and, after multiplication in the lymphoid tissue of the tonsils or Peyer's patches (gut-associated lymphoid tissue, GALT) and the local lymph nodes, it enters the blood and then the CNS. The paralytic effect of poliovirus is due to destruction of motor neurone cells in the anterior horns of the spinal cord or bulbar regions. Once within the brain or spinal cord, virus can spread directly to neighbouring cells, or indirectly via the CSF.

The viraemic phase marks the end of the incubation period, and is manifest in the patient by fever and generalized symptoms; it is followed by a period of about 48 h of relative well-being (the disease is biphasic) while the virus is invading nerve tissue and then the signs of paralysis appear. If antibody is present in blood, virus can be prevented from reaching the CNS.

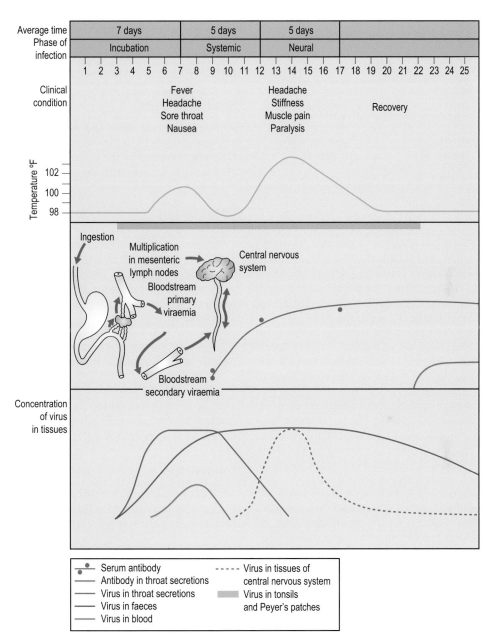

| Average time | 7 days | 5 days | 5 days | |
|---|---|---|---|---|
| Phase of infection | Incubation | Systemic | Neural | |

1 2 3 4 5 6 7 8 9 10 11 12 13 14 15 16 17 18 19 20 21 22 23 24 25

| Clinical condition | Fever Headache Sore throat Nausea | Headache Stiffness Muscle pain Paralysis | Recovery |
|---|---|---|---|

Temperature °F
102
100
98

Ingestion

Multiplication in mesenteric lymph nodes

Central nervous system

Bloodstream primary viraemia

Bloodstream secondary viraemia

Concentration of virus in tissues

- ●— Serum antibody
- —— Antibody in throat secretions
- —— Virus in throat secretions
- —— Virus in faeces
- —— Virus in blood
- - - - Virus in tissues of central nervous system
- ▬ Virus in tonsils and Peyer's patches

**Fig. 48.1** Pathogenesis of paralytic poliomyelitis.

Enteroviruses are lytic, destroying the infected cell within a few hours to days. Cell damage will trigger an inflammatory response; the resultant oedema may affect neurones other than those infected with the virus. As the oedema resolves, function will recover in these uninfected cells, thereby explaining the apparent improvement in the degree of paralysis in the weeks to months after the acute stage.

## LABORATORY DIAGNOSIS (Table 48.6)

### Culture

Virus isolation was the most useful method for establishing a diagnosis but has been superseded by RT-PCR for RNA detection in CSF. Examination of CSF is an essential part of the laboratory diagnosis of

**Table 48.6** Laboratory diagnosis of picornaviruses

| | Sample | Timing | Laboratory method |
|---|---|---|---|
| Enterovirus | CSF | Acute <5 days | Cell culture, PCR |
| | Faeces | | Cell culture, PCR |
| | Throat | | Cell culture, PCR |
| | Blood | | IgM[a] |
| Poliovirus | CSF | Acute <5 days | Cell culture, PCR |
| | Throat | | Cell culture, PCR |
| | Faeces | | Cell culture, PCR |
| Rhinovirus | Respiratory secretions | Acute <5 days | Cell culture, PCR |

[a]Including hepatovirus.

meningitis. Faecal samples should also be submitted, although isolation can be made from rectal and throat swabs (in virus transport medium, VTM). As virus excretion can be intermittent, two specimens should be collected on successive days, as early as possible in the illness, ideally within 5 days of the onset.

In paralytic poliomyelitis, the virus can be found in faeces for a few days preceding the onset of acute symptoms, and is present in more than 80% of cases in faeces during the first 4 days of symptoms. Only a few patients continue to excrete the virus after the 12th week although prolonged excretion may occur in the immunocompromised host. The virus can be isolated from the oropharynx of many patients for a few days before and after the onset of the illness. Isolation from the CSF is seldom successful in cases of paralytic poliomyelitis.

Echoviruses, coxsackie B viruses and coxsackie A9 virus are readily isolated from nose and throat swabs, stools or CSF; they are present in 80% of cases in faeces for at least 2 weeks after the onset. Identification is by neutralization, now carried out in reference laboratories. The clinical relevance of virus isolation from faeces is not always clear, as enteroviruses can be excreted for some time after asymptomatic infection and may, thus, only be an incidental finding.

### Polymerase chain reaction

Nucleic acid amplification tests have become the most common approach to enterovirus detection. Identification of conserved sequences within the 5′ non-coding region of the enterovirus genome has resulted in the development of PCR primers that allow the detection of most enteroviruses. Many studies have confirmed that enterovirus RT-PCR is more sensitive (and specific) than culture for the detection of enteroviruses. The current 'gold standard' of diagnosis is to detect the enterovirus genome in CSF by RT-PCR.

Molecular analysis of amplified targets provides further insight (e.g. for epidemiological purposes) and can distinguish live-attenuated vaccine from wild-type virus.

### Serological tests

Although specific IgM and IgG enzyme immuno-sorbent assays (EIA) for enteroviruses are available, their use is limited by the heterotypic and anamnestic responses associated with infections.

## TREATMENT

Treatment is symptomatic. A number of antiviral agents (e.g. *pleconaril*, an inhibitor of viral attachment to cell receptors and of uncoating) were investigated years ago for the treatment of paralytic poliomyelitis, but were of no practical value owing to the rapid emergence of drug resistance.

## EPIDEMIOLOGY AND TRANSMISSION

The only natural source of poliovirus is man. The virus is spread from person to person, and no intermediate host is known. Echovirus and coxsackievirus have a similar epidemiology.

### Transmission

All enteroviruses are excreted in large numbers from the gut and are ingested to cause infection. This can be achieved in the following ways:

- by direct transfer on fingers (faecal–oral transfer)
- on eating utensils
- through contamination of food or drink
- by entry through the conjunctiva (rare).

Outbreaks are often seen in closed communities (e.g. military establishments) and schools. In the acute phase of infection, virus is present in the throat and, although droplet spread could occur, the faecal–oral route is the usual means of transmission. After the acute phase, it is the only possible route. Cases are most infectious late in the incubation period, but infection can be transmitted at any time during virus excretion in faeces.

Infection rates can reach 100% in closed communities and households, particularly where children are present. Social factors, such as standards of hygiene and overcrowding, are also important. Sewage can contain polioviruses, particularly when there is infection in a community. Enteroviruses can survive for several months in river water, but are unlikely to survive in chlorine-treated water or swimming pools where the recommended level of chlorination (without protein contamination) is achieved. Flies and cockroaches have been found to harbour the viruses, but their role in transmission is minimal.

## PREVENTION AND CONTROL

After natural infection, immunity is long lasting. Virus-neutralizing antibodies are formed early during the disease (often before the 7th day) and persist for several decades. Secretory IgA is produced in the gut. In the clinical setting, standard infection control precautions (including adequate hand hygiene) are critical in preventing spread.

### Immunization

Polio is a vaccine preventable disease. There are two types of polio vaccine: inactivated and live-attenuated.

#### Inactivated polio vaccine (Salk vaccine)

Developed by Jonas Salk (USA) and introduced in 1956 for routine immunization, this vaccine contains strains of the three types of virus grown in monkey kidney cell culture and inactivated by exposure to formaldehyde. The batches of vaccine are tested for the presence of residual live poliovirus and must be free of contaminants. Inactivated poliovaccines are used widely, and with many countries achieving acceptance rates in excess of 90% (e.g. the Nordic countries), such regions have eliminated poliovirus infection despite the fact that inactivated vaccine does not induce much secretory IgA in the alimentary tract or afford protection to individuals that are not vaccinated. A high rate of immunization is necessary and antibody levels need to be maintained as the outcome of exposure to virus is directly related to the level of antibody at the time of exposure. For example, an outbreak in Finland was due to a poorly immunogenic type 3 component in the vaccine. From 2004, in the UK, the inactivated vaccine replaced the live attenuated one for routine immunization and forms a component of the current multivalent childhood vaccine schedule. The vaccine should be administered by deep subcutaneous or intramuscular injection. A primary course of three injections given with an interval of 1 month between each dose is recommended for infants of 2 months of age, followed by booster doses

at 1–3 years after the primary course and at 5–10 years after the first booster. The vaccines can be given at the same time as other vaccines but should be given at a separate site, ideally in a different limb.

#### Live-attenuated polio vaccine (Sabin vaccine)

This replaced the Salk vaccine for routine use in the UK in 1962 and is used extensively in many other countries. Developed by Albert Sabin (USA) in 1959, it contains live but attenuated strains of poliovirus types 1, 2 and 3, grown in cultures of either monkey kidney cells or human diploid cells. The strains were obtained by growing less virulent polioviruses and, after passage, selecting strains that had lost their neurovirulence.

The vaccine is administered orally and thus mimics natural infection with stimulation of circulating IgG and local secretory IgA in the pharynx and alimentary tract, thereby producing local resistance to subsequent infection with wild-type polioviruses. Herd immunity is important in preventing the circulation of the wild-type virus and high levels of immunization uptake are necessary. The wide circulation of vaccine virus, which helps to maintain immunity in the community, aids this. However, vaccine strains are not completely stable, and studies of sequential isolates of virus from vaccine recipients show very rapid reversion to neurovirulence with multiple rounds of replication in the vaccinee and after transmission to contacts. Vaccine-associated poliomyelitis has been reported in oral vaccine recipients at a rate of 1 in 2 million doses, and it has also been seen in contacts of recipients. It is not possible to predict who will be affected, although the extended replication, which occurs in the immunocompromised host, should be avoided as the rate of vaccine-associated poliomyelitis in such patients is 10 000 times greater than in immunocompetent individuals. Non-immunized parents and household contacts of children receiving primary immunization should be immunized against poliomyelitis at the same time as the children.

In the UK, oral polio vaccine was recommended up until 2004 for infants from 2 months of age. The primary course consists of three separate doses given at the same time as the then used diphtheria/tetanus/pertussis vaccine. Each dose contains all three poliovirus strains. In infants, three drops are dropped from a spoon directly into the mouth. Breast-feeding does not interfere with the antibody response and should continue. A reinforcing dose is given to children at school entry and prior to leaving school, but it is not necessary for adults unless they are at special risk, for instance through travel or occupational exposure. The last cases of indigenous polio infection were notified in England in 1984 and in Scotland in 1994, the latter being associated with the vaccine itself.

When a case of paralytic poliomyelitis is diagnosed, a dose of oral live-attenuated poliovirus vaccine should be given to all immunocompetent persons in the immediate vicinity of the case, whether or not they have a history of previous vaccination against polio (immunocompromised contacts should receive the inactivated vaccine). This should be followed by completion of the primary course in those not immunized. If the source of the outbreak is uncertain, it should be assumed to be wild-type virus until proven otherwise. Such circumstances necessitate co-ordinated efforts of the relevant health-care and public health bodies to ensure a prompt and appropriate response.

### Global eradication

The World Health Organization (WHO), through an expanded programme on immunization, has increased the rate of polio immunization, chiefly with the use of oral live-attenuated vaccine. In 1988, the World Health Assembly (WHA; the governing body of the WHO) set a target date of the year 2000 for the global eradication of poliomyelitis (the Global Polio Eradication Initiative, GPEI). The programme has been extremely successful, but the virus is still circulating in a handful of countries and a new target date of end-2012 has been set.

The GPEI strategy relies on using the oral live-attenuated polio vaccine on national immunization days (NIDs) with the aim of immunizing all young children (less than 5 years of age) in a particular region in a short period of time followed by repeat session(s) to break polio transmission. Using this strategy, the Americas were declared free of indigenous poliovirus in 1994, the western Pacific region in 2000, and Europe in 2002. Currently, endogenous poliovirus is circulating in India, Pakistan, Afghanistan and Nigeria but other countries have also notified re-importation of the virus and outbreaks are currently underway in Africa (e.g. Angola and the Congo) that threaten national and international spread. Difficulties associated with the vaccination campaign, some of which are specific to the use of live attenuated vaccine, include interference from other enteroviruses leading to poor responses, malnutrition, inhibitory factors in the gut, social/cultural resistance to polio vaccination, problems in maintenance of the 'cold chain', delivery of vaccine in war zones, and programme funding. No decision will be made to discontinue immunization against polio until all countries are free of wild-type poliovirus infections. In countries where no such virus

is reported, surveillance systems must be introduced that are effective at detecting wild-type poliovirus infections, and all cases of paralytic illness must be investigated. Only then is a country certified poliovirus-free. Currently, the main obstacle to achieving the WHO's goal of global polio eradication is funding, but recent data show that completing this task within the next 5 years may translate into a net benefit of £25–35 billion for the world community.

### Prospects for the future

Routine and mass administration of oral live-attenuated polio vaccine since 1961 has prevented many millions of cases of paralytic poliomyelitis; however, when the incidence of poliomyelitis falls dramatically, as in the USA for example, the proportion of paralytic cases attributable to vaccine, although very low, becomes increasingly significant. Furthermore, recombination of live-attenuated vaccine and wild-type virus in areas of poor vaccine coverage as well as long-term excretion of vaccine virus in immunocompromised individuals pose additional oral vaccine- related problems. There is, thus, a considerable rationale for shifting to use of the inactivated vaccine. In the long-term, whilst eradication of poliovirus may be achievable, some problems will remain. Re-emergence of wild-type polio from stored stocks (e.g. laboratory virus, stored clinical samples) is a possibility that needs to be addressed, and a decision made whether the oral vaccine should still be manufactured to deal with such an occurrence or, alternatively, emphasis placed on the inactivated vaccine (that requires inoculation).

## PARECHOVIRUSES

Sixteen human parechovirus types (1–16) have been described so far within the human parechovirus species of the *parechovirus* genus. Two of these (human parechovirus 1 and 2) were originally counted amongst the enteroviruses (echovirus 22 and 23, respectively). Generally, parechoviruses cause a similar range of clinical disease as members of the closely related *enterovirus* genus. In particular, human parechoviruses cause mild *respiratory* or *gastrointestinal illness* in young children as well as being associated with *aseptic meningitis, encephalitis* and *myocarditis*. These viruses are ubiquitous, and infection occurs early in life with most children having acquired parechoviruses by 5 years of age. Laboratory diagnosis is by genome detection (RT-PCR). There is no vaccine available against parechovirus infection.

## HEPATOVIRUSES

## HEPATITIS A VIRUS

Hepatitis A has a worldwide distribution and occurs in epidemics as well as sporadically. The virus was first detected by electron microscopical (EM) examination of faeces. The genus *hepatovirus* consists of hepatitis A virus (HAV) as its only species.

HAV is the causative agent of *infectious hepatitis*. It has similar polypeptides to the four major polypeptides of the enteroviruses, and shares the same properties of resistance to physical and chemical agents. Recently, it has been adapted to cell culture; it will grow only in cells of primate origin.

### Clinical features

Although the incidence has fallen in the past decade, HAV is still responsible for almost 60% of acute viral hepatitis in the USA. The illness is usually mild and occurs after an incubation period of 3–6 weeks. There is a prodrome of malaise, muscle pain and headache, and there may be a low-grade fever. The symptoms improve and disappear as jaundice develops. Serological tests show that many patients have a subclinical illness, and *fulminant* hepatitis and liver failure are rare. HAV does not cause chronic infection although the immunocompromised state may support longer-term excretion. Infection is mildest in young children, often accompanied only by nausea and malaise. Of children aged under 3 years, only 5% develop jaundice, but this rises progressively to more than 50% in adults. The fatality rate also rises with age, to 2% in adults. Some patients develop diarrhoea and some appear to have a relapse a few weeks after the onset. Arthritis and aplastic anaemia are rare complications. Treatment is supportive (e.g. replacement of fluid). There are no specific antiviral drugs. Severe cases of fulminant liver failure can be considered for receipt of a *liver transplant*.

### Pathogenesis

Like the enteroviruses, hepatitis A virus probably infects cells in the gut initially and then spreads to the liver via blood. The histopathological appearance shows periportal necrosis and infiltration of mononuclear cells. Viral antigens are seen in the cytoplasm of the hepatocytes. Virus is excreted via the bile into the gut 1–2 weeks before the onset of jaundice and excretion then declines rapidly over the next 5–7 days.

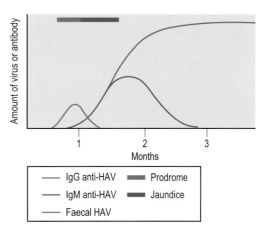

**Fig. 48.2** Events in hepatitis A infection.

Virus is also present in urine of clinical and subclinical cases during the same period.

### Laboratory diagnosis

Although the virus has been grown in cell culture, it is not possible to do this routinely from faeces of patients. Diagnosis relies on the demonstration of specific IgM antibody which develops very early in the course of infection and is generally present by the time the patient is investigated. It is detectable in the serum for 2–6 months after the onset of symptoms (Fig. 48.2). IgG antibody usually persists for many years and is a useful indicator of immunity. Virus can be detected in stool samples by EIA or RT-PCR.

### Epidemiology

Only one major type of HAV has been recognized. Molecular typing is now available to investigate outbreaks and link sporadic cases with common source outbreaks. Serological studies confirm that virus is prevalent in countries where sanitation is poor (consistent with faecal–oral route of spread) and children are infected early in childhood. Even in developed countries, more than half of the population has been infected with the virus. However, with increasing use of vaccine, lower rates are seen. This can result in increased numbers of acute cases in young adults and older patients who may have a history of recent travel to an endemic area.

Outbreaks of HAV infection have been associated with food. Shellfish have often been incriminated, particularly when they are harvested from coastlines adjacent to sewage outlets. When shellfish are eaten raw, or only partially cooked, the virus retains its ability to infect. Contaminated raspberries were incriminated in another notorious outbreak in which uncooked frozen raspberries were eaten many months after picking. Infection is assumed to have come from an infected raspberry picker. The infectious dose is low – less than 100 virus particles. Because there is only a transient viraemic phase, only a few infections have been recognized after blood transfusion.

## Prevention and control

A highly effective and immunogenic vaccine was licensed for use in the UK in 1991. It is a formaldehyde-inactivated vaccine prepared from virus grown in human diploid cells. A primary course of two doses (or, more recently, a single dose) of vaccine given intramuscularly produces good levels of neutralizing antibody that are known to persist for at least 10 years. The vaccine is now preferred to human normal immunoglobulin (HNIG) for frequent travellers, for those with potential occupational exposure, and to protect contacts of cases. Recent vaccine formulations may combine hepatitis A and B antigens in the same vaccine.

## RHINOVIRUSES

Although other viruses can give a similar illness, viruses belonging to the human rhinovirus species A and B of the genus *enterovirus* are responsible for the most frequent of all human infections, the 'common cold'. Most people suffer from two to four colds every year and, although the primary infection is not a severe one, the symptoms of secondary bacterial infection often follow and may be more severe. Sinusitis and otitis media are quite common. Rhinoviruses have also been associated with acute exacerbations of asthma. These viruses are of major economic significance because they cause the loss of many million man-hours of work each year, accounting for up to half of upper respiratory tract infections. The recently discovered human rhinovirus species C appears ubiquitous and associated with upper and lower respiratory tract disease in young children, but the features of this species are still being characterised.

## PROPERTIES

As the name rhinovirus implies, the viruses are associated with the nose. Rhinoviruses can be distinguished from other enteroviruses by their acid lability;

**Fig. 48.3** Human rhinovirus. This virus is indistinguishable in appearance from other picornaviruses. Approximate size 25–30 nm. (From Madeley CR, Field AM 1988 *Virus Morphology*, 2nd edn. Churchill Livingstone, Edinburgh.)

consequently, they do not infect the intestinal tract. There are over 100 serotypes of rhinoviruses; all are fastidious in cell culture. EM cannot differentiate them from other family members (Fig. 48.3). Some non-human primates may be susceptible to human rhinoviruses, and there are related viruses in cattle, cats and horses. The genomes of some rhinoviruses have 45–60% homology with polioviruses in hybridization tests.

The capsid of rhinoviruses appears to be less rigid than that of other enteroviruses. This loose packaging is consistent with its greater buoyant density and sensitivity to acid.

## Cultivation

Rhinoviruses show a distinct preference for cells of human origin, especially fetal lung and kidney. They are divided into major (90%) and minor (10%) groups according to their cell receptors.

## Stability

Inactivation of rhinoviruses occurs below pH 6.0 and is more rapid the lower the pH. Complete inactivation occurs at pH 3.0.

Some rhinoviruses may survive heating at 50°C for 1 h. They are relatively stable in the range of 20–37°C, and can survive on environmental surfaces such as doorknobs for several days. They can be preserved at −70°C.

Rhinoviruses are resistant to 20% ether and 5% chloroform, but are sensitive to aldehydes and hypochlorites.

## REPLICATION

Most (*major group*) rhinoviruses attach to the same intercellular adhesion molecule 1 (ICAM 1) cell receptors on HeLa cells (90%). The minor group (10%) attaches to members of the low-density lipoprotein receptor (LDLR) family. The viruses replicate in the cytoplasm of infected cells to give a cytopathic effect (CPE) that coincides with release of the virus. If the infected cultures are incubated at 37°C, the yield is reduced to 30–50% of that at 33°C.

## CLINICAL FEATURES AND PATHOGENESIS

The typical illness is generally referred to as the common cold. The onset, after contact with infection, is usually within 2–3 days, sometimes as long as 7 days. The symptoms are:

- clear watery nasal discharge, which often becomes mucoid, or purulent due to secondary bacterial infection
- sneezing and coughing
- sore throat
- headache and malaise.

The symptoms are most severe for 2–3 days when nasal virus titres are maximal and, although recovery is usually complete within a week, symptoms can persist for 2 weeks or longer. The ratio of symptomatic to asymptomatic infection is about 3:1, and the illness is generally worse in cigarette smokers. Rhinoviruses have frequently been isolated from patients during acute exacerbation of chronic obstructive airway disease and are the most common viruses to be associated with wheeze in pre-school children.

It should be remembered that all respiratory viruses may cause symptoms of the common cold, and dual infections with rhinovirus and another respiratory agent are not uncommon. In the immunocompetent individual, colds are mostly trivial and an inconvenience. Conversely, rhinovirus infection of an immunocompromised host can cause serious respiratory disease.

In organ cultures, the virus settles on the ciliated nasal epithelial cells, enters, infects and spreads from cell to cell in the epithelium. The cilia become immobilized, and both cilia and cell degenerate as the virus replicates. Bacterial invasion of the damaged epithelium can then occur. Interferon is usually detectable shortly after the peak of virus shedding and probably plays a part in recovery. Virus shedding ceases when antibody is detected in nasal secretions suggesting that this may be the main factor leading to recovery. Little is known of the importance of cell-mediated immunity. The symptoms probably relate to the local inflammatory response and interferon release. Rhinoviruses have been recovered in pure culture from sinus fluids collected from patients with acute sinusitis, but secondary bacterial infection is thought to be the usual cause. *Acute otitis media* is the most common complication in children suffering upper respiratory tract infection, and rhinoviruses can be detected (by RT-PCR) in the middle ear in up to 40% of such cases.

Lower respiratory tract infection may occur on some occasions since:

- patients with colds may also have lower respiratory tract symptoms with abnormal lung function
- children who develop colds may develop wheeze
- adults with colds may suffer exacerbation of chronic obstructive airway disease (e.g. asthma).

### Immunity

After the acute illness, neutralizing antibody can be detected in both serum and nasal secretions. It can continue to rise in titre for 4–5 weeks after infection and may persist for up to 4 years, although some infections may provoke only a poor response leaving the patient susceptible to the same serotype after a few weeks or months. New virus types continue to emerge by a process of immune selection and random mutation.

## LABORATORY DIAGNOSIS

Nose and throat swabs (in VTM) are the specimens of choice for the recovery of virus from all age groups. Nasopharyngeal aspirates (NPA) are excellent specimens from young (<2 years old) children. Specimens should be taken as early in the illness as possible, preferably within the first 3 days.

Cell cultures of human origin, such as MRC5 or WI38, are preferred for the isolation of rhinoviruses. Organ cultures are not used routinely. Cultures are incubated at 33°C and observed microscopically for a characteristic CPE. The majority of isolates are apparent within 2 weeks of inoculation, although some may take longer. Acid lability is a further aid to identification of an isolate as a rhinovirus.

## Serology

Serological methods cannot be used in the routine diagnosis of rhinovirus infections because of the multiplicity of serotypes and the lack of a common antigen.

## Nucleic acid detection

Culture is slow and cumbersome and serology inadequate, so nucleic acid amplification (usually PCR-based) of respiratory samples is used for diagnosis.

## EPIDEMIOLOGY AND TRANSMISSION

Rhinoviruses can be isolated from patients with respiratory illnesses throughout the year, but in temperate climates, the incidence of colds due to rhinoviruses increases in autumn and spring, and is lowest in the summer months. In the tropics, the peak incidence occurs in the rainy season. Although deliberate exposure of volunteers to wet and chilling conditions does not *per se* cause colds, the association is notable. Rhinoviruses may be transmitted by inhalation of droplets expelled from the nose of a patient and also by hand-to-surface contact. During the acute phase of the illness, high concentrations of virus are present in nasal secretions and may contaminate the fingers and thereafter the contaminated fingers may touch the eye or nasal mucosa. The incidence of rhinovirus infections is highest in pre-school children, who often introduce colds to their homes, and therefore people who are in contact with young children are at increased risk of infection.

## TREATMENT AND CONTROL

Although inactivated vaccines can be produced, there remains the considerable problem of deciding on the antigenic composition. Much effort has been devoted to the development of suitable antiviral therapy. Pleconaril is one such drug showing some activity against rhinoviruses and other enteroviruses (see above) but it is not available in the UK. Isolation of the infected person, although perhaps desirable, is not always a practical method of preventing the spread of infection. Good infection control practices, including adequate hand washing, reduces spread of infection in the hospital (and community) setting.

RECOMMENDED READING

Knipe DM, Howley PM, editors: Picornaviridae. In *Fields Virology*, ed 5, Philadelphia, 2007, Lippincott Williams & Wilkins, pp 795–948.

Logan SAE, MacMahon E: Viral meningitis, *The British Medical Journal* 336:36–40, 2008.

Mahy BWJ, Ter Meulen V, editors: Picornaviridae. In *Topley & Wilson's Microbiology & Microbial Infections: Virology*, ed 10, London, 2005, Hodder Arnold, pp 857–887, 1160–1188.

Nathanson N, Kew OM: From Emergence to Eradication: The epidemiology of poliomyelitis deconstructed, *American Journal of Epidemiology* 172:1213–1229, 2010.

Obregón R, Chitnis K, Morry C, et al: Achieving polio eradication: A review of health communication evidence and lessons learned in India and Pakistan, *Bulletin of the World Health Organization* 87: 624–630, 2009.

Rhoades RE, Tabor-Godwin JM, Tsueng G, Feuer R: Enterovirus infections of the central nervous system, *Virology* 411:288–305, 2011.

Zuckerman AJ, Banatvala JE, Schoub BD, et al, editors: *Principles and Practice of Clinical Virology*, ed 6, Chichester, 2009, Wiley-Blackwell, 273–279, pp 489–510, 601–624.

### Websites

Global Polio Eradication Initiative: http://www.polioeradication.org/

UK Department of Health: UK hepatitis A immunisation policy. http://www.dh.gov.uk/prod_consum_dh/groups/dh_digitalassets/@dh/@en/documents/digitalasset/dh_124297.pdf

UK Department of Health: UK polio immunisation policy. http://www.dh.gov.uk/prod_consum_dh/groups/dh_digitalassets/@dh/@en/documents/digitalasset/dh_108823.pdf

# 49 Orthomyxoviruses

## Influenza

*M. Zambon*

## KEY POINTS

- Influenza viruses cause respiratory infections worldwide; there are three types: A, B and C.
- Influenza A is found in aquatic birds, poultry and pigs, and these play important roles in the epidemiology of human infections.
- Influenza viruses are segmented RNA viruses that regularly undergo genetic change.
- The surface proteins, the haemagglutinin and the neuraminidase, can show gradual change (*antigenic drift*) and sudden major change (*antigenic shift*).
- In humans, influenza A results in high morbidity and mortality rates in the winter months in temperate zones, but throughout the year in more tropical climates.
- The spread pattern may be pandemic, epidemic or sporadic/zoonotic.
- Pandemic influenza typically arises when a new virus from an animal host emerges into a susceptible human population. The impact of pandemics may be mild, moderate or severe, depending on the virulence properties of the virus.
- Zoonotic influenza A infections in humans may have a high case fatality and different clinical manifestations compared with seasonal influenza A.
- Since 1997, H5 avian influenza has been a major problem in the Far East, with strains from domestic poultry occasionally infecting humans directly, resulting in high mortality rates; this virus could become adapted to humans.
- Vaccines have been available for many years, recommended for annual boosting of high-risk groups in interpandemic periods to reduce mortality, morbidity and hospital admission rates.
- Antiviral drugs act to inhibit viral replication, and are clinically useful in treatment and prophylaxis.

The Orthomyxoviridae family comprises four genera: *influenza A, B* and *C* and *thogotoviruses*, within the negative sense RNA virus order *Mononegavirales.* All of these are small enveloped viruses with a segmented genome. The thogotoviruses are the most recently discovered genus and are found in mosquitoes, ticks and the banded mongoose, but are not so far associated with human disease and are not discussed further.

## INFLUENZA A, B AND C HOST RANGE

Influenza B and C have limited genetic diversity and occur almost exclusively in humans, which are the natural animal reservoir. Occasional transmission of influenza B to mammalian species such as seals and influenza C to pigs has been described. In contrast, there are many different subtypes of influenza A viruses, all of which naturally infect water-based wild birds, usually with very little disease. Influenza A viruses have a broad host range with the potential to infect a wide range of animal species. Viral subtypes are distinguished according to their surface proteins, the haemagglutinin (HA) and neuraminidase (NA). Sixteen HA subtypes and 9 NA subtypes are found in varying combinations circulating in wild birds. Only a limited number of influenza A subtypes have adapted to circulation in mammalian species, including humans, horses and swine (Fig. 49.1).

Avian influenza A subtypes are transmitted through a faeco–oral route and virus can be shed in high quantity in the environment following replication in the gastrointestinal tract. There is frequent spillover of avian influenza A subtypes into domestic poultry reservoirs, as a result of their shared habitat with wild birds. Replication in poultry may be associated with disease of varying severity or may be asymptomatic, depending on the viral subtype and the poultry species.

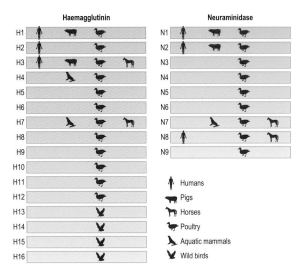

**Fig. 49.1** Natural hosts for different influenza subtypes.

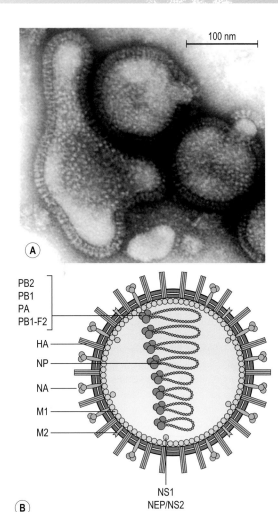

**Fig. 49.2** (A) EM of influenza virus. (B) Schematic representation of virus particle and internal composition.

## Nomenclature

The World Health Organization (WHO) system of nomenclature for influenza A includes the host of origin, geographical origin, strain number and year of isolation; then, in parentheses, the antigenic description of the haemagglutinin and neuraminidase is given, e.g. A/swine/Iowa/3/70 ($H_1N_1$). If isolated from a human host the origin is not given: e.g. A/Scotland/42/89 ($H_3N_2$).

## Physical characteristics

In common with many enveloped viruses, influenza A, B and C are relatively labile and easily destroyed by common household cleaning agents and detergents. In the environment, influenza A virus can survive in cold seawater for several days, and is detectable in dust beyond one week although the infectivity of such material is not well understood.

## THE VIRUSES

Influenza virions are spherical, 80–120 nm in diameter, but may be filamentous and up to one hundred fold longer (Fig. 49.2A). They have a helical nucleocapsid comprising, in A and B, eight segments of single-stranded RNA and, in C, seven segments. Also present within the virion particle is the viral RNA-dependent RNA polymerase enzyme; this is essential for infectivity as the viral RNA is of negative sense and therefore has to be transcribed to produce viral

messenger RNA. The nucleocapsid is surrounded by the M1 protein shell, immediately exterior to which is a lipid envelope derived from the host cell. The viral M2 protein projects through the envelope to form ion channels, which assist virus entry through an endosomal route which involves pH changes. Two types of spike project from the lipid envelope, the *haemagglutinin* (HA) and the *neuraminidase* (NA) enzyme (Fig. 49.2B). The HA, so-called because the virus agglutinates certain species of erythrocyte, is about 10 nm in length and consists of trimers of identical glycoprotein subunits, each consisting of two polypeptide chains, $HA_1$ and $HA_2$ joined by a linkage site that may be a single basic amino acid, usually arginine, or a string of basic amino acids (Fig. 49.3).

Influenza viruses bind to cells by the HA interacting with cell membrane receptors containing

Fig. 49.3 Schematic of HA1 and HA2 monomer.

Fig. 49.4 Host virus receptor configuration in avian and human viruses, leading to differences in receptor binding preferences.

*N*-acetylneuraminic acid (sialic acid). The amino acid residues involved in receptor binding show variability according to host of origin. Differences in viral receptor binding characteristics have important biological significance for the transmission properties of the virus. Human influenza viruses recognize receptors that contain sialic acid attached to the penultimate sugar (usually lactose) via an α(2,6)-linkage, whereas avian strains prefer receptors with an α(2,3)-linkage (Fig. 49.4).

Between the HA spikes on the virus surface are the mushroom-shaped NA spikes. The NA protein is assembled from four subunits attached by a stalk containing a hydrophobic region which is anchored in the viral lipid envelope. The NA enzyme catalyses the cleavage of sialic acid and an adjacent sugar residue from glycoproteins found in mucus. This action allows the virus to permeate through the mucin overlying host epithelial surfaces. Neuraminidase activity is also important in the release of new virus particles from infected cells. Sialic acid is always present in newly synthesized virions, and its removal by NA prevents the new virus particles clumping through the binding to viral HA, thus assisting the spread of the virus from the original site of infection.

## Virus variability

All influenza viruses replicate via virally encoded RNA dependent RNA polymerase enzymes. Such enzymes lack a proof reading (error correction) function, leading to high rates of mutation during replication, particularly for influenza A. Viruses carrying mutations which do not provide a severe replication disadvantage therefore evolve rapidly, a feature described as *genetic drift*. Genetic recombination between diverse influenza A viral subtypes occurs when more than one subtype infects a single host, creating new combinations of viral gene segments (reassortment) and altering the replication and virulence properties of the progeny virus. Together, the combination of genetic drift and segment reassortment provide the mechanism for generation of genetic diversity amongst influenza A viruses. These genetic mechanisms generate adaptive flexibility, which is reflected in the wide variety of animal species (host range) that can be infected. Different genetic lineages of influenza B and C also show some evidence of segment reassortment, but this is very much more limited than for influenza A and is not associated with significant biological diversity.

## EPIDEMIC AND PANDEMIC INFLUENZA

Major epidemics that may have been caused by influenza viruses have been described for more than 2000 years. Historically, it was rationalized that such unexpected events occurred under the influence of the stars, hence the term *influenza* (Italian for influence). It is well recognized that epidemics vary in severity. Occasionally infection arising from a new strain spreads throughout the world and causes very significant marked waves of illness; such *pandemics* have been recognized at irregular intervals.

Pandemics occurred in 1918, 1957 and 1968 with the emergence of $H_1N_1$ Spanish influenza, $H_2N_2$ and $H_3N_2$ respectively, and most recently in 2009, with the emergence of $H_1N_1$ from swine ($H_1N_1$ 2009pdm) into the human population. The great pandemic of 1918–1919 was particularly severe, killing 20–40 million people as it spread over a few years. In 1957, the emergence of $H_2N_2$ as a pandemic virus displaced circulating $H_1N_1$, which disappeared until 1977, when it re-emerged after 20 years (Fig. 49.5). The emergence of new influenza A viruses in humans which are able to transmit person to person and cause a global pandemic, is likely to have arisen from an initial rare event involving a novel influenza A virus with the capacity of replicating in humans and transmitting. Virus isolation studies from 1933 onwards, and analysis of isolates, have given an understanding of how the epidemic and pandemic behaviour relates to changes in the virus.

Major pandemics are associated with *antigenic shifts* – when the viral HA or NA (or both) is changed. Antigenic shift results from the acquisition of a complete new RNA segment 4 and/or 6, either as a result of reassortment or infection of humans with an animal virus. Until 1977, when $H_1N_1$ reappeared, it was considered that when a 'new' pandemic virus appeared the 'old' one disappeared, but since that time two influenza A subtypes have been circulating concurrently, namely $H_3N_2$ and $H_1N_1$ (Fig. 49.5). $H_1N_1$ viruses in 1977 were antigenically very similar to $H_1N_1$ viruses from before the 1957 pandemic, and may have been reintroduced from frozen laboratory sources, as there is no evidence of latent or persistent infection of humans. The most recent pandemic of 2009 exemplifies the emergence of an influenza strain from an animal reservoir ($H_1N_1$ from swine reservoir), to cause widespread disease in humans of all age groups. Although $H_1N_1$ has been circulating since 1918, $H_1N_1$ swine viruses were sufficiently different to $H_1N_1$ viruses circulating in humans, so that pre-existing immunity in the population was insufficient to prevent widespread transmission, especially in younger age groups. The impact of $H_1N_1$ in the population was mild to moderate overall, partly due to the lower intrinsic virulence of the strain, and partly due to the pre-existing immunity in the adult and elderly population, although susceptible groups such as pregnant women had an increased risk of serious outcome. At the time of writing, $H_1N_1$ 2009pdm has almost completely displaced the previously circulating $H_1N_1$ strain.

Epidemics occurring regularly in winter months between pandemics are associated with genetic drift in the HA antigen. Amino acid changes arising as a result of genetic mutation provide a selection advantage for the virus if they occur on the globular head of the HA protein, where host antibody binds (Fig. 49.3). Mutation at these sites allows the virus to infect despite the presence of antibody to previous strains, a phenomenon known as *antigenic drift*.

**Fig. 49.5** Influenza viruses first isolated in 1933. Co-circulation of different viruses during the 20th and 21st centuries. Oval symbol denotes sporadic incidents and outbreaks with avian influenza viruses.

The wild bird reservoir for influenza A is globally dispersed and mobile, creating a natural milieu for relentless evolution of genetic diversity. Consequently, there is a continuous threat to humans of the emergence of a new influenza A virus, capable of adapting to human transmission, causing a pandemic of disease in a globally susceptible population. The criteria for the establishment of a new pandemic of influenza in humans include:

- a novel virus, with a new haemagglutinin (HA) subtype (*antigenic shift*)
- association with disease
- susceptible population
- ability of virus to transmit person to person.

Sporadic zoonotic infections of influenza A are therefore closely monitored, in view of the potential they have to create a new pandemic influenza strain. All of the HA and NA subtypes are found in aquatic birds

(both seabirds and ducks), but in these animals the viruses vary little. Viral factors govern the ability to transmit and replicate in humans. These include receptor characteristics, replication competence and ability of virus to be shed directly into bodily secretions, which can be transmitted. In the laboratory it is easy to show that, if a cell is infected with two different strains, viruses arise with RNA segments derived from each parent through reassortment of segments.

Pigs have receptors for both human and avian strains, and this mammalian host has long been considered a key 'mixing vessel' for reassortment following simultaneous infection with human and avian viruses. The conditions in South East Asia, where there are high densities of people, poultry and pigs, favour such an outcome (Fig. 49.6). The importance of the pig host in the generation of diversity is emphasized by the 2009 pandemic.

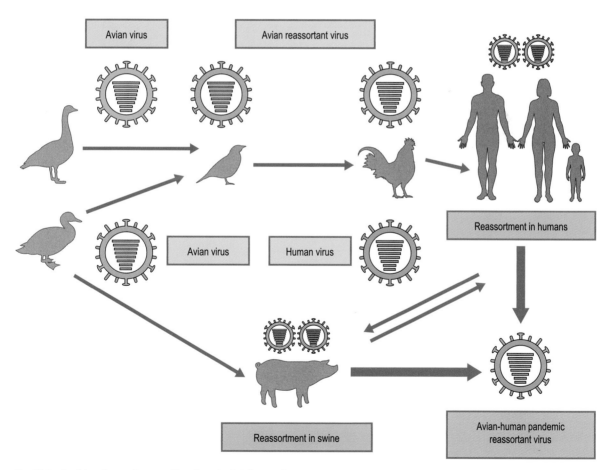

**Fig. 49.6** Possible pathways for generation of pandemic influenza viruses.

## CROSS SPECIES INFLUENZA A INFECTION

In recent years, influenza A viruses have been detected in a variety of mammalian species including dogs, mink, tigers, whales, cats and civets, usually arising from occasional transmission events from avians which may cause a range of disease symptoms in the new host, depending on the infecting virus subtype. Influenza A infection in mammalian species is usually associated with viral replication in the respiratory tract leading to respiratory illnesses with some systemic features, and occasionally extra respiratory replication. Sporadic infection events have usually involved only limited transmission in the new host. Diseased poultry and domestic ducks usually serve as the source of infection for avian influenza in mammalian hosts (Fig. 49.6). Infection arises through a variety of routes including contact with contaminated water, avian faecal material or contact with carcasses of infected birds. However, adaptation to dogs in North America has occurred, as a result of transmission of H7 from horses, creating a new animal reservoir of endemic influenza A (Fig. 49.7).

## Zoonotic transmission to humans

Sporadic zoonotic infection of humans with influenza A viruses should be distinguished from epidemic human influenza A seasonal infection, which occurs during the winter months and is attributable to subtypes of influenza A ($H_3N_2$ and $H_1N_1$) which normally transmit between humans causing seasonal respiratory illness along with influenza B or C.

Human cases of infection with avian influenza viruses involving $H_5$, $H_7$, $H_{10}$ or $H_9$ subtypes have usually been acquired as a result of exposure to domestic poultry, material containing avian influenza virus or other mammalian species infected as an intermediate host with an avian influenza virus. The outcome of sporadic human infection ranges from severe disease of the respiratory system, which may also lead to multi-organ failure and death, to milder respiratory infection or simple conjunctivitis. The spectrum of disease is dependant on the nature of the infecting avian influenza A virus, e.g. $H_5$ infections are associated with severe respiratory infections with a high case fatality rate; $H_7$ infections are associated with conjunctivitis and milder respiratory infections.

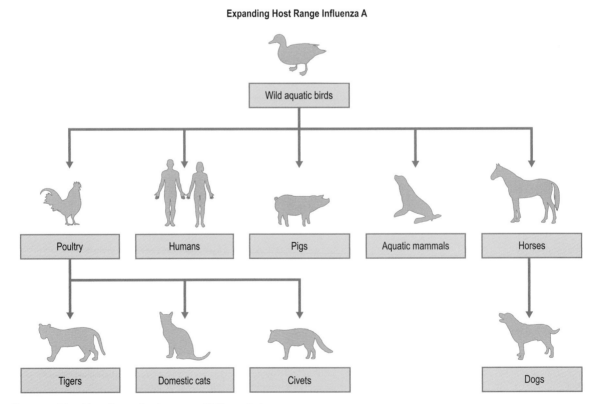

**Fig. 49.7** Adaptable and expanding host range of influenza A viruses.

Risk factors for the acquisition of zoonotic avian or non human influenza A include:

- close or direct contact with diseased poultry or other domestic fowl
- close or direct contact with other mammalian species infected with unusual influenza A viruses (swine, seals)
- inhalation, ingestion or mucosal contact with infectious material.

Risk factors for severe human disease outcome following zoonotic infection of influenza A include:

- $H_5$ subtype (50% case fatality rate)
- young age
- pre-existing lung disease
- pathogenicity of infecting virus in poultry reservoir

## Human seasonal influenza A, B and C infections

As can be seen from the foregoing discussion, influenza A virus subtypes circulating in humans ($H_1N_1$ and $H_3N_2$) were ultimately derived from an animal reservoir. Several influenza A subtypes co-circulate globally in humans in varying proportion, causing respiratory disease during the winter months in temperate climates, and during months of highest humidity in dry climates. In tropical climates, distinct seasonality is less evident, with patterns of influenza transmission throughout the year. Influenza B viruses co-circulate globally with influenza A viruses and contribute to the burden of seasonal influenza (Fig. 49.5), but are not usually associated with such severe morbidity and mortality. Influenza B viruses do not undergo antigenic shift as there is no animal reservoir and, although epidemics do occur at 3–6-year intervals, they never reach pandemic proportions. The antigenic changes in influenza B result from genetic drift, as seen in influenza A after the appearance of 'new' virus strains. Influenza C viruses are associated with much milder illness, with limited generation of genetic diversity and sporadic pattern of circulation.

## Clinical features in human seasonal influenza A infection

Influenza is an acute infection of the human respiratory tract. Disease is characterized by the sudden onset of fever, chills, headache, muscle pain and extreme fatigue. Other common symptoms include a dry cough, sore throat and stuffy nose. For otherwise healthy individuals, influenza is an unpleasant but usually self-limiting disease with recovery usually within two to seven days. The illness may be complicated by (and may present as) bronchitis, secondary bacterial pneumonia or with otis media (ear infection) in children.

Serious illness and mortality are highest among newborns, older people and those with underlying disease, particularly chronic respiratory or cardiac disease, or those who are immunosuppressed.

In classical seasonal influenza A infection:

- the incubation period is short, 2 days, but may vary from 1–4 days
- the illness is characterized by a sudden onset of systemic symptoms such as chills, fever, headache, myalgia and anorexia
- respiratory symptoms are also common but take second place to the systemic effects, especially early in the illness.

Many patients have both upper and lower respiratory tract infection, often with a troublesome, dry cough. The main physical finding is pyrexia, which rises rapidly to a peak of 38–41°C within 12 h of onset. Fever usually lasts for 3 days, but may be present for 1–5 days. During the second and third days of the illness the systemic effects diminish, and by the fourth day, the respiratory symptoms and signs are predominant. In adults, systemic illness without respiratory symptoms is common. Some symptoms are age-specific, for example febrile convulsions and otitis media in children and dyspnoea in the elderly. About one-third of patients suffer only a common cold-like illness, and as many as 20–30% of cases are subclinical (asymptomatic). A long convalescence is common, and cough, lassitude and malaise may last for 1–2 weeks after the disappearance of other manifestations. Many other respiratory viruses can cause typical influenza-like illnesses, although the severity of the systemic symptoms is usually greatest with influenza virus.

## Complications of human seasonal influenza

- Primary influenza pneumonia is an unusual complication that may occur at any age and carries a case fatality rate of 1–5%, depending on age and underlying conditions. This can be fatal, especially in young adults during an outbreak, after a very short illness of sometimes less than 1 day. A similar rapid illness can occur in the elderly.
- More commonly a bacterial pneumonia caused by *Staphylococcus aureus*, *Streptococcus pneumoniae* or *Haemophilus influenzae* occurs

late in the course of the illness, often after a period of improvement, resulting in a classical biphasic fever pattern.
- Very rare complications include myocarditis, encephalitis or meningoencephalitis.

The incidence of chest complications is related to the age of the patient, increasing progressively after the age of 60 years. Severe infections and sudden death can occur, especially if there is some underlying disease, such as cerebrovascular, cardiovascular or chronic respiratory disease.

In the immunocompromised, symptoms may last longer and viral excretion may go on for weeks to months. Excess mortality was reported in pregnant women during the 1918 and 1957 pandemics, and even in non-pandemic outbreaks an increase in hospital admission due to cardiorespiratory disease is seen in the second and third trimesters. Susceptibility of pregnant women to severe influenza was also evident in the 2009 pandemic.

### Clinical features in zoonotic influenza A infections

There is a spectrum of illness associated with the presentation of zoonotic avian influenza A virus infection, which is associated with the infecting subtype. Conjunctivitis was a feature of $H_7N_7$ outbreak cases in the Netherlands. $H_5N_1$ infections are associated with illness onset up to seven days post exposure, in contrast to the shorter incubation time of seasonal influenza, with associated delayed viral shedding. The early stages of infection may be difficult to distinguish from seasonal influenza or other respiratory infections which share many common presenting symptoms. The predominant clinical features include high temperature, cough and shortness of breath. Although the majority of cases have been respiratory in presentation, a handful of cases present atypically with fever, gastrointestinal disturbance and diarrhoea. Early clinical signs include alteration in liver function tests, particularly elevated aminotransferase enzymes, lymphopenia and evidence of interstitial pneumonia on chest X-ray. Progression of disease predominantly involves the respiratory tract and can lead to acute respiratory distress syndrome, with death most frequently being due to respiratory failure, often associated with multi organ failure. Limited autopsy evidence from fatal $H_5$ cases is consistent with respiratory failure and primary viral interstitial pneumonia, but with little evidence of extra respiratory spread of virus to account for the multisystem dysfunction. The latter may be attributable to immune dysregulation leading

to a 'cytokine storm' (uncontrolled release of tissue damaging immune response molecules); there is some autopsy evidence for haemophagocytic syndrome, but the overall understanding of pathogenesis is limited. Recovery from $H_5$ infection occurs from about 7–10 days post illness onset, and is associated with a rise in neutralizing antibody titres.

### Clinical features in human seasonal influenza B infection

Symptoms closely resemble those associated with seasonal influenza A infections, consisting of a 3-day febrile illness with predominantly systemic symptoms. Overall, the infection is somewhat milder.

### INFLUENZA C

Clinically, influenza C causes an afebrile upper respiratory tract infection usually confined to young children; outbreaks are not recognized.

### SEASONAL INFLUENZA A EPIDEMICS

An individual throughout life can expect to experience multiple influenza infections. Viruses bearing mutations accumulated during error prone replication (*genetic drift*) may have a replication advantage because they can evade the existing human immune response, giving a selection advantage due to *antigenic drift* in circulating strains. Over a period of several years, antigenic variants gradually predominate, displacing older strains, and cause epidemic disease.

Influenza virus is transmitted is by aerosol, droplets or direct contact with respiratory secretions of someone with the infection, for example sneezing and coughing. Influenza spreads rapidly, especially in closed communities. Most influenza cases in temperate countries tend to occur during a twelve to sixteen-week period during the winter. The timing, extent and severity of 'seasonal' influenza can all vary according to country. Winter activity is therefore unpredictable. Influenza A viruses cause outbreaks most years in most countries, and it is these viruses that are the usual cause of seasonal epidemics. More severe epidemics occur intermittently, often associated with the emergence of an antigenic drift variant. Influenza B tends to cause less severe disease and smaller outbreaks, although in children the severity of illness may be similar to that associated with influenza A.

High rates of infection are generally found in preschool children; thereafter the rates are lower, even in the elderly. However, elderly patients in residential homes, if not protected, are at particular risk from acute illness and sudden death. Thus, even if the attack rate is low, the case fatality rate is high. Staff, visitors or other patients may introduce the virus, and this is an important consideration when planning intervention measures.

## Pathogenesis

Inhaled virus is deposited on the mucous membrane lining the respiratory tract or directly into the alveoli, the anatomical location depending on the size of the droplets inhaled. The virus is exposed to mucoproteins containing sialic acid that can bind to the virus, thus blocking virus attachment to respiratory tract epithelial cells. However, the action of viral neuraminidase allows the virus to break any bonds formed. Specific local secretory immunoglobulin (Ig) A antibodies, if present from a previous infection, may neutralize the virus before attachment occurs, provided the antibody corresponds to the infecting virus type. If not prevented by one of these immune defence mechanisms, virus attaches to the surface of a respiratory epithelial cell and the intracellular replication cycle is initiated.

The major site of infection for seasonal influenza in humans is the ciliated columnar epithelial cell. New viruses bud from the apical membrane, the cilia are lost and viruses spread to other areas of the respiratory tract. The cell damage initiates an acute inflammatory response with oedema and the attraction of phagocytic cells. The earliest response is the synthesis and release of interferons from the infected cells: these can diffuse to and protect both adjacent and more distant cells before the virus arrives. It appears that interferons released in this way cause many of the systemic features of the 'flu-like' syndrome. Although viral components are absorbed and trigger the immune system, the virus itself is confined to the epithelium of the respiratory tract. Specific antibody helps to limit the extracellular spread of the virus, whereas T cell responses are directed against the viral glycoproteins on the surface of infected cells, leading to their destruction by cytotoxic T cells and also by antibody-dependent cell cytotoxicity. The pathogenesis of severe sporadic influenza A zoonotic infections in humans can involve multisystem failure, but evidence of extra respiratory virus replication is rare. It is considered likely that aberrant innate immune responses (cytokine storm arising from massive unregulated production of cytokines and chemokines) contribute to poor outcome in severe cases, possibly arising from different respiratory cell tropism.

The pathogenicity of influenza viruses is multifactorial and may involve viral, host and environmental factors. Pathogenicity is best understood with influenza A in birds. Host cell receptors are determinants of tropism in birds. Virus infectivity is dependent on host protease activity, cleaving HA into $HA_1$ and $HA_2$. There is a clear molecular correlate of pathogenicity associated with the presence of a string of polybasic amino acids at the $HA_1$–$HA_2$ cleavage site in certain $H_5$ or $H_7$ avian strains, as the HA protein containing such an insert can now be cleaved by a much wider range of host protease enzymes. In turn, virus dissemination within the avian host is enhanced, and replication occurs in a much wider range of tissues outside the gastrointestinal tract.

Understanding of pathogenesis in mammals is much less complete, but is recognized to be multifactorial involving several genes, including viral HA, NA, polymerase proteins and NS1. Receptor binding preference is an important determinant of tissue and cell tropism which may influence innate immune responses. Polymerase replication proteins may influence the ability of virus to replicate efficiently, and the NS1 non-structural protein may also influence pathogenicity by its role in antagonism of innate immune responses.

## Immunity

After an attack of influenza, immunity to the particular strain of infecting virus is of long duration. It is related to the amount of local antibody (IgA) in the mucous secretions of the respiratory tract together with specific IgG serum antibody concentration. Immunity to infection, especially with influenza A, is subtype specific, giving little or no protection against subtypes possessing immunologically distinct H or N proteins. Once recovered from an initial influenza infection, exposure to more recent related strains will boost IgG levels to the earlier strains, the so-called *original antigenic sin* phenomenon.

## Laboratory diagnosis

Prior to the 21st century, laboratory diagnosis of influenza depended on virus isolation through culture methods, or through detection of viral proteins in respiratory epithelial cells by immunofluoresence (IF) or enzyme linked immunosorbent assays (ELISA).

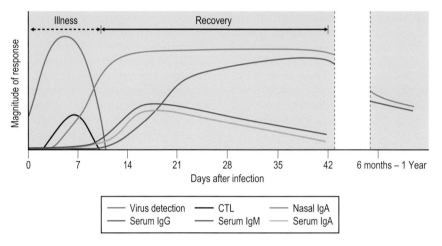

**Fig. 49.8** Diagnostic detection of influenza infections in humans. CTL, cytotoxic T cell response.

The application of reverse transcription PCR to respiratory clinical material to detect viral genomic material has transformed the time taken to provide accurate and reliable diagnosis from days to within a matter of hours. Rapid diagnosis of respiratory infections has increased in importance, particularly in hospital or care facilities, such as homes for the elderly. Antiviral drugs given early in infection can be used to control disease and limit transmission. The best specimens for rapid diagnosis are nasal aspirates or nasal washes, but nasal or throat swabs containing epithelial cells are satisfactory if taken in the first few days of illness (Fig. 49.8).

In zoonotic influenza A infection ($H_5$ or $H_7$), virus shedding peaks several days after illness onset, and slightly later than in seasonal influenza, but may continue for up to 10 days, and declines in the recovery phase. In fatal cases, viral shedding may continue at very high levels. $H_5$ virus replication occurs predominantly in the lower respiratory tract. Detection of virus genomic material by RT-PCR is optimal if secretions from the lower respiratory tract are obtained. Detection of infected airway epithelial cells using direct IF is an insensitive technique, and if undertaken, should be recognized as a suboptimal diagnostic test.

Whilst it is now possible to make a diagnosis of influenza without a virus isolate, it is important in the early stages of an outbreak or in sporadic cases that viruses should be isolated and analyzed antigenically to provide the best possible information for vaccine production. For primary isolation the most suitable cells are Madin–Darby canine kidney (MDCK) cells.

## Serology

Serological confirmation of a clinical diagnosis is by demonstration of a four-fold or greater rise in functional strain specific antibody titre. Strain differences can be demonstrated by means of haemagglutination inhibition (HI) and neutralization antibody assays. Specific neutralizing antibody can be detected from about 10–14 days post infection, and reaches a plateau at around 28 days (Fig. 49.8). Complement fixation tests are still occasionally used. This test uses nucleocapsid antigens that are type-specific and can distinguish A from B and C infections, but cannot distinguish between different influenza A infections.

## Treatment

Oral amantadine hydrochloride was introduced in the early 1980s, followed by a derivative, rimantadine. These drugs work by blocking the M2 ion channels in the envelope, thus preventing the pH changes that precede the membrane fusion step essential for nucleocapsid release. Unfortunately, these compounds have activity only against influenza virus type A. Amantadine is effective when given prophylactically, and also therapeutically in patients treated within 24 h of onset of illness. Viruses resistant to amantadine and rimantadine may appear within a few days of drug administration; however, resistant strains show no increased pathogenicity or transmissibility. In recent years, most circulating $H_3N_2$ and approximately 10% of $H_1N_1$ viruses have been naturally resistant to amantadine. Therefore, amantadine is not the drug of first choice, and it is essential to know which virus subtype is circulating prior to prescribing amantadine.

More recently two neuraminidase inhibitors (NIs), zanamivir and oseltamivir, have been licensed for therapeutic use in both influenza A and B infections, and other drugs with a similar mode of action are in development (e.g. peramivir). They act to prevent the release of viral particles through the action of viral neuraminidase enzymes which are conserved across all viral NA subtypes. They can reduce the duration of symptoms by 1–3 days if given within 36 h of the onset of illness. Zanamivir has poor bio-availability and is administered by inhalation of a dry powder twice daily for 5 days. Oseltamivir is given by mouth as a pro-drug and has excellent bio-availability, although nausea and vomiting may occur in some patients. Twice-daily dosage for 5–7 days has been used in those with normal renal function; once-daily dosage is recommended when renal function is impaired.

Both drugs have been licensed since 1999–2000 and a decade of global use indicates that mutations in viral NA are the major source of drug resistant variants. Resistant viruses have usually had a fitness deficit which compromises their transmissibility. Oseltamivir has been used much more extensively in this time, and as a consequence most available data on the emergence of antiviral resistance is related to oseltamivir use. Some key principles have become evident about the emergence of NI drug resistance.

Influenza A virus NAs are classified into group I and group II NAs, which differ in configuration of the enzyme active site. Group I NAs e.g. $N_1$, have an active site cleft for substrate binding which is broader, so that the most common oseltamivir resistance mutation in $N_1$ NA at position 275 is readily tolerated and inhibits drug action. Such mutations in $H_1N_1$ viruses arise during treatment, most commonly in younger or immunocompromised individuals where viral shedding is higher, and in $H_5N_1$ viruses where viral replication is not controlled by human immune responses. The spontaneous emergence and transmission of resistant $H_1N_1$ virus due to H275Y mutation during the northern hemisphere winter of 2007–2008 was a demonstration of the genetic evolution of influenza viruses. Compensatory mutations in the viral NA or other parts of the viral genome, arising from genetic drift have overcome the fitness deficit normally associated with mutation at position 275, enabling an otherwise disadvantaged virus to outcompete sensitive strains and predominate globally. Over a period of approximately 12 months, virtually all seasonal $H_1N_1$ viruses have become naturally oseltamivir resistant.

The patterns of mutations conferring drug resistance are subtype and drug specific. Although H275Y resistance is most common in N1 subtype containing viruses, such viruses remain susceptible to zanamivir (but not peramivir). N2 NAs fall into group 2 NA, for which the active site is narrower, and mutation at position 275 does not have the same effect. In $H_3N_2$, the most common mutation conferring NI resistance is at position 119 or position 272. As a consequence of the emergence of significant antiviral resistance, it is now important to ensure global surveillance of drug resistance and a rapid analysis of circulating subtypes so as to direct appropriate antiviral therapy.

During a pandemic there is a major role for the prophylactic use of anti-influenza drugs such as oseltamivir and zanamivir in those at high risk, in healthcare staff and in staff in long-term care facilities who have not been protected by an appropriate vaccine. Early studies have identified protection rates of over 80% with such chemoprophylaxis.

## Control measures

The presence of a large global mobile animal reservoir of influenza A virus suggests that eradication of avian influenza A as a zoonotic infection of humans will be impossible. Control strategies focus on limiting the opportunities for cross species transmission of novel subtypes. For example:

- housing domestic poultry in shelters to avoid contact with over-flying migrating birds
- eliminating wild bird markets
- segregating different species of birds in markets
- housing aquatic birds and domestic poultry separately
- slaughtering domestic flocks infected with highly pathogenic influenza A viruses.

These measures may achieve some success in preventing zoonotic transmission of influenza A to humans, and have certainly reduced the circulation of $H_5$ in domestic poultry in Hong Kong since 1997. However, they have little impact on the annual cycle of avian influenza in the wild bird population. Transmission of avian influenza by migrating birds is responsible for extending the geographical range of evolving avian influenza strains, as has been seen in 2005 and 2006 with the detection of $H_5N_1$ in birds and poultry in parts of Europe and Africa and the Middle East, whereas hitherto it was confined to South East Asia.

**Fig. 49.9** Inactivated vaccine preparations. (A) Whole virus. (B) Split vaccine preparation, with some internal components. (C) Subunit vaccine, highly purified surface proteins.

## Infection control

Exposure to heat for 30 min at 56°C is sufficient to inactivate most strains. The viruses are inactivated by a variety of substances, detergents, soaps, and other household compounds as well as 20% ethanol, halogens and phenolic compounds. These biological properties are the basis of most infection control advice and practices surrounding the management of noscomial influenza infection and exposure of individuals to influenza viruses.

## Immunization

A key control strategy for reduction of morbidity and mortality due to influenza is immunization. The aim is to produce haemagglutination inhibiting or neutralizing antibody in all vaccinees. This protects against infection, but only with strains closely related to those in the vaccine, and limits transmission. Whole virus, split and subunit inactivated influenza vaccines for intramuscular injection have been widely available for many years (Fig. 49.9), and live attenuated vaccines have been available more recently for use in children in the USA. Inactivated vaccines are trivalent and contain the H and N subunits from two type A strains and one type B strain. The strains are updated annually on the recommendation of the WHO and, in the UK, are recommended for use in people aged over 65 years, and in those of any age who suffer from chronic cardiorespiratory problems, diabetes, renal or liver failure or an immunosuppressive illness. In interpandemic years, with the elderly given annual boosting, the mortality rate can be reduced by 75% and the rate of hospital admission with complications by about 50%.

Intervention during a pandemic is more difficult, often for logistic and vaccine supply reasons. Vaccine delivery may be delayed, and the risk groups for vaccination may differ from those normally vaccinated during seasonal influenza, as was noted during the pandemic of 2009, where the key risk groups were children and pregnant women. The interval from isolation of a potential pandemic strain to release of an inactivated vaccine made by current methods using eggs is 4–6 months. Such vaccines rely on adequate quantities of virus with the appropriate H and N antigens being produced in cells or eggs inoculated with seed virus. Reassortment of two strains, one a high-yielding laboratory-adapted strain and the other containing the required H and N antigens, may be designed for growth in eggs so that vaccine is prepared as quickly as possible. More recently using the newer process of reverse genetics, vaccine seed strains can be generated without using traditional reassortment methods. Appropriate vaccine strains are developed by cloning of relevant genes and this is a successful innovation to speed up vaccine production, which is gradually being introduced in the vaccine industry.

Vaccine seed strains need to be grown in cell or egg substrates to make inactivated vaccines. Separated whole virus particles are inactivated by either formalin or β-propiolactone, and may be used at this stage as 'whole virus vaccines'. Whole virus vaccine should not be given to those who are allergic to egg protein. The H and N antigens may be separated from the whole virus by treatment with detergent, and such subunit or split-virus vaccines are better tolerated, especially by young children. Other types of vaccines have been tried, such as cold-adapted live-attenuated vaccines given intranasally. These have been generally effective in provoking a good local (IgA) antibody response and are particularly good at developing protective efficacy in children, though less so in adults, but are not widely used at present.

Clinical trials as part of pandemic vaccine development programmes have demonstrated an important role for vaccine adjuvants such as MF59 and ASO3 in antigen sparing, enabling reduced quantities of vaccine to go further and providing excellent immune responses, particularly in young children. Such vaccines were used for the first time as part of the response to the 2009 pandemic. Future vaccine development will concentrate on ensuring better understanding of human immune responses, improving immunogenicity of existing vaccines and developing processes and substrates for a more rapid response.

## Global surveillance

The WHO Global Influenza Programme with its network of reference laboratories plays a very important role in monitoring the evolution of influenza viruses, selecting and developing prototype pandemic vaccine strains, and developing and updating WHO diagnostic reagents. Recent changes in International Health Regulations have increased the obligation in countries worldwide to have the capacity for preventive measures and to be able to detect and respond to infections of international concern. The emergence of the 2009 pandemic demonstrated the unpredictability of influenza virus evolution and the continuing threat to human health posed by this viral infection. Responses to the pandemic were the most sophisticated ever known following the emergence of a new virus, which despite its mildness still presented formidable challenges to health care systems in developed and developing world countries. As a result of the global experiences during the first waves of the pandemic, incremental improvements in surveillance and vaccine production may be expected. An enhanced search for antiviral combination therapies and new antiviral targets to provide better counter measures for future epidemic and pandemic influenza A strains, which will inevitably emerge, are required.

### RECOMMENDED READING

Bright RA, Medina MJ, Xu X, et al: Incidence of amantadine resistance among influenza A (H3N2) viruses isolated worldwide from 1994–2005: a cause for concern, *The Lancet* 366:1175–1181, 2005.

Capua I, Alexander DJ: The challenge of avian influenza to the veterinary community, *Avian pathology* 35:189–205, 2006.

de Jong M, Thanh TT, Khank TH, et al: Oseltamivir resistance during treatment of influenza H5N1, *The New England Journal of Medicine* 353:2667–2672, 2005.

Fiore AE, Bridges CB, Cox NJ: Seasonal influenza vaccines, *Current Topics in Microbiology and Immunology* 333:43–82, 2009.

Garten RJ, Davis CT, Russell CA, et al: Antigenic and genetic characteristics of swine-origin 2009 A(H1N1) influenza viruses circulating in humans, *Science* 325:197–201, 2009.

Hardelid P, Andrews NJ, Hoschler K, et al: Assessment of baseline age-specific antibody prevalence and incidence of infection to novel influenza AH1N1 2009, *Health Technology Assessment* 14:115–192, 2010.

Koopmans M, Wilbrink B, Conyn M, et al: Transmission of H7N7 avian influenza A virus to human beings during a large outbreak in commercial poultry farms in the Netherlands, *The Lancet* 363: 587–593, 2004.

Russell CA, Jones TC, Barr IG, et al: The global circulation of seasonal influenza A (H3N2) viruses, *Science* 320:340–346, 2008.

Stephenson I, Nicholson KG, Wood JD, et al: Confronting the avian influenza threat: vaccine development for a potential pandemic, *The Lancet Infectious Diseases* 4:499–509, 2004.

Wright PF, Neumann G, Kawaoka Y: Orthomyxoviruses. In Fields BN, Knipe DM, Howley PM, editors: *Virology*, ed 5, Philadelphia, 2007, Lippincott-Raven, pp 1691–1740.

Writing Committee of the World Health Organisation (WHO) Consultation of Human Influenza: Avian influenza A (H5N1) infection in humans, *The New England Journal of Medicine* 353:1374–1385, 2005.

Writing Committee of the World Health Organisation (WHO) Consultation on Clinical Aspects of Pandemic (H1N1): Influenza 2010 Clinical Aspects of Pandemic 2009 Influenza A (H1N1) virus infection, *The New England Journal of Medicine* 362:1708–1719, 2009.

Zambon M, Potter CW: Influenza. In Zuckerman AJ, Banatvala JE, Schoub BD, et al, editors: *Principles and Practice of Clinical Virology*, ed 6, Chichester, 2009, Wiley.

### Websites

World Health Organization. Influenza. http://www.who.int/csr/disease/influenza/en/

Health Protection Agency (UK). Influenza. http://www.hpa.org.uk/Topics/InfectiousDiseases/InfectionsAZ/Influenza/

Neuraminidase Inhibitor Susceptibility Network. http://www.nisn.org/l_influenza_resources.html

International Society for Influenza and Respiratory Viruses. http://www.isirv.org/

# 50 Paramyxoviruses

## Respiratory infections; mumps; measles; Hendra/Nipah disease

*J. S. M. Peiris and C. R. Madeley*

## KEY POINTS

- Respiratory syncytial virus, parainfluenza viruses and human metapneumovirus are important and frequent causes of respiratory tract infections, especially in children.
- Seasonality of respiratory viruses is variable depending on the geographical region.
- Measles remains a serious disease, especially in the immunocompromised in whom it may be 'spotless' and often fatal, and in less developed countries where it contributes to significant morbidity and mortality.
- Measles is well-controlled with vaccine, but reappears quickly when the levels of herd immunity drop.
- Vaccines are available for measles and mumps viruses, but not for other paramyxoviruses.
- There are no reliable antiviral drugs for any of the paramyxoviruses other than for RSV.

The paramyxoviruses are a family of enveloped viruses containing negative sense single-stranded RNA as a single piece. They resemble the orthomyxoviruses in both morphology and their affinity for sialic acid receptors on mammalian cells, but they are larger and more fragile (Fig. 50.1A).

Within the family Paramyxoviridae there are four genera, each with several members that cause disease in man or animals (Table 50.1).

## STRUCTURE AND REPLICATION

Originally, these viruses were classified together because they were thought to be similar in structure and function. Neither property is constant throughout the family but there are strong similarities.

## Structure

Parainfluenza, mumps, measles, NDV and simian virus 5 are indistinguishable when seen in the electron microscope (and as described below), whereas the pneumoviruses (respiratory syncytial virus and metapneumovirus) have slightly longer surface spikes and are more difficult to visualize. The helical nucleocapsids have a herring-bone or 'zipper-like' appearance (Fig. 50.1B), which is more easily recognized than the complete particle when sought using electron microscopy.

Functionally there are other differences. Parainfluenza viruses (1–4a, b), Newcastle disease virus (NDV) and mumps virus have a surface haemagglutinin and neuraminidase located on the same spike; measles virus spikes have haemagglutinin but no neuraminidase activity; while pneumoviruses have neither. In addition, measles virus has a haemolysin not possessed by the others. Respiratory syncytial (RS) virus has a large surface glycoprotein, G, which has a cell-attaching function similar to that of a haemagglutinin; other surface spikes carry fusion (F) proteins, and all envelopes have matrix (M) proteins. In all members, the RNA is complexed with protein to form the nucleocapsid.

## Replication

The replication of paramyxoviruses follows a common theme. After attachment, the F protein fuses the viral envelope to the cell membrane, becoming part of it and releasing the nucleocapsid into the cell. The negative-sense genome cannot act as messenger RNA (mRNA), making it necessary for the virus to carry its own RNA-dependent RNA polymerase. This polymerase produces subgenomic-sized mRNA transcripts, which are translated to produce some of the early virus-specific polypeptides. These include a second RNA polymerase, which copies the genome into full-length positive complementary strands that are, in turn, copied back into negative strands both

**Fig. 50.1** (A) Electron micrograph of a typical paramyxovirus. (B) Separate internal helical nucleocapsid. Negative contrast, 3% potassium phosphotungstate, pH 7.0, magnification ×200 000.

**Table 50.1** Classification and important pathogens of the paramyxoviruses

| Genus | Human viruses | Animal viruses |
|---|---|---|
| *Paramyxovirus* | *Paramyxovirus*<br>  Parainfluenza viruses types 1, 3<br>*Rubulavirus*<br>  Mumps virus<br>  Parainfluenza viruses types 2, 4a, 4b | Newcastle disease virus (NDV) (poultry), simian virus 5 |
| *Morbillivirus* | Measles virus | Canine distemper virus, rinderpest virus, equine morbillivirus, morbilliviruses of seals, dolphins and porpoises |
| *Pneumovirus* | Respiratory syncytial (RS) virus<br>Human metapneumovirus (hMPV) | Turkey rhino-tracheitis virus (avian metapneumovirus) |
| *Henipavirus* | Hendra virus[a]<br>Nipah virus[a] | Hendra virus<br>Nipah virus |

[a]These viruses cause disease in animals but can cause serious zoonotic human disease (see text).

for transcription into later mRNA (coding for structural proteins) and for incorporation into new virions. The virus haemagglutinin is incorporated into the cell membrane allowing the virus to bud off from the cell surface. Red blood cells will adsorb to the cell surface expressing the viral haemagglutinin (called haemadsorption) and this is used in the laboratory to identify virus-infected cells (see Ch. 7).

In the 1990s, two new paramyxoviruses, Hendra and Nipah, were discovered in Australia and Malaysia respectively; they are animal viruses occasionally transmitted to man. As they are genetically distinct from the other members of this family, they are classified as a separate genus. Their ecology is still being investigated and their full significance as human pathogens is not yet clear.

## PARAINFLUENZA VIRUSES

### CLASSIFICATION

The paramyxoviruses are subdivided into two subgenera, *Paramyxoviruses* and *Rubulaviruses* (see Table 50.1), but the distinction is not clinically relevant. There are four types of parainfluenza viruses (1–4) that are antigenically distinct. Nevertheless, there are conserved antigenic epitopes on the paramyxovirus envelope proteins, which cause the serological cross-reactions that are found between the parainfluenza viruses, mumps virus and simian virus 5. Type 4 has two subtypes, 4a and 4b, which can be distinguished only by neutralization or haemadsorption inhibition tests.

NDV is a typical paramyxovirus. It infects chickens and other domestic birds. The severity of infection varies considerably from inapparent to fatal, depending on the strain of virus. Because some strains can cause major outbreaks with high mortality, an effective live chicken vaccine based on a virulent strain has been developed. Simian virus 5 (SV5) is often present in normal uninfected monkey kidney cell cultures but does not appear to reduce their sensitivity to other viruses and does not cause human illness. Additional parainfluenza viruses are natural pathogens for cattle and other domestic species; they are not known to infect man.

### CLINICAL FEATURES AND PATHOGENESIS

The parainfluenza viruses are mostly associated with:

- *croup*, a harsh brassy cough in children familiar to many parents as a middle-of-the-night irritant caused by a combination of tracheitis and laryngitis
- minor upper respiratory tract illness
- some cases of *bronchiolitis*.

They are responsible for 6–9% of respiratory infections for which a virus cause can be identified. The incubation period is 3–6 days, during which the virus spreads locally within the respiratory tract.

Many infections occur in infants in the presence of circulating maternal antibody that appears neither to be protective nor to make the illness worse.

NDV may cause a mild conjunctivitis in man, usually as a result of a laboratory accident.

### LABORATORY DIAGNOSIS

Molecular methods (e.g. reverse transcription-polymerase chain reaction, RT-PCR) have been developed for detection of parainfluenza virus RNA; some of these assays have been incorporated into multiplex nucleic acid amplification tests to detect any of a number of respiratory viruses within a single reaction tube.

A rapid diagnosis may be made by immunofluorescent staining of exfoliated respiratory cells separated from well-taken nasopharyngeal secretions. There are monoclonal antibody reagents for immunofluorescent detection of parainfluenza virus types 1, 2 and 3, but reagents for type 4 are less widely available.

Similar antiviral antibodies may also be used in enzyme immuno-assays to identify viral antigen in specimens from the patient. They have the advantage of requiring only antigen to be present in the specimen, whereas other assays require intact infected cells (for immunofluorescence) or infective virus (for culture). However, enzyme immuno-assays give no information on the quality of the specimen, nor the extent of infection.

Virus may be isolated in monkey kidney cell cultures, when available. Visible cytopathic effects in the cell sheets are minimal and it is usually necessary to show infection of the cells by the haemadsorption of 1% guinea-pig or human group O red blood cells. The infecting virus can be typed (or subtyped) by coating the cell cultures with type-specific antisera before adding the red cells. Only the appropriate antibody will inhibit the haemadsorption. The typing can be confirmed by a neutralization test or by immunofluorescence.

Serology is not used routinely in diagnosis. Commonly available tests, such as complement fixation, are difficult to interpret because of cross-reactions between parainfluenza viruses and with mumps virus and, possibly, simian virus 5 as well (see above). Type-specific antibodies may be detected by neutralization or haemadsorption inhibition but these tests are too complex for routine use.

### EPIDEMIOLOGY AND TRANSMISSION

In temperate regions, parainfluenza type 1 infections are more frequent in the winter, whereas type 3 is a summer infection, with small epidemics appearing reliably each year. Type 2 and 4a and 4b infections are more infrequent, in Newcastle upon Tyne at least, although elsewhere in Britain type 2 can be another summer visitor. Type 4 infections are underdiagnosed because of a lack of suitable reagents, and reported figures are too low for epidemiological patterns to be clear. The reasons for these differing individual epidemiological patterns are unknown.

Numerically, parainfluenza infections are far fewer than those due to RS virus, and most diagnosed infections are in pre-school and primary school children. Reinfections occur but fatalities are rare. The viruses are present in respiratory secretions and are expelled during coughing and sneezing. Infection is acquired by inhalation of infected droplets and by person-to-person contact.

No vaccine is yet available for routine use.

## MUMPS VIRUS

### DESCRIPTION

Mumps virus is a typical paramyxovirus, indistinguishable in EM appearance from parainfluenza viruses, measles virus and NDV, with a similar ribonucleocapsid, which may be the only virus-like material seen by electron microscopy. There is only one serotype, although monoclonal antibodies have shown minor variations in the various surface antigenic epitopes.

### CLINICAL FEATURES AND PATHOGENESIS

Mumps is an 'iceberg' disease which, although common as a childhood infection, is often subclinical. Although the salivary glands are often involved, inapparent or minor infections are more common. The advent of MMR (mumps, measles, rubella) vaccine as a universal vaccine of childhood has resulted in a significant age-shift, with most clinical cases in the UK now occurring in university-age adults.

Infection is probably acquired by inhalation of droplets into the respiratory tract. The incubation period is 14–18 days, and is followed by a generalized illness with later localization in the salivary glands, usually the parotids. The generalized phase is the usual 'flu-like' illness with fever and malaise, followed by developing pain in the parotid glands, which then swell rapidly. Much of the swelling is due to blockage of the efferent duct of the parotid gland, and sucking a lemon in front of a sufferer is a refined form of torture although likely to be diagnostic!

Neurological involvement is common in mumps (in more than 50% of infections), although the majority

of cases are not clinically apparent. However, clinical meningitis remains the most common serious complication of mumps, occurring in 1–10% of patients with mumps parotitis. Meningitis (like any other complication of mumps) can occur before, during, after or even in the absence of salivary gland involvement. Before the widespread use of the MMR vaccine, mumps virus and the enteroviruses (see Ch. 48) accounted for most of the cases of aseptic meningitis in the UK. Mumps meningitis is rarely fatal and complete recovery is usual. Meningo-encephalitis has been described, but is much rarer, carries a poorer prognosis and may result in long-term neurological sequelae or death. Deafness and tinnitus have also been described as complications, but are very rare.

In prepubertal children the acute illness usually subsides in 4–5 days, with complete recovery. The best known complication, in postpubertal males, is *orchitis*. This, although painful and causing softening and atrophy of the affected testicle, is usually unilateral and rarely causes sterility. *Oophoritis* also occurs in girls, and should be distinguished from a ruptured ovarian cyst or acute appendicitis. Both orchitis and oophoritis usually develop as the parotitis resolves, and a history of previous parotid pain and swelling usually provides the clue.

The role of mumps in pancreatitis is difficult to establish. There may be abdominal pain in acute mumps but the levels of serum amylase do not correlate with the clinical picture. High levels may provide supportive evidence but are not diagnostic. Although uncomfortable, it is not fatal.

### LABORATORY DIAGNOSIS

#### Detection and isolation

Typical mumps does not always require laboratory confirmation, but mild cases with little parotid swelling may not be noticed until complications develop. Demonstration of mumps virus RNA by genome amplification (e.g. RT-PCR) is the most sensitive test and should be considered for virus detection, especially in the cerebrospinal fluid (CSF) of patients with possible mumps meningitis. Isolation of the virus in cell culture (usually in monkey kidney or HEp2 cells) from throat swabs, saliva, urine or the CSF is possible, although not as sensitive as RT-PCR testing, and the virus may take up to a week to grow to detectable levels. Virus presence can be reliably confirmed by indirect immunofluorescent staining of cultured cells. Alternatively, neutralization or haemadsorption, which can be inhibited by specific antiserum, may be used to confirm the presence and identity of the virus.

The detection of nucleocapsid helix in CSF by electron microscopy (EM) is diagnostic of mumps; however, the small quantities of CSF usually taken for all assays make routine EM diagnosis of mumps meningitis impractical.

## Serology

Serological confirmation of mumps in a child is most easily accomplished by testing salivary fluid (or serum) for the presence of mumps-specific IgM. In older adults, especially those with a history of MMR vaccination, there may not be an IgM response, but high titres of IgG are strongly suggestive if the clinical picture fits. There are a number of ELISA-based and complement fixation tests available; neutralization and haemagglutination inhibition tests are more complex and do not offer any advantages in routine diagnosis.

## EPIDEMIOLOGY

Mumps is a worldwide disease, with man the only known reservoir. In the absence of vaccination, most infections are in children of school age but, where MMR has been introduced, most infections occur in adults around 20–25 years of age. Infections in adults may be more severe and more likely to lead to complications. Although epidemics occur, mumps is less infectious than measles or chickenpox. Initial infection appears to confer lifelong immunity, and second infections do not occur.

## CONTROL

Some, but not very reliable, protection can be given by passive immunization, which may prevent severe orchitis even when given at the stage of parotitis.

Mumps vaccine, based on the *Jeryl Lynn* or *Urabe* strains, has been available as a monovalent vaccine for some time, particularly in the USA, but is now widely incorporated into the triple MMR vaccine. All three components are live-attenuated viruses, and the mumps component induces good antibody levels, lasting long enough to suggest that the recipients will not become susceptible as adults. A few cases of mild post-vaccine meningitis have been described but have not caused serious concern.

## MEASLES VIRUS

### DESCRIPTION

Measles virus, a *morbillivirus*, is morphologically indistinguishable in the EM from other members of the group. The ribonucleoprotein helix is readily released from the virion and may, as with the others, be the only identifiable virus structure seen by electron microscopy. The virion structure differs from other paramyxoviruses:

- spikes carry a haemagglutinin but not a neuraminidase function
- the F protein is also a haemolysin.

There is only one serotype of measles virus and no subtypes have yet been recognized, although monoclonal antibodies show that there may be minor differences between wild and cultivated strains.

Human morbilliviruses are related to a number of animal strains. *Canine distemper* and *rinderpest* in cattle are well-known relatives, although a global campaign for the eradication of rinderpest has recently come to a successful conclusion. In the past few years other similar viruses have been isolated from seals (of several species), dolphins and porpoises, and an equine morbillivirus has reappeared that has apparently been transmitted to man in contact, fatally in one case. All are distinct and can cause serious illness in their natural species, although survivors develop solid immunity. There is partial cross-protection experimentally in ferrets between measles and canine distemper viruses.

### CLINICAL FEATURES AND PATHOGENESIS

Measles is an acute febrile illness, usually in childhood, after an incubation period of 10–12 days. The onset is 'flu-like', with high fever, cough and conjunctivitis. *Koplik's spots* (red spots with a bluish-white centre on the buccal mucosa) may be present at this stage. After 1–2 days the acute symptoms decline, with the appearance of a widespread maculopapular rash. Viral antigen, but not infectious virus, may be found in the spots. The rash can be inhibited by local injections of immune serum, but does not appear at all in those who are severely immunocompromised ('spotless measles' – usually rapidly fatal), and this has been thought to point to an immunopathological (T cell-mediated) component of the rash.

Over the next 10–14 days recovery is usually complete as the rash fades, with considerable desquamation. Complications include:

- giant cell pneumonia, more common in adults
- otitis media
- post-measles encephalitis.

The pneumonia is due to direct invasion by virus, but the role of virus in the other two complications is uncertain. Measles encephalitis can cause severe and permanent mental impairment in those it does not kill. It is rare but disastrous.

The mortality rate associated with uncomplicated measles in immunocompetent, well-nourished children is low but rises rapidly with malnourishment (particularly in Africa), in the immunocompromised and, to a much lesser extent, with age. The virus has also been devastating in isolated populations (such as the Inuit in Greenland some years ago) into which it was introduced as a 'new' disease.

One further complication of measles is *subacute sclerosing panencephalitis* (SSPE), which occurs in children or early adolescents who have had measles early in life, usually when under 2 years of age. It is a progressive and inevitably fatal degenerative disease. Within infected cells is a defective form of measles virus, which, because it is unable to induce the production of a functional M protein, is not released from the cells as complete virus. Patients deteriorate over several years, losing intellectual capacity before motor activities. Oligoclonal antibodies to measles virus proteins appear in the CSF, but the virus cannot be cultivated unless it is 'rescued' by co-cultivating neuronal cells with a susceptible cell type.

The virus has been linked with multiple sclerosis, Paget's disease of bone and Crohn's disease. In each disease, tubular structures resembling measles nucleocapsids have been seen by thin-section electron microscopy, and immunofluorescence has been used to demonstrate measles 'antigens' in biopsy material. Serum from about 50% of adults aged over 50 years, however, will fix complement with measles antigen, although the individuals give no history suggestive of recent measles, and it is possible that auto-antibodies to a measles-like protein can be induced with age. If so, its significance is unknown but must be a factor in assessing measles virus involvement in older patients with chronic diseases. The evidence linking measles virus to the aetiology of these diseases is not compelling.

## LABORATORY DIAGNOSIS

The widespread use of vaccine has made the disease rarer in the community, and consequently fewer clinicians are familiar with it. There are also a number of other diseases which produce morbilliform rashes in children. Clinical diagnosis of measles therefore has a low sensitivity and specificity. Laboratory confirmation is best done by demonstration of measles-specific IgM in a venous blood or salivary sample (avoiding the need for venesection). It may also be possible to amplify the viral genome from a throat swab or other respiratory tract specimen using RT-PCR. In hospital, and particularly in immunocompromised patients in whom the disease is often rashless (and where the diagnosis may not be suspected at first), the diagnosis may be made rapidly by immunofluorescence on exfoliated respiratory cells in well-taken nasopharyngeal secretions. The presence of a large number of giant cells, particularly in patients on cytotoxic drugs, is a bad prognostic sign.

The virus may be isolated, though not readily, from blood or nasopharyngeal aspirates during the prodrome and until day 2 of rash, in human fibroblasts, primary monkey kidney cells and Vero cells. The virus can then be identified by neutralization or immunofluorescence.

## EPIDEMIOLOGY

Transmission is from person to person, probably by respiratory droplets, but the associated conjunctivitis may also be a source. Measles epidemics occur every 2 years in developed countries in the absence of widespread use of the vaccine. This periodicity is absent in isolated populations too small to maintain transmission (<400 000), in poverty and overcrowding, and following the widespread use of vaccine. The disease is ubiquitous throughout the world and, although a candidate for eradication, this may be difficult to achieve due to the likely high cost and the logistic challenges such a programme poses.

In tropical areas, particularly Africa, children become infected under the age of 1 year, and the mortality rate rises in consequence, up to 42% in children under 4 years of age. Malnutrition is one of the main underlying causes of this excess mortality. The attack rate is also very high in isolated populations that have not experienced the disease for some years. In the Faroe Islands in the 1840s, three-quarters of the population were infected, although the mortality rate was low. Most of those who were not infected were aged over 65 years, the interval since the last time the disease had been present in the islands, and confirms that infection gives prolonged immunity.

## CONTROL

The first measles vaccine was a formalin-inactivated one. Although inducing circulating antibody, it was found that vaccinees exposed to natural measles were likely to develop atypical disease. The rash was more peripheral, involving the palms and soles, and pneumonia was common. It was later recognized that the vaccine had failed to induce adequate levels of antibody to the haemolytic F protein, and the immune response it induced did not inhibit cell-to-cell spread of the virus. Consequently it was withdrawn and replaced with a live-attenuated vaccine, containing the *Edmonston B* or *Schwarz* strains, which have given a seroconversion rate of over 90%. So far (over about 30 years) the immunity induced by the vaccine has persisted and may be lifelong.

Measles vaccine is now combined with those against mumps and rubella to form the MMR vaccine. This combination of three attenuated viruses has been shown to induce good immunity to all three. Introduced initially in the USA, it is now the preferred vaccine in the UK for administration to children aged between 12 and 18 months, with a preschool booster.

The attenuated measles vaccine, alone or in combination with mumps and rubella, has been shown to be effective and safe. Unfortunately, vaccine uptake fell in the UK due to fears over its safety, particularly as a possible cause of autism. These fears have now been shown to be unsubstantiated but measles reappeared when levels of herd immunity dropped.

Elimination of measles has been attempted in the USA; the number of cases was reduced from over 500 000 per year to about 2000 (a reduction of over 99%), but outbreaks in immigrants and high-school students have emphasized the problems of preventing cases from being imported into the country and of keeping up a high level of immunization.

Immunization in the regions of Africa with high levels of endemic measles still presents problems, however. Because many infants are infected before their first birthday, the vaccine has to be given to babies aged around 9 months to have any effect. Passively-transferred maternal antibody often interferes with the immune response to a live vaccine, and such early immunization does not always produce adequate and long-lasting immunity. A second dose at 12–13 months is then probably necessary, but

adds to the cost and the logistic difficulties. Solutions to both will have to be found before progress is made towards substantial measles reduction in the developing world.

## RESPIRATORY SYNCYTIAL VIRUS

## DESCRIPTION

Superficially, RS virus resembles other paramyxoviruses, with a similar pleomorphic envelope studded with surface spikes that may be defined more clearly on electron microscopic images than those on the parainfluenza viruses, mumps and measles. The spikes may also be slightly longer, but neither the complete virus particles nor the nucleoprotein helix are easy to visualize in the electron microscope. However, individual particles are generally larger than other paramyxoviruses (Fig. 50.2).

RS virus is placed in a separate genus – *pneumovirus* – because of these minor physical differences and the lack of a haemagglutinin, haemolysin or neuraminidase. It has a G lipoprotein, a receptor for cell attachment (but not to red blood cells), which differs in chemical composition from the haemagglutinin/

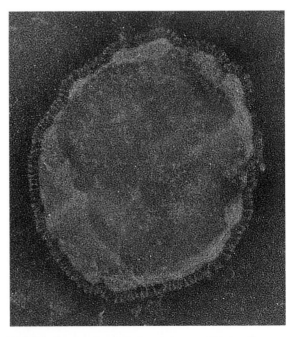

**Fig. 50.2** Electron micrograph of respiratory syncytial virus. Human metapneumovirus is indistinguishable in appearance. Negative contrast, 3% potassium phosphotungstate, pH 7.0, magnification ×200 000.

neuraminidase (HN) protein of other paramyxoviruses. The F protein induces the syncytia in cell cultures from which the virus gets its name, and is probably responsible for both virus penetration and spread in the host. The virus is relatively fragile and may not survive even snap-freezing to –70°C. Specimens for isolation should therefore never be frozen.

For most purposes there is only one serotype, although the advent of monoclonal antibodies has confirmed that there are two subtypes, A and B. In Newcastle upon Tyne, strains of subgroup A have been prevalent every year since 1974, but subgroup B strains have been more erratic and have not been isolated every winter. The reason for this is unknown. Analysis of the genome has revealed further minor differences that appear to be unimportant in diagnosis (i.e. do not represent major antigenic variations) but which have allowed various strain lineages to be recognized.

RS virus is also a significant pathogen in cattle and infects chimpanzees readily – early isolates were termed *chimpanzee coryza agent.* Both goats and sheep may be infected naturally, and there is evidence that several other domestic and rodent species are susceptible, either naturally or after some adaptation.

## CLINICAL FEATURES AND PATHOGENESIS

The most serious illness caused by RS virus is *bronchiolitis* in young babies, in whom the bronchiolar inflammation acts as a one-way valve leading to hyperinflation of the lungs (very characteristic on radiography), but the virus is also associated with minor upper tract infections. It usually presents with fever, wheezing, crepitations and increased transparency on chest X-ray. The peak incidence is in babies under 1 year of age. This infection is potentially life-threatening, particularly in those with bronchopulmonary dysplasia or congenital heart defects, or in those who are immunosuppressed or immunodeficient. In normal babies it is rarely fatal where medical staff have the experience and facilities for appropriate management. RS virus has been recovered from some victims of the *sudden infant death syndrome* (SIDS). Although it may have contributed to the death, other factor(s) are more significant.

While the main clinical feature is bronchiolitis, the upper respiratory tract is also infected, and this makes it possible to confirm the diagnosis with nasopharyngeal aspirates or nasopharyngeal swabs. If RS virus is present in the nasopharynx and there is clinical evidence of lower respiratory tract involvement, RS virus is likely to be responsible.

It is not uncommon for a diagnosis of 'failure to thrive' to accompany a respiratory specimen from which RSV can be recovered. Whether a failure to thrive makes the child more susceptible to the virus or whether the resultant loss of the ability to suck from the infection causes a failure to thrive is debatable but it is worth investigating such apparently unpromising specimens.

Recovery is apparently complete, although it has been suggested that the infection predisposes to chronic respiratory tract disease (e.g. asthma, bronchiectasis, etc.). This has yet to be confirmed.

The sequelae to the use of an inactivated vaccine (see below) have led to the suggestion that some of the severity of bronchiolitis is due to hypersensitivity induced by an earlier infection. Studies in various centres have neither confirmed this theory nor fully excluded it.

In older children and adults, the virus causes only minor infections, possibly because their air passages are larger. Re-infections are common due to poor RNA copying leading to antigenic drift of the immunogenic surface proteins, and in adults the virus may cause no more than a 'cold'. However, this drift emphasizes the difficulty of producing a vaccine.

There have been reports of severe illness, with some fatalities, in old people's homes as well as in the elderly living in the community. The under-recognition of RS virus in these groups may be due to the difficulty in confirming a virological diagnosis in adults and the elderly (see below).

## LABORATORY DIAGNOSIS

### Detection and isolation

During the acute phase of illness virus may be readily demonstrated in nasopharyngeal secretions (which are usually copious) by RT-PCR, immunofluorescence, enzyme immunoassays or culture.

Rapid diagnosis in less than 1 h with commercially available, directly conjugated, monoclonal antibodies can be made reliably by immunofluorescence, provided an adequate number of desquamated respiratory cells are collected in the secretions. Generally, similar results can be obtained with enzyme immunoassays. Such assays may be less sensitive compared with culture, but the virus grows slowly and positive results will come too late to influence management. Although antigen detection and culture methods are good for diagnosing RS virus infections in infants and young children, they are less reliable in adults and the elderly because the levels of virus or antigen are lower in adult secretions compared with those in infants, and taking adequate specimens from adults may be difficult as the process is uncomfortable.

As with other respiratory viruses, molecular methods such as RT–PCR, either for a single virus or multiplexed to detect a panel of respiratory viruses (see under Parainfluenza viruses) can be used and may be more sensitive, especially with adult patients.

## Serology

Serological assessment using complement fixation is generally not helpful. Many of the patients are too young to respond reliably and even adults do not always produce a detectable rise in serum antibody levels. However, immunoassays for the G and F proteins may be more reliable in adults where the other options are limited.

## TREATMENT

Appropriate management includes use of oxygen, if indicated, and tube feeding to maintain energy intake if the baby has difficulty in suckling. Most babies can be managed symptomatically by these measures. The only specific antiviral drug available for chemotherapy is ribavirin when given as a small-particle inhalation aerosol. However its clinical efficacy remains controversial, possibly because the most affected parts of the lungs are also the least well aerated and therefore least accessible to the aerosolized drug. At present, ribavirin is only recommended for use in at-risk infants (i.e. those with lung, cardiac or immune system abnormalities) and immunocompromised patients (especially haematopoetic stem cell transplant recipients) with RSV pneumonia.

Hyperimmune RS virus immunoglobulin and humanized monoclonal antibodies have become available for the prevention and/or treatment of RS infections. These preparations are very expensive and their use may be difficult to justify except in groups at very high risk, such as very premature babies or those with pre-existing bronchopulmonary dysplasia.

## EPIDEMIOLOGY

In temperate climates in both the northern and southern hemispheres, RS virus causes a substantial winter epidemic every year. In the Newcastle upon Tyne/Tyne and Wear conurbation (total population about 1 million), the annual number of virologically confirmed diagnoses regularly exceeds 500. Similar figures are obtained elsewhere where adequate facilities for diagnosis exist.

Why RS virus induces this epidemic every autumn/winter is unknown. In other regions of the world the pattern can be markedly different. In tropical regions there is an equally clear epidemic, but it occurs in the hot and humid months of the summer. Therefore, RS virus epidemics do not always correspond to the same variations in climatic factors (temperature, humidity, etc.), and sporadic cases occur anyway throughout the year. Moreover, this apparent climatic paradox is found with other respiratory viruses as well. The virus is distributed all over the world, but its activities in tropical, overcrowded and poor areas are under-recorded so far.

The significance, if any, of subtypes in explaining these RS virus phenomena is still under investigation.

## CONTROL

A formalin-inactivated, crude, whole-virus vaccine was tried in the 1960s. It induced good levels of circulating antibody but failed to protect the recipients, who actually became more ill than placebo controls when subsequently exposed to RS virus. As with measles, this may have been due to the vaccine failing to induce the right protective antibodies. Subsequently, several live vaccines based on cold adaptation, temperature-sensitive mutants or administration by a different route (intramuscularly) were tried but none has yet proved satisfactory.

A major obstacle in developing a good vaccine is that the peak of disease occurs within the first year of life, and thus a safe vaccine immunogenic to such young and immunologically immature recipients is difficult to prepare. The increasing recognition that RS virus causes morbidity in the elderly may stimulate the preparation of an adult vaccine – possibly an easier challenge to meet.

## HUMAN METAPNEUMOVIRUS

## DESCRIPTION

Human metapneumovirus (hMPV) was discovered in the Netherlands in 2001 as an additional cause of respiratory infections, closely mimicking RSV in both the disease caused and the age-group affected. It is indistinguishable from RSV in the electron microscope (see Fig. 50.2).

It has a 13.4 kilobase genome, similar to RS virus, although slightly smaller. The order of the genes is different, resembling more closely that of an avian virus, turkey rhinotracheitis virus. The genes, however, code for similar structural and non-structural proteins. Genetic analysis indicates that at least two separate lineages circulate world-wide; antigenic studies confirm that there may be more than one subtype (A & B), although further work is needed to clarify this.

Like RS virus, hMPV has no haemagglutinin, haemolysin and neuraminidase functions on the surface spikes. It can be cultured in tertiary monkey kidney cells, but grows slowly, and these cells are becoming less available.

## CLINICAL FEATURES AND PATHOGENESIS

Clinically hMPV causes a very similar spectrum of disease to RS virus. It affects mostly young children in whom it causes a bronchiolitis with fever of up to 39°C, wheezing, crepitations, and changes on chest radiography, but all ages may be affected. There is some evidence that the virus may precipitate attacks of asthma. The proportion of respiratory patients infected with hMPV has been reported to be about 12%, and there are yearly variations in the activity of this virus.

## LABORATORY DIAGNOSIS

Routine diagnosis is becoming more widely available. Molecular detection using RT-PCR is the method most often used. Culture is only possible in primary or secondary primate cell cultures which are not widely available. Although specific monoclonal antibodies are available, reliable antigen detection tests and serology are not routinely available.

## TREATMENT AND CONTROL

As yet, there is no specific drug treatment, although animal models are being developed with the aim of exploring both treatment and vaccine prevention. It is likely that very similar obstacles to those found with RS virus will present the same difficulties.

## EPIDEMIOLOGY

The epidemiology of hMPV is still being researched. Serological studies in the Netherlands have shown that the virus has been circulating there for more than 50 years, indicating that this is not a 'new' human virus. The seasonality of infections, where data are available, has shown similar patterns to those of other respiratory viruses, and RS virus in particular.

## NIPAH AND HENDRA VIRUSES

During 1998–1999, an outbreak of respiratory disease in pigs was associated with encephalitis in humans in Malaysia. There were more than 200 human cases, with 105 deaths. The causative agent was found to be a paramyxovirus given the name Nipah. Other outbreaks of Nipah virus have been reported in India and Bangladesh without obvious involvement of pigs as an intermediate host. In some of these outbreaks there is also some evidence of limited human-to-human transmission and nosocomial infection. It is distinct genetically from all the other paramyxoviruses and most closely related to Hendra virus, another paramyxovirus discovered in 1994 causing epidemic fatal respiratory disease in horses that can be transmitted to man, resulting in fatal encephalitis. Both viruses continue to be active, with human cases occurring from time to time in Asia and Australia.

These new viruses are now officially classified as paramyxoviruses, but in a separate genus within the Paramyxoviridae. Fruit bats appear to be the natural reservoir of both viruses, with transmission to other mammals (including man) an exceptional event. Nevertheless, these discoveries underline the fact that new pathogens capable of causing human disease continue to emerge.

RECOMMENDED READING

Field HF, Mackenzie JS, Daszak P: Henipaviruses: emerging paramyxoviruses associated with fruit bats, *Current Topics in Microbiology and Immunology* 315:133–159, 2007.
Mandell GL, Bennett JE, Dolin R: *Principles & Practice of Infectious Diseases*, ed 7, Philadelphia, 2009, Churchill Livingstone.
Peiris JSM, Tang W-H, Chan K-H, et al: Children with respiratory disease associated with metapneumovirus in Hong Kong, *Emerging Infectious Diseases* 9:628–633, 2003.

Wild TF: Henipaviruses: a new family of emerging paramyxoviruses, *Pathologie Biologie (Paris)* 57:188–196, 2009.
Zuckerman AJ, Banatvala JE, Griffiths PD, et al, editors: *Principles & Practice of Clinical Virology*, ed 6, Chs 17, 18, 22 & 24 Chichester, 2009, Wiley-Blackwell: 409–40, 441–62, 533–60.

# 51 Arboviruses: alphaviruses, flaviviruses and bunyaviruses

Encephalitis; yellow fever; dengue; haemorrhagic fever; miscellaneous tropical fevers; undifferentiated fever

*A. D. T. Barrett and S. C. Weaver*

## KEY POINTS

- Arboviruses are transmitted biologically by arthropod vectors (mosquitoes, ticks and biting flies).
- There are three major types of clinical disease caused by these viruses: central nervous system, visceral organs/haemorrhagic fever, and febrile infections, with many progressing from the latter to the former syndromes. Many arboviruses are highly pathogenic and require a high level of biocontainment.
- There are more than 500 recognized arbovirus species classified in six virus families: Togaviridae, Flaviviridae, Bunyaviridae, Rhabdoviridae, Reoviridae and Orthomyxoviridae.
- In the UK arboviruses are overwhelmingly of concern to travellers. Yellow fever and dengue viruses are two widely distributed flaviviruses of global concern, but numerous other agents must be considered in specific locations.
- The *Hantavirus* genus of the Bunyaviridae contains many pathogens associated with haemorrhagic fever with renal syndrome or hantavirus pulmonary syndrome. Hantaviruses are transmitted by rodents, not arthropods.
- Commercial vaccines are available only for yellow fever, Japanese encephalitis and tick-borne encephalitis, but a number of experimental vaccines show promise.
- The only effective antiviral treatment is ribavirin, which has efficacy only against selected bunyaviruses and alphaviruses.

The name 'arbo' (arthropod-borne) virus denotes viruses transmitted biologically by arthropod (mainly insect and tick) vectors. Arboviruses are found in many different taxa, and over 500 individual arbovirus species that are now officially classified in six virus families. Many arboviruses are highly pathogenic and are classified at biosafety level 3 or 4. As there are many similarities in their transmission cycles and in the diseases that they cause, they are considered together in this chapter.

Arboviruses were defined by a World Health Organization Scientific Group as 'viruses that are maintained in nature principally, or to an important extent, through biological transmission between susceptible vertebrate hosts by haemotophagous arthropods or through transovarian and possible venereal transmission in arthropods; the viruses multiply and produce viraemia in the vertebrates, multiply in the tissues of arthropods, and are passed on to new vertebrates by the bites of arthropods after a period of extrinsic incubation.'

Certain viruses within the six families containing arboviruses are not transmitted by arthropods, but are maintained in nature within rodent reservoirs that may transmit infection directly to man. These include the *Hantavirus* genus of the family Bunyaviridae.

## DESCRIPTION

### Classification

Most arboviruses are members of the families Togaviridae, Flaviviridae and Bunyaviridae; some are assigned to the families Reoviridae (genera *Coltivirus* (e.g. Colorado tick fever virus) and *Orbivirus* (e.g. Bluetongue viruses)), Orthomyxoviridae (e.g. Thogoto virus) and Rhabdoviridae (members of the genera *Vesiculovirus* (e.g. vesicular stomatitis virus) and *Lyssavirus*) (Table 51.1). Within the Togaviridae, only one (*Alphavirus*) of the two genera contains arthropod-borne viruses; the other genus, *Rubivirus*, contains rubella virus, which is not arthropod-borne, as its sole member (see Ch. 59). The Flaviviridae contain three genera (*Flavivirus, Pestivirus* and *Hepacivirus*), but only the *Flavivirus* genus contains arthropod-borne viruses. Pestiviruses infect only vertebrate animals (e.g. bovine viral diarrhoea virus), and hepatitis C

**Table 51.1** Characteristic properties of arboviruses

| Property | Arbovirus family (principal genus) | | | | | |
| --- | --- | --- | --- | --- | --- | --- |
| | Togaviridae (*Alphavirus*) | Flaviviridae (*Flavivirus*) | Bunyaviridae (*Orthobunyavirus*)[a] | Rhabdoviridae (*Rhabdovirus*)[b] | Reoviridae (*Reovirus*)[c] | Orthomyxoviridae |
| Symmetry[d] | Cubic | Cubic | Helical | Bullet-shaped | Cubic | Cubic |
| Total diameter (nm) | 70 | 40–60 | 80–120 | 180 × 85 | 60–80 | 15–120 |
| Nucleic acid | (+)ssRNA | (+)ssRNA | (−)ssRNA and antisense | (−)ssRNA | dsRNA | (−)ssRNA |
|   Molecular weight (×10$^6$) (Da) | 4.2–4.4 | 4.2–4.4 | 0.3–3.1 | 3.5–4.6 | 0.2–3.0 | |
|   No. of molecules | 1 | 1 | 3 | 1 | 10–12 | 6–7 |
| No. of viruses | 29 | 68 | 318 | 63 | 77 | 2 |
| Inactivation by diethyl ether or sodium deoxycholate | + | + | + | + | − | + |

ssRNA, single-stranded RNA; dsRNA, double-stranded RNA.
[a]Other important genera: *Nairovirus, Phlebovirus* (arthropod-borne), *Hantavirus* (not arthropod-borne).
[b]See Chapter 58.
[c]See Chapter 54.
[d]All have enveloped virions (except Reoviridae).

virus is described in Chapter 52. The Bunyaviridae consist of five genera (*Orthobunyavirus, Hantavirus, Nairovirus, Phlebovirus* and *Tospovirus*), containing a total of over 300 species, and is the largest virus family. The *Tospovirus* genus contains plant viruses that are transmitted by vectors (thrips), whereas the *Hantavirus* genus contains viruses that are transmitted by rodents rather than arthropods.

The classification of arboviruses into individual species is now made on the basis of polythetic criteria including genetic as well as antigenic and other phenotypic characteristics. Clusters of viruses that show antigenic overlap are termed serogroups or antigenic complexes. Table 51.2 lists some of the important members.

## Properties

Arboviruses share common biological attributes (see Table 51.1):

1. Most induce fatal encephalitis 1–10 days after intracerebral inoculation of mice aged less than 48 h; some also induce fatal encephalitis after intracerebral inoculation of weaned mice aged 3–4 weeks.
2. Haemagglutination. Most arboviruses can agglutinate erythrocytes, an ability that is inhibited by antiserum against viruses within the same serogroup. Seroreactivity against viruses from dissimilar serogroups is generally weak.
3. Many arboviruses multiply in continuous polyploid tissue cultures of mammalian cells

incubated at 37°C, such as grivet monkey kidney (Vero) and baby hamster kidney (BHK).
4. Many arboviruses, such as dengue and Ross River viruses, multiply in continuous cultures of mosquito cells when incubated at 34°C or lower temperatures; *Aedes albopictus* C6/36 mosquito cells are often used. In general, mosquito-borne viruses do not replicate in tick cell cultures and vice versa.
5. Mosquito-borne arboviruses multiply after oral feeding or intrathoracic injection of several *Aedes* and *Culex* mosquito species after incubation at 4–28°C (depending on the mosquito species). Intrathoracic susceptibility of mosquitoes to dengue and California serogroup viruses is 10 to 100 times higher than that of mammalian tissue cultures or suckling mice. Some arboviruses, including members of the *Orthobunyavirus* and *Phlebovirus* genera of the Bunyaviridae, *Flavivirus* genus of the Flaviviridae, *Alphavirus* genus of the family Togaviridae and some members of the *Vesiculovirus* genus of the family Rhabdoviridae, are also transmitted transovarially by vectors. Ticks do not normally transmit mosquito-borne arboviruses and vice versa. Sandfly-borne viruses are transmitted only by sandflies (Phlebotomus spp. and Lutzomyia spp.).
6. Tick-borne arboviruses multiply after oral feeding to larval or nymphal ixodid ticks (hard ticks of the genera *Dermacentor* and *Ixodes*). The virus is transferred trans-stadially to the next developmental stage (nymph or adult, respectively), which then transmits virus by biting susceptible vertebrates.

**Table 51.2** Some important arboviruses

| Family and genus | No. of members | Some important members | Comments |
|---|---|---|---|
| **Togaviridae** | | | |
| *Alphavirus* | 29 | Western equine encephalitis virus | Mosquito-borne |
| | | Eastern equine encephalitis virus | |
| | | Venezuelan equine encephalitis virus | |
| | | Chikungunya virus | |
| | | Ross River virus | |
| **Flaviviridae** | | | |
| *Flavivirus* | 68 | St Louis encephalitis virus | Mosquito-borne |
| | | Japanese encephalitis virus | |
| | | Murray Valley encephalitis virus | |
| | | Yellow fever virus | |
| | | Dengue virus | |
| | | West Nile virus | |
| | | Louping ill virus | Tick-borne |
| | | Powassan virus | |
| | | Tick-borne encephalitis virus | |
| | | Kyasanur Forest virus | |
| | | Omsk haemorrhagic fever virus | |
| **Bunyaviridae** | 318 | | |
| *Orthobunyavirus* | 172 | La Crosse virus | California (CAL) serogroup |
| | | Snowshoe hare virus | |
| | | Oropouche virus | |
| *Phlebovirus* | 51 | Rift Valley fever virus | |
| | | Punta Toro virus | |
| | | Sandfly fever virus | |
| | | Toscana virus | |
| *Nairovirus* | 34 | Crimean–Congo haemorrhagic fever virus | |
| *Hantavirus* | 15 | Sin Nombre virus (not arthropod-borne) | |

## REPLICATION

The replication of the various arboviruses differs significantly and is one of the major criteria used in their classification (see Ch. 7 for a general account).

## Alphaviruses

Alphaviruses are 70 nm in diameter and enter cells by receptor-mediated endocytosis but co-receptors or other factors probably also contribute to entry and cell specificity. The virion fuses with an endosomal membrane via a fusion peptide in the E1 envelope glycoprotein. The nucleocapsid is released and binds to ribosomes, and the non-structural proteins are translated directly from the genomic RNA. RNA replication occurs in complexes comprised of the non-structural proteins and cellular proteins in association with cytoplasmic membranes. Genomic RNA is messenger sense (positive strand) and serves as a template for full-length negative sense RNA synthesis; these negative-sense RNAs are templates for the production of positive-sense genomic RNA, as well as a subgenomic mRNA that encodes the structural proteins. Both of these RNAs are capped at the 5′ end and polyadenylated at the 3′ end. Regulation of positive- versus negative-strand synthesis occurs via changes in the non-structural protease activity mediated by different cleavage patterns of the non-structural polyprotein. The subgenomic message is translated to yield a polyprotein comprised of the capsid and envelope glycoproteins. The capsid is cleaved co-translationally in the cytoplasm via its own protease activity, and the remaining polyprotein enters the endoplasmic reticulum, where it is processed through the secretory pathway to yield glycosylated E2 and E1 protein heterodimers in the plasma membrane. Genomic RNA combines in the cytoplasm with 240 copies of the capsid protein to form a nucleocapsid, and nucleocapsids interact with the cytoplasmic tail of the E2 envelope protein to mediate budding, whereby 240 E2/E1 protein heterodimers and a portion of the plasma membrane are incorporated into the mature virion.

## Flaviviruses

Flavivirus virions are 50 nm in diameter and have three structural proteins; the genome is encapsidated by a small core protein and there are two proteins, the membrane (M) and envelope (E), on the outside of the virus particle. The E protein is the major protein of the virus. It is normally glycosylated, has haemagglutination activity, and is the target of neutralizing antibodies. The NS3 protein (see below) contains the majority of T cell epitopes. The virus genome is one single-stranded, positive-sense RNA molecule. Flavivirus RNA is not polyadenylated. The 5' one-third of the genome encodes the three structural proteins, and the remaining two-thirds encodes seven non-structural (NS) proteins involved in virus replication, including an RNA-dependent RNA polymerase. Flaviviruses replicate in the cytoplasm of cells. The input virion RNA is translated as a single open reading frame to generate a polyprotein precursor that is rapidly co- and post-translationally processed by viral and cellular proteases to yield the structural and NS proteins. Flavivirus particles assemble by budding through Golgi vesicles and contain prM, a precursor to M protein, as a chaperone for the E protein. Mature virions are produced at the cell surface where the 'pr' portion of prM is cleaved by the cell enzyme furin to yield the mature M protein found in virions.

## Bunyaviruses

The Bunyaviridae are icosahedral enveloped viruses, with diameters of 100–120 nm. They have tripartite RNA genomes of negative sense, termed the large (L), medium (M) and small (S) segments. The L RNA encodes the RNA-dependent RNA polymerase carried in the virion. The L protein of Crimean–Congo haemorrhagic fever virus encodes an ovarian tumour-like cysteine protease motif, suggesting that the L polyprotein is cleaved autoproteolytically. The M RNA encodes two glycoproteins, Gc and Gn, found on the surface of virions. The S RNA encodes a nucleocapsid (N) protein.

The *Orthobunyavirus* genus also contains a non-structural protein, NSs, which is an interferon antagonist that also inhibits host cell protein synthesis. The tripartite genome enables bunyaviruses to undergo genetic reassortment that occurs naturally between closely related bunyaviruses and contributes to genetic variation and evolution. The *NSm* gene of the *Tospovirus* genus and the *NSs* gene of the *Phlebovirus* and *Tospovirus* genera are encoded as genes in the positive-sense orientation. Thus, the S- and M-RNA segments of tospoviruses and the S-RNA of phleboviruses are termed ambisense RNAs.

Bunyaviruses replicate in the cytoplasm of cells and assemble by budding through Golgi vesicles.

## PATHOGENESIS

Natural vertebrate infection by arboviruses is initiated when mosquitoes or other arthropods deposit saliva in extravascular tissues and blood vessels while blood-feeding. For some alphaviruses, murine model systems using needle inoculations indicate that the initial site of replication is the Langerhans cell. Alphavirus replication appears to stimulate both the migratory response of these cells to, and the accumulation of leucocytes in, the draining lymph nodes, where local replication produces viraemia. Arboviruses induce high titres of viraemia in many susceptible vertebrates 1–4 days after parenteral inoculation or following bites by infected arthropods, resulting in the potential for infection of additional vectors. Invasion of the central nervous system (CNS) via the olfactory nervous tract may ensue in some infections, whereas other viruses cross the blood–brain barrier. In alphavirus infections accompanied by rash and arthritis, virus replication and necrosis occur in the epidermis and possibly the muscles, tendons and connective tissue. Infection of macrophages may mediate musculoskeletal pathology via the release of inflammatory mediators. Wild bird and mammal reservoir hosts regularly exhibit viraemia without symptoms.

Antibodies are first detected when the fever subsides, usually within 5–10 days after infection, and may persist for many years. Antibodies are of the immunoglobulin (Ig) M class for 1–7 weeks after infection; subsequently they are of the IgG class, which appears 2–3 weeks after infection.

Arboviruses cause a spectrum of disease ranging from inapparent infection (often the most likely outcome) to acute encephalitis. Within the CNS, arboviruses multiply in and induce necrosis of neurones, which in turn become surrounded by microglia, forming glial knots. There is also evidence of apoptosis for some virus infections. An age dependence of CNS disease has been observed for many arboviruses, and animal model systems indicate that age-dependent apoptosis of neurones may explain this phenomenon. Perivascular cuffing with mononuclear cells affects many cerebral blood vessels. Usually there is concomitant meningitis with accumulation of mononuclear cells in the subarachnoid space and hyperaemia of adjacent capillaries. Invasion of the CNS appears to be a critical determinant in the pathogenesis and is due in some cases to the level of viraemia. The role of the immune system is not clear, although it may be involved in the pathogenesis of dengue haemorrhagic fever and dengue shock syndrome. Antigen–antibody complex formation may underlie the syndrome, which is associated with increased capillary permeability and shock, often with haemorrhage. It is known that the uptake of virus into macrophages is enhanced in the presence of non-neutralising antibody, as the virus–antibody complexes bind to Fc receptors, so there is likely to be a great increase in the uptake and release of virus from macrophages.

Some arboviruses including alphaviruses (e.g. Ross River virus), flaviviruses (e.g. West Nile virus) and bunyaviruses (e.g. Bunyamwera virus) can disrupt the activation of specific innate immunity antiviral pathways, including interferon induction, to enhance their replication.

## CLINICAL FEATURES

The tissue tropism of arboviruses can be divided into three categories:

1. the CNS (e.g. encephalitis, aseptic meningitis)
2. visceral organs (e.g. hepatitis and haemorrhagic fevers)
3. febrile infections.

Human arbovirus infections become clinically manifest according to the target organ principally infected (Table 51.3). These include the following syndromes.

### Encephalitis

For many arboviruses, encephalitis is most common in children and/or the elderly. Illness typically has an abrupt onset within 1 week of infection, with headache, fever, myalgia and dysthesias, and sometimes lethargy, chills, dizziness, nausea, vomiting and prostration. Inflammation of the throat, cervical lymphadenitis and abdominal tenderness are also common. Signs and symptoms usually subside after several days, but may recrudesce. Progression to encephalitis may occur rapidly, or a prodromal illness may last for 1 week or more. Severe CNS disease is accompanied by neck stiffness, motor weakness and paralysis, meningismus, cranial nerve palsy, confusion, convulsions and somnolescence, leading to coma. Rigidity or weakness of the limbs may occur with reduction in reflexes. White blood cells, predominantly lymphocytes, and raised glucose levels may occur in the cerebrospinal fluid, which can exhibit increased pressure. Peripheral blood cell counts may be raised, with a left shift.

During most outbreaks of arboviral encephalitis, a proportion of patients develop aseptic meningitis alone, without significant neuronal involvement, whereas up to 50% of patients recover from acute encephalitis to suffer from neuropsychiatric sequelae varying from physiological impairment to mental disorder, which may last from months to years.

### Yellow fever

Yellow fever is caused by a mosquito-borne flavivirus that is found in tropical South America and Africa. The disease has an incubation period of 3–6 days, characterized by the sudden onset of headache and fever (temperatures may exceed 39°C), with generalized myalgia, nausea and vomiting. Jaundice may appear by the third day of illness, but frequently is mild or absent. Haematemesis, melaena, epistaxis and bleeding gums may also be noted. Albuminuria and oliguria may also begin suddenly during the first week of illness. In severe cases, death may occur 3–6 days after the onset of illness, and mid-zonal necrosis is observed in the liver. The case fatality rate is estimated as 20–50%.

### Dengue

Dengue is caused by four serologically related flaviviruses called dengue-1, -2, -3 and -4. These viruses are found in most tropical parts of the world. Dengue presents as an acute febrile illness with chills, headache, retro-ocular pain, body aches and arthralgia in more than 90% of apparent cases, with nausea or vomiting and a maculopapular rash resembling measles lasting for 2–7 days in about 60% of cases. Illness persists for 7 days, fever remitting after 3–5 days, followed by relapse ('saddleback fever') and pains in the bones, muscles and joints sufficiently severe to earn the epithet 'breakbone fever'. Rash occurs more commonly in patients aged less than 14 years. Complete recovery is the rule. The incubation period is 5–11 days.

### Dengue haemorrhagic fever

This is a less common manifestation of dengue, with about 500 000 cases per year and a case fatality rate of 15%, mainly affecting children. It is occasionally accompanied by a shock syndrome, known as dengue shock syndrome, with a case fatality rate of 50%. These two severe forms of dengue are observed in patients who undergo successive infection with two different dengue viruses (e.g. a primary dengue-1 infection followed by a secondary infection with dengue-2 virus). After an acute onset, fever of 40°C, accompanied by vomiting and anorexia, enlarged liver

**Table 51.3** Clinical syndromes associated with selected arboviruses and their geographical distribution

| Syndrome | Genus | Serogroup (vector) | Causative | Arbovirus serotype | Geographical distribution |
|---|---|---|---|---|---|
| Encephalitis or aseptic meningitis | *Alphavirus* | (mosquito) | EEEV | Eastern equine encephalitis | Eastern Canada, USA, Caribbean |
| | | | VEEV | Venezuelan equine encephalitis | North, Central and South America |
| | | | WEEV | Western equine encephalitis | North, Central and South America, Caribbean |
| | *Flavivirus* | (mosquito) | JEV | Japanese encephalitis | Orient (Japan to Malaysia) |
| | | | MVEV | Murray Valley encephalitis | Australia |
| | | | SLEV | St Louis encephalitis | Canada, USA, Central America |
| | | (tick) | LIV | Louping ill | Scotland, Northern Ireland |
| | | | POWV | Powassan | Canada, Northern USA |
| | | | TBEV | Tick-borne encephalitis complex | Central and northern Europe, Siberia |
| | *Orthobunyavirus* | CAL (mosquito) | LACV | La Crosse | USA |
| | | | SSHV | Snowshoe hare | Canada |
| Yellow fever | *Flavivirus* | (mosquito) | YFV | Yellow fever | Tropical Africa, Caribbean, tropical South America |
| Dengue | *Flavivirus* | (mosquito) | DENV | Dengue (four types) | Entire tropical zone |
| Haemorrhagic fever | *Alphavirus* | (mosquito) | CHIKV | Chikungunya | East Africa, India, South-East Asia |
| | *Flavivirus* | (mosquito) | DENV | Dengue (four types) | India, Philippines, South-East Asia, Oceania |
| | | (tick) | KFDV | Kyasanur Forest disease | India |
| | | | OMSKV | Omsk haemorrhagic fever | Siberia |
| | *Nairovirus* | CCHF (tick) | CCHFV | Crimean–Congo haemorrhagic fever | Central and southern Africa, Asia, Europe |
| Miscellaneous tropical fevers | *Alphavirus* | (mosquito) | CHIKV | Chikungunya | East Africa, India, South-East Asia |
| | | | RRV | Ross River[a] | Australia, Oceania |
| | *Flavivirus* | (mosquito) | ILHV | Ilheus | Caribbean, South America |
| | | | WNV | West Nile | Central and northern Africa, Europe, North, Central and South America, Caribbean |
| | *Orthobunyavirus* | SIM (mosquito) | OROV | Oropouche | Caribbean, South America |
| | *Phlebovirus* | PHL (mosquito) | RVFV | Rift Valley fever | Northern, eastern and southern Africa |
| | | PHL (sandfly) | PTV | Punta Toro | Central America |
| | | PHL (sandfly) | SFNV | Sandfly fever – Naples | Mediterranean |
| | *Vesiculovirus* | VS (sandfly) | VSIV | Vesicular stomatitis – Indiana | USA, Central America |
| Undifferentiated fever | *Coltivirus* | CTF (tick) | CTFV | Colorado tick fever | Western USA |

[a]Ross River virus infections frequently exhibit polyarthralgia.

and petechiae persists for 5–10 days. This is followed by a complete recovery unless shock supervenes, as occurs in 7–10% of patients 2–7 days after onset, usually accompanied by haematemesis and melaena.

## Miscellaneous tropical fevers

These comprise an increased temperature to above 39°C with any combination of headache, myalgia, malaise, nausea or vomiting, and sometimes accompanied by maculopapular rash or polyarthralgia, that is, a dengue-like syndrome but without haemorrhagic manifestations or the shock syndrome. Tropical fevers arise from infection with a wide variety of arboviruses (see Table 51.3) and clinical diagnosis is impossible without access to serological tests for diagnosis. Many of the Old World alphaviruses such as Ross River, chikungunya, o'nyong-nyong and Sindbis viruses cause an arthritic syndrome accompanied by rash, which can persist for months. Chronic or relapsing arthritic symptoms may be caused by inflammation associated with periodic increase in replication within peristently infected synovial macrophages, which persist despite neutralizing antibodies and antiviral cytokine responses. Inhibition of cytokine responses by virus–antibody complexes binding to Fc receptors, and interleukin-10 induction, may facilitate persistence.

## Undifferentiated fever

A US example is Colorado tick fever (genus *Coltivirus*) in which symptoms of chilliness, headaches, retro-orbital pain and generalized aches, especially in the back and limbs, appear 3–6 days after bites by infected *Dermacentor andersoni* ticks in wooded areas of the Rocky Mountain region. Fever of 39–40°C often shows a biphasic course, with eventual defervescence within 1 week, followed by complete recovery.

## Hantavirus pulmonary syndrome

This syndrome, due to the hantavirus Sin Nombre, was first recognized in south-western USA during 1993. Sudden onset of fever, myalgia, headache, cough, and nausea or vomiting is accompanied by rapid respirations exceeding 20 per minute, temperature above 38°C and hypotension. Extensive interstitial and alveolar infiltrates are observed in the lungs, accompanied by reduced oxygen saturation. Fatal cases develop progressive pulmonary oedema with hypoxia and severe hypotension, and die 2–16 days after onset of symptoms; the case fatality rate may exceed 50%. Patients with non-fatal infection usually recover within 1–3 weeks.

## LABORATORY DIAGNOSIS

Diagnosis of arbovirus infections depends on:

- the isolation of virus from blood, cerebrospinal fluid or tissues
- detection of arbovirus-specific RNA in blood, cerebrospinal fluid or tissues
- antigen detection by indirect immunofluorescence, commonly used as a rapid diagnostic method
- serology – haemagglutination inhibition and enzyme-linked immunosorbent assays (ELISAs) and neutralization tests can be used to detect serum antibodies from patients. However, these assays are dependent on availability of virus and/ or antigens.

## Virus isolation

Virus isolation is an important diagnostic tool, but is normally a slow process and unlikely to generate results until after an acute disease. The causative virus can often be isolated from blood collected during the initial 3–4-day febrile illness when viraemia titres peak. Some arboviruses can also be isolated from cerebrospinal fluid or brain biopsy, or from brain at autopsy of fatal encephalitis cases. Liver may yield virus isolation from fatal cases of yellow fever.

## Arbovirus–specific RNA detection

Detection of virus-specific RNA, by reverse transcriptase–polymerase chain reaction (RT-PCR) and the more sensitive real-time RT-PCR, are rapid approaches to diagnosis but depend on the availability of specific oligonucleotide primers. Given the large number of arboviruses, there must be significant differential diagnosis before selection of appropriate primers. Genus-reactive primers have been described for alphaviruses, flaviviruses and bunyaviruses.

After amplification of extracted RNA, the product is analysed by restriction enzyme digestion and/or determination of the nucleotide sequence of the PCR product and comparison with sequences in Genbank or other nucleotide sequence databases.

## Serology

Serological testing is often the only available means of laboratory diagnosis of encephalitis. The detection of a four-fold or greater rise of antibody titre by haemagglutination inhibition tests or ELISAs on paired sera collected during the initial week and several days later may provide good, but not definitive, evidence of concurrent infection. Antibodies detected by complement fixation testing first appear 2 weeks or more after onset and become undetectable by 3 years. Haemagglutination inhibition and complement fixation test results are usually not as specific as those obtained by neutralization. Virus-specific IgM antibody may be detected within 1 day of onset of clinical symptoms using an IgM capture ELISA. IgM antibody generally wanes 1–3 months after onset and is replaced by IgG antibodies beginning 2–3 weeks after infection. IgM antibodies are indicative of a recent infection.

## TREATMENT

Currently, no specific anti-arboviral therapeutic agent is available. Patients with encephalitis are managed supportively, using anticonvulsants as required, and ice packs are applied when indicated to reduce hyperthermia. Raised intracranial pressure can also be treated, and airway protection may be needed in unconscious patients, with hyperventilation accompanied by anaesthesia and sedation. Brain swelling can be minimized by regulating serum sodium levels and osmolarity. Nosocomial infections, especially pneumonia, should be prevented and treated aggressively when they occur. Similarly, in dengue and haemorrhagic fevers, supportive measures may include careful maintenance of fluid and electrolyte balance. Ribavirin shows activity against some bunyaviruses (and in combination with interferon-$\alpha$), but has not been well evaluated and is not therapeutic in many arbovirus infections.

## EPIDEMIOLOGY

### Natural cycles

Arboviruses are maintained in natural transmission cycles involving reservoir hosts and arthropod vectors, typically:

- ticks
- mosquitoes
- other biting flies.

Except for dengue virus and chikungunya virus in some locations, arboviruses are zoonotic pathogens that utilize wild animals as reservoir hosts. Many arboviruses also use non-human animals as amplification hosts during epidemics, and human beings are often tangentially infected, *dead-end hosts* during these outbreaks. Mosquitoes or other arthropods become infected by engorging on a viraemic vertebrate. In mosquitoes, infection begins in the midgut epithelium and spreads to the haemocele or open body cavity, where it may disseminate to other tissues and organs including the salivary glands. This extrinsic incubation period is completed when replication in salivary gland acinar cells leads to virus release into the apical cavities and salivary ducts. Transmission may then occur upon a subsequent blood meal, when mosquitoes deposit saliva in extravascular tissues while probing to locate a venule, or intravascularly. Infection of the vertebrate then leads to viraemia and the opportunity for infection of additional vectors. Nonviraemic transmission, where by an infected vector transmits to an uninfected vector feeding at the same time on the same host before replicative viraemia can occur, has been described for tick-borne viruses and West Nile virus (WNV).

Examples of natural cycles are:

- human–mosquito cycle, as in DENV, CHIKV and urban YFV (Fig. 51.1)
- mosquito–bird cycle, as in SLEV and WNV (Fig. 51.2)
- mosquito–mammal cycle, as in Venezuelan equine encephalitis virus (VEEV; Fig. 51.3).

Epidemiological aspects of arbovirus infections with major impact on human health are described according to syndrome and infecting serotype (see also Table 51.2).

## Alphaviruses

### Western equine encephalitis virus

Western equine encephalitis virus (WEEV) has caused periodic outbreaks of equine and human encephalitis in the western half of North America, as well as in Brazil and Argentina. Although massive outbreaks occurred during the mid-20th century in western North America, only one human case has been documented since 1998. In North America, cases occur only during June to September, when mosquitoes are abundant. Outbreaks of infection occur at intervals of a few years and are preceded by epizootic peaks of encephalitis among horses. The principal mosquito vector species in Canada and the western USA is *Culex tarsalis*. Passerine birds constitute the principal reservoirs. Human beings and equids are considered dead-end hosts because they produce little viraemia. Although all age groups may be involved, encephalitis due to WEEV (and California serogroup agents) commonly affects children, in whom the disease is often severe.

### Eastern equine encephalitis virus

Eastern equine encephalitis virus (EEEV) causes human and horse cases in Atlantic coastal areas extending from Massachusetts and New Jersey to Florida and Texas and northeastern Mexico, and in a few inland locations such as Michigan and Wisconsin. Occasionally, disease extends northwards into Canada. In the United States, an average of 6 human cases of EEEV are reported annually. Illness affects mainly those aged less than 14 years and more than 55 years, with overall case fatality rates as high as 69%. Surviving patients usually have severe neurological sequelae. Most human cases occur during late August and September, about 3 weeks after the peak of horse cases. Distinct forms of EEEV occur

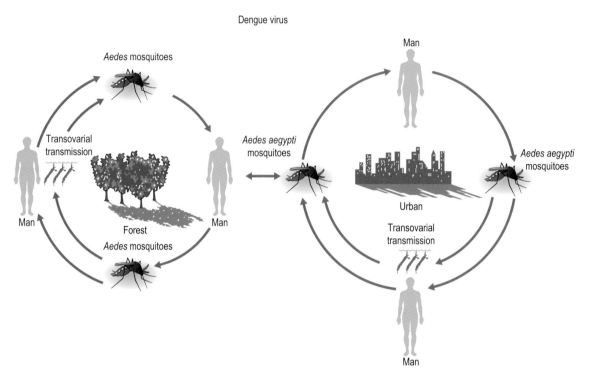

**Fig. 51.1** Natural cycle of arbovirus infection: human–mosquito cycle (e.g. dengue and urban yellow fever).

throughout South and Central America, but are rarely associated with human disease. In North America, EEEV is maintained enzootically in hardwood swamp habitats, where the mosquito *Culiseta melanura* transmits among passerine birds. During years of hyperenzootic transmission, horses and human beings residing near the swamp habitats become infected via bridge vectors such as *Aedes* spp. (*Cs. melanura* feeds primarily on birds). Equids and humans are considered dead-end hosts because they develop little viraemia, and outbreaks are therefore confined to regions of enzootic activity.

### Venezuelan equine encephalitis virus

Venezuelan equine encephalitis virus (VEEV) causes outbreaks involving up to hundreds of thousands of human beings and equids, primarily in northern South America, with one outbreak extending as far north as Texas in the USA in 1971. During outbreaks, VEEV is transmitted among equids by a variety of mosquitoes such as *Aedes* and *Psorophora* spp. Equids are extremely effective amplifying hosts because they develop high-titred viraemia and are attractive to mosquitoes. Antigenically related viruses occur in sylvatic and swamp habitats through much of the

Neotropics and subtropics, as far north as Florida, USA, and as far south as northern Argentina. These viruses can cause febrile illness and sometimes fatal encephalitis in human beings that enter these foci, and one antigenic subtype (designated ID) can mutate to become capable of initiating widespread outbreaks. Rates of encephalitis in apparent infections (generally 5–15% of symptomatic cases) and mortality (around 0.5%) are generally lower than for EEEV, with most fatal cases occurring in young children. Attack rates can exceed 50% and neurological sequelae are common.

### Ross River virus

Ross River virus (RRV) infection, known in Australia as epidemic polyarthritis, has also occurred in the South Pacific. In Australia, disease occurs primarily during the summer and autumn as sporadic cases and small outbreaks. An average of 5000 cases is reported each year, mostly involving vacationers and others in rural areas. RRV is maintained in a zoonotic vertebrate–mosquito cycle, with *Culex annulirostris* and *Aedes vigilax* serving as the principal vectors, and flying foxes and marsupials implicated as reservoir hosts. Human infections have also been documented

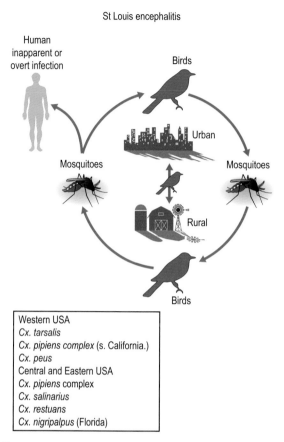

St Louis encephalitis

Human inapparent or overt infection

Birds

Urban

Mosquitoes

Mosquitoes

Rural

Birds

Western USA
*Cx. tarsalis*
*Cx. pipiens* complex (s. California.)
*Cx. peus*
Central and Eastern USA
*Cx. pipiens* complex
*Cx. salinarius*
*Cx. restuans*
*Cx. nigripalpus* (Florida)

**Fig. 51.2** Natural cycle of arbovirus infection: bird–mosquito cycle (e.g. St Louis encephalitis).

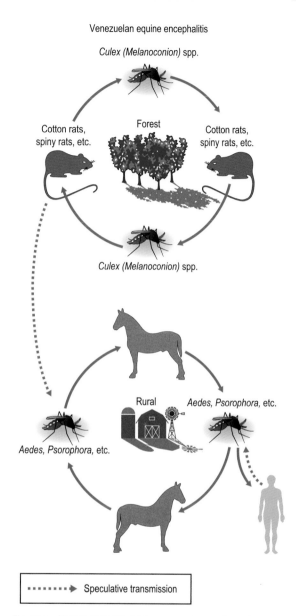

Venezuelan equine encephalitis

*Culex (Melanoconion)* spp.

Cotton rats, spiny rats, etc.

Forest

Cotton rats, spiny rats, etc.

*Culex (Melanoconion)* spp.

Rural

*Aedes, Psorophora*, etc.

*Aedes, Psorophora*, etc.

┅┅┅► Speculative transmission

**Fig. 51.3** Natural cycle of infection: mammal–mosquito cycle (e.g. Venezuelan equine encephalitis).

in New Guinea, the Solomon Islands, New Caledonia, Fiji, American Samoa and the Cook Islands. During 1979–1980 a large, explosive epidemic of Ross River polyarthritis swept across the South Pacific, with 40–60% of the population affected on some islands. *Aedes polynesiensis* was implicated as the vector, and epidemiological studies suggested a man–mosquito–man transmission cycle.

## Chikungunya virus

Chikungunya virus (CHIKV), named after a Swahili word meaning 'that which bends up', referring to the posture of patients with severe joint pains, has probably occurred sporadically in India and South-East Asia for at least 200 years. However, it has its enzootic ancestry in sub-Saharan Africa where a sylvatic transmission cycle occurs between wild primates and arboreal *Aedes* mosquitoes. Urban CHIKV epidemics in the Indian Ocean, India and South-East Asia, causing hundreds of thousands of cases, involve *Ae. aegypti*

and/or *Ae. albopictus* transmission in a man–mosquito–man cycle. Unlike dengue, which is endemic in many of these Asian cities, CHIKV may disappear and reappear at irregular intervals. However, CHIKV infection is often overlooked because it is clinically indistinguishable from dengue fever. Since March 2005, epidemics have taken place in the Indian Ocean, Asia and Africa involving millions of people with some fatalities. Disability-adjusted life year (DALY) estimates during the 2006 Indian Ocean epidemic exceeded 265 per million in some regions, accounting for up to 69% of the total DALYs, and case-fatality rates have been estimated at ca. 0.1%. Transmission in many locations has been enhanced by the adaptation of newly emerged strains to *Ae. albopictus* mosquitoes via a mutation in the E1 envelope glycoprotein gene. The ability of this vector to mediate epidemic transmission in a temperate region of an industrialized nation (Italy), underscores the direct risk of CHIKV to many parts of the world including Europe and the Americas. Like dengue, CHIK intervention using vector control has been ineffective, even in highly regulated and industrialized nations like Singapore.

## O'nyong-nyong virus

O'nyong-nyong virus (ONNV), derived from the description by the Acholi tribe, meaning 'joint breaker', was first isolated during a 1959–1962 epidemic affecting 2 million people in Uganda, Kenya, Tanzania, Mozambique, Malawi and Senegal. Another major outbreak involving an estimated 1 million cases occurred in 1996 in Uganda and northern Tanzania. Attack rates are generally high and all age groups are affected during ONNV epidemics. The transmission cycle involves *Anopheles funestus* and *Anopheles gambiae* mosquitoes; ONNV is the only known alphavirus with *Anopheles* vectors. The reservoir and amplification hosts are unknown.

## Flaviviruses: mosquito-borne

### St Louis encephalitis virus

St Louis encephalitis virus (SLEV) was first isolated from the brain of a person dying from acute encephalitis in St Louis, Missouri. SLEV activity is widely distributed throughout the USA. The largest outbreak in recent times occurred in 1975, when 1815 (86%) of 2113 confirmed cases of arbovirus encephalitis were due to SLEV. Mosquito vectors in California, the Rocky Mountains and plains states comprise mainly *Cx. tarsalis*, but *Cx. pipiens* and *Cx. quinquefasciatus* are important along the Mississippi Valley and eastwards. The salt marsh mosquitoes *Cx. restuans* and *Ae. sollicitans* may be important vectors in some localities. SLE virus is seen most often in persons aged 55 years or more.

### Japanese encephalitis virus

Japanese encephalitis virus (JEV) was first isolated from the brain of a patient with fatal encephalitis in Tokyo in 1935. It continues to cause epidemics of encephalitis, affecting children, particularly in India, Korea, China, South-East Asia and Indonesia, with case fatality rates often exceeding 20%. JEV has recently emerged in the Torres Straits and the tip of northern Australia. Approximately 50 000 cases occur each year, of which 15 000 are fatal. The ratio of apparent to inapparent infection is 1 : 50–400, depending on the geographical area. *Cx. tritaeniorhynchus* mosquitoes are the principal vectors, and maximal virus isolation rates from mosquitoes occur during late July, simultaneously with human and equine epidemics. Important vertebrate reservoirs are black-crowned night herons and other water birds, and pigs are considered to be an amplifying host.

## West Nile virus

West Nile virus (WNV) was first isolated from a febrile patient in the West Nile district of Uganda in 1937. The virus has a wide geographical distribution, including southern Europe, Africa, central and south Asia, and Oceania. Genetic studies have shown that the related Kunjin virus, found in Australasia, is a subtype of West Nile virus. Although the virus infects a wide variety of animals, including horses, cattle and man, the major vertebrate hosts are wild birds, and migratory birds are important in the spread of the disease owing to long-term high-titre viraemia. The principal vectors are considered to be mosquitoes of the *Culex* genus. Both sylvatic and urban transmission cycles have been reported, with *Cx. pipiens* implicated as the major urban vector. WNV usually causes a febrile illness, but encephalitis is seen in patients over 50 years of age. Epidemics vary in size, with the largest reported in Israel and South Africa, including an epidemic of 3000 clinical cases in South Africa in 1974 and over 400 cases in Russia in 1998, and an equine epidemic in North Africa in 1998. In the late summer of 1999, the first outbreak of WNV infection was reported in the western hemisphere, in New York. A total of 62 clinical cases was reported, mostly in the elderly, including seven deaths.

Since then WNV has spread across the USA with at least 4161 human cases (277 fatalities) and more than 14 000 equine cases reported in 2002. This is the largest recorded epidemic of arboviral meningoencephalitis in the USA. Overall, in the USA there had been more than 29 500 human cases and over 1150 deaths by the end of 2009. As of 2006, the distribution of the virus has expanded to include the continental USA and seven Canadian provinces, as well as Mexico, El Salvador and many of the Caribbean Islands. During 2006 the virus spread as far south as Argentina, causing disease in equines. WNV has infected at least 308 species of birds, 30 other vertebrate species and 60 species of mosquitoes. In addition, cases of WNV infection have been imported into European countries from endemic areas.

## Usutu virus

Usutu virus, isolated in Africa, is a member of the Japanese encephalitis serogroup of the *Flavivirus* genus and was not known to cause disease. In 2001 the virus emerged in Austria, in Vienna and surrounding districts, and was responsible for a large epizootic with high mortality in birds, especially Eurasian blackbirds (*Turdus merula*) and owls. The virus has continued to cause epizootics in birds plus some human cases.

## Murray Valley encephalitis virus

Murray Valley encephalitis virus (MVEV) was first isolated from the brain of a patient with fatal encephalitis at Mooroopna, Victoria, Australia. MVEV caused epidemics of encephalitis in irrigated farming regions of the Murray–Darling River basin during the summer months (January to March) of 1951 and 1974, with case fatality rates approaching 40%. MVE virus was isolated from *Cx. annulirostris* mosquitoes only during 1974 but not during intervening years, which suggests epidemic introduction of virus into this dry temperate region. In the tropical irrigated Ord River region of Western Australia, the virus is endemic and encephalitis cases occurred in 1974, 1978, 1981 and 1986. Another endemic focus exists in the Gulf of Carpentaria region of Queensland. Natural cycles of transmission of MVEV involve *Cx. annulirostris* as the principal mosquito vector and water birds as reservoirs.

## Yellow fever virus

Yellow fever virus (YFV) was first isolated in Ghana from the blood of a male patient with fever, headache, backache and prostration. YFV is found mostly in tropical Africa and tropical South America. There are two epidemiological patterns. In the sylvatic cycle, virus is transmitted among monkeys by mosquitoes (*Haemagogus* and *Sabethes* species in South America and *Aedes* species in Africa). Humans are infected incidentally when entering the area, for example to work as foresters. In the urban cycle, person-to-person transmission is via *Ae. aegypti*, which uses larval habitats close to human habitation in water, pits and scrap containers such as oil drums.

In the Americas, the majority of YFV cases are reported in Brazil, Peru and Bolivia, and involve males aged 15–45 years who are agricultural and forest workers. YFV usually occurs from December to May, and peaks during March and April, when populations of *Haemagogus* mosquitoes are highest during the rainy season.

YFV is endemic in many parts of West, Central and East Africa, principally between latitudes 15°N and 15°S, extending northwards into Ethiopia and Sudan. Continuing activity has been encountered in parts of West Africa. There are relatively few outbreaks in East Africa with the last major outbreaks in Sudan in 2003 and 2005. *Ae. africanus* is the principal vector in Africa.

## Dengue viruses

Dengue virus (DENV) infection is endemic in all tropical regions between latitudes 23.5°N and 23.5°S. Four serologically related viruses termed dengue-1, -2, -3 and -4 cause the disease *dengue*. The febrile clinical symptoms associated with dengue are similar to those of other arboviruses from other families; this has resulted in confusion in the diagnosis of dengue. In particular, the high incidence of dengue has resulted in the misdiagnosis of some arbovirus outbreaks as discussed above. Serological studies are needed to differentiate these.

DENV are thought to have originated in Asia in a sylvatic cycle involving arboreal mosquitoes and monkeys. However, endemic viruses have evolved and are now maintained in nature by a cycle involving man as both reservoir and amplification host, and domestic mosquitoes, principally *Ae. aegypti*, as vectors.

Dengue virus has caused numerous outbreaks throughout the south-west Pacific region since it was first recognized among servicemen during the Second World War. Subsequently, in the south-west Pacific, multiple dengue viruses have affected Tahiti, with haemorrhagic dengue first encountered in 1971. In addition to *Ae. aegypti* other species have been implicated as vectors, including *Ae. scutellaris hebrideus* in New Guinea, *Ae. polynesiensis* in Tahiti and *Ae. cooki* in Niue. Hawaii was dengue-free from 1944 to 2001 until, in 2001–2002, there was a DENV-1 outbreak involving at least 122 cases and *Ae. albopictus* as the vector.

DENV activity continues in many tropical countries of the Pacific rim, including northern Australia. Most South-East Asian countries, including Indonesia, Malaysia, Thailand, Vietnam, China, the Philippines and India, experience repeated epidemics of dengue caused by all four viruses, with most cases occurring between June and November. Mostly children are affected; in some outbreaks up to 25% may develop haemorrhagic fever. Most epidemics occur in urban areas and villages where *Ae. aegypti* is abundant, but not in rural environments. Up to 100 million infections may occur each year, mostly in children; this is a major public health problem.

Dengue is endemic throughout tropical Africa, including Nigeria in the west and Mozambique in the east, and also in Middle Eastern countries such as Saudi Arabia. Dengue disease is seldom severe in Africa and dengue haemorrhagic fever is rare.

Caribbean countries have been involved in epidemic waves of dengue since 1827, with little evidence of clinical dengue during interepidemic periods. All four DENV have been implicated in outbreaks affecting residents of Caribbean islands and adjacent areas of Central and South America. Each year cases of dengue are imported into continental USA and Europe following visits to dengue-endemic countries. Although most infections in the USA occur among travellers returning from the Caribbean, small numbers of cases (less than 30 per year) of indigenous dengue occur regularly among residents of southern Texas who live near the border with Mexico. The semi-tropical climate in this area allows *Ae. aegypti* to flourish during the nine warmer months of each year. Recently, a small epidemic was detected in the Florida Keys, another subtropical area inhabited by *Ae. aegypti*. In 1985, *Ae. albopictus* was introduced from Asia into the Americas via used motor tyre casings that had been imported for retreading into Texas, from Japan, South Korea and several South-East Asian countries. The mosquito rapidly established itself in Texas and spread into mid-western, north-eastern and north-western states of the USA, and also into Mexico and other countries. A peri-domestic mosquito, *Ae. albopictus*, was first identified as a dengue vector in Malaysia during the 1960s, and it transmits dengue both in the human–mosquito cycle and by transovarial transfer. However, to date, there have been few reports of dengue virus transmission in the Americas by *Ae. albopictus*.

## Zika virus

Zika virus (ZIKV) is a flavivirus related to yellow fever virus that until recently has been considered endemic to Africa and Southeast Asia, but human cases are rare. In 2007 ZIKV caused an outbreak of 49 confirmed, and 59 probable cases, of a relatively mild disease characterized by rash, arthralgia, and conjunctivitis on Yap Island, Federated States of Micronesia, in the southwestern Pacific Ocean.

Serologic studies suggest that 73% of Yap Island residents aged 3 or older had been recently infected with ZIKV. This was the first time that ZIKV was detected outside of Africa and Asia. The emergence of ZIKV outside of its previously known geographic range demonstrates another example of an emerging viral disease.

## Flaviviruses: tick–borne

### Powassan virus

Powassan virus, the sole North American tick-borne flavivirus, was first isolated from the brain of a fatal human case of encephalitis in Powassan, Ontario, Canada. To date, it has caused approximately 40 cases of encephalitis and four deaths among residents of forested areas of Ontario, Quebec and Nova Scotia in Canada, as well as Massachusetts, New York State and Pennsylvania in the USA. All of these cases occurred between May and October. Principal tick vector species in Ontario are *Ixodes cookei*, which feeds on groundhogs, and *I. marxi*, which feeds on tree squirrels; both of these mammals serve as reservoirs.

### Tick-borne encephalitis viruses

Tick-borne encephalitis virus (TBEV) is used to describe a serocomplex of related viruses that are transmitted by ticks and cause similar diseases. These include central European (also known as the western subtype) TBEV that causes central European encephalitis and Russian spring–summer encephalitis (also known as the Far Eastern subtype of TBEV). In addition, a third subtype, Siberian TBEV, has been described mainly on the basis of genetic studies. Russian spring–summer encephalitis occurs in eastern Europe and parts of Asia, including northern Japan, and causes a more severe disease than the central European encephalitis found in western Europe and Scandinavia. The case fatality rate of central European encephalitis is usually below 10%, whereas it can reach 30% for Russian spring–summer encephalitis. In Britain and Ireland and some parts of France and Scandinavia, a mild form of tick-borne encephalitis is caused by a related virus called 'louping ill'. The latter virus also infects sheep and grouse and gets its name from the leaping gait in infected sheep; the virus rarely infects man.

Human infections with TBEV may range in severity from mild biphasic meningo-encephalitis, which is characteristic of the central European TBEV and louping ill virus, to a severe form of polio-encephalomyelitis that is characteristic of Russian spring–summer encephalitis virus.

Natural cycles involve *I. ricinus* ticks as vectors, and mice, shrews and other small rodents as reservoirs, with infection transferred tangentially to sheep or other farm animals, and also to human beings. In Siberia, *I. persulcatus* ticks serve as vectors. Recently, additional viruses have been described from Spain, Turkey and Bulgaria that are related to louping ill virus and are members of the TBEV complex and cause TBEV-like disease symptoms in sheep and other animals.

The TBEV complex contains three viruses associated with haemorrhagic fever: Omsk haemorrhagic fever (OHF) and Kyasanur Forest disease (KFD) and Alkhumra viruses. OHF was identified during the Second World War in Omsk and the virus causes occasional outbreaks in Russia, whereas KFD is found only in India and causes regular outbreaks of haemorrhagic fever. Alkhumra virus was isolated in 1995, and subsequently in 2001 in Saudia Arabia; it caused haemorrhagic fever with a fatal outcome in 25% of patients. Genetic studies suggest that Alkhumra virus is a subtype of KFD virus.

## Bunyaviruses: *Bunyavirus* genus
### California (CAL) serogroup

There are at least 14 viruses related antigenically to the prototype California encephalitis virus. In the USA, encephalitis and aseptic meningitis arise commonly from infections with La Crosse virus, first isolated from the brain of a patient with fatal encephalitis in La Crosse, Wisconsin. Other viruses occasionally associated with aseptic meningitis are snowshoe hare virus, isolated from the blood of a snowshoe hare in Montana, and Jamestown Canyon virus (JCV), isolated from *Culiseta inornata* mosquitoes collected at Jamestown Canyon, Colorado. In central Europe, febrile illness, sometimes with aseptic meningitis, arises from infection with Tahyna virus, isolated from *Ae. caspius* mosquitoes collected near Tahyna, in the former Czechoslovakia.

Currently, CAL serogroup viruses are the most common arboviruses associated with encephalitis in the USA. The highest attack rates occur in states adjoining the Great Lakes, affecting mainly children aged less than 15 years. Abundant tree holes in wooded areas provide optimal breeding sites for the principal mosquito vector *Ae. triseriatus*, but rainwater collected in disused motor tyres is a suitable breeding ground for *Ae. triseriatus* in suburban locations. As adult mosquitoes die in winter, CAL serogroup

viruses survive through transovarial transmission. Principal vertebrate reservoirs are tree squirrels and chipmunks.

### Oropouche (ORO)

This virus is the only human pathogen in the Simbu serogroup; it was isolated in Trinidad in 1955. Outbreaks of oropouche fever, a febrile illness, have occurred in Brazil since 1961, involving urban transmission by the midge *Culicoides paraensis*. An outbreak was reported in Panama in 1989, and cases of oropouche fever have been reported in Peru since 1992.

### Garissa virus

In 1997–1998 Garrisa virus was described as a reassortant bunyavirus. It was isolated from patients with acute haemorrhagic fever during an epidemic of Rift Valley fever in Kenya and southern Somalia. Acute sera from patients with haemorrhagic fever yielded either virus isolation or PCR evidence of infection. Initial studies indicated that the sequences of the L and S RNA segments were nearly identical to those of Bunyamwera virus, whereas the sequence of the M segment was very different (33% nucleotide and 28% amino acid differences). Very recent studies have shown that Garissa and Ngari virus M segments are nearly identical in sequence, whereas the L and S segments of Bunyamwera virus are similar to those of both Ngari and Garissa virus. These data indicate that Garissa virus is not a reassortant but an isolate of Ngari virus, which is a reassortant of Bunyamwera virus. Previously Ngari virus had not been considered a cause of haemorrhagic fever; further studies are required to investigate the pathogenesis and epidemiology of Ngari virus.

## Bunyaviruses: *Phlebovirus* genus
### Rift Valley fever virus

Rift Valley fever virus (RVFV) was first isolated in 1930 from sheep during an epizootic causing abortion and death in the Rift Valley near Lake Niavasha, Kenya, but is present from South Africa to Egypt. The virus infects many large domestic animals and a wide variety of mosquito species, with sheep, cattle, buffaloes and rodents as reservoirs. RVFV is epizootic with long inter-epizootic periods. Outbreaks of Rift Valley fever occurred in Egypt during 1977 involving an estimated 200000 human cases and 600 deaths. Subsequently, Rift Valley fever has been reported during 1998–1999 in Mauritania and Senegal, and in Yemen and south-west Saudi Arabia in 2000–2001, involving over 2000 clinical cases and a mortality rate of 14%. Genetic studies of the virus are consistent with the theory that infection came from East Africa.

### Sandfly fever group

These viruses are distributed throughout the European and North African countries surrounding the Mediterranean Sea, extending eastward through Israel and Iran to West Pakistan and central India. Sandfly fever (Naples and Sicilian) viruses were first isolated from the sera of US servicemen during an outbreak in the Second World War.

Epidemics of dengue-like fever occur during the sandfly season (June to September) and affect mainly visitors rather than residents. Natural vectors are *Phlebotomus papatasi* and other phlebotomine sandflies. Isolation of virus from male sandflies collected during July suggests transovarial transfer of virus. The natural cycle of sandfly fever appears to involve solely human beings, as definitive host and reservoir, with sandflies as vectors.

### Toscana virus

Toscana virus was first isolated from sandflies collected in Tuscany, Italy; it is transmitted by *Phlebotomus perniciosus* sandflies, and can be transferred transovarially. Natural reservoirs of Toscana virus appear to be small rodents (*Apodemus sylvaticus*).

## Bunyaviruses: *Nairovirus* genus
### Crimean–Congo haemorrhagic fever virus

Crimean–Congo haemorrhagic fever virus (CCHFV) was originally described as two separate viruses: Crimean haemorrhagic fever virus, isolated from the serum of a man with fatal haemorrhagic fever near Samarkand, Uzbekistan, and Congo virus isolated from the serum of a child with fever and arthralgia in Zaire. Antigenic and genetic studies show that the two viruses are identical. CCHFV is distributed widely throughout tropical Africa, from Mauritania to Uganda and Kenya, the Middle East and West Pakistan, and southwards to South Africa. It is also found in Asia, including parts of China. The geographical distribution of CCHFV corresponds to that of *Hyalomma* sp. ticks, from which the virus can be isolated. Human infection is rare but mortality rates of up to 50% have been reported.

## Bunyaviruses: *Hantavirus* genus

Unlike the other genera in the Bunyaviridae, members of the *Hantavirus* genus are rodent-associated viruses. They are zoonotic viruses of rodents (mainly mice or voles) that excrete virus in urine for prolonged periods. Virus is transmitted to man by contact with aerosols of rodent urine.

### Hantaan and Puumala viruses

These viruses induce either (1) a severe illness, termed *haemorrhagic fever* with *renal syndrome*, due to Hantaan virus in Japan, Korea, China and Siberia and Puumala virus in Scandinavia, or (2) a mild illness, termed *nephropathia epidemica*, due to Puumala virus in Scotland, France, Belgium and Germany, the Balkans and Greece. Hantaan virus was first identified in soldiers serving in Korea in 1951 and named after the area where it was detected. Principal vertebrate reservoirs comprise *Apodemus agrarius* rodents in Asia and *Clethrionomys glareolus* (bank vole) in Europe.

### Sin Nombre virus

Sin Nombre virus induces hantavirus pulmonary syndrome, a severe acute respiratory illness with a case fatality rate exceeding 50%. Initially encountered in May 1993 in the Four Corners region of the USA (Arizona, Colorado, New Mexico and Utah), cases have since occurred elsewhere in the USA, Canada and many countries in South America. The principal rodent reservoir is considered to be *Peromyscus maniculatus* (deer mouse), but each hantavirus pulmonary syndrome-causing virus occupies a geographical region defined by the rodent species that carries it. Thus, Black Creek Canal virus found in cotton rats (*Sigmadon hispidus*) in Florida is related to viruses found in South America, with a distinct rodent host.

This was the first occasion on which molecular methods identified an unknown arbovirus before the virus was isolated. Hantavirus group antibodies were detected in sera from human cases and rodents. RNA from lung and liver of fatal human cases and seropositive rodents was amplified by RT-PCR; positive bands were detected using primers for Prospect Hill (North American) and Puumala virus-like hantaviruses, but not Hantaan and Seoul-like (Asian) hantaviruses. This was achieved within 3 weeks after death of the initial human cases. Several months later, Sin Nombre virus, genomically distinct from Prospect Hill and other hantaviruses, was isolated from tissue suspensions, initially from *P. maniculatus* and subsequently from man.

## CONTROL

Strategies for the prevention of arbovirus infections depend on either vector control or active immunization with vaccine.

### Vector control

Suppression of populations of vector mosquito species can halt virus transmission in urban and suburban localities as follows:

1. Use of insecticides to kill adult mosquitoes ('adulticiding'), for instance aerial sprays of malathion; however, nontarget insects may also be affected. The use of persistent insecticides on the interiors of houses has decreased due to environmental concerns.
2. Removal of domestic larval development sites for *Ae. aegypti* such as tin cans and tyres that could contain rainwater, both near human habitations and in public parks and drainage systems; this has prevented the occurrence of dengue in Singapore and urban yellow fever in metropolitan areas in Caribbean countries.
3. Chemical control of larvae (barricading) by applying insecticides or oil to small larval sites; this has reduced mosquito vector populations substantially in irrigated localities in California and elsewhere.
4. Biological control of larvae by microbiological agents such as *Bacillus thuringiensis israeliensis*, larvivorous fish, flatworms or mermethid nematodes, or insect growth regulators such as the juvenile hormone that mimics methoprene.
5. Personal protection against bites by mosquitoes involving a combination of protective clothing, preferably impregnated with permethrin, screening of dwellings to prevent entry of vectors and frequent application of repellants such as *N,N*-diethyl-*m*-toluamide (DEET) or picaridin to exposed skin. For tick-borne viruses, protective clothing should be worn outdoors, followed by rigorous inspection to remove attached ticks from the skin.

### Vaccines

To date relatively few vaccines have been developed to control arbovirus diseases.

#### Alphaviruses

There are no licensed vaccines for use in man. However, formalin-inactivated vaccines for WEEV, EEEV and VEEV are used to immunize horses, researchers who work with the viruses, and military personnel. A live VEE vaccine, known as TC-83, is also administered to horses and researchers. TC-83 is associated with significant adverse reactions and lack of seroconversion in many human vaccinees, and is not suitable for use in the general population.

#### Flaviviruses

Vaccines have been licensed against yellow fever, Japanese encephalitis and TBE viruses. A live yellow fever vaccine, 17D, was developed in the 1930s by 176 passages of wild-type strain Asibi through chicken tissue. One dose of vaccine administered subcutaneously and containing 5000–200 000 plaque-forming units of virus gives protective immunity 10 days after immunization; immunity lasts for at least 10 years. The World Health Organization recommends immunization every 10 years to maintain immunity; the vaccine can be given to children over 9 months of age. Immunization is contra-indicated in immunocompromised individuals and pregnant women. More than 550 million doses of vaccine have been administered, leading to only a few cases of yellow fever associated neurotropic disease (YEL-AND) and yellow fever associated viscerotropic disease (YEL-AVD).

Both live and killed vaccines have been developed to control Japanese encephalitis. Formalin-inactivated vaccines were developed in the 1940s based on virus grown in mouse brain but were recently discontinued due to the risk of allergic reaction following immunization. Killed vaccines based on virus grown in Vero cell culture are now being used. Two doses of killed vaccine given 7–28 days apart are required for protective immunity. A booster is given at 1 year and subsequently every 3–4 years to maintain immunity. A live vaccine has been developed: SA14-14-2 was generated in the People's Republic of China by 126 passages of wild-type strain SA14 in primary hamster kidney cell culture. It is given as two doses and has been administered to more than 300 million people in China without any reports of adverse reactions. To date the vaccine has been used in seven other Asian countries. In addition, a live vaccine is used to immunize pigs.

A formalin-inactivated TBE vaccine using virus grown in chicken eggs was developed in the 1970s to control central European tick-borne encephalitis virus. The vaccine was improved by transferring manufacture to primary chick embryo fibroblast cell culture. Two doses are given, 2 weeks to 3 months apart, followed by a booster given 9 months to 1 year later. Boosters are recommended every 3 years. The vaccine has proved to be very effective, with few adverse reactions, and has resulted in the near elimination of tick-borne encephalitis in Austria. The effectiveness of the vaccine against Russian spring–summer encephalitis is uncertain.

There are no vaccines available to prevent dengue. However, a number of candidate live vaccines are currently undergoing human trials.

## Bunyaviruses

Although there are no commercially available vaccines against diseases caused by bunyaviruses, a number of experimental live and killed vaccines have been developed against Rift Valley fever. In addition, experimental deoxyribonucleic acid (DNA)-based vaccines have been developed against several hantaviruses and show promise in preclinical studies.

RECOMMENDED READING

Barrett ADT: Japanese encephalitis. In Service MW, editor: *The Encyclopedia of Arthropod-Transmitted Infections*, Wallingford, UK, 2001, CAB International, pp 239–246.

Elliott RM, editor: *The Bunyaviridae*, New York, 1996, Plenum Press.

Karabatsos N: *International Catalogue of Arboviruses Including Certain Other Viruses of Vertebrates*, ed 3, San Antonio, 1985, American Society for Tropical Medicine and Hygiene

Ksiazek TG, Peters CJ, Rollin PE, et al: Identification of a new North American hantavirus that causes acute pulmonary insufficiency, *American Journal of Tropical Medicine and Hygiene* 52:117–123, 1995.

Monath TP, editor: *The Arboviruses: Ecology and Epidemiology*, Vols 1–5, Boca Raton, 1988, CRC Press.

US Department of Health and Human Services: *Biosafety in Microbiological and Biomedical Laboratories*, ed 5, Washington, DC, 2007, US Government Printing Office.

Weaver SC: Eastern equine encephalitis. In Service MW, editor: *The Encyclopedia of Arthropod-Transmitted Infections*, Wallingford, UK, 2001, CAB International, pp 151–159.

Weaver SC, Barrett AD: Transmission cycles, host range, evolution and emergence of arboviral disease, *Nature Reviews Microbiology* 2:789–801, 2004.

Weaver SC, Ferro C, Barrera R, et al: Venezuelan equine encephalitis, *Annual Reviews of Entomology* 49;141–174, 2001.

Weaver SC, Reisen WK: Present and future arboviral threats, *Antiviral Research* 85:328–345, 2009.

# 52 Hepaciviruses and hepeviruses

## Hepatitis C and E viruses; non-A, non-B hepatitis

*P. Simmonds*

## KEY POINTS

- Hepatitis C virus (HCV) is principally transmitted by parenteral routes. The development of serological and PCR-based methods for the diagnosis of HCV infection is of major value in blood donor screening and investigation of clinical hepatitis.
- HCV infection is persistent in a large proportion of those exposed. Significant liver disease develops slowly (20–30 years) and can lead to cirrhosis, end-stage liver failure and hepatocellular carcinoma.
- Chronic HCV infection can be successfully treated in a proportion of individuals by combination therapy with pegylated interferon-α and ribavirin.
- Hepatitis E virus produces an acute infection prevalent in South-East Asia, north and central Africa, India and Central America, transmitted by faecal contamination, often affecting water supplies and caused by a single-stranded, non-enveloped RNA virus.
- Most cases are recognized in those aged 15–40 years. Large outbreaks occur; a severe form with fulminant hepatitis may be seen in the third trimester of pregnancy.

## HEPATITIS C VIRUS

Hepatitis C virus (HCV), discovered in 1989, was the long sought-after and highly elusive causative agent of post-transfusion non-A, non-B hepatitis. This hugely important discovery allowed rapid development of serological screening assays for HCV infection and their adoption for blood donor screening. Consequently transmission of HCV by blood transfusion has been virtually eliminated, as has the occurrence of transfusion-associated hepatitis.

Infection with HCV is widespread throughout the world, and is particularly associated with risk groups for parenteral (blood-borne) exposure. Amongst these, drug users sharing needles are numerically the most significant in Western countries. HCV infection is frequently persistent, and leads to the development of significant liver disease, such as cirrhosis and hepatocellular carcinoma (HCC), but only after a long asymptomatic carrier phase. There are currently intensive efforts to develop effective antiviral treatment for chronic infection, and protective vaccines.

## PROPERTIES

### Structure

HCV is a small, enveloped virus with a single stranded RNA genome of positive (coding) polarity (Fig. 52.1). HCV has been visualized in the plasma of HCV-infected individuals as small (50 nm), round particles. The surface of the virus particle contains a number of small projections thought to be formed from complexes of the virally encoded envelope glycoproteins, E1 and E2. The RNA genome is approximately 9400 bases in length, of which over 98% contains protein-coding sequence. In common with many other small RNA viruses, the gene sequences of HCV are translated in a single block to produce a large (>3000 amino acid) polyprotein. During and after translation, proteases cleave this precursor into a total of 9 mature proteins, which are involved in virus replication (NS2–NS5B), or form structural components of the virus particle (core, E1 and E2).

### Replication

Information on the replication of HCV and its assembly into infectious virus particles remains limited because it still remains problematic to culture the virus in vitro. However, investigation of individual HCV-encoded proteins and comparison with related viruses have allowed the functions of most to be

537

**Fig. 52.1** Organisation of HCV genome, showing (A) the structural (core, E1 and E2) and non-structural genes (NS2–NS5B), and (B) the proteins produced from them by proteolytic cleavage of the translated polyprotein. Properties and functions of the HCV proteins, where known are summarised below. ER, endoplasmic reticulum; UTR, untranslated terminal region.

ascertained (Fig. 52.1). For example, NS5B is the RNA polymerase required by HCV for replication of its genetic material through a negative-stranded intermediate. NS3 contains protease and helicase activities; the former is required for the majority of cleavage reactions in the processing of the polyprotein after translation. The three proteins at the left hand end of the genome are structural proteins. Multiple copies of the core protein assemble to form a nucleocapsid that packages the viral RNA, while E1 and E2 are synthesized on internal membranes within the infected cell, become heavily glycosylated and form the HCV envelope as the nucleocapsid buds out of the cell.

The extreme ends of the HCV genome are non-coding, and play a number of roles in the transcription and translation of the virus genome. Details of the factors that initiate and regulate HCV transcription remain unclear at present, although the non-coding ends are likely to be involved in protein complexes with NS5B, NS3 and other HCV and cellular proteins

to mediate binding and initiation of RNA copying. The 5′ untranslated region (5′UTR) plays an important role in directing the translation of the HCV polyprotein from an internal (methionine) codon. RNA secondary structure formation allows direct binding of the host cell ribosome to internal sequences in the 5′UTR (known as the internal ribosomal entry site, or IRES), bypassing the conventional attachment to the (capped) end of the RNA molecule, as is found in translation of cellular mRNAs.

Hepatocytes are the principal sites of HCV replication in vivo, although there may be extrahepatic sites of replication including haemopoietic cells such as B lymphocytes, and stem cells in the bone marrow. The entry mechanism of HCV into hepatocytes (and other cell types) is complex and incompletely understood. A variety of cellular proteins are involved in the initial attachment of HCV to the cell (e.g. the LDL receptor, heparin sulphate, DC-SIGN, L-SIGN). Interaction with other host factors such as CD81, the scavenger receptor B-1 (SRB-1), claudin 1 and occludin leads to viral internalisation through endocytosis of the bound virion in a clathrin-coated endosome, and fusion of viral and endosomal membranes. *In vivo*, this likely occurs on the basolateral membrane surface of hepatocytes to allow concentration of the virion. On entering the cytoplasm, the RNA genome is released from the viral capsid and translated. The newly synthesized RNA replicating and unwinding enzymes, such as NS5B, NS5A and NS3, subsequently initiate transcription of the genomic RNA into a full-length negative-polarity copy, which in turn acts as the template for the production of multiple positive-stranded RNA copies. These can be used for further rounds of transcription, or used for the production of further viral proteins. Factors that regulate negative- and positive-strand synthesis and the use of the latter transcripts for translation remain undetermined, and are likely to be complex.

Replication of HCV takes place in membranous webs associated with the NS4B protein and cellular endoplasmic reticulum (ER). The core protein, however, remains within the cytoplasm after cleavage from E1, E1 and E2 are embedded in the ER membrane, and their extracellular domains are glycosylated. Details of the subsequent stages of capsid assembly and maturation, the insertion of HCV RNA, and the budding of HCV through the ER into extracytoplasmic space and release from the cell await further studies.

## Classification

HCV shows the greatest similarity in structure, size and genome organization with the flaviviruses. Together, these viruses are classified as members of the Flaviviridae (Table 52.1), currently divided into four named genera. The *Hepacivirus* genus contains HCV, a recently discovered canine homologue of HCV (canine hepacivirus; CHV) and GB virus-B, originally isolated from a captive tamarind, in which it causes acute hepatitis and liver disease similar to that of HCV in humans. Both GBV-B and CHV are currently under evaluation as possible experimental models for HCV vaccines and antiviral treatment.

Human pegivirus (HPgV, originally described as GB virus C or hepatitis G virus) is classified as a member of the recently described *Pegivirus* genus. This virus is widely distributed in humans and was originally thought to be a further agent involved in post-transfusion and chronic hepatitis of unexplained aetiology. This association has subsequently been disproved, and infection appears to be entirely asymptomatic, despite being persistent in a significant proportion of those it infects. Its genome shows a number

**Table 52.1** Members of the Flavivirus family

| Genus | Examples |
| --- | --- |
| *Hepacivirus* | Hepatitis C virus<br>Canine hepacivirus<br>GB virus B |
| *Pegivirus* | Human pegivirus (formerly GB virus C, hepatitis G virus)<br>Simian pegivirus (formerly GBV-A) and other homologues in non-human primates<br>Bat pegivirus (described as GBV-D) |
| *Pestivirus* | Bovine viral diarrhoea virus, types I and II<br>Swine vesicular disease virus (formerly hog cholera virus)<br>Border disease virus + less well characterized variants in other ruminant species |
| *Flavivirus* (examples of the 68 members) | Yellow fever virus<br>Dengue virus, serotypes 1–4<br>Tick-borne encephalitis virus, louping ill virus<br>Japanese encephalitis virus |

of similarities to that of HCV, including a 5'UTR that has similar ribosomal binding and internal initiation (although a different RNA secondary structure), while the coding region contains homologues to HCV structural and non-structural proteins. However, it lacks a protein corresponding to the core protein of HCV that forms the nucleocapsid. Viruses similar to HPgV are widely distributed in a range of non-human primate species (simian pegiviruses; formerly described as GBV-A) and in bats (bat pegivirus; originally described as GBV-D). The *pestivirus* genus contains viruses which are structurally similar to HCV and infect a number of domestic and wild species of ruminants such as pigs, sheep and cows.

## Genetic variation

Nucleotide sequences of HCV frequently show substantial differences from each other. This has led to the current genotypic classification of HCV, in which variants from a variety of geographical locations can be classified into 6 main genotypes and a very rare genotype 7, and a number of subtypes (Fig. 52.2). Genotypes show approximately 30% sequence divergence from each other, differences that greatly modify their antigenic properties, and their biology (see Treatment).

Some HCV genotypes (types 1a, 2a, 2b) show a broad worldwide distribution, while others such as

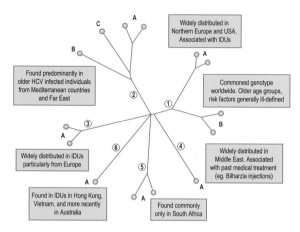

**Fig. 52.2** Comparison of complete genome sequences of the common genotypes of HCV plotted as a phylogenetic tree, showing the 6 main genetic groups (genotypes 1–6) and a number of the commoner subtypes (A, B, C). The distribution of the different genotypes in the principal risk groups for HCV infection is indicated.

type 5a and 6a are only found in specific geographical regions (South Africa and South East Asia respectively). HCV infection in blood donors and patients with chronic hepatitis from countries in Western Europe and the USA frequently involves genotypes 1a, 1b, 2a, 2b and 3a. The relative frequencies of each may vary geographically, such as the trend for more frequent infection with type 1b in southern and Eastern Europe, and the association of genotype 1a and 3a infection with infection through drug use. HCV genotypes can be identified by analysis of sequences from the 5'UTR or from coding regions. Methods for rapid genotyping of HCV have been developed, and play a role in the pre-treatment assessment of patients receiving antiviral treatment (See Treatment).

## Virus stability

HCV is inactivated by exposure to chloroform, ether and other organic solvents and by detergents. The effectiveness of a number of virus-inactivating procedures have been demonstrated by studies of the infectivity of products manufactured from plasma such as the factor VIII and IX concentrates used to treat haemophiliacs. For example, dry-heat treatment at 80°C or wet-heat treatment at 60°C, organic solvents (*n*-heptane) and detergents have been shown to efficiently remove HCV infectivity.

## LABORATORY DIAGNOSIS

Chronic infection with HCV is associated with the presence of both plasma viraemia and antibody to HCV. Methods to detect both antibody and HCV directly are used for diagnosis of HCV infection.

The technical simplicity of antibody testing has favoured its use for general screening and diagnostic testing. Antibody tests for HCV are based upon cloned HCV RNA sequences of HCV genotype 1a originally derived from an experimentally infected chimpanzee. Recombinant proteins expressed from these clones have formed and remain the basis for almost all assays for antibody to HCV since then. Current assays incorporate antigens from the core, NS3, NS4 and NS5 regions to produce assays of high sensitivity and specificity for antibody to HCV of all HCV genotypes.

Testing for antibody to HCV is normally carried out as a two stage procedure. An ELISA format is used for initial testing of serum or plasma from patients or blood donors. Repeatedly reactive samples are then re-tested by a second ELISA in a different format or by a supplementary assay such as the recombinant immunoblot assay (RIBA) that contains a number of separate HCV antigens. Currently used serological tests for anti-HCV are now highly sensitive and specific in most patient groups, although individuals who are immunosuppressed, such as those co-infected with HIV, on renal dialysis, or transplant patients, and those with congenital immunodeficiencies can produce false-negative serological test results. In these cases, direct detection methods for viral RNA or antigen are required.

## Direct detection methods

While current screening and supplementary serological tests will detect the vast majority of infections, there remains a considerable window period in HCV infection between exposure and development of antibody detectable by the best current ELISAs (Fig. 52.3). Also, the presence of antibodies to HCV does not allow distinction between past, cleared infection and current infection. For these reasons, further direct methods for the detection of HCV antigens or RNA sequences are required for the effective diagnosis of HCV infection in acute hepatitis, for diagnosis of HCV infection in immunosuppressed individuals who do not mount a detectable antibody response, and to identify current, as opposed to past, infection. Genome detection methods have also been widely adopted in addition to serological tests for the routine screening of blood donors for HCV in most Western countries.

Direct detection methods are based upon either the detection of HCV RNA sequences by the polymerase chain reaction (PCR) or other nucleic acid amplification methods, or of viral antigens by ELISA.

**Fig. 52.3** Virological and biochemical markers of acute HCV infection. HCV RNA (red line) and abnormal ALT levels (blue line) appear approximately 4–6 weeks after exposure to HCV in a typical individual. The subsequent development of chronic hepatitis is indicated by persistent viraemia and by fluctuating abnormal ALT levels. Antibody to HCV first appears after the onset of acute hepatitis, in this example leading to 'window periods' of around 100–150 days for the first generation serological assay (containing only NS3 and NS4 proteins) and approximately 60–80 days for second and third generation assays (containing additional NS3, NS5 and core proteins).

Reverse transcriptase PCR is the most commonly used method for direct detection of HCV. Diagnostic PCR methods are commercially available and are capable of high sensitivity and specificity for the detection of HCV RNA sequences in plasma (or liver biopsy) specimens. Alternative, non-PCR-based methods, such as transcript-mediated amplification, have recently been developed and provide comparable sensitivity. An alternative to nucleic acid detection is the use of ELISA-based methods for the detection of HCV core protein in plasma, and more recently combined antibody/antigen detection methods.

Direct virus detection is the only reliable method of monitoring the effect of treatment with antiviral drugs in patients with chronic infection since normalization of liver biochemistry is not always associated with virus clearance, and chronic HCV infection with associated disease may arise in patients with normal liver functions tests. Quantitation of the virus genome titre is now increasingly possible with commercial tests based on real-time PCR, other amplification methods or hybridization, and is used as a predictor for response to antiviral therapy (see Treatment).

## EPIDEMIOLOGY

In Western Europe, Australia and North America, most HCV-infected patients have a history of parenteral exposure to the virus, and the majority are, or have been, injecting drug users (IDUs). The infection rate of IDUs has been estimated at 20% per year, so long-term drug users are almost invariably HCV-infected. Drug use was uncommon before the 1960s and so infected drug users tend to be younger than patients infected by blood transfusion or other routes. Most drug users have asymptomatic infection with no

history of jaundice but have chronic hepatitis; few have overt clinical signs or symptoms of liver disease or liver failure.

Other blood-borne routes of HCV transmission include blood transfusion before 1991 (when universal donor screening was initiated), and receipt of pooled plasma products such as factor VIII, and immunoglobulin manufactured before 1986 (when virus-inactivation procedures for plasma-derived blood products became widely used). Other at-risk groups include transplant recipients, haemodialysis patients, and healthcare workers from needle-stick injuries. Tattooing and acupuncture may also be responsible for some percutaneous exposure, and in countries of high prevalence, the use of unsterilized needles for cultural rituals, medical treatment or vaccination programmes may result in HCV infection.

The lowest frequencies of HCV infection are found in Scandinavian and other Northern European countries such as the United Kingdom (0.3–0.4%), with slightly higher prevalences in North America (1%) and Australia. Prevalence is intermediate in Eastern and Southern European countries, higher in Japan, and most prevalent in the Middle East; frequencies of HCV infection of up 30% have been recorded in areas of Egypt. In this latter case, bilharzia treatment using reusable and unsterile needles in the 1960s has been identified as the main source of infection.

There is little evidence for non-parenteral transmission of HCV. For example, there is little convincing evidence for transmission by sexual contact where compounding factors have been removed. Mother-to-child transmission of HCV occurs at frequencies between 3–10% in the majority of studies. Transmission occurs generally at birth, presumably through contact with blood (some evidence suggests that elective Caesarian section may prevent transmission).

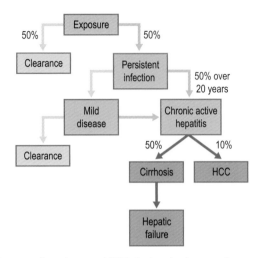

**Fig. 52.4** Natural course of HCV infection, showing approximate frequencies and time course of persistence, and of progression to clinically significant disease.

## CLINICAL FEATURES

Hepatitis C infection causes an indolent and slowly progressive liver disease that is asymptomatic until the development of cirrhosis and decompensated liver disease, or liver cancer (Fig. 52.4).

### Acute hepatitis

Exposure to HCV usually results in an asymptomatic infection without jaundice, with only 25–50% patients clearing the infection spontaneously – the remainder become chronically infected. Most studies have reported an interval of around 8 weeks to the development of abnormal liver function tests (such as alanine aminotransferase (ALT) levels) (Fig. 52.3). Clinically, hepatitis caused by HCV is indistinguishable from that caused by other hepatitis viruses; jaundice may develop, but more usually symptoms are non-specific such as fatigue, anorexia and nausea. Viraemia can be detected in the early stages of acute hepatitis, appearing at the same time or slightly earlier than abnormal ALT levels, while seroconversion for antibody may be delayed for several weeks or months after the onset of hepatitis. Histologic features of acute HCV are similar to those associated with acute HAV and HBV infection; liver biopsy is rarely indicated to make a diagnosis of acute HCV infection.

### Chronic hepatitis

The frequency of chronic infection following exposure to HCV is between 50 and 75% (Fig. 52.4). Chronic infection with HCV is generally associated with persistent and progressive hepatitis, with fluctuating or continuously abnormal ALT levels. Although viraemia is invariably detected in patients with chronic hepatitis, there is no correlation between level of viraemia and the severity of liver disease, ALT levels or other biochemical abnormalities associated with hepatitis.

HCV infection causes a range of characteristic histological changes in the liver, although few allow a specific diagnosis of HCV infection to be made. These include lymphoid follicles within the portal tracts, a dense periportal inflammatory process, bile duct damage, and lobular hepatitis, with lymphocyte infiltration within sinusoids surrounding the hepatocytes. Chronic infection with genotype 3 HCV is particularly associated with the development of fatty change in the liver (steatosis). There are a variety of 'scoring systems' or histological activity indices (HAI) available (e.g. Knodell, Ishak, Metavir), designed to assess the degree of liver damage as seen on biopsy.

The percentage of chronically infected individuals who progress to cirrhosis and liver failure is not known. When chronic hepatitis does progress to clinically significant liver damage, then progression is almost invariably very slow, although faster progression may be associated with risk factors such as alcohol ingestion, older age, and immunodeficiency. Particularly aggressive HCV-associated liver disease has been observed in immunosuppressed organ transplant recipients, and in patients with inherited immunodeficiency states. Cirrhosis is rarely observed within 10 years of infection, but around 20% of infected patients have cirrhosis after 20 years follow-up. Cirrhosis may be complicated by liver failure (decompensated cirrhosis), manifested as jaundice, portal hypertension and variceal bleeding; these manifestations of liver failure are shared with other forms of cirrhosis. Hepatocellular carcinoma (HCC) frequently complicates chronic hepatitis C, although HCC is rare within 15 years of initial infection. In many Western countries such as Spain and Italy, and, in Japan, HCV infection is found in 60–90% cases of HCC.

### Extrahepatic manifestations

In a minority of infected patients, HCV may be responsible for extrahepatic clinical manifestations and disease. These include certain types of vasculitis and glomerulonephritis caused by immune complex deposition. Associations between HCV infection and Sjogren's syndrome, essential mixed cryoglobulinaemia and membranoproliferative glomerulonephritis type 1 have been suggested.

## TREATMENT AND CONTROL

Interferon-α (IFN-α) covalently linked to polyethylene glycol (PEG-IFN), combined with oral Ribavirin (RBV) is the current standard treatment for chronic HCV infection. Pegylation prolongs the half-life of the interferon, so dosing is restricted to once weekly injection. Response to therapy is monitored by quantitative PCR for detection of viral RNA. Three patterns are observed – non-response, response but with relapse after cessation of therapy, and sustained virological response (SVR, see Fig. 52.5). Duration of therapy, and likelihood of a successful outcome, are governed by viral genotype (see below). Overall, around 50% of patients achieve an SVR, i.e. viral RNA is not detectable 6 months after the end of therapy, which equates to having been cured. In an attempt to improve response rates, and to avoid the unnecessary treatment of potential non-responders, clinical and virological features associated with SVR have been defined. The most important factors follow.

*HCV genotype.* Sensitivity to current standard-of-care therapy varies significantly between genotypes. Six months therapy in patients infected with genotypes 2a, 2b and 3a results in SVR rates of the order of 75–80%, whereas even prolonged (12 months) therapy in patients infected with genotypes 1 or 4 still only results in around 45% achieving SVR. Limited data indicates an intermediate response rate for genotypes 5 and 6. The mechanism by which different genotypes differ in their susceptibility to treatment remains unknown, particularly as the mechanisms of action of PEG-IFN and RBV are unknown in this

context. It is unlikely that the greater response rates achieved with types 2 and 3 are simply secondary to differences in disease severity. Pre-treatment assessment of genotype is essential in order to specify the dose and duration of therapy likely to give the best chance of obtaining a sustained clearance of viraemia.

*IL-28B genotype.* Recent genome-wide association studies have identified a series of linked single nucleotide polymorphisms close to IL-28B (also known as interferon Lambda-3), a recently characterised antiviral cytokine distantly related to type I IFNs and IL-10, that are associated with treatment response. The frequencies of the 'good' and 'bad' responder alleles differ markedly in populations of different ethnic origins, which largely accounts for the observation that response rates in Caucasians are invariably higher than those in, say, black African-Americans. These polymorphisms are also associated with differences in spontaneous clearance of HCV infection after exposure. They likely represent, or are closely genetically linked to, key factor(s) governing infection outcomes of HCV.

*Immunosuppression.* Subjects co-infected with HIV-1 (even when controlled with anti-retroviral therapy) and immunosuppressed individuals (genetic immunodeficiencies, iatrogenic, those with systemic disease such as leukaemia) all show reduced response rates to therapy, emphasising the necessary role of the adaptive immune system in virus clearance.

*Disease progression.* Patients with advanced HCV-related disease such as cirrhosis or decompensated liver disease respond poorly to therapy; the latter are best referred for transplant (see below).

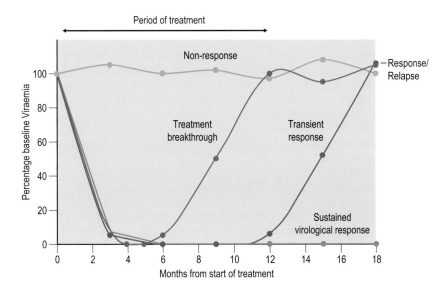

**Fig. 52.5** Outcomes of combination therapy with pegylated interferon and ribavirin in chronic hepatitis C. Non-responders (NR) are those where HCV RNA remains detectable at high levels during and after cessation of treatment. Among those initially achieving virus clearance, a proportion will relapse during therapy (treatment breakthrough) and many more will relapse at conclusion of therapy. These patients are collectively referred to as responder/relapsers (RR). The desired outcome is a sustained virological response (SVR), where individuals remain non-viraemic for 6 months (and longer) from the cessation of treatment.

*Baseline viral load and early treatment response.* High viral loads are associated with a reduced likelihood of achieving a sustained response to treatment. Monitoring of viral loads early in treatment is also predictive of outcome; rapid reduction, particularly if associated with clearance of detectable viraemia by 4 weeks of therapy, a so-called rapid virological response (RVR), is the best single predictor of eventual SVR. Patients with a low pretreatment viral load who achieve an RVR may be given shortened duration of therapy (e.g. only 6 months for genotype 1, or 16 weeks for genotype 2 or 3) without altering their chances of eventual success.

A new generation of drugs with specific antiviral actions against HCV are under active development. The first two of these agents, telaprevir and boceprevir, were licensed for clinical use in 2011 as an adjunct to PEG-IFN-α/RBV therapy of genotype 1 infections. The three main classes of anti-HCV drugs currently leading in development are inhibitors of the viral NS3/4A protease (e.g. Telaprevir, Boceprevir), inhibitors of the NS5B RNA polymerase (e.g. Mericitabine), and inhibitors of the multi-functional NS5A protein (e.g. Alisporivir, BMS-790052). Analogous to the antiretrovirals used for HIV therapy, polymerase inhibitors are either nucleoside analogues that cause chain termination of RNA transcripts, or non-nucleoside protein binding inhibitors of RNA polymerase. Also analogous to HIV therapy is the potential for rapid development of antiviral resistance during therapy through mutations in the genes encoding the target viral proteins.

To date, almost all trials have evaluated the additive effect of antiviral drugs to the efficacy of PEG-IFN-α/RBV therapy. For example, addition of Telaprevir increases the clearance rate in genotype 1-infected trial subjects from around 50% to nearly 80%. Addition of protease inhibitors additionally substantially increases the effectiveness of re-treatment in those who had previously failed with conventional therapy. In the longer term, it may perhaps be possible to treat with multiple antiviral drug combinations (without interferon) to suppress virus replication sufficiently before drug resistance develops. HCV genotypes respond differently to certain classes of antivirals; for example, genotypes 1 and 4 are more effectively inhibited by current protease inhibitors than genotypes 2 and 3. This differential susceptibility is opposite to the genotype-associated differences in responsiveness to PEG-IFN/RV therapy described above.

*Liver transplantation.* Liver transplantation is indicated for patients with decompensated HCV cirrhosis, and for some patients with hepatocellular carcinoma complicating HCV infection. Liver transplantation does not cure HCV infection, and re-infection of the graft, with subsequent rapidly progressive liver disease, is frequently encountered.

## Prevention

Screening of blood donors has proved to be effective at preventing transmission of HCV infection through blood transfusion. A combination of blood donor screening and virus inactivation has virtually eliminated HCV transmission by blood products such as clotting factor concentrates and immunoglobulins.

The main continuing risks for HCV transmission are injecting drug use and the use of unsterile needles for medical and dental procedures, tattooing and other percutaneous exposures. Much of this could be prevented by education, greater availability of disposable needles, and for drug users by needle exchange programmes. Many of the public health measures adopted to prevent transmission of HIV by parenteral routes will assist efforts at controlling HCV.

## Immunization

The development of a vaccine for HCV faces a series of formidable obstacles, amongst which viral heterogeneity, and the difficulty in evaluating candidate vaccines in suitable animal models, are the most acute. Recombinant envelope proteins (E1 and E2) have been shown to induce a short-lived specific anti-E1 and E2 response in immunized chimpanzees, and transient protection from challenge with the same virus strain. There is, however, little prospect of an effective vaccine for human use in the coming decade.

Infection with HCV is a growing medical problem worldwide. A combination of public health preventative measures, improved diagnosis, screening, antiviral treatment and immunization will undoubtedly all be required to combat its spread in the future.

## HEPATITIS E VIRUS

### DESCRIPTION

Hepatitis E virus was characterized in 1991. The virion is non-enveloped, with a genome of single-stranded RNA of positive sense. It is classified as a *Hepevirus*. Virion structure and genome organization resemble those of the caliciviruses; there is also some similarity with rubella and other togaviruses. There is a single serotype with strong cross-reactions among the four known human species (HEV-1, -2, -3 and -4) and also with other unidentified viruses of mammals as well as an avian virus.

## CLINICAL FEATURES

The disease has an incubation period of 15–60 days (average 40 days). The clinical features are those of acute hepatitis with anorexia, fever, abdominal pain, nausea and vomiting. The urine darkens and the stools lighten. Liver function tests show hepatocellular damage, and jaundice develops.

Most clinical cases occur in those aged 15–40 years. Infections in younger patients are mostly mild and anicteric.

The virus is acquired by the oral route; virus excretion can be detected about 4 weeks after infection and persists for about 2 weeks. Evidence of liver damage can be found after about 3 months. The overall mortality rate is 1–3%, but can reach 15–25% in the third trimester of pregnancy.

Chronic infection has been described recently in the context of heavily immunosuppressed patients e.g. liver transplant recipients or HIV-infected individuals.

## LABORATORY DIAGNOSIS

Antibodies to the virus can be measured and show the usual profile of IgM and IgG responses. Reverse transcriptase–PCR can be used to detect viral RNA, although it is not widely available.

## EPIDEMIOLOGY AND TRANSMISSION

The virus is acquired orally and outbreaks, often involving many thousands of cases, are linked to faecal contamination of water supplies or food. Unlike hepatitis A, there is little evidence of person-to-person transmission. Several large water-borne outbreaks have been recognized in Africa, India, China and Mexico. Infection is endemic in undeveloped areas of the world, and HEV is the cause of more than 50% of cases of sporadic hepatitis. In the developed world the prevalence of antibody to the virus is less than 2%, and most cases are seen in travellers returning from endemic areas, although there is good evidence that there are endemic HEV strains within the UK and other Western European countries, as several cases of acute infection have been described in individuals with no travel history.

Antibody studies suggest that several animal species, including primates, pigs, cows, sheep, goats and rodents, may be infected with HEV or related viruses. Strains from swine are related to human strains 3 and 4. The virus may be maintained in endemic areas by person-to-person transmission or in a non-human reservoir.

## TREATMENT AND CONTROL

There is no specific therapy, although ribavirin has been shown to be effective in cases of chronic infection. Prevention requires the provision of safe clean water and raising standards of food hygiene. Travellers should take the same precautions as recommended for protection from any faecal–oral infection.

Passive immunization is not available. Studies to develop a vaccine are under way.

### RECOMMENDED READING

Alter MJ: Epidemiology of hepatitis C virus infection, *World Journal of Gastroenterology* 13:2436–2441, 2007.

Dalton HR, Bendall R, Ijaz S, Banks M: Hepatitis E: an emerging infection in developed countries, *Lancet Infectious Diseases* 8:698–709, 2008.

Hofmann WP, Zeuzem S: A new standard of care for the treatment of chronic HCV infection, *Nature Reviews Gastroenterology & Hepatology* 8:257–264, 2011.

Houghton M, Abrignani S: Prospects for a vaccine against the hepatitis C virus, *Nature* 436:961–966, 2005.

Lindenbach BD, Rice CM: Unravelling hepatitis C virus replication from genome to function, *Nature* 436:933–938, 2005.

Poenisch M, Bartenschlager R: New insights into structure and replication of the hepatitis C virus and clinical implications, *Seminars in Liver Disease* 30:333–347, 2010.

Vermehren J, Sarrazin C: New HCV therapies on the horizon, *Clinical Microbiology and Infection* 17:122–134, 2011.

# 53 Arenaviruses and filoviruses

## Viral haemorrhagic fevers

*D. Safronetz, H. Feldmann and D. Falzarano*

## KEY POINTS

- Members of the arenavirus and filovirus families can cause a spectrum of clinical symptoms with the most severe form being a viral haemorrhagic fever (e.g. Lassa, Junin and Machupo viruses (arenaviruses) and Marburg and Ebola viruses (filoviruses)).
- Viral haemorrhagic fever initially presents with non-specific symptoms such as fever, headache, and muscle and joint pain; pharyngitis; and later nausea, vomiting and diarrhoea. There follows increasing fever, abdominal pain, oedema and enlarged lymph nodes with bleeding from gums, nose, vagina and into the gut; however, overt bleeding is typically not the cause of death.
- The reservoirs for arenaviruses are certain rodent species; while the reservoirs for filoviruses may be multiple species of fruit bats.
- Person-to-person transmission typically requires close contact and/or exposure to contaminated body fluids or tissues. This transmission route is notorious for hospital-acquired infections.
- Experimental data suggests that vaccines against members of both the arenaviruses and filoviruses are possible; however, the only approved vaccine is for Junin and is only available for use in Argentina.
- Convalescent plasma and ribavirin appear to be possible treatments for certain arenavirus infections but efficacy has not been demonstrated for filoviruses.

# ARENAVIRUSES

## INTRODUCTION

The family Arenaviridae consists of a single genus (*Arenavirus*) which is currently comprised of 23 unique viral species, as recognized by the International Committee for Taxonomy of Viruses, at least 10 of which are associated with human disease. Arenaviruses are categorized into two complexes based largely on antigenic properties, and more recently genetic analysis. These groups correspond in general to the geographic distribution of the viruses and rodent reservoirs, and are therefore classified as either 'Old' or 'New World' arenaviruses (Fig. 53.1, Table 53.1). The prototype arenavirus, Lymphocytic choriomeningitis (LCM) virus, was initially discovered in 1933, and although classified as an 'Old World' virus, has a worldwide distribution due to the global movement of its rodent reservoir, the common house mouse (*Mus musculus*). In addition to LCM virus, the 'Old World' lineage contains several African arenaviruses, the most prevalent of which is Lassa virus. The 'New World' arenaviruses are divided into three clades (A, B and C). The most prominent lineage is clade B which contains the highly pathogenic arenaviruses responsible for South American haemorrhagic fevers. By comparison, clades A and C are much smaller and are mainly comprised of viruses currently believed to be non-pathogenic to humans. Recently, genetic analysis of arenaviruses isolated from North America has suggested the presence of a fourth recombinant (rec) clade (A/rec), which is comprised of viruses with genetic characteristics of both clade A and B viruses. Recent advances in genetic sequencing techniques, coupled with increased surveillance, is accelerating new arenavirus discoveries, as evidenced by the recent identification of Lujo virus, the first pathogenic arenavirus discovered in Africa in nearly four decades.

## PROPERTIES

Members of the family Arenaviridae contain a genome of two segments of single-stranded, negative sense RNA (Fig. 53.2A). Each segment contains two non-overlapping open reading frames of opposite polarity

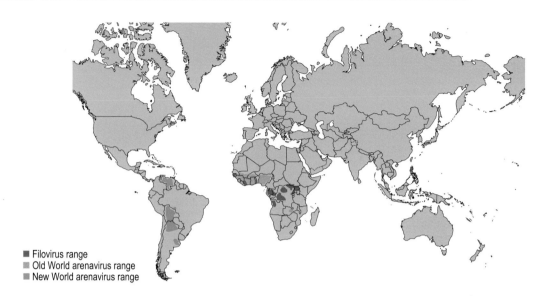

- Filovirus range
- Old World arenavirus range
- New World arenavirus range

**Fig. 53.1** Approximate geographic distributions of arenaviruses and filoviruses. The potential geographic range of the 'Old World' and 'New World' arenaviruses and the filoviruses is indicated based on known human cases and host reservoir sampling. LCM virus has a predicted worldwide distribution and is not indicated.

**Table 53.1** Members of the arenaviridae and filoviridae

|  | Year first isolated | Human disease | Natural host | Distribution |
|---|---|---|---|---|
| **Old World** | | | | |
| Lymphocytic choriomeningitis | 1933 | Mild to severe meningitis | *Mus musculus, Mus domesticus* | Worldwide |
| Lassa | 1975 | Asymptomatic to severe VHF | *Mastomys natalensis* | West Africa |
| Ippy | 1970 | Not known | *Arvicanthus* spp. | Central African Republic |
| Mopeia | 1977 | Not known | *Mastomys natalensis* | Eastern Africa |
| Mobala | 1983 | Not known | *Praomys jacksoni* | Central African Republic |
| Kodoko | 2007[a] | Not known | *Mus minutoides* | Guinea |
| Lujo | 2008 | VHF | Not known | Southern Africa |
| Morogoro | 2009 | Not known | *Mastomys* spp. | Tanzania |
| Merino Walk | 2010 | Not known | *Myotomys unisulcatus* | South Africa |
| **New World (clade)** | | | | |
| Junín (B) | 1958 | Argentinian VHF | *Callomys musculinus* | Argentina |
| Machupo (B) | 1965 | Bolivian VHF | *Callomys callosus* | Bolivia |
| Tacaribe (B) | 1963 | Not known | *Artibeus* bat | West Indies |
| Amapari (B) | 1966 | Not known | *Oryzomys goeldi, Neacomys guianae* | Brazil |
| Paraná (A) | 1970 | Not known | *Oryzomys buccinatus* | Paraguay |
| Tamiami (A/rec)[b] | 1970 | Asymptomatic | *Sigmodon hispidus* | USA |
| Cupixi (B) | 1970 | Not known | *Oryzomys capito* | Brazil |
| Pichinde (A) | 1971 | Not known | *Oryzomys albigularis* | Columbia |
| Latino (C) | 1973 | Not known | *Callomys callosus* | Bolivia |
| Flexal (A) | 1977 | VHF[c] | *Oryzomys* spp. | Brazil |
| Guanarito (B) | 1989 | Venezuelan VHF | *Sigmodon alstoni, Zygodontomys brevicauda* | Venezuela |
| Sabiá (B) | 1994 | Brazilian VHF | Not known | Brazil |
| Oliveros (C) | 1996 | Not known | *Necromys benefactus* | Argentina |
| Pirital (A) | 1997 | Not known | *Sigmodon alstoni* | Venezuela |
| Allpahuayo (A) | 1997 | Not known | *Oecomys bicolor, Oecomys paricola* | Peru |

**Table 53.1** Continued

| | Year first isolated | Human disease | Natural host | Distribution |
|---|---|---|---|---|
| Whitewater Arroyo (A/rec) | 2000 | VHF, suspected[d] | *Neotoma albigula, Neotoma mexicana* | USA |
| Bear Canyon (A/rec) | 2002 | Not known | *Netotoma macrotis, Peromyscus californicus* | USA |
| Chapare (B) | 2004 | VHF | Not known | Bolivia |
| Catarina (A/rec) | 2007 | Not known | *Neotoma micropus* | USA |
| Pinhal (C) | 2007[a] | Not known | *Calomys tener* | Brazil |
| Skinner Tank (A/rec) | 2008 | Not known | *Neotoma mexicana* | USA |
| **Filoviruses** | | | | |
| Lake Victoria marburgvirus | 1967 | VHF | *Rousettus aegyptiacus, Hypsignathus monstrosus* | Angola, DRC[e], Kenya, Uganda, Zimbabwe |
| Zaire ebolavirus | 1976 | VHF | *Epomops franqueti, Hypsignathus monstrosus, Myonycteris torquata, Micropteropus pusillus, Mops condylurus, Rousettus aegyptiacus* | DRC, RC[f], Gabon |
| Sudan ebolavirus | 1976 | VHF | Not known | Sudan, Uganda |
| Reston ebolavirus | 1989 | Not known | Not known | Philippines |
| Côte d'Ivoire ebolavirus | 1994 | VHF | Not known | Côte d'Ivoire |
| Bundibugyo ebolavirus | 2007 | VHF | Not known | Uganda |
| Lloviu cuevavirus | 2010[a] | Not known | *Miniopterus schreibersii* | Spain |

Names underlined indicate the viral species currently classified as members of the *Arenaviridae* and *Filoviridae* by the International Committee for Taxonomy of Viruses. Non-underlined names indicates recently discovered viruses whose taxonomic status remains to be determined.
VHF, viral haemorrhagic fever.
[a] Identification based on nucleotide sequence only, virus has yet to be isolated.
[b] Recently identified arenaviruses in North America appear to have genetic characteristics of both lineage A and B, and therefore represent a fourth recombinant lineage (A/rec).
[c] Moderate laboratory-associated infection described.
[d] A causal relationship between Whitewater Arroyo and three fatal cases has yet to be proven.
[e] Democratic Republic of the Congo.
[f] Republic of the Congo.

separated by a short hairpin configuration (ambisense coding strategy). The large (L) segment (approximately 7200 nucleotides) encodes in the genomic sense the viral polymerase and in the antigenomic sense the zinc-binding matrix protein (Z). The small (S) segment (approximately 3400 nucleotides) encodes in the genomic sense the nucleoprotein (NP) and in the antigenomic sense the glycoprotein precursor (GPC), which is post-translationally cleaved by cellular proteases into two envelope proteins, GP1 and GP2. The 5′ and 3′ terminal ends of both segments contain conserved complementary nucleotides, allowing for pan-handle formation resulting in the appearance of circular genomic segments (Fig. 53.2B). The virions are pleomorphic, enveloped particles with diameters ranging from 50–300 nm (typically between 110–130 nm) on electron microscopy and enclose a helical nucleocapsid (Fig. 53.2C). Virions contain not only virus genome but also host ribosomes (both 28S and 18S ribosomal RNA) which give the virus its characteristic grainy morphology and the family name (arena is derived from the Latin word for sand). The lipid envelope is derived from the host plasma membrane and T-shaped GP spikes extend 7–10 nm from its surface. Virions are relatively unstable and infectivity is abolished by ultraviolet or gamma irradiation, heating to 56°C, exposure to detergents or other lipid solvents, and pH outside the range 5.5–8.5.

## REPLICATION

Arenaviruses can replicate in a number of mammalian hosts and in many tissues. Most 'Old World' and clade C 'New World' arenaviruses use α-dystroglycan as a cellular receptor, whereas the haemorrhagic 'New World' arenaviruses (Junin, Machupo, Guanarito and Sabia) have been shown to use human transferrin receptor 1. Attachment is mediated by GP1, after which viral particles are taken up by endocytosis.

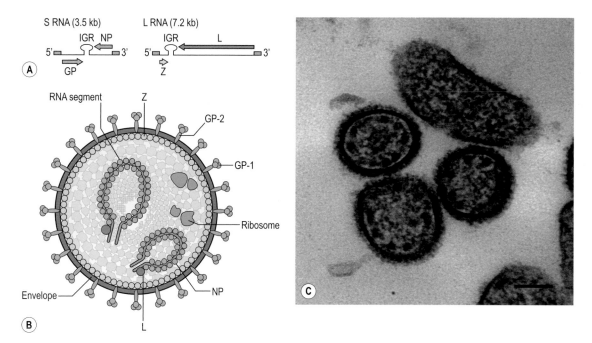

**Fig. 53.2** Particle structure and genome organization of arenaviruses. (A) Schematic diagram of the arenavirus genome. (B) An arenavirus particle. (C) Electron micrograph of Lassa virus particles.

Acidification of the endocytotic vesicle results in conformational changes in GP1/GP2 and allows the viral envelope to fuse with the vesicle membrane, releasing the nucleocapsid. Viral transcription and replication is restricted to the cytoplasm of infected cells and utilizes a cap-snatching mechanism. The NP and viral polymerase mRNAs are transcribed from genomic RNA, whereas GP and Z mRNAs are transcribed only from antisense transcripts of the genome. The intergenic stem-loop hairpins on both L and S segments serve as transcription terminators. The RNA polymerase (molecular weight 250 kDa) catalyses the production of both RNA transcripts and new genome RNA. The Z protein (11 kDa) is involved in viral transcription and serves as a structural protein, perhaps linking the glycoproteins to the nucleocapsid. The NP (63 kDa) is the most abundant protein with 1500–2000 copies per virion. The surface glycoproteins GP1 and GP2 are produced as a glycoprotein precursor on the rough endoplasmic reticulum. The precursor protein is glycosylated and cleaved by signal peptidase and SKI-1/S1P protease (or a closely related protease) to GP1 (43 kDa) and GP2 (35 kDa) in the Golgi apparatus prior to delivery to the cell surface. Together they form the T-shaped spikes with an estimated 650 copies of each per virion. The assembled virus, together with host ribosomes, is released by budding.

## CLINICAL FEATURES AND PATHOGENESIS

### Lymphocytic choriomeningitis virus

LCM virus is focally distributed throughout the world, though infection in humans is rare and typically mild or asymptomatic, except in immunocompromised individuals. Most infections are acquired by contact with laboratory mice or hamsters, though fatal infections have occurred after transplantation of infected tissues from LCM positive donors. During pregnancy, LCM virus infection can be severe and is associated with developmental defects in the fetus.

LCM infection, although rare, may present as:

- an undifferentiated febrile illness
- aseptic meningitis
- encephalitis.

The incubation period is 1–2 weeks and the illness is normally of short duration. It can vary from a mild disease with headache and fever to neck stiffness, myalgia and photophobia. Long-term effects including persistent headache, paralysis and psychological changes have been described. Although persistent infection and T cell reactivity to epitopes on GP2 associated with disease manifestation have been described in mice, there is no evidence of either in human infections.

## Lassa fever

Lassa fever was first documented in 1969 and is now known to be endemic in West Africa, especially Nigeria, Liberia, Sierra Leone and Guinea. Lassa virus has also been described in Mali, Ivory Coast and surrounding countries, suggesting a larger region of endemicity than previously thought. Throughout West Africa as many as 500 000 people are infected annually, with approximately 3000–5000 deaths. In addition, several imported cases of Lassa fever have been diagnosed in Europe and North America over the last few decades, making Lassa virus a prominent aetiological agent of viral haemorrhagic fever with a high impact on public health systems worldwide. Similar to other arenaviruses, contact with infected rodent hosts (*Mastomys natalensis*), or ingestion/inhalation of virus laden particles is a common source of human infection, however person-to-person transmission is also well documented and can result in outbreaks, especially in hospital settings.

The majority of Lassa virus infections are asymptomatic or mild in nature; however, approximately 20% of infections demonstrate moderate to severe disease, and can be associated with haemorrhagic manifestations and multi-organ failure. The incubation period is 1–3 weeks with a gradual onset of fever, headache, and muscle and joint pain. Pharyngitis with a non-productive cough is a common feature. In severe cases there is vomiting, diarrhoea, increased levels of liver enzymes (ALT and AST) and a raised haematocrit. Abdominal and retrosternal pain, oedema of the face and neck, enlarged lymph nodes and/or haemorrhage in the conjunctiva or mucosal surfaces are particularly indicative of a poor prognosis. Recovery takes 1–3 weeks and can be associated with hearing loss.

In fatal cases the fever is maintained and rapid deterioration occurs over the first 2 weeks, associated with:

- hypovolaemia, hypotension, pleural effusion, ascites and anuria
- bleeding from the gums, nose, intestine or vagina, linked to platelet dysfunction
- acute neurological changes varying from unilateral or bilateral deafness (in one-third of patients), to signs of encephalopathy including generalized seizures, dystonia and neuropsychiatric changes.

Infection in pregnancy (especially the third trimester) is particularly severe with maternal mortality rates of approximately 20% and fetal mortality rates near 100%. In children, infection is associated with a 'swollen baby' syndrome consisting of widespread oedema, abdominal distension and bleeding. Blood platelet and lymphocyte counts fall early in the illness. Endothelial cell damage leads to extravascular fluid loss and thus oedema and, together with platelet loss and dysfunction, to the haemorrhagic manifestations. Viraemia can persist for weeks and reaches high levels in severe and fatal cases.

Until recently, Lassa virus was the only arenavirus associated with haemorrhagic fever in Africa. However, in 2008 a small outbreak of unexplained haemorrhagic fever occurred in South Africa after a severely ill patient was medically evacuated from Zambia. A novel arenavirus was isolated and named Lujo virus. In total, Lujo infected 5 people, 4 of whom contracted the virus through secondary or tertiary transmission, and resulted in 4 deaths.

## South American haemorrhagic fever

Argentinian, Bolivian, Venezuelan and Brazilian haemorrhagic fevers are caused by Junin, Machupo, Guanarito and Sabia viruses, respectively. Of these, Argentinian haemorrhagic fever (AHF) represents the most significant public health concern, with cases occurring annually in a constantly expanding endemic region. AHF is seasonal (from April to June) and cases or epidemics occur every year, with several hundred cases being reported annually. In untreated individuals the mortality rate ranges from 15–30%. Approximately 80% of Junin infections demonstrate mild to moderate symptoms. Following a 1–2 week incubation period, AHF begins with a gradual onset of nondescript symptoms (e.g. fever, muscle ache, dizziness, lymph node swelling, flushing of the face neck and upper chest). After 6–10 days, 20–30% of patients progress to more serious, multi-system disease with neurological and haemorrhagic manifestations. Cardiovascular and renal involvements are uncommon, but can occur. In severe disease petechiae develop and there can be bleeding from the gastrointestinal tract. Leakage of fluid through damaged vascular endothelium leads to hypotension, oliguria and hypovolaemic shock; encephalopathy occurs in many patients. Raised levels of tumour necrosis factor (TNF)-$\alpha$ and thrombopoietin are proportional to disease severity.

Severe AHF is associated with:

- neurological symptoms including confusion, ataxia and tremors which can progress to convulsions and coma
- haemorrhagic manifestations, resulting from thrombocytopenia, which can include hematomas,

blood in vomit, sputum and urine as well as bleeding from gums, nose, vagina and gastrointestinal tract
- secondary bacterial infections, especially pneumonia and septicaemia, are common and complicate recovery.

In contrast to Junin infections, Machupo and Guanarito viruses are typically associated with sporadic outbreaks with similar clinical manifestations and mortality rates as AHF. To date, Sabia virus has been associated with one confirmed naturally occurring infection (initially thought to be yellow fever virus (YFV)) and two laboratory acquired infections.

In 2004, a novel arenavirus, subsequently named Chapare virus, was isolated from a fatal case associated with a small outbreak of haemorrhagic fever in Bolivia. Due to the remote location, the scope of the original outbreak remains unknown, as does the incidence and detailed manifestations of disease. Flexal and Tacaribe viruses have caused laboratory-acquired haemorrhagic fever and, in 2000, a variant (approximately 89% similar) of Whitewater Arroyo virus is suspected to have caused three fatal cases of viral haemorrhagic fever in California, USA.

Despite the initial isolation of LCM virus over 80 years ago, arenaviruses remain emerging viruses which are often considered among the most neglected pathogens studied worldwide. Over the last several years the genus *Arenavirus* has continued to expand with discoveries of several novel arenaviruses, a few through outbreak investigations and many more from ecological studies of rodent hosts. The pathogenic potential of many of the new arenaviruses remains to be determined and therefore they cannot be ruled out as human pathogens.

## DIAGNOSIS

Diagnosis depends upon an initial clinical suspicion of infection and involves obtaining a history of potential contact associated with travel or with confirmed cases. Specific diagnosis depends on detection of the virus, its antigens and/or genome. A specific immune response may provide retrospective diagnosis or information on seroprevalence rates in given populations. With the exception of LCM virus, diagnosis of arenaviral infections should involve a national or international reference laboratory to provide recommendations for specimen collection, storage and transport as well as appropriate diagnostic tests.

## Genome detection

Genome detection by reverse transcriptase–polymerase chain reaction (RT-PCR) amplification either by conventional or real-time methods is commonly utilized for diagnosis of RNA viruses. RT-PCR is highly sensitive and specific, and is particularly valuable for early diagnosis; however, appropriate assays must be carefully selected. For example, the genetic diversity associated with Lassa virus is detrimental to the development of a specific real-time RT-PCR assay. Rather, conventional multiplex RT-PCR assays, targeting conserved regions of 'Old' and/or 'New World' arenaviruses have been developed to detect, and in some cases differentiate, these viruses.

## Antigen detection

Antigen detection from blood by antigen capture enzyme-linked immunosorbent assay (ELISA) or immunofluorescence assay (IFA) is useful for early diagnosis and for providing information on prognosis. Immunohistochemistry can be useful for laboratory confirmation of arenaviruses in tissue samples collected from fatal cases; however, this is rarely done due to the highly infectious nature of these agents and the risks associated with performing post-mortems.

## Serology

Antibody detection by ELISA is the most useful serological test and can be adapted to detect specific immunoglobulin (Ig) M responses in acute sera as well as IgG in convalescent serum samples. Care should be taken however when interpreting apparently negative results in acute samples since with some arenaviruses, most particularly Lassa virus, the development of specific IgM and IgG antibody responses can be delayed.

## Virus isolation

Arenaviruses that cause viral haemorrhagic fever are all considered category A, biosafety level 4 agents and culture from confirmed cases should not be attempted except in designated high containment facilities. Arenaviruses can be isolated from:

- blood or serum in acutely infected patients
- throat swabs, breast milk, cerebrospinal fluid, urine or a variety of tissues taken by biopsy/autopsy.

Cell culture (BHK-21, Vero E6 or Vero 76 cells) is the most convenient and efficient mode of isolation.

Animals (suckling mice, guinea-pigs, hamsters) have also been used with limited success.

## TREATMENT

For AHF (Junin virus), infusion of high-titre convalescent plasma is beneficial; especially if given within the first week of illness and can reduce mortality rates to as low as 1%. However, approximately 10% of those receiving immunotherapy develop a neurological syndrome 4–6 weeks later, which is generally reversible. Intravenous ribavirin, a broad spectrum nucleoside analogue antiviral, is effective against Lassa virus infections and has been shown to reduce mortality rates in cases of severe disease from 55% to 5% if administered early in the infection (within 6 days). There is also anecdotal evidence of ribavirin being beneficial in the treatment of Junin, Sabia and Lujo virus infections, therefore ribavirin therapy should be considered early after symptom onset of any suspected arenavirus infection. Short of specific treatments, supportive care, including maintaining fluid, electrolyte and osmotic balance is critical for increasing survival rates.

## EPIDEMIOLOGY AND TRANSMISSION

All arenavirus infections are zoonotic and the animal reservoir hosts are thought to be largely unaffected following infection. Rodent-to-rodent transmission likely occurs via both horizontal (i.e. between two animals not in a parent/offspring relationship) and vertical (i.e. mother-to-child) routes and results in persistent infections with excretion of the virus in excreta and secreta. Human infection usually occurs by inhalation/ingestion of particles contaminated with urine or saliva from infected rodents and rarely by direct methods (e.g. bites). Introduction of virus through open wounds and ingestion of infected rodent tissues also seems possible. In addition, laboratory acquired infections have been documented for several pathogenic arenaviruses and nosocomial transmission can be common when proper containment and infection control practices are not followed.

In general, arenaviruses persistently infect two of the rodent families:

1. The *Muridae* (house mice, *Mastomys* and *Praomys*) inhabit the same ecosystem as man.
2. The *Cricetidae* (voles, deer-mice, gerbils) inhabit open grasslands and it is only when they invade human territory, or vice versa, that human infections occur.

Tacaribe virus is the only arenavirus isolated from outside these two rodent families, being excreted by the fruit-bat *Artibeus*.

## CONTROL

As with all rodent-borne diseases, controlling reservoirs/vectors of disease is extremely difficult for arenaviruses. Therefore, medical interventions are paramount to controlling and preventing human illness; however, few approved vaccines or therapeutics currently exist. An effective Junin virus vaccine (Candid no. 1) is in use in Argentina. Experimental Lassa fever vaccines, including recombinant Vaccinia and Vesicular-stomatitis viruses expressing structural proteins of Lassa virus, have been shown to be highly effective in non-human primate models. Prophylaxis with oral ribavirin in contacts has also shown some benefit. In the absence of specific therapeutics and treatments, educational campaigns targeting rodent avoidance have become essential in infection control of arenaviruses. Suspected and confirmed cases of arenavirus hemorrhagic fever must be cared for in strict isolation in designated hospitals to prevent exposure of the attendant staff to the high levels of virus present in acutely ill patients. For imported cases, contact tracing is often carried out to assess the possibility of secondary transmission.

## FILOVIRUSES

## INTRODUCTION

Ebola (EBOV) and Marburg (MARV) viruses belong to the family Filoviridae (filamentous or thread-like viruses) in the order *Mononegavirales*. The genus *Ebolavirus* is further subdivided into 4 defined species based on serological cross-reactivity and genetic differences: *Zaire ebolavirus* (ZEBOV), *Sudan ebolavirus* (SEBOV), *Cote d'Ivoire ebolavirus* (CIEBOV), and *Reston ebolavirus* (REBOV) (see Table 53.1). A fifth species, *Bundibugyo ebolavirus* (BEBOV), has recently been proposed. This virus was isolated during an outbreak of haemorrhagic fever in Uganda in 2007. Lake Victoria marburgvirus (MARV) is currently the only recognized species in the *Marburgvirus* genus. Sequence data derived from bats in Spain identified a new filovirus, Lloviu cuevavirus, representing a tentative new genus, *Cuevavirus*, within the family Filoviridae; however, the actual virus has yet to be isolated. Currently, the most widely investigated isolates are

Zaire ebolavirus strain Mayinga, and Lake Victoria marburgvirus strain Musoke. Infection with either EBOV or MARV can result in severe haemorrhagic fever in humans and non-human primates, with case-fatality rates in humans as high as 90%.

## PROPERTIES

The non-segmented negative-sense RNA genome of filoviruses is approximately 19 kb in length with the following gene order: 3' leader, nucleoprotein (NP), virion protein (VP) 35, VP40, glycoprotein (GP), VP30, VP24, polymerase protein (L) and the 5' trailer (Fig. 53.3B). Virus particles are filamentous and can appear as U-shaped, 6-shaped, circular or branched (Fig. 53.3C). While they are uniformly 80 nm in diameter, they can vary in length from 800 to 14 000 nm, with peak infectivity ranging between 970 and 1200 nm. Virus particles possess a helical central core, known as the ribonucleoprotein complex (RNP), composed of NP, VP35, VP30, L and the viral RNA (Fig. 53.3A). The surface consists of a cell-derived lipid envelope containing the membrane-anchored glycoprotein ($GP_{1,2}$), which projects approximately 10 nm from the surface. The matrix proteins VP40 and VP24 underlie the membrane and it appears that VP40 is the driving force behind virus particle formation.

## REPLICATION

*In vitro* and *in vivo* studies have indicated that most cell types, with the exception of lymphoid cells, can be infected by filoviruses. The spike glycoprotein, $GP_{1,2}$, is the sole protein on the surface of the virion and mediates binding and entry into target cells. $GP_1$ is thought to interact with attachment factors and/or the virus receptor(s) to initiate entry, while the $GP_2$ subunit modulates membrane fusion. A number of different molecules have been shown to enhance infection; however, a definitive receptor has not been identified. Following attachment, the current paradigm is that EBOV is taken up by macropinocytosis in a glycoprotein-dependent manner. Subsequent release of the virus from the endosome requires membrane fusion. For EBOV it is predicted that a structural rearrangement of GP occurs following a decrease in pH in addition to cleavage of $GP_1$ by endosomal proteases. This allows $GP_2$ to insert its hydrophobic fusion peptide into the host membrane allowing the release of the ribonucleoprotein (RNP) complex into the cytoplasm. While not extensively studied, it is assumed that similar mechanisms are responsible for the entry of MARV.

Following the release of the RNP into the cytoplasm, transcription is the first event to occur. Due to the similar genome organization among all members of the *Mononegavirales*, transcription and replication are assumed to follow common mechanisms. The viral polymerase complex, consisting of at least L and VP35, produces polyadenylated, monocistronic mRNAs that are likely capped at the 5' end for each viral gene in a 3' to 5' direction. Similar to other members of the order, there seems to be a gradual decrease in mRNA levels from the 3' to the 5' end of the genome. Transcription requires NP, VP35, L and VP30 for EBOV, but can proceed in the absence of VP30 for MARV. The genome ends are predicted to form stem-loop structures at the 3' and 5' ends of genomic and antigenomic RNAs that are important for replication, similar to other negative sense RNA viruses. Replication proceeds from the *cis*-acting promoter at the 3' end of the genomic RNA, resulting in the synthesis and encapsidation of antigenomic RNA molecules. These in turn serve as templates for the genomic RNA which is also encapsidated. The balance between transcription and replication is thought to be regulated by the quantity of NP. The glycoprotein gene of EBOV undergoes transcriptional editing which allows for the production of at least three different glycoprotein products: the soluble glycoprotein (sGP) and its cleavage product (Δ-peptide), the full-length glycoprotein ($GP_{1,2}$) and the small secreted glycoprotein (ssGP). The full-length glycoprotein is only produced following the insertion of an additional adenosine residue into the editing site making this the only example of an edited viral glycoprotein; however, transcriptional editing has also been observed in the phosphoprotein gene from members of the Paramyxovirinae subfamily, family Paramyxoviridae.

Virus assembly and budding requires the major matrix protein VP40. When expressed alone, it is capable of forming virus-like particles (VLPs) that resemble authentic particles. During the production of viral proteins, NP induces the formation of inclusion bodies, which accumulate the other viral proteins of the RNP complex. RNPs are likely assembled in these inclusions when sufficient levels of viral proteins and negative-sense genomes are reached. Interactions between RNPs and VP40 direct the transport of RNPs to the plasma membrane via host cell proteins, where VP40 most likely initiates the assembly process. VP24 also associates with the plasma membrane and may play a role in particle formation. Once all the virus structural components are together in one location, VP40 octamers (which encompass the RNP via interactions with viral RNA) are tightly associated with $GP_{1,2}$ lipid rafts, allowing the entire complex to be

**Fig. 53.3** Particle structure and genome organization of filoviruses. (A) Schematic diagram of a filovirus particle and (B) a filovirus genome. (C) Electron micrograph of a filovirus particle.

enveloped and extruded from the host cell as infectious virions.

## CLINICAL FEATURES AND PATHOGENESIS

Following an incubation period of 2–21 days there is sudden onset of relatively non-specific symptoms including:

- fever (>38.3°C)/chills
- general malaise
- myalgia
- headache
- nausea
- vomiting
- sore throat
- diarrhoea
- abdominal and/or chest pain.

In approximately 50% of cases a maculopapular rash associated with varying degrees of erythema will develop, primarily on the trunk. In fatal cases, disease progression may include other signs of bleeding such as:

- conjunctival injections/haemorrhage
- bruising
- bleeding from mucosal membranes and/or venipuncture sites
- melaena and haematuria.

Increased D-dimers, which are highly suggestive of coagulation abnormalities, were observed in nearly all patient plasma analyzed during an outbreak of SEBOV in Uganda in 2000; however, observations during a ZEBOV outbreak noted clinical manifestations of coagulation disorders in less than 45% of patients. Profuse bleeding is rare and when present is primarily restricted to the gastrointestinal tract. The later stages of the disease are characterized by severe nausea, obtundation, tachypnoea, vomiting, prostration, increased respiratory rate, anuria and decreased body temperature indicative of the onset of shock. The specific cause of death is unclear; however, impairment of cardiovascular regulation leading to a lack of control of blood pressure, coagulation/anticoagulation and fluid distribution coupled with the inability to mount an appropriate immune response, together contribute to multi-organ failure leading to shock and death. An elevation of liver enzymes has also been noted. Individuals who survive frequently have prolonged myelitis, arthralgia, headache, lethargy, psychosis, recurrent hepatitis and ocular disorders in addition to psycho-social difficulties integrating back into their community.

The case-fatality rate and severity of symptoms appear to be viral species dependent: ZEBOV (60–90%), MARV (25–90%), SEBOV (50–60%), BEBOV (25%), CIEBOV (0%) and REBOV (0%). In fatal cases, viremia can reach $10^9$ genome copies/mL, while survivors generally have lower levels of viremia (<$10^7$ genomes/mL). Viral antigen can be found systemically, but is most abundant in the spleen and liver.

The initial targets for filovirus replication are monocytes/macrophages and dendritic cells.

Infection results in the activation of monocytes/ macrophages with the systemic release of cytokines, chemokines and other mediators such as tissue factor. Infection of dendritic cells leads to impaired functioning including a decreased ability to secrete pro-inflammatory cytokines, a lack of up-regulation of co-stimulatory molecules, a decreased ability to stimulate T cells and a decreased ability to produce type I interferon (IFN). Together, these processes result in increases in vascular permeability, disseminated intravascular coagulation and impaired immune responses. An effective IFN response may be the most useful mechanism to control filovirus replication and early IFN-$\alpha$ production has been associated with survival. Unfortunately for the host, the IFN response is usually suppressed, resulting in the inability to control infection. For EBOV, VP35 and VP24 have been characterized as interferon antagonists, while for MARV, VP35 and VP40 appear to function as interferon antagonists.

Trafficking of the initial infected target cells to regional lymph nodes, liver and spleen, where resident macrophages and dendritic cells are subsequently infected, is thought to aid in the dissemination of the virus. Following replication in the initial target sites, the liver and adrenal cortex are important secondary sites with both showing evidence of extensive virus replication and necrosis. While liver impairment itself is not considered to be significant enough to be the sole cause of death, it probably contributes to overall pathogenesis by exacerbating coagulation abnormalities through the decreased synthesis of coagulation factors and other plasma proteins as a result of liver damage. Impairment of the adrenal cortex likely contributes to hypotension and sodium loss with hypovolemia. Late in infection, extensive necrosis is observed in parenchymal cells of many organs, including the liver, spleen, kidney and gonads with little infiltration of immune cells into infected tissues. Tissue damage correlates with the presence of viral antigens and nucleic acid. Though not directly infected, lymphocytes are depleted as a result of infection. The mechanism remains unknown but several reports have suggested that lymphocytes undergo apoptosis; however this has not been observed in all studies.

Poorly maintained fluid distribution and uncontrolled coagulation are hallmarks of filovirus infection. This is manifested as systemic oedema and disseminated intravascular coagulation (DIC). Disruption of the endothelium seems to occur indirectly as a result of mediator-induced inflammatory responses from primary target cells (i.e. monocytes/macrophages). Coagulation and fibrinolysis are also severely disrupted during filovirus infection and can be observed as thrombocytopenia, consumption of clotting factors and increased levels of fibrin degradation products. This pro-coagulant state enhances inflammation, which subsequently induces further coagulation. Fibrin deposition results in the development of microvascular thrombi in various organs leading to ischemia and impaired organ perfusion, which contributes to multi-organ failure.

## DIAGNOSIS

As filovirus outbreaks occur sporadically, typically in isolated regions of Africa, initial diagnosis is usually based on clinical symptoms. It is quite likely that single cases of filovirus infection are misdiagnosed as the symptoms can be similar to other diseases, such as malaria or haemorrhagic measles. When possible, international reference laboratories should be involved in sample collection, storage and transport, especially when potential cases occur in non-endemic countries.

### Genome detection

Currently the most frequently used method to identify filovirus infections is RT-PCR on blood samples. Nucleic acid can be detected in blood as early as 3 days post-onset of symptoms. Most laboratories favour RT-PCR because of its sensitivity, specificity and rapidity. It has been successfully implemented in the mobile laboratory setting and has proven accurate and effective in both Ebola and Marburg haemorrhagic fever outbreaks. Due to the seriousness of a positive test for filoviruses, the diagnosis of index cases or of single imported cases should not be solely based on a single assay. Confirmation by an independent assay and/or laboratory should always be attempted.

### Antigen detection

Viral antigen detection is performed using ELISA-based methods. Typically this is performed to confirm results from RT-PCR. Classically, antigen detection was performed on formalin-fixed tissue samples by immunofluorescence assay (IFA).

### Serology

Antibody detection can be performed by ELISA-based methods on both acute (IgM) and convalescent (IgG) serum. These assays are typically used to confirm diagnosis and for surveillance efforts.

## Virus Isolation

Filoviruses can be isolated from blood and tissue samples by cell culture, typically on Vero or VeroE6 cells. These viruses are considered category A agents and require biosafety level 4 for virus isolation.

## TREATMENT

Currently, there is no specific treatment for either Ebola or Marburg haemorrhagic fever other than supportive care, which is directed towards the maintenance of effective blood volume and electrolyte balance. Due to the remote location of the outbreaks and limited resources available in the affected regions, treatment options have not been tested in patients. A post-exposure vesicular stomatitis virus-based vaccine platform has been demonstrated to protect non-human primates from either EBOV or MARV when given up to 48 h post-infection. This was the treatment of choice following an accidental laboratory EBOV exposure in 2009. Stable nucleic acid-lipid particles (SNALPs) have also been shown to be effective in protecting non-human primates from EBOV when given 30 mins post-infection. Monoclonal antibody treatments have proven successful in rodent models but have failed in preliminary nonhuman primate studies. Other treatments (interferon, activated protein C, recombinant nematode anticoagulant protein C2, etc.) have shown partial or limited protection. To date, there are no approved treatment options available. Ribavirin, which is used to treat other viral haemorrhagic fevers, does not appear to be effective for either EBOV or MARV.

## EPIDEMIOLOGY AND TRANSMISSION

With the exception of REBOV, all human filovirus infections have an origin linked to tropical Africa (Table 53.2). The initial MARV outbreaks occurred in Germany and the former Yugoslavia (now Serbia) in 1967 following contact with infected monkey tissues imported from Uganda. Imported cases have also occurred in South Africa (MARV, 1975 and ZEBOV, 1996) where persons became infected in other African countries and, following travel, subsequently infected health care providers. In 2008, there were two imported cases of MARV, one in the United States and the other in the Netherlands, in individuals who had travelled to Uganda. While imported cases of MARV and EBOV are uncommon, this nevertheless demonstrates that filoviruses have the potential to cause disease outside of Africa and that they need to be considered in travelers returning from regions where exposure is possible. When known, transmission has occurred as a result of direct contact with blood, secretions or tissues from infected patients or animals, such as gorillas and chimpanzees. EBOV has been found in saliva, stool, semen, breast milk, tears and blood as well as nasal and skin swabs from infected individuals. While aerosol exposure has only been conclusively demonstrated in experimentally-infected animals, an airborne route has been suggested in a limited number of human cases as the mode of transmission.

The filovirus reservoir has not been definitely indentified but there is a strong association with multiple African fruit bat species. Comparisons with other viruses that cause haemorrhagic fever, such as members of the 'Old World' arenaviruses, suggest that chronic infection of an animal reservoir might be responsible for maintenance of filoviruses in nature. Both viral RNA and antibodies (IgG) against EBOV and MARV have been detected in several species of fruit bats, suggesting these species may be a natural reservoir. Despite many attempts, only MARV has actually been isolated (from five bats of the species *Rousettus aegyptiacus*). Two other bat species (*Hypsignathus monstrosus* and *Epomops franqueti*) were strongly associated with the start of an outbreak of EBOV in the Democratic Republic of the Congo (DRC) in 2007. While contact with monkeys, typically as a source of food, has probably served as the route of infection in a number of outbreaks, they are not considered the reservoir.

The only species of EBOV that has not appeared in tropical Africa is REBOV, which was identified in imported cynomolgus macaques in 1989 at a quarantine facility in Virginia, USA. Importation of REBOV-infected monkeys from one holding facility in the Philippines has subsequently occurred multiple times. In 2008, during an investigation regarding high swine mortality at multiple farms in the Philippines, a number of pigs that had died tested positive for REBOV; however, it is unclear if REBOV coinfection was the cause of death. While virulent in monkeys, to date there has been no apparent pathogenicity in humans despite at least 25 laboratory confirmed infections.

## CONTROL

In the early outbreaks, nosocomial spread was a major route of infection. The use of barrier nursing techniques, isolation of potentially infected patients, contact tracing and a rapid response from

**Table 53.2** Occurrences of filovirus infections[a]

| Virus | Country | Year | No. of cases (CFR[b]) | Epidemiology |
|---|---|---|---|---|
| MARV | Germany/Serbia (former Yugoslavia) | 1967 | 32 (22%) | Contact with imported vervet monkeys and their tissues |
| | Zimbabwe/South Africa | 1975 | 3 (33%) | Index infected in Zimbabwe, two secondary cases in companion and nurse |
| | Kenya | 1980 | 2 (50%) | Traveller to the area that was the source of vervet monkeys in 1967; secondary infection in doctor who survived |
| | Kenya | 1987 | 1 (100%) | Traveller to Mount Elgon Cave (bat infested) |
| | DRC[c] | 1998–2000 | 154 (83%) | Community outbreak lasting more than 2 years |
| | Angola | 2005 | 252 (90%) | Outbreak in an urban setting |
| | Uganda | 2007 | 4 (25%) | Contact with workers or worked in mine (containing bats) |
| | Netherlands | 2008 | 1 (100%) | Imported from Uganda (visited cave containing bats) |
| | USA[d] | 2008 | 1 (0%) | Imported from Uganda (visited same cave as above) |
| ZEBOV | DRC (former Zaire) | 1976 | 318 (88%) | Unknown origin, nosocomial spread by needlestick |
| | DRC (former Zaire) | 1977 | 1 (100%) | Sporadic case |
| | Gabon | 1994 | 52 (60%) | Workers in gold-mining camps, identified retrospectively |
| | DRC | 1995 | 315 (81%) | Index worked in forest, close contact, nosocomial transmission |
| | Gabon | 1996 | 37 (57%) | Butchering dead chimpanzee, close contact transmission |
| | Gabon | 1996 | 60 (75%) | Index case a hunter, close contact transmission |
| | South Africa | 1996 | 2 (50%) | Index treated patients in Gabon, attending nurse in South Africa died |
| | Gabon/RC | 2001–2004 | 302 (84%) | Multiple outbreaks, contact with dead monkeys |
| | RC[e] | 2005 | 12 (83%) | Butchering a chimpanzee |
| | DRC | 2007 | 264 (71%) | Unknown origin |
| | DRC | 2008–2009 | 13 (69%) | Unknown origin |
| SEBOV | Sudan | 1976 | 284 (53%) | Linked to bat infested cotton factory, nosocomial transmission |
| | Sudan | 1979 | 34 (65%) | Index linked to same cotton factory as 1976, nosocomial transmission |
| | Uganda | 2000–2001 | 425 (53%) | Unknown source, nosocomial and community transmission |
| | Sudan | 2004 | 17 (41%) | Index butchered monkeys, nosocomial and close contact transmission |
| REBOV | USA | 1989 | epizootic | Imported monkeys (Philippines), 4 potential asymptomatic human infections |
| | USA | 1990 | | Imported monkeys (Philippines), no human infections |
| | Italy | 1992 | | Imported monkeys (Philippines), no human infections |
| | USA | 1996 | | Imported monkeys (Philippines) |
| | Philippines | 1996 | | Quarantine facility for all previous occurrences of REBOV |
| | Philippines | 2008 | | Large outbreak in pigs, presumed asymptomatic human infections |
| CIEBOV | Côte d'Ivoire | 1994 | 1 (0%) | Performed autopsy on dead chimpanzee infected with CIEBOV |
| | Liberia | 1995 | 1 (0%) | Serological diagnosis only |
| BEBOV | Uganda | 2007 | 149 (25%) | Unknown origin, community transmission |

[a]All known incidents of naturally-acquired filovirus infections are listed including date and country of infections, in addition to the number of cases, the case-fatality rate and the available epidemiological data.
[b]Case-fatality rate.
[c]Democratic Republic of the Congo.
[d]United States of America.
[e]Republic of the Congo.

international agencies remains the primary mechanism of control of both MARV and EBOV. The potential reservoir(s) (i.e. bats) are not well defined, regardless population control of bats does not seem to be a feasible option. Multiple methods are available for disinfection including UV light, gamma irradiation and heat (>60°C for 30 mins); however, virus infectivity is quite stable at room temperature, particularly in clinical specimens.

There are no approved vaccines against filoviruses despite multiple vaccine platforms demonstrating success in non-human primates. The most important antigen component in vaccines appears to be the filovirus glycoprotein, which has been expressed in both non-replicating vaccines (DNA, recombinant adenovirus serotype 5 and virus-like particles) and replication competent vaccines (recombinant human parainfluenza virus 3 and recombinant vesicular stomatitis virus). Recently blended vaccines (i.e. containing antigens from more than one species) have been demonstrated to provide protection against multiple filovirus species.

## RECOMMENDED READING

Buchmeier MJ, de la Torre J-C, Peters, CJ: Arenaviridae: The viruses and Their Replication. In Knipe DM, Howley PM, editors: *Fields Virology*, Philadelphia, 2007, Wolters Kluwer Health/Lippincott Williams & Wilkins, pp 1792–1827.

Feldmann H, Geisbert TW: Ebola hemorrhagic fever, *The Lancet* 377:849–862, 2011.

Feldmann H, Geisbert TW, Jahrling P, et al: Filoviridae. In Van Regenmortel MHV, Fauquet CM, Mayo MA et al: editors: *Virus Taxonomy, Eighth report of the International Committee on Taxonomy of Viruses*, San Diego, 2005, Elsevier, pp 645–653.

Hartmann AL, Towner JS, Nichol ST: Ebola and Marburg hemorrhagic fever, *Clinics in Laboratory Medicine* 30:161–177, 2010.

Kuhn J, Calisher CH, editors: *Filoviridae: A compendium of 40 Years of epidemiological, clinical, and laboratory studies*, New York, 2008, Springer.

Moraz ML, Kunz S: Pathogenesis of arenavirus hemorrhagic fevers, *Expert Review of Anti-Infective Therapy* 9:49–59, 2011.

Salvato MS, Clegg JCS, Buchmeier MJ, et al: Family Arenaviridae. In Van Regenmortel MHV, Fauquet CM, Mayo MA, et al, editors: *Virus Taxonomy, Eighth report of the International Committee on Taxonomy of Viruses*, San Diego, 2005, Elsevier, pp 725–733.

Sanchez A, Geisbert TW, Feldmann H: Filoviridae: Marburg and Ebola Viruses. In Knipe DM, Howley PM, editors: *Fields Virology*, 2007, Philadelphia, Wolters Kluwer Health/Lippincott Williams & Wilkins, pp 1410–1447.

# 54 Reoviruses

## Gastroenteritis

*N. A. Cunliffe and O. Nakagomi*

## KEY POINTS

- The Reoviridae comprise four genera which infect humans; they are characterized by the possession of 10–12 segments of double-stranded RNA encased within an unenveloped capsid of icosahedral symmetry.
- When viewed under the electron microscope, the characteristic wheel-shaped virus particles measure 70–75 nm in diameter.
- Group A rotaviruses are the major cause of acute gastroenteritis in infants and young children worldwide.
- A unique feature of rotavirus replication is the transient acquisition of an envelope during the process of budding into the endoplasmic reticulum.
- Rotaviruses produce NSP4, the first described viral enterotoxin.
- Diagnosis of rotavirus gastroenteritis is usually made by the detection of viral antigen (VP6) using enzyme-linked immunosorbent and immunochromatographic assays.
- A distinct winter seasonality of rotavirus infection is evident in temperate countries; infection is year-round in tropical countries.
- Rehydration and restoration of electrolyte balance are the primary aims of treatment of acute rotavirus gastroenteritis.
- Two live oral rotavirus vaccines are entering childhood immunization schedules and promise to substantially reduce the global rotavirus disease burden.

The family Reoviridae comprises a diverse collection of viruses that infect man, many mammals, other vertebrates (including birds), plants and insects. The genus *Rotavirus* is the most important cause of severe infantile gastroenteritis throughout the world, and is a recognized aetiological agent of diarrhoea in the young of many animal species. Viruses in the genera *Orbivirus* and *Coltivirus* infect various species of insects and can be transmitted to vertebrates including man, and can thus be described as arboviruses (see Ch. 51).

## CLASSIFICATION

Four of the nine genera of the Reoviridae family infect humans:

- *Orthoreovirus* – reovirus types 1, 2 and 3
- *Orbivirus* and *Coltivirus* – various serogroups
- *Rotavirus* – of seven species, formerly called serogroups (A–G), *Rotavirus A–Rotavirus C* have been detected in humans. Multiple genotypes exist within *Rotavirus A*.

The virion has icosahedral symmetry and is triple-layered (the double-shelled capsid surrounds a core); it does not possess an envelope and measures 70–75 nm in diameter under negative-stain electron microscopy. The RNA genome consists of 10 to 12 segments of double-stranded RNA.

## REPLICATION

The virus replicates in the cytoplasm of infected cells. Attachment is via a specific protein component of the outer capsid (e.g. σ1 of orthoreoviruses or viral protein (VP) 4 of rotaviruses) to a cellular receptor; orthoreoviruses use sialic acid for binding and junctional adhesion molecule-A as a post-binding receptor, whereas rotaviruses use both sialic acid and α2β1 integrin for binding and α2β1 and other integrins, and heat shock protein 70 as post-binding receptors. The viral protein–receptor interaction leads to a conformational change in the viral capsid, which enables orthoreoviruses to enter the cell by receptor-mediated endocytosis. The multistep attachment and entry process for rotaviruses is complex and involves a remarkable conformational change in the structure of VP4 induced by proteolytic cleavage, exposing additional attachment sites. When crossing the cell membrane, the outer capsid is removed, but the viral particle is never completely uncoated, leaving the viral genomic RNA in the core of the double-layered particle (subviral particle). RNA is transcribed by the virion-associated, RNA-dependent RNA polymerase complex to produce messenger RNA (mRNA) molecules from each genomic RNA segment. The mRNA molecules, which are capped but not polyadenylated, leave the subviral particle through channels penetrating the outer and inner capsids, and are then translated to generate the various viral proteins. They also act as templates for RNA replication, which is completed by the RNA polymerase complex, and packaged within new core structures. The whole replication events occur within electron-dense structures (viroplasms) in the cytoplasm, which are localized adjacent to the nucleus and the endoplasmic reticulum (ER). Nascent double-layered particles, after binding to an intracellular viral receptor (NSP4), bud from viroplasms into the ER in a unique process during which double-layered particles transiently acquire an envelope. At the same time the outer capsid proteins, VP7 and VP4, are incorporated into newly synthesized particles, which become mature, triple-layered particles by losing their envelope. These are then released from the apical surface of enterocytes after vesicular transport from the ER by a pathway bypassing the Golgi apparatus.

## ASSOCIATION WITH CLINICAL ILLNESS

The first human isolates of the Reoviridae were recovered from both respiratory secretions and faeces, but could not be associated with disease – hence the name *reo*virus (*r*espiratory *e*nteric *o*rphan). However, orthoreoviruses cause systemic disease (meningitis and encephalitis) in mice, and this virus–host system has been used extensively to study viral pathogenesis. Although most of the human population is exposed to and develops antibodies against orthoreoviruses from an early age, there is still no clear link between these viruses and illness.

The orbiviruses include several serogroups that infect man and are transmitted by a variety of insects (ticks, midges and mosquitoes). In the blood the virus is associated with erythrocytes, and thus is hidden from immune responses. Clinically, patients experience a febrile illness, with rashes in 10% and leucopenia in two-thirds of cases. Infections of the central nervous system leading to meningitis or encephalitis are seen in 3–7% of laboratory-confirmed cases.

The coltiviruses are also transmitted by insects (ticks, mosquitoes), and rodents are considered to be the main animal reservoir. Infection is spread to man by insect bite. A febrile illness develops with gastrointestinal symptoms (20%), rash (10%), and meningitis or encephalitis (3–7%) (see Ch. 51).

Rotaviruses are the main cause of acute gastroenteritis in infants and young children, as well as in the young of many animal species.

## ROTAVIRUSES

Infection with rotavirus can result in a wide spectrum of clinical outcomes, ranging from asymptomatic infection to severe, life-threatening gastroenteritis. More severe disease outcomes are typically encountered among children in developing countries. Rotavirus also causes diarrhoea in the young of a wide variety of avian and mammalian species including cattle, sheep, goat, horses, pigs, dogs, cats and mice, rabbits, monkeys and many others.

### Description and classification
#### *Morphology*

The virion measures 75 nm in diameter and has characteristic sharp-edged, double-shelled capsids, which in electron micrographs look like spokes grouped around the hub of a wheel (the Latin word, *rota*, means wheel); this appearance is diagnostic (Fig. 54.1). Cryo-electron microscopy has shown that the

**Fig. 54.1** Negatively stained electron micrograph of rotavirus particles in a faecal specimen. Potassium phosphotungstic acid stain. Bar = 100 nm.

triple-layered particle is penetrated by 132 large channels and that the virion has 60 spikes on its surface that consist of trimers of VP4 (Fig. 54.2) (see below).

## Genome and gene-coding assignments

The 11 segments of double-stranded RNA can be extracted easily from rotaviruses and separated by polyacrylamide gel electrophoresis. This has been used to establish so-called 'electropherotypes' of rotavirus isolates (Fig. 54.2). As well as 'long' and 'short' electropherotypes (differing in the rates of relative migration of RNA segments 10 and 11), various minor differences in the migration of corresponding segments have been recognized and utilized extensively in epidemiological studies.

Generally, each genome segment codes for only one virus-specific protein (VP). The gene-coding assignments have been established (Fig. 54.2). RNA segments 1, 2 and 3 code respectively for the inner core proteins VP1 (which functions as the viral polymerase), VP2 (the main scaffolding protein) and VP3 (the capping enzyme). RNA segment 6 codes for the middle layer protein, VP6, which is the single most abundant rotavirus protein and which interacts with the core protein VP2 and the outer capsid proteins VP7 and VP4 (see below). VP6 carries epitopes specifying groups and subgroups. To date, seven different group antigens (A–G) have been identified; for groups A–E a complete lack of serological cross-reactivity has been shown.

- *Rotavirus A* is responsible for the vast majority of human rotavirus infections in infants and young children, and may also cause disease in adults.
- *Rotavirus B* was initially discovered as the cause of outbreaks of acute diarrhoea among all age groups in China, and is now endemic in several countries including China, India, Bangladesh, Myanmar and Nepal.
- *Rotavirus C* causes occasional episodes of gastroenteritis in older children.

The outer capsid (third layer) is formed by two proteins: VP7, a glycoprotein (encoded by RNA 7, 8 or 9, depending on the strain, and determining the G serotype), and VP4 (encoded by RNA 4, and determining the P serotype). Each of these surface proteins carries neutralization epitopes that define the virus serotype. VP4 is cleaved post-translationally into VP5* and VP8* (an asterisk is to denote post-translational product); this proteolytic cleavage is essential for infectivity. Six non-structural proteins are coded for by RNAs 5 (NSP1), 7, 8 or 9 (NSP2 and NSP3, depending on the strain), and 10 or 11 (NSP4,

NSP5 and NSP6, depending on the strain). NSP2 is proposed to act as a molecular motor to drive replicating mRNA into the nascent viral particles and so maintain nucleotide pools in viroplasms during replication. Both NSP2 and NSP5 are involved in viroplasm formation. NSP3 functions as polyadenylic acid-binding protein (rotavirus mRNA is not polyadenylated), and binds to the 3′ end of viral mRNA and to cellular eIF4G, thus enhancing the translation of viral mRNA. While NSP4 is an intracellular viral receptor playing an important role in viral morphogenesis (see above), it also functions as a viral enterotoxin (see below).

## Antigenic and genetic diversity

*Rotavirus A* is genetically diverse in each of the 11 genome segments (called genotypes), and a nucleotide sequence-based, complete genome classification system is used; the genome of individual rotavirus strains is given the complete descriptor of Gx-P[x]-Ix-Rx-Cx-Mx-Ax-Nx-Tx-Ex-Hx (Fig. 54.2). Of these eleven genotypes, the G and P genotypes, corresponding to the G serotype and the P serotype, respectively, have been extensively investigated because of their importance in protective immunity. There are thus far 26 G genotypes and 35 P genotypes reported among human and animal rotaviruses. Reverse transcriptase–polymerase chain reaction (RT-PCR) with gene- and type-specific primers has been widely applied as a reliable typing procedure. Although the correlation between G serotypes (determined by neutralization assays) and G genotypes (determined by molecular methods) is absolute, not all P types have as yet been confirmed as serotypes, and therefore the P-serotype designation differs from the P-genotype designation (which is included in a square bracket). For example, strain Wa is designated as P1A[8]G1, where P1A represents the P-serotype; [8] represents the P-genotype; and G1 represents the G-genotype/serotype.

At the molecular level, several factors have been identified that can explain the genomic and antigenic variability of co-circulating rotavirus strains.

- Like other viruses that depend on virion-associated, RNA-dependent RNA polymerases for their replication, rotavirus genomes undergo frequent point mutations that accumulate over time and give rise to multiple lineages and sublineages (when this occurs in the neutralization proteins, *antigenic drift* will result).
- Rotaviruses, like other segmented RNA viruses, undergo extensive reassortment in doubly infected cells. This has been shown to occur both in vitro

| | | |
|---|---|---|
| 1 — VP1 | RNA polymerase: R2 |
| 2 — VP2 | Core protein: C2 |
| 3 — VP3 | Methylase (capping): M2 |
| 4 — VP4 | P type: P[4] |
| 5 — NSP1 | Interferon antagonist: A2 |
| 6 — VP6 | Innercapsid: I2 |
| 7 — NSP3 | Poly A binding protien: T2 |
| 8 — VP7 | G type: G2 |
| 9 — NSP2 | Molecular motor: N2 |
| 10 — NSP5/6 | Viroplasm formation: H2 |
| 11 — NSP4 | Intracellular viral receptor Enterotoxin: E2 |

Long RNA pattern   Short RNA pattern

**Fig. 54.2** Schematic diagram showing the relationships between the structure of a rotavirus virion (derived from cryo-electron microscopy images and computer image processing) and the genomic double-stranded RNA segments separated by polyacrylamide gel electrophoresis. Two RNA patterns, long and short, are shown. The cut-away representation of the reconstructed virion shows the triple-layered icosahedral architecture and the locations of the various structural proteins. Note that coding assignment is slightly different between long and short RNA pattern strains. RNA segment 10 of the short RNA strain is the result of rearrangement of RNA segment 11 of the long RNA pattern. The outer (VP7 and VP4), middle (VP6) and inner (VP2) layers are shown in orange, blue and green, respectively. The flower-like structures inside the VP2 layer represent VP1–VP3 complexes, which function as RNA polymerase and capping enzymes. The genotype of each RNA segment of the short RNA strain (strain DS-1) is shown in blue. The corresponding genotypes of the long RNA strain (strain Wa) are G1-P[8]-I1-R1-C1-M1-A1-N1-T1-E1-H1. (The 3D image structure of reconstructed rotavirus virion was conceived by B. V. V. Prasad, Baylor College of Medicine, Houston, Texas, USA.)

and in vivo. If RNA segments coding for serotype-specific proteins are involved, major antigenic changes can result (*antigenic shift*).

- Rotaviruses may be transferred to man from animal species either as whole virions or by reassortment of genome segments. The result is that in such cases, the genome of human group A rotavirus isolates is related to that of animal rotaviruses (e.g. cat, cow, pig), either in whole or in part.
- Rotaviruses that establish chronic infections in immunodeficient hosts may undergo various forms of genome rearrangement, resulting in highly atypical RNA profiles.

## PATHOGENESIS AND IMMUNITY

Rotaviruses replicate exclusively in the differentiated epithelial cells at the tips of the small intestinal villi and the crypts, which contain undifferentiated enterocyte stem cells, are spared. Progeny virus is produced after 10–12 h, and released in large numbers into the intestinal lumen ready to infect other cells. Biopsies show atrophy of the villi and mononuclear cell infiltrates in the lamina propria. The pathogenesis of rotavirus diarrhoea includes both malabsorptive and secretory components. Malabsorption may be consequent upon damage to mature absorptive enterocytes resulting in malabsorption of nutrients, electrolytes and water; virus-induced down-regulation of the expression of absorptive enzymes; and functional changes in tight junctions between enterocytes leading to paracellular leakage. Secretory mechanisms include those mediated by activation of the enteric nervous system and the effect of NSP4, the latter being via activation of cellular Cl⁻ channels (different from the cystic fibrosis transmembrane regulator), leading to increased Cl⁻ and consequently water secretion.

Rotavirus infection was previously thought to be limited to the intestine, but rotavirus causes viraemia for at least a short period in the acute phase of infection in immunocompetent infants as well as in experimentally infected animals. The clinical significance of this systemic spread of rotavirus is unclear, however.

Studies of the natural history of rotavirus infection show that immunity acquired following primary infection results predominantly in protection against the development of subsequent severe disease, but that protection against asymptomatic infection or mild disease is much less. Such post-infection immunity is believed to be mediated by both humoral and cell-mediated immune responses. Rotavirus-specific immunoglobulin (Ig) A antibodies on the enteric mucosal surface are thought to be the primary mediator of protective immunity.

The role of the innate immune system in rotavirus infection has captured recent attention. NSP1 functions as a viral ubiquitin ligase, interacting with and promoting the degradation of IFN regulatory factor (IRF) 3 and IRF7 through a ubiquitination-proteasome mechanism. NSP1 also inhibits activation of nuclear factor-κB. Thus, rotavirus counteracts the production of INFβ by host cells.

## Clinical features

The onset of symptoms is abrupt after a short incubation period of 1–2 days. Fever, vomiting and watery diarrhoea are seen in the majority of infected children, lasting for 2–6 days. If body fluids are not replaced, dehydration ensues that may range in severity from mild to life threatening. There is little evidence that illness severity is related to virus serotype. Rotavirus infection can cause gastroenteritis in older children and adults, although severe disease is less common. Outbreaks of gastroenteritis due to rotavirus infection have been observed in the elderly, in whom severe dehydration can result. In the immunodeficient host, a persistent infection may occur with severe chronic diarrhoea associated with rotavirus excretion that can last for many months.

## Laboratory diagnosis

At the peak of infection, as many as $10^{11}$ virus particles per millilitre of faeces are present, and can be detected by a variety of methods. Electron microscopy will easily detect the characteristic virus particles (Fig. 54.1). In the majority of cases there are sufficient numbers of virions in faeces to allow identification of

RNA profiles (Fig. 54.2). Antigen detection tests, targeted on the middle-layer protein VP6, include enzyme-linked immunosorbent assays and immuno-chromatographic assays. The diagnosis of rotavirus infection can also be made by genome detection (RT-PCR), although such assays are much less frequently applied in the diagnostic laboratory than are rotavirus antigen detection tests.

## Epidemiology

Rotavirus infections occur worldwide, but the vast majority of deaths occur in children in developing countries (Fig. 54.3). Thus, an estimated 2 million children under the age of 5 years die from diarrhoeal disease in developing countries each year, and rotavirus accounts for about 40% of these deaths (an estimated 527 000 rotavirus-associated deaths in 2004, the last year before the introduction of rotavirus vaccine). In industrialized countries rotavirus accounts for 40–50% of hospital admissions due to diarrhoeal disease. Most symptomatic infections are seen in children between 6 months and 2 years of age in industrialized countries, although in developing countries symptomatic rotavirus infection below 6 months of age is common. By the age of 5 years, virtually all children have been infected with rotavirus. In temperate countries rotavirus infections display marked seasonality, with distinct peaks during the winter months and few infections identified outside this period (Fig. 54.4). In contrast, rotavirus infections occur year-round in most tropical countries. Transmission of rotavirus within families to siblings and parents is well recognized. The release of enormous numbers of virions during the acute phase contributes to the easy transmission of the virus. Only a few virus particles are sufficient to cause disease in the susceptible host.

Among group A rotaviruses, five genotype combinations comprise more than 85% of rotaviruses detected in humans, including P[8],G1, P[4],G2, P[8],G3, P[8],G4, and P[8],G9 (Fig. 54.5). However, strains with G12 emerged globally over the last decade, and G8 has been commonly reported in many African countries.

## TREATMENT

Although no specific anti-rotaviral treatment is available routinely, probiotic therapy (e.g. with *Lactobacillus* GG) has been shown in clinical trials to shorten the duration of symptoms of gastroenteritis. In selected clinical situations, anti-rotaviral immunoglobulin

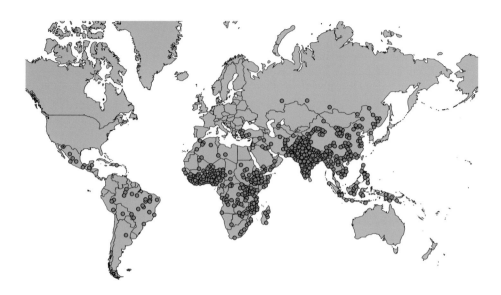

**Fig. 54.3** Estimated distribution of deaths due to rotavirus disease among children < 5 years of age, by country. Each dot represents 1000 deaths. (Adapted from Parashar UD, Burton A, Lanata C et al 2009 Global mortality associated with rotavirus disease among children in 2004. *Journal of Infectious Diseases* 200: S9–15.)

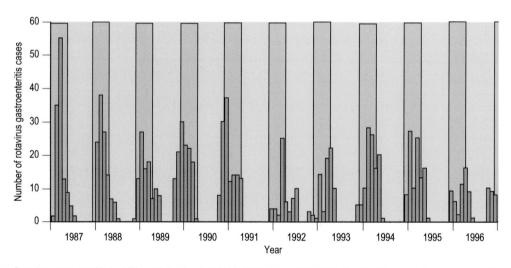

**Fig. 54.4** Rotavirus gastroenteritis in children admitted to hospital in Akita, Japan, 1987–1996. The light blue shaded area represents the winter season (December to March).

therapy has been used as prophylaxis against, and as treatment of, rotavirus gastroenteritis. However, the mainstay of therapy consists of oral rehydration with fluids of specified electrolyte and glucose composition (see Table 30.1, p. 318). Intravenous rehydration therapy is reserved for patients with severe dehydration, shock or reduced level of consciousness.

## CONTROL

Attention to hygienic measures such as handwashing, safe disposal of faeces and disinfection of contaminated surfaces is essential in reducing the risk of transmission. However, universal vaccination of

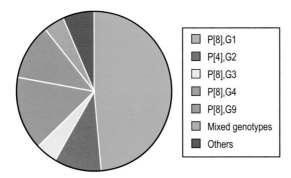

**Fig. 54.5** Distribution of combined P and G types in Europe between 2006 and 2009. (Adapted from Iturriza-Gómara M, Dallman T, Bányai K et al 2011 Rotavirus genotypes co-circulating in Europe between 2006 and 2009 as determined by EuroRotaNet, a pan-European collaborative strain surveillance network. *Epidemiology and Infection* 139: 895–909.)

infants is the most important preventive strategy. The rotavirus vaccines that have been developed are live-attenuated, orally administerable strains. Attenuation of virulence has been achieved either by repeated passage in cell culture or by substitution through genetic reassortment of serotype-determining gene segment(s) of a human rotavirus into the backbone of an animal rotavirus (which is both naturally attenuated for humans and attenuated through repeated cell culture passage).

The first licensed rotavirus vaccine, a Rhesus monkey rotavirus-based tetravalent human reassortant vaccine (RotaShield), was withdrawn after this live oral vaccine was associated with the development of intestinal intussusception in approximately 1 in 10 000 vaccine recipients in the USA. Two further live-attenuated oral rotavirus vaccines were developed and extensively evaluated, and have now entered childhood immunization programmes following recommendation by the World Health Organisation. These are the monovalent P1A[8]G1 human rotavirus vaccine Rotarix, and the pentavalent human–bovine reassortant rotavirus vaccine RotaTeq, which includes the world's most common human serotypes G1, G2, G3, G4 and P[8] on a bovine rotavirus background. Both vaccines have demonstrated efficacy against severe rotavirus disease caused by globally common rotavirus strains. The administration of Rotarix (2 doses) and Rotateq (3 doses) needs to be completed by 32 weeks of age to minimize any potential risk of intusscusception. In the USA, the number of hospitalizations and emergency visits due to rotavirus infection has dramatically fallen following national introduction of rotavirus vaccination. The greatest potential for impact on child morbidity and mortality lies in the developing countries in Africa and Asia, where both vaccines have recently been evaluated. Although vaccine efficacy was lower than observed in industrialized settings, universal rotavirus vaccination in such countries would result in a large decrease in the number of severe rotavirus episodes because of the high incidence of disease.

## RECOMMENDED READING

Dormitzer PR: Rotaviruses. In Mandell GL, Bennett JE, Dolin R, editors: *Principles and Practice of Infectious Diseases*, ed 7, Philadelphia, 2010, Elsevier, pp 2105–2115.

Estes M, Kapikian A: Rotaviruses. In Knipe DM, Howley PM, Griffin DE, et al, editors: *Fields Virology*, ed 5, Philadelphia, 2007, Kluwer Health/ Lippincott, Williams and Wilkins, pp 1917–1974.

Greenberg HB, Estes MK: Rotaviruses: from pathogenesis to vaccination, *Gastroenterology* 136:1939–1951, 2009.

Lopez S, Arias CF: Multistep entry of rotavirus into cells: a Versaillesque dance, *Trends in Microbiology* 12:271–278, 2004.

Matthijnssens J, Ciarlet M, Rahman M, et al: Recommendations for the classification of group A rotaviruses using all 11 genomic RNA segments, *Archives of Virology* 153:1621–1629, 2008.

Santosham M: Rotavirus vaccine – a powerful tool to combat deaths from diarrhea, *New England Journal of Medicine* 362:358–360, 2010.

# 55 Retroviruses

## Acquired immune deficiency syndrome; HTLV-1

### Y. A. Taha

### KEY POINTS

- Some retroviruses, including HTLV-I, the cause of human T-cell leukaemia, cause tumours in natural hosts.
- HIV-1 is the cause of the acquired immune deficiency syndrome (AIDS), a persistent infection leading to loss of CD4+ T cells, immunodeficiency and many opportunistic infections.
- Disease status can be measured by sequential changes in CD4 count and viral load in plasma (HIV RNA copy number).
- HIV has a global distribution; it is spread by sexual intercourse, mother-to-child transmission and via blood and blood products. The greatest incidence is in sub-Saharan Africa and South-East Asia.
- HIV replication can be inhibited by drugs that block co-receptor binding, membrane fusion, reverse transcription, integration and protein cleavage during maturation.
- Combination antiretroviral therapy (cART) reduces the appearance of drug resistance and, combined with control of opportunistic infections, substantially improves survival.

The family Retroviridae contains many viruses from widely different host species. They have been studied for many years, initially because a wide variety of tumours including leukaemias and lymphomas, sarcomas, breast and brain tumours are caused by oncogenic members of this family. Other retroviruses are associated with a plethora of neurologic, autoimmune and blood disorders. The host species include birds, mice, cattle, pigs and several primates. The first human retrovirus was isolated from T cells of patients with T cell leukaemia – human T-cell lymphotropic virus type I or HTLV-I – in 1980. The acquired immune deficiency syndrome (AIDS) is caused by a different retrovirus, also with a predilection for T cells that is referred to as human immunodeficiency virus type 1 or HIV-1. Infection with this virus has become pandemic and remains a major cause of morbidity and mortality in sub-Saharan Africa and other developing countries. HIV-2 infection is restricted largely to West Africa and is less pathogenic.

## DESCRIPTION

All retroviruses have an outer envelope of lipid and viral proteins; the envelope encloses the core, consisting of other viral proteins, within which lie two molecules of viral RNA (positive single-stranded) and the enzyme reverse transcriptase, an RNA-dependent DNA polymerase. The virions have a diameter of about 100 nm (Fig. 55.1) and, in thin section, characteristic differences can be seen in the appearance and position of the core (e.g. C-type and D-type particles), a feature that was previously used to classify retroviruses. The typical genome size is approximately 10 kilobases (kb) or less.

## CLASSIFICATION

The Retroviridae family was originally divided into the subfamilies Oncovirinae, Spumavirinae and Lentivirinae, based on their biological properties and appearances in cell cultures. However, nucleotide sequencing of a large number of human and animal retroviruses has revealed that viruses cluster in two subfamilies, the Spumavirinae and Orthoretrovirinae, with the latter comprising 6 distinct genera, the *Alpha-*, *Beta-*, *Delta-*, *Epsilon-* and *Gamma-retroviruses* and the *Lentivirus* genus (Fig. 55.2).

The spumaviruses have been detected in various species, including cats, cattle and primates, but are not associated with disease. The name is derived from the foamy (vacuolated) appearance of infected cells in culture. There is no evidence for pathogenic human infection with spumaviruses.

The human retroviruses HTLV-I and HTLV-II belong to the genus *Deltaretrovirus* (formerly termed *Oncovirus*). They are related to the simian viruses STLV-I and -II, which are widely distributed in Old and New World monkeys. STLV-I shows approximately 90% similarity to HTLV-I at the sequence level. A more distantly related virus is found in cows (Bovine Leukaemia Virus). The recent identification of two new HTLV types (HTLV-III and HTLV-IV) in a few bush meat hunters in central Africa is believed to represent isolated incidents of primate-to-human virus transmission rather than an established human infection.

The other two human retroviruses HIV-1 and HIV-2 are lentiviruses, closely related to lentiviruses that infect Old World primates. HIV-2 is almost identical to simian immunodeficiency virus ($SIV_{sm}$) found in sooty mangabeys. It is believed that human infection originated through cross-species transmission. Similarly, HIV-1 corresponds closely to $SIV_{cpz}$ variants that infect chimpanzees in Central Africa, the probable source of the human virus. The genus *Lentivirus* also includes feline and bovine immunodeficiency viruses and Visna-Maedi of sheep, the first lentivirus to be recognized. Lentiviruses are distinguished from Deltaretroviruses by their molecular

**Fig. 55.1** Electron micrograph of HIV. Thin section of infected T lymphocyte. There are numerous virions lying outside the cell membrane.

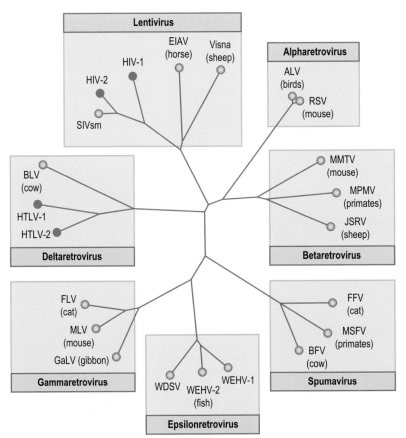

**Fig. 55.2** Tree of sequences from the retroviral *pol* gene showing relatedness of retroviruses infecting man and a range of animal species. Sequences form seven main genera, in which human retroviruses (HTLV and HIV; shown in blue) are found in two. For animal retroviruses (red), the host species and names of familiar viruses are indicated. ALV, avian leukosis virus; BFV, Bovine foamy virus; BLV, bovine leukaemia virus; EIAV, equine infectious anaemia virus; FFV, feline foamy virus; FLV, feline leukaemia virus; GaLV, Gibbon ape leukaemia virus; JSRV, Jaagsiekte sheep retrovirus; MLV, murine leukaemia virus; MMTV, mouse mammary tumour virus; MPMV, Mason–Pfizer monkey virus; MSFV, Macaque simian foamy virus; RSV, Rous sarcoma virus; SIV, simian immunodeficiency virus; WDSV, walleye dermal sarcoma virus; WEHV, walleye epidermal hyperplasia virus.

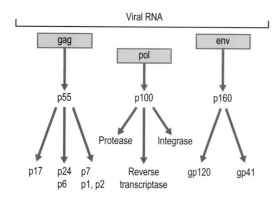

**Fig. 55.3** The genomic organization of HIV structural genes and their protein products.

**Fig. 55.4** Diagram of HIV to show location of structural proteins.

structure and lack of oncogenic capability; however both genera are capable of establishing prolonged asymptomatic infection.

Both HIV-1 and HIV-2 show considerable sequence variability, allowing their classification into a number of subtypes with marked differences in geographical distribution and association with risk groups. HIV-1 variants are classified into three genetic groups: major (M), outlier (O) and non-M, non-O (N). Group M viruses which dominate the pandemic are further classified into subtypes A, B, C, D, F, G, H, J and K and several 'circulating recombinant forms' (CRF) that comprise more than one subtype, e.g. CRF01-A/E. Subtype B is most frequently found in western countries, whereas other genotypes such as C (Africa, parts of Asia), E (Thailand) and F (South America) are the main subtypes responsible for the recent epidemic spread. HIV-1 diversity is greatest in sub-Saharan African countries such as the Congo, where there is wide co-circulation of most of the current subtypes.

Human endogenous retroviruses, often replication-defective, are present in the human germ line and have not been shown to cause disease.

### Genome and gene coding assignment

The genome organization is similar for all retroviruses as their genomes contain in the same order the genes *gag*, *pol* and *env* coding for three groups of structural and enzymatic proteins (Figs 55.3 & 55.4). The long terminal repeat sequences (LTR) at both ends of the genome contain promoter and enhancer sequences. However, there are important differences between the viruses in the accessory genes involved in the regulation of replication which are found only in *Complex* retroviruses (Δ-, ε-, lenti- and spumaviruses). *Simple* retroviruses (α-, β- and γ-retroviruses) encode only for *gag*, *pol* and *env* genes products. Studies of HTLV

genes and gene products provided the basis for understanding of the functional homologues subsequently found in HIV, despite the lack of significant sequence homology between the two viruses. The HIV transactivating gene, *tat*, which stimulates the synthesis of all viral proteins and *rev*, the gene that mediates the transport of unspliced viral mRNA from the nucleus to the cytoplasm are homologues of the HTLV genes *tax* and *rex*, respectively.

The six proteins coded for by the *gag* gene, of HIV, are all found in the virion (see Figs. 55.3 and 55.4). The *pol* gene products are the protease, reverse transcriptase and integrase enzymes; all required during replication. The *env* gene codes for a large protein that is glycosylated and cleaved to gp41, the transmembrane protein and gp120, present on the envelope as a trimer with many glycosylation sites.

### REPLICATION

Retroviruses replicate and produce viral RNA from a DNA copy of the virion RNA (hence their name).

Initial attachment of HIV to target cells is by the interaction of the external envelope glycoprotein gp120 with part of the CD4 molecule of T helper lymphocytes and other cells; the HIV envelope then interacts with a second (co-) receptor. These include the chemokine receptors, CCR5 and CXCR4 expressed on a wide range of lymphoid and non-lymphoid cells, whose ligands are chemotactic cytokines such as CCL3 (formerly known as macrophage inflammatory protein-1α). After this second binding step, entry of the virus occurs by fusion of the viral envelope with the cellular membrane, which requires exposure of a hydrophobic domain in gp41. Once the RNA is released into the cytoplasm, the reverse transcriptase acts to form the double-stranded DNA copy, which is transported to the nucleus and is spliced into the host cell DNA (see Ch. 7) in which

Exposure

PHI

Asymptomatic

AIDS-related features

Remains asymptomatic

AIDS

**Fig. 55.5** Stages of infection with HIV. PHI, primary HIV infection.

| Table 55.1 | Staging of laboratory confirmed human immunodeficiency virus infection (Communicable Disease Centre, CDC) | | |
|---|---|---|---|
| Stage | CD4+ T cell count (or CD4+ T cell %) | | Clinical evidence |
| 1 | >499 cells/µL (or >28%) | AND | No AIDS-defining condition |
| 2 | 200-499 cells/ µL (or 14-28%) | AND | No AIDS-defining condition |
| 3* (AIDS) | <200 cells/ µL (or <14%) | OR | confirmed AIDS-defining condition |
| Unknown | No information on CD4+ count (%) | | No clinical information |

*CDC stage 3 is equivalent to the WHO Clinical Stage 4

state it is referred to as the *provirus*. Once inserted into the host DNA, infection with HIV is permanent. The virus may stay latent or enter a productive cycle. Transcription of mRNA from the provirus is by the host RNA polymerase II to produce viral mRNA and RNA. Proteins are synthesized and processed to form the virion components (see Figs 55.3 & 55.4). Virions are assembled at the cell membrane where envelope and core proteins have located. The internal structure of the virion matures as it buds from the cell; the entire replicative cycle is completed in approximately 24 hours. In the productive growth cycle the host cell is frequently destroyed.

## HIV INFECTION

### CLINICAL FEATURES

The different stages of HIV infection are summarized in Figure 55.5. These stages are generally reflected in CDC (Table 55.1) and WHO surveillance case definitions that utilize clinical and immunological evidence to classify established HIV infections. Both schemes may provide reliable information on the stage of the epidemic within populations in which combination antiretroviral therapy (cART) is not universally used, however their usefulness is somewhat limited in the cART era. Patients are assigned a stage according to the lowest CD4 positive T lymphocyte cell count (CD4+) or worst clinical stage they have ever reached.

Symptomatic *primary HIV infection* (PHI), often referred to as acute seroconversion illness, occurs within 10–30 days of initial exposure to the virus and resolves in the majority of infected individuals within a month. Features described include fever, pharyngitis, headache, malaise, generalized lymphadenopathy and non-pruruitic maculopapular rash. Although up to 70% of patients experience some symptoms, only 5–10% show the full picture. Even fewer have a rare aseptic meningoencephalitis presentation.

Following resolution of primary infection symptoms, a prolonged, largely asymptomatic phase ensues. This may last as long as 10 years during which the virus continues to replicate resulting ultimately in significant damage to the immune system in untreated individuals. *Persistent generalized lymphadenopathy* is present in 30–70% of patients who are otherwise asymptomatic. The rate of progression of patients to AIDS is no greater in these patients than in those without adenopathy.

The inexorable decline in immune function eventually predisposes the patient to the development of the *acquired immune deficiency syndrome* (AIDS). This may present in many ways, all due to loss of the ability to respond appropriately to infectious agents and to control tumours. There are over 20 AIDS-defining conditions reflecting the specific agents involved; a diagnosis of AIDS is made if one (or more) of the conditions listed in Box 55.1 is present.

The occurrence of an AIDS-defining illness may be preceded by non-specific features such as fever, adenopathy and weight loss and minor opportunistic infections such as reactivation of latent herpes viruses (e.g. herpes zoster), oral candidiasis and oral *hairy leucoplakia* (secondary to Epstein–Barr virus infection). The latter condition in which the margins of the tongue show white ridges of fronds on the epithelium appears to be unique to HIV-infected patients.

> **Box 55.1** AIDS defining clinical conditions
>
> - Bacterial infections, multiple or recurrent in child aged less than 13 years
> - Candidiasis of oesophagus, bronchi, or lungs
> - Cervical cancer
> - Coccidiomycosis, disseminated
> - Cryptococcosis, extrapulmonary
> - Cytomegalovirus retinitis
> - Encephalopathy, HIV related
> - Herpes simplex virus for more than 1 month; or bronchi, lung or oesophagus involved
> - Histoplasmosis, extrapulmonary or disseminated
> - Isosporiasis, chronic
> - Kaposi's sarcoma
> - Lymphoma, non-Hodgkin's or primary in brain
> - Lymphoid interstitial pneumonia/pulmonary lymphoid hyperplasia in child less than 13 years
> - *Mycobacterium tuberculosis*, any site
> - *Mycobacterium* (other species), extrapulmonary or disseminated
> - *Pneumocystis jirovecii* pneumonia
> - Progressive multifocal leuco-encephalopathy
> - *Salmonella* septicaemia, recurrent
> - Toxoplasmosis of the brain
> - Wasting syndrome

Without treatment, such patients progress rapidly to AIDS.

*Pneumocystis jirovecii* pneumonia was the presenting illness in many of the first AIDS patients. Salient features include fever, unproductive cough and progressive shortness of breath. Radiological examination classically shows bilateral lung infiltrates radiating out of the peri-hilar region on plain chest film and/or ground-glass lung opacities on high resolution CT scan. Diagnosis is confirmed by detection of fungal cysts in deep respiratory specimens and increasingly by fungal DNA detection by PCR (see Ch. 61).

*Toxoplasma gondii* remains the most common cause of AIDS complications affecting the brain. Toxoplasma encephalitis (TE), which is almost always caused by a reactivation of latent toxoplasma gondii cysts, classically presents with headache, confusion and fever, developing subacutely over a few days to a month. Seizure and focal neurological signs such as hemiparesis are often present and head MRI (or CT) scans show multiple, ring enhancing brain lesions in most cases. The imaging findings are characteristic but not diagnostic of TE.

*Kaposi's sarcoma* was one of the earliest diseases used to define AIDS. This previously rare tumour had been known for many years; it usually occurred at a single site and was not aggressive. In patients with AIDS the tumour arises in many sites, including the skin, mouth, gut and eye. The tumours arise from endothelial cells of blood vessels, causing bluish-purple, raised, irregular lesions. The aetiological agent is human herpesvirus 8 (see Ch. 43). The tumours were mainly seen in homosexual men, presumably reflecting sexual transmission of the causative agent; the incidence has now declined.

In developing countries, whilst many of the same infections are seen, there is also an emphasis on local problems. *Mycobacterium tuberculosis* infections are an enormous problem in many regions, with the development of strains of the organism resistant to many antibiotics. Many patients show profound weight loss, perhaps accompanied by chronic diarrhoea; the term 'slim disease' has been given to this presentation.

Paediatric patients with AIDS suffer from many of the same problems as adults. However, children infected early in life or at birth are at risk of recurring bacterial infections as they have not acquired immunity to micro-organisms. Lymphoid interstitial pneumonia and pulmonary lymphoid hyperplasia are presentations seen only in young children.

HIV associated clinical manifestations, regardless of whether they are AIDS-defining or not, are diverse and affect all body organ systems. The advent of combination antiretroviral therapy has dramatically decreased the overall incidence of opportunistic infections (OI) owing to the improvement attained in immune function. However, immune recovery may paradoxically worsen underlying OI. This phenomenon, referred to as immune reconstitution inflammatory syndrome (IRIS) is not fully understood. IRIS clinical features vary with the pathogen and the organ system involved (e.g. *Cryptococcus neoformans* in the brain).

## PATHOGENESIS OF HIV INFECTION AND AIDS

The major virological and immunological features of the acute and persistent stages of HIV infection are shown in Figure 55.6. The incubation period in the acute stage is 1–2 months. This is preceded by a period of intense, unrestrained viral replication, reflected in the presence of high numbers of viral RNA genomes and p24 antigen in the circulation. After entering the body, virus is taken up by cells such as dendritic cells that express viral receptors. Within 24–48 h infected cells are present in the regional lymph nodes; virus can be detected in the blood and circulating lymphocytes by 5 days; the number of circulating CD4+ T lymphocytes is decreased. As the immune system responds, both p24 antigen and RNA copy number (usually referred to as *viral load*) decrease, so that by 6–12 months p24 antigen is usually undetectable and the

**Fig. 55.6** Events in HIV infection. PHI, primary HIV infection.

RNA load has stabilized at a lower level (referred to as the set-point); in some it may be undetectable. The HIV viral load set-point, an indirect reflection of the rate of CD4+ cell death, is a strong predictor of the rapidity of progression to AIDS. Temporary increases in viral load can be seen during intercurrent infections, immunizations and pregnancy. CD4+ cell counts recover, albeit partially, and remain more or less within the normal ranges until progression to AIDS occurs, the counts then being less than 200/μL.

In peripheral blood, lymphoid tissue and other tissues such as brain where HIV replication occurs, HIV targets CD4+ T cells and cells of the monocyte–macrophage lineage; the latter may act as a reservoir of virus. Macrophages are also important in carrying the virus into the central nervous system across the blood–brain barrier.

Destruction of CD4+ T cells is caused by:

- viral replication
- syncytium formation via membrane gp120 binding to cell CD4 antigen
- cytotoxic T cell lysis of infected cells
- cytotoxic T cell lysis of CD4+ cells carrying gp120 released from infected cells
- natural killer cells
- increased susceptibility of CD4+ cells (infected and un-infected) to apoptosis.

The proportion of infected CD4+ cells and the quantity of circulating virus rise as the infection progresses, until the patient becomes symptomatic.

Analysis of viral genomes from an individual patient shows that there are several different viral sequences present at any time and that these change with time. Virus isolated in culture may be different from the predominant variants in the blood. Viruses isolated in the later stages of infection have been shown to grow more rapidly, to higher titres and to form syncytia (giant cells) more readily than virus isolated in the early stages. The switch to syncytium-inducing variants is accompanied by a change in co-receptor use from CCR5 to CXCR4. Regions of the envelope glycoproteins show most variation and this could affect the ability of antibody to react with the viruses. Although this could be relevant to the progression of the infection, it also has important implications for the development of vaccines.

## Disease progression

There are host genetic differences influencing the risk of disease progression; for example, human leucocyte antigen (HLA) haplotype A1B8DR3 has been linked to rapid progression to severe disease. There is also an age effect, with evidence of fast progression in some infants and in the elderly. Conversely, other host genetic factors, such as HLA B*5701 and heterozygosity for a 32-bp deletion in the chemokine receptor CCR5 (*CCR5-Δ32*) and immune response factors, such as effective CTL responses, are strongly linked to long-term non-progression or even resistance to HIV infection. Box 55.2 lists a number of laboratory markers that are associated with progression. The most useful marker in assessing the state of a patient's immune system is the absolute CD4+ cell count. Although this can vary, a downward trend is indicative of progression: when the count reaches 200/μL the patient is severely compromised and the diagnosis of AIDS is made even in the absence of an AIDS-defining clinical illness (Table 55.1). The median time from infection onset to AIDS is approximately 10 years, although the use of cART has fundamentally changed the outlook for HIV-infected patients.

## Paediatric infection

In most paediatric cases, infection arises from mother-to-baby transmission in the perinatal period when the child's immune system is immature. This results in a major difference from the picture seen in older children and adults as the initial replicative phase is not limited by the immune response and high levels of viral RNA persist. RNA viral loads are often greater than $10^5$ copies/mL at 2 months of age. About 75% of children show a steady decline thereafter; however, by age 9–16 years a third are still asymptomatic and show little impairment of immune function. The other 25% of children have high levels of viral RNA and develop early-onset disease, with death by 20–24 months without treatment. These babies may have been infected before birth by a mother with advanced disease. This group can be identified by detection within peripheral blood of proviral DNA, viral RNA (and culture if available) within 48 h of birth. Analysis of the child's RNA may show that it differs from that of the mother, suggesting that replication has occurred by the time of sample collection or that a minor maternal variant has been transmitted to the baby.

## LABORATORY DIAGNOSIS

HIV infection can be diagnosed through detection of antibodies to the virus (anti-HIV), or of the virus itself (e.g. HIV p24 antigen, RNA or proviral DNA) in a peripheral blood sample.

### Tests for anti-HIV

The main approach to the diagnosis of infection in patients and for screening populations (e.g. blood donors) has been by testing for anti-HIV. Many different testing formats are available, most using enzyme-linked immunoassay (EIA). All current tests use HIV antigens derived from cloned recombinant HIV *gag, pol* and *env* genes expressed in *Escherichia coli*, or synthetic peptides. Western or immunoblotting has been used extensively as a confirmatory assay. Most current assays can detect antibody to both HIV-1 and HIV-2 antigens. A first positive result must be confirmed by at least two other different assays with different viral antigens and a second serum sample checked to confirm that the original sample was identified correctly. At least one of the confirmatory assays should distinguish between antibodies to HIV-1 and to HIV-2. Most patients will seroconvert within 1–2 months (see Fig. 55.6). Thus there is a window before antibody tests can detect infection. Rapid tests are now available to detect antibody in blood and saliva; this format is very useful for point of care testing.

### Combination assays

Reliable and highly sensitive methods to detect anti-HIV and p24 antigen in a single EIA are now available (so-called 4th generation assays); these allow improved diagnostic sensitivity of diagnosis of primary HIV infections by approximately 1 week. Although less sensitive than RT-PCR for HIV RNA, the combination test is of value for diagnosis and for large-scale screening (e.g. blood donors).

### PCR

Direct detection methods are required when serological tests are inappropriate, such as during the early acute stage and in infants who still carry maternal anti-HIV, and for monitoring progression.

Both HIV RNA and DNA sequences can be detected in blood. RNA sequences are found in extracellular virus particles in plasma, and the RNA can be accurately quantified as the number of RNA copies to indicate the extent of virus replication in the patient. Measurement of plasma virus load is now essential for monitoring disease progression and the response to antiretroviral therapy. A number of commercial assays have been developed to provide accurate and standardized viral load measurements in clinical laboratories.

HIV proviral DNA is present in infected cells and can be detected in peripheral blood mononuclear cells. This method is used principally to diagnose infection in infants born to HIV-infected mothers. The standard procedure involves analysis of serial blood samples collected at birth, 6 weeks and 3 months. The absence of proviral DNA at 3 months of age (or any time later) excludes HIV infection in babies who are not being breastfed.

## TREATMENT

Currently used multiple drug regimens (previously referred to as *highly active antiretroviral therapy*, or HAART; now known as combination antiretroviral therapy, or cART) have achieved remarkable success in halting the progression to AIDS, and have helped to transform HIV from a deadly infection to a treatable chronic condition in industrialized countries with access to therapy.

The aim of antiretroviral therapy is to arrest and reverse the damage to the immune system. This will in turn avert the risks of HIV-related clinical problems, reduce infectivity and prolong survival. The decision to commence treatment is dependent on specific clinical and immunological factors (Box 55.3). cART is not recommended, at the present time, in asymptomatic patients who display no clinical or laboratory features of definite or imminent immunodeficiency.

Antiretroviral drugs exert their effects by inhibiting specific steps in the virus replicative cycle that range from virus entry and reverse transcription to integration and protein processing in budding virus (see Ch. 5). To maximize effect and delay or prevent the emergence of viral resistance, three drugs, from at least two different classes, are prescribed together.

The objective of therapy is to achieve continuous suppression of plasma viral RNA to a level below the limits of detection afforded by modern molecular assays, usually around 40 copies/mL. In a patient who has not been treated before, a combination of two nucleoside/nucleotide reverse transcriptase inhibitors (NRTI, e.g. tenofovir/emtricitabine, abacavir/lamivudine, zidovudine/lamivudine) plus either a nonnucleoside reverse transcriptase inhibitor (NNRTI, e.g. efavirenz, nevirapine) or a ritonavir boosted protease inhibitor (PI/r, e.g. darunavir/ritonavir, lopinavir/ritonavir, atazanavir/ritonavir) is currently recommended. The two NRTI agents, often referred to as 'the backbone' are preferably given as a co-formulated preparation.

The management of HIV infection can be difficult and is ideally delivered by a specialist team with access to a clinical laboratory. Specific clinical guidelines on timing, components and monitoring of cART are available from many national bodies, including the British HIV Association (BHIVA). The World Health Organization makes similar recommendations for patients in 'resource-limited settings', taking account of local conditions such as the need for a cold chain to deliver the drugs to the patients and how they are administered.

A patient on combination therapy will have to adhere to a strict regimen. This may be a problem in very young and adolescent patients. The drugs chosen may have side effects in a particular patient or interactions with therapy for other conditions and infections such as hepatitis B and C viruses, herpesviruses, tuberculosis, toxoplasmosis and *P. jirovecii*. Therapy to prevent or treat these infections, if indicated, must be maintained.

Knowledge of previous antiretroviral therapy is also essential as drug resistance may have arisen. It is now standard practice to test the patient's virus population for drug resistance using genotyping methods, before initiation of cART and in situations of virological failure (see below).

## Monitoring progress

The CD4 count and the plasma viral load should be assayed when therapy is started and at 1-month and 3–4-month intervals thereafter. If there is a response, the RNA load will decrease within a few days, will drop by 1 $\log_{10}$ at 2–8 weeks and be less than 40 copies/mL by 4–6 months. If these objectives are not achieved, or the viral load increases after a time on therapy, or the clinical state deteriorates, a new combination regimen should be started (assuming patient compliance with the prescribed regimen). The resistance pattern of the patient's virus should be tested before selecting new drugs. Genotypic resistance testing is accomplished by sequencing of viral target genes and comparing the sequences against an extensive repository of possible resistance mutations such as the *Stanford University Drug Resistance Database*. The locus and nature of any identified mutations will allow determination of which drug(s) within the combination regimen are failing and therefore rational drug switches/substitution(s) by the attending physician.

It is important to note that drug-related toxicity, a largely unpredictable phenomenon, and potential drug–drug interactions remain significant problems despite the progress made over the past decade in improving drug efficacy and tolerability.

The prophylaxis of perinatal infection and accidental exposure is described below.

## TRANSMISSION AND EPIDEMIOLOGY

Virus is present in the blood, semen, and cervical and vaginal secretions, and these sources are important in transmission. Virus may also be present in cerebrospinal fluid, saliva, tears and urine, but at lower titres than in blood. There is no epidemiological evidence that these are significant sources for transmission. Free virus is present at high titre during the early stage of infection and increases in titre in the blood in the later stages of the disease; there is evidence of a greater risk of transmission from such patients.

To transmit, virus has to reach susceptible cells at the point of entry (e.g. Langerhan's cells in mucous membranes) or after entering the circulation.

The three important routes of transmission of HIV are:

1. by unprotected, penetrative sexual intercourse
2. from mother to child
3. by blood and blood products.

### Sexual intercourse

Heterosexual transfer of virus is the route by which the great majority of infections are spread, accounting for 90% of the global total, mostly in the developing world. Overall the estimated risk of transmission from one unprotected exposure is 0.1–0.2% for vaginal intercourse. The probability of transfer is increased if either partner has ulcerative genital or other sexually transmitted disease. Any trauma during intercourse will also facilitate transfer, by allowing direct access of the virus to susceptible cells and the circulation. Transmission may be more likely from male to female.

AIDS was first recognized in men who have sex with men in the USA. Most early studies established that unprotected anal intercourse was a particular risk, especially to the passive, receptive partner. The estimated risk from a single exposure is 0.1–0.3%.

Transmission during oral sexual contact has been documented, but is not a major route.

### Mother to child

Most transmission occurs late in pregnancy or during birth (perinatal). The most likely source is cells and virus in the cervix and vagina, as the baby passes through the birth canal. Maternal plasma viral load is the strongest predictor of the risk of virus transmission from mother to infant; the transmission rate is estimated to be 2% or less in mothers with a viral load of less than 1000 copies/mL. Clinical factors known to influence the risk of transmission include, primary or advanced HIV disease, co-infection with other sexually transmitted diseases and prolonged and difficult labour, Breast milk is another source that is responsible for as many as 40% of new HIV infections in infants occurring in the postnatal period.

### Blood and blood products

All blood for transfusion and the preparation of products such as factor VIII for haemophiliacs is screened by sensitive assays. This eliminates almost all the risk, but it is important to ask donors about possible exposure to risk. Preparation of blood products from large pools of donations was a major factor in contaminating the product as even one infected donation could introduce virus to all the material. Transplanted organs have been implicated in a few cases.

Intravenous drug use is a risk factor in about one-quarter of patients with AIDS in the USA and to a varying extent elsewhere in the world. The risk rises with the volume of blood injected and the frequency of sharing contaminated equipment. The withdrawal of blood before injection increases contamination. By sharing syringes, the virus can spread very rapidly so that most IV drug users in an area become infected in a few months. Those infected in this way can spread the virus to their sexual partners or children. Drug and sexual routes merge when IV drug users support their habit by prostitution.

Occupational exposure of health-care workers to infected patients has resulted in transmission in a small number of cases. The route is via accidental penetrating injuries with needles and sharps contaminated with blood. The risk from a needlestick is 1 in 200–300; contamination of eyes and mucous membranes has a lower risk of transmission. Transmission from health-care workers to patients has been suspected in only a few cases.

HIV-2 is transmitted by the same routes as HIV-1.

### General

The majority of infected individuals have a recognized exposure to a known source of infection. In some this may be difficult to establish, but there is no evidence that HIV can spread by casual contact or inhalation.

Studies of people exposed to the virus on many occasions (e.g. sex workers in sub-Saharan Africa) have shown that a few develop no evidence of infection, and remain negative for anti-HIV. How these individuals are resistant to infection is of great interest in understanding protective immunity.

## EPIDEMIOLOGY OF HIV

The extent of spread of infection can be measured by the numbers of cases identified clinically and by serological testing. Much more evidence can be obtained from seroprevalence surveys of particular groups or the general population. Surveys have been performed on patients attending hospitals, antenatal clinics, sexually transmitted disease clinics and blood donors. Specific groups such as IV drug users and commercial sex workers can be targeted; noninvasive sampling (e.g. collecting saliva or dried blood spots) may make these studies more feasible. Repeat testing over time will give an indication of the trend of infection in that population. Such studies are important in monitoring the effect of intervention strategies and forecasting the demand for health services.

HIV was isolated in the early 1980s, but the first identified cases date to the 1960s. During the 1970s, the virus began to spread widely in some populations and groups by the routes described above.

The scale of the HIV-1 epidemic is monitored by coordinated surveillance by the Joint United Nations Programme on HIV/AIDS (UNAIDS). For 2009, it is estimated that there were 33.3 million individuals living with HIV worldwide, 2.6 million newly infected individuals and 1.8 million AIDS-associated deaths, of whom 370 000 were children under 15 years of age. Although the global number of annual new infections has declined by 19% in comparison to 1999, owing to the impact of preventative efforts and the natural course of the HIV epidemic, the total number of individuals living with HIV has actually increased by 27% since 1999. This is contributed to by the significant reductions in annual AIDS-associated deaths brought about by the increased availability of antiretroviral drugs and care afforded to infected patients in developing countries. Ominously, over 7000 new HIV infections occur every day, a third of whom are young people between 15 and 24 years old. The social and economic consequences of this epidemic have been devastating, with the loss of parents and wage earners.

Frequencies of HIV infection remain highest in sub-Saharan Africa (with a mean 5% overall population prevalence) where most AIDS-related deaths have occurred. Exceptional effort is clearly required, at all levels, to curtail the ruinous effects of the epidemic in this region. In North and South America, Europe and Australia, at least 30–40% of cases are in men who have sex with men (MSM). Parenteral drug users are the other major risk group in these areas. The other cases are in the heterosexual partners of bisexual men, IV drug users, and men and women infected in other areas of the world. The numbers of infections in risk groups can change as health education programmes are introduced; however, the success of programmes varies and advice may be ignored if the perception of risk changes.

HIV was introduced into South and South-East Asia later than in the rest of the world; infection is spreading rapidly. The earliest infections were in IV drug users, but this did not lead to wide spread outside the risk group. Some 1–10% of antenatal patients may be infected. Without effective intervention large numbers of cases and deaths will occur, with all the expected human and socio-economic consequences. It is of concern that the number of new HIV infections is increasing in Eastern Europe, North Africa and the Middle East.

The existence of different subtypes of HIV, and recombinants, is important for two reasons. Firstly, assays for anti-HIV and viral nucleic acid must be able to recognize all types. Secondly, vaccine developers must take account of the various types and establish the spectrum of protection of candidate vaccines.

The Global Fund to fight AIDS (tuberculosis and malaria), a public/private partnership established following the United Nations' pivotal Declaration of Commitment on HIV/AIDS in 2001, spearheads the efforts to mobilize and provide funds for national and regional HIV/AIDS programmes. Despite the unprecedented expansion of access to antiretroviral treatment that has occurred since 2001, up to two thirds of people in need of therapy still have no access to the drugs. The United Nations General Assembly adopted a new declaration on HIV/AIDS on 10 June 2011, reaffirming the 2001 commitment and emphasizing the urgent need to scale up significantly the efforts towards the goal of universal access to comprehensive preventative schemes, treatment, care and support. The target of the new strategy is to halt and reverse the spread of HIV by 2015.

## CONTROL

Until a vaccine is available, the emphasis in controlling the spread of infection must be on risk reduction. Antiretroviral therapy is expected to play an important part in attempts to contain the spread of HIV-1.

### Sexual transmission

The emphasis is on risk reduction by avoiding unprotected penetrative intercourse with partners of unknown status. Despite knowledge of the major routes of infection, there has been only limited success in reducing sexual transmission. Globally the problem is enormous and efforts are hampered by the poverty and lack of resources of the countries worst affected. The use of condoms and vaginal antiseptics could have an impact, but they need to be available and acceptable to the local population.

In the areas of the world with low levels of infection, early efforts to encourage safe practices had an effect on the spread of the virus among MSM in the

Americas, Europe and Australia, but this was not always maintained as the perception of the risks changed as a result of declining rates of infection and, more recently, as the latest therapies appeared to be succeeding and prolonging survival. In addition, it is difficult to persuade the heterosexual majority that safe practices are relevant to them.

Male circumcision has been shown to confer a protective effect against HIV in men, possibly through reduction in surface area of disrupted foreskin epithelium teeming with cells permissive for HIV infection, including CD4+ T lymphocytes. Modeling indicates that the population level impact will be greater than the individual level gain if a large proportion of men get circumcised. This may have an impact on HIV prevalence at least in endemic areas where heterosexual transmission is the dominant route.

## Mother to child transmission

Overall, around 25% of HIV-infected pregnant women transmit the virus to their infants. Rational strategies, based on improved understanding of disease pathogenesis and availability of better antiretroviral drugs and reliable laboratory monitoring methods, have almost eliminated the risk of mother-to-child transmission (MTCT) in high income nations. The main components of current recommendations are universal antenatal HIV testing to identify infected mothers, use of cART to suppress plasma viral load, planning caesarian delivery when indicated and avoidance of breast feeding. Although low cost drugs have increasingly become available, the above strategy is not entirely applicable in low income countries where most MTCT occurs.

The limited therapy available in resource-poor countries such as sub-Saharan Africa can also still play a major preventive role although better approaches are urgently needed. Zidovudine alone given to the mother before delivery and to the baby for 6 weeks can reduce transmission three-fold even if the mother has advanced disease and single doses of nevirapine given to the mother at the onset of labour and to the neonate within the first 3 days after birth reduce the rate of transmission by more than 50%. However, several concerns, including recruitment of drug-resistant viral strains and increased risk of perinatal transmission or progression in infected babies, remain.

Breast-feeding is another possible route of transmission. Exclusive bottle-feeding may reduce risk of virus transmission however that may occur at the expense of increased infant mortality from diarrheal and respiratory infection in developing countries. Where alternative nutrition to breast milk is available, avoidance of breast-feeding is sensible.

## Exposure to blood

Drug injectors can avoid risk by not injecting, or can reduce risk by using only clean equipment. Screening of all blood donors should eliminate almost all possibility of transmission through receipt of blood transfusion. Factor VIII and other blood products are heat treated, if possible, to inactivate HIV. All organ donors must be screened.

Occupational risk in the health-care setting can be controlled by the implementation of safe working practices to prevent accidental injury and contamination with blood and body fluids. The use of gloves, masks and eye protection is important in situations such as surgical procedures where bleeding and spattering are possible. The risk must be assessed in other situations. Safe disposal of used needles, scalpel blades and other sharps is an essential requirement. The sensitivity of HIV to heat and various disinfectants is described below.

HIV is inactivated by:

- heat, in an autoclave or hot-air oven
- glutaraldehyde (2%)
- hypochlorite (10 000 ppm); 1 in 10 dilution of domestic bleach
- other disinfectants, including alcohols.

The chemicals will inactivate at least $10^5$ units of virus within a few minutes, but disinfectants are inactivated in the presence of organic material.

HIV can survive for up to 15 days at room temperature and for 10–15 days at 37°C. At temperatures greater than 60°C, virus is inactivated 100-fold each hour.

If an accidental exposure occurs, any wound should be washed with soap and water, or mucous membranes flushed with water. The accident must be reported so that, if necessary, post-exposure prophylaxis (PEP) can be started as soon as possible. The risk must be assessed through knowledge of the circumstances:

- The HIV status of the source patient; if unknown, can the source be tested?
- Any particular risk of infection of the source patient.
- The nature of the exposure (e.g. penetrating injury or contamination of skin or mucous membranes).

The risk of infection from splashing on to mucous membranes or skin is hard to quantify, but is certainly less than with penetrating injuries. An intact skin is an effective barrier, but abrasions and diseases such as eczema may impair this protection.

If a sharp injury is reported the nature of the injury has to be assessed.

- Needlestick or cut with sharp instrument.
- Depth of penetration.
- Volume of blood involved.
- Whether the needle had entered a blood vessel.

If there is an indication of risk, PEP must be started within 1–2 h, and not later than 48–72 h. If no professional advice is available, for instance at night, prophylaxis should be started and advice obtained. A decision should made about continuing with the drugs preferably within 12–24 h. The victim should be involved in the decision, with discussion of the risks and the possible side effects of the drugs.

Zidovudine alone can reduce the transmission rate, but should now be combined with another reverse transcriptase inhibitor (e.g. lamivudine) and a protease inhibitor. Alternative triple agent combinations can be used or specifically selected with knowledge of any drug resistance in the source. Therapy should be continued for 4 weeks and the victim followed with testing for virus for the next 6 months. A few cases of transmission have been seen in cases despite appropriate PEP.

## Vaccines

Much effort has been devoted to the development of a vaccine to provide protection against infection (prophylactic vaccine) or to boost the immune system of those infected (therapeutic vaccine). Major problems arise because of the antigenic variability of HIV and the difficulty of developing immunogens that elicit protective responses to all variants. In addition, HIV may be transferred by blood-borne or mucosal routes, through transfer of free virus or infected cells. To protect, therefore, it is likely that both cell-mediated and humoral responses need to be stimulated. Whether an HIV vaccine could ever induce fully protective immunity is subject to some doubt, because the immune response, although highly active during acute infection, is never capable of fully clearing infection, and life-long persistence is the norm.

Most efforts have been directed to the development of vaccines containing the viral Env proteins gp160, gp120 or gp41 prepared by recombinant DNA cloning and expression, or synthetic peptides known to be important epitopes for induction of neutralizing antibodies. To date, human trials have shown no evidence of protection from infection by sexual transmission and injecting drug use.

## HTLV–I AND II INFECTION

### CLINICAL FEATURES

Primary HTLV-I infection is not associated with a recognizable clinical syndrome or seroconversion illness. Like HIV, up to 8 weeks may elapse following initial exposure for antibody to become detectable. Seroconversion is followed by an asymptomatic period that can last from years to decades. Clinical disease may eventually develop as a direct result of cell transformation by the virus, in 1–4% of cases (*adult T-cell leukaemia/lymphoma*, ATL), or as a manifestation of immunological responses to it, in 1–2% (*human T-cell lymphotropic virus-associated myelopathy*, HAM; or *tropical spastic paraparesis*, TSP).

ATL was first recognized in Japan. It is an aggressive T cell proliferative malignancy; the features are leukaemia, generalized lymphadenopathy and hepatosplenomegaly, skin lesions, and metabolic disorders, especially hypercalcaemia (*acute ATL*). A distinct, aggressive T-cell lymphoma clinical type has also been identified (*lymphoma/leukaemia ATL*). The two forms have poor prognosis with median survival time of 6.2 and 10 months, respectively. Other less dramatic forms exist, including a variant that runs a slow course, associated with adenopathy and splenomegaly (*chronic ATL*) and an indolent form with skin lesions but no visceral involvement (*smoldering ATL*). Males are at greater risk than females of developing ATL. The period of latency until ATL arises lasts for many years, often decades. The T cells involved carry the CD4 antigen.

HTLV-I is also the cause of HAM/TSP, a slowly progressive myelopathy with spastic or ataxic features. Pathologically, areas of demyelination with lymphocytic inflammation and perivascular cuffing are seen.

There are several other recognized virus-associated diseases, notably a form of uveitis in otherwise asymptomatic carriers and infective dermatitis in children born to HTLV-I positive mothers.

HTLV-II has not conclusively been shown to cause a particular disease however evidence showing a link to HAM/TSP and possibly other neurologic manifestations is accumulating.

### PATHOGENESIS

During the latent period viral proteins are expressed, as there are steady high antibody titres to various proteins, particularly the *gag* proteins. The virus is genetically stable and little cell-free virus is produced. However, during the latent period, virus is present as integrated provirus and is replicated with the cellular DNA as the cell divides. The tumour cells contain monoclonally integrated HTLV-I provirus at random sites. There are no transforming genes. The T cell proliferation is the result of the action of the viral *tax* gene, which can activate transcription of cellular genes including those for interleukin-2 and its receptor, and cause cell proliferation. It is not known what triggers this effect after the long latency in the 1–4% of those infected who develop disease. Antibody to the tax protein can block the stimulation of cell division; loss or decay of immune control may be important. Interactions with tumour-suppressor genes such as p53 and promotion of S-phase in the cell cycle are other probable mechanisms of oncogenesis.

## LABORATORY DIAGNOSIS

Current serological assays, incorporating recombinant or synthetic viral peptides, for the detection of antibody to HTLV-I and HTLV-II are highly sensitive and specific. As with HIV, confirmation is achieved by other assays or immunoblotting (e.g. Western blot) although interpretation can be difficult. Confirmatory tests are able to distinguish between antibodies to HTLV-I and HTLV-II. Detection of HTLV proviral sequences by PCR can also be used as a confirmatory test, and to distinguish between types.

## TREATMENT

There is no indication for treatment of asymptomatic HTLV carriers. ATL patients are treated with conventional anti-cancer chemotherapy or, when appropriate, haematopoietic stem cell transplantation. Interferon and inhibitors of reverse transcriptase (e.g. zidovudine) and lamivudine may have a complementary role in treatment of HTLV-related diseases but further evaluation is needed.

## TRANSMISSION AND EPIDEMIOLOGY

There are three lineages of HTLV-I strains, which are linked to Melanesia, Central Africa and various countries (the Cosmopolitan group). The latter includes viruses from Japan, North and West Africa and the Caribbean, which can be distinguished. HTLV-I and the simian virus, STLV-I, are closely related and it is proposed that human infection occurred many thousands of years ago in Africa and that the presence of the virus in many different parts of the world is related to the migration of ancient peoples. The slave trade may account for foci found in the West Indies and the southern USA.

The virus is endemic in certain communities. In parts of Japan, the prevalence of antibody can be as high as 27%, with a rising trend from 7–8% in the 20–39-year age group to 52% in females and 32% in males by 80 years. In the Caribbean, the rates are in the range of 5–10%, with clusters in communities and families. In other regions, infection has been found in parenteral drug users and sex workers.

The virus is cell associated in the host, so transmission will occur when infected cells are transferred. This can occur during sexual intercourse, blood transfusion and through sharing injecting equipment by IV drug users. In contrast to HIV, breast-feeding appears to be the dominant route of mother-to-child transmission; maternal retroviral load is the major predictor of transmission. HTLV-II is transmitted by the same routes. The strains found in IV drug users in different countries are related.

RECOMMENDED READING

Pillay D, Geretti AM, Weiss RA: Human immunodeficiency viruses. In Zuckerman AJ, Banatvala JE, Schoub BD, et al editors: *Principles and Practice of Clinical Virology*, ed 6, Chichester, 2009, Wiley-Blackwell, pp 897–938.

Taylor GP: The human T-lymphotropic viruses. In Zuckerman AJ, Banatvala JE, Schoub BD, et al editors: *Principles and Practice of Clinical Virology*, ed 6, Chichester, 2009, Wiley-Blackwell, pp 875–896.

UK Health Departments: *Guidance for Clinical Health Care Workers; Protection Against Infection with Blood-Borne Viruses. Recommendations of the Expert Advisory Group*, London, 1998, HMSO.

Volberding PA, Deeks SG: Antiretroviral therapy and management of HIV infection, The *Lancet* 376:49–62, 2010.

### Websites

British HIV Association (BHIVA). http://www.bhiva.org/ClinicalGuidelines.aspx

Joint United Nations Programme on HIV/AIDS (UNAIDS). http://www.unaids.org/en/dataanalysis/

Stanford University Drug Resistance Database. http://hivdb.stanford.edu/

# 56 Caliciviruses and astroviruses
## Diarrhoeal disease

*W. D. Cubitt*

## KEY POINTS

- Caliciviruses (noroviruses and sapoviruses) and astroviruses are common causes of diarrhoeal disease transmitted worldwide by the faecal–oral route and via fomites. Diagnosis is established by RT-PCR, enzyme immune assays or electron microscopy.
- They cause diarrhoea and vomiting with an incubation period of 12–72 h (3–4 days for astroviruses). Illness lasts for 1–4 days, and virus may be shed for up to 2 weeks.
- The very young and elderly are most at risk and may require rehydration. Prolonged excretion occurs in some immunocompromised patients.
- Cold foods are an important source, as are shellfish harvested from contaminated seawater.

The introduction of electron microscopy for the examination of faecal samples led, in the 1970s, to the discovery of a number of viruses that cause diarrhoeal disease in man and animals. The viruses discussed here are the *noroviruses* and *sapoviruses* that form two distinct genera of the Caliciviridae, and viruses belonging to the family Astroviridae, genus *mamastroviruses*. Epidemiological surveys, human volunteer experiments and laboratory investigations have confirmed that they cause diarrhoeal disease. Noroviruses are a major cause of food- and water-associated outbreaks of diarrhoea and vomiting, throughout the world. Sapoviruses are generally associated with sporadic cases of diarrhoea and vomiting, and astroviruses have been associated with extensive outbreaks of food-borne infection in Japan.

## DESCRIPTION

The properties of the viruses are summarized in Table 56.1.

## Morphology

Sapoviruses have a non-enveloped viral capsid with icosahedral symmetry and display a characteristic surface morphology (Fig. 56.1), formed by the 32 cups or 'calices'. Three distinct appearances can be observed depending on the orientation of the particles (Fig. 56.2). Factors such as freezing and thawing, the presence of proteolytic enzymes or incorrect staining can affect the appearance of the particles, which may then be indistinguishable from 'small round structured viruses'. The morphology may also be masked by the presence of antibodies. Noroviruses have a similar structure when studied by cryo-electron microscopy, but the tips of the capsomeres are bent and partially obscure the hollows, resulting in an amorphous surface structure with a ragged outline (Fig. 56.3). Complete virions measure 35–39 nm in diameter with a solid inner shell at a radius of 11.5–15.5 nm surrounding the RNA.

Astroviruses can be recognized by a five- or six-pointed star on their surface (Fig. 56.4), although this is generally evident on only a minority of particles in a preparation. The particles have a diameter of 28–35 nm and are surrounded by a hair-like fringe.

## Physicochemical and physical properties

The buoyant density of the noroviruses and sapoviruses are identical (see Table 56.1) and both genera are stable to acid pH 4.5–7. Astroviruses have similar properties but appear to be more resistant to inactivation, withstanding acid (pH 3.0), 50°C for 1 h and 60°C for 5 min.

## Genome organization

Morphologically typical human caliciviruses and many small round structured viruses contain positive sense single stranded RNA and have been classified within the Caliciviridae. Based on differences in their

**Table 56.1** Properties of human caliciviruses and human astroviruses

| | Sapovirus | Norovirus | Astrovirus |
|---|---|---|---|
| Nucleic acid | +ssRNA | +ssRNA | +ssRNA |
| | 7.3 Kb | 7.3–7.7 Kb | 6.8–7.9 Kb |
| Structural Proteins | VP1 (major,capsid), VP2 (minor) | VP1 (major,capsid), VP2 (minor) | VP34, VP29, VP26 |
| Lipid | None | None | None |
| Buoyant density (g/cm³) | 1.38–1.4 | 1.38–1.41 | 1.36–1.38 |
| Morphology | See Figs 56.1 & 56.2 | See Fig. 56.3 | See Fig. 56.4 |
| Diameter (nm) | 35–39 | 35–39 | 28–35 |
| Antigenic strains | >4 | Numerous | 8 |
| Genotypes | GI, II, IV, V | GI, GII | G1–8 |
| Replication | Cytoplasm | Cytoplasm | Cytoplasm and nuclear |
| Host range | Man | Man | Man |
| Transmission | Faecal–oral | Faecal–oral, air–borne, contaminated food and water | Faecal–oral, air–borne, contaminated food and water |

ssRNA, single–stranded ribonucleic acid.

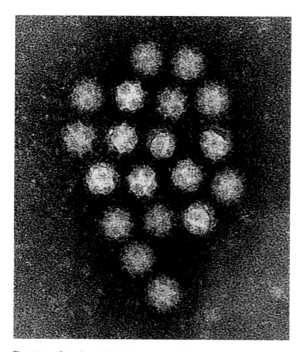

**Fig. 56.1** Sapovirus, displaying characteristic cupped surface morphology. Original magnification ×300 000. (From Cubitt WD, Blacklow NR, Herrmann JE et al 1987 Antigenic relationships between human caliciviruses and Norwalk virus. *Journal of Infectious Diseases* 156: 806–814.)

genomic organization (Fig. 56.5A), human caliciviruses have been characterized within two genera, the sapoviruses and the noroviruses. The nomenclature that has been adopted is similar to influenza, i.e. Calicivirus/genus/place/date/country.

• *Sapoviruses* (SV, e.g. human calicivirus/SV/Manchester/93/UK)

• *Noroviruses* (NV, e.g. human calicivirus/NV/Norwalk/68/US).

Caliciviruses contain a single molecule of linear positive sense, single stranded RNA (see Table 56.1). The sapoviruses contain two or possibly three open reading frames (ORF). ORF1 encodes non-structural proteins and the major structural (capsid) protein (VP1). The Manchester strain (Fig 56.5A) is thought to contain an ORF2 that encodes a putative protein with unknown function. The genomic organization of noroviruses differs (Fig 56.5A); ORF1 encodes a polyprotein that is subsequently cleaved into a set of non-structural proteins during replication; ORF2 encodes the major structural (capsid) protein and ORF3 is thought to encode for a minor structural protein (VP2).

Caliciviruses possess highly conserved regions within ORF1, encoding a helicase (2C), a protease (3C) and the RNA-dependent RNA polymerase (3D). These serve as suitable sites to direct primers for reverse transcriptase–polymerase chain reaction (RT-PCR). Primers have also been designed to amplify regions that encode the antigenic domains. Phylogenetic analyses of the caliciviruses that infect humans have shown that there are at least four distinct clades within the sapoviruses, GI, GII, GIV and GV, and two major clades, GI and GII, within the noroviruses. Sequencing of calicivirus genomes in the regions encoding the RNA polymerase and major capsid protein have shown that recombinants of sapoviruses and noroviruses exist.

Astroviruses have a unique genomic arrangement (Fig. 56.5B) and constitute a separate family, the Astroviridae comprising two genera, the *Mamastroviruses* that infect animals and the *Avastroviruses* which

Fig. 56.2 Electron micrograph showing sapovirus morphology when viewed along the (A) two-, (B) five- and (C) three-fold axes of symmetry. Original magnification ×450 000. (From Cubitt WD, Blacklow NR, Herrmann JE et al 1987 Antigenic relationships between human caliciviruses and Norwalk virus. *Journal of Infectious Diseases* 156: 806–814.)

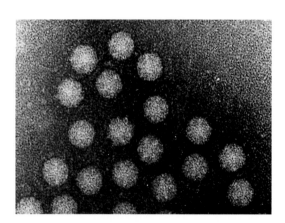

Fig. 56.3 Norovirus. Original magnification ×300 000. (From Cubitt WD, Blacklow NR, Herrmann JE et al 1987 Antigenic relationships between human caliciviruses and Norwalk virus. *Journal of Infectious Diseases* 156: 806–814.)

Fig. 56.4 Astroviruses, showing surface star. Original magnification ×280 000.

infect birds. The genome encodes three open reading frames ORFs 1a, 1b and 2. ORF1a encodes transmembrane helices (MB), a 3C-like serine protease (Pro) and a nuclear localization signal (NLS) and ORF1b encodes an RNA dependent RNA polymerase (Pol). A 70-nucleotide region between ORF1a and 1b is highly conserved among astrovirus serotypes and contains a signal and downstream stem loop structure indicative of ribosomal frameshifting. ORF2 encodes a 79-KDa structural polyprotein which is cleaved by cellular proteases to generate the viral capsid proteins, Vp34, Vp29 and Vp26.

Recombinant strains of human astrovirus have been identified.

## Antigenic properties

At least four antigenically distinct strains of sapovirus have been identified: Saporo, Houston, London and

**Fig. 56.5** (A) Genomic organization of the two genera of human caliciviruses: *Sapovirus* (Manchester strain) and *Norovirus* (Norwalk strain). (B) Genomic arrangement of astrovirus. HuCV, human calicivirus. (From Murphy et al 1995 by kind permission of Springer-Verlag.)

Stockholm. These correspond with the four genotypes that infect humans GI, GII, GIV and GV.

The use of immune electron microscopy and enzyme immuno-assays has demonstrated that there are numerous strains of norovirus.

Eight strains of astrovirus can be identified with specific antisera which correspond with the eight human astrovirus genotypes. The use of a monoclonal antibody has shown that all serotypes share a group antigen.

## Host range

In vivo studies with strains of sapoviruses and noroviruses suggest that they are not readily transmitted to or from other species, although other caliciviruses have been identified in primates, domestic and farm animals, birds, fish, reptiles, amphibians and insects, and some are known to cross species barriers. There are two reports suggesting that primates can undergo subclinical infection when fed with a Sapo-like virus

or Norwalk virus. In both of these cases, animals showed a significant antibody response and were found to be excreting small numbers of virus particles in faeces. Similar experiments have not been conducted with human astroviruses.

Human volunteer studies with several strains of norovirus and astrovirus have shown that some adults can be infected with faecal filtrates containing virus. Pre-existing antibody to Norwalk virus did not confer immunity to subsequent challenge. A person's ABO and secretor (functional fucosyltransferase enzyme (FUT-2)) phenotype determine whether or not they are susceptible to norovirus infection. Approximately 20% of caucasians/Europeans do not secrete the enzyme and are resistant to infection.

## Replication

Attempts to propagate human caliciviruses in vitro have been unsuccessful.

Astroviruses can be propagated readily in a human intestinal cell line, Caco-2, and in HT-29 cells provided trypsin is incorporated in the medium. Immunofluorescence studies show that replication occurs within the cytoplasm and that a protein is present in the nucleolus at an early stage in the replication cycle. Electron microscopic examination of thin sections of infected cells shows the presence of crystalline arrays of particles adjacent to cytoplasmic vacuoles.

## PATHOGENESIS AND CLINICAL FEATURES

Human volunteer studies with Hawaii and Norwalk viruses have shown that replication occurs in the jejunum. Light microscopy showed that the villi in the proximal part of the small intestine were broadened and blunted, and the enterocytes covering the damaged villi were cuboidal and vacuolated. At the same time the numbers of intraepithelial lymphocytes and neutrophils were increased. Electron microscope studies showed that epithelial cells remained intact but the microvilli were disarranged and reduced in length. A similar histopathological picture has been found in calves infected experimentally with a bovine calicivirus ('Newbury agent 2').

Limited data on astrovirus infection in man come from the examination of duodenal and jejunal biopsies obtained from infants with symptoms of gastroenteritis. Histopathological examination showed blunting of the villi, non-specific alterations in epithelial cells, and a mixed lamina propria inflammatory infiltrate. In the jejunum, viral antigen was present in surface epithelia near the villus tips (Fig.

**Fig. 56.6** (A) Duodenal and (B) jejunal biopsies from a bone marrow transplant recipient with astrovirus infection stained with anti-astrovirus monoclonal antibody, demonstrating progressively more extensive staining of surface epithelial cells near the villus tips. (From Sebire NJ, Malone M, Shah N et al 2004 Pathology of astrovirus associated diarrhoea in a paediatric bone marrow transplant recipient. *Journal of Clinical Pathology* 57: 1001–1003.)

**Table 56.2** Clinical features recorded in outbreaks

| Virus | No. of cases | Cases presenting with symptom (%) | | | | | | |
|---|---|---|---|---|---|---|---|---|
| | | Vomiting | Diarrhoea | Fever | Abdominal pain | Nausea | Aching limbs | Headache |
| HuCV/Norwalk | 30 | 66 | 83 | 47 | 70 | 100 | 73 | 83 |
| HuCV/Snow Mountain | 59 | 71 | 70 | 32 | 67 | 72 | NS | 68 |
| HuCV/UK | 181 | 52 | 66 | 65 | 60 | NS | 56 | NS |
| HuCV/UK | 9 | 100 | 22 | NS | 33 | NS | NS | NS |
| HuCV/Sapporo | 250 | 42 | 96 | 18 | 77 | NS | NS | NS |
| Astrovirus | 14 | 74 | 30 | 30 | 49 | NS | NS | NS |

HuCV, human calicivirus; NS, not stated.

56.6). Electron microscopic examination of jejunal enterocytes showed the presence of paracrystalline arrays of virus.

In vitro studies using experimentally infected Caco-2 cells showed that astrovirus coat protein disrupts tight junction proteins and decreases the number of actin fibres resulting in increased intestinal barrier permeability in the absence of viral replication which would result in symptoms of diarrhoea in vivo.

## Clinical features

The clinical features of infection with calicivirus and astrovirus are shown in Table 56.2. The symptoms are similar, but vomiting, sometimes projectile, is more frequently reported in calicivirus infections. In some outbreaks of calicivirus infection involving adults, the illness resembles 'gastric flu' (i.e. diarrhoea, headache, fever, aching limbs and malaise). Patients

of all age groups are affected by norovirus and in outbreaks attack rates are often greater than 70%.

The incubation period for caliciviruses is between 12 and 72 h, and slightly longer (3–4 days), for astrovirus. Illness typically lasts for 1–4 days, with excretion of detectable numbers of particles for the same period. Application of RT-PCR has shown that virus may continue to be shed for up to 2 weeks. Occasionally, symptoms persist for up to 2 weeks.

In patients with severe combined immune deficiency disease, persistent excretion of caliciviruses, astroviruses and rotaviruses can occur, either individually or simultaneously; in one report a patient was found to be excreting five different enteric viruses over a period of several weeks before he died.

Symptoms of illness are generally mild and seldom require admission to hospital. However, when outbreaks occur among debilitated elderly patients or infants with other underlying problems, intravenous rehydration may be necessary; fatalities are extremely rare.

## LABORATORY DIAGNOSIS

### Specimens required

Faecal samples should be collected as soon as possible and stored at 4°C.

### Laboratory tests

For many years the only widely available test for the diagnosis of calicivirus and astrovirus infections was electron microscopy. All of the viruses are small and often difficult to recognize. The sensitivity of electron microscopy and virus particle recognition are increased by solid-phase immune electron microscopy (IEM) or conventional IEM, in which virus reacts with antibodies in a fluid phase, resulting in aggregates of particles, provided that the particles are not masked by excess antibody. IEM can also be used to measure antibody responses.

### Enzyme immuno–assays

Commercial assays are available to detect some strains of norovirus; human astroviruses share a group antigen and a commercial enzyme immuno-assay is available that detects all eight serotypes. An enzyme immuno-assay for sapovirus is not available.

### RT–PCR

The success in obtaining the complete sequence of several human caliciviruses enabled primers to be designed, directed to the highly conserved RNA polymerase region, the VP1 region or the area bridging the two regions. RT-PCR is now the most widely used method for diagnosing norovirus and sapovirus infections, but there is a lack of agreement about which primers are best, because of the extreme genetic diversity of these viruses. The predominant strain circulating in the community often changes from year to year. A number of commercial real-time PCR assays are now available for detection and quantification of noroviruses.

RT-PCR has been applied for the diagnosis of astrovirus infection using primers directed to conserved regions within ORF2. Primers have been designed that are group-specific and others that can differentiate between the genotypes.

The sensitivity of RT-PCR has enabled the technique to be used increasingly for environmental monitoring of water, shellfish and control of infection in hospitals.

## EPIDEMIOLOGY

### Age distribution

Tests for antigen and sero-epidemiological surveys indicate that caliciviruses and astroviruses have a worldwide distribution. All age groups can be affected, but outbreaks of sapovirus and astrovirus infection most commonly involve:

• infants
• schoolchildren
• the elderly.

In contrast, noroviruses cause extensive outbreaks, particularly among adults and the elderly, although there are increasing reports of episodes in children.

### Modes of transmission

The various routes of transmission are shown in Figure 56.7. Epidemiological studies can identify two characteristic epidemic curves for an outbreak. In one

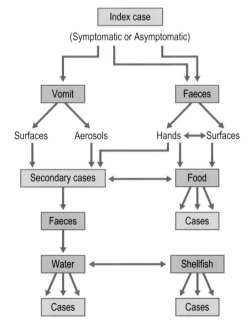

**Fig. 56.7** Routes of transmission of viruses associated with gastroenteritis.

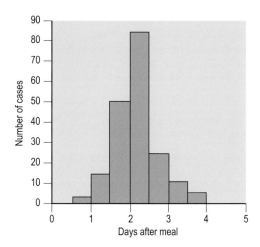

Fig. 56.8 Distribution of cases of norovirus infection following a meal, indicative of a point source of infection.

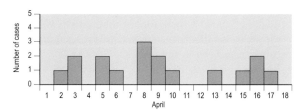

Fig. 56.9 Distribution of cases of astrovirus infection in a geriatric ward, indicative of person-to-person spread.

| Table 56.3 | Food- and water-borne infections with noroviruses | |
|---|---|---|
| Source | Origin | Attack rate |
| Asymptomatic food handler; salads | USA | 220/383 (57%) |
| Asymptomatic food handler; melon | UK | 239/280 (85%) |
| Caterers; cold foods | Japan | 835/3000 (28%) |
| Oysters | UK | 500/1700 (29%) |
| Oysters | Japan | 63/121 (52%) |
| Cockles and mussels | UK | >130/>300 |
| Drinking water | USA | 495/647 (76%) |
| Secondary home contacts | | 719/1740 (41%) |

(Fig. 56.8), when most cases appear at about the same time, this usually results from a *point source*, such as contaminated food or water. In the other (Fig. 56.9), cases occur in smaller numbers over a longer period, often with short intervals between the occurrence of new cases. This is characteristic of person-to-person spread.

## Faecal–oral route

Affected individuals may excrete large numbers of particles in their faeces and/or vomit (>$10^9$ particles per gram). Volunteer studies indicate that virus can remain viable for several years and that the infectious dose is 10–100 particles. Therefore, even minor contamination of hands, work surfaces, taps, carpets, etc. can be a major source of infection. This is illustrated by the number of people who can become ill when food is contaminated by a single handler (Table 56.3).

## Respiratory route

There is strong epidemiological evidence that inhalation of aerosols of vomit or faecal material, from bed-linen or nappies, can result in infection. There is no evidence that virus replicates in the respiratory tract.

## Cold foods

Cold foods that undergo extensive handling during preparation are a major source of outbreaks of norovirus infection. The foods involved, such as sandwiches, iced cakes, melons and salads, are not generally considered as potential vehicles of food poisoning; the true extent of the problem may not be recognized.

## Shellfish

Numerous outbreaks of gastroenteritis due to noroviruses and, occasionally, astroviruses have been caused by the consumption of bivalve shellfish (i.e. oysters, clams, mussels, cockles and scallops). These are harvested from estuarine or coastal waters polluted with faecal material, which is greatly concentrated by the filter-feeding bivalves. Methods to cleanse them prior to consumption (i.e. holding them in tanks of ultraviolet-irradiated, circulating filtered water), although successful in removing bacteria, are ineffective in freeing them of viruses. A further problem is that shellfish are frequently eaten raw or after minimal cooking.

## Water

Outbreaks of norovirus and astrovirus infection associated with the consumption of untreated water, contaminated municipal drinking water or ice have been reported in the USA, UK and Australia. In the developing world, where water is often untreated, the problem is likely to be far greater.

## Asymptomatic excretors

Epidemiological investigation and volunteer trials have shown that asymptomatic excretion of noroviruses and astroviruses is not uncommon. Such individuals may serve as an important reservoir of infection, particularly in situations such as hospitals or the catering industry.

## TREATMENT

At present there is no specific treatment for infections with these agents. Severe dehydration in infants or elderly debilitated patients should be managed in hospital with parenteral fluid replacement.

### Control of food-borne outbreaks

The following guidelines for the management of an outbreak associated with food are provided by the Health Protection Agency in the UK:

- Staff who develop or have had symptoms such as diarrhoea and/or vomiting should be excluded from work until 48 h after recovery.
- If kitchen or adjacent areas have been fouled (e.g. by vomit) then (a) the area should be thoroughly cleaned and disinfected with a 10 000-ppm hypochlorite solution, and (b) all food to be eaten uncooked should be destroyed.
- The importance of hygienic practices, particularly hand-washing, should be reinforced.
- High-risk foods such as bivalve shellfish should be excluded from the kitchen, and other foods that require much handling (e.g. salads and

sandwiches) should be bought in or obtained from other branches if at all possible.
- Unnecessary kitchen traffic should be stopped: the kitchen should not be used as a short cut for other staff, particularly during an outbreak.

### Management and prevention of hospital outbreaks

- Ensure that both bacteriological and virological investigations are instigated at the same time.
- Whenever possible, affected patients should be isolated and infected nursing, medical and support staff excluded from work.
- All staff and patients on an affected ward should be screened as asymptomatic infections are common.
- Particular attention should be paid to hand-washing; 70–90% methanol or ethanol has been shown to be effective against astroviruses and rotaviruses even in the presence of faeces.
- Bed-pan washers need to be examined to ensure they are working efficiently.
- In some outbreaks it may be necessary to close wards to new admissions until all patients have stopped excreting virus and no new cases have occurred for a period of 72 h.
- Staff movement from affected to unaffected wards should be restricted, group activities stopped and visits by children discouraged.

RECOMMENDED READING

Brievogel B: Diary of a Norwalk virus. Following an outbreak in long-term care, *Assisted Living Success* 3:1–9, 2003.

Butot S, Le Guyader S, Krol J, et al: Evaluation of various real time RT-PCR assays for the detection and quantification of human noroviruses, *Journal of Virological Methods* 167:90–94, 2010.

Gallimore CI, Taylor C, Gennery AR, et al: Contamination of the hospital environment with gastroenteritis viruses: comparison of two paediatric wards over a winter season, *Journal of Clinical Microbiology* 46:3112–3115, 2008.

Glass RI, Parashar UD, Estes MK: Norovirus gastroenteritis, *New England Journal of Medicine* 36:1776–1785, 2009.

Green KY: Norovirus and Sapovirus. In Mahy BWJ, van Regenmortel MHV, editors: *Desk Encyclopedia of Human and Medical Virology*, Oxford, 2009, Elsevier Ltd, pp 208–213.

Kroneman A, Vennema H, van Duijinhoven Y, et al: High number of Norovirus outbreaks associated with a GII.4 variant in the

Netherlands and elsewhere: does this herald a worldwide increase? *Eurosurveillance* 10:51–52, 2005.

Moser LA, Carter MJ, Schultz-Cherry S: Astrovirus increases epithelial barrier permeability independently of viral replication, *Journal of Virology* 81:11937–11945, 2007.

Svraka S, Vennema H, van der Veer B, et al: Epidemiology and genotype analysis of emerging sapovirus-associated infections across Europe, *Journal of Clinical Microbiology* 48:2191–2198, 2010.

Tan M, Jiang X: Norovirus gastroenteritis, carbohydrate receptors, and animal models, *PLoS Pathogens* 6:e1000983, 2010.

### Websites

Institute for Animal Health: Caliciviridae. http://www.caliciviridae.com/
International Committee for Taxonomy of viruses: Virus taxonomy. http://www.ictvonline.org/

# 57 Coronaviruses

*J. S. M. Peiris*

## KEY POINTS

- Coronaviruses are widespread among mammals and birds, affecting many organ systems and causing a range of diseases.
- Human coronaviruses 229E and OC43 are major causes of the 'common cold'. These, as well as the newly discovered HCoV NL-63 and HKU1, can cause both upper respiratory tract infection and sometimes lead to lower respiratory tract infections in all age groups.
- SARS CoV emerged from bats, adapted in other small wild mammals (e.g. civet cats) and acquired efficient human transmission leading to a global outbreak of a novel disease. However, unusual features of its pathophysiology allowed public health measures to interrupt virus transmission in humans.
- No vaccines or antivirals are in routine clinical use for any HCoV.

Coronaviruses were discovered in the early 1930s when an acute respiratory infection of domesticated chickens was shown to be caused by a virus now known as avian infectious bronchitis virus (IBV). The first human coronaviruses (HCoV) were discovered in the 1960s. Research with human volunteers at the Common Cold Unit near Salisbury, UK, showed that colds could be induced by nasal washings that did not contain rhinoviruses. Subsequent in-vitro experiments, where nasal swabs from these volunteers were inoculated onto organ cultures of the respiratory tract, revealed the presence of enveloped viruses with the characteristic morphology of coronaviruses as previously described for IBV. The term *coronavirus* (Latin: corona, crown) was adopted for these agents, reflecting their characteristic fringed appearance in the electron microscope after negative staining. Coronaviruses are now recognized in a range of animal species causing respiratory, gastrointestinal,

neurological and systemic diseases (Box 57.1). Until the emergence of SARS in 2003, only two, HCoV 229E and OC43, were recognized as human pathogens. Both were causes of the common cold, considered a mild and insignificant illness and thus not a high priority for intensive research. Following the recognition that SARS was caused by a novel coronavirus, two other new HCoVs, NL63 and HKU-1, were found in association with respiratory disease. The renewed interest in this group of viruses has led to the discovery of a plethora of other animal coronaviruses in diverse species and stimulated research on their capacity to cross species-barriers to infect new animal species.

## TAXONOMY

*Coronaviruses* and *toroviruses* are two virus genera within the virus family Coronaviridae, order Nidovirales. Coronaviruses are well-established pathogens of humans and animals while the toroviruses are recognized as causes of animal diarrhoea. Toroviruses have also been found in human faeces but their aetiological role remains unclear.

Coronaviruses are classified into three groups, initially based on antigenic relationships of the spike (S), membrane (M) and nucleocapsid (N) proteins and now re-enforced by viral genetic phylogeny (Box 57.1). The HCoVs 229E and NL63 are group 1 coronaviruses, while OC43, HKU-1 and SARS coronaviruses are classified in group 2. Group 3 coronaviruses are found in avian species. Genetic recombination readily occurs between members of the same and of different coronavirus groups providing opportunity for increased genetic diversity.

Efforts to identify the animal reservoir of SARS coronavirus led to the discovery of diverse bat coronaviruses in both group 1 and 2 that are closely related phylogenetically to different mammalian coronaviruses. It has been proposed that bat coronaviruses

**Box 57.1    Classification of coronaviruses**

**Group 1**
- Human coronavirus (HCoV) 229E
- Human coronavirus NL63
- Porcine transmissible gastro-enteritis virus (TGEV)
- Canine coronavirus (CCoV)
- Feline infectious peritonitis virus (FIPV)
- Porcine epidemic diarrhoea virus (PEDV)
- Bat coronaviruses (e.g. 1A, HKU2)

**Group 2**
- Human coronavirus (HCoV) OC43
- Human coronavirus HKU1
- SARS coronavirus
- Rat coronavirus (RCoV)
- Rat sialodacro-adenitis virus (SDAV)
- Porcine haemagglutinating encephalomyelitis virus (HEV)
- Bovine coronavirus (BCoV)
- Mouse hepatitis virus (MHV)
- Bat coronaviruses (e.g. SARS-like coronavirus Rp3, HKU4, 229E like bat coronavirus)

**Group 3**
- Avian infectious bronchitis virus (IBV)
- Turkey coronavirus (TcoV)

**Fig. 57.1** Particles of HCoV serogroup 229E grown in human fibroblast cells and stained with 1.5% phosphotungstic acid. Bar = 100 nm.

may indeed have been the ancestors of many mammalian coronaviruses. It is noteworthy that recent studies on the comparative evolution of animal and human coronaviruses have led to the conclusion that HCoV 229E and OC43, the causes of the common cold which are now globally endemic in humans, crossed species from their animal reservoirs (bats and cattle, respectively) to humans within the last 200 years, illustrating the fact that coronaviruses continue to cross species barriers and cause novel diseases.

## PROPERTIES

### Morphology and structure

Coronaviruses are pleomorphic and enveloped, varying between 60–220 nm in diameter in negatively stained virus particles. Club-shaped surface projections or peplomers (composed of trimers of spike (S) protein) of approximately 20 nm in length are seen in all species, giving the particles their characteristic fringed appearance (Fig. 57.1). Some group 2 coronaviruses (OC43, bovine coronavirus) have an additional shorter haemagglutinin-esterase protein on the virus surface which forms a distinct inner fringe of short peplomers.

Coronaviruses have a non-segmented single-stranded positive-sense RNA genome of approximately 30 kb, making these the largest known RNA virus genomes. In the virion, viral RNA is complexed with nucleoprotein (N) in an extended helical nucleocapsid 9–11 nm in diameter. This is enclosed within a lipid-bilayer membrane envelope in association with a transmembrane protein (M), which is the most abundant virus structural protein. The spike (S) glycoprotein, smaller amounts of a non glycosylated envelope (E) protein, and in some group 2 viruses, also the haemagglutinin-esterase (HE) protein, are also found on the virus envelope.

The S protein is the major inducer of neutralizing antibody, although when it is present, the haemagglutinin esterase protein is also a target for neutralizing antibody. Monoclonal antibodies raised against M protein can neutralize infectivity in the presence of complement. Antigenic variation is a feature of the S protein, whereas the N protein is relatively conserved.

## REPLICATION

Coronaviruses attach to their glycoprotein receptors on host cells via their S (and when present, the HE) proteins. The tissue tropism of coronaviruses is mainly determined by the S1 part of the S protein and by the type and distribution of respective receptors on the cell surface. An illustrative example comes from veterinary virology. Transmissible gastroenteritis virus

(TGEV) and porcine respiratory coronavirus (PRCV) are common causes of disease in pigs, the former causing gastrointestinal disease and the latter being a cause of respiratory disease. It has been found that PRCV arose from TGEV through a deletion in part of the S protein that dramatically altered the tropism of the virus from the gastrointestinal to the respiratory tract. Group 1 coronaviruses 229E and NL63 bind to the metalloproteases, human aminopeptidase N and angiotensin converting enzyme 2 (ACE-2) respectively. Group 2 coronaviruses bind to 9-O-acetylated neuraminic acid molecules on the cell surface. SARS coronavirus also uses ACE-2 as the receptor for virus binding and entry. The receptors for OC43 and HKU-1 have not been yet identified. Viral entry is mediated by fusion of the viral envelope with the host cell membrane or by receptor mediated endocytosis. The fusion of the viral and cell membranes (either at the cell surface or within the endocytic vesicle) is mediated by the S2 portion of the virus spike protein which functions as a class 1 fusion protein.

Once the viral RNA is released into the cytoplasm, an RNA-dependent RNA polymerase translated from the plus-stranded viral genomic RNA makes a negative strand template from which it then synthesizes a series of 3′ co-terminal nested genomic mRNAs. The viruses replicate in the cytoplasm with a growth cycle of 10–12 h. Newly forming virions bud into the rough endoplasmic reticulum (where the M protein localizes) and accumulate into intracytoplasmic vesicles (Fig. 57.2). These newly formed virions are transported via the Golgi apparatus to the plasma membrane where they are released by exocytosis. Viral infection may result in cell lysis or fusion of adjacent cells may lead to the formation of syncytia.

## PATHOGENESIS

Infection with the common-cold coronaviruses leads to loss of ciliary action (ciliostasis) and degenerative changes affecting the cilia of epithelial cells of the respiratory tract. Direct cell cytolysis is not prominent although this may also contribute to pathogenesis. The mechanisms of pathogenesis of HKU-1 and NL63 are not yet well studied. SARS CoV targets type 1 and type 2 alveolar epithelial cells of the lung and also differentiated bronchial epithelial cells. The desquamation of alveolar epithelial cells leads to hyaline membrane formation within the alveoli and diffuse alveolar damage, the histological hallmark of acute respiratory distress syndrome (ARDS). Patients with SARS have elevated levels of pro-inflammatory cytokines (IL-6, IL-12) and chemokines (IL-8, CCL-2,

CXCL10) in the plasma but whether these mediators drive disease pathogenesis or are simply the consequence of the lung pathology remains unresolved. However, viral load in the upper respiratory tract peaks around days 7–10 of the disease and falls thereafter, while the lung pathology appears to progress through the second week of illness, suggesting that the lung pathology continues to be driven by mechanisms other than viral replication alone. The severity of SARS infection in humans increased with age, and interestingly, a similar phenomenon is also observed in SARS CoV infected mice and primates. The SARS CoV also infects the intestinal epithelium and virus is shed in the faeces. The diarrhoea associated with SARS infection may be related in part to direct infection of the intestinal tract.

A possible link between multiple sclerosis and coronaviruses has been investigated for some time. The genomes of Coronavirus 229E and OC43 have been detected in the brain tissue of patients with multiple sclerosis. However, these virus genomes are also detected in persons dying of non-neurological causes and thus the aetiological link between coronaviruses and neurologic disease in humans seems unclear. Some animal coronaviruses, such as variants of mouse hepatitis virus, can cause demyelinating CNS disease following experimental infection in the mouse.

## TRANSMISSION

The primary route of transmission of human coronaviruses is via the respiratory tract. Experimental transmission of disease was demonstrated by the intra-nasal inoculation of adult human volunteers with 229E and OC43. These viruses have also caused outbreaks of nosocomial disease. Implementing contact and droplet precautions reduced its transmission in health care settings suggesting that respiratory droplets and direct or indirect contact was the major route of transmission. SARS CoV was found to retain infectivity on smooth surfaces for longer than some other human respiratory coronaviruses or other respiratory viruses suggesting the potential importance of fomites and indirect contact in its transmission. However, there was also evidence of small-particle aerosol (long-range) airborne transmission associated with aerosol generating procedures (e.g. use of nebulizers, intubation, high-flow oxygen therapy). SARS coronavirus was also excreted in faeces. Aerosolized faecal material from a faulty sewage system has been proposed as the mechanism of spread in one high-rise housing estate in Hong Kong where one index case led to many hundreds of secondary cases.

## EPIDEMIOLOGY

Studies using virus detection or serology have shown that HCoV 229E, OC43 and NL63 occur worldwide. Although data on HKU1 is more limited, it too has a global distribution and has been found wherever it has been diligently sought. Initial infections occur early in life but re-infection continues to occur at all ages. There is no cross-protection between different types of coronavirus and immunity to the same virus type is also short lived with re-infection being documented within a few months. They have a winter-spring seasonality in temperate and sub-tropical climates. In contrast to viruses such as influenza or RSV which cause predictable annual outbreaks, the contribution of each HCoV may vary widely from year to year, for example 229E contributing as little as 1% to acute respiratory infections in the community in one year and up to 35% in the next. Furthermore, activity may be hetrogeneous in different geographic regions of the same country.

### SARS coronavirus

The epidemiology of SARS CoV deserves special mention, because it highlights the emergence and control of a novel human infectious disease. SARS CoV emerged from a precursor virus which is endemic in insectivorous bats. The close proximity of different animal species (including bats) within large live game-animal markets which service the restaurant trade for exotic food in southern China allowed the bat SARS CoV-like precursor virus to adapt to other mammalian species (civet cats, raccoon dogs) and subsequently, to humans. Initial infections in late 2002 were asymptomatic and did not lead to onward transmission but the virus finally adapted to efficient human transmission leading to large outbreaks of disease in Guangdong Province, China, in February 2003. One infected patient from Guangdong travelled to Hong Kong and stayed one day at a hotel there leading to the infection of 15 other guests who travelled onwards to Toronto, Singapore, Hanoi and elsewhere, seeding chains of secondary transmission in different parts of the world. Within months, the outbreak had spread to 29 countries and regions causing over 8000 human cases and almost 800 deaths.

SARS was characterized by explosive outbreaks of disease in the community as well as in healthcare settings, 21% of all cases worldwide being nosocomially acquired. While many patients did not transmit infection at all, a few patients (so called 'super-spreading events') were responsible for large numbers of secondary cases. Such outbreaks appeared to be associated with a constellation of factors related to host, environment and circumstance and was not explained solely by host factors such as viral load in the patient's respiratory tract. The 'super-spreader' phenomenon has been described also in other infectious diseases.

By July 2003, determined and coordinated global public health measures had interrupted transmission in humans. SARS was unusual in two respects of its pathophysiology that allowed its transmission to be interrupted by public health measures. Unlike other respiratory viruses where the viral load in the upper respiratory tract and transmission is maximal early in the disease, in SARS, peak viral titres in the upper respiratory tract and maximal transmission typically occurred in the second week. This allowed early case-detection and isolation to interrupt community transmission. Furthermore, most infected persons manifested clinically overt disease, and thus, once symptomatically ill patients were detected and isolated, there was little asymptomatic infection in the community to sustain virus transmission. Other respiratory viral pathogens such as influenza are transmitted soon after, or even before, the manifestation of clinical symptoms and much of the infection remains mild or asymptomatic. Thus, while the spread of SARS was interruptible by public health measures, the influenza pandemic of 2009 was not.

New zoonotic infections of SARS emerged from the live game-animal markets in Guandong Province, China in December 2003 and January 2004. But these were caused by viruses poorly adapted to human transmission. Action to remove the potential animal sources of infection avoided a re-emergence of SARS. There were four other instances of human infection with human-adapted SARS CoV arising from laboratory accidents. In one of these instances, there was secondary transmission to contacts in the community, but prompt detection and case-isolation prevented a major outbreak.

## CLINICAL FEATURES

229E and OC43 are associated with around 25% of common colds and are second only to rhinoviruses as the cause of this syndrome. Human volunteer studies have established that the incubation period is around 2 days with peak symptoms occurring at three to four days post infection. Subclinical or mild infections are common. The symptoms of nasal discharge, mild sore throat, sneezing, sometimes together with headache and general malaise lasts for 6-7 days. Fever and cough are found in a minority of cases. Around 10% of children with otitis media have evidence of coronavirus infection. Coronaviruses have also been found in some patients with lower respiratory tract infections but as they may also be found in a proportion of asymptomatic controls, their aetiological role is difficult to establish. HCoV 229E, OC43, NL63 and HKU1 have all been identified in bronchoalveolar lavages in immunocompromised patients with lower respiratory tract disease suggesting that they contribute to severe respiratory illness in these patients. Serological studies have shown an association between coronavirus infections and exacerbations of respiratory symptoms in adults with underlying respiratory diseases or asthma. HCoV infections in the elderly with underlying respiratory disease may lead to lower respiratory tract disease although rarely severe enough to warrant hospitalization.

NL63 and HKU1 have been associated with a range of symptoms including fever, cough, rhinorrhoea, pharyngitis, bronchiolitis, pneumonia and febrile seizures. NL63 has also been strongly implicated as a cause of croup. Between 50–80% of patients with HKU1 infections had other underlying diseases.

## SARS coronavirus

Although SARS CoV is not presently transmitting in the human population, the clinical features of SARS are instructive as an example of a severe viral respiratory disease. The incubation period of SARS was estimated to be 2–14 days. The disease presented as fever, myalgia, chills and a dry cough of acute onset leading to a rapidly progressing viral pneumonia. Upper respiratory symptoms of rhinorrhoea and sore throat were less common. Some patients had a watery diarrhoea. Ground glass opacities and focal consolidation predominantly involving the lung periphery and lower lobes was seen on radiographic examination. Some patients progressed to increasing tachypnoea, oxygen desaturation and respiratory distress syndrome. Moderate liver dysfunction and marked lymphopenia was seen. Central nervous system manifestations were reported but rare. The overall case fatality rate was 9.6%. The severity of disease increased with age and with the presence of underlying co-morbidities.

## Gastrointestinal disease caused by coronaviruses and toroviruses

Coronavirus-like particles have been detected by electron microscopy in stool from diarrhoeal as well as healthy subjects and their role in diarrhoeal disease has remained controversial. A few human enteric coronaviruses (HECoV) have been successfully cultured in human embryonic intestinal organ culture. They appear to be endemic throughout the world, with a higher prevalence in developing countries. In western countries the prevalence is high in travellers from developing countries and in low socio-economic groups, and is markedly higher in male homosexuals than in the normal population. There is strong circumstantial evidence that HECoV are spread by the enteric or faecal–oral route. The observed high prevalence among western male homosexuals may be explained by oral–anal–genital contact.

More recently, HKU1 has been detected in stool as well as the respiratory tract of patients with diarrhoeal syndromes by molecular methods and it is possible that this virus disseminates beyond the respiratory tract.

Toroviruses (a distinct genus within the family coronaviridae; see section on Taxonomy) have also been found in association with gastroenteritis in humans. Clinically these cases were less likely to manifest with vomiting and more likely to have a bloody diarrhoea and were more common in the immunocompromised.

## LABORATORY DIAGNOSIS

Respiratory specimens are the specimens of choice but some coronaviruses (HKU1, SARS CoV, enteric coronaviruses) can also be detected in stool specimens. Prior to the emergence of SARS, coronaviruses were regarded as insignificant pathogens and routine laboratory diagnosis was not regarded as important. Furthermore, isolation of coronaviruses from clinical specimens is technically challenging, some of them requiring inoculation onto organ cultures of human embryonic trachea (e.g. OC43-like viruses) or special cell-lines (e.g. human embryonic lung fibroblasts, HUH7, LLC-MK2, Vero-E6) together with multiple sub-passages for their detection, procedures not readily amenable to routine diagnostic practice. The human hepatoma cell-line HUH7 has been recently used for primary isolation of OC43, 229E and HKU-1 viruses from clinical specimens and NL63 has been isolated in LLC-MK2 and Vero B4 cells. Some avian and mammalian (not human) coronaviruses can be cultivated readily in embryonated eggs. Some coronaviruses have the ability to haemagglutinate red blood cells, a property that has been used to detect their growth in cell cultures. Direct antigen detection of virus infected cells in clinical specimens has been shown to be feasible, but validated reagents are not widely available and the method is not frequently used.

Detection of viral RNA by RT-PCR is the widely used method in recent times. Specific primers for detecting 229E, OC43, NL-63 and HKU have been reported. However the limited sequence data available on non-SARS coronaviruses needs to alert us to the possibility that PCR primers designed on the basis of currently available viral genetic data may not encompass the full genetic diversity of these viruses. There are also consensus coronavirus-specific primers that are broadly reactive with many human and animal coronavirus types and these have been used to detect novel coronaviruses (e.g. HKU1) but they are typically less sensitive than good type-specific primers.

Electron microscopy of negatively stained stool specimens is useful for the detection of enteric coronaviruses and toroviruses. The two types of viruses are similar in size and may be difficult to distinguish by electron microscopic morphology but toroviruses typically exhibit a doughnut-like or rod-like appearance unlike typical coronaviruses.

Complement fixation, ELISA assays, immunofluorescence or virus neutralization tests have been used for serological diagnosis and for sero-epidemiology of coronavirus infections.

## Discovery of a new human pathogen, SARS coronavirus

SARS presented as a severe progressive 'atypical pneumonia' with no pathognomonic features except a propensity to lead to clusters of disease in close contacts including healthcare workers. Initial investigations of suspected cases did not find conclusive evidence of known respiratory pathogens. The WHO set up a worldwide network of virological laboratories investigating SARS cases which discussed their results in daily teleconferences. Approaches taken to identify a novel pathogen included virus isolation (including cell-lines not typically used to grow respiratory pathogens) and electron microscopy (EM) on respiratory specimens including lung tissue obtained at open-lung biopsy or autopsy. Immunological methods for virus detection require specific antibodies reactive with the virus and PCR or RT-PCR methods predicate knowledge of the viral genetic sequence upon which PCR primers are based, information and reagents not available in the context of the emergence of a novel pathogen. However, consensus primers targeting regions of the viral genome conserved across viral genera or families, low stringency PCR and PCR using random primers are feasible approaches to detect novel pathogens and were deployed in the hunt for the aetiological agent of SARS. The initial findings independently came from three laboratories within the WHO network isolating a cytopathic-effect causing agent in fetal rhesus kidney cell-lines or Vero-E6 cells. Thin section

EM revealed that these cells were indeed infected with a virus (Fig. 57.2A) and immunofluoresence tests showed that this agent was not reactive with antibodies to previously known respiratory pathogens. EM of negatively strained preparations of ultracentrifuged deposits of infected cells showed particles that were compatible in size and morphology to coronaviruses. EM of lung-biopsy tissue also revealed virus-like particles of comparable size. PCR amplicons generated by random primer based RT-PCR assays on infected and non-infected cells were compared and those unique to virus infected cells were genetically sequenced. Some sequences were found to have homology to those of the coronavirus family. In immunofluorescent tests using virus infected cells, sera collected early in the course of illness from these patients (acute sera) failed to react whereas convalescent sera from patients with suspected-SARS gave a strong reaction (Fig. 57.2B), suggesting sero-conversion to the novel virus in patients with this novel disease. Control sera from an uninfected population had no antibody to this newly isolated virus. Taken together, these provided strong circumstantial evidence of an association between the coronavirus isolated in cell culture and SARS. The partial virus genetic sequence was then used to design specific RT-PCR assays and the virus infected cells were used as substrates for serological diagnosis in immunofluoresence tests and enzyme linked immunosorbent (ELISA) assays. Koch's postulates were fulfilled by infecting macaques with the isolated virus and reproducing a disease similar to SARS. A short while later, the full genome of the novel pathogen was elucidated, confirming thereby that the aetiological agent of SARS was indeed a novel pathogen within group 2 of the Coronaviridae.

This experience demonstrates the importance of 'classical' virological methods (cell culture, electron microscopy), which are 'catch-all' methods indispensible for detecting novel pathogens. Such methods should not be completely replaced by newer PCR based molecular diagnostics. The sharing of information in 'real-time' within the WHO laboratory network allowed rapid progress to be made in identifying the new pathogen, in establishing consensus, in validating reliable diagnostic tests to diagnose SARS and in disseminating credible information about the disease and its diagnosis.

## CONTROL

Given the sheer number of 'common cold' episodes, their inconvenience and economic impact, prophylactic strategies that target coronaviruses and

**Fig. 57.2** (A) Thin section transmission electron microscopy of cells infected with SARS CoV showing virus particles in intracellular vesicles and on cell surface. Bar = 500 nm. (Courtesy of Dr JM Nicholls.) (B) Immunofluoresence reaction of a serum from a patient with SARS on SARS CoV infected cells. (Courtesy of Dr KH Chan.)

rhinoviruses (the two common aetiological agents of this syndrome) would be attractive. However, there are no validated antiviral drugs or vaccines to contain coronavirus infections so far.

## TREATMENT

During the outbreak of SARS, given its severity and high mortality rates, a number of therapeutic options including ribavirin, interferon alpha, lopinavir/ritonavir, and nucleoside analogue protease inhibitor combination therapy were all tried. While there is evidence of activity in-vitro, these drugs were not evaluated in controlled clinical trials and their therapeutic benefit remains uncertain.

## PREVENTION

Attempts to control transmissible gastroenteritis virus of pigs and feline coronavirus of cats through the use of vaccines have not been successful although vaccines for the avian disease infectious bronchitis virus has been modestly effective. The fact that natural infections with 229E or OC43 do not provide long-lasting immunity is instructive in this regard. Thus, so far, there is no vaccine for a HCoV that is in clinical use. The severity of SARS led to a concerted effort to develop vaccines for SARS CoV and range of vaccine strategies including inactivated whole virus vaccines, spike-subunit vaccines, DNA vaccines and vaccinia or parainfluenza virus type 3 vectored vaccines have all been tried in experimental animal models, with some providing evidence of efficacy. It has been established that antibody to the spike protein is the key correlate of protection in animal models. However, as there is perceived to be no imminent public health threat from SARS, few of these vaccines have been taken to human clinical trials. Passive immunotherapy using monoclonal antibodies that neutralize SARS CoV has also been developed and evaluated in experimental animal models of SARS.

### RECOMMENDED READING

Bradburne AF, Bynoe ML, Tyrrell DA: Effects of a 'new' human respiratory virus in volunteers, *British Medical Journal* 3:767–769, 1967.

Falsey AR, Walsh EE, Hayden FG: Rhinoviruses and coronavirus infection-associated hospitalization among older adults, *Journal of Infectious Diseases* 185:1338–1341, 2002.

Gillim-Ross L, Subbarao K: Emerging respiratory viruses: challenges and vaccine strategies, *Clinical Microbiology Reviews* 19:614–636, 2006.

McIntosh K, Peiris JSM: Coronaviruses. In Richman DD, Whitley RJ, Hayden FG, editors: *Clinical Virology*, ed 3, Washington DC, 2009, ASM Press, pp 1155–1171.

Peiris JSM, Guan Y, Poon LLM: Severe acute respiratory syndrome (SARS). In Scheld WM, Hooper DC, Huges JM, editors: *Emerging Infections*, ed 7, Washington DC, 2007, ASM Press, pp 23–50.

van der Hoek L: Human coronaviruses: What do they cause? *Antiviral Therapy* 12:651–658, 2007.

# 58 Rhabdoviruses

*D. M. Healy, A. C. Banyard and A. R. Fooks*

## KEY POINTS

- Rabies has the highest case-fatality (100%) rate of any infectious disease once clinical symptoms are observed. There are at least 55 000 cases annually worldwide.
- Over 99% of human rabies infections are due to bites from a rabid dog. Most of these occur in developing countries and the majority in children under the age of 15.
- Pre- and post-exposure vaccination is available and both are extremely effective.
- A paradigm shift is required to focus rabies control efforts towards the elimination of rabies in domestic dogs.
- Reducing the risk of rabies transmission to humans means implementation of vaccination schemes for both domestic animals and wildlife.
- The number of reported human rabies cases due to bat bites is on the increase worldwide.
- Vaccination of people in high-risk groups (laboratory workers, animal handlers and those travelling to rabies endemic areas) is recommended.

The rhabdoviruses belong to the order *Mononegavirales*, family Rhabdoviridae, and as such each of the viruses contains a single strand of non-segmented, negative sense RNA as its genome. This diverse group of over 150 viruses includes those that infect mammals, reptiles, birds, fish, insects and plants. Within this virus family there are six different genera including: the *vesiculoviruses*, *ephemeroviruses* and *lyssaviruses* that infect mammals; the *cyto-* and *nucleorhabdoviruses* that infect plants; and the *novirhabdoviruses* that infect fish. Only the lyssaviruses and the vesiculoviruses are recognised as viral agents able to infect both animals and humans and cause clinical disease. Of these two genera the lyssaviruses include one of the most notable viral infections known to man: rabies.

First described in Mesopotamia in 2300 BC, rabies has been recognized in humans and animals for many centuries as an almost invariably fatal disease once clinical signs have been observed. Disease usually occurs with the onset of an acute encephalomyelitis, often preceded by periods of excitement or agitation, and quickly followed by coma and death. Hypersalivation, hydrophobia and aerophobia are also prominent features.

## VIRUS STRUCTURE AND LIFECYCLE

### Virion morphology

The *lyssavirus* genus includes rabies virus and ten other defined species differentiated according to their genomic sequence. Two further isolates, Shimoni bat virus (SHIBV) and Bokeloh bat virus (BBLV), are awaiting official classification (Table 58.1). First established by Louis Pasteur as a transmissible agent, the rabies virion is 'bullet-shaped' in appearance, with an average diameter of approximately 75 nm (60–110 nm), an average length of 180 nm (130–200 nm), and has helical symmetry (Fig. 58.1).

### Virus genome structure

The rabies virus genome is composed of approximately 12 000 nucleotides, although variations in length exist between rabies virus strains (Fig. 58.2). The genomic RNA contains all the information necessary to produce the five different viral proteins: nucleoprotein (N), phosphoprotein (P), matrix protein (M), glycoprotein (G) and the large polymerase protein (L). The viral ribonucleoprotein (RNP) core consists of the viral RNA encapsidated by N proteins and associated with the P and L proteins. This RNP is the minimal replicative unit for these viruses. The other viral proteins, M and G are involved in virion structure and attachment to cellular receptors, respectively. The intergenic region (G-L) is approximately

450 nucleotides in length and does not appear to encode any polypeptides. Studies on the G-L region of a wide range of RABV isolates have shown that these viruses do not have the first termination signal identified in the Pasteur virus (PV) strain but instead have a second termination signal, conserved in all RABV genomes, and closer to the beginning of the L-gene.

## Virus adsorption and cell entry

Infection is initiated as soon as the virus envelope glycoprotein (G) attaches to the host cell. This process of adsorption involves the interaction of the glycoprotein spikes, the major determinants for virus neuropathogenicity, with cell surface receptors. The mechanisms by which rabies virus targets cells for infection, the nature of the cell receptor(s) and the determinants of cell fusion remain unclear. Neuron-specific receptors for the virus including p75 neurotrophin receptor (p75NTR), the nicotinic acetylcholine receptor (nAChr) and the neuron adhesion molecule (NCAM), may promote efficient entry into neurons. However, it is unlikely that these are the only receptors utilised by the virus, as efficient viral replication may occur in a number of different cell lines including chick or duck embryo cells, baby hamster kidney cells, mouse neuroblastoma cells, human diploid lung fibroblasts, chick embryo fibroblasts, and Vero cells, although with minimal cytopathic effects. Therefore, cell receptors must exist on a number of different cell types that lyssaviruses can exploit and use for cell entry and replication.

## Virus penetration and uncoating

After the virion has bound to its cellular receptor, viral entry (internalization) usually proceeds by fusion of the viral envelope with the cellular membrane. The

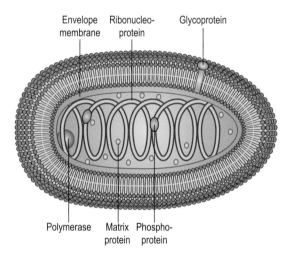

Fig 58.1  A pictorial representation of RABV. (Adapted from an image designed by Dr AR Fooks, AHVLA-UK and produced by A Featherstone, Research Graphix, UK.)

Fig 58.2  Schematic representation of rabies virus genome, with approximate genome sizes (in nucleotides) for representatives of 7 lyssavirus species. ∇ indicates the intergenic region (G-L).

| | N | P | M | G | L |
|---|---|---|---|---|---|
| Species 1 | 1353 | 894 | 609 | 1575 | 6428 |
| Species 2 | 1353 | 918 | 609 | 1569 | 6384 |
| Species 3 | 1353 | 897 | 609 | 1602 | 6384 |
| Species 4 | 1356 | 894 | 609 | 1575 | 6384 |
| Species 5 | 1356 | 897 | 609 | 1575 | 6384 |
| Species 6 | 1356 | 894 | 609 | 1575 | 6384 |
| Species 7 | 1353 | 894 | 609 | 1578-81 | 6384-87 |

**Table 58.1**  Lyssaviruses

| Serotype/genotype | Species | Distribution | Species from which isolated |
|---|---|---|---|
| 1 | Classical rabies virus (RABV) | Worldwide | Wide range of mammals and human(s) |
| 2 | Lagos bat virus (LBV) | Africa | Fruit bat, dog and cat |
| 3 | Mokola virus (MOKV) | Africa | Shrew, cat, dog, rodent and human |
| 4 | Duvenhage virus (DUVV) | Africa | Insectivorous bat and human |
| 5 | European bat lyssavirus type-1 (EBLV-1) | Europe | Insectivorous bat, sheep, stone marten and human |
| 6 | European bat lyssavirus type-2 (EBLV-2) | Europe | Insectivorous bat and human |
| 7 | Australian bat lyssavirus (ABLV) | Australia | Fruit and insectivorous bat, and human |
| 8 | Aravan virus (ARAV) | Eurasia | Insectivorous bat |
| 9 | Khujand virus (KHUV) | Eurasia | Insectivorous bat |
| 10 | Irkut virus (IRKV) | Eurasia | Insectivorous bat |
| 11 | West caucasian bat virus (WCBV) | Eurasia | Insectivorous bat |
| Unclassified | Shimoni bat virus (SHIBV) | Africa | Insectivorous bat |
| Unclassified | Bokeloh bat virus (BBLV) | Germany | Insectivorous bat |

virus may also enter the cell through coated pits and uncoated vesicles (viropexis or pinocytosis), which often incorporate several virions at once. Following internalization, the viral glycoprotein mediates fusion of the viral envelope with the endosomal membrane and releases the viral RNP in an endosomal vesicle. The endosome then fuses with a lysosome where the enzymes allow the ribonucleocapsid to discharge into the cytoplasm.

## Transcription

The RNP complex contains all of the components required to activate viral transcription. Complete uncoating of the nucleocapsid is not necessary as the viral RNA polymerase is capable of copying the virus RNA while it is still in the RNP form. This provides the genomic RNA with protection from cellular ribonucleases. Each of the five viral proteins is encoded on individual monocistronic messenger RNAs (mRNA). These mRNAs are capped, methylated and polyadenylated by the enzymes packaged in the virion. Transcription proceeds following attachment of the polymerase complex to the genome promoter at the terminal 3′ end of the genome. The transcriptase complex then produces transcripts of each virus gene with a transcriptional gradient being produced through polymerase 'fall-off' at each gene boundary where intergenic gene start and stop signals exist. This results in a much greater expression of 3′ proximal genes. This transcriptional gradient is seen in many non-segmented negative strand viruses and is thought to be an evolutionary mechanism to ensure appropriate expression of each gene.

## Translation

Following transcription, the individual viral mRNAs are processed using the host cell translation system. Free polyribosomes, present in the cytoplasm, translate the N, P, M and L mRNAs, and the G protein is constructed as a transmembrane molecule in the rough endoplasmic reticulum (RER), followed by transportation via the Golgi apparatus to the plasma membrane of the cell. In neuronal cells, visible changes are sometimes apparent and large accumulations of viral protein occur with the continuation of the transcription translation process. These dense areas of protein are referred to as 'Negri bodies'.

## Replication, assembly and budding

Once the mRNAs have been translated into proteins a change in composition of the viral polymerase

complex occurs that leads to a switch from transcription to replication. This switch is thought to be associated with the accumulation of N protein in the cell but the exact mechanism remains unclear. Once the polymerase is in a replicative mode, the complex initially drives the production of a full-length antigenome (positive-) sense strand of RNA, with the viral polymerase ignoring transcriptional signals present at each of the gene boundaries. The antigenome strand serves as an intermediate for the formation of nascent genome (negative-) sense RNA.

The negative sense genomic RNA is then encapsulated by the M protein which forms a matrix surrounding the RNP core. Interactions between M and the RNP are thought to enable migration of the RNP to areas of the plasma membrane in which the glycoprotein is embedded. Condensation and coiling of the RNPs is then initiated by the matrix protein. Once associated with the glycoprotein, the condensed M-RNP forms a complete virion which buds from the plasma membrane and is released from the cell.

## EPIDEMIOLOGY

### Rabies virus

Rabies infection in man is generally acquired from the bite of an infected animal. The domestic dog (*Canis familiaris*) is the most important vector, although bat rabies continues to cause human infection across much of Central and South America. Extensive vaccination campaigns in dog and terrestrial wildlife populations have reduced the incidence of rabies across the globe. However the virus still remains endemic across much of the developing world, where the majority (99%) of human deaths due to rabies occur, mainly in Africa and Asia. The World Health Organisation (WHO) estimates an annual toll of 55 000 deaths following human infection with rabies virus, although this is likely to be a gross underestimate. Despite having a devastating impact on human life, rabies infection is preventable either through pre-immunisation, or in the event of exposure, post exposure prophylaxis (PEP) involving vaccination and the administration of rabies immunoglobulin. Importantly, a high proportion of infections occur in children under the age of 16, often in poor rural areas where vaccine and PEP are not readily available.

The UK is currently classified as 'rabies free', with 25 human cases of rabies reported between 1946 and 2010. The majority of these cases were acquired in countries other than the UK. However, the death of a bat worker in Scotland in 2002 due to infection with an indigenous bat rabies virus, European bat lyssavirus type-2 (EBLV-2), was a notable exception. Of the human cases reported in the UK, 19 had not received any PEP, two had started PEP, and three had no known history of pre- or post-exposure vaccination.

In endemic areas, urban rabies occurs among scavenger dogs and cats living in close proximity to human populations, and poses a more immediate threat. Sylvatic rabies, which refers to the spread of disease amongst wildlife, poses less of an immediate threat to the human population. The main focus of sylvatic spread is confined to different species depending on the region in which an outbreak occurs. Examples include: fox rabies in continental Europe, Canada and northern parts of the USA; rabid racoons along the US eastern seaboard; rabies in skunk populations in the US mid-western states; rabies in coyotes in the southern states of the USA; and rabies in the mongoose populations of the West Indies and in Africa. As there is limited contact between these wild species and humans, spread is mostly to other susceptible wildlife.

Control of the spread of rabies in dogs has been achieved using surveillance projects and the initiation of vaccination programmes. These approaches have been successful in the USA and many European countries, resulting in a concomitant reduction in the number of rabies cases in humans in these countries. The red fox (*Vulpes vulpes*) was the principal reservoir of sylvatic rabies virus in many of these countries but oral vaccination campaigns have eliminated the virus across Western Europe and the USA. However, reintroduction from areas of endemicity in Eastern Europe and the Americas has occurred; in France in 2008 after importation of a rabid dog, and in Italy in 2008 when rabies was isolated from red foxes. Both Italy and France had been classified as rabies free since 1997 and 1998, respectively, and remained so up until these recent re-introductions.

Despite elimination of terrestrial rabies, lyssaviruses present in bat populations continue to pose a further, albeit low risk, threat to human life. In 1916, in Brazil, a number of cattle and also humans were diagnosed with rabies following bites from infected haematophagus vampire bats. Further infection was then reported in many Central and South American countries, and also in the West Indies, with considerable mortality in cattle. Numerous reports have shown that many species of insectivorous and fruit-eating bats may harbour rabies virus, with excretion and transmission occurring at different rates. Exposure appears to occur readily in some bat colonies from the close contact among large numbers congregating together, evidenced by the presence of rabies virus neutralising antibodies in bat populations.

While rabies virus has a worldwide distribution, other species appear to be restricted to particular geographic regions and hosts. Lagos bat virus (LBV), first isolated from a fruit bat colony on the island of Lagos in Nigeria, is distributed throughout Africa and has been isolated from domestic cats and dogs, but not from humans. Mokola virus, distributed across Africa, has been isolated from shrews and humans, but not from bats. Duvenhage virus (DUVV), first isolated in South Africa, has been shown to cause disease in both bats and humans.

In Europe, four related lyssaviruses exist within bat populations. European bat lyssavirus type-1 (EBLV-1) is present in Europe as two distinct genetic lineages, EBLV-1a and EBLV-1b. EBLV-1a is thought to be the most recently introduced strain from North Africa via southern Spain, and it exhibits an east–west European division. The distribution of EBLV-1b follows a north-south division. EBLV-1a and EBLV-1b have only been reported together in France and the Netherlands. Most of the EBLV-1 cases in European bats have been identified in one bat species, *Eptesicus serotinus,* which habituates both the UK and mainland Europe, and should be regarded as the host species for EBLV-1. European bat lyssavirus type-2 (EBLV-2) was first isolated in 1985 from a Swiss bat biologist who had been working with bats in Finland, Switzerland and Malaysia. A year later this virus was isolated from bats in Denmark (*Myotis daubentonii* and *M. dasycneme*) and from *M. daubentonii* in Germany, the only known natural wild hosts of this virus (apart from a single case in *N. noctula*). In total, there are only 19 records of this virus (17 in bats, two in humans) from Denmark, Finland, Germany, the Netherlands, Ukraine, Switzerland and the UK. Both EBLV-1 and EBLV-2 have been shown to cause disease in mammals including companion animals, wildlife and domestic livestock. EBLV-1 has been shown to cause disease in sheep, foxes, a stone marten, ferrets, cats and dogs. In contrast, EBLV-2 has not been detected naturally in mammals other than bats and humans.

West caucasian bat virus (WCBV) was isolated in 2002 from *Miniopterus schreibersii* bats in southeastern Europe. This is the only isolation of this virus. Antigenically this isolate represents the most divergent member of the lyssaviruses, and shows a lack of serological cross reactivity to the other lyssavirus species. Bokeloh bat virus (BBLV) a new 'putative' bat lyssavirus isolated in Bokeloh, Germany, in 2010 from a *Myotis nattereri* bat, has yet to be classified.

## Virus transmission

The inability of rabies virus to penetrate intact skin means that it has to gain entry to the body through broken skin (often as a result of a biting incident) or through the mucous membranes (eyes, nose and mouth). In many developing countries, where canine immunisation programs are minimal or non-existent, the predominant source of human infection is from dogs (99% of cases worldwide). In regions of the world where canine rabies has been controlled by vaccination, wild animal bites represent the main source of human infection. Bat bites are also a source of concern throughout the world, as these bites are often small and may go unnoticed.

There have also been reports of rabies infection due to aerosolised virus, either following potential exposure to virus in caves containing large numbers of potentially infected bats, or following accidental laboratory exposure. Experimental aerosol transmission has been reported using a murine model. Transfer of infection via infected corneal transplants has been reported on at least eight occasions in five different countries. A number of organ recipients have acquired rabies having received organs from infected donors. In 2004 in the USA, transplantation of kidneys, liver and an arterial segment from a donor who died from unexplained encephalitis, resulted in the deaths of the transplant recipients from rabies virus. A history of bat bite was subsequently identified in the donor. A similar situation occurred in Germany in 2005. Even though virus has been shown to be excreted in both saliva and conjunctival exudates, direct transmission of virus from person-to-person spread is extremely rare, although possible transmission from mother-to-child has been reported.

## LABORATORY DIAGNOSIS

It can often be difficult to diagnose a case of unidentified encephalitis as rabies infection, especially if there is no recorded history of animal bite or travel to a rabies endemic area. A number of diagnostic techniques can be used to test for the presence of virus neutralising antibodies, virus genome or live virus. Tests on CSF, saliva and on skin biopsy from the nape of the neck (nuchal skin biopsy) are the only reliable assays that can be used ante-mortem. Post-mortem diagnosis of rabies virus infection in brain samples is reliable and is used as a confirmatory test.

## Diagnostic methods

### Rabies virus antigen detection techniques

The 'gold standard' Office International des Epizooties (OIE) and WHO approved diagnostic test is the fluorescent antibody test (FAT), which detects virus antigen in brain samples (hippocampus, brainstem or cerebellum) using fluorescently labelled anti-rabies antibodies. This is reliable and can provide results within 2 h. Sensitivity, however, is dependent upon the quality of the sample received.

Rabies virus nucleocapsid can also be detected using the enzyme-linked immunosorbent assay (ELISA), which has the added advantage of being able to detect virus in autolysed samples. A number of variations of this technique are available.

### Rabies virus isolation

The mouse inoculation test (MIT) involving inoculation of sample into mouse brain and observation of the animal for a period of 28 days or until clinical signs developed, was the gold standard for rabies virus isolation. This has now been superseded and replaced by tissue culture methods.

The rabies tissue culture isolation test (RTCIT) is used to isolate lyssaviruses in a range of clinical specimens from a number of host species, including dogs, cats, bats, wild carnivores and humans. Samples are inoculated onto a neuroblastoma monolayer. Following a 4-day incubation period, the plates are fixed and stained using fluorescein-labelled monoclonalantibodies (mAbs) and the presence or absence of virus is determined.

### Histopathological examination

Histopathological analysis of tissue samples is often used post-mortem as a confirmatory test. The sample is fixed, blocked and stained with eosin and haemotoxylin before application of a rabies specific antibody, which detects the presence of rabies virus nucleoprotein.

*In situ* hybridisation can also be used to detect both messenger and genomic viral RNA. This assay uses a digoxigenin labelled riboprobe to detect lyssavirus RNA in brain samples.

### Serological assays

The presence of rabies virus neutralising antibodies can be detected using the fluorescent antibody virus neutralisation assay (FAVN), a rapid fluorescent focus inhibition test (RFFIT) or an ELISA-based detection system. The FAVN is the current method of choice when assessing both human and animal antibody titres following pre-exposure vaccination. The basic premise for both the RFFIT and FAVN is that a known quantity of virus is mixed with different dilutions of the test serum and the neutralising limit dilution is determined. The non-neutralised virus is then detected using a fluorescence-conjugated virus specific antibody. The results are then calibrated from standard reference sera and expressed as international units (IU). Due to the use of live virus in these assays each test must be undertaken in high containment facilities.

More recently, a virus neutralisation assay using a rabies virus-pseudotyped lentivirus has been developed. This approach uses lentiviral expression of the viral glycoprotein as a surrogate for live lyssavirus. The pseudotype assay has a number of advantages over serological assays based on the use of live virus. Although it requires tissue culture facilities, it does not need to be performed in a high containment facility and is therefore more feasible in rabies endemic areas that may lack such facilities; also the assay requires lower volumes of serum, which is of importance where only small volumes of serum are available.

### Molecular methods for the detection of rabies virus RNA

The use of molecular based assays to detect the presence of virus nucleic acid is becoming more commonplace as these techniques become more widely available and accessible. These techniques are not currently accepted as prescribed diagnostic techniques by the OIE or WHO, but are useful as screening tools and for the generation of sequence data for phylogenetic analysis of samples.

The reverse transcriptase polymerase chain reaction (RT-PCR) is one of the most widely used tools in rabies virus detection and research. The hemi-nested RT-PCR and various other similar techniques are utilised routinely in laboratories worldwide for rabies virus detection. Other assays that have recently been developed include the Taqman PCR, a real time assay that can distinguish between lyssavirus species, and also a PCR ELISA.

The detection of rabies virus ante-mortem is more difficult, as the virus is only excreted intermittently in saliva samples and antibodies are not always detectable in CSF. The use of nucleic acid sequence based amplification (NASBA) is more sensitive that RT-PCR when assessing ante-mortem samples. This technique amplifies viral RNA directly in an isothermal reaction, and therefore does not require expensive thermocycling equipment.

Other techniques are currently being investigated. Microarray utilises oligonucleotide probes designed to bind to the different lyssavirus species. While this technique currently has limited sensitivity when using clinical samples, in the future it could prove a useful tool in the diagnosis of viral diseases of the CNS, for which rabies virus detection will form part of the differential diagnosis

## TREATMENT

### Vaccination

It was the French scientist Louis Pasteur who first introduced vaccination following rabies virus exposure. The original vaccine was a crude extract of infected rabbit spinal cord, which had been desiccated and passaged several times to produce a 'fixed' strain of the virus. The success of this vaccination regime in cats and dogs was announced at the *Academies des Sciences* in 1885. The successful treatment of a young boy who experienced multiple bites from a rabid animal subsequently established this approach. The Semple vaccine, a modification of Pasteur's original vaccine, was a suspension of 4% inoculated rabbit brain attenuated with 5% phenol. This was used in the UK from 1919–1966, but due to the high rate of allergic encephalitis following its administration, was replaced by a duck embryo-derived vaccine in 1966. This was not produced in neuronal cell-lines and there was a decrease in the incidence of adverse reactions following its introduction. This type of vaccine has since been replaced by cell culture-derived inactivated vaccines, several types of which are currently available, including: human diploid cell vaccine (HDCV), purified chick embryo cell vaccine (PCEV) and Vero cell vaccine. While each of these current vaccines has proven to be both safe and immunogenic, they are not necessarily available in developing countries, and they do not protect against all lyssavirus species.

### Pre-exposure prophylaxis

In the UK, the HDCV and PCEV vaccines are licensed and available. These are normally administered to those who require pre-exposure vaccination, e.g. laboratory staff working directly with the virus. For those people travelling to rabies-endemic countries, pre-exposure vaccination may be recommended depending on the local incidence of rabies in the country to be visited, the availability of appropriate anti-rabies biologicals, and the intended activity and duration of stay of the traveller. The protocol requires administration of three intramuscular doses of vaccine at days 0, 7 and 28, following which the levels of neutralising antibody are assessed using a certified test. Response to these vaccines can persist for at least two years post-vaccination. These vaccines are safe and well tolerated, with adverse reactions being extremely rare.

There are a number of different animal vaccines available, mostly live-attenuated preparations that would not be acceptable for use in humans. The animal is generally inoculated intramuscularly, with boosters required every 1–3 years depending on the vaccine type.

### Post-exposure prophylaxis

Wound cleansing and immunizations, undertaken as soon as possible after suspected contact with an animal and following WHO recommendations, can prevent the onset of rabies in virtually 100% of exposures, although some exceptions to this have been recorded. The wound should be washed immediately with copious amounts of water and preferably cleansed with soap. Alcohol, quaternary ammonium compounds, iodine or povidone should be used, if available. The level of treatment or care required depends on the category of the contact as outlined by the WHO (category 1, 2 or 3, see Table 58.2). Post-exposure anti-rabies vaccination should always include administration of both passive antibody (human rabies immunoglobulin, HRIG) and vaccine in patients without any history of rabies pre-vaccination, for both bite and non-bite exposures, regardless of the interval between exposure and initiation of treatment. HRIG provides immediate availability of neutralising antibodies at the site of exposure before the patient elicits an endogenous antibody response following vaccination.

Depending on vaccine type, the post-exposure schedule requires four to five intramuscular doses over four weeks. According to the WHO, two intramuscular doses of a cell-derived vaccine separated by three days are sufficient for rabies-exposed patients who have previously undergone complete pre-vaccination or PEP with cell-derived rabies vaccines. Rabies immune globulin treatment is not necessary in such cases.

There have been seven reports of recovery from rabies once clinical signs have developed, five of whom had received pre-exposure vaccination, and two of whom had no pre-exposure vaccination, but were treated according to variations of the Milwaukee protocol. The first was a 15-year-old girl who developed clinical rabies one month after she had been bitten by a bat. A 'therapeutic' coma was induced allowing an immune response to be elicited. A cocktail of drugs including ketamine, midazolam, ribavirin and amantadine was then used as part of the treatment regimen. Lumbar puncture after 8 days showed a raised level of anti-rabies antibodies and the girl was brought slowly out of the coma. Signs of paralysis and sensory denervation were observed. After nearly 5 months following initial hospitalisation she was alert and communicative but with involuntary movements, difficulty speaking and an unsteady gait. The second was reportedly in Brazil in 2008; a young boy was treated following a similar protocol and survived. Similar regimens have been attempted for at least 12 other rabies patients without success.

### CONTROL

Control of the spread of rabies would require elimination of infection from all reservoir species throughout the world, which is unlikely due to its broad host range, and its urban as well as sylvatic spread. Methods such as shooting and gassing animals have short-term effects. Therefore the principal aim of current strategies is to eliminate rabies in domestic dogs worldwide, thus breaking the transmission cycle and reducing the risk of human infection acquired from dogs.

A number of countries, mainly islands, have been classified as terrestrial rabies free including Australia, New Zealand, Hawaii, Ireland and Great Britain since the early 1900s, and Switzerland, Belgium, Finland, Luxemburg and the Netherlands since 2001. This has been achieved by a combination of strict quarantine laws and vaccination programmes. Although achieving a rabies-free status is more difficult in countries that share borders with rabies endemic regions, the

| Table 58.2 | WHO categories of rabies exposure | |
| --- | --- | --- |
| Category | Exposure | Treatment |
| 1 | Touching, feeding of animals or licks on unbroken skin | No treatment if history is reliable |
| 2 | Minor scratches or abrasions without bleeding or licks on broken skin and nibbling of uncovered skin | Treat with vaccine |
| 3 | Single or multiple transdermal bites, scratches or contamination of mucous membrane with saliva (i.e. licks) | Treat with immunoglobulin and vaccine |

control of sylvatic (wildlife) rabies throughout Eastern Europe and North America is underway. This has largely been possible through the vaccination of domestic animals (dogs and cats) likely to come into contact with these species, as well as oral bait vaccination schemes for wild animals. As most cases of rabies in humans are due to contact with a rabid dog or cat, these vaccination programmes, together with PEP for those individuals exposed in specific incidents to suspected rabid animals, have notably reduced the number of human fatalities due to rabies virus infection in the developed world. This approach, together with vaccination of specific individuals who may come into contact with rabies virus, or rabid animals during the course of their work (e.g. laboratory workers, those individuals handling animals at quarantine centres, veterinarians, animal health inspectors, bat handlers and travellers to areas where rabies is still endemic) has reduced the number of incidents in developed countries who have adopted this scheme.

RECOMMENDED READING

Baer GM: Rabies – an historical perspective, *Infectious Agents and Disease* 3:168–180, 1994.
Department of Health: *Memorandum on Rabies: Prevention and Control,* London, 2000, Department of Health.
Jackson AC, Wunner WH: *Rabies,* ed 2, London, 2007, Elsevier: Academic Press.
Rupprecht CE, Barrett J, Briggs D, et al: Can rabies be eradicated? *Developmental Biology (Basel)* 131:95–121, 2008.
Rupprecht CE, Dietzschold B, Koprowski H, editors: *Lyssaviruses,* Geneva, 1994, Springer-Verlag.
Schnell MJ, McGettigan JP, Wirblich C, Papaneri A: The cell biology of rabies virus: using stealth to reach the brain, *Nature Reviews Microbiology* 8:51–61, 2010.
Tordo N, Marianneau MP: Viruses and bats: rabies and Lyssavirus, *Bulletin et Memoires de l Academie Royale de Medecine de Belgique (Brussels)* 164:7–15, 2009.
Wunner WH, Briggs DJ: Rabies in the 21st Century, *PLoS Neglected Tropical Diseases* 4:e591, 2010.

## Websites

Department of Health: Memorandum on Rabies: Prevention and Control. http://www.dh.gov.uk/prod_consum_dh/groups/dh_digitalassets/@dh/@en/documents/digitalasset/dh_4080657.pdf
Department for Environment, Food and Rural Affairs: Disease factsheet: Rabies. http://archive.defra.gov.uk/foodfarm/farmanimal/diseases/atoz/rabies/
Eurosurveillance: http://www.eurosurveillance.org/
Global alliance for rabies control (GARC): http://www.rabiescontrol.net/
OIE – World Organisation for Animal Health: http://www.oie.int/
World Health Organization: Human and animal rabies. http://www.who.int/rabies/
World Health Organization. Rabies Bulletin Europe: http://www.who-rabies-bulletin.org/
World Health Organization: Rabnet. http://www.who.int/rabies/rabnet/
World Health Organization: Immunization, vaccines and biologicals. http://www.who.int/immunization/topics/rabies/en/index.html

# 59 Togaviruses

## Rubella

*L. M. Hesketh*

## KEY POINTS

- Rubella (German measles) is caused by infection with a single-stranded, enveloped RNA virus of a single antigenic type. It is characterized by a widespread macular rash.
- In the first 3 months of pregnancy, rubella can infect the fetus, causing the congenital rubella syndrome in 70% of cases and leading to abnormalities of the eye, ear and heart, as well as a range of other problems including mental handicap and purpura.
- Clinical diagnosis is unreliable. Serological detection of specific IgM is the investigation of choice.
- Rubella is now uncommon in the UK owing to widespread immunization with a live-attenuated vaccine included in the MMR preparation.

The Togaviridae comprise of two genera, the *Alphavirus* genus which contains arthropod-borne viruses (see Chapter 51) and the *rubivirus* genus, which contains rubella virus as its sole member.

In the mid eighteenth century, two German physicians described the disease now known as rubella or German measles. Commonly considered to be a mild disease with few complications, little attention was paid to rubella until the mid 1940s. However, in 1941, an Australian ophthalmologist, Sir Norman Gregg, described the association between maternal rubella in pregnancy and congenital abnormalities in the infant. He noted an increased incidence of congenital cataracts in children. When questioned, the mothers gave a history of having had rubella in early pregnancy when there had been an epidemic in Australia. Since then the importance of maternal rubella for the fetus has been confirmed by many studies.

## DESCRIPTION

Rubella virus is classified as a member of the togavirus family, and is the only member of the genus *Rubivirus*. It has a single stranded positive sense RNA genome and replication occurs in the cytoplasm of infected cells. It has a lipid containing envelope and a pleomorphic shape with a diameter of 60–70 nm and the nucleocapsid has icosohedral symmetry. The envelope is acquired by the virions by budding from cell membranes into intracellular vesicles or to the exterior. There are 3 major virion polypeptides: C, and the envelope glycoproteins E1 and E2. The virus envelope carries a haemagglutinin (E1), present as 5–6-nm projections, which agglutinates the erythrocytes of 1-day-old chicks, pigeons, sheep and human beings, a characteristic that is utilized in the haemagglutination inhibition test for specific antibodies.

Several chemical agents such as detergents and organic solvents inactivate rubella. The virus is stable at 4°C for over 7 days.

Rubella virus was first isolated in cell culture in 1962 in primary vervet monkey kidney and primary human amnion cultures from throat washings, blood and urine. The virus can be isolated in a variety of primary and continuous cell lines (e.g. Vero, RK13, and baby hamster kidney-21 cells) but only certain lines display a cytopathic effect (e.g. RK13). In other cell lines, the presence of virus is demonstrated by immunofluorescence with specific antibody or resistance to superinfection with another unrelated virus such as echovirus 11.

There is only one antigenic type of rubella virus (although there are minor differences between strains). The World Health Organisation has subdivided rubella virus into two clades and thirteen genotypes. In the laboratory, rubella virus can be transmitted to rhesus monkeys, rabbits and some other animals but man is the only naturally infected species.

**Fig. 59.1** Rubella rash.

## CLINICAL FEATURES

### Postnatal primary rubella

The incubation period for postnatal primary rubella is 12–21 days, with an average of 16–17 days. Virus may be excreted in the throat for up to a week before and after the rash, and this covers the period of infectivity. High concentrations of virus may be excreted but close and personal contact is needed for onwards transmission. Infection has several characteristic clinical features.

- A macular rash (Fig. 59.1), which usually appears first on the face and then spreads to the trunk and limbs. Particularly in childhood, the rash may be fleeting and perhaps 50% of infections in children are asymptomatic. In adults, asymptomatic rubella is less common.
- General features such as minor pyrexia, malaise and lymphadenopathy also occur, with the suboccipital nodes being those most commonly enlarged and tender.
- Arthralgia is uncommon in children but may occur in up to 60% of women. The joints commonly involved are the fingers, wrists, ankles and knees, and, although arthralgia usually lasts for only a few days, it may occasionally persist for some months.
- Encephalitis and thrombocytopenia are rare complications of rubella and recovery is usually complete.

The clinical features of rubella in an immunocompromised patient are similar to those seen in normal individuals.

Rubella is difficult to diagnose clinically as other virus infections such as some enteroviruses and erythroviruses can present with identical clinical features.

Hence laboratory investigation is essential. In the UK, rubella is a notifiable infection; if a doctor suspects a patient has rubella s/he has a legal duty to report it.

### Rubella reinfection

Some patients who have had natural infection or have been successfully immunised can display an increase in rubella antibodies, usually only discovered following investigation of a rubella contact. This reinfection is seldom clinically apparent, but laboratory diagnosis is important. Asymptomatic reinfection in pregnancy presents a negligible risk to the fetus whereas clinically apparent reinfection, although rare, may present a risk similar to that of primary infection.

### Congenital rubella

If the fetus is infected during a primary maternal infection, a wide spectrum of abnormalities may occur. The classical congenital rubella syndrome (CRS) triad consists of abnormalities of the eyes, ears and heart.

- Abnormalities of the eyes, which may be bilateral or unilateral, include cataracts, micro-ophthalmia, glaucoma and pigmentary retinopathy, which may result in blindness.
- Bilateral or unilateral sensorineural deafness may be present at birth, although not detected until later in life; it may increase in severity as the child gets older.
- There are many possible heart defects, with patent ductus arteriosus, pulmonary artery and valvular stenosis and ventricular septal defect being the most common.

The baby often has a low birth weight due to intrauterine growth retardation. There may be a purpuric rash due to thrombocytopenia but this usually resolves, as does hepatosplenomegaly. Microcephaly, psychomotor retardation and behavioural disorders can occur. Rarely there may be a persistent infection of the central nervous system (*progressive rubella subacute panencephalitis*) similar clinically to subacute sclerosing panencephalitis due to measles virus infection. Other problems that may present later in life include pneumonitis, diabetes mellitus, growth hormone deficiency, and thyroid function abnormalities.

Some fetuses may be so severely affected that intrauterine death or stillbirth occurs. Many babies are born with no abnormalities; the risk is associated with the gestational age.

- If maternal infection occurs in the first trimester, the risk of CRS is at least 70%, and many babies have multiple developmental defects.
- In the fourth month of pregnancy the risk reduces to around 20%, and the only abnormality likely to be seen is sensorineural deafness.
- After the 16th week of pregnancy, although fetal infection still occurs, congenital abnormalities are infrequent and the risk is no more than in an apparently uncomplicated pregnancy.

## PATHOGENESIS

### Postnatal rubella

The virus is transmitted by the airborne route. The virus first replicates in the epithelium of the buccal mucosa and the lymphoid tissue of the nasopharynx and upper respiratory tract. Towards the end of the incubation period a viraemia occurs and seeds target organs such as skin and joints. Most of the clinical features are probably due to the host's immune response, e.g. virus can be demonstrated in both unaffected skin and the macules of the rash, suggesting that the presence of virus *per se* is not sufficient to cause the rash.

### Congenital rubella

During viraemia the virus infects and crosses the placenta (in early gestation this is an ineffective barrier to infection) to infect the differentiating cells of the fetus. If such fetal infection occurs in early pregnancy a persistent infection is likely. The fetus cannot mount an immune response in early gestation.

The congenital abnormalities arise from a number of effects of rubella infection. Cell division is slowed, cell differentiation becomes disordered and damage to small blood vessels can occur. Such effects may lead to the abnormalities seen at birth but the persistence of infection may result in the clinical problems presenting later in life, possibly due to direct damage such as in late-onset deafness or because of immunopathological mechanisms such as in pneumonitis. Virus can persist for many years in babies infected during early gestation, but persistent infection is rare in later pregnancy, when the babies are not damaged.

## DIAGNOSIS

### Postnatal rubella

Given the unreliability of clinical diagnosis, laboratory investigation is required to diagnose rubella and

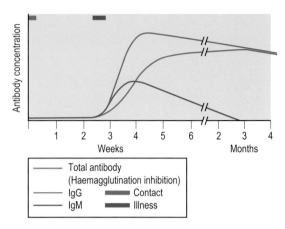

**Fig. 59.2** Serological response in primary rubella.

this is of paramount importance for the pregnant patient. As subclinical rubella may occur pregnant women should also be investigated if they are in contact with someone who has possible rubella.

Virus isolation has low sensitivity and is time consuming and so has no role to play. Serology is the method of choice. Assays to detect total rubella antibody or rubella specific immunoglobulin G (IgG) and M (IgM) are used together. The assays chosen should have a high level of sensitivity and specificity.

In primary rubella, specific antibody becomes detectable at about the time of the rash, although there may be a delay of 7–10 days, and rapidly increases in concentration (Fig. 59.2). Specific IgM usually (but not always) precedes specific IgG by 1–2 days.

IgG persists for life but IgM generally is only detectable for 1–3 months. If a serum obtained soon after contact but prior to illness is examined in parallel with a sample soon after the appearance of the rash, primary infection can be demonstrated by the development of specific IgM.

Problems in diagnosis can arise if serum is collected after the rash appears or more than 12–14 days after contact as any total rubella antibody or specific IgG may be from recent infection or infection many years prior. Again IgM testing must be performed in order to delineate recent infection. Rubella IgG avidity (the tightness of the bond between antibody and antigen) can also be used to differentiate between recent (low avidity) and remote (high avidity) rubella.

The diagnosis of recent rubella can now also be made by using a genome amplification technique such as Reverse Transcriptase Polymerase Chain Reaction (RT-PCR) on specimens such as throat washings and oral fluids.

## Congenital rubella

Most babies with CRS excrete large amounts of virus for the first few months of life (and are very infectious to their carers). Virus isolation was used historically from throat swabs or urine but this has largely been superseded by molecular tests such as RT-PCR, or serology. Maternal IgM does not cross the placenta, so the detection of rubella-specific IgM in a newborn baby is diagnostic of intrauterine infection. Specific IgG crosses the placenta so its detection in the first few months of life is of no help. Maternal IgG has a half-life in the infant of 3–4 weeks, however, so persistence to the age of 9–12 months is diagnostic of congenital rubella. Occasionally, requests are made to diagnose congenital rubella in an older infant, e.g. one who presents with deafness. However, the reliable diagnosis of congenital infection in older children is impossible as any rubella-specific IgM generated by congenital infection will have disappeared, and rubella-specific IgG in the patient's serum may have arisen from postnatal infection or immunisation.

## Screening for rubella antibody

Screening for rubella antibodies in pregnant women performs the function of identifying those individuals who are susceptible and offering them vaccine postpartum. Blood is usually obtained at the first antenatal clinic visit and serum samples routinely stored for one year. This could be important if an infant is delivered with congenital abnormalities as the maternal serum collected in early pregnancy can be examined together with a later maternal one and also the infant's blood. This allows investigation of not only rubella but other important pathogens such as cytomegalovirus later in pregnancy. Sometimes, preconceptual screening is performed especially in those undergoing *in vitro* fertilization.

Rubella antibody screening is most usually performed by enzyme immunoassay, a format which is sensitive and easily automated.

Negative results in an EIA test should be confirmed by a different assay such as latex agglutination. Some women do not produce protective levels of antibody (defined in the UK as >10 IU/mL) even after several vaccinations and they should be considered immune if they have had two documented doses of vaccine.

## EPIDEMIOLOGY

Rubella has a worldwide distribution and infection is endemic in all countries that have not had a successful immunisation policy. Outbreaks usually occur in spring and early summer with major epidemics occurring every 4–8 years. Infection is common in childhood. Currently only 2–3% of young adult females are susceptible in the UK due to immunisation: many of those who are susceptible come from areas of the world such as the Indian subcontinent, where immunisation is uncommon. It is of paramount importance that the prevalence of pregnant women susceptible to rubella is monitored; should it decrease substantially immunisation protocols may have to change.

## CONTROL

### Passive prophylaxis

There is little evidence that administering normal human immunoglobulin after contact reduces the risk of maternal rubella and fetal infection, although it may attenuate the illness.

### Active prophylaxis

Attenuated live rubella vaccines have been available since the early 1970s. They are safe and only have minimal side effects such as a transient rash and arthralgia. Seroconversion occurs in over 95% of susceptible vaccinees and protection is of more than 20 years duration. Vaccine virus can be isolated from the throat of vaccinees but there is no evidence of onward transmission to susceptible contacts. It is advisable that all women of childbearing age are screened for rubella antibody before immunisation so that only susceptible women are offered vaccine. The vaccine is live and therefore contraindicated in pregnancy, and pregnancy should be avoided in the month after vaccination. However, although vaccine virus has been shown to infect the fetus, there is no evidence of teratogenicity. Thus, if a susceptible woman is immunised inadvertently whilst pregnant, she can be reassured that any risk to the baby is very remote.

The objective of rubella immunisation is to eradicate congenital rubella. Historically in the UK there have been two approaches. In the 1970s vaccination was targeted at girls aged 11–14 years and susceptible adult women, identified by screening for rubella antibody in situations such as antenatal care and family planning clinics. The reasons for this policy were twofold: firstly there were uncertainties about the duration of protection of the vaccine, and secondly it was thought natural rubella, acquired by around 50% of teenage girls, would afford women greater protection.

There was also the consideration of exposure to natural rubella boosting vaccine immunity.

However, by the late 1980s it was apparent that this approach was not achieving the aim of eradicating congenital rubella, as there were still 10–20 cases of CRS and 100–200 terminations of pregnancy per annum in the UK. This was because the small number of women who were susceptible to rubella were becoming infected via their own or other people's young children. This led to a different approach, commencing in October 1988, whereby all children were offered vaccine in an attempt to eradicate circulating rubella from the community and thus avoid exposure of any susceptible pregnant women. In order to make the vaccine more attractive to parents it was combined with measles and mumps (the MMR vaccine) and offered to both girls and boys at around 15 months of age. There was also a preschool 'catch-up' programme. In the late 1990s a second dose of MMR was introduced at 3–5 years to boost immunity of those who had received only one dose and to reach some of the children who had missed their first dose. This approach, similar to that adopted in the USA, has now almost eliminated congenital rubella. However there have been recent concerns in the UK about the safety of MMR vaccine and this has led to a fall in immunisation rates to below 95%, which may lead to a resurgence of rubella.

## RECOMMENDED READING

Banatvala JE, Brown DWG: Rubella, *The Lancet* 363:1127–1136, 2004.

Best JM, Icenogle JP, Brown DWG: Rubella. In Zuckerman AJ, Banatvala JE, Schoub BD, et al, editors: *Principles and Practice of Clinical Virology*, ed 6, Chichester, 2009, Wiley-Blackwell, pp 561–592.

Miller E, Cradock-Watson JE, Pollock TM: Consequences of confirmed maternal rubella at successive stages of pregnancy, *Lancet* ii:781–784, 1982.

### Websites

Health Protection Agency (UK). Rubella (German Measles). http://www.hpa.org.uk/Topics/InfectiousDiseases/InfectionsAZ/Rubella/

# 60 Prion diseases (transmissible spongiform encephalopathies)

Creutzfeldt–Jakob disease; Gerstmann–Sträussler–Scheinker syndrome; fatal familial insomnia; iatrogenic Creutzfeldt–Jakob disease; kuru; variant Creutzfeldt–Jakob disease; bovine spongiform encephalopathy; scrapie

*J. W. Ironside*

## KEY POINTS

- Prion diseases are fatal neurodegenerative disorders with very lengthy incubation periods caused by unconventional agents. They are transmitted by inoculation or ingestion; the intracerebral route of transmission results in the shortest incubation period.
- Prion diseases occur in mammals, including scrapie in sheep, bovine spongiform encephalopathy (BSE) in cattle and Creutzfeldt–Jakob disease (CJD) in man.
- The infectious agents are known as prions, which are thought to lack nucleic acid and appear to consist entirely of a modified host-encoded protein, the prion protein.
- Prion diseases do not elicit conventionally detectable immune responses. Asymptomatic or subclinical infections are very difficult to detect.
- Human prion diseases occur in sporadic, familial and acquired forms, all of which are rare diseases. In 1996, a new form of human prion disease known as variant CJD was identified, which results from infection with the BSE agent, probably via the oral route.

Prion diseases, or transmissible spongiform encephalopathies (TSEs), are a unique group of fatal neurodegenerative disorders occurring in human beings and animals that possess two major characteristics:

1. All are transmissible to a variety of mammals, either experimentally or by natural exposure. The precise nature of the transmissible agents involved is unknown (see below), but they possess physical and chemical properties that are quite distinct from those of conventional viruses and bacteria. There is increasing evidence to support the prion hypothesis, which states that the infectious agent is composed entirely of protein, without any nucleic acid, for which the term *prion* (**pro**teinaceous **in**fectious particle) is used. No evidence of a conventional host immune reaction has been found in prion diseases.

2. The diseases caused by these agents are characterized in all species by neurodegeneration in the central nervous system (CNS), usually with spongiform change. This consists of numerous small vacuoles (10–200 μm) that are formed within neuronal cell bodies and their processes (Fig. 60.1A), probably through dilatation of neuronal lysosomal, Golgi and endoplasmic reticulum structures. Spongiform change may be reversible in its early stages. Ultimately, neuronal death occurs accompanied by reactive proliferation of astrocytes and microglia. The normal cellular form of the prion protein ($PrP^C$) is converted by misfolding into an abnormal disease-associated form ($PrP^{Sc}$) and accumulates within the CNS, usually as diffuse deposits, but occasionally in the form of amyloid plaques.

## The transmissible agent: a prion?

Although the precise nature of prions is uncertain, they are subviral in size and notoriously resistant to inactivation by many physical and chemical agents, including:

- heat
- exposure to ionizing or ultraviolet radiation
- deoxyribonuclease (DNAase) and ribonuclease (RNAase)
- formaldehyde and glutaraldehyde.

Prions have been studied by experimental transmission to mice and hamsters; this has identified around 20 strains of scrapie, a naturally occurring TSE in sheep. These strains are defined by their biological properties, particularly the disease incubation period and the nature and distribution of the pathology in

**Fig. 60.1** (A) Spongiform change in the cerebral cortex in a case of sporadic CJD consists of numerous small cyst-like spaces that tend to coalesce in the neuropil and around neurones (centre). Haematoxylin and eosin stain, original magnification ×400. (B) In this case of sporadic CJD, prion protein (PrP) accumulation in the cerebellum has occurred in the form of numerous amyloid plaques that stain intensely on immunohistochemistry for PrP. Original magnification ×200.

the CNS. Incubation periods range from 60 days to more than 2 years, which is close to the natural lifespan of mice and hamsters, and cases of asymptomatic infection have been recorded in inoculated animals dying from unrelated causes after a prolonged period. The incubation period is influenced by:

- the route of inoculation – intracerebral inoculation is the most efficient mode of infection; oral or parenteral routes are often less efficient
- the dose of the injected inoculum and its infective titre
- host genetic factors, particularly polymorphisms in the prion protein gene.

$PrP^C$ is expressed in a variety of cells, including neurones in the CNS, where it may act as a copper-binding protein, and is thought to play a role in synaptic function. This protein has a molecular weight of 33–35 kDa and is highly conserved through a wide range of species, but its amino acid sequence varies from one species to another. This variation is thought to influence the species barrier, a factor that regulates the success of disease transmission from one species to another under experimental and natural conditions.

During prion infection, $PrP^C$ appears to undergo a conformational change to convert to $PrP^{Sc}$. This abnormal isoform has a relatively high beta-pleated sheet conformation, which renders it partially resistant to digestion with proteinase K and allows it to aggregate as amyloid fibrils in the brain. In the prion hypothesis, conversion of the $PrP^C$ to $PrP^{Sc}$ occurs by a direct interaction, which sparks off a catalytic conversion. This has been replicated experimentally using recombinant prion protein, which has been misfolded in a cell-free system to produce infectious $PrP^{Sc}$. These

findings support the prion hypothesis; however, it is not known whether this biochemical change alone accounts for all the biological properties of prions. For example, the mechanisms by which the various strains of scrapie agent have different biological properties are unclear, and some research groups believe that a second (as yet unidentified) molecule determines the strain of the infectious agent.

### Pathogenesis

Transmission of prions to experimental hamsters and mice can be achieved by inoculation of infected brain tissue into a number of sites. After oral inoculation, spread of infection may occur along either the vagus nerve to the brainstem, or along sympathetic nerve fibres that connect via the splanchnic nerve complex to the spinal cord. Infection then spreads to the brain at a rate of around 1 mm/day, probably within neurones. Peripheral inoculation of the agent may be followed by a phase of accumulation and replication in the lymphoid tissues, mainly in follicular dendritic cells. In the spleen, there is a postulated 'neuroimmune' connection that allows access to the splanchnic plexus and then to the CNS.

### HUMAN PRION DISEASES

The most common form of human prion disease was first described in the 1920s and is known as *Creutzfeldt–Jakob disease* (CJD) after the authors of the early reports. Since then, an ever-widening spectrum of human prion diseases has been identified (Table 60.1), with three main subgroups, comprising:

| **Table 60.1** Human spongiform encephalopathies classified by aetiology | |
| --- | --- |
| Aetiology | Encephalopathy |
| Idiopathic disorders | Sporadic CJD (around 90% of all cases) |
| Familial disorders | Familial CJD (around 10% of all cases) |
| | Gerstmann–Sträussler–Scheinker syndrome |
| | Fatal familial insomnia |
| Transmitted from person-to-person | Kuru |
| | Iatrogenic CJD (less than 1% of all cases) |
| Transmitted from bovines to man | Variant CJD |
| CJD, Creutzfeldt–Jakob disease. | |

- idiopathic disorders, where the cause is unknown
- familial disorders, occurring as autosomal dominant disorders
- acquired disorders, following accidental infection by inoculation or ingestion.

The identification of the prion protein and sequencing of the human prion protein gene on chromosome 20 have greatly increased our understanding of human transmissible spongiform encephalopathies.

## DIAGNOSIS

The diagnosis of human prion diseases requires a range of clinical, biochemical, genetic and pathological studies. Careful assessment of the clinical features (see below) by an experienced neurologist allows a presumptive diagnosis of CJD to be made with a high level of accuracy (at least 70%). Analysis of the prion protein gene is essential to identify cases of familial CJD associated with a pathogenic mutation. Genetic studies have also demonstrated a naturally occurring polymorphism at codon 129 in the prion protein gene, which is important in determining disease susceptibility (see below). At present, there is no form of screening test for human prion diseases and no specific treatment is available. A definitive diagnosis depends on examination of the brain at autopsy. Brain biopsy is not a routine investigation, as the procedure can compromise an already ill patient and the neurosurgical instruments used have to be destroyed if the diagnosis is confirmed, to prevent accidental iatrogenic infection via subsequent neurosurgical procedures.

## NEUROPATHOLOGY

It is recommended that all suspected CJD cases should be investigated by autopsy, with appropriate

**Fig. 60.2** Western blot analysis of prion protein (PrP) in post-mortem CJD brain. PrP from CJD brain occurs in three glycoforms resulting in diglycosylated, monoglycosylated or non-glycosylated PrP, which can be separated by western blotting into distinct bands. Proteinase K treatment (+) destroys the normal form of the prion protein, but in CJD it only partly denatures the disease-associated protein, which has an increased mobility (shown in A). Two main subtypes of the abnormal protein can be identified: (B) types 1 and 2 are found in sporadic CJD (s) irrespective of the genotype at codon 129. Examples of two types (MM1 and VV2) are shown here. All cases of variant CJD (v) thus far tested are methionine homozygotes (MM) and have had a type 2 PrP characterized by the predominance of the diglycosylated glycoform (*), termed type 2B. The type 2 cases found in sporadic CJD, in which the monoglycosylated glycoform predominates, are termed type 2A.

permission for retention and examination of the brain to allow confirmation of the clinical diagnosis and accurate subclassification of the case. The principal neuropathological features of human prion diseases are:

- spongiform change (Fig. 60.1A)
- neuronal loss
- astrocytosis
- accumulation of PrP$^{Sc}$
- amyloid plaque formation (Fig. 60.1B).

A range of techniques is now available to detect PrP$^{Sc}$ accumulation within the CNS. PrP$^{Sc}$ can be detected by immunocytochemistry in the CNS in a variety of patterns, including amyloid plaques (see Fig. 60.1B), perivacuolar and perineuronal and axonal deposition. PrP$^{Sc}$ can also be detected by western blot techniques, which allow further study of the PrP$^{Sc}$ isotype in terms of its glycosylation and molecular weight following digestion with proteinase K (Fig. 60.2).

## SPORADIC CJD

CJD occurs most commonly as a sporadic disorder, affecting around one person per million population per year worldwide. Sporadic CJD usually presents as a rapidly progressive dementia of less than 1 year's duration, often accompanied by other neurological abnormalities, including cerebellar dysfunction, pyramidal and extrapyramidal signs, cortical blindness and akinetic mutism. Many of these features evolve as the disease progresses, and electro-encephalography often shows characteristic diffuse, periodic, synchronous discharges. The peak incidence is in the seventh decade of life, but the disease has been described in teenagers and even in the ninth decade. The disease is untreatable and invariably fatal; most patients survive for only 4 months after the onset of major symptoms.

The naturally occurring methionine/valine polymorphism at codon 129 in the prion protein gene is of major influence in determining susceptibility to sporadic CJD (Table 60.2). The mechanism for this influence is unclear. The precipitating event leading to development of sporadic CJD remains unknown; it might possibly reflect selective exposure to an unidentified ubiquitous agent, perhaps causing disease only in genetically susceptible individuals, or a somatic mutation involving the prion protein in the CNS (Fig. 60.3). No occupational or dietary risk factors exist for sporadic CJD. The global distribution of sporadic CJD is markedly different from that of scrapie, particularly in Australia, where scrapie has been eradicated for many decades, but sporadic CJD occurs at a similar frequency to that in the UK, where scrapie is endemic.

## FAMILIAL PRION DISEASES

Around 10% of cases of CJD occur as autosomal dominant inherited disorders; these are associated with mutations or insertions in the open reading frame of the human prion protein gene on chromosome 20 (see Fig. 60.3). *Gerstmann–Sträussler–Scheinker syndrome* (GSS) is the best known example of an inherited human prion disease. In this very rare disorder, which affects middle-aged adults, cerebellar ataxia, nystagmus and gait abnormalities are prominent clinical features, with dementia occurring only towards the end of the illness. Numerous multicentric PrP amyloid plaques are present throughout the CNS. GSS was the first human disease linked to a mutation in the PrP gene; a codon 102 proline-to-leucine mutation was identified in 1989 and has subsequently been found in several GSS families, including the original kindred described in 1936. *Fatal familial insomnia* is an extremely rare inherited disorder, characterized clinically by disturbances of sleep and autonomic function with relative intellectual preservation in middle age. This disorder is associated with a unique PrP genotype (codon 178 asparagine, 129 methionine/methionine), and neuropathological changes mainly in the thalamus. The relationship between the genotype, neuropathology and clinical features of this enigmatic disorder await further study.

## ACQUIRED PRION DISEASES

### Iatrogenic CJD

CJD can occur by accidental transmission from one person to another (see Fig. 60.3). *Iatrogenic CJD* was first described in 1974 in a corneal graft recipient. Other examples of iatrogenic CJD have involved accidental inoculation of contaminated CNS tissue from a CJD patient to another patient, for example following the implantation of inadequately decontaminated intracerebral electrodes, or via human dura mater grafts. In the UK, the most common form of iatrogenic CJD occurs in recipients of human growth hormone derived from cadaveric pituitary glands, at an approximate incidence of 1 in 10000 at-risk individuals, with an average age at death of 25 years and an incubation period of up to 20 years.

### Kuru

Kuru was a disease occurring in the Fore tribe of Papua New Guinea, apparently in association with practices related to ritualistic cannibalism. The brain was handled and apparently eaten, particularly by females and children, who went on to develop this disorder. The name *kuru* means shivering or trembling in the local dialect, and reflects the predominant clinical manifestations of a progressive cerebellar

| Table 60.2  Prion protein gene codon 129 polymorphism in CJD | | | |
|---|---|---|---|
| Codon 129 genotype | Methionine/ methionine | Methionine/ valine | Valine/ valine |
| Normal population | 37% | 51% | 12% |
| Sporadic CJD | 75% | 11% | 14% |
| Variant CJD | 100% | 0% | 0% |
| CJD, Creutzfeldt–Jakob disease. | | | |

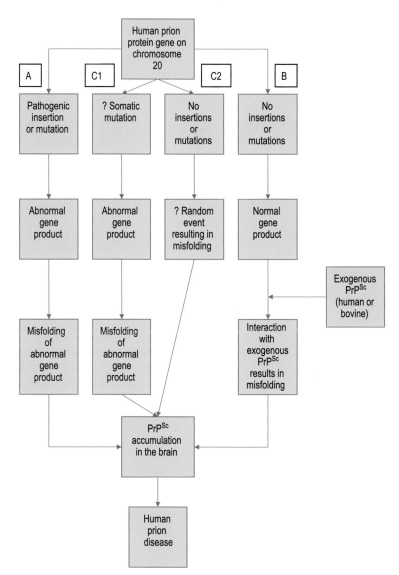

**Fig. 60.3** Postulated mechanisms of PrP$^{Sc}$ accumulation in CJD. (A) An inherited PrP gene mutation results in an unstable form of prion protein that misfolds to cause familial CJD. (B) Exogenous PrP$^{Sc}$ interacts with the normal host prion protein, resulting in PrP$^{Sc}$ accumulation. This mechanism is thought to operate in iatrogenic CJD (exposure to human PrP$^{Sc}$) and variant CJD (exposure to bovine PrP$^{Sc}$). The cause of sporadic CJD is unknown, but proponents of the prion hypothesis have suggested that a somatic mutation in a neurone (C1) might initiate the process of PrP$^{Sc}$ accumulation in the brain, or alternatively a rare random event results in spontaneous misfolding of the normal prion protein (C2). These 'rare events' might also explain the low incidence of sporadic CJD.

syndrome with dementia. The incubation period was variable, ranging from around 5 to over 40 years. There was no evidence of mother-to-child transmission. Its increasing prevalence made it the primary cause of death in most individuals within the tribes in the 1960s. The disease is now extinct since cannibalistic practices were abandoned.

## Variant CJD

The emergence of *bovine spongiform encephalopathy* (BSE) as a new epidemic in UK cattle raised the possibility that this disorder might be transmitted to man through the food chain. A National CJD Surveillance Unit was established for the UK in May 1990, based in Edinburgh. In 1996, the Unit identified a new form of human prion disease, now known as *variant CJD*, which by 2010 has affected more than 170 people in the UK, and 47 in other countries including France, Ireland, the Netherlands, Spain, Portugal, USA, Canada, Japan and Saudi Arabia.

- The age of onset is unusually young (mean 28 years), with a range from 12–74 years.
- The clinical illness is prolonged, with an average duration of 14 months (range 6–39 months).

**Fig. 60.4** The cerebral cortex in variant CJD contains numerous aggregates of PrPSc in the form of fibrillary amyloid plaques (centre), surrounded by spongiform change. Haematoxylin and eosin stain, original magnification ×200.

**Fig. 60.5** Section of a tonsil from a patient with variant CJD stained to show the prion protein by immunohistochemistry. The dark stain demonstrates accumulation of the prion protein in the follicular dendritic cells within germinal centres of the tonsil. Accumulation of prion protein in lymphoid tissues does not occur in sporadic CJD. Original magnification ×100.

- The clinical features are also unusual, with psychiatric and sensory symptoms at onset, followed by ataxia and myoclonus, with dementia only in the final stages of the illness.
- So far, all patients with definite variant CJD are methionine homozygotes at codon 129 in the prion protein gene (see Table 60.2).

The neuropathological features are relatively uniform and consist of massive accumulations of PrPSc throughout the brain, with the formation of multiple amyloid plaques surrounded by spongiform change, known as florid plaques (Fig. 60.4). Variant CJD differs from other forms of human prion disease in that PrPSc can be detected in lymphoid tissues (in follicular dendritic cells) both during the clinical illness (Fig. 60.5) and in the late preclinical illness. This is consistent with variant CJD being acquired by the oral route (see below) and has implications for the possible transmission of the variant CJD agent by surgical instruments used on lymphoid tissues (e.g. in tonsillectomies).

The variant CJD prion is also present in the blood of individuals in the preclinical incubation phase of the illness. Four cases of variant CJD transmission by blood transfusion have been reported in the UK. Many steps have been taken in the UK to prevent further transmission by this route, including filtration of whole blood to remove white cells (which may carry the highest levels of infectivity), sourcing of plasma products from overseas, and banning recipients of blood transfusions from themselves becoming blood donors.

Experimental strain typing studies in mice have shown that the transmissible agent in variant CJD is identical to the BSE agent. Furthermore, biochemical analysis of PrPSc from cases of variant CJD shows a similar banding pattern in western blot preparations to PrPSc from BSE in cattle, which is distinct from sporadic CJD (see Fig. 60.2). These findings provide strong support for the hypothesis that variant CJD is causally linked to BSE, and there is epidemiological evidence that dietary exposure through beef products is the most likely route of infection.

Recently, a decrease in the incidence and death rate for variant CJD has been reported in the UK. However, continuing surveillance is required, since the incubation period for variant CJD is unknown and future cases may emerge in other genetic subgroups (relating to the codon 129 polymorphism in the PRNP gene) in the UK population.

## BOVINE SPONGIFORM ENCEPHALOPATHY AND OTHER ANIMAL PRION DISEASES

Prion diseases have been recorded in an increasing number of captive or domesticated animals (Table 60.3), the most significant of which is BSE. This was identified in 1985 in the UK and spread rapidly throughout the cattle population to affect around 1% of all adult cattle by 1992. It appears that this epidemic resulted from:

- oral ingestion of a prion (possibly a novel strain of scrapie) via contaminated meat and bone meal in cattle feed

**Table 60.3** Animal diseases caused by scrapie and related agents

| Disease | Occurrence | Hosts |
| --- | --- | --- |
| Scrapie | Common in many countries worldwide | Sheep and goats |
| Transmissible mink encephalopathy | Very rare, mostly in farms in the USA | Mink |
| Chronic wasting disease | Spreading from Colorado and Wyoming | Mule deer and elk |
| Bovine spongiform encephalopathy | Widespread epidemic in dairy cattle in the UK; smaller outbreaks in other countries | Domestic cattle |
| Unnamed spongiform encephalopathy | Small number of exotic ungulates in zoos | Nyala, gemsbok, greater kudu, Arabian oryx, eland |
| Feline spongiform encephalopathy | Small numbers of domestic cats in the UK and a few large cats in zoos | Domestic cats, cheetah, lion, puma, ocelot, tiger |

- changes in the rendering processes by which this feed was produced in the 1980s, allowing the BSE agent to persist as a contaminant
- recycling of contaminated cattle carcasses in the meat and bone meal fed to cattle appears to have fuelled the epidemic.

The incidence of BSE is now declining markedly as a result of a ban on the use of bovine organs as foodstuffs for other animals. Experimental studies on BSE indicate that it represents a single prion strain. This strain was also transmitted by foodstuff to domestic cats, large cats and exotic ungulates in zoos (see Table 60.3). There is good evidence that the BSE agent has also spread to man, giving rise to variant CJD (see above).

## SCRAPIE

The first animal spongiform encephalopathy to be described was *scrapie*, an endemic disorder of sheep and goats that has been present in Europe for at least two centuries. Affected animals become ataxic and wasted, and often rub or scrape the fleece off the sides of their bodies, hence the name. The first experimental transmission of scrapie from affected to healthy sheep by intra-ocular injection of spinal cord homogenate was reported in 1936. Natural transmission is thought to occur at parturition, or by scarification or via the oral (alimentary) route. The placenta from an infected ewe is one known source of infection that can contaminate the farm environment. There is no epidemiological evidence that scrapie is pathogenic to man.

RECOMMENDED READING

Bruce ME, Will RG, Ironside JW, et al: Transmissions to mice indicate the 'new variant' CJD is caused by the BSE agent, *Nature* 389:498–501, 1997.

Collinge J, Clarke A: A general model of prion strains and their pathogenicity, *Science* 318:930–936, 2007.

Ironside JW, Ghetti B, Head MW, et al: Prion Diseases. In Love S, Louis DN, Ellison DW: *Greenfield's Neuropathology*, ed 8, vol 2, London, 2008, Hodder Arnold, pp 1197–1273.

Ironside JW, Head MW, Bell JE, et al: Laboratory diagnosis of variant Creutzfeldt–Jakob disease, *Histopathology* 37:1–9, 2000.

Peden AH, Head MW, Ritchie DL, et al: Preclinical vCJD after blood transfusion in a PRNP codon 129 heterozgous patient, *Lancet* 364:527–529, 2004.

Prusiner SB: Prions, *Proceedings of the National Academy of Sciences of the USA* 95:13363–13383, 1998.

Wadsworth JD, Collinge J: Update on human prion disease, *Biochimica et Biophysica Acta* 1772:598–609, 2007.

Ward HJT, Everington D, Cousens SN, et al: Risk factors for variant Creutzfeldt–Jakob disease: A case-control study, *Annals of Neurology* 59:111–120, 2006.

Will RG, Ironside JW, Zeidler M, et al: A new variant of Creutzfeldt–Jakob disease in the UK, *Lancet* 347:921–925, 1996.

### Websites

Health and Safety Executive: BSE – Occupational guidance. http://www.hse.gov.uk/pubns/web22.pdf

Health Protection Agency: CJD Incidents Panel. http://www.hpa.org.uk/web/HPAweb&Page&HPAwebAutoListName/Page/1204031511121

Department of Health: Guidance from the ACDP TSE Risk Management Subgroup. http://www.dh.gov.uk/ab/ACDP/TSEguidance/index.htm?ssSourceSiteId=en

Medical Research Council Prion Unit: http://www.prion.ucl.ac.uk/

UK Creutzfeldt–Jakob Disease Surveillance Unit: http://www.cjd.ed.ac.uk/

# PART 5

## FUNGAL PATHOGENS, PARASITIC INFECTIONS AND MEDICAL ENTOMOLOGY

# 61 Fungi

## Superficial, subcutaneous and systemic mycoses

*D. W. Warnock*

## KEY POINTS

- Most infections are caused by fungi that grow as saprobes in the environment. *Superficial*, *subcutaneous* and *systemic* patterns of infection are recognized.
- Fungi take the form of *yeasts*, which grow by *budding* and *moulds*, which grow as filamentous extensions called *hyphae*, forming a *mycelium*, or *dimorphic* fungi, which can grow as yeast or mould forms.
- Pathogenic fungi can establish an infection in all exposed individuals; others are opportunist pathogens that cause disease only in a compromised host.
- Many fungal diseases have a global distribution, but some are endemic to specific geographical regions.
- Subcutaneous fungal infections are acquired by traumatic implantation; systemic infections are usually acquired by inhalation.
- Only dermatophytosis, a common superficial infection of the skin, nails and scalp hair, is truly contagious.
- Some yeasts are human commensals and cause endogenous infection when there is some imbalance in the host.
- The most frequently encountered fungal agents in the UK are *Candida albicans*, dermatophytes, *Aspergillus* spp., *Cryptococcus neoformans* and *Pneumocystis jirovecii*.
- Diagnosis of fungal infections is based on a combination of clinical observation and laboratory investigation, which may include direct microscopy, histology, culture, PCR and serology. Early recognition of systemic infections in immunocompromised persons is a major challenge.

Fungi constitute a large, diverse group of heterotrophic organisms, most of which are found as saprobes in the soil and on decomposing organic matter. They are eukaryotic, with a range of internal membrane systems, membrane-bound organelles, and a well-defined cell wall composed largely of polysaccharides (glucan, mannan) and chitin. They show considerable variation in size and form, but can be divided into three main groups:

1. *Moulds (multicellular filamentous fungi)*, which are composed of branching filaments, termed hyphae, that grow by apical extension to form an intertwined mass, termed a mycelium. In most fungi the hyphae have regular cross-walls (septa) but in lower fungi these are usually absent. Moulds reproduce by means of spores produced, often in large numbers, by an asexual process (involving mitosis only) or as a result of sexual reproduction (involving meiosis, preceded by fusion of the nuclei of two haploid cells). Many fungi can produce more than one type of spore, depending on the growth conditions. The precise method of spore production and the type(s) of spore produced are unique to each individual fungal species. In some higher fungi the sexual spores are produced in macroscopic structures such as mushrooms and toadstools. In laboratory cultures, moulds produce mainly asexual spores.

2. *Yeasts*, which are predominantly unicellular and oval or round in shape. Most propagate by an asexual process called budding in which the cell develops a protuberance, which enlarges and eventually separates from the parent cell. Some yeasts produce chains of elongated cells (pseudohyphae) that resemble the hyphae of moulds; some species also produce true hyphae. A small number of yeasts reproduce by fission.

Yeasts are neither a natural nor a formal taxonomic group, but are a growth form shown by a wide range of unrelated fungi.

3. *Dimorphic fungi*, which are capable of changing their growth to either a mycelial or yeast phase, depending on the growth conditions.

The fungal kingdom is currently divided into seven phyla which include the Ascomycota, Basidiomycota and Glomeromycota. Historically, fungal classification has largely been based on the method of sexual spore production. In some fungi, however, asexual spore production has proved so successful as a means of rapid dispersal to new habitats that sexual reproduction has disappeared, or, at least, has not been discovered. Even in the absence of the sexual stage it is now often possible to assign these fungi to the phyla Ascomycota or Basidiomycota on the basis of DNA sequence analysis. There is no longer any separate formal grouping for those fungi that appear to be strictly asexual. Nonetheless, mycologists continue to employ the asexual reproductive characteristics of moulds, at least for routine identification purposes. Yeasts are identified primarily according to their ability to ferment sugars and to assimilate carbon and nitrogen compounds.

## FUNGAL DISEASES OF MAN

### FUNGAL PATHOGENS

There are at least 100 000 named species of fungi. However, fewer than 500 have been recognized to cause disease (*mycosis*) in man or animals. Most are moulds, but there are a number of pathogenic yeasts and some are dimorphic. Dimorphic fungi usually change from a multicellular mould form in the natural environment to a budding single-celled yeast form when causing infection. In the laboratory, the tissue form can be induced by culture at 37°C on rich media such as blood agar, whereas the mould form develops when incubated at a lower temperature (25–30°C) on a less rich medium such as Sabouraud dextrose agar.

Some fungi, such as the systemic pathogens *Histoplasma capsulatum* and *Blastomyces dermatitidis*, can establish an infection in all exposed individuals. Others, such as *Candida* and *Aspergillus* species, are opportunist pathogens that ordinarily cause disease only in a compromised host. In some mycoses the form and severity of the infection depend on the degree of exposure to the fungus, the site and method of entry into the body, and the level of immunocompetence of the host.

Some fungi may cause serious, occasionally fatal, toxic effects in man, either following ingestion of poisonous toadstools or consumption of mouldy food that contains toxic secondary metabolites (*mycotoxins*). Allergic disease of the airways may result from inhalation of fungal spores.

## EPIDEMIOLOGY

Most human fungal infections are caused by fungi that grow as saprobes in the environment. Infection is acquired by inhalation, ingestion or traumatic implantation. Some yeasts are human commensals and cause endogenous infections when there is some imbalance in the host. Only dermatophyte infections are truly contagious.

Many fungal diseases have a worldwide distribution, but some are endemic to specific geographical regions, usually because the causal agents are saprobes restricted in their distribution by soil and climatic conditions.

## TYPES OF INFECTION

### Superficial mycoses

Diseases of the skin, hair, nail and mucous membranes are the most common of all fungal infections and have a worldwide distribution.

* Dermatophytosis (ringworm) is a complex of diseases affecting the outermost keratinized tissues of hair, nail and the stratum corneum of the skin; it is caused by a group of closely related mould fungi called *dermatophytes*, which can digest keratin. Dermatophyte infections occur in both man and animals.
* Yeast infections affect the skin, nail and mucous membranes of the mouth and vagina, and are usually caused by commensal *Candida* species, notably *Candida albicans*. Infection is generally endogenous in origin but genital infection can be transmitted sexually. The yeast *Malassezia furfur*, a skin commensal, can cause an infection of the skin called *pityriasis versicolor*.

### Subcutaneous mycoses

Mycoses of the dermis, subcutaneous tissues and adjacent bones that show slow localized spread occur mainly in the tropics and subtropics; they usually result from the traumatic inoculation of saprobic fungi from soil or vegetation into the subcutaneous tissue. The principal subcutaneous mycoses are mycetoma, chromoblastomycosis and sporotrichosis.

## Systemic mycoses

Deep-seated fungal infections generally result from the inhalation of air-borne spores produced by the causal moulds, present as saprobes in the environment. Initially there is a pulmonary infection, but the organism may become disseminated to other organs. The organisms that cause systemic mycoses can be divided into two distinct groups: the true pathogens and the opportunistic pathogens. The first of these groups is comprised mostly of dimorphic fungi and infections occur mainly in the Americas. The principal diseases are:

- blastomycosis (caused by *Blastomyces dermatitidis*)
- coccidioidomycosis (*Coccidioides immitis* and *C. posadasii*)
- histoplasmosis (*H. capsulatum*)
- paracoccidioidomycosis (*Paracoccidioides brasiliensis*).

Systemic mycoses caused by opportunistic pathogens such as *Aspergillus, Candida* and *Cryptococcus* species have a more widespread distribution. These infections are being seen with increasing frequency in patients compromised by disease or drug treatment. In transplant patients, for example, these fungi are among the most frequent causes of death due to infection.

## INCIDENCE

The incidence of all the mycoses is related directly to factors that affect the degree of exposure to the causal fungi, such as living conditions, occupation and leisure activities.

- Dermatophytosis of the foot (*athlete's foot*), with associated infections of nails and groin, occurs most commonly in swimmers, sportspersons and industrial workers who use communal bathing facilities.
- Animal dermatophytosis is an occupational hazard for farmers, veterinarians and others closely associated with animals.
- Agricultural workers in warm climates who wear little protective clothing frequently contract subcutaneous infections following minor injuries from vegetation.
- In developed countries the incidence of infections due to opportunistic fungal pathogens has increased following major advances in healthcare

that have led to increases in the size of the population at risk.
- In many developing countries the acquired immune deficiency syndrome (AIDS) pandemic has been associated with a marked increase in the rate of opportunistic fungal infections. High mortality rates have been reported from countries where adequate treatment is often unavailable.
- The incidence of several of the systemic mycoses that are endemic in the Americas has increased as a result of urban development and changing land use in the endemic areas. Increased international travel and tourism has also led to a rise in the number of cases of disease among individuals who normally reside in countries far from the endemic areas.

## DIAGNOSIS

Diagnosis of fungal infections is based on a combination of clinical observation and laboratory investigation.

## Clinical investigation

Superficial and subcutaneous mycoses often produce characteristic lesions, but they may also closely resemble and be confused with other diseases. In addition, the appearance of lesions may be modified beyond recognition by previous therapy, for example with topical steroids.

The first indication that a patient may have a systemic mycosis is often their failure to respond to antibacterial antibiotics. As early diagnosis considerably increases the chances of successful treatment, it is important that the possibility of fungal involvement be considered from the outset, particularly in those known to be at risk of developing a fungal infection. Computed tomography is widely used to help diagnose *Aspergillus* infections and other invasive mycoses.

## Laboratory diagnosis

Laboratory diagnosis depends on:

- recognition of the pathogen in tissue by microscopy
- isolation of the causal fungus in culture
- the use of serological tests
- detection of fungal DNA by the polymerase chain reaction (PCR).

It is important that the correct type of specimen, together with adequate clinical data, is sent to the laboratory so that the appropriate investigations can be carried out. Information on factors such as travel or residence abroad, animal contacts and the occupation of the patient enable the laboratory staff to direct their investigations towards a particular fungus or group of fungi when appropriate.

## Types of specimen

Skin scales, nail clippings and scrapings of the scalp that include hair stubs and skin scales are the most suitable specimens for the diagnosis of ringworm; these are collected into folded paper squares for transport to the laboratory. Swabs should be taken from suspected *Candida* infections from the mucous membranes and preferably sent to the laboratory in 'clear' transport medium. For subcutaneous infections the most suitable specimens are scrapings and crusts, aspirated pus and biopsies. In suspected systemic infection, specimens should be taken from appropriate sites.

## Direct microscopy

Most specimens can be examined satisfactorily in wet mounts after partial digestion of the tissue with 10–20% potassium hydroxide. Addition of Calcofluor white and subsequent examination by fluorescence microscopy enhances the detection of most fungi as the fluorescent hydroxide–Calcofluor binds to the fungal cell walls. Gram films may also be used for the diagnosis of yeast infections of mucous membranes. Giemsa staining of smears is advised for detection of the yeast cells of *H. capsulatum* because of their small size.

## Histology

Invasive procedures are required to obtain specimens for histological examination. Although sometimes necessary to provide firm evidence of invasive disease, such procedures are often impracticable on patients who are already seriously ill. Haematoxylin and eosin staining is seldom of value for demonstrating fungi in tissue, and specific fungal stains such as periodic acid–Schiff and Grocott–Gomori methenamine–silver are widely used.

## Culture

Most pathogenic fungi are easy to grow in culture. Sabouraud dextrose agar and 4% malt extract agar are most commonly used. These may be supplemented with chloramphenicol (50 mg/L) to minimize bacterial contamination and cycloheximide (500 mg/L) to reduce contamination with saprophytic fungi. Many fungal pathogens have an optimum growth temperature below 37°C. Consequently, cultures are incubated at 25–30°C and at 37°C. With some dimorphic pathogens, enriched media such as brain–heart infusion or blood agar are used to promote growth of the yeast phase.

Many fungi develop relatively slowly and cultures should be retained for at least 2–3 weeks (in some cases up to 6 weeks) before being discarded; yeasts usually grow within 1–5 days. Moulds are identified by their macroscopic and microscopic morphology. Yeasts are identified by sugar fermentation and their ability to assimilate carbon and nitrogen sources. Commercial kits are available for the identification of medically important yeasts.

Culture may provide unequivocal evidence of fungal infection when established pathogens are isolated or when fungi are recovered from normally sterile sites. However, when commensals such as *Candida* species are isolated, results must be interpreted according to the quantity of the fungus isolated, the source and clinical evidence.

## Serology

The most common tests for fungal antibodies are:

- immunodiffusion
- countercurrent immuno-electrophoresis (CIE)
- whole cell agglutination
- complement fixation
- enzyme-linked immunosorbent assay (ELISA).

For antigen detection the following are used:

- latex particle agglutination
- ELISA.

## Polymerase chain reaction

Detection of fungal DNA in clinical material, principally blood, serum, broncho-alveolar lavage fluid and sputum, is increasingly used for diagnosis.

## TREATMENT

There are relatively few therapeutically useful antifungal agents compared with the large number of antibacterial agents that are available (see Chs 5 & 67). As fungi and human beings are both eukaryotes, most substances that kill or inhibit fungal pathogens are also toxic to the host. Antifungal agents vary considerably in their spectrum of activity (see Table 5.4, p. 61). Most exploit differences in the sterol composition of the fungal and mammalian cell membranes, although the echinocandins (anidulafungin, caspofungin and micafungin) interfere with β-glucan synthesis in the fungal cell wall.

Most antifungal agents are available only for topical use. Relatively few can be administered systemically.

- Amphotericin B and the echinocandins are given parenterally because of poor absorption from the gastrointestinal tract.
- Fluconazole, itraconazole, posaconazole, voriconazole and flucytosine are available for oral and/or parenteral administration.
- Terbinafine and griseofulvin are usually administered orally.
- Amphotericin B has long been the treatment of choice in life-threatening disease, despite its toxicity; liposomal and lipid complex formulations are less toxic but much more expensive.
- A combination of amphotericin B and flucytosine reduces the likelihood of the emergence of resistance to flucytosine. Combinations of azole drugs and amphotericin B are seldom used therapeutically.
- New antifungals are being evaluated for use in systemic mycoses. Posaconazole appears to be effective in histoplasmosis and mucormycosis, but it is not yet licensed for these indications.

Antifungal prophylaxis is often used to help prevent opportunistic infections in patients undergoing solid-organ, blood or marrow transplants and in those with haematological malignancies. Oral or topical antifungals are also used to prevent recurrent vaginal candidosis.

Primary or acquired resistance is not a major problem. Resistance to azole antifungals is sometimes encountered, especially after prolonged fluconazole therapy of oropharyngeal *Candida* infections in persons with AIDS. Some yeast species (e.g. *Candida krusei, Candida glabrata*) are inherently resistant to triazoles such as fluconazole. Consequently, susceptibility testing is often carried out for fluconazole and for any drug that fails to produce the expected therapeutic response.

**Fig. 61.1** Microscopical appearance of infected skin scrapings showing the development of arthroconidia. (Reproduced with permission from Richardson MD, Warnock DW, Campbell CK 1995 *Slide Atlas of Fungal Infection: Superficial Fungal Infections.* Blackwell Science, Oxford.)

also referred to as ringworm or as *tinea*, a name that is qualified by the site affected, for example *tinea pedis* or *tinea capitis* for infections of the feet or scalp, respectively. These infections are caused by about 20 species of fungi that are grouped into three genera: *Trichophyton, Microsporum* and *Epidermophyton*. Some species are worldwide in distribution, whereas others are restricted to, or are more common in, particular parts of the world.

Many dermatophyte species produce two types of asexual spore: multi-celled macroconidia and single-celled microconidia. Classification into the three genera *Trichophyton, Microsporum* and *Epidermophyton* is based on the morphology of the macroconidia, although the identification of species is also based on the shape and disposition of the microconidia and the macroscopic appearance of the colonies.

The clinical appearances of dermatophyte infections are the result of a combination of direct tissue damage caused by the fungus and of the immune response of the host. The damage to tissue is due to a combination of mechanical pressure and enzymatic activities. In tissue the dermatophytes take the form of branching hyphae, which may eventually break up into arthroconidia, particularly in infected hair (Fig. 61.1).

### Epidemiology

The dermatophytes can be divided into three groups depending on whether their normal habitat is the soil (geophilic species), animals (zoophilic species) or man (anthropophilic species). Members of all three groups can cause human infection, but their different natural

## SUPERFICIAL INFECTIONS

### DERMATOPHYTOSIS

Dermatophyte infections are common diseases of the stratum corneum of the skin, hair and nail; they are reservoirs have important epidemiological implications in relation to the acquisition, site and spread of human disease.

Although geophilic dermatophytes occasionally cause infection in both animals and man, their normal habitat is the soil. Members of the anthropophilic and zoophilic groups are thought to have evolved from these and other keratinophilic soil-inhabiting fungi, different species having adapted to different natural hosts. Individual members of the zoophilic group are often associated with a particular animal host, for instance *M. canis* with cats and dogs and *T. verrucosum* with cattle. However, these organisms can also spread to man. The anthropophilic species are the most highly specialized group of dermatophytes. They rarely infect other animals and often show a strong preference for a particular body site, only occasionally being found in other regions. For instance, *M. audouinii* commonly infects scalp hair, whereas *E. floccosum* is usually found on the skin.

Infections are spread by direct or indirect contact with an infected individual or animal. The infective particle is usually a fragment of keratin containing viable fungus. Indirect transfer may occur via the floors of swimming pools and showers or on brushes, towels and animal grooming implements. Dermatophytes can remain viable for long periods of time and the interval between deposition and transfer may be considerable. In addition to exposure to the fungus, some abnormality of the epidermis, such as slight peeling or minor trauma, is probably necessary for the establishment of infection.

In industrialized countries, tinea capitis is relatively uncommon, and is caused by dermatophytes of both human and animal origin, although infections with the anthropophilic species *T. tonsurans* are on the increase among urban populations in Europe and the Americas. However, the use of communal bathing facilities has resulted in a considerable increase in the incidence of tinea pedis and associated nail and groin infections. These now comprise about 75% of all dermatophyte infections diagnosed in temperate zones.

In developing countries, particularly in warm climates, scalp, body and groin infections predominate, with *T. rubrum* and *T. violaceum* among the most common causes.

## Clinical features

Lesions vary considerably according to the site of the infection and the species of fungus involved. Sometimes there is only dry scaling or hyperkeratosis, but more commonly there is irritation, erythema, oedema and some vesiculation. More inflammatory lesions

**Fig. 61.2** Tinea corporis due to *Microsporum canis.*

with weeping vesicles, pustules and ulceration are usually caused by zoophilic species.

In skin infections of the body, face and scalp, spreading annular lesions with a raised, inflammatory border are usually produced (Fig. 61.2). Lesions in body folds, such as the groin, tend to spread outwards from the flexures. In tinea pedis, infection is often confined to the toe clefts, but it can spread to the sole; sometimes, painful secondary bacterial infection occurs in the toe clefts.

In nail infection, the nail becomes discoloured, thickened, raised and friable; most nail infections are due to *T. rubrum* and involve the toenails (Fig. 61.3).

In scalp infections there is scaling and hair loss, the extent of which depends on the causal fungus. Some zoophilic species give rise to a highly inflammatory, raised, suppurating lesion called a *kerion*; kerions may also occur in the beard area of adults. It is important that tinea capitis is recognized and treated promptly because it can lead to scarring and permanent hair loss.

**Fig. 61.3** Toenail infection due to *Trichophyton rubrum.* (Reproduced with permission from Richardson MD, Warnock DW, Campbell CK 1995 *Slide Atlas of Fungal Infection: Superficial Fungal Infections.* Blackwell Science, Oxford.)

**Fig. 61.4** Tinea capitis (favus) due to *Trichophyton schoenleinii.* (Reproduced with permission from Richardson MD, Warnock DW, Campbell CK 1995 *Slide Atlas of Fungal Infection: Superficial Fungal Infections.* Blackwell Science, Oxford.)

In scalp infection the fungus invades the hair shaft and the hyphae then break up into chains of arthroconidia. In some species (e.g. *T. tonsurans, T. violaceum*) the arthroconidia are retained within the hair shaft (endothrix invasion), whereas in others (e.g. *Microsporum* species, *T. verrucosum*) they are produced in a sheath surrounding the hair shaft (ectothrix invasion). The pattern of hair invasion affects the clinical appearance of the lesion.

- In endothrix infection the hair breaks off at, or just below, the mouth of the follicle to give what is described as a 'black dot' appearance.
- In ectothrix infection the hair usually breaks off 2–3 mm above the mouth of the follicle, leaving short stumps of hair.
- In favus, caused by *T. schoenleinii*, fungal growth within the hair is minimal. The hair remains intact, but intense fungal growth within and around the hair follicle produces a waxy, honeycomb-like crust on the scalp (Fig. 61.4).

Infections of the groin, hands and nails are nearly always secondary to infection of the feet and are usually (except in developing countries) caused by *T. rubrum, T. mentagrophytes* or *E. floccosum*. Mixed infections also occur.

Occasionally, patients with inflammatory infections develop a secondary rash known as an *id reaction*, which is thought to be an immunological reaction to fungal antigens. In patients with tinea pedis this takes the form of a vesicular eczema of the hands, whereas patients with tinea capitis (especially kerion) develop a follicular rash, usually on the trunk or limbs. These secondary lesions do not contain viable

fungus and they disappear spontaneously when the infection subsides.

## Laboratory diagnosis

Dermatophyte infections may be reliably diagnosed in the laboratory by direct microscopical examination and culture of skin, crusts, hair and nail.

### Collection of samples

Skin, hair and nail samples are best collected into folded squares of black paper or card, which can be fastened with a paper clip. The use of paper allows the specimen to dry out, which helps reduce bacterial contamination and provides conditions under which specimens can be stored for 12 months or more without appreciable loss in viability of the fungus.

Nail samples should be collected by taking clippings from any discoloured, dystrophic or brittle parts of the nail and, importantly, by scraping material from underneath the nail. The sample should be taken from as far back as possible from the free edge of the nail.

Scales from skin lesions should be collected by scraping outwards with a blunt scalpel from the edges of the lesions, where most viable fungus is likely to be. Specimens from the scalp should include hair stubs, the contents of plugged follicles and skin scales. Infected hairs are usually easy to pluck from the scalp with forceps. Cut hairs are unsatisfactory because the focus of infection is usually below or near the surface of the scalp.

## Wood's lamp

This is a source of long-wave ultraviolet light that can be used to detect fluorescence in infected hair. It is especially useful for the detection of inconspicuous scalp lesions, and to select infected hairs for laboratory investigation.

## Hairbrush sampling

Adequate material from minimal lesions may be obtained by brushing the scalp with a sterilized plastic hairbrush or scalp massage pad; this is then used to inoculate an appropriate culture medium by pressing the brush or pad spines into the agar.

## Processing of specimens

If there is insufficient material for both microscopy and culture, the sample should be used for culture, since this is generally the more sensitive procedure (except for nails).

The specimen should first be examined macroscopically; hair samples are examined under a Wood's lamp. Material from representative parts, and any fluorescent hairs, are divided up into 1–2-mm fragments with a sterile scalpel blade before microscopical examination and culture.

## Direct microscopy

Microscopy of wet mounts of keratinous material in potassium hydroxide is simple and reliable. The preparation is allowed to stand for 15–20 min to digest and 'clear' the keratin. Dermatophytes are seen in skin and nail as branching hyphae, which often appear slightly greenish in colour and run across the outlines of the colourless host cells. With Calcofluor (see above) the cell outlines fluoresce white.

## Culture

Small fragments of keratinous material are planted or scattered on Sabouraud dextrose or 4% malt extract agar and incubated at 28–30°C for up to 2 weeks; room temperature is adequate but the dermatophytes grow more slowly. Only *T. verrucosum* grows well at 37°C.

Identification is based on colonial appearance and colour, pigment production, and the micromorphology of any spores produced. Special tests exist for differentiating certain morphologically similar species. Thus, the ability of *T. mentagrophytes* to produce urease within 2–4 days distinguishes it from *T. rubrum*, and the ability to grow on rice grains distinguishes *M. canis* from *M. audouinii*.

## Treatment and prevention

Topical therapy is satisfactory for most skin infections, although oral antifungals are required to treat infections of the nail and scalp, and severe or extensive skin infections.

Topical agents include azole compounds, terbinafine, amorolfine and ciclopirox olamine. Oral griseofulvin is useful for scalp, skin and fingernail infections, but gives poor results in toenail infections, even after 18 months' therapy. Terbinafine and itraconazole have largely replaced griseofulvin for the treatment of nail infections because of their much better cure rates and shorter periods of treatment (around 85% cure for toenails after 3 months' therapy).

Relatively little has been done to control the spread of dermatophyte infections. The prophylactic use of antifungal foot powder after bathing helps to reduce the spread of infection among swimmers. Foot-baths containing antiseptic solutions, which are commonplace in swimming pools, are of no value.

## SUPERFICIAL CANDIDOSIS

Superficial *Candida* infections involving the skin, nails and mucous membranes of the mouth and vagina are very common throughout the world. *Candida albicans* accounts for 80–90% of cases, but other species, notably *C. glabrata*, *C. parapsilosis*, *C. tropicalis*, *C. krusei* and *C. guilliermondii*, may occur.

On Sabouraud dextrose agar *Candida* species grow predominantly in the yeast phase as round or oval cells, 3–8 mm in diameter. A mixture of yeast cells, pseudohyphae and true hyphae is found in vivo and under micro-aerophilic growth conditions on nutritionally poor media. *C. glabrata* does not form either hyphae or pseudohyphae.

## Epidemiology

*Candida* species, usually *C. albicans*, are found in small numbers in the commensal flora (mouth, gastrointestinal tract, vagina, skin) of about 20% of the normal population. The carriage rate tends to increase with age and is higher in the vagina during pregnancy. Commensal yeasts are more prevalent among patients in hospital. Yeast overgrowth and infection occur when the normal microbial flora of the body is altered or when host resistance to infection is lowered by disease.

In most cases, infection is derived from an individual's own endogenous reservoir. In some instances, however, transmission from person to person can occur; for example neonatal oral candidosis is more common in infants born of mothers with vaginal candidosis. The hands of healthcare workers are another potential source of neonatal infection.

Individuals colonized with *Candida* species possess numerous non-specific and immunological defences to prevent infection. In superficial candidosis the non-specific inhibitory factors include inhibitors in serum, such as unsaturated transferrin, and epithelial proliferation. Specific defence largely depends on the development of active T cell-mediated immunity.

Both general and local predisposing factors are important in the development of oropharyngeal candidosis. Debilitated and immunosuppressed individuals, such as persons with diabetes mellitus, stem cell transplant recipients and those with human immunodeficiency virus (HIV) infection, are more susceptible to infection. Local factors, such as xerostomia and trauma from unhygienic or ill-fitting dentures, are also important. Local tissue damage is also a critical factor in the development of cutaneous forms of candidosis. Most infections occur in moist, occluded sites and follow maceration of tissue.

*Candida* vaginitis is more common during pregnancy. The lower prevalence of this infection after menopause emphasizes the hormonal dependence of the infection. Most cases of vaginal candidosis in older women are associated with uncontrolled diabetes mellitus or the use of exogenous oestrogen replacement treatment.

## Clinical features

### Mucosal infection

This is the most common form of superficial candidosis. Discrete white patches develop on the mucosal surface, and may eventually become confluent and form a curd-like pseudomembrane (Fig. 61.5).

In oropharyngeal candidosis white flecks appear on the buccal mucosa, tongue, and the hard and soft palate; although these are adherent, they can be removed. The surrounding mucosa is red and sore. This form of oropharyngeal candidosis occurs most frequently in infancy and old age, or in severely immunocompromised patients, including those with AIDS. Other forms of oral candidosis occur:

**Fig. 61.5** Pseudomembranous oral candidosis with associated angular cheilitis.

- lesions in the occluded area under the denture in those who wear dentures
- painful infection of the tongue in some individuals receiving antibiotic therapy
- chronic infection with extensive leucoplakia and infection of the angles of the mouth (angular cheilitis).

In vaginal candidosis, itching, soreness and a non-homogeneous white discharge accompany typical white lesions on the epithelial surfaces of the vulva, vagina and cervix. Sometimes the mucosa simply appears inflamed and friable. The perivulval skin may become sore and small satellite pustules may appear around the perineum and natal cleft. Some women suffer recurrent episodes.

Chronic, intractable oropharyngeal candidosis, which may extend to give oesophageal infection, is common in persons with HIV infection, although the use of combinations of antiretroviral drugs has reduced its incidence. The appearance of this infection can be the indicator of the transition from HIV-positive status to AIDS.

### Skin and nail infection

Cutaneous candidosis is less common than dermatophytosis. The lesions usually develop in warm, moist sites such as the axillae, groin and submammary folds. In infants, *Candida* species are often secondary invaders in napkin dermatitis. Infection of the finger webs, nail folds and nails is associated with frequent immersion of the hands in water.

### Chronic mucocutaneous candidosis

This is a rare form of candidosis that usually becomes apparent in childhood and takes the form of a

**Fig. 61.6** Microscopical appearance of *Candida albicans* yeast cells and pseudohyphae in a Gram-stained vaginal smear.

persistent, sometimes granulomatous, infection of the mouth, scalp, hands, feet and nails. In some cases, disfiguring hyperkeratotic lesions develop on the scalp and face. Some of those who develop this condition have subtle defects in lymphocyte function.

## Laboratory diagnosis

Specimens of skin and nail are collected in the same way as for suspected dermatophytosis. For infections of the mouth or vagina, scrapings taken with a blunt scalpel or a spatula from areas with white plaques or erythema are better than swabs if the material is to be processed immediately. However, swabs are more convenient for transport to the laboratory, and they are better for collecting vaginal discharge. Swabs should first be moistened with sterile water or saline before taking the sample and should be sent to the laboratory in 'clear' transport medium.

In Gram-stained smears of mucous membrane samples the fungus is seen as budding Gram-positive yeast cells; pseudohyphae are usually present except in the case of *C. glabrata* (Fig. 61.6). Contrary to popular belief, the presence of *Candida* pseudohyphae in clinical material does not confirm infection with the organism, particularly as it may have developed in the period between collection and processing of the sample.

*Candida* species grow well on Sabouraud medium or on blood agar at 25–37°C; typical yeast colonies appear within 1–2 days. *C. albicans* isolates can be identified by the germ tube test: after incubation in serum at 37°C for 1.5–2 h, *C. albicans* produces short hyphae known as germ tubes. Other yeasts may be identified with one of the commercial kits, or by fermentation and assimilation tests.

Quantification of growth, especially in the case of vulvovaginal samples, may help the clinician to distinguish between commensal carriage and infection.

## Treatment and prevention

Most superficial infections respond well to topical therapy with an imidazole. In oral candidosis, nystatin, amphotericin B or miconazole may be effective in lozenge or gel form. Most patients with vaginal candidosis can be treated successfully with a single application of a topical imidazole, or with oral fluconazole or itraconazole. Intermittent prophylaxis with an oral azole or vaginal pessaries is of benefit in controlling recurrent vaginal candidosis.

Treatment of chronic paronychia involves a combination of antifungal therapy, nail care and avoidance of prolonged exposure to water by use of protective gloves; patients should dry their hands carefully after washing. Regular application of an azole lotion or an azole given orally, sometimes in conjunction with a topical steroid and an antibacterial agent, is the most appropriate therapy but it may take several months to cure the condition; antifungal creams or ointments are less effective.

Oral therapy is essential for the treatment of intractable chronic *Candida* infections; treatment is given until remission is achieved but in some patients, for instance those with AIDS, relapse is common, and intermittent or prolonged therapy may be required. This may, however, lead to the development of resistance, as occasionally happens with fluconazole.

## PITYRIASIS VERSICOLOR

This is a common, mild and often recurrent infection of the stratum corneum that produces a patchy discoloration of the skin caused by lipophilic yeasts of the genus *Malassezia*. These organisms require lipids for growth and special media containing Tween and lipid supplements have been developed.

On normal skin and in conditions such as dandruff and seborrhoeic dermatitis (in which its precise role is uncertain), *Malassezia* occurs as an oval or bottle-shaped yeast, which characteristically produces buds on a broad base. In pityriasis versicolor the organism produces predominantly round yeast cells and short hyphae.

## Epidemiology

*Malassezia* species are common members of the normal skin flora and most infections are thought to be endogenous. The incidence of skin colonization rises from around 25% in children to almost 100% in adolescents and adults. Disease is probably related to host and environmental factors. It is very common in hot, humid tropical climates, where 30–40% of adults may be affected.

## Clinical features

Small patches of well demarcated, non-inflammatory scaling are usually present on the upper trunk or neck; these may appear hypopigmented or hyperpigmented, depending on the degree of pigmentation of the surrounding skin. The lesions tend to spread and coalesce, and occasionally they spread to other sites.

## Laboratory diagnosis

The diagnosis can be confirmed reliably by direct microscopy of skin scales; culture is unnecessary. Demonstration of clusters of the characteristic round yeast cells (5–8 μm in diameter) with short, stout hyphae, which may be curved and occasionally branched, is diagnostic.

## Treatment

Pityriasis versicolor responds well to topical therapy with 2% selenium sulphide or azoles such as ketoconazole in cream, lotion or a shampoo. Oral azole therapy is sometimes used for recalcitrant or widespread infections. Relapse is common, particularly in hot climates.

## OTHER SUPERFICIAL INFECTIONS

### Skin and nail

Certain non-dermatophyte moulds may cause infection of skin and nail. It is important that these are recognized because they are often resistant to the agents used to treat dermatophytosis and superficial candidosis.

In the UK, about 5% of fungal nail infections are caused by non-dermatophyte moulds. *Scopulariopsis brevicaulis*, a ubiquitous saprophyte of soil, is the most common, although other saprophytic moulds such as *Fusarium, Aspergillus* and *Acremonium* species are also occasionally implicated. There is some debate as to whether these moulds are primary pathogens of nails – infection usually follows trauma and in many cases they are found in nails along with a dermatophyte.

Non-dermatophyte mould infections do not respond to existing antifungal agents. Attempts may be made to remove the nail with topical 40% urea paste.

## Otomycosis

About 10–20% of chronic ear infections are due to fungi. The disease has a worldwide distribution but is more common in warm climates. Topical antibiotics and steroids are predisposing factors. The most common causes are species of *Aspergillus*, in particular *A. niger*. The fungi are easy to see in material from swabs or scrapings and grow readily in culture.

Treatment with topical antifungals is usually successful, although relapse is common. Any concurrent bacterial infection or other underlying abnormality should also be treated.

## Mycotic keratitis

Fungal infections of the cornea usually follow traumatic implantation of spores. Topical antibiotics and steroids are important predisposing factors. These infections occur most often in hot climates and are caused by common saprophytic moulds, in particular *Aspergillus* and *Fusarium* species. Culture results should be interpreted with care as these opportunist pathogens are also encountered as contaminants. Superficial swabs are of no value for laboratory investigation, and scrapings should be taken from the base or edge of the ulcer. The branched, septate hyphae may be rather sparse in potassium hydroxide mounts and some of the material should also be stained with periodic acid–Schiff or Grocott–Gomori methenamine–silver.

Management entails surgical debridement of infected tissue, discontinuation of topical corticosteroids, and topical or oral treatment with an antifungal drug. Topical treatment with natamycin is often successful, but oral treatment with an azole drug is required in patients with severe or worsening lesions. Even with intensive treatment, corneal perforation can occur.

## SUBCUTANEOUS INFECTIONS

## MYCETOMA

Mycetoma is a chronic granulomatous infection of the skin, subcutaneous tissues, fascia and bone that most often affects the foot or the hand. It may be caused

**Fig. 61.7** Microscopical appearance of *Madurella grisea* in a stained mycetoma grain. (Reproduced with permission from Richardson MD, Warnock DW, Campbell CK 1995 *Slide Atlas of Fungal Infection: Subcutaneous and Unusual Fungal Infections*. Blackwell Science, Oxford.)

**Fig. 61.8** Mycetoma of the foot.

by one of a number of different actinomycetes (actinomycetoma) (see Ch. 20) or moulds (eumycetoma). The disease is most prevalent in tropical and subtropical regions of Africa, Asia, and Central and South America.

A large number of organisms have been implicated in this disease, including species of *Madurella, Leptosphaeria, Acremonium, Pseudallescheria, Actinomadura, Nocardia* and *Streptomyces*. Within host tissues the organisms develop to form compacted colonies (grains) 0.5–2 mm in diameter, the colour of which depends on the organism responsible; for example, in unstained preparations *Madurella* grains are black and *Actinomadura pelletieri* grains are red (Fig. 61.7).

## Epidemiology

Infection follows traumatic inoculation of the organism into the subcutaneous tissue from soil or vegetation, usually on thorns or wood splinters. Consequently, the disease occurs most frequently in agricultural workers, in whom minor penetrating skin injuries are common.

## Clinical features

Localized swollen lesions that develop multiple draining sinuses are usually found on the limbs, although infections occur on other parts of the body (Fig. 61.8). There is often a long period between the initial infection and formation of the characteristic lesions; spread from the site of origin is unusual but may occur, particularly from the foot up the long bones of the leg.

## Laboratory diagnosis

The presence of grains in pus collected from draining sinuses or in biopsy material is diagnostic. The grains are visible to the naked eye and their colour may help to identify the causal agent. Grains should be crushed in potassium hydroxide and examined microscopically to differentiate between actinomycetoma and eumycetoma; material from actinomycetoma grains may be Gram stained to demonstrate the Gram-positive filaments. Samples should also be cultured, at both 25–30°C and 37°C, on brain–heart infusion agar or blood agar for actinomycetes and on Sabouraud agar (without cycloheximide) for fungi. The fungi that cause eumycetoma are all septate moulds that appear in culture within 1–4 weeks, but their identification requires expert knowledge.

## Treatment

The prognosis varies according to the causal agent, so it is important that the identity is established. Actinomycetoma responds well to medical treatment: combinations of streptomycin with co-trimoxazole or dapsone are often effective, but an average of 9 months' therapy is required. In eumycetoma, chemotherapy is ineffective and radical surgery is usually necessary. However, some antifungals have yet to be properly evaluated in this condition.

## CHROMOBLASTOMYCOSIS

This disease, also known as *chromomycosis*, is a chronic, localized infection of the skin and subcutaneous tissues, characterized by slow-growing verrucous lesions usually involving the limbs. The disease is encountered mainly in the tropics, in Central and South America, and Madagascar. The principal causes are *Fonsecaea pedrosoi, F. compacta, Phialophora verrucosa* and *Cladophialophora carrionii*. Like mycetoma, infection follows traumatic inoculation of the organism into the skin or subcutaneous tissue, and is seen most often among those with outdoor occupations.

## Laboratory diagnosis

The characteristic clusters of brown-pigmented, thick-walled fungal cells are relatively easy to see on microscopical examination of skin scrapings, crusts and pus. Culture on Sabouraud agar at 25–30°C yields slow-growing, greenish grey to black, compact, folded colonies. Cultures should be incubated for 4–6 weeks. Specific identification of these closely related fungi is usually left to a reference laboratory.

## Treatment

There is no ideal treatment for this disease, but promising results have been obtained with terbinafine and itraconazole, both of which can be combined with flucytosine in difficult cases. Early, solitary lesions may be excised.

## SPOROTRICHOSIS

Sporotrichosis is a chronic, pyogenic, granulomatous infection of the skin and subcutaneous tissues that may remain localized or show lymphatic spread. It is caused by *Sporothrix schenckii*, which is found in the soil and on plant materials, such as wood and sphagnum moss. The disease is worldwide in distribution, but occurs mainly in Central and South America, parts of the USA and Africa, and Australia; it is rare in Europe.

*S. schenckii* is a dimorphic fungus. In nature and in culture at 25–30°C, it develops as a mould with septate hyphae. The yeast phase is formed in tissue and in culture at 37°C, and is composed of spherical or cigar-shaped cells (1–3 × 3–10 μm).

## Epidemiology

Minor trauma, such as abrasions or wounds due to wood splinters, is often sufficient to introduce the organism. Infection occurs mainly in adults, and is more common among individuals whose work or recreational activities bring them into contact with soil or plant materials, such as gardeners and florists.

**Fig. 61.9** Sporotrichosis of the hand showing local lymphatic spread.

## Clinical features

Sporotrichosis presents most frequently as a nodular, ulcerating disease of the skin and subcutaneous tissues, with spread along local lymphatic channels (Fig. 61.9). Typically, the primary lesion is on the hand with secondary lesions extending up the arm. The primary lesion may remain localized or disseminate to involve the bones, joints, lungs and, in rare cases, the central nervous system. Disseminated disease usually occurs in debilitated or immunosuppressed individuals.

## Laboratory diagnosis

Diagnosis is confirmed by isolation of the causative organism by culture of swabs from moist, ulcerated lesions or pus aspirated from subcutaneous nodules; biopsy specimens may be necessary in some cases. Direct microscopy is of little value as so few of the small *S. schenckii* yeast cells are present in diseased tissue. The mycelial phase develops within 7–10 days on Sabouraud agar or blood agar at 25–30°C; the yeast phase develops in 2 days at 37°C. Identification depends on the micromorphology of the mould phase and its conversion to the yeast phase at 37°C.

## Treatment

Prolonged therapy is usually required. For the lymphocutaneous form, treatment with potassium iodide or itraconazole is satisfactory. In disseminated disease, intravenous amphotericin B is required.

## OTHER SUBCUTANEOUS MYCOSES

Phaeohyphomycosis is a general term used to describe solitary subcutaneous lesions caused by any brown-pigmented mould. If left untreated these lesions slowly increase in size to form a painless abscess. Diagnosis is often made at surgery, and treatment is by excision.

Several other fungi, including *Lacazia loboi*, *Basidiobolus ranarum* and *Conidiobolus coronatus*, occasionally cause subcutaneous infections, usually in the tropics. Surgical excision is often curative in *L. loboi* infections; antifungal therapy may be of use for the other infections, but the newer drugs have not been properly evaluated.

## SYSTEMIC MYCOSES

## COCCIDIOIDOMYCOSIS

This is primarily an infection of the lungs caused by *Coccidioides immitis* and *C. posadasii*, two closely related dimorphic fungi found in the soil of semi-arid regions of the western hemisphere. In the USA, the endemic region includes parts of California, Arizona, New Mexico and Texas. The endemic region extends southwards into the desert regions of northern Mexico, and parts of Central and South America.

In culture and in soil *Coccidioides* grows as a mould, producing large numbers of barrel-shaped arthroconidia (4 × 6 μm diameter), which are easily dispersed in wind currents (Fig. 61.10). In the lungs the arthroconidia form spherules (up to 120 μm in diameter) which contain numerous endospores (2–4 μm in diameter) (Fig. 61.11). Endospores are released by rupture of the spherule wall and develop to form new spherules in adjacent tissue or elsewhere in the body. In culture the mould colonies are initially moist and white but change within 5–12 days to become floccose and pale grey or brown.

## Epidemiology

Infection is acquired by inhalation; the incubation period is 1–3 weeks. The major risk factor for infection is environmental exposure. Outbreaks have been associated with ground-disturbing activities, such as building construction and archaeological excavation, as well as with natural events that result in the generation of dust clouds, such as earthquakes and dust storms. The most serious disseminated forms of the disease are more common among those of black, Asian or Filipino ethnicity, and among pregnant women in the third trimester.

## Clinical features

*Coccidioides* causes a wide spectrum of disease, ranging from a transient pulmonary infection that resolves without treatment, to chronic pulmonary infection, or to more widespread disseminated disease. About 40% of newly infected persons develop an acute symptomatic and often severe influenza-like illness. However, most otherwise healthy persons recover without treatment, their symptoms disappearing in a few weeks. In some cases primary infection may result in chronic, cavitating, pulmonary disease.

Fewer than 1% of infected individuals develop disseminated coccidioidomycosis. This is a progressive disease that usually develops within 3–12 months of the initial infection, although it can occur much later following reactivation of a quiescent infection in an immunosuppressed individual. The clinical manifestations range from a fulminant illness that is fatal within a few weeks if left untreated, to an indolent chronic disease that persists for months or years. One or more sites may be involved, but the skin, soft tissue, bones, joints and the central nervous system are most commonly affected. Meningitis is the most serious

**Fig. 61.10** Microscopical appearance of *Coccidioides* arthroconidia.

**Fig. 61.11** Microscopical appearance of *Coccidioides* spherules in tissue.

complication of coccidioidomycosis, occurring in 30–50% of patients with disseminated disease. Without therapy, it is almost always fatal.

## Laboratory diagnosis

Microscopical examination of sputum, pus and biopsy material is helpful as the relatively large size and numbers of mature spherules present makes their detection and identification comparatively straightforward. Material for culture should be inoculated on to screw-capped slopes of Sabouraud agar and incubated at 25–30°C for 1–2 weeks. The fungus can be identified by its colonial morphology and the presence of numerous thick-walled arthroconidia formed in chains from alternate cells of the septate hyphae.

The arthroconidia are highly infectious and are a serious danger to laboratory staff. Consequently, Petri dishes should never be used for isolation of the organism and all procedures should be carried out in a biological safety cabinet under Category 3 containment. Preparations for microscopy should be made only after wetting the colony to reduce spore dispersal.

Serological tests play an important part in diagnosis. The immunodiffusion test is most useful for detection of early primary infection or exacerbation of existing disease; antibodies appear 1–3 weeks after infection but are seldom detectable after 2–6 months, or in patients with disseminated coccidioidomycosis. The latex agglutination test gives similar results to the immunodiffusion test, but is less specific. Complement-fixing antibodies appear 1–3 months after infection and persist for long periods in individuals with chronic or disseminated disease. In most cases the titre is proportional to the extent of infection; failure of the titre to fall during treatment of disseminated coccidioidomycosis is an ominous sign.

## Treatment

The historical standard of treatment is intravenous amphotericin B, but oral fluconazole is now used to treat many patients with skin, soft tissue, bone or joint infections. Itraconazole is also effective, but less well tolerated. Because oral fluconazole is so much more benign than intrathecal amphotericin B, it is now the drug of choice for coccidioidal meningitis.

## HISTOPLASMOSIS

This disease is caused by *H. capsulatum*, a dimorphic fungus found in soil enriched with the droppings of

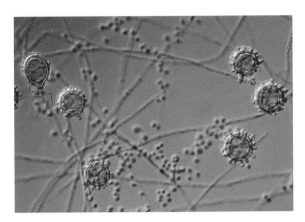

**Fig. 61.12** Microscopical appearance of *Histoplasma capsulatum* microconidia and macroconidia.

birds and bats. Histoplasmosis is the most common endemic mycosis in North America, but also occurs throughout Central and South America. In the USA, the disease is most prevalent in states surrounding the Mississippi and Ohio Rivers. Other endemic regions include parts of Africa, Australia, India and Malaysia. *H. capsulatum* var. *duboisii* is restricted to the continent of Africa.

*H. capsulatum* var. *capsulatum* grows in soil and in culture at 25–30°C as a mould and as an intracellular yeast in animal tissues. The small oval yeast phase cells (2–4 μm diameter) can also be produced in vitro by culture at 37°C on blood agar or other enriched media containing cysteine. In culture the mould colonies are fluffy, white or buff-brown; the mycelium is septate and two types of unicellular asexual spores are usually produced: large round, tuberculate macroconidia (8–15 μm in diameter) are most prominent and are diagnostic, but smaller, broadly elliptical, smooth-walled microconidia (2–4 μm in diameter) are also present in primary isolates (Fig. 61.12). *H. capsulatum* var. *duboisii* is morphologically identical to *H. capsulatum* var. *capsulatum* in its mycelial phase, but the yeast phase has larger cells (10–15 μm in diameter).

## Epidemiology

Infection results from the inhalation of spores; the incubation period is 1–3 weeks. The major risk factor is environmental exposure; longer and more intense exposures usually result in more severe pulmonary disease. Most reported outbreaks have been associated with exposures to sites contaminated with *H. capsulatum* or have followed activities that disturbed accumulations of bird or bat guano, such as building demolition, soil excavation and caving.

The most serious disseminated forms of the disease are more common among individuals with underlying cell-mediated immunological deficiencies, such as persons with HIV infection, transplant recipients, and those receiving immunosuppressive treatments.

## Clinical features

There is a wide spectrum of disease, ranging from a transient pulmonary infection that subsides without treatment, to chronic pulmonary infection, or to more widespread disseminated disease. Many healthy individuals develop no symptoms when exposed to *H. capsulatum* in an endemic setting. Higher levels of exposure result in an acute symptomatic and often severe flu-like illness, with fever, chills, non-productive cough and fatigue. The symptoms usually disappear within a few weeks, but patients are frequently left with discrete, calcified lesions in the lung.

Disseminated histoplasmosis may range from an acute illness that is fatal within a few weeks if left untreated (often seen in infants, persons with AIDS and solid organ transplant recipients) to an indolent, chronic illness that can affect a wide range of sites. Hepatic infection is common in non-immunosuppressed individuals and adrenal gland destruction is a frequent problem. Mucosal ulcers are found in more than 60% of these patients; central nervous system disease occurs in 5–20% of patients.

The clinical features of *H. capsulatum* var. *duboisii* infection differ from those of var. *capsulatum* infection. The illness is indolent in onset and the predominant sites affected are the skin and bones. Those with more widespread infection involving the liver, spleen and other organs have a febrile wasting illness that is fatal within weeks or months if left untreated.

## Laboratory diagnosis

Microscopy of smears of sputum or pus should be stained by the Wright or Giemsa procedure. Blood smears may be positive for *H. capsulatum*, especially in persons with AIDS. Liver or lung biopsies stained with periodic acid–Schiff or Grocott–Gomori methenamine–silver may provide a rapid diagnosis of disseminated histoplasmosis in some patients. *H. capsulatum* is seen as small, oval yeast cells, often within macrophages or monocytes (Fig. 61.13).

Specimens should be cultured on Sabouraud agar at 25–30°C to obtain the mycelial phase. Mycelial colonies develop within 1–2 weeks but cultures should be retained for 4 weeks before discarding. The fungus is identified by its colonial morphology and the presence of the characteristic macroconidia and

**Fig. 61.13** Microscopical appearance of *Histoplasma capsulatum* yeast cells in tissue.

microconidia. Culture at 37°C for the yeast phase is not used for primary isolation, although conversion from the mould to yeast phase is useful to confirm the identity of isolates. Mould cultures of *H. capsulatum* are a hazard to laboratory staff and consequently screw-capped slopes rather than Petri dishes should be used for isolation.

Serological tests are useful, but cross-reactions can occur, mainly with *Coccidioides*. Antibody tests fail to detect antibodies in up to 50% of immunosuppressed individuals. Tests for antigen detection in the urine by ELISA are useful in disseminated histoplasmosis but are not widely available outside the USA.

## Treatment

Intravenous amphotericin B is recommended for treatment of the most severe forms of disseminated histoplasmosis. Itraconazole is widely used in non-immunocompromised patients with milder forms of disseminated disease and for the continuation of treatment in those who have responded to amphotericin B.

## BLASTOMYCOSIS

This disease is caused by *B. dermatitidis*, a dimorphic soil-inhabiting fungus. The largest number of cases of blastomycosis has been reported from North America, but the disease is also endemic in Africa, and parts of Central and South America. In the USA, the organism is most commonly found in states surrounding the Mississippi and Ohio Rivers; in Canada, the disease occurs in the provinces that border the Great Lakes.

In culture at 25–30°C *B. dermatitidis* grows as a mould with a septate mycelium. The colony varies in

**Fig. 61.14** Microscopical appearance of *Blastomyces dermatitidis* yeast cells in tissue, showing broad-based budding.

texture from floccose to smooth and from white to brown in colour. Asexual conidia are produced on lateral hyphal branches of variable length; the oval or pear-shaped conidia are 2–10 μm in diameter. In tissue and in culture at 37°C the fungus grows as a large round yeast (5–15 μm in diameter) that characteristically produces broad-based buds from a single pole on the mother cell (Fig. 61.14).

## Epidemiology

Infection results from inhalation of spores; the incubation period is 4–6 weeks. The disease is more commonly seen in adults than in children, and often occurs in individuals with an outdoor occupation or recreational interest.

## Clinical features

Acute pulmonary blastomycosis usually presents as a nonspecific influenza-like illness, similar to that seen with histoplasmosis or coccidioidomycosis. Most otherwise healthy persons recover after 2–12 weeks of symptoms, but some return months later with infection of other sites. Other patients with acute blastomycosis fail to recover and develop chronic pulmonary disease or disseminated infection.

The skin and bones are the most common sites of disseminated disease. The skin is involved in more than 70% of cases; the characteristic lesions are typically raised, with a well-demarcated edge. It is from these skin lesions that the diagnosis is most often made. Osteomyelitis occurs in about 30% of patients, with the spine, ribs and long bones being the most common sites of infection. Arthritis occurs in about 10% of patients. Meningitis is rare, except in immunocompromised individuals.

## Laboratory diagnosis

Direct microscopy of pus, scrapings from skin lesions, or sputum usually shows thick-walled yeast cells 5–15 μm in diameter that characteristically produce buds on a broad base; the buds remain attached until they are almost the size of the parent cell, often forming chains of three or four cells. In biopsy material the yeasts are best seen in stained sections.

*B. dermatitidis* will grow in culture on Sabouraud agar (or blood agar) without cycloheximide, to which the fungus is sensitive. The mycelial phase develops slowly at 25–30°C and cultures must be retained for 6 weeks before discarding. Test-tube slopes rather than Petri dishes are used for culture. Identification is usually confirmed by subculture at 37°C to convert it to the yeast phase.

The most useful serological test is the immunodiffusion test using the A antigen of *B. dermatitidis*. However, a negative result does not rule out the diagnosis because the sensitivity ranges from 30% for localized infections to 90% for cases of disseminated blastomycosis.

## Treatment

Intravenous amphotericin B is used to treat all forms of blastomycosis and is the drug of choice in serious life-threatening infection. Itraconazole follow-on therapy is given once the patient improves. Itraconazole is also the drug of choice in less serious infection that does not involve the central nervous system.

## PARACOCCIDIOIDOMYCOSIS

This is a chronic granulomatous infection caused by the dimorphic fungus *P. brasiliensis* that may involve the lungs, mucosa, skin and lymphatic system. The disease may be fatal if untreated. Although *P. brasiliensis* has been isolated from soil, understanding of its precise environmental reservoir remains limited. The endemic region extends from Mexico to Argentina, but the disease is seen most frequently in Brazil, Colombia and Venezuela.

*P. brasiliensis* grows in the mycelial phase in culture at 25–30°C and in the yeast phase in tissue or at 37°C on brain–heart infusion or blood agar. The mould colonies are slow growing with a variable colonial morphology, although most are white and velvety to floccose in texture with a pale brown reverse. Spore production is usually sparse and best seen in 4–6-week-old cultures. Asexual conidia may be produced but are not characteristic, and identification

**Fig. 61.15** Microscopical appearance of *Paracoccidioides brasiliensis* yeast cells in sputum, showing multipolar budding.

depends on conversion from the mycelial to the yeast phase. The yeast phase consists of oval or globose cells 2–30 µm in diameter, with small buds attached by a narrow neck encircling the parent cell (Fig. 61.15).

## Epidemiology

Infection is usually acquired by inhalation; the incubation period is unknown. More than 90% of cases of symptomatic disease occur in men, most of whom have agricultural occupations; oestrogen-mediated inhibition of the mould to yeast transformation could help to account for this.

## Clinical features

The lungs are the usual initial site of *P. brasiliensis* infection, but the organism then spreads through the lymphatics to the regional lymph nodes. In most cases the primary infection is asymptomatic. There is evidence of prolonged latent infection before overt disease develops, and a mild, self-limiting pulmonary form of paracoccidioidomycosis probably exists. Children and adolescents sometimes present with an acute disseminated form of infection in which superficial and/or visceral lymph node enlargement is the major manifestation. This presentation is also seen in immunocompromised patients. It has a poor prognosis.

In adults, paracoccidioidomycosis usually presents as an ulcerative granulomatous infection of the oral and nasal mucosa and adjacent skin. In 80% of cases the disease involves the lungs. In some, the liver and spleen, intestines, adrenals, bones and joints, and central nervous system are also involved. The disease is slowly progressive, and may take months or even years to become established.

## Laboratory diagnosis

Microscopy of sputum or pus, crusts and biopsies from granulomatous lesions usually reveals numerous yeast cells showing the characteristic multipolar budding, which is diagnostic. In culture the mycelial and yeast phases both develop slowly and cultures must be retained for 6 weeks before discarding. The mould phase can be isolated on Sabouraud agar supplemented with yeast extract at 25–30°C, but colonies may take 2–4 weeks to appear. Serological tests are useful for diagnosis and for monitoring the response to therapy.

## Treatment

The choice of therapy depends on the site of infection and its severity. Oral itraconazole is the drug of choice, although amphotericin B remains useful for severe or refractory infections. Oral ketoconazole is almost as effective, but less well tolerated than itraconazole.

## ASPERGILLOSIS

There are more than 200 species of *Aspergillus* but fewer than 20 have been implicated in human disease; the most important are *A. fumigatus*, *A. flavus*, *A. terreus*, *A. niger* and *A. nidulans*. In immunocompromised individuals, inhalation of spores can give rise to life-threatening invasive infection of the lungs or sinuses and dissemination to other organs often follows (*invasive aspergillosis*). In non-immunocompromised persons, these moulds can cause localized infection of the lungs, sinuses and other sites. Human disease can also result from non-infectious mechanisms: inhalation of spores can cause allergic symptoms in both atopic and non-atopic individuals.

*Aspergillus* species are ubiquitous in the environment, growing in the soil, on plants, and on decomposing organic matter. These moulds are often found in the outdoor and indoor air, in water, on food items, and in dust. All grow in nature and in culture as moulds with septate hyphae and distinctive asexual sporing structures, termed conidiophores, that bear long chains of conidia (Fig. 61.16).

## Epidemiology

Inhalation of *Aspergillus* conidia is the usual mode of infection; less frequently, infection follows the traumatic implantation of spores as in corneal infection (see p. 626), or inadvertent inoculation as in endocarditis.

Invasive aspergillosis has emerged as a major problem in several groups of immunocompromised patients, including those with acute leukaemia, stem-cell and solid organ transplant recipients, and children

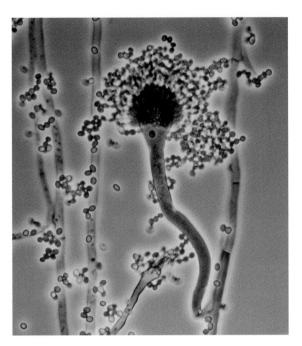

**Fig. 61.16** Microscopical appearance of an *Aspergillus fumigatus* conidiophore. (Reproduced with permission from Richardson MD, Warnock DW, Campbell CK 1995 *Slide Atlas of Fungal Infection: Systemic Fungal Infections*. Blackwell Science, Oxford.)

**Fig. 61.17** Radiological appearance of an aspergilloma. (Reproduced with permission from Richardson MD, Warnock DW, Campbell CK 1995 *Slide Atlas of Fungal Infection: Systemic Fungal Infections*. Blackwell Science, Oxford.)

with chronic granulomatous disease. The likelihood of aspergillosis developing in these individuals depends on a number of host factors, the most important of which is the level of immunosuppression. The mortality rate is high, ranging from 50–100% in almost all groups of immunocompromised patients.

## Clinical features

### Invasive aspergillosis

This form occurs in severely immunocompromised individuals who have a serious underlying illness. *A. fumigatus* is the species most frequently involved. The most common initial presentation in the neutropenic patient is an unremitting fever (>38°C), without any respiratory tract symptoms, that fails to respond to broad-spectrum antibiotics.

The lung is the sole site of infection in 70% of patients, but dissemination of infection to other organs often occurs; the central nervous system is involved in 10–20% of cases. There is widespread destructive growth of *Aspergillus* species in lung tissue and the fungus invades blood vessels, causing thrombosis and infarction; septic emboli may spread the infection to other organs. Invasive aspergillosis has a poor prognosis; early diagnosis is essential for successful management.

### Aspergilloma

In this form of aspergillosis, also referred to as *fungus ball*, the fungus colonizes pre-existing (often tuberculous) cavities in the lung and forms a compact ball of mycelium, eventually surrounded by a dense fibrous wall (Fig. 61.17).

Aspergillomas are usually solitary. Patients are either asymptomatic or have only a moderate cough and sputum production. Occasional haemoptysis may occur, especially when the fungus is actively growing, and haemorrhage following invasion of a blood vessel is one of the fatal complications. Surgical resection is most often used to treat this condition.

### Sinusitis

*Aspergillus* species, particularly *A. flavus* and *A. fumigatus*, may colonize and invade the paranasal sinuses; the infection may spread through the bone to the orbit of the eye and brain. Acute invasive sinusitis is a rapidly progressive disease, most commonly seen in immunocompromised persons. There are also several forms of slowly progressive chronic *Aspergillus* sinusitis that occur in immunocompetent individuals.

### Allergic bronchopulmonary aspergillosis

Allergy to *Aspergillus* species is usually seen in atopic individuals with raised immunoglobulin (Ig) E levels; about 10–20% of asthmatics react to *A. fumigatus*. The condition is a form of asthma with pulmonary eosinophilia that manifests as episodes of bronchial obstruction and lung consolidation; the fungus grows in the airways to produce mucous plugs of fungal mycelium that may block off segments of lung tissue and that, when coughed up, are a diagnostic feature.

## Laboratory diagnosis

The value of the laboratory in diagnosis varies according to the clinical form of aspergillosis; the diagnosis of invasive disease is particularly difficult.

### Direct microscopy

In potassium hydroxide preparations (preferably with Calcofluor to enhance detection) of sputum the fungus appears as non-pigmented septate hyphae, 3–5 μm in diameter, with characteristic dichotomous branching and an irregular outline; rarely the characteristic sporing heads of *Aspergillus* species are present.

- In allergic aspergillosis there is usually abundant fungus in the sputum and mycelial plugs may also be present.
- In aspergilloma, fungus may be difficult to find on microscopy.
- In invasive aspergillosis, microscopy is often negative.

Biopsy may provide a definitive diagnosis, although many clinicians are reluctant to undertake this procedure because of the associated risk in immunosuppressed patients. In tissue sections *Aspergillus* species are best seen after staining with periodic acid–Schiff or methenamine–silver.

### Culture

*Aspergillus* species grow readily at 25–37°C on Sabouraud agar without cycloheximide; colonies appear after 1–2 days. Isolates can be identified by their colonial appearance and micromorphology. The ability of *A. fumigatus* to grow well at 45°C can be used to help identify this species or to isolate it selectively.

As aspergilli are among the most common laboratory contaminants, quantification of the amount of fungus in sputum helps to confirm the relevance of a positive culture. However, all isolates from immunocompromised patients must be taken seriously and acted upon.

Large quantities of fungus are usually recovered from the sputum of patients with allergic aspergillosis, but cultures from those with aspergilloma or invasive disease are commonly negative or yield only a few colonies. Blood cultures are negative in invasive disease.

### Skin tests

Skin tests with *A. fumigatus* antigen are useful for the diagnosis of allergic aspergillosis. All patients give an immediate type I reaction and 70% of those with pulmonary eosinophilia also give a delayed type III Arthus reaction.

### Serological tests

Immunodiffusion, CIE and ELISA are widely used for the detection of antibodies in the diagnosis of all forms of aspergillosis, particularly aspergilloma and allergic bronchopulmonary aspergillosis. Tests for *Aspergillus* antibodies are seldom helpful in the diagnosis of invasive infection in immunocompromised patients.

Antigen detection has also been used successfully for diagnosis of invasive aspergillosis by techniques such as ELISA and latex agglutination. However, nucleic acid amplification methods are now being developed for diagnosis of invasive aspergillosis.

## Treatment

In invasive aspergillosis, the historical standard of treatment is intravenous amphotericin B (conventional or liposomal). Voriconazole proved superior to amphotericin B in a large clinical trial, and is now used to treat many patients with this disease.

Aspergilloma is treated by surgical excision because antifungal therapy is of little value, but because of the significant morbidity and mortality with this procedure it is reserved for patients with episodes of life-threatening haemoptysis. Allergic forms of aspergillosis are treated with corticosteroids.

## INVASIVE CANDIDOSIS

In addition to causing mucosal and cutaneous infections (see p. 655–57), *Candida* species can cause acute or chronic invasive infections in immunocompromised or debilitated individuals. This may be confined to one organ or become widespread (disseminated candidosis).

### Epidemiology

In most cases invasive candidosis is endogenous in origin, but transmission of organisms from person to person can also occur. Hospital outbreaks of infection have sometimes been linked to contaminated medical devices, such as vascular catheters, and/or parenteral nutrition. There are also reports of cross-infection due to hand carriage by healthcare workers.

Invasive candidosis is a significant problem in several distinct groups of hospitalized patients:

- neutropenic cancer patients
- stem cell and liver transplant recipients
- patients receiving intensive care.

Invasive candidosis is now more common in patients in intensive care than among neutropenic individuals. The reduced incidence of the disease among the latter group has been attributed to the widespread use of fluconazole prophylaxis. The predominant pathogen in all groups is still *C. albicans*, but the proportion of serious infections due to less azole-susceptible species, such as *C. glabrata*, has increased.

Many risk factors for invasive candidosis have been identified. These can be divided into host-related and healthcare-related factors:

- underlying immunosuppression
- low birth-weight
- intravascular catheterization
- broad-spectrum antibiotic use
- total parenteral nutrition
- haemodialysis.

Among adult patients cared for in surgical intensive care units, *Candida* bloodstream infection has a case fatality rate of about 40%.

## Clinical features

Infection may be localized, for instance in the urinary tract, liver, heart or meninges, or may be widely disseminated and associated with a septicaemia (*candidaemia*). Invasive candidosis is difficult to diagnose and treat, and for some forms the prognosis is poor.

Disseminated infection is most commonly seen in seriously ill individuals who usually have one or more indwelling vascular catheters, although these are not necessarily the source of the infection. Many cases are thought to arise from translocation of organisms across the wall of the intestinal tract.

Adults with candidaemia usually present with a persistent fever that fails to respond to broad-spectrum antibiotics, but with few other symptoms or clinical signs. One sign of invasive candidosis is the presence of white lesions within the eye (*Candida* endophthalmitis) (Fig. 61.18). These are found in up to 45% of patients in the intensive care unit, but are seldom seen in neutropenic individuals. Other useful signs are the nodular cutaneous lesions that occur in about 10% of neutropenic individuals with disseminated *Candida* infection. Other manifestations include:

**Fig. 61.18** Fundoscopic appearance of *Candida* endophthalmitis. (Reproduced with permission from Richardson MD, Warnock DW, Campbell CK 1995 *Slide Atlas of Fungal Infection: Systemic Fungal Infections*. Blackwell Science, Oxford.)

- meningitis
- renal abscess
- myocarditis
- osteomyelitis
- arthritis.

Invasive candidosis is a common complication in infants of low birth-weight (<1000 g) requiring prolonged neonatal intensive care. Meningitis occurs more frequently than in older patients and is sometimes associated with arthritis and osteomyelitis.

## Laboratory diagnosis

*Candida* species may be present as commensals in the absence of infection, so that isolation from clinical material, except from sites that are normally sterile, is of little significance. Similarly, antibodies to *Candida* species can be detected in uninfected individuals because of their exposure to commensal yeasts, although a rise in antibody titre or high titres may be of diagnostic significance. In suspected invasive candidosis, samples from as many sources as possible should be examined by direct microscopy and culture. Results should always be interpreted in the light of clinical findings.

### Direct microscopy

Appropriate samples are examined microscopically in potassium hydroxide or after Gram staining. In tissue sections, the fungus is seen best in stained preparations. Hyphae are often abundant, but their presence in sputum or urine does not confirm that the yeast is present as a pathogen.

## Culture

*Candida* species grow readily in culture at 37°C on common isolation media, such as Sabouraud dextrose agar. Blood cultures provide the most reliable evidence of invasive infection, although repeated attempts to isolate the organism may be required.

Isolation of the yeast from otherwise sterile sites provides reliable evidence for the diagnosis, but cultures obtained from urine, faeces and sputum are of less value unless done quantitatively over a period of time. Cell counts of the yeast in urine in excess of $10^4$ per mL are usually taken to indicate urinary tract infection, except in those with an indwelling urinary catheter. As *Candida* species multiply rapidly in clinical material it is important that specimens are processed as soon as possible after collection.

## Serological tests

Currently available tests lack specificity and sensitivity, and the results must be interpreted with care. A positive test does not necessarily indicate infection because the antigens used do not differentiate between antibodies formed during mucosal colonization and those produced during deep infection. Similarly, a negative antibody test does not necessarily rule out the possibility of invasive candidosis in immunocompromised patients who are incapable of mounting an adequate antibody response.

Antigen tests, based mainly on ELISA or latex agglutination, that detect cell wall mannan or cytoplasmic components have been developed and are used for diagnosis. Nucleic acid detection methods are increasingly being used to diagnose invasive candidosis, although their place in diagnosis is still being evaluated.

## Treatment

The treatments of choice for most forms of invasive candidosis are:

- intravenous echinocandin (anidulafungin, caspofungin or micafungin)
- intravenous amphotericin B (conventional or liposomal)
- intravenous or oral fluconazole.

Amphotericin B can be used in combination with flucytosine, but flucytosine is not used alone as resistance may develop during treatment. Voriconazole has also been used successfully. Removal of existing intravenous catheters is desirable if feasible, especially in non-neutropenic patients.

The choice of antifungal treatment depends on both the clinical status of the patient and the species of infecting organism.

- All *Candida* species are susceptible to echinocandins.
- *C. albicans*, *C. parapsilosis* and *C. tropicalis* are susceptible to amphotericin B and fluconazole.
- *C. glabrata* often becomes resistant to fluconazole during therapy.

## CRYPTOCOCCOSIS

Cryptococcosis, caused by the encapsulated yeasts *Cryptococcus neoformans* and *C. gattii*, is most frequently recognized as a disease of the central nervous system, although the primary site of infection is the lungs. The disease occurs sporadically throughout the world but it is currently seen most often in persons with AIDS.

There are four serotypes of *Cryptococcus* (A–D) that represent two distinct species of the organism, namely, *C. neoformans* (A & D) and *C. gattii* (B & C). Most infections are caused by *C. neoformans*, which is commonly found in the droppings of wild and domesticated birds throughout the world. Pigeons carry *C. neoformans* in their crops, but do not appear to become infected, probably because of their high body temperature. *C. gattii* has been isolated from decaying wood in various species of trees including Eucalyptus. These trees are indigenous to Australia, but have been planted in numerous other countries. *C. gattii* infection has been reported from subtropical regions and from temperate parts of the world, including western Canada and the Pacific North West Region of the USA.

## Epidemiology

Infection is acquired by inhalation; the incubation period is unknown. The likelihood that an infection with *C. neoformans* will develop after inhalation depends largely on host factors. Even before the advent of AIDS, infections with *C. neoformans* tended to occur in individuals with abnormalities of T lymphocyte function, such as are found in persons with lymphoma, and those receiving corticosteroid therapy. The major risk factor for development of infection with *C. gattii* appears to be environmental exposure, although there is indirect evidence that unidentified host factors contribute to the higher incidence of disease in Australian Aboriginals.

With the advent of the AIDS epidemic, cryptococcosis became the most common cause of meningitis in hospitals in which persons with HIV infection are treated. Although the incidence of the disease has declined in developed countries where combination antiretroviral treatment is available, the incidence is rising in many developing countries afflicted with large epidemics of HIV infection.

## Clinical features

A mild self-limiting pulmonary infection is believed to be the most common form of cryptococcosis. In symptomatic pulmonary infection there are no clear diagnostic features. Lesions may take the form of small discrete nodules, which may heal with a residual scar or may become enlarged, encapsulated and chronic (*cryptococcoma* form). An acute pneumonic type of disease has also been described.

The meningeal form of cryptococcosis can occur in apparently healthy individuals, but occurs most frequently in immunocompromised persons. Chronic meningitis or meningo-encephalitis develops insidiously with headaches and low-grade fever, followed by changes in mental state, visual disturbances and eventually coma. The disease may last from a few months to several years, but the outcome is always fatal unless it is treated. Patients with AIDS and cryptococcosis generally develop a chronic meningeal form with milder symptoms.

Although predominantly a disease of the central nervous system, lesions of the skin, bones and other deep sites may also occur; in its disseminated form, the disease may resemble tuberculosis. Rarely, lesions of skin and bones may occur without any evidence of infection elsewhere.

## Laboratory diagnosis

*Cryptococcus* is readily demonstrated in cerebrospinal fluid (CSF) or other material by direct microscopy, culture or serological tests for capsular antigen. The yeast load is generally higher in patients with AIDS. The cellular reaction and chemical changes in CSF usually resemble those seen in tuberculous meningitis. The yeast cells of *Cryptococcus* are round, 4–10 μm in diameter and surrounded by a mucopolysaccharide capsule. The width of the capsule varies and is greatest in vivo and on rich media in vitro.

In unstained wet preparations of CSF mixed with a drop of Indian ink or nigrosine, the capsule can be seen as a clear halo around the yeast cells (Fig. 61.19).

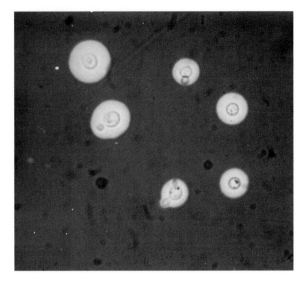

**Fig. 61.19** Microscopic appearance of encapsulated *Cryptococcus* cells in an Indian ink preparation of CSF. (Reproduced with permission from Richardson MD, Warnock DW, Campbell CK 1995 *Slide Atlas of Fungal Infection: Systemic Fungal Infections.* Blackwell Science, Oxford.)

Capsulate yeasts are seen in the CSF of about 60% of patients with cryptococcosis (higher in AIDS), but the capsule may be difficult to visualize in some cases. Sputum, pus or brain tissue should be examined after digestion in potassium hydroxide and here the capsulate yeasts are often delineated by the cellular debris. For examination of tissue sections it is best to use a specific fungal stain such as periodic acid–Schiff; alcian blue and mucicarmine stain the capsular material, enabling the organisms to be differentiated from *H. capsulatum* and *B. dermatitidis.*

The yeast is easily cultured from CSF although large volumes or multiple samples may be required in some cases; in patients with AIDS it is also useful to culture blood. On Sabouraud agar (without cycloheximide) cultured at 25–30°C and 37°C, colonies normally appear within 2–3 days, but cultures should not be discarded for 3 weeks. In culture, *Cryptococcus* appears as creamy white to yellow–brown colonies, which are mucoid in strains with well developed capsules and dry in strains that lack prominent capsules. Buds appear at any point on the cell surface but hyphae or pseudohyphae are not normally produced. Preliminary identification depends on demonstration of the capsule but this may be absent or difficult to see. *Cryptococcus* can be identified with commercial kits or distinguished from other yeasts by its lack of fermentative ability, its ability to produce urease, to grow at 37°C and to assimilate inositol.

The latex agglutination test for the detection of cryptococcal polysaccharide antigen in CSF or blood is highly sensitive and specific for the diagnosis of cryptococcal meningitis and disseminated forms of the disease, and gives better results than microscopy and culture. In AIDS, the test is positive in well over 90% of infected patients; titres of over $10^6$ may be detected.

### Treatment

Intravenous amphotericin B in combination with flucytosine is usually the treatment of choice for individuals with meningeal or disseminated cryptococcosis. Oral fluconazole is widely used for the continuation of treatment in those who have responded to amphotericin B. Patients with AIDS commonly relapse after the initial course of therapy and many require lifelong maintenance treatment with fluconazole.

## MUCORMYCOSIS

Mucormycosis, formerly known as *zygomycosis*, is a relatively rare, opportunistic infection caused by saprophytic mould fungi, notably species of *Rhizopus* and *Lichtheimia* (*Absidia*). These moulds are ubiquitous in the soil and on decomposing organic matter. They are characterized by having broad, aseptate hyphae, with large numbers of asexual spores inside a sporangium which develops at the end of an aerial hypha.

### Epidemiology

Most infections follow inhalation of spores; less frequently, infection follows traumatic inoculation into the skin and soft tissue. Major risk factors include:

- prolonged or profound neutropenia
- uncontrolled diabetes mellitus
- other forms of metabolic acidosis
- burns.

Certain predisposing conditions seem to be more commonly associated with particular clinical forms of disease; for example, persons with diabetic ketoacidosis often develop rhinocerebral mucormycosis, whereas neutropenic individuals often develop pulmonary or disseminated disease.

### Clinical features

The best known form of the disease is rhinocerebral mucormycosis. There is rapid and extensive tissue

**Fig. 61.20** Necrotic palatal lesion in a case of rhinocerebral mucormycosis. (Reproduced with permission from Richardson MD, Warnock DW, Campbell CK 1995 *Slide Atlas of Fungal Infection: Systemic Fungal Infections.* Blackwell Science, Oxford.)

destruction, most commonly spreading from the nasal mucosa to the turbinate bone, paranasal sinuses, orbit and brain (Fig. 61.20). The condition is fatal if untreated and, although the prognosis has improved over recent years, many diagnoses are still made at necropsy.

Pulmonary and disseminated infections can occur in severely immunocompromised individuals. Primary cutaneous infections have also been reported; these are uncommon but often result in extensive necrotizing fasciitis or disseminated disease. They usually occur in patients with burns or other forms of local trauma.

### Laboratory diagnosis

Recognition of the fungus in tissue by microscopy is considerably more reliable than culture, but material such as nasal discharge or sputum seldom contains much fungal material and examination of a biopsy is usually necessary for a firm diagnosis. Direct examination of curetted or biopsy material in potassium hydroxide may reveal the characteristic broad, aseptate, branched and sometimes distorted hyphae. However, they are seen much more clearly when stained with methenamine–silver; the hyphae of these fungi do not stain with periodic acid–Schiff (Fig. 61.21).

The fungi are readily isolated on Sabouraud dextrose agar at 37°C, but isolation is of little diagnostic significance in the absence of strong supporting clinical evidence of infection. There are no established serological tests.

**Fig. 61.21** Microscopic appearance of mucormycosis. (Reproduced with permission from Richardson MD, Warnock DW, Campbell CK 1995 *Slide Atlas of Fungal Infection: Systemic Fungal Infections.* Blackwell Science, Oxford.)

## Treatment

Successful treatment depends on early diagnosis of the infection to allow prompt therapy with high doses of intravenous amphotericin B (conventional or liposomal), control of any underlying disorder, such as diabetes, and aggressive surgical intervention.

## PNEUMOCYSTOSIS

*Pneumocystis* is an opportunistic pathogen with some of the features of protozoa, but comparative DNA sequence analysis showed it to be more closely related to the fungi. The organism was originally described as a cause of atypical pneumonia in malnourished infants, but came to prominence in the 1980s as a common cause of pneumonia, which was commonly fatal, in patients with AIDS. With the advent of reliable antiretroviral therapy, the incidence of the disease in HIV-positive individuals has declined.

Based on its morphology, which is similar to that of protozoa, the life cycle of *Pneumocystis* is divided into three stages:

1. the cyst, a spherical or crescent-shaped form (5–7 μm in diameter)
2. the sporozoite, up to eight of which develop within each cyst
3. the trophozoite, found outside the cyst.

When openings appear in the cyst wall, the excysted sporozoites become trophozoites. All of these forms reside within the alveoli of the lungs. As the organism is not cultivatable in vitro, its life cycle has not been fully elucidated.

The finding that *Pneumocystis* organisms from different mammalian hosts are genetically quite dissimilar has led to a name change from *P. carinii* (which infects rats) to *P. jirovecii* for the organisms that infect man.

## Epidemiology

Infection is probably acquired by inhalation. Serological and PCR studies indicate that most human beings become subclinically infected with *Pneumocystis* during childhood and that this infection is usually well contained by an intact immune system. The occurrence of clinical disease is related to the extent of immunosuppression, especially impairment of cell-mediated immunity. It may be due to primary infection, re-infection or reactivation. Pneumocystosis has a global distribution.

## Clinical features

The clinical presentation of *Pneumocystis* pneumonia is non-specific. Symptoms include:

- fever
- non-productive cough
- dyspnoea
- shortness of breath.

Patients with AIDS have a more indolent course with longer duration of symptoms than patients receiving immunosuppressive drugs. Without treatment the course is progressive and usually ends in death.

In addition to pneumonia, *Pneumocystis* infection may disseminate to the lymph nodes, liver, spleen, bone marrow, adrenal gland, intestines and meninges. Extra-pulmonary disease occurs predominantly in patients with advanced HIV infection and in those not taking co-trimoxazole prophylaxis or receiving aerosolized pentamidine.

## Laboratory diagnosis

Diagnosis usually depends on the identification of typical octonucleate cysts or trophozoites in tissues or body fluids. Organisms are detected by immunofluorescent staining of broncho-alveolar lavage fluid or induced sputum smears. Molecular diagnosis by PCR methods is being introduced in some centres.

## Treatment

Co-trimoxazole and intravenous pentamidine are the most effective therapies. The former is as potent as the latter, but less toxic. Other regimens include atovaquone, trimetrexate, the combination of trimethoprim and dapsone, and the combination of clindamycin and primaquine.

Co-trimoxazole is the preferred prophylactic agent, but patients with AIDS or those undergoing solid-organ or bone marrow transplantion may suffer unacceptable side effects to the high doses used. Aerosolized pentamidine is also used for prophylaxis.

## OTHER OPPORTUNIST FUNGI

*Penicillium marneffei* causes serious disseminated disease with characteristic papular skin lesions in patients with AIDS in South-East Asia. The fungus is dimorphic, forming yeast-like cells that are often intracellular, resembling histoplasmosis, in infected tissues. Treatment is with amphotericin B, followed by itraconazole to prevent relapse.

Almost any fungus may invade a severely immunocompromised host, and infections with many common fungi, including *Fusarium* species, *Trichosporon asahii* and *Pseudallescheria boydii*, have been reported. Diagnosis is made by culture of the causative organism from clinical specimens and serological tests play little part. Tissue sections are often not very helpful, either because the causal fungi have no special features to enable identification or because they resemble other fungal pathogens.

Infections are usually treated speculatively, and sometimes successfully, with amphotericin B.

---

RECOMMENDED READING

Anaissie EJ, McGinnis MR, Pfaller MA, editors: *Clinical Mycology*, ed 2, New York, 2009, Elsevier.

Dismukes WE, Kauffman C, Pappas PG, Sobel JD, editors: *Clinical Mycology*, ed 2, New York, 2010, Springer.

Hospenthal DR, Rinaldi MG, editors: *Diagnosis and Treatment of Human Mycoses*, Totowa, New Jersey, 2008, Humana Press.

Richardson MD, Johnson EM: *Pocket Guide to Fungal Infection*, ed 2, Oxford, 2006, Wiley Blackwell.

Richardson MD, Warnock DW: *Fungal Infection: Diagnosis and Management*, ed 3, Oxford, 2003, Blackwell Science.

### Websites

The Aspergillus Website: http://www.aspergillus.org.uk/

Doctor Fungus: http://www.doctorfungus.org/

University of Adelaide: Mycology Online. http://www.mycology.adelaide.edu.au/

World of Dermatophytes: A Pictorial. http://www.provlab.ab.ca/mycol/tutorials/derm/dermhome.htm

# 62 Protozoa

Malaria; toxoplasmosis; cryptosporidiosis; amoebiasis; trypanosomiasis; leishmaniasis; giardiasis; trichomoniasis

*D. Greenwood*

---

## KEY POINTS

- Protozoa are unicellular eukaryotic organisms.
- Most protozoal infections require laboratory confirmation for diagnosis; toxoplasmosis is diagnosed serologically.
- Malaria kills over 750 000 people each year.
- Acute malaria is a medical emergency demanding immediate diagnosis and treatment; quinine or artemisinin derivatives, usually in combination with other antimalarial drugs, are effective.
- African trypanosomiasis (sleeping sickness) is treated with toxic arsenical drugs; the West African form responds to eflornithine.
- South American trypanosomiasis (Chagas' disease) is a chronic condition that is difficult to treat.
- Leishmaniasis takes various forms; the most dangerous is visceral leishmaniasis (kala azar). Antimonial compounds, antifungal drugs or miltefosine are used for treatment.
- Amoebiasis, giardiasis and trichomoniasis occur worldwide; they usually respond to 5-nitroimidazole drugs such as metronidazole.

Infection with pathogenic protozoa exacts an enormous toll of human suffering, notably, but not exclusively, in the tropics. Numerically the most important of the life-threatening protozoan diseases is malaria, which is responsible for at least 750 000 deaths a year, mostly in young children in Africa.

Pathogenic protozoan parasites are conveniently dealt with by placing them in four groups: *sporozoa, amoebae, flagellates* and a miscellaneous group of other protozoa that may cause human disease (Table 62.1).

## SPOROZOA

This group includes the malaria parasites and related coccidia, which exhibit a complex life cycle involving alternating cycles of asexual division (*schizogony*) and sexual development (*sporogony*). In malaria parasites, the sexual cycle takes place in the female anopheline mosquito (Fig. 62.1).

## MALARIA PARASITES

### Description

Four species are commonly encountered in human disease: *Plasmodium falciparum*, which is responsible for most fatalities; *P. vivax* and *P. ovale*, both of which cause *benign tertian malaria* (febrile episodes typically occurring at 48-h intervals); and *P. malariae*, which causes *quartan malaria* (febrile episodes typically occurring at 72-h intervals). The appearances of trophozoites of the four species as seen in Romanowsky-stained films of peripheral blood are illustrated in Figures 62.2–62.7. *P. knowlesi*, a parasite of long-tailed macaque monkeys may also affect man. Human infection in south-east Asia, where the parasite is found, may be more common than has been supposed as the blood forms can be confused with *P. falciparum* or *P. malariae*.

### Life cycle

When an infected mosquito bites, *sporozoites* present in the salivary glands enter the bloodstream and are carried to the liver, where they invade liver parenchyma cells. They undergo a process of multiple nuclear division, followed by cytoplasmic division (*schizogony*); when this is complete, the liver cell ruptures, releasing several thousand individual parasites (*merozoites*) into the bloodstream. The merozoites

**Table 62.1** Principal protozoan pathogens of man

| Group | Species | Disease |
|---|---|---|
| Sporozoa | *Plasmodium falciparum* | Malignant tertian malaria |
| | *P. vivax* | Benign tertian malaria |
| | *P. ovale* | Benign tertian malaria |
| | *P. malariae* | Quartan malaria |
| | *Toxoplasma gondii* | Toxoplasmosis |
| | *Isospora belli* | Diarrhoea |
| | *Cryptosporidium parvum* | Diarrhoea |
| | *Cyclospora cayetanensis* | Diarrhoea |
| Amoebae | *Entamoeba histolytica* | Amoebic dysentery; liver abscess |
| | *Naegleria fowleri*[a] | Meningo-encephalitis |
| | *Acanthamoeba* spp.[a] | Keratitis |
| | *Balamuthia mandrillaris*[a] | Encephalitis |
| | *Blastocystis hominis*[b] | Pathogenicity doubtful |
| Flagellates | *Giardia lamblia* | Diarrhoea, malabsorption |
| | *Trichomonas vaginalis* | Vaginitis, urethritis |
| | *Trypanosoma brucei gambiense* | Sleeping sickness |
| | *T. brucei rhodesiense* | Sleeping sickness |
| | *T. cruzi* | Chagas' disease |
| | *Leishmania* spp. | See Table 62.4 |
| Others | *Babesia microti*[a] | Babesiosis |
| | *B. divergens*[a] | Babesiosis |
| | *Balantidium coli*[a] | Balantidial dysentery |
| | *Encephalitozoon cuniculi*[a] | Microsporidiosis |
| | *Enterocytozoon bieneusi*[a] | Microsporidiosis |
| | *Nosema connori*[a] | Microsporidiosis |

[a]Organisms rarely encountered in human disease.
[b]Taxonomic status uncertain.

**Fig. 62.2** Stages in the erythrocytic cycle of *Plasmodium vivax*.

**Fig. 62.3** Ring form trophozoites of *P. falciparum*.

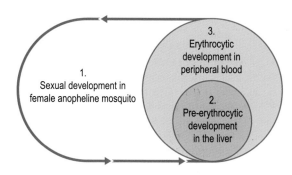

**Fig. 62.1** Schematic representation of the life cycle of malaria parasites.

**Fig. 62.4** Trophozoites of *P. falciparum*. Note peripheral location of the parasites (*appliqué* or *accolé* forms) and light stippling of the red cells (*Maurer's spots*).

**Fig. 62.5** Amoeboid trophozoites of *P. vivax*. Note the marked enlargement of the parasitized red cells and the intense stippling (*Schüffner's dots*).

**Fig. 62.6** Trophozoite of *P. ovale*. Note the fimbriate, oval-shaped red cell and marked stippling (*James' stippling*).

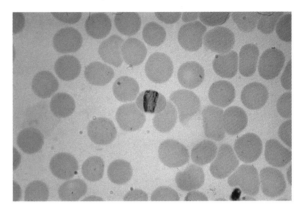

**Fig. 62.7** Band-form trophozoite of *P. malariae*.

penetrate red blood cells and adopt a typical 'signet-ring' morphology (see Fig. 62.3).

In the case of *P. vivax and P. ovale*, some parasites in the liver remain dormant (*hypnozoites*) and the cycle of pre-erythrocytic schizogony is completed only after a long delay. Such parasites are responsible for the relapses of tertian malaria that may occur, usually within 2 years of the initial infection.

In the bloodstream, the young ring forms (*trophozoites*) develop and start to undergo nuclear division (*erythrocytic schizogony*). Depending on the species, about 8 to 24 nuclei are produced before cytoplasmic division occurs, and the red cell ruptures to release the individual merozoites, which then infect fresh red blood cells (see Fig. 62.2).

Instead of entering the cycle of erythrocytic schizogony, some merozoites develop within red cells into male or female *gametocytes*. These do not develop further in the human host, but when the insect vector ingests the blood, the nuclear material and cytoplasm of the male gametocytes differentiate to produce several individual gametes, which give it the appearance of a flagellate body (*exflagellating male gametocyte*). The gametes become detached and penetrate the female gametocyte, which elongates into a zygotic form, the *ookinete*. This penetrates the mid-gut wall of the mosquito and settles on the body cavity side as an *oocyst*, within which numerous sporozoites are formed. When mature, the oocyst ruptures, releasing the sporozoites into the body cavity, from where some find their way to the salivary glands.

*P. falciparum* differs from the other forms of malaria parasite in that developing erythrocytic schizonts form aggregates in the capillaries of the brain and other internal organs, so that normally only relatively young ring forms or gametocytes (which are typically crescent shaped) are found in peripheral blood.

---

---

**Table 62.2** Differential characteristics of human malaria parasites as seen in Romanowsky-stained thin films of peripheral blood (see also Figs 60.2–60.7)

| Species | Morphology of trophozoite | Morphology of red cell | Stippling of red cell | Morphology of gametocyte | No. of merozoites in mature schizont |
|---|---|---|---|---|---|
| P. falciparum | Ring forms only | Normal | Maurer's spots[a] | Crescentic | (16–24)[b] |
| P. vivax | Rings, becoming amoeboid during development | Enlarged | Schüffner's dots | Large, round | 16–24 |
| P. ovale | Rings, becoming compact during development | Slightly enlarged; sometimes oval with fimbriate edge | James's stippling[c] | Round | 8–12 |
| P. malariae | Rings, becoming compact, stretched across red cell | Normal or slightly shrunken | (Ziemann's dots)[d] | Small, round | 8–12 |

[a]Maurer's spots (or clefts) are relatively scanty and accompany more mature ring forms.
[b]Mature schizonts of P. falciparum are rarely seen in peripheral blood.
[c]James's stippling is similar to the intense stippling of Schüffner's dots.
[d]Ziemann's dots are rarely seen, except in intensely stained preparations.

The cycle of erythrocytic schizogony takes 48 h, except in the case of *P. malariae*, in which the cycle occupies 72 h. Since febrile episodes occur shortly after red cell rupture, this explains the characteristic periodic fevers. However, with *P. falciparum*, the cycles of different broods of parasite do not become synchronized as they do in other forms of malaria, and typical tertian fevers are not usual in falciparum malaria.

## Laboratory diagnosis

Acute falciparum malaria is a medical emergency that demands immediate diagnosis and treatment. To establish the diagnosis, a drop of peripheral blood is spread on a glass slide. The smear should not be too thick; a useful criterion is that print should be just visible through it. The smear is allowed to dry thoroughly and stained by Field's method. This is an aqueous Romanowsky stain, which stains the parasites very rapidly and haemolyses the red cells, so that the parasites are easy to detect despite the thickness of the film.

With experience, the species of malaria can usually be determined from a thick blood film, but some of the characteristic features used to establish the identity of the parasites (Table 62.2), such as the typical stippling of the red cell that accompanies infection with *P. vivax* or *P. ovale*, are better observed in a conventional thin blood film stained by one of the many modifications of Giemsa's or Leishman's stain. The water used to dilute the stain should be at pH 7.2 (not 6.8 as used for haematological purposes).

Various other diagnostic tests have been devised for the rapid diagnosis of malaria including simple 'dipstick' tests, which are sufficiently reliable to be used by inexperienced staff (perhaps even by patients themselves) or in field conditions where microscopy is not available. Tests that detect *P. falciparum* alone or discriminate between *P. falciparum* and *P. vivax* are available. They are not foolproof, and may remain positive for some time after successful treatment. Visualization of the parasites in Romanowsky-stained peripheral blood films remains the most reliable method.

## Pathogenesis

Malaria is characterized by severe chills, high fever and sweating, often accompanied by headache, muscle pains and vomiting. Falciparum malaria, unlike the other forms, may progress (especially in primary infections) to coma, convulsions and death. This condition, *cerebral malaria*, is associated with the adherence of parasitized red blood cells to the endothelium of brain capillaries. However, the precise mechanism for the pathological sequelae that follow, including the marked increase in the production of tumour necrosis factor that occurs, is not known with certainty.

Falciparum malaria is notoriously varied in its presentation, so that a definitive laboratory diagnosis is most important. Various systems may be affected. Severe anaemia and renal failure are common complications, and hypoglycaemia, pulmonary oedema and gastroenteritis may be present.

Individuals that are homozygous or heterozygous for the sickle cell gene have a much-reduced susceptibility to infection with *P. falciparum*, and this has provided a selective advantage for the maintenance of sickle cell disease in holo-endemic areas. Similarly, individuals whose red cells lack the antigen known as the *Duffy factor* are protected from infection with

*P. vivax*. In parts of tropical Africa, where most of the population are Duffy factor negative, *P. vivax* is rare, although the related *P. ovale* is found, especially in West Africa.

## Treatment

For many years the standard treatment for acute malaria was chloroquine. However, resistance to that drug in *P. falciparum* (and, less commonly, in *P. vivax*) is now widespread and other agents have to be used. Derivatives of artemisinin (a natural product from the plant *Artemisia annua*), including artemether and sodium artesunate, are quick acting and effective. They have become the drug of choice for treatment of uncomplicated falciparum malaria in endemic areas; combination therapy with other antimalarial agents that target different functions in the parasite are recommended.

Alternatively, quinine (or quinidine), which has been available for centuries in the form of cinchona bark, remains effective. Some antibiotics, including tetracyclines and clindamycin, exhibit antimalarial activity and are used as an adjunct to quinine therapy. Mefloquine and halofantrine are active against chloroquine-resistant strains, but resistance to them is increasing in prevalence and both are associated with occasional problems of toxicity. The combination of atovaquone and proguanil offers a safer alternative.

Treatment of acute malaria with chloroquine, quinine or other antimalarials will not eliminate parasites in the liver. For this purpose the 8-aminoquinoline drug primaquine is used. This agent carries the risk of precipitating haemolysis in individuals who are deficient in the enzyme glucose-6-phosphate dehydrogenase.

## Prophylaxis

Antimalarial prophylaxis is essential for non-immune travellers to malarious areas. Chloroquine and the antifolate drugs pyrimethamine (often combined with sulfadoxine or dapsone) and proguanil were formerly used widely, but the widespread occurrence of resistance to these agents has made it difficult to offer definitive advice to travellers, particularly those going to regions in which *P. falciparum* is prevalent. Common recommendations include:

- the combination of atovaquone and proguanil daily
- the combination of daily proguanil and weekly chloroquine
- mefloquine, once a week.

Others recommend daily doxycycline or even primaquine. Whatever prophylactic guidance is given, it should be combined with advice to bring any fever to medical attention; to avoid exposure to mosquito bites by wearing long clothing in the evening when the insects are most active; to use insect repellents; and to sleep under mosquito netting impregnated with insecticide.

Because parasites in the pre-erythrocytic stage of development escape the action of most prophylactic drugs, prophylaxis should continue for at least 4 weeks after leaving a malarious area. This will effectively prevent the development of falciparum malaria, although relapses of other types may occur up to 2 years after exposure.

An effective vaccine has long been sought, but is still awaited.

## COCCIDIA

The coccidia are related to malaria parasites and share alternating sexual and asexual phases of development. They are not, however, transmitted by insects and infection is usually acquired by ingesting mature oocysts.

### *Toxoplasma gondii*

This is a coccidian parasite of the intestinal tract of the cat that is transmissible to many other mammals. It occurs worldwide. Serological evidence suggests that human infection is common, presumably as a transient febrile illness or a subclinical attack. Occasionally, more severe infection occurs.

- Intra-uterine toxoplasmosis is an important cause of stillbirth and congenital abnormality.
- Ocular disease is a rare but serious condition.
- Cerebral toxoplasmosis sometimes occurs in immunocompromised patients, probably through reactivation of latent infection.

Mature oocysts excreted by infected cats contain two sporocysts, within which *tachyzoites* develop. On ingestion the tachyzoites pass to the bloodstream and lymphatics to invade macrophages, in which they multiply (Fig. 62.8). As the immune response develops, other cells are infected and tissue cysts containing slowly metabolizing *bradyzoites* are formed. Infection is acquired by ingestion of oocysts, or of tissue cysts in undercooked meat. Intra-uterine infection is acquired transplacentally.

It is difficult to find toxoplasmas in clinical material. Diagnosis of acute infection is made by

**Fig. 62.8** Tachyzoites of *Toxoplasma gondii* in a macrophage (top left) and lying free (bottom right.)

demonstration of a rising titre of serum antibodies to *Tox. gondii*. The *Sabin–Feldman dye exclusion test* recognizes the ability of serum antibody to kill viable toxoplasmas. Other serological tests, including an enzyme-linked immunosorbent assay (ELISA), are available and have the advantage that they avoid the use of live toxoplasmas. The polymerase chain reaction (PCR) is useful in the diagnosis of intra-uterine and cerebral infections.

The combination of pyrimethamine and a sulphonamide is effective against active tachyzoites. Spiramycin is also effective and may be preferred during pregnancy. Clindamycin, azithromycin and atovaquone, usually in combination with pyrimethamine, offer alternatives in patients with cerebral toxoplasmosis.

### Isospora belli

This coccidian parasite usually causes mild self-limiting diarrhoea, but is occasionally associated with more severe infection, particularly in patients with acquired immune deficiency syndrome (AIDS). It is more common in areas of poor sanitation. The characteristic oocysts can be seen in faecal 'wet' mounts, but are poorly refractile and easily missed. Co-trimoxazole is usually effective if antimicrobial treatment is necessary.

### Cryptosporidium parvum

Cryptosporidia are common animal parasites. One species, *Cryptosporidium parvum*, commonly causes diarrhoea in humans, especially infants. Infection is usually water-borne or acquired directly from animals or infected cases. Large numbers of oocysts are often present in faeces; they are partially acid-fast and can be demonstrated by modifications of the Ziehl–Neelsen method (see p. 217).

The infection usually responds to symptomatic treatment, with fluid replacement if necessary. In severely immunocompromised patients, cryptosporidia may cause severe life-threatening diarrhoea for which nitazoxanide or macrolides such as azithromycin may offer some benefit.

### Cyclospora cayetanensis

Unlike cryptosporidia, cyclospora develop intracellularly in the gut mucosa. The immature oocysts are excreted in the faeces as round bodies about 10 μm in diameter, with a characteristic 'mulberry' appearance. They are more variably acid-fast than are cryptosporidia.

*Cyclospora cayetanensis* causes diarrhoea and is associated with poor sanitation. As with other coccidian parasites, infection is more severe in the immunocompromised. Mild infection is treated symptomatically, with rehydration if necessary. Co-trimoxazole appears to be effective in serious infection.

### Sarcocystis species

The animal parasites *Sarcocystis bovihominis* and *S. suihominis* occasionally invade the human intestinal tract or muscle. Infection is usually subclinical and discovered accidentally.

## AMOEBAE

### ENTAMOEBA HISTOLYTICA

This is the most important amoebic parasite of man. The amoebae invade the colonic mucosa, producing characteristic ulcerative lesions and a profuse bloody diarrhoea (*amoebic dysentery*). Systemic infection may arise, leading to abscess formation in internal organs, notably the liver. Such disease may arise in the absence of frank dysentery.

### Laboratory diagnosis

In acute amoebiasis, blood-stained mucus or colonic scrapings from ulcerated areas are examined by direct

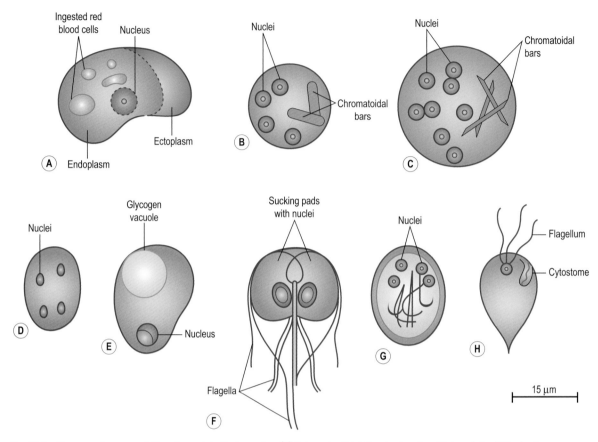

**Fig. 62.9** Diagrammatic representation of some intestinal parasites: (A) *Entamoeba histolytica*, trophozoite with ingested red blood cells; (B) *E. histolytica*, mature cyst; (C) *E. coli*, mature cyst; (D) *Endolimax nana*, mature cyst; (E) *Iodamoeba bütschlii*, mature cyst; (F) *Giardia lamblia*, trophozoite; (G) *G. lamblia*, mature cyst; (H) *Chilomastix mesnili*, trophozoite.

microscopy. The material should be examined within 2 h of collection. *Entamoeba histolytica* may be recognized by its active movement, pushing out fingerlike pseudopodia and, sometimes, progressing across the microscope field. If mucosal invasion has occurred, the amoebae usually contain ingested red blood cells, but these may be absent if infection is confined to the gut lumen. The nucleus is not usually visible in unstained 'wet' preparations, but in fixed smears stained with haematoxylin it is seen as a delicate ring of chromatin with a central karyosome (Fig. 62.9A).

Typical amoebic trophozoites may also be seen in aspirates of liver abscess. The pus often has a distinctive red–brown 'anchovy sauce' appearance. As the amoebae actively multiply in the walls of the abscess, they are most likely to be found in the last few drops of pus drained from the lesion.

In the intestinal carrier state, active amoebae are usually absent, but the encysted form, by which infection is spread, may be found. They are spherical,

about 10–15 μm in diameter, and contain one to four of the nuclei typical of *Entamoeba* species – a circular ring with a central dot. Young uninucleate cysts may also contain a large glycogen vacuole and, in fresh specimens, cysts of all stages of development may exhibit one or more thick, blunt-ended *chromatoidal bars* (Fig. 62.9B).

Although demonstration of active amoebae or cysts is the best way to make a definitive diagnosis, serology is also sometimes helpful, particularly in systemic disease. Various immunodiagnostic tests have been described, but they are usually performed only in reference centres. Culture of *E. histolytica* is unhelpful as a diagnostic procedure.

## Treatment

Metronidazole and tinidazole have superseded older drugs such as emetine and dehydroemetine for the treatment of amoebic dysentery and amoebic liver abscess.

**Table 62.3** Differential characteristics of intestinal amoebae

| Species | Trophozoites | | Cysts | | | |
|---|---|---|---|---|---|---|
| | Size (μm) | Ingested red blood cells | Size (μm) | No. of nuclei[a] | Chromatoidal bars | Nuclear morphology |
| Entamoeba histolytica[b] | 10–40 | + | 10–15 | 4 | Solid, blunt-ended | Fine ring of chromatin with central karyosome |
| E. hartmanni | 4–10 | – | 6–10 | 4 | As above | As above |
| E. coli | 10–40 | – | 15–25 | 8 | Slender, pointed | As above, but karyosome may be eccentric |
| E. gingivalis[c] | 10–25 | – | No cyst stage | | | |
| Iodamoeba bütschlii | 10–20 | – | 10–15 | 1 | None | Chromatin massed at one end of ring |
| Endolimax nana | 5–12 | – | 5–8 | 4 | None | Small shadowy masses of chromatin |
| Dientamoeba fragilis | 5–10 | – | No cyst stage | | | Ring containing several chromatin granules |

[a]Refers to mature cyst.
[b]Including E. dispar.
[c]E. gingivalis is a commensal of the mouth.

Not all strains of *E. histolytica* are invasive and some (now classified as *E. dispar*) never cause disease. However, since cysts of pathogenic and non-pathogenic strains are indistinguishable, it is prudent to treat all asymptomatic cyst excreters, particularly if they are food handlers, at least in areas of the world in which amoebiasis is uncommon. For this purpose, diloxanide furoate is often used.

## NON-PATHOGENIC INTESTINAL AMOEBAE

Although there are occasional reports of diarrhoea associated with other intestinal amoebae, notably *Dientamoeba fragilis* (an amoeba flagellate) most are commensals and are important only because of potential confusion with *E. histolytica*. The differential characteristics of non-pathogenic intestinal amoebae are compared with those of *E. histolytica* in Table 62.3. The greatest opportunity for confusion arises with the other intestinal *Entamoeba* species, *E. hartmanni* and *E. coli*. *E. hartmanni* is morphologically identical to *E. histolytica*, but is smaller and the trophozoite never contains ingested red blood cells. *E. coli* is somewhat larger than *E. histolytica*, particularly in the cyst form. The trophozoites are more sluggish than those of *E. histolytica*, and mature cysts contain up to eight nuclei; chromatoidal bars, if present, are fine and pointed, rather like slivers of broken glass (Fig. 62.9C).

*Blastocystis hominis*, an organism commonly found in faeces and formerly thought to be a yeast, is probably an amoeba. Any pathogenic role is the subject of dispute, but it has been associated with diarrhoea in the absence of other known pathogens. Metronidazole is said to be useful if true infection is suspected.

## FREE-LIVING AMOEBAE

Environmental amoebae belonging to the genus *Naegleria* (usually *N. fowleri*) are occasionally implicated in meningo-encephalitis. Rare cases of granulomatous encephalitis caused by *Balamuthia mandrillaris* and *Acanthamoeba* species have also been described, often, but not exclusively, in immunocompromised patients. The outcome in all kinds of amoebic encephalitis is ordinarily fatal, although amphotericin B has been successfully used in infections with *N. fowleri*.

*Acanthamoeba* spp. more commonly cause keratitis, sometimes following use of contaminated cleaning fluids for soft contact lenses. Optimal antimicrobial chemotherapy remains to be defined, but topical treatment with propamidine, biguanides or voriconazole have been used.

## FLAGELLATES

### *GIARDIA LAMBLIA (*SYN. *G. INTESTINALIS, G. DUODENALIS)*

This intestinal parasite lives attached to the mucosal surface of the upper small intestine. Vast numbers may be present, and their presence may lead to mal-absorption of fat and chronic diarrhoea. Young infants may be particularly severely affected. Infection is usually water-borne.

The trophozoite is kite-shaped, with two nucleated sucking pads and four pairs of flagella (Fig. 62.9F). Trophozoites may be found in duodenal aspirate, but examination of faeces usually reveals the cyst form by which the disease is transmitted. This is oval, about $10 \times 8$ μm, and contains up to four nuclei as well as the remains of the skeletal structure of the trophozoite (Fig. 62.9G).

Cysts of other, non-pathogenic, intestinal protozoa, including *Chilomastix mesnili*, *Enteromonas hominis* and *Retortamonas intestinalis*, may be mistaken for *G. lamblia*, but they are usually smaller and lack the regular oval shape and characteristic internal morphology. These non-pathogenic protozoa may also be found as trophozoites during microscopy of diarrhoeic faeces, but the most common intestinal flagellate is *Trichomonas hominis*, which is recognizable by its undulating membrane. There is no cyst form.

Giardiasis can be treated with 5-nitroimidazoles such as metronidazole or, on the rare occasions when this fails (and re-infection is excluded), with albendazole or mepacrine (quinacrine).

## TRICHOMONAS VAGINALIS

*T. vaginalis* is a flagellate protozoon with four anterior flagella and one lateral flagellum which is attached to the surface of the parasite to form an undulating membrane. There is no cyst form; the parasite is transmitted by sexual intercourse.

As the name suggests, *T. vaginalis* is predominantly a vaginal parasite, although urethritis may occur in the male consorts of infected women. The organism is responsible for a mild vaginitis, with discharge, which ordinarily responds to treatment with metronidazole or tinidazole.

*T. vaginalis* is readily identified by its characteristic motility in untreated 'wet' films of vaginal discharge and can be cultivated in appropriate culture media.

## TRYPANOSOMES

In contrast to the flagellates already described, trypanosomes have a complex life cycle involving an insect vector. The diseases that are caused in man, African trypanosomiasis (*sleeping sickness*) and South American trypanosomiasis (*Chagas' disease*), are restricted in distribution according to the habitat of the insect host.

## African trypanosomiasis

African sleeping sickness is caused by trypanosomes that are subspecies of *Trypanosoma brucei*, an important aetiological agent of the fatal disease *nagana* in cattle in tropical Africa. Tsetse flies (see p. 672) act as the insect vector. The human parasites are *T. brucei gambiense*, which occurs in riverine areas of west and central Africa, and *T. brucei rhodesiense*, a parasite of the savannah plains of east Africa, where cattle and wild antelope act as reservoirs of infection.

### Pathogenesis

Following the bite of an infected tsetse fly, a localized *trypanosomal chancre* may appear transiently, but invasion of the bloodstream rapidly occurs. The parasites multiply in blood, and at this stage there may be non-specific symptoms with occasional febrile episodes and some lymphadenitis. Swollen lymph glands in the posterior triangle of the neck (*Winterbottom's sign*) are often present in *T. brucei gambiense* infection. If untreated, the disease progresses inexorably to involve the central nervous system with the classical signs of sleeping sickness and, ultimately, death.

Infection with *T. brucei rhodesiense* tends to follow a more acute, fulminating course over a period of a few months, whereas *T. brucei gambiense* infection usually progresses slowly, sometimes over several years.

### Laboratory diagnosis

During the parasitaemic stage, sparse trypanosomes may be found in peripheral blood in unstained 'wet' mounts or in smears stained by the Giemsa or Leishman methods. Examination of lymph node exudate may be helpful. Once the disease has progressed to involve the central nervous system, examination of cerebrospinal fluid reveals a lymphocytic exudate, often with *morula cells* (plasma cells) and sparse motile trypanosomes.

The parasites have a characteristic morphology: they are elongated, about 20–30 μm in length, with a single anterior flagellum arising via an undulating membrane from a basal body situated near a posteriorly placed kinetoplast (Figs 62.10 & 62.11).

In-vitro cultivation is unreliable, but animal inoculation is sometimes useful, particularly with *T. brucei rhodesiense*, which infects laboratory mice more readily than *T. brucei gambiense*. Various immunodiagnostic tests have been described, but they are not as reliable as direct microscopy in establishing a definitive diagnosis.

Fig. 62.10  Trypomastigotes of *Trypanosoma brucei rhodesiense* in mouse blood.

## Treatment

In the early parasitaemic stage, the infection is amenable to treatment with suramin or pentamidine, but once the disease has progressed to sleeping sickness the trivalent arsenicals, melarsoprol or tryparsamide, are used. Less toxic alternatives are clearly required; eflornithine is effective in *T. brucei gambiense* infections, but not in disease caused by *T. brucei rhodesiense*.

## South American trypanosomiasis

Chagas' disease, caused by *T. cruzi*, is quite different from African trypanosomiasis. The insect vectors are various species of reduviid bugs (see p. 669). The trypanosomes are present in the bug's faeces, which the unwitting sleeper rubs into the bite wound. They do not multiply in the bloodstream, but invade cells of the reticulo-endothelial system and muscle, where they lose their flagellum and associated undulating membrane and adopt a more rounded shape (Fig. 62.11). This morphological form is called an *amastigote*, and suggests a phylogenetic relationship with *Leishmania* species (see below). The amastigotes multiply in muscle and are liberated from ruptured cells as trypanosomal forms (*trypomastigotes*), which disseminate the infection and provide the parasitaemia needed to infect fresh reduviid bugs when they next feed.

Trypomastigotes are shorter than those of the *T. brucei* group and have a characteristically large kinetoplast (Fig. 62.12). The appearance of amastigotes in heart muscle is shown in Figure 62.13.

## Pathogenesis

Chagas' disease is a chronic condition characterized by extensive cardiomyopathy, sometimes with gross

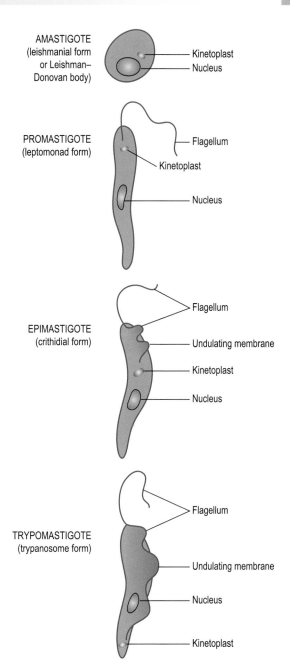

Fig. 62.11  Forms that may be adopted by *Leishmania* and *Trypanosoma* spp. In parentheses are given the terms for the forms under the old nomenclature now superseded.

distension of other organs (e.g. mega-oesophagus and megacolon). Death is usually from heart failure.

## Laboratory diagnosis

PCR methods and various immunoassays have been described for serological diagnosis and are now

Fig. 62.12 Trypomastigote of *T. cruzi* in blood. Note the prominent kinetoplast and the 'C' shape adopted by the parasite.

Fig. 62.14 Amastigotes of *Leishmania tropica* in a ruptured macrophage from a cutaneous lesion (*oriental sore*).

Fig. 62.13 Amastigotes of *T. cruzi* in heart muscle.

Fig. 62.15 Promastigotes of *L. tropica* from laboratory culture in Novy, MacNeal and Nicolle's (NNN) medium.

preferred to older tests. These include: direct microscopy of peripheral blood, in which small numbers of trypomastigotes may be found; culture in the rich blood agar medium also used to isolate leishmania (see below); mouse inoculation; and *xenodiagnosis*, in which uninfected reduviid bugs are allowed to feed on the patient and after about 3–4 weeks the gut contents of the bug are examined for trypanosomes.

### Treatment

There is no reliable chemotherapy for Chagas' disease. The nitrofuran derivative nifurtimox and the imidazole compound benznidazole have been used with modest success.

## Leishmania species

*Leishmania* species are intracellular parasites of the reticulo-endothelial system. They are related to

trypanosomes, but exist in only two morphological forms: *amastigotes* (non-flagellate forms), which occur in the infected lesion, and *promastigotes* (flagellate forms that lack an undulating membrane), which occur in the insect vector or in laboratory culture (Figs 62.11, 62.14 & 62.15).

The parasites are transmitted by sandflies (see p. 671) in various parts of the world, including the Middle East, India, South America, the Mediterranean littoral and parts of Africa.

### Pathogenesis

Several distinct types of disease are recognized (Table 62.4), although they are caused by morphologically identical parasites. *Cutaneous leishmaniasis (oriental sore)* is the least troublesome, causing a boil-like swelling on the face or other exposed part of the body. The central part of the lesion may become secondarily infected with bacteria, but the leishmania organisms

**Table 62.4** Leishmania species involved in human disease

| Species | Form of disease | Common names | Main geographical distribution |
|---|---|---|---|
| *Leishmania tropica* | Cutaneous | } Oriental sore, Baghdad boil, Delhi boil, etc. | Middle East, central Asia |
| *L. major* | Cutaneous | | Africa, Indian subcontinent, central Asia, Ethiopia, Kenya |
| *L. aethiopica* | Cutaneous, DCL | | |
| *L. donovani* | Visceral | } Kala azar, Dum-dum fever | Middle East, Africa, Indian subcontinent |
| *L. infantum*[a] | Visceral | | Mediterranean coast, Middle East, China |
| *L. chagasi* | Visceral | | Tropical South America |
| *L. mexicana complex* | Cutaneous, DCL | Chiclero's ulcer | Central America, Amazon basin |
| *L. braziliensis complex* | Mucocutaneous | Espundia | Tropical South America |
| *L. peruviana* | Cutaneous | Uta | Western Peru |

DCL, disseminated cutaneous leishmaniasis.
[a]*L. infantum* may be a subspecies of *L. donovani.*

reside in the raised, indurated edge of the lesion. The sore usually heals spontaneously, leaving a scar, but with some species a more severe *disseminated cutaneous leishmaniasis* may occur. Parasites of the *Leishmania mexicana* complex may cause a destructive lesion of the outer ear (*Chiclero's ulcer*).

In *mucocutaneous leishmaniasis (espundia)*, which is associated with the *L. braziliensis* complex, disfiguring lesions of the mouth and nose may be caused. However, the most serious form of leishmaniasis is *visceral leishmaniasis (kala azar)*, which is a life-threatening disease involving the whole of the reticuloendothelial system. There are estimated to be around 500 000 cases a year in the world, with the greatest burden in north east India and Bangladesh. A late complication of kala azar, *post-kala azar dermal leishmaniasis*, may be confused with leprosy or other skin conditions.

### Laboratory diagnosis

In the cutaneous or mucocutaneous form of the disease, typical intracellular amastigotes may be recognized in Giemsa-stained smears of material obtained from tissues at the margin of the lesion (Fig. 62.14). Free amastigotes are commonly seen because of rupture of the macrophage host cell. Material should also be cultured in Novy, MacNeal and Nicolle's (NNN) medium or a modification thereof. This is a rabbit blood agar containing antibiotic to prevent bacterial contamination and a buffered salt overlay solution in which the parasites grow as promastigotes (Fig. 62.15). Incubation is maintained for up to 3 weeks at room temperature (*not* 37°C).

In kala azar, spleen puncture is the most reliable method of diagnosis, but sternal marrow aspirate is safer and is usually preferred. Smears and cultures are made and examined as for cutaneous leishmaniasis. Various serological tests have been designed, but demonstration of the parasite by microscopy or culture is preferable whenever possible.

### Treatment

The pentavalent antimony compounds, sodium stibogluconate and meglumine antimoniate, have been used traditionally in all forms of leishmaniasis, but they are toxic and therapy often fails. Amphotericin B is effective, but poorly tolerated, and the less toxic lipid-based formulations are preferred. Antifungal azoles and paromomycin (aminosidine) have been used with some success in cutaneous forms of disease. A phosphocholine derivative, miltefosine, offers considerable promise in kala azar.

## OTHER PATHOGENIC PROTOZOA

## *BABESIA* SPECIES

Babesiae are predominantly animal parasites related to the piroplasmas that cause theileriasis in wild and domestic animals in many parts of the world. They are intracellular parasites living within red blood cells and are transmitted by ixodid ticks (see p. 673–4). In stained blood films they superficially resemble young ring forms of plasmodia.

Human infection is uncommon. European cases have mostly been in patients whose resistance was impaired by lack of a functioning spleen; the causative parasite was usually *Babesia divergens*. In contrast, babesiosis caused by *B. microti* has been reported in otherwise healthy persons in parts of the USA.

In immunocompetent individuals the disease is usually self-limiting, so that specific treatment is not required. Optimal treatment for more serious cases has not been properly defined, but the combination of quinine with clindamycin has been used successfully.

## *BALANTIDIUM* COLI

The ciliate protozoon *Balantidium coli* is a common parasite of the pig, and human infections have usually been traced to contact with these animals. The infective form is a large (about 50 μm in diameter) thick-walled cyst. The trophozoite inhabits the lumen of the gut and may attack the colonic mucosa in much the same way as *E. histolytica*, to cause balantidial dysentery. Many highly motile ciliate trophozoites are readily seen in untreated 'wet' films of diarrhoeic faeces. Tetracyclines and metronidazole are said to offer effective treatment.

## MICROSPORIDIA

These animal and insect parasites are now thought to be fungi and are represented by several genera, including *Encephalitozoon*, *Enterocytozoon* and *Nosema*. They are, on rare occasions, implicated in opportunistic infections of immunocompromised patients, especially those with AIDS. Infections of the eye, meninges and other organs have been reported. Albendazole may be useful in treatment, but is not always curative.

RECOMMENDED READING

Cook GC, Zumla A, editors: *Manson's Tropical Diseases*, ed 22, London, 2008, Elsevier: Saunders.
Croft SL: Kinetoplastida: new therapeutic strategies, *Parasite* 15:522–527, 2008.
Farthing MJ: Treatment options for the eradication of intestinal protozoa, *Nature Clinical Practice. Gastroenterology & Hepatology* 3:436–445, 2006.
Greenwood BM, Bojang K, Whitty CJM, Targett GAT: Malaria, *Lancet* 365:1487–1498, 2005.
Guerrant RL, Walker DH, Weller PF: *Tropical Infectious Diseases*, ed 3, Philadelphia, 2011, Elsevier: Saunders.
Jacquerioz FA, Croft AM: Drugs for preventing malaria in travellers, *Cochrane Database Systematic Review* 4:CD006491, 2009.
Nosten F, White NJ: Artemisinin-based combination treatment of falciparum malaria, *American Journal of Tropical Medicine and Hygiene* 77:181–192, 2007.
Peters W, Pasvol G: *Atlas of Tropical Medicine and Parasitology*, ed 6, London, 2006, Elsevier: Mosby.
Rosenblatt JE: Laboratory diagnosis of infections due to blood and tissue parasites, *Clinical Infectious Diseases* 49:1103–1108, 2009.
Stanley SL: Amoebiasis, *Lancet* 361:1025–1034, 2003.
World Health Organization: *Basic Laboratory Methods in Medical Parasitology*, Geneva, 1991, WHO.

### CD-ROMs

Wellcome Trust: 2007 *Malaria*, ed 3, (Topics in International Health series).

Wellcome Trust: 2007 *Human African Trypanosomiasis* (Topics in International Health series).
Wellcome Trust: 2000 *Leishmaniasis* (Topics in International Health series).
The above CD-ROMs are available from Wellcome Trust, London (http://www.wellcome.ac.uk/tih/) and (for developing countries) from TALC (Teaching-aids at Low Cost; http://www.talcuk.org/)

### Websites

Centers for Disease Control and Prevention: Division of Parasitic Diseases, Professional Information. http://www.cdc.gov/parasites
Malaria Centre, London School of Hygiene and Tropical Medicine: http://malaria.lshtm.ac.uk/
National Travel Health Network and Centre: http://www.nathnac.org/travel/index.htm
World Health Organization: Basic Laboratory Methods in Medical Parasitology. http://whqlibdoc.who.int/publications/9241544104_%28part1%29.pdf
World Health Organization: Malaria Rapid Diagnostic Tests. http://www.wpro.who.int/sites/rdt/home.htm
World Health Organization: World Malaria Report 2010. http://www.who.int/malaria/world_malaria_report_2010/worldmalariareport2010.pdf

# 63

# Helminths

Intestinal worm infections; filariasis; schistosomiasis; hydatid disease

*D. Greenwood*

## KEY POINTS

- Helminths are multicellular parasitic worms that often have complex life cycles.
- Intestinal nematodes (roundworms) are extremely common, especially in conditions of poor hygiene.
- Heavy infections with hookworm can give rise to severe anaemia; benzimidazoles offer effective therapy.
- Serious infections caused by tissue nematodes include bancroftian filariasis (elephantiasis) and onchocerciasis (river blindness); they are treated with ivermectin or diethylcarbamazine.
- Trematodes (flukes) cause schistosomiasis (bilharzia) and other diseases such as Chinese liver fluke infection.
- Cestodes (tapeworms) are often several metres long, but usually cause little pathology.
- Most trematode and cestode infections respond to praziquantel.
- Hydatid disease is caused by a dog tapeworm. Treatment is by surgery.

Medical helminthology is concerned with the study of parasitic worms. These creatures are responsible for an enormous burden of infection throughout the world and, although few helminthic infections are life-threatening, their impact on human health is incalculable. Most helminths have no independent existence outside the host and are therefore truly parasitic. As they rely on the host for sustenance, it is not in their interest to cause the host harm; consequently they do not usually exhibit great virulence and are characterized more by the novel methods that they have evolved to prevent rejection by the host defences. The pathogenic manifestations of helminthic disease, which can none the less be considerable, are ordinarily due to physical factors related to the location of the worms, their lifestyle or their size (see Ch. 11).

There are two major groups of helminth: *nematodes*, or roundworms, and *platyhelminths*, or flatworms. Flatworms are, in their turn, represented by two classes: *trematodes* (flukes) and *cestodes* (tapeworms).

## NEMATODES

The principal nematode parasites of man are conveniently considered under two headings: intestinal nematodes and tissue nematodes.

## INTESTINAL NEMATODES

Infection with intestinal roundworms (Table 63.1) is generally associated with conditions of poor hygiene. Such infections are extremely common, particularly throughout the tropics and subtropics, although several are also found in temperate regions. Low worm burdens are generally asymptomatic, but heavy infections may cause problems, especially in young children in whom they have been associated with impaired development.

### Ascaris lumbricoides

This is the common roundworm, which infects more than a billion people in the world. The adults are large and fleshy and, as with many nematodes (other than the hookworm group), the smaller male can be recognized by his characteristically crooked tail. The eggs (ova) are produced in huge numbers; they are thick-walled, bile-stained and typically exhibit a corrugated albuminous coat (Fig. 63.1A). In the absence of a male worm, the female produces infertile eggs, which are more elongated and irregular than the fertile variety (Fig. 63.1B).

In warm, moist conditions, infective larvae develop within fertile eggs, but do not hatch. Such eggs can

**Table 63.1** Principal intestinal nematodes of man

| Species | Common name | Relevant examination |
|---|---|---|
| *Ancylostoma duodenale* | Hookworm | Stool concentration (ova) |
| *Ascaris lumbricoides* | Common roundworm | Stool concentration (ova) |
| *Enterobius vermicularis* | Threadworm | Peri-anal swab (ova), adult worms on stool |
| *Necator americanus* | Hookworm | Stool concentration (ova) |
| *Strongyloides stercoralis* | – | Stool concentration (larvae) or culture |
| *Toxocara canis*[a] | Dog roundworm | Serology |
| *Trichostrongylus* spp. | Hookworm | Stool concentration (ova) |
| *Trichuris trichiura* | Whipworm | Stool concentration (ova) |

[a]Not an intestinal parasite of man; causes visceral larva migrans (see text).

**Fig. 63.1** Eggs of intestinal helminths: (A) *Ascaris lumbricoides* (fertile eggs); (B) *A. lumbricoides* (infertile egg); (C) *Trichuris trichiura*; (D) hookworm; (E) *Strongyloides stercoralis* (larva); (F) *Enterobius vermicularis*.

survive for long periods in soil. If ingested, the eggs hatch in the duodenum and the larvae penetrate the gut mucosa to reach the bloodstream. They are carried to the pulmonary circulation, where they gain access to the lung and undergo two moults before migrating via the trachea to the intestinal tract. Having completed their round trip, they mature in the gut lumen and live for several years.

*Ascaris lumbricoides* is a well-adapted parasite that is usually not pathogenic in the ordinary sense. However, pneumonic symptoms may accompany the migratory phase, and the adult worms may invade the biliary and pancreatic ducts. Moreover, heavy

infection with these large worms can cause intestinal obstruction. Allergy is also sometimes a problem.

The dog ascarid, *Toxocara canis*, may accidentally infect man. Larvae hatch in the small intestine and penetrate the gut wall, but they are unable to complete their migratory phase. Instead, they find their way to remote parts of the body, a condition known as *visceral larva migrans*. Occasionally the larvae reach the eye and cause serious retinal lesions. Larvae of several other roundworms, including *Angiostrongylus*, *Gnathostoma* and *Anisakis* species, are occasionally implicated in visceral larva migrans in some parts of the world.

## Trichuris trichiura

This is the common whipworm, often found together with ascaris. The adults live with the head (the 'whip' end of the worm) embedded in the colonic mucosa. Each female lays thousands of characteristic 'tea-tray' eggs (Fig. 63.1C) every day. Like those of ascaris, they develop infective larvae in warm, moist conditions, but the ova do not hatch outside the body. However, after ingestion and hatching, there is no migratory phase and adult worms develop directly in the large intestine.

Infection is usually trivial, although massive infections can cause rectal prolapse in young children, and a form of dysentery is described.

## Hookworm

The two human hookworms, *Ancylostoma duodenale* and *Necator americanus*, are widely distributed throughout the tropics and subtropics. The two species produce indistinguishable thin-walled eggs (Fig. 63.1D) that hatch in soil. Infection is usually acquired by walking barefoot in soil contaminated with human faeces. The larvae undergo several moults before infective larvae are produced. These are capable of penetrating unbroken skin, and in this way they gain access to the bloodstream to begin a migratory phase similar to that of ascaris. When they reach the gut they attach by their mouthparts to the mucosa of the small intestine. The adult worms, which are about 1-cm long, are similar, but the buccal capsule of *A. duodenale* bears two pairs of teeth, whereas *N. americanus* has two so-called 'cutting plates'. Unlike most nematodes, the tail of male hookworms has a membranous *bursa* used for attachment to the female during copulation.

Hookworms ingest blood and move from site to site in the gut mucosa, leaving behind small bleeding lesions. These two facts are responsible for the chief pathological manifestation of heavy infection with hookworms: iron deficiency anaemia.

Larvae of animal hookworms, notably the dog hookworm, *A. caninum*, may penetrate human skin, but do not migrate further. They do, however, cause local irritation by wandering through subcutaneous tissue, a condition called *cutaneous larva migrans*.

## Trichostrongylus species

Various species of *Trichostrongylus* have been associated with human disease, particularly in the Middle East. Like the hookworms, they are bursate nematodes with similar, but more elongated, eggs.

## Strongyloides stercoralis

This parasite is also related to the hookworms but differs in several important respects. There is a distinct free-living phase in the life cycle, during which males and females reproduce. Human infections arise after penetration of infective larvae through skin and there is a migratory phase involving the lungs. However, human infection appears to be restricted to female worms, which attach to the gut mucosa and produce eggs that contain fully developed larvae; these hatch within the intestinal lumen so that larvae, not eggs, are found in faecal samples (Fig. 63.1E). Infection can persist for many years, probably because some larvae can develop sufficiently within the body to initiate a fresh cycle of development and cause auto-infection.

Symptoms are usually benign, but in debilitated individuals larvae may be activated to penetrate the gut wall and invade other organs, a serious condition known as *hyperinfection*.

## Enterobius vermicularis

This is the common threadworm, which infects children throughout the world. It has the simplest life cycle of all intestinal worms. Adults live in the large intestine and are occasionally found in the appendix. Mature, gravid females crawl through the anus at night and lay their eggs in the peri-anal area. The eggs are characteristically flattened on one side (Fig. 63.1F) and usually contain fully developed larvae. Ingestion of these eggs initiates a fresh infection. Symptoms are restricted to itching (*pruritus ani*) associated with the deposition of eggs.

As eggs are not discharged by the worm into faeces, faecal examination is not appropriate in the laboratory diagnosis of threadworm infection. The diagnosis is established by finding the characteristic 'threads' on the surface of formed stools, or by examination of swabs (or Sellotape impressions) of unwashed perianal skin for the characteristic ova.

## Treatment of intestinal nematode infections

In endemic areas, the need to treat intestinal worm infections has to be balanced against the severity of symptoms (if any), the inevitability of re-infection, and the use of scarce medical resources. In the industrially developed world, where the infections are less common and mostly imported, a more liberal approach to treatment can be adopted.

The range of options is listed in Table 63.2. Most effective (and expensive) are the benzimidazole derivatives, especially albendazole and mebendazole.

**Table 63.2** Spectrum of activity of drugs used in the treatment of intestinal nematode infections

| Drug | Ancylostoma duodenale | Necator americanus | Ascaris lumbricoides | Strongyloides stercoralis | Trichuris trichiura | Enterobius vermicularis |
|---|---|---|---|---|---|---|
| Piperazine | – | – | +++ | – | – | +++ |
| Levamisole | ++ | ++ | +++ | – | – | – |
| Pyrantel pamoate | ++ | ++ | +++ | + | ++ | +++ |
| Tiabendazole | ++ | ++ | ++ | ++ | – | ++ |
| Mebendazole | ++ | ++ | +++ | + | ++ | +++ |
| Albendazole | +++ | ++ | +++ | ++ | ++ | +++ |

+++, highly effective; +, poorly effective; –, no useful activity.
From Greenwood D, Finch RG, Davey PG, Wilcox MH 2007 *Antimicrobial Chemotherapy*, 5th edn. Oxford University Press, Oxford.

**Table 63.3** Principal tissue nematodes of man

| Species | Intermediate host | Geographical distribution | Relevant examination |
|---|---|---|---|
| *Wuchereria bancrofti* | Mosquitoes | Tropical belt | Night blood |
| *Loa loa* | *Chrysops* spp. | West and Central Africa | Day blood |
| *Brugia malayi* | Mosquitoes | South-East Asia | Night blood |
| *Mansonella perstans* | *Culicoides* spp. | Tropical Africa, South America | Blood |
| *M. ozzardi* | *Culicoides* spp. | West Indies, South America | Blood |
| *Onchocerca volvulus* | *Simulium* spp. | Tropical Africa, Central America | Skin shavings |
| *M. streptocerca* | *Culicoides* spp. | West and Central Africa | Skin shavings |
| *Dracunculus medinensis* | Water fleas | Africa, Indian subcontinent | Adult worm when mature |
| *Trichinella spiralis* | None[a] | Worldwide | Muscle biopsy, serology |

[a]Pork forms the chief reservoir.

## TISSUE NEMATODES

This group includes the filarial worms, the Guinea-worm (*Dracunculus medinensis*) and *Trichinella spiralis* (Table 63.3).

## Filarial worms

Filarial worms have a complex life cycle involving developmental stages in an insect vector. They vary considerably in their pathogenic effects, but some are responsible for disabling diseases that have a major impact on communities living in endemic areas.

### Wuchereria bancrofti

This worm is transmitted by the bite of various species of mosquito throughout the tropical belt of the world. Over 100 million people are thought to be infected. The larvae invade the lymphatics, usually of the lower limbs, where they develop into adult worms. The presence of adult worms causes lymphatic blockage and gross lymphoedema, which sometimes leads to the bizarre deformities associated with bancroftian filariasis, *elephantiasis*.

Embryonic forms (*microfilariae*) are liberated into the bloodstream. They retain the elastic egg membrane as a sheath, which covers the whole larva (Fig. 63.2A). Microfilariae remain in the pulmonary circulation during the day, emerging into the peripheral circulation only at night, to coincide with the biting habits of the insect vector. The physiological basis of this nocturnal periodicity is not understood, but it can be reversed by altered sleep patterns in, for example, night-shift workers. Moreover, strains of *Wuchereria bancrofti* encountered in some Pacific islands do not exhibit a nocturnal periodicity. Aside from these exceptions, blood for examination for *W. bancrofti* must be taken during the night, optimally between midnight and 2 a.m.

### Loa loa

This worm is restricted in distribution to central and western parts of tropical Africa, where it is transmitted by biting flies (*Chrysops* species; see p. 672). The adult worms live in subcutaneous tissue and wander round the body, provoking localized reactions known

**Fig. 63.2** Sheathed microfilariae of (A) *Wuchereria bancrofti* and (B) *Loa loa*; (C) Tail of microfilaria of *W. bancrofti* showing tip devoid of somatic nuclei; (D) Tail of microfilaria of *L. loa* showing nuclei extending to tip of tail.

as *Calabar swellings* and sometimes migrating across the front of the eye.

The sheathed microfilariae of *Loa loa* (Fig. 63.2B) exhibit diurnal periodicity, so that, unlike those of *W. bancrofti*, they appear in peripheral blood only during the day.

## Brugia malayi

This parasite is probably related to *W. bancrofti*. It is transmitted by mosquitoes in parts of India, the Far East and South-East Asia. Adult worms inhabit the lymphatics and, like *W. bancrofti*, can cause elephantiasis. Microfilaraemia usually shows a nocturnal periodicity.

## Onchocerca volvulus

This filarial worm is common in parts of tropical Africa and Central America. It is transmitted by *Simulium damnosum* and related species of black-fly (see p. 672). Adult worms develop in subcutaneous and connective tissue, and often become encapsulated in nodules, which form on bony parts of the body such as the hip, elbow and (particularly in Central America) the head. The microfilariae are not found in blood, but live in the superficial layers of the skin causing itching and, in heavy chronic infections, gross thickening of the skin. The eye is commonly invaded by microfilariae, which may cause corneal and retinal lesions that lead to blindness. Because the vector breeds by rivers, the condition is known as *river blindness*.

**Table 63.4** Differential features of human microfilariae

| Species | Site in human host | Periodicity | Sheath | Nuclei in tip of tail | Length (µm) |
|---|---|---|---|---|---|
| *Wuchereria bancrofti* | Blood | Nocturnal[a] | Present | Absent | 250–300 |
| *Loa loa* | Blood | Diurnal | Present | Present | 250–300 |
| *Brugia malayi* | Blood | (Nocturnal)[b] | Present | Present[c] | 200–250 |
| *Mansonella perstans* | Blood | Non-periodic | Absent | Present | 150–200 |
| *M. ozzardi* | Blood | Non-periodic | Absent | Absent | 180–220 |
| *Onchocerca volvulus* | Skin | Non-periodic | Absent | Absent | 250–300 |
| *M. streptocerca* | Skin | Non-periodic | Absent | Present | 180–240 |

[a]Subperiodic forms occur in the Pacific Islands.
[b]Partial nocturnal periodicity.
[c]Two small, well separated nuclei in the tip of the tail.

If nodules are present, diagnosis can be made by finding macroscopic worms within an excised nodule. Otherwise, superficial slivers of skin, taken from calves, buttocks and shoulders, are suspended in a drop of saline and examined microscopically for motile microfilariae.

## Mansonella *species*

*Mansonella perstans* is widespread throughout tropical Africa and parts of South America; the related *M. ozzardi* is restricted to parts of the West Indies and South America. They are transmitted by biting midges (*Culicoides* species; see p. 671). The unsheathed microfilariae appear in the bloodstream and exhibit no periodicity. They are generally regarded as non-pathogenic.

*M. streptocerca* causes skin infections similar to those of *O. volvulus*, although the symptoms are usually milder. It is restricted to parts of western and central Africa.

## Differential characteristics of microfilariae

The microfilariae of filarial worms can be differentiated in stained preparations of clinical material by various criteria, the most useful of which are the presence or absence of a sheath and the disposition of the somatic nuclei in the tip of the tail (Table 63.4 & Fig. 63.2). Giemsa stain is suitable for the demonstration of somatic nuclei, but hot (60°C) haematoxylin is necessary to stain the sheath.

## Treatment of filariasis

Diethylcarbamazine (DEC) has been used for many years for the treatment of all forms of filariasis. It effectively kills microfilariae, but is not reliably lethal to adult worms. It is relatively non-toxic, but death of the microfilariae is often accompanied by a severe allergic reaction (*Mazzotti reaction*), especially in onchocerciasis. Suramin kills the adult worms, but is much more toxic than DEC.

The treatment of onchocerciasis has been revolutionized by use of the veterinary anthelminthic ivermectin. This drug is effective in a single oral dose and is less likely than DEC to elicit a severe reaction. Periodic administration of ivermectin, together with vector control measures, has had an important impact on onchocerciasis in endemic areas.

Ivermectin and albendazole are effective in other forms of filariasis, although neither drug kills adult worms. As they exhibit activity against intestinal nematodes, including *A. lumbricoides*, these may be incidentally expelled during treatment. Albendazole is being used, alone or in combination with ivermectin, in campaigns aimed at eradicating lymphatic filariasis.

Surprisingly, tetracyclines also have an effect in filariasis, apparently by inhibiting endosymbiotic bacteria (*Wohlbachia* species) that are essential for the fertility of the worms.

## Dracunculus medinensis

This is the *Guinea-worm*. The infective larvae develop within water fleas of the genus *Cyclops*, and human infection is normally acquired through infected drinking water. The larvae penetrate the gut mucosa and grow to maturity in connective tissue, usually of the lower limbs. The male is small and insignificant, but the female may reach a length of 1 m. After fertilization, the female worm incubates the larvae to maturity and, when ready to give birth, emerges to the skin surface to provoke an intensely irritating blister. When the sufferer immerses the blister in water, the uterus of the female worm bursts, liberating up to 1 million larvae, which are ingested by water fleas to continue the cycle.

**Fig. 63.3** Larvae of *Trichinella spiralis* in muscle.

Attempts can be made to wind out the dead worm over several days, but breakage of the worm often occurs, and pyogenic cocci may be carried into the tissues to cause a cellulitis. Chemotherapy is not usually helpful, other than to treat secondary bacterial infection. Prevention is the best approach; health education campaigns and the provision of safe water have much reduced the prevalence of this disease, and complete eradication is now possible.

### Trichinella spiralis

Unlike most parasitic worms, *Trichinella spiralis* has an extremely wide host range. Human infections are usually acquired by eating undercooked pork products, although other meat, including bear and walrus meat, has been incriminated. The infected larvae lie dormant in skeletal muscle (Fig. 63.3) and are released when the meat is digested. Male and female worms develop to maturity attached to the mucosa of the small intestine. The female is viviparous, producing numerous larvae during a lifespan of only a few weeks. The larvae penetrate the gut wall and migrate to skeletal muscle, where they enter the quiescent phase. Most of the symptoms of trichinosis, which can be severe – even life threatening – are associated with the migration of larvae.

Mebendazole is said to be effective against the adult worms and the larvae, but treatment is unsatisfactory. Symptoms usually develop only during the invasive stage, and measures to control the sequelae of invasion are more important than anthelminthic therapy.

## TREMATODES

The flukes (Table 63.5) are a diverse group of worms that share a similar life cycle involving a snail host and, often, a second intermediate host that provides the vehicle for the transmission of infection. Most flukes have a restricted geographical distribution that reflects the habitat of the appropriate type of snail.

Most trematodes are hermaphrodite, but the most important human flukes, the schistosomes, are differentiated into separate sexes.

### Life cycle

When excreted, trematode eggs often contain a fully developed ciliated organism called a miracidium, although in some species immature eggs are produced that require a period of development before the miracidium is formed. In water, the miracidium escapes, either through a lid-like *operculum* in the egg shell or (in the case of the schistosomes) by osmotic rupture of the egg. The miracidium penetrates the appropriate species of snail and undergoes several stages of asexual reproduction before emerging as a free-swimming body called a *cercaria*. The cercariae encyst in the muscle of fish (*Clonorchis sinensis*), crabs and crayfish (*Paragonimus westermani*), water chestnuts (*Fasciolopsis buski*) or vegetation (*Fasciola hepatica*), and man becomes infected by ingesting the encysted metacercariae. In the case of *Schistosoma* species, the cercariae remain in water and penetrate unbroken skin to gain access to the body.

### Clonorchis sinensis (syn. Opisthorchis sinensis)

This is the Chinese liver fluke. Infection is acquired from uncooked freshwater fish, notably carp. The metacercariae excyst in the small intestine and pass into the bile ducts, where they mature. Typical small, flask-shaped eggs with a prominent operculum (Fig. 63.4A) are excreted in large numbers into the faeces.

Infection is commonly asymptomatic, but fibrosis of the bile ducts with impairment of liver function may occur in heavy, chronic infections. As with most fluke infections, praziquantel is the drug of choice for treatment.

A closely related fluke, *Opisthorchis felineus*, which is a parasite of the cat, has been associated with human disease in parts of eastern Europe.

**Table 63.5** Principal trematode parasites of man

| Species | Common name | Intermediate host First[a] | Intermediate host Second | Geographical distribution | Relevant examination |
|---|---|---|---|---|---|
| *Clonorchis sinensis* | Chinese liver fluke | *Bithynia* sp. | Freshwater fish | Far East | Stool concentration |
| *Fasciola hepatica* | Sheep liver fluke | *Lymnaea* sp. | Vegetation | Worldwide | Stool concentration, serology |
| *Fasciolopsis buski* | Giant intestinal fluke | *Segmentina* sp. etc. | Water chestnut | Far East | Stool concentration |
| *Paragonimus westermani* | Lung fluke | *Semisulcospira* sp. | Crabs and crayfish | Chiefly Far East | Sputum |
| *Schistosoma mansoni* | Bilharzia | *Biomphalaria* sp. | None (water) | Africa, West Indies, South America | Stool concentration, rectal biopsy |
| *S. haematobium* | Bilharzia | *Bulinus* sp. | None (water) | Africa | Terminal urine (midday) |
| *S. japonicum* | Bilharzia | *Oncomelania* sp. | None (water) | Far East | Stool concentration, rectal biopsy |

[a]The first intermediate host is a snail in each case.

**Fig. 63.4** Eggs of trematodes: (A) *Clonorchis sinensis*; (B) *Fasciola hepatica*; (C) *Paragonimus westermani*; (D) *Schistosoma mansoni*; (E) *S. haematobium*; (F) *S. japonicum*.

## Fasciola hepatica

This is the cosmopolitan liver fluke of sheep. Human infections have usually been associated with eating wild watercress from infected sheep pastures. The adult worm is larger than *C. sinensis*, and lighter infections can cause biliary fibrosis and obstructive jaundice. The large, immature eggs with an indistinct operculum (Fig. 63.4B) may be found in faeces, but are usually sparse.

Unlike other trematode infections, fascioliasis does not reliably respond to praziquantel, and treatment with the veterinary anthelminthic triclabendazole or the more toxic chlorophenol derivative bithionol may be required.

## Paragonimus westermani

This is the lung fluke, which is found in parts of the Far East. Closely related species have occasionally been implicated in human disease in parts of Africa and South America. Human infection follows ingestion of raw, infected muscle of freshwater crabs and crayfish. The metacercariae penetrate through the gut wall and diaphragm to reach the lung, where they develop to maturity. Occasionally the larvae find their way to the brain. Pulmonary infection usually provokes the production of sputum, in which the characteristic large eggs (Fig. 63.4C) can be found, often associated with flecks of altered blood. Praziquantel is used for treatment.

## Intestinal flukes

Several genera of intestinal flukes cause human infection, particularly in the Far East. *Fasciolopsis buski* is found in restricted foci in China and South-East Asia. Infection is often acquired by the habit of opening water chestnuts with the teeth. The adult flukes live attached to the wall of the small intestine and produce a large number of eggs that resemble those of *F. hepatica*.

Other intestinal flukes include *Gastrodiscoides hominis*, *Heterophyes heterophyes*, *Metagonimus yokogawai* and various species of *Echinostoma*. Infection is usually asymptomatic unless the worm burden is large. Such evidence as exists suggests that praziquantel is effective in these cases.

## *Schistosoma* species

The schistosomes, or *blood flukes*, also known as *bilharzia* after the discoverer, Theodor Bilharz, are the most important of the pathogenic trematodes. At least 200 million people are infected, principally in Africa, where *Schistosoma mansoni* and *S. haematobium* are widespread, and *S. intercalatum* is encountered in some areas. *S. mansoni* is also found in parts of the West Indies and South America; *S. japonicum* and the related *S. mekongi* are restricted to the Far East.

Human infection follows exposure to cercariae in water harbouring infected snails. The cercariae penetrate the skin, often causing a transient dermatitis, called *swimmer's itch*. Once in the bloodstream, the schistosomula migrate to the liver, where they develop into mature male and female worms. The integument of the mature male worm is adapted in the form of two long flaps, the *gynaecophoral canal*, in which the female is held. The mature worms migrate to the small veins of the rectum (*S. mansoni, S. intercalatum, S. japonicum* and *S. mekongi*) or the bladder (*S. haematobium*). Eggs, which contain a fully developed miracidium, are passed through the rectal mucosa on to the surface of colonic faeces or through the bladder wall into the urine.

The ova of *S. mansoni* (Fig. 63.4D) are large (about 140 µm long) and possess a characteristic lateral spine, whereas those of *S. haematobium* (Fig. 63.4E) and *S. intercalatum* have a terminal spine. The smaller, more rounded, eggs of *S. japonicum* and *S. mekongi* do not have a prominent spine, but may exhibit a rudimentary nipple-like appendage (Fig. 63.4F).

### Pathogenesis

The adult worms adopt the subterfuge of coating themselves with host antigens to evade attack by host defences; in themselves, the adults are innocuous. Most of the serious manifestations of schistosomiasis arise from the deposition of eggs, with the formation of granulomata and fibrotic lesions of the liver, bladder or other organs. Such effects may herald malignant changes. Heavy infection with *S. mansoni* may give rise to *schistosomal dysentery*, whereas *S. haematobium* infections are commonly accompanied by a marked haematuria (visible in Fig. 63.4E).

### Laboratory diagnosis

Ova of rectal schistosomes can be sought on the surface of formed faeces. Blood-stained mucus should be examined, if present. Alternatively, microscopical examination of snips of rectal mucosa teased out in a drop of saline on a microscope slide may reveal viable or calcified eggs.

For the diagnosis of infection with *S. haematobium*, the last few drops of urine at the end of micturition (*terminal urine*) are most likely to be rich in ova. Excretion is said to be maximal around midday.

To test for viability of the eggs after treatment, the ova can be hatched in water (the motile miracidia can be seen with the help of a hand-lens) or the eggs can be examined microscopically for the characteristic flickering movement of excretory 'flame cells'.

Various serodiagnostic tests, including enzyme-linked immunosorbent assay (ELISA), are available, but are no substitute for demonstration of the ova. Antigen detection methods have also been developed.

### Treatment

Praziquantel is effective against all the human schistosomes and is the drug of choice. Because of its lack of toxicity and simplicity in administration. praziquantel has been used, together with molluscicides and water purification, in control programmes.

Other compounds are more selective in their action: metrifonate (an organophosphate compound) is active against *S. haematobium*; oxamniquine is effective in *S. mansoni* infection.

## CESTODES

The species of tapeworm most commonly involved in human infection are listed in Table 63.6.

### Taenia species

*Taenia saginata*, the *beef tapeworm*, is much more prevalent than the related *T. solium*, the *pork tapeworm*. Both have a relatively simple life cycle, alternating between man and the intermediate host. Human infection is acquired by eating raw or undercooked beef or pork containing the encysted larval stage, the *cysticercus*. The larvae hatch in the small intestine and attach to the mucosal surface by four suckers on the head (*scolex*) of the worm. The scolex of *T. solium* additionally carries a crown of hooklets. The worm grows backwards from the head, first producing immature segments (*proglottids*), which continue to develop as they become more distant from the head. When sexually mature, the proglottids, which exhibit both male and female characteristics, cross-fertilize one another, and eggs start to be produced in the uterine canal. This becomes grossly distended as more eggs are produced, so that the fully gravid segments at the end of the worm become nothing more than bags full of eggs. The complete chain of segments is known as a *strobila*, and may measure 10 m or more.

Eggs are not laid. They are retained within the proglottids, which become detached from the end of the worm and are passed with the faeces. Animals become infected by ingesting the eggs from pastures contaminated with inadequately treated sewage or by the droppings of birds that scavenge in untreated sewage.

Considering the size of the worm, infection is usually remarkably asymptomatic. However, in the case of *T. solium*, eggs may hatch in the human host and form cysticerci. When these lodge in the brain, they may cause a serious epileptiform disease, *cerebral cysticercosis*.

### Laboratory diagnosis

Taenia infection is usually diagnosed by finding the typical segments in faeces. Since eggs are not laid, faecal examination for ova is inappropriate. *T. saginata* can usually be differentiated from *T. solium* if the segment is pressed between two microscope slides and examined macroscopically. In the case of *T. saginata*, numerous branchings of the central uterine canal are evident, whereas there are usually far fewer branchings with *T. solium* (Fig. 63.5). The eggs (Fig. 63.6A) are thick walled and contain an *oncosphere* with six hooklets. The eggs of *T. saginata* and *T. solium* are indistinguishable.

### Treatment

A single dose of praziquantel is usually successful. Niclosamide is also used, but this drug causes the worm to disintegrate, with the consequent theoretical (but unproven) risk of auto-infection in the case of *T. solium* through the intraluminal release of eggs. Treatment of cerebral cysticercosis is problematical, but albendazole and praziquantel have been used successfully.

### Diphyllobothrium latum

This is the *fish tapeworm*, which is prevalent in lakeland areas where freshwater fish is eaten raw. A few cases caused by the related *D. nihonkaiense* have been reported, mainly from Japan. The life cycle is reminiscent of that of the trematodes. The mature adult worm, which may attain a length of 10 m, lays

| Table 63.6 Principal cestode parasites of man | | | |
|---|---|---|---|
| Species | Common name | Intermediate host | Relevant examination |
| *Taenia saginata* | Beef tapeworm | Cattle | Mature segments on stool |
| *T. solium* | Pork tapeworm | Pig | Mature segments on stool |
| *Diphyllobothrium latum* | Fish tapeworm | *Cyclops* spp./fish | Ova in stool |
| *Hymenolepis nana* | Dwarf tapeworm | None | Ova in stool |
| *Echinococcus granulosus*[a] | Hydatid worm | Sheep, man | Radiology; serology |

[a]Dog tapeworm; man is one of the intermediate hosts.

**Fig. 63.5** Segments of (A) *Taenia saginata* and (B) *T. solium*. The uterine canal has been injected with Indian ink to show the branchings.

**Fig. 63.6** Eggs of cestodes: (A) *Taenia* species; (B) *Diphyllobothrium latum*; (C) *Hymenolepis nana*.

numerous operculate eggs within which a ciliated body called a *coracidium* develops. This hatches in water and is ingested by the water flea (*Cyclops* species). After a period of development, the larva awaits ingestion by a freshwater fish in which it invades the muscle as an infective *plerocercoid larva* or *sparganum*.

Human infection is usually asymptomatic, although a form of pernicious anaemia caused by competition for dietary vitamin $B_{12}$ has been described.

The characteristic immature eggs have an indistinct operculum (Fig. 63.6B) and are usually present in large numbers in faeces. Occasionally, a length of the worm may break off and be passed in the stool.

Niclosamide or praziquantel is used for treatment.

### Hymenolepis nana

In contrast to the enormous length of *Taenia* species and *D. latum*, *Hymenolepis nana* is only 2–4 cm long, and is consequently known as the *dwarf tapeworm*.

It has a very simple life cycle with no known intermediate host. The characteristic 'poached egg' ova (Fig. 63.6C) are directly infective, and it is surprising that infection is not more common.

Infection is usually asymptomatic; heavy infections can be treated with praziquantel or niclosamide.

A slightly larger species, *H. diminuta*, is occasionally found in man. This is a parasite of small rodents and is transmitted by their fleas.

### Echinococcus granulosus

This is the tapeworm of the dog and other canine species, and, unusually, man is an intermediate host. It is a small worm, consisting usually of just four segments and measuring less than a centimetre. Sheep are the usual intermediate hosts. Other animals, including man, may become infected, especially in sheep-farming areas, where the cycle of transmission is maintained between sheep and dogs.

After ingestion of the eggs, which resemble those of *Taenia* species, larvae hatch in the small intestine, penetrate the gut mucosa and are carried by the bloodstream to various organs (commonly the liver), where they are filtered out. The larva starts to grow, eventually forming a cystic cavity, the *hydatid cyst*. The inner wall of the cyst contains the *germinal layer*, from which develop *brood capsules* that bud off and fall into the cyst cavity. Within these brood capsules new scolices develop, and some of these may initiate the formation of daughter cysts within the main cavity. The young cyst may die and calcify, but it often continues to grow inexorably, eventually seriously compromising the function of the organ in which it is situated.

In certain parts of the world, notably the arctic regions of North America and Siberia, infection with a related canine tapeworm, *E. multilocularis*, is encountered. The hydatid cyst infiltrates the surrounding tissue, making it difficult to remove surgically.

**Fig. 63.7** Scolices of *Echinococcus granulosus* from hydatid cyst.

## Laboratory diagnosis

The diagnosis is usually made on clinical and radiological evidence. Examination of the cyst fluid (*hydatid sand*) reveals the typical invaginated scolices (Fig. 63.7), but diagnostic puncture of cysts is not recommended because of the risk of spillage (see below).

Imaging techniques supported by serological tests offer the best means of diagnosis. ELISA is the preferred laboratory method, but other serodiagnostic tests are also available. A skin test with antigen derived from hydatid fluid (*Casoni test*) was formerly used, but is unreliable.

## Treatment

Cysts of *E. granulosus* can often be removed surgically, but accidental spillage of viable scolices into body cavities may cause an anaphylactic reaction and, moreover, is likely to lead to the development of fresh cysts. For this reason the hydatid cyst is first injected with a scolicidal agent, such as hypertonic saline or ethanol.

The relative impermeability of the cyst militates against successful chemotherapy, but some success has been obtained with benzimidazole derivatives, notably albendazole, and with praziquantel.

## RECOMMENDED READING

Cook GC, Zumla A, editors: *Manson's Tropical Diseases*, ed 22, London, 2008, Elsevier: Saunders.

Crompton DWT: How much helminthiasis is there in the world? *Journal of Parasitology* 85:397–403, 1999.

Guerrant RL, Walker DH, Weller PF: *Tropical Infectious Diseases*, ed 3, Philadelphia, 2011, Elsevier: Saunders.

Peters W, Pasvol G: *Atlas of Tropical Medicine and Parasitology*, ed 6, London, 2006, Elsevier: Mosby.

Taylor MJ, Hoerauf A, Bockarie M: Lymphatic filariasis and onchocerciasis, *Lancet* 376:1175–1185, 2010.

World Health Organization: *Basic Laboratory Methods in Medical Parasitology*. Geneva, 1991, WHO.

## CD-ROM

Wellcome Trust 1998 *Schistosomiasis* (Topics in International Health series).

Available from Wellcome Trust, London (www.wellcome.ac.uk/tih) and (for developing countries) from TALC (Teaching-aids at Low Cost; www.talcuk.org)

## Websites

Centers for Disease Control and Prevention. DPDx – CDC Parasitology Diagnostic Website. http://www.dpd.cdc.gov/dpdx/

World Health Organization: Basic Laboratory Methods in Medical Parasitology. http://whqlibdoc.who.int/publications/9241544104 _%28part1%29.pdf

# 64 Arthropods

Arthropod–borne diseases; ectoparasitic infections; allergy

*R. C. Russell*

## KEY POINTS

- Medically important arthropods include insects (bugs, flies, gnats, lice and fleas) and arachnids (spiders, ticks and mites).
- Many arthropods act as accidental or obligatory vectors of bacteria, viruses, protozoa or helminths.
- Certain fleas, lice and mites are human parasites.
- Some arthropods cause allergies (e.g. house dust mites); others may cause painful bites or stings.
- Myisais is a condition caused by invasion of the body by insect larvae.

Arthropods are invertebrate animals with jointed legs, segmented bodies and chitinous exoskeletons. They are hugely diverse and incredibly numerous – more than 850 000 species have been described (probably only one-tenth of the true number). Strictly speaking, the term 'arthropod' includes the crustaceans (e.g. lobsters and crabs), the myriapods (e.g. millipedes and centipedes) and some minor groups, but these seldom cause much serious mischief, and most medical interest centres on the insects (e.g. mosquitoes, fleas and lice) and the arachnids (e.g. mites, ticks and spiders). A simplified classification and relevance scheme is shown in Table 64.1.

## MEDICAL IMPORTANCE OF ARTHROPODS

Insects and other arthropods are mainly of importance in human disease in three ways:

1. as vectors of the agents of bacterial, viral or parasitic infection
2. as parasites in their own right, spending part or all of their lifespan on humans
3. as instigators of allergic responses that vary in severity.

In addition, many arthropods have a considerable nuisance effect because of their biting or stinging habits, and these occasionally give rise to serious, even life-threatening, reactions.

The larvae (maggots) of some common flies that feed on decomposing matter have been used for centuries to treat infected lesions. There is renewed interest in this phenomenon as wound therapy, as the maggots not only scavenge dead tissue, but also appear to secrete factors conducive to wound healing.

Abnormal fear of insects or other arthropods (e.g. arachnophobia; excessive fear of spiders) is well recognized, as are delusions of infestation with these creatures. The mere mention of head lice can make people scratch their scalps. Distinguishing between the real and the imaginary can test the diagnostic acumen of the attending physician. Persistent cases may need psychiatric referral.

## Arthropods as disease vectors

### Mechanical transmission

Insects such as flies, ants and cockroaches that are attracted by food can transmit pathogenic microorganisms passively. The common housefly, *Musca domestica*, is a particular nuisance because of its predilection for decaying matter, its mobility and its habit (shared by a number of other flies) of regurgitating gut contents and defecating on food. While such flies can undoubtedly play a role in the transmission of enteric diseases, and also trachoma, along with cockroaches they are of lesser importance in modern urban settings than in poorer communities where lower standards of sanitation and hygiene prevail.

### Intermediate hosts

A wide variety of arthropods act as obligatory hosts in the transmission of viral, bacterial, protozoal and

**Table 64.1** Simplified classification of arthropods of medical importance

| Class | Members of class | Medical importance |
|---|---|---|
| Insects | Ants, bees, wasps (Hymenoptera) | Venomous bites and stings |
| | Beetles (Coleoptera) | Some secrete fluids causing blisters |
| | Bugs (Hemiptera) | Bites; vectors of Chagas' disease |
| | Butterflies and moths (Lepidoptera) | Urticaria (caterpillars) |
| | Cockroaches (Dictyoptera) | Mechanical vectors of disease |
| | Fleas (Siphonaptera) | Ectoparasites; vector of plague |
| | Flies and gnats (Diptera) | Vectors of many viral and parasitic diseases; myiasis |
| | Lice (Phthiraptera) | Ectoparasites; vectors of typhus, trench fever, relapsing fever |
| Arachnids | Spiders and scorpions | Venomous bites and stings |
| | Ticks | Vectors of rickettsiae, borreliae |
| | Mites | Scabies; allergy; vectors of scrub typhus, rickettsial pox |
| Pentastomes | Tongue worms | Animal parasites; human infestations rare |
| Myriapods | Centipedes and millipedes | Some cause painful bites or secrete fluids causing blisters |
| Crustacea | Crabs, crayfish | Intermediate host of lung fluke |
| | Copepods | Intermediate host of fish tapeworm and guinea-worm |

helminthic agents of human disease. Their association with particular vectors is mentioned below and their role in individual diseases is dealt with in appropriate chapters elsewhere in the book.

## Arthropods as ectoparasites

Many insects, ticks and mites pester humans to obtain a blood meal, or spend part or all of their life in association with human beings. Several fleas, lice and mites are among those that are adapted in various ways for life on humans. Occasionally, humans act as the host of the larval stages of certain insects, and this invasive condition is known as *myiasis*.

## Arthropods as allergens

Stinging insects and other venomous arthropods can give rise to severe reactions in hypersensitive individuals, and anaphylactic reactions need immediate treatment with adrenaline (epinephrine). The hairs of several caterpillar species found in various parts of the world are irritating and may give rise to urticaria if brushed against. The irritating reactions to the bites of mosquitoes, midges, fleas and some other insects are immunological reactions to the salivary secretions that are injected at the bite site. However, the degree of reaction can vary remarkably between individuals, from little or no reaction to quite severe dermal and systemic affects and may need medical attention in the latter cases.

Various domestic arthropods, such as dust mites and cockroaches have been incriminated as a cause of asthma in atopic subjects; their allergens can be present in dead bodies as well as in the live individuals, and also secreted in the faeces.

## INSECTS

Insects are the most numerous and familiar form of arthropod life. They are characterized by having six legs and segmented bodies. The legs (and wings, if present) are carried on the thoracic segment between the head, which bears sucking or biting mouthparts, and the abdomen. Most insects of medical importance, apart from lice and bugs, undergo complete metamorphosis, developing from eggs to adults through morphologically distinct active larval but often inactive pupal stages inside which the adult is developing.

## Ants, bees and wasps (Hymenoptera)

These insects have little medical relevance apart from their propensity to retaliate to disturbance with defensive bites or stings. These can be serious if the subject is hypersensitive, but are usually trivial. Particularly notorious are the African honey bees (*Apis mellifera scutellata*), the European wasp (*Vespula germanica*) and the South American fire ants (*Solenopsis* spp.), all of which have been introduced into various countries, and also the Bull ants (*Myrmecia* spp.) of Australia. Other ants also forage in urban areas wherever food is to be found and frequently infest kitchens and food stores; they have some potential to transfer pathogenic organisms (particularly in hospitals).

## Beetles (Coleoptera)

Some beetles act as intermediate host of the dwarf tapeworm *Hymenolepis diminuta*, an uncommon human parasite of minor importance (see p. 665). Otherwise, their only real medical significance lies in the fact that the body fluids of certain beetles (e.g. Meloid and Staphylinid species) can cause blistering of the skin. One such beetle, 'Spanish fly', is the source of cantharidin, a vesiculating agent.

## Bugs (Hemiptera)

The bugs of importance in human medicine are blood-sucking species. Most familiar throughout the world is the common bed bug, *Cimex lectularius*, which in recent years has been undergoing a widespread international resurgence in distribution and abundance. There is also a tropical species, *C. hemipterus*, which is confined to warmer climes. They have a body that is flattened dorsoventrally and from a distance they resemble brown lentils. Bed bugs live in cracks and crevices of walls, floorboards and furniture, from where they emerge to take a periodic blood meal whenever it is on offer. The adults are long-lived and can survive up to a year without a blood meal. They are usually spread between premises in infested furniture or personal baggage. There is no evidence that they transmit disease.

Reduviid bugs (colloquially known as *kissing bugs* or *assassin bugs*) transmit the trypanosome protozoan that causes Chagas disease in Central and South America (see p. 651). Various species of *Triatoma, Rhodnius* and *Panstrongylus* are implicated. They are about 2.5 cm in length, much larger than bed bugs and, unlike them, they have wings (Fig. 64.1). They are usually active at night, settling on the face of an unsuspecting sleeper to take a blood meal and to defecate on site. The infective trypanosomes are in the hindgut and the bitten person becomes infected by rubbing the bug's faeces into the irritating bite wound or mucous membranes.

## Butterflies and moths (Lepidoptera)

Adult butterflies and moths are of no great medical significance (although there is one species that feeds on the blood of large mammals in Southeast Asia, and

**Fig. 64.1** A reduviid bug feeding on human skin. These insects transmit Chagas disease in South America. (Photograph courtesy of Dr H-J Grundmann.)

some that feed on the discharge from the eyes of mammals, including humans) but hairs of certain caterpillars can cause skin rashes, through contact with either fine urticarial spines or stronger hollow spines that contain a venom.

## Cockroaches (Blattaria)

Cockroaches are of little medical significance. They can harbour various pathogens (viruses, bacteria and protozoans) but, as with houseflies, they are of lesser significance in modern urban settings than in developing regions with less sanitary conditions. In modern cities, however, they are also known to be responsible for allergy-related conditions including asthma.

## Fleas (Siphonaptera)

Fleas are small blood-sucking parasites. Their laterally flattened bodies and lack of wings enable them to negotiate the hairs and feathers of their animal hosts. Well-developed hind legs enable them to jump from host to host (Fig. 64.2). Many fleas will feed on humans if given the opportunity, as those who have been attacked by the common cat flea *Ctenocephalides felis* can bear witness. However, the species that is adapted for life on humans is the human flea, *Pulex irritans*, which is still common throughout the world. Female fleas of another species, *Tunga penetrans*, known as *chigoes* or *jiggers*, attack humans by burrowing into the underside skin of the foot, or under the toenails, and the abdomen of the gravid female becomes grossly distended with eggs, causing pain, irritation and, sometimes, secondary infection. These

**Fig. 64.2** The rat flea *Xenopsylla cheopis*, vector of plague.

**Fig. 64.3** *Pthirus pubis*, the human 'crab' louse.

fleas are common in dry, sandy soil, mainly in Africa and parts of Central and South America.

Human or cat fleas are seldom implicated in the transmission of disease, but some other species are important disease vectors. Most notorious is the rat flea, *Xenopsylla cheopis*, which is the most important, but not the sole, vector of the bacterium that is responsible for plague (see p. 350 and Fig. 64.2). Some forms of rickettsial typhus are also transmitted by rodent fleas (see Table 40.1, p. 391).

## Lice (Anoplura)

Lice are wingless insects that undergo incomplete metamorphosis during their development. The ones that parasitize humans are blood-sucking species with flattened bodies and short legs that are adapted to cling to hairs or clothing. Body lice and head lice are variants of the same species, *Pediculus humanus*. Although the body louse, *P. humanus corporis*, is somewhat larger than the head louse, *P. humanus capitis*, and there are other minor differences, they are not readily distinguishable. A third species, *Pthirus pubis*, is quite distinct morphologically, living up to its common description as the 'crab' louse (Fig. 64.3). Head lice are usually confined to the hairs of the scalp, but body lice live in clothing covering the body, rather than on the skin itself. *P. pubis*, as the name suggests, is usually found on pubic hairs, but may also infest other hairy parts, including body and axillary hair in adults and eyelashes in children. All types attach their characteristic eggs (often called *nits*) to body hairs (head and crab louse) or clothing fibres (body louse), and effective treatment involves removal of the eggs as well as dealing with the adults.

Body lice are the classic vectors of the rickettsia that causes epidemic typhus (see p. 393) and the spirochaete that causes relapsing fever (see p. 371), but head and pubic lice are generally not involved as vectors of pathogens. Lice also cause irritation, and continuous scratching may lead to various forms of infective dermatitis.

Lice are very common throughout the world and head lice, in particular, often spread quickly between school children, even in affluent areas. Treatment with insecticides such as permethrin, malathion and carbaryl may be effective, but chemical resistance is widespread, and there are also fears about the possible neurotoxicity of malathion and the mutagenic potential of carbaryl, so unnecessary repeat treatments should be avoided. Repeated 'wet-combing' with a fine-tooth comb after shampooing the hair and applying conditioner can succeed in eliminating an infestation, although reinfection from untreated family members or school contacts is common. The same insecticidal treatments can be effective against pubic lice but all body hair should be treated and, as the infestation is transmitted by intimate contact, sexual partners should also be treated.

## Flies (Diptera)

Dipterous insects are usually active flyers as adults, with a pair of wings used for flying and an additional vestigial pair, known as *halteres*, which are used as organs of balance. The developmental cycle from egg to adult fly involves complete metamorphosis. As well as being among the most annoying of insect pests, many biting flies have an obligate role in the transmission of a wide variety of important infections (Table 64.2). The larvae of certain flies may also infest wounds and others are able to penetrate skin, causing myiasis (see below).

## Mosquitoes

Mosquitoes are readily recognized by a long needle-like proboscis (Fig. 64.4). Adult males and females both feed on plant juices, but the female needs blood for the development of her eggs, and is a voracious predator on a wide variety of vertebrate animals throughout the world. Mosquitoes of importance in human medicine are divided into two broad types: *anopheline* mosquitoes, numerous *Anopheles* species of which transmit the protozoans that cause malaria in humans and result in great mortality in tropical countries (see p. 674), and *culicine* mosquitoes (e.g. *Culex* and *Aedes* spp.), which are the vectors of many so-called *arboviruses* (arthropod-borne viruses), such as yellow fever, dengue, West Nile, Japanese encephalitis, chikungunya, Ockelbo and Ross River viruses, that can cause various encephalitis, haemorrhagic and polyarthritic symptoms in both tropical and temperate regions (see Ch. 51). Both anopheline and culicine mosquitoes also act as the intermediate hosts of certain nematodes that cause lymphatic filariasis (see Ch. 63).

Female mosquitoes lay their eggs on water or on surfaces that will be flooded; larvae and pupae are both aquatic. Most *Anopheles* and *Culex* mosquitoes prefer relatively permanent water bodies that do not dry up, but *Aedes* spp. will utilize temporary habitats, such as created by flood- and tidal-waters, and also small pockets of water, such as in rock-pools, tree-holes, discarded containers, water butts, etc. Some adults can disperse widely and may be found several kilometres from their breeding ground, while others are very limited in their range.

**Table 64.2** Principal infections associated with biting flies, mosquitoes and midges

| Type of insect | Diseases transmitted |
|---|---|
| Biting midges (*Culicoides* spp.) | Filariasis (*Mansonella* spp.) |
| Black-flies (*Simulium* spp.) | Onchocerciasis |
| Deer flies (*Chrysops* spp.) | Loiasis |
| Mosquitoes: | |
|   Anopheline (*Anopheles* spp.) | Malaria; bancroftian filariasis |
|   Culicine (*Culex, Aedes, Mansonia* spp.) | Bancroftian and brugian filariasis; yellow fever, dengue and other arbovirus infections |
| Sandflies (*Phlebotomus, Lutzomyia* spp.) | Leishmaniasis; Oroya fever; sandfly fever |
| Tsetse flies (*Glossina* spp.) | African trypanosomiasis |

## Biting midges

Biting midges are tiny flies that are able to cause a nuisance out of all proportion to their size. They arise from mostly aquatic or semi-aquatic habitats and the females attack in swarms, usually in the evening, and may give rise to painful and intensely itchy reactions. These midges are more important in veterinary than human medicine as vectors of arboviruses, although some *Culicoides* spp. transmit filarial nematodes of *Mansonella* spp. to humans in parts of Africa and Central/South America (see p. 660).

## Sandflies

Sandflies are small enough to penetrate most mosquito netting. They have terrestrial (not aquatic) habitats and utilise dark, humid natural hollows areas, such as rodent burrows or termite mounds, but are often also found in or around human earthen dwellings and associated animal shelters. Female flies suck blood, usually at night, but have limited flight range, so that the diseases they transmit – notably the visceral (kala azar) and cutaneous (e.g. oriental sore) forms of leishmaniasis (see p. 652), bacterial bartonellosis (see p. 347) and viral sandfly fever (see p. 534) – tend to be localized in distribution. Species

**Fig. 64.4** A female anopheline mosquito, the vector of human malaria. (Photograph courtesy of Dr S Doggett, Westmead Hospital, Sydney, Australia.)

associated with disease transmission in Africa, the Middle East, Asia and the Mediterranean littoral belong to the genus *Phlebotomus*, while in Central and South America the vectors of the various pathogens are species of *Lutzomyia*.

### Other biting flies

Although flies that are capable of inflicting a painful bite, such as the stable-fly *Stomoxys calcitrans*, various black-flies and tabanids are found throughout the world and can be serious nuisance pests in temperate regions, species that are important vectors of human disease are restricted in distribution to areas of the tropics.

Black-flies (*Simulium* species) are the vectors of the filaria that causes onchocerciasis (*river blindness*; see Ch. 63) in parts of tropical Africa, and also Central and South America, and are associated with flowing rivers where the immature stages are attached to vegetation or rock substrates. The adults are small hump-backed flies that often attack in swarms but only the females feed on blood. Species in the *Simulium damnosum* complex and the *S. neavei* group are important vectors in western and eastern regions of Africa, respectively, while other species such as *S. ochraceum* and *S. metallicum* transmit the infection in the Americas.

Tsetse-flies, *Glossina* spp., are large flies found only in Africa, where they transmit the protozoans that are responsible for trypanosomiasis ('sleeping sickness') in humans as well as in cattle and other animals (see p. 650). The immature stages are associated with dry terrestrial habitats where mature larvae are deposited on friable soil that they penetrate for pupal development and, unusually, both male and female adults feed on blood. The vectors of human trypanosomiasis in areas of West Africa are riverine species belonging to the *Glossina palpalis* group, whereas species in the *G. morsitans* group, which prefer savannah plains and woodlands, are the principal vectors in the eastern part of the continent.

Tabanids (sometimes known as *deer-flies*) are large flies that can act as vectors of the filarial worm *Loa loa* (see p. 658) in tropical West and Central Africa, where *Chrysops dimidiatus* and *C. silaceus* breed in aquatic or semi-aquatic muddy or marshy areas of the rainforests. Other tabanid species, known throughout the world by various common names such as horse-flies, clegs and March-flies, have very painful bites but generally are not involved in disease transmission (although some have been associated with tularaemia and anthrax).

### Myiasis

Given the chance, many common flies that usually lay their eggs or larvae on carrion, will deposit eggs or first stage larvae on exposed human tissues of ulcers and sores, which consequently become infested with the maggots. The condition is known as *semi-specific* or *facultative myiasis* to distinguish it from *specific* or *obligatory myiasis*, in which humans and other animals act as obligate hosts for the larval stage of development of certain species. *Accidental myiasis* is said to occur when larvae are ingested with food, or incidentally invade orifices such as the urogenital tract.

Myiasis is of great economic importance in animal husbandry throughout the world, but human infestation is largely a problem of the tropics. Obligatory myiasis in Africa is most commonly caused by *Cordylobia anthropophaga* (the *tumbu fly*) or *C. rodhaini* (*Lund's fly*). In Central and South America *Dermatobia hominis* (the *human bot fly*) is the usual culprit. *Cordylobia* lays its eggs in soil or dust contaminated with urine or faeces and humans are infested when contacting that substrate, but *Dermatobia* attaches its eggs to other insects (including mosquitoes) that are attracted to humans. When the larvae hatch they burrow into the skin of the individual with whom they are in contact and remain there, breathing through spiracles at the posterior end until they are ready to pupate and emerge. This is also termed cutaneous myiasis and is a transient condition resulting in boil-like lesions in the skin. The body of the larva is furnished with spines (Fig. 64.5), which make it difficult to remove, but covering the lesion (and thus the posterior spiracles) with a gel substance (such as petroleum jelly, vaseline) prevents the larva from breathing and encourages it to emerge with the help of digital pressure. There should be no subsequent problem with the lesion, providing care is taken not to allow it to become secondarily infected.

Larvae of another African fly, *Auchmeromyia luteola* (the *Congo floor maggot*), also 'parasitize'

**Fig. 64.5** Larva of *Dermatobia hominis*, from a case of human myiasis.

humans, but they do not penetrate the skin, preferring instead to suck the blood of unsuspecting sleepers.

## ARACHNIDS

Of most importance in this group are spiders, scorpions, ticks and mites. Unlike insects, the adult forms have eight legs and are invariably wingless. They have two main body regions – cephalothorax and abdomen – which in mites and ticks are fused to give the appearance of a single segment. They develop by incomplete metamorphosis, and immature forms resemble small versions of adults. However, ticks and mites acquire the full complement of eight legs only as they mature from larvae to nymphs during their progression to adulthood.

### Mites

Despite their name, mites are variable in size, although many, including those commonly implicated in human disease, are so small as to be almost invisible to the naked eye. The only strictly human parasites are *Sarcoptes scabiei* (the *itch mite*), *Demodex folliculorum* and *Demodex brevis* (the *follicle mites*).

The human itch mite, *Sarcoptes scabiei*, is related to mites causing mange in various animals (Fig. 64.6). It is the cause of scabies, an infestation of the skin that is still very prevalent in many countries. After fertilization on the surface of the skin, the gravid female mite burrows into the epidermis, eventually leaving behind a trail of about 40 eggs. The larvae usually hatch in 3–4 days, leave the burrow and pass through nymphal stages to reach adulthood in hair follicles. Burrowing females cause intense itching. There may be a rash on the trunk but this is unrelated to the

**Fig. 64.6** Scabies mite (*Sarcoptes scabiei*), female with eggs/embryos.

distribution of the mites, which are most often found in folds of thin skin, especially between the fingers, often on the wrists and elbows, the axillae, and penis in men and breasts in women. There may be secondary bacterial infection that complicates diagnosis and treatment, and elderly and immunocompromised patients may develop a severe keratotic crusting infestation known as *crusted* (previously *Norwegian*) *scabies*, which can cause outbreaks in institutions and may be misdiagnosed as psoriasis. Application of an aqueous solution of malathion or permethrin is often successful therapy, but household contacts should also be treated. Crusted scabies can be treated systemically with the anthelminthic agent ivermectin, which is widely used in animal husbandry for the control of ectoparasites.

*Demodex* spp., the follicle (or blackhead) mites have an elongated body adapted for its life in hair follicles and sebaceous glands on the face, commonly around the nose, on the cheeks or eyelashes. They seldom cause much pathology (although they have been associated with acne and other skin conditions), but can be treated with permethrin application or sulphur preparations.

Other species that impact on human health occupy a wide variety of habitats that humans enter or entertain, and human contact with certain species in their environment may lead to an intense pruritus or dermatitis. Mites associated with commensal birds and rodents (*Ornithonyssus* spp.), and stored grains or dry foodstuffs (e.g. *Tyrophagus putrescentiae* and related spp.), can cause serious dermatological irritation.

Dust mites (*Dermatophagoides* spp. and *Euroglyphus* spp.) have attracted considerable attention as a precipitating cause of atopic disease, including asthma and eczema (see above). The *Dermatophagoides* species (usually *D. pteronyssinus* in Europe and more commonly *D. farinae* in North America) flourish in centrally heated homes with wall-to-wall carpeting. They feed on flakes of skin and have been incriminated as a cause of asthma in atopic subjects. The allergens are present in the dead bodies and also secreted in the mites' faeces.

The most important mite-borne pathogenic disease is scrub typhus (see p. 393), a potentially fatal rickettsial infection with a localized but widespread distribution in eastern and southeastern Asia to northern Australia.

### Ticks

Ticks are essentially large mites, but they are much more important as vectors of human disease. They are

**Fig. 64.7** *Dermacentor andersoni*, the vector of Rocky Mountain spotted fever and a cause of tick paralysis. These are known as 'hard ticks' because of the presence of the dorsal scutum, prominent in the male (right), but much reduced in the female (left).

conveniently classified into two main families: *hard (ixodid) ticks*, which have a chitinous shield (*scutum*) on the back (Fig. 64.7), and *soft (argasid) ticks*, which lack this feature. In addition, the head parts of soft ticks are hidden on the ventral surface and are not visible from above. Ticks are obligate blood-feeders. They parasitize a very wide variety of animals in nature and many species will attack humans, given the opportunity. The initial bite is usually painless, but it can give rise to a serious reaction and, in some countries (notably Canada, the USA and Australia), ixodid ticks are responsible for *tick paralysis*, a potentially fatal condition caused by a neurotoxin injected while the tick feeds.

Ixodid ticks also transmit many rickettsiae of the spotted fever group (see p. 393), as well as the agents of rickettsial Q fever, spirochaetal Lyme disease (see p. 372), bacterial tularaemia (see p. 357), protozoan babesiosis (see p. 653) and arboviruses (see Ch. 51) that can cause encephalitis. Adults, especially the females, gorge on blood for long periods, and efforts to remove them manually often leave the head embedded in the skin. However, the developmental stages (larvae, nymphs and adults) may not remain on the same host and some of the most important species involved in disease transmission, such as *Dermacentor andersoni* and *Ixodes ricinus*, are known as *three host ticks*. Larvae that acquire micro-organisms remain infected through the nymphal and adult stages (*transstadial transmission*); the adult can, in turn, pass on infection to the next generation through the eggs (*transovarial transmission*). Thus, spread of infection to new hosts may be very efficient.

Argasid ticks tend to be 'nest ticks', preferring to attack a resting or sleeping host at night, and do not remain attached to the host after feeding.

They are relatively long-lived and inhabit dry, dusty environments, mainly in hot countries. The most important species from a medical point of view is *Ornithodoros moubata*, the main vector of tick-borne borreliosis (relapsing fever) in tropical Africa (see p. 371). Other species of *Ornithodoros* transmit American forms of relapsing fever and some are notorious for their voracious feeding habits and extremely painful bites.

## Spiders and scorpions

Although all spiders kill their prey by injecting venom, the toxin is usually innocuous to humans, and the mouthparts (*chelicerae*) are seldom robust enough to allow penetration of human skin. The sting of scorpions, which is carried at the end of an elongated extension of the abdomen, can penetrate human skin, but the venom is usually of low potency (although it can be sufficient to make children ill).

Some spiders and scorpions have painful bites or stings and a few can cause serious, occasionally fatal, illness by virtue of powerful neurotoxins. The most dangerous spider is the Australian funnel web spider, *Atrax robustus*, but species of *Latrodectus* (including types of *black widow spider*, found in many areas of the world, and the Australian *redback spider*) can also inflict a serious bite. The venom of some *Loxosceles* spiders encountered in the USA and South America may cause tissue necrosis.

The most dangerous scorpions belong to the large Buthidae family. Buthid scorpions with dangerous stings are most commonly found in parts of Africa, the Middle East, the southern states of the USA and Central America. They are nocturnal creatures and sting as a defensive reaction. Most human cases of scorpion bite occur when the arthropod seeks shelter in shoes or other clothing.

Spider and scorpion wounds seldom need more than supportive treatment. Antivenoms are sometimes available in areas where the more dangerous species are prevalent.

## Other arthropods

Some centipedes can inflict a painful bite and some millipedes can secrete a fluid capable of raising blisters. Crustaceans (crabs and crayfish) are of interest in human medicine mainly as intermediate hosts of *Paragonimus westermani*, the lung fluke (see p. 663). Copepods (*water fleas*) are similarly important only as hosts of the guinea-worm, *Dracunculus medinensis* (see p. 664–5) and the fish tapeworm, *Diphyllobothrium latum* (see p. 664–5).

## RECOMMENDED READING

Goddard J: *Physician's Guide to Arthropods of Medical Importance*, ed 5, Boca Raton, 2007, CRC Press.

Kettle DS: *Medical and Veterinary Entomology*, ed 2, Wallingford, 1995, CABI publications.

Mullen G, Durden L: *Medical and Veterinary Entomology*, ed 2, Burlington, 2009, Academic Press.

Service MW: *Medical Entomology for Students*, ed 4, Cambridge, 2008, Cambridge University Press.

## Website

Iowa State University Entomology Index of Internet Resources: http://www.ent.iastate.edu/list/directory/114/vid/5

# PART 6
## DIAGNOSIS, TREATMENT AND CONTROL OF INFECTION

# Infective syndromes

*R. C. B. Slack*

Throughout this book, infections have been dealt with as appropriate according to the micro-organisms involved. In this chapter, the study of infection is considered by syndromes associated with the major organs in order to emphasize the variety of microbes that may attack different body systems. The subject is presented in broad outline, and the reader should refer back to earlier chapters for a more extensive account of specific themes.

In infectious diseases, as in other branches of clinical practice, a diagnosis may be obvious and require little investigation, e.g. a case of chickenpox during an epidemic, or may be established only after laboratory and radiological examination, as with a patient with pyrexia of unknown origin (PUO). Figure 65.1 shows a flow diagram of a rational approach to diagnosis and management of a patient with infection. In practice, treatment is often started before isolating and identifying the pathogen and in many viral conditions the exact cause can only be determined during convalescence, either by serological tests or after prolonged growth in tissue culture. The availability of rapid laboratory methods and new chemotherapeutic agents has made the accurate diagnosis of infectious disease even more important.

## SPECIFIC SYNDROMES

### UPPER RESPIRATORY TRACT

The upper respiratory tract is frequently the site of general and localized infections. Indeed, this group of ailments is amongst the most common presenting to domiciliary practice. It is the primary site of infection for most viral diseases, which are spread by sneezing, coughing or direct contact with materials contaminated by respiratory secretions. Although the majority of such symptoms are viral in origin, secondary bacterial infection may often follow, particularly in the very young and malnourished. Resident bacteria in the upper respiratory tract such as *Haemophilus influenzae, Streptococcus pyogenes* and *Str. pneumoniae* are the most common causes. Figure 65.2 shows the anatomical sites of respiratory infection and the appropriate specimens which may be taken for microbiology.

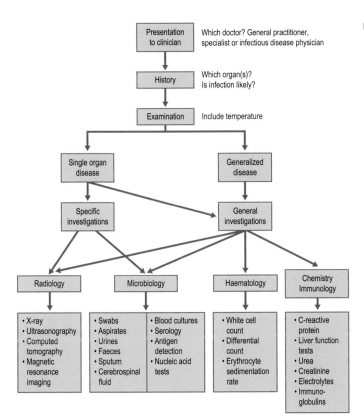

**Fig. 65.1** Flow diagram for the diagnosis of infection.

Presentation to clinician — Which doctor? General practitioner, specialist or infectious disease physician

History — Which organ(s)? Is infection likely?

Examination — Include temperature

Single organ disease

Generalized disease

Specific investigations

General investigations

Radiology
- X-ray
- Ultrasonography
- Computed tomography
- Magnetic resonance imaging

Microbiology
- Swabs
- Aspirates
- Urines
- Faeces
- Sputum
- Cerebrospinal fluid
- Blood cultures
- Serology
- Antigen detection
- Nucleic acid tests

Haematology
- White cell count
- Differential count
- Erythrocyte sedimentation rate

Chemistry Immunology
- C-reactive protein
- Liver function tests
- Urea
- Creatinine
- Electrolytes
- Immuno-globulins

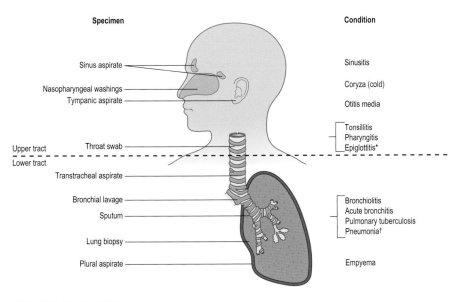

**Fig. 65.2** Microbial infections of the respiratory tract and the appropriate specimens for laboratory investigation.

Specimen

Condition

Sinus aspirate — Sinusitis

Nasopharyngeal washings — Coryza (cold)

Tympanic aspirate — Otitis media

Tonsillitis
Pharyngitis
Epiglottitis*

Upper tract — Throat swab

Lower tract

Transtracheal aspirate

Bronchial lavage

Sputum

Bronchiolitis
Acute bronchitis
Pulmonary tuberculosis
Pneumonia†

Lung biopsy

Plural aspirate — Empyema

*Take a blood culture to diagnose
†Blood culture and serology may be useful

## Sore throat

Bacterial acute tonsillitis or pharyngitis is commonly due to *Str. pyogenes* (group A), and a few are caused by groups C and G. Viruses are even more common causes of sore throats, especially the milder, non-exudative forms. However, it is important to make a definitive diagnosis of streptococcal pharyngitis for two reasons:

1. *Str. pyogenes* remains sensitive to penicillin, which should be used for treatment.
2. Group A β-haemolytic streptococci, if untreated, may give rise to septic complications such as a peritonsillar abscess, or to immune complex disease (e.g. glomerulonephritis, rheumatic fever).

On the other hand, since Str. *pyogenes* may account for only 20% of patients presenting with typical symptoms, many courses of antibiotics would be prescribed unnecessarily if all suspected cases were treated. Even in experienced hands it is difficult to predict on clinical grounds alone which cases are streptococcal. This has led to three approaches:

1. Treat all children with a penicillin, or erythromycin if allergic. Adults are treated if the throat looks very inflamed or if there is pus on the tonsils.
2. Swabs are taken for culture of streptococci and antibiotics are started as above but stopped if *Str. pyogenes* is not found.
3. Swabs are taken for rapid diagnosis (by antigen detection) and penicillin commenced only if the throat swab is positive.

There are pros and cons to each method. One drawback to the early use of antibiotics is that the patient may react to the drug. If ampicillin is used, there is a strong chance of a skin reaction if the sore throat is the harbinger of glandular fever. In defence of the antibiotic lobby, there is no doubt that complications of streptococcal disease are seen far less commonly where there is access to medical service and pharmacies. However, these improvements have occurred in concert with better housing and social conditions.

There was less need to make a virological diagnosis as specific therapy was limited. However, epidemiological studies of patients with throat symptoms have revealed how common and varied are the viruses in the respiratory tract. With the advent of antivirals active against specific viruses, interest has increased in using tests for influenza and RSV.

In the severely ill child with toxaemia and a membrane, diphtheria must be considered and treatment should not await laboratory confirmation. Moreover, the laboratory needs to do special tests to isolate and identify *Corynebacterium diphtheriae*, and communication (by telephone, if possible) between the clinician and laboratory is essential. Other corynebacteria such as *C.ulcerans* and *Arcanobacterium haemolyticum* may rarely cause ulcerated sore throats. In the sexually active, gonococcal pharyngitis should not be missed and again the laboratory needs to be told as they will use special selective media for *Neisseria gonorrhoeae*.

## Common cold (coryza)

This common complaint, characterized by a nasal discharge (acute rhinitis) that is usually watery with scanty cells, afflicts humans of all ages who congregate together. Since there are many types of rhinoviruses, coronaviruses, adenoviruses, etc., and since immunity may be short-lived, individuals in a crowded environment, such as at school and university or travelling on public transport, may suffer three or four clinical infections a year. Most of these do not seek medical help knowing that there is little to offer. This is a condition for which many 'alternative' remedies are tried, from garlic to peppermint and vitamin supplements.

Bacterial superinfection with pneumococci and *H. influenzae* can occur in the nasopharynx but is only symptomatic when the sinuses or middle ear are involved. Pharyngitis and, occasionally, tracheobronchitis may occur with a cold or develop in more susceptible individuals. Respiratory syncytial virus (RSV) may cause upper respiratory symptoms in children and adults, but in those contracting the virus for the first time (usually infants under 1 year of age) acute bronchiolitis is common.

## Sinusitis and otitis media

Direct extension of a viral or bacterial infection from the nasopharynx into frontal and maxillary sinuses in adults and into the middle ear in children is not uncommon. Obtaining adequate material for microbiology is difficult and requires the expertise of ear, nose and throat specialists. In most cases of acute sinusitis or otitis media the microbial cause is not found. It is assumed that severe pain and discharge of pus from the nose or ear is suggestive of bacterial infection and antibiotics are usually given to cover streptococci (mainly *Str. pneumoniae*) and *H. influenzae*. In adults with recurrent or chronic sinusitis, anaerobes (peptostreptococci or bacteroides) are often found in sinus washings.

## LOWER RESPIRATORY TRACT

### Epiglottitis

Although situated in the upper part of the respiratory tract, *epiglottitis* behaves like a serious systemic infection which requires urgent admission to hospital and treatment. The diagnosis should be made clinically in a toxic child (usually under 5 years old) with respiratory obstruction and stridor. The most useful investigation is blood culture, which invariably grows *H. influenzae* type b unless antibiotics have been given or the child immunized. The epiglottis, which is swollen and cherry-red in appearance, should only be examined by skilled paediatricians prepared for a respiratory arrest. A lateral radiograph shows a soft tissue swelling in the throat.

### Laryngotracheobronchitis

In adults, some viral infections cause acute laryngitis with voice loss or tracheitis with a dry cough. Respiratory tract infection in children is usually generalized and presents as *croup*. This may lead to respiratory obstruction and, as with haemophilus epiglottitis, urgent admission to hospital is necessary. The condition may be caused by a variety of respiratory viruses, with para-influenza viruses, adenoviruses and enteroviruses the most common. RSV can also cause croup, but more commonly this virus attacks infants in the first few months of life. In the UK there are winter epidemics of *acute bronchiolitis* due to RSV. This clinical syndrome which starts as a cold, followed by wheezing. In older children, asthmatic attacks are often precipitated by viral respiratory infections.

### Whooping cough

Pertussis may be confused with croup, and, as special specimens need to be taken, the laboratory must be informed. A pernasal swab in special transport medium is required, and *Bordetella pertussis* will only grow on enriched culture media in conditions of high humidity.

### Acute bronchitis

Acute exacerbation of chronic obstructive pulmonary disease (COPD) is the most common adult lower respiratory infection. It is invariably due to pneumococci, non-encapsulated haemophili, or both. Sometimes, acute bronchitis follows a viral infection. Although often examined, expectorated sputum from ambulatory patients with COPD is almost always a waste of effort.

Cystic fibrosis patients have frequent exacerbations and, in those situations, sputum examination is valuable because the causative bacteria (*Staphylococcus aureus, H. influenzae, Pseudomonas aeruginosa* or *Burkholderia cepacia*) may show variable antimicrobial resistance and appropriate therapy is essential.

### Acute pneumonias

It is sometimes possible on clinical and radiological grounds to distinguish between *lobar pneumonia* (pneumococcal), *bronchopneumonia* (staphylococcal and klebsiellal) and *'atypical' pneumonias* (mycoplasmal and chlamydial). This division is of importance in guiding primary treatment, but should not give the clinician a blinkered view in investigation, as some cases will invariably not follow a textbook! Expectorated sputum is often poorly collected and may not yield the pathogen. Blood cultures should always be taken from pneumonia patients but may not yield an organism, especially if antibiotics have been started. *Antigen detection* in urine or sputum by fluorescent antibodies, immuno-electrophoresis, latex agglutination or enzyme-linked immunosorbent assay (ELISA) is a useful method for rapid diagnosis but may lack sensitivity. New amplified DNA detection methods are likely to improve diagnostic accuracy in respiratory infections. At present most cases of 'atypical' pneumonia are diagnosed by obtaining acute and convalescent sera, and by finding a significant titre or a rising titre of antibodies. *Legionnaires' disease* may be diagnosed by culture of *Legionella pneumophila* from sputum or a biopsy, but this has too low a sensitivity. Urine antigen detection by ELISA or DNA amplification of respiratory secretions have become more widely available methods of diagnosis. However, as with most pneumonias treatment must often be given on clinical suspicion.

### Chronic chest disease

Tuberculosis must always be considered in any patient with fever, prolonged cough and weight loss. Again, a request for examination for mycobacteria in sputum must be included on the request card. Blood tests examining for interferon produced by peripheral lymphocytes are of value in detecting latent tuberculosis but are of limited value in diagnosis of the a ctive disease.

In the immunocompromised, various opportunist pathogens may give rise to respiratory infection. *Pneumocystis carinii* is demonstrated by fluorescent antibody staining of bronchial lavage. Fungal infections are diagnosed by growth of the pathogen or by serology. Special investigations are required for all these situations and unless the diagnosis is considered the laboratory cannot assist the clinician.

## GASTROINTESTINAL INFECTION

Acute diarrhoea with or without vomiting is a common complaint. Microbial causes, either by multiplication in the intestine or from the effects of preformed toxin, are the most important reasons for acute gastrointestinal upset in an otherwise healthy individual. The aetiology of inflammatory bowel disease such as ulcerative colitis has not been established, although a patient may present with symptoms similar to an infectious diarrhoea but usually the natural history and chronicity of the condition make the distinction obvious.

Although many new causes of bowel infection have been discovered in the past 25 years the majority of food-related and short-lived episodes do not yield a microbial cause. In part this is due to the wide range of viruses, bacteria and protozoa which may be sought (Table 65.1). A search for all causes involves extensive and expensive laboratory effort, and this is often considered unnecessary for a condition which is usually self-limiting and relatively harmless.

Toxin-mediated disease of microbial origin ranges in severity from relatively trivial episodes of food poisoning caused by:

- enterotoxin-producing strains of *Staph. aureus*
- *Clostridium perfringens*
- *Bacillus cereus*;

to the life-threatening systemic diseases:

- botulism caused by *Cl. botulinum*
- severe *pseudomembranous colitis* caused by *Cl. difficile* (often antibiotic-associated).

**Table 65.1** Common microbial causes of infectious intestinal disease (see individual chapters for details)

| Viruses | Bacteria | Protozoa |
|---------|----------|----------|
| Norovirus (SRSV) | *Salmonella enterica* serotypes | *Cryptosporidium parvum* |
| Rotavirus | *Campylobacter* spp. | *Entamoeba histolytica* |
| Astrovirus | *Clostridium difficile* | *Giardia lamblia* |
| Calicivirus (SRSV) | *Shigella* spp. | |
| | *Escherichia coli* (ETEC, VTEC) | |
| | *Vibrio cholerae* | |
| | *V. parahaemolyticus* | |
| | *Yersinia enterocolitica* | |

ETEC, enterotoxigenic *E. coli*; SRSV, small round structured viruses; VTEC, verotoxigenic *E. coli*.

There are, in addition, many non-microbial causes of food poisoning, such as that due to the ingestion of certain toadstools, undercooked red kidney beans or various types of fish (*ciguatera toxin, scombrotoxin*); most notorious is the puffer fish which, during part of its reproductive cycle, produces a neurotoxin that is responsible for more than 100 deaths a year in Japan, where the delicacy *fugu* is enjoyed.

It may be possible on clinical grounds to distinguish between patients with dysentery, in which bloody diarrhoea and mucus are found, and those with watery diarrhoea, due to the toxic effects of the pathogen on the small intestinal mucosa, leading to accumulation of fluid in the bowel. Some conditions, such as staphylococcal food poisoning and some viral illnesses, present largely with vomiting. A specific cause is also suspected if there is a history of foreign travel, if the case forms part of an outbreak that is food- or water-associated, or if the individual has a relevant food history.

*Travellers' diarrhoea* encompasses many clinical and microbial causes, but the most common organisms implicated are enterotoxigenic strains of *Escherichia coli* (ETEC). However, a host of microbes must be considered. Some, such as salmonellae, are found worldwide; others, such as vibrios, have a more limited distribution.

More chronic intestinal infections contracted in warmer climates usually do not present with diarrhoea but with vague abdominal symptoms. Many helminths and protozoa are found on screening faeces for other pathogens.

## URINARY TRACT INFECTIONS

The diagnosis of urinary tract infection cannot be made without bacteriological examination of the urine because many patients with the frequency–dysuria syndrome have sterile urine and, conversely, asymptomatic bacteriuria is a common condition. Infection is most commonly caused by members of the Enterobacteriaceae (Table 65.2), but there are great variations in antimicrobial susceptibility, and control of chemotherapy requires laboratory examination. Occasionally, *Mycobacterium tuberculosis* invades the kidney and appropriate tests must be carried out if this is suspected.

Infection in the urinary tract may be confined to particular anatomical sites, e.g. urethritis or renal abscess. Alternatively, the urine may become infected and, in cases of obstruction or reflux, bacteria may ascend from the bladder to give rise to kidney infections. *Urethritis* is really a genital infection and is most

**Table 65.2** Common causes of urinary tract infection (approximate %)

| Organism | Domiciliary (%) | Hospital (%) |
|---|---|---|
| *Escherichia coli* | 70–80 | 50 |
| *Proteus mirabilis* | 10 | 1–5 |
| *Klebsiella* spp. | 1–5 | 5–10 |
| *Staphylococcus saprophyticus* | 10–15 | 0 |
| *Staph. epidermidis* | 1–5 | 10–20 |
| Enterococci | 1–5 | 10–20 |
| Other coliforms | <1 | 5–10 |
| *Pseudomonas aeruginosa* | 1–2 | 5–10 |

**Table 65.3** Causes of aseptic meningitis

| | |
|---|---|
| Viruses | Enteroviruses (echoviruses, polioviruses, coxsackieviruses)<br>Mumps (including post-immunization)<br>Herpes (herpes simplex and varicella-zoster)<br>Arboviruses |
| Spiral bacteria | Syphilis (*Treponema pallidum*)<br>Leptospira (*Leptospira canicola*) |
| Other bacteria | Partially treated with antibiotics<br>Tuberculous (*Mycobacterium tuberculosis*)<br>Brain abscess |
| Fungi | *Cryptococcus neoformans* |
| Protozoa | *Acanthamoeba, Naegleria, Toxoplasma gondii* |
| Non-infective | Lymphomas, leukaemias<br>Metastatic and primary neoplasms<br>Collagen-vascular diseases |

commonly due to sexually transmitted organisms such as chlamydiae or *N. gonorrhoeae*. Confirmation depends on obtaining, by swabbing or scraping, a sample of urethral discharge for microscopy and culture. *Metastatic abscesses* in the kidney and *perinephric abscesses* cannot usually be diagnosed by urine examination, although pyuria may be present. Specific radiological or surgical exploration is necessary, as with any localized infection.

Throughout most of their lifespan women suffer far more attacks of urinary tract infection than men. In young adult women who become sexually active, frequency and dysuria are common reasons for seeking medical attention. Only about one-half of these yield an organism in 'significant' numbers, usually defined as above $10^7$ organisms per litre. The most common cause by far is *E. coli* (Table 65.2), some strains of which possess specific uropathogenic determinants. It has been suggested that many of the culture-negative infections are due to coliforms which are present in small numbers in urine. Infection of the urine is common and may be asymptomatic in many elderly patients.

## INFECTIONS OF THE CENTRAL NERVOUS SYSTEM

### Meningitis

Meningeal irritation may occur in association with other acute infections (*meningism*) or with non-infective conditions such as subarachnoid haemorrhage. In the early stages of meningococcal disease, signs of meningitis may be absent, yet examination of the cerebrospinal fluid (CSF) yields *N. meningitidis*. Thus, CSF and blood cultures should be examined from all suspected cases. There are contra-indications to performing a lumbar puncture in any patient with raised intracranial pressure because of the danger of herniation through the foramen magnum (*coning*). Thus, lumbar puncture should only be carried out in hospital. In fulminating disease, especially if it is meningococcal, it is prudent to give penicillin as soon as the diagnosis is suspected and before admission. This has led to a greatly reduced yield by culture of suspected cases. Antigen and DNA detection have become increasingly important in confirming the diagnosis.

It is often possible to consider the likely pathogen on clinical and epidemiological grounds. *H. influenzae* type b occurs almost always in infants from 6–24 months-of-age, although use of the Hib vaccine in many countries has almost made this a disease of the past. *Str. pneumoniae* is seen generally in the very young and the elderly. *Meningococcal meningitis* is characteristically a disease of children and young adults. In the neonate, coliforms (mainly *E. coli* K1), *Listeria monocytogenes*, group B streptococci and pneumococci may be found. In infants a few months old, salmonella meningitis is an important condition in some countries with a warm climate.

If no readily cultivated organism is found, but the CSF shows an increase in cells, the syndrome of *aseptic meningitis* is present. Table 65.3 shows some of the causes of this condition. If the symptoms are short in duration, viruses are most likely. If the child has been unwell for more than 1 week, *tuberculous meningitis* must be considered. This is one of the most difficult and important microbiological diagnoses to make. Interferon assays of activated lymphocytes from peripheral blood of patients with tuberculosis have been shown to be a useful adjunct to the clinical diagnosis in such situations.

In the immunocompromised, listeria meningitis may be seen in the adult and *Cryptococcus neoformans* in all age groups, but particularly those with human immunodeficiency virus (HIV) infection.

**Table 65.4** Causes of neurological damage in HIV-infected patients

| | |
|---|---|
| Direct HIV infection | Subacute encephalomyelitis (AIDS-dementia complex) |
| **Opportunist infections** | |
| Viruses | Cytomegalovirus |
| | Herpes simplex |
| | Varicella-zoster |
| | Papovavirus |
| Bacteria | *Treponema pallidum* (syphilis) |
| Fungi | *Cryptococcus neoformans* |
| Protozoa | *Toxoplasma gondii* |
| **Malignancy** | |
| Primary | Brain lymphoma |
| Secondary | Kaposi's sarcoma |
| | Systemic lymphoma |

Central nervous system disease in patients with acquired immune deficiency syndrome (AIDS) is a very complicated differential diagnosis (Table 65.4).

## Cerebral infections

*Encephalitis* may extend into the meninges with signs and CSF findings of an aseptic meningitis. Many viral infections may, however, only infect the brain cortex and clinical symptoms may be vague: loss of consciousness, fits, localized paralysis. This can also occur in toxaemia, cerebral malaria, electrolyte disturbances or vascular accidents.

In western Europe, herpes simplex or varicella–zoster viruses are the most common causes of encephalitis, but in many parts of the world arboviruses such as Japanese B encephalitis virus are important (see Ch. 51).

*Abscesses* in the brain or subdural space may arise from haematogenous spread during bacteraemia or by direct extension, either through the cribriform plate from the nasopharynx or from sinuses or the middle ear. They may be clinically silent or present as a space-occupying lesion accompanied by fever and systemic upset. Scanning by computerized axial tomography (CAT) or magnetic resonance imaging (MRI) and early neurosurgical intervention will reduce complications and with appropriate systemic antibiotics given for a prolonged period, the success rate is nowadays good.

## SKIN AND SOFT TISSUE INFECTIONS

Human skin acts as an excellent barrier to infection. Some parasites, such as hookworm larvae and schistosome cercariae, can penetrate skin to initiate infection. This may also be true of some bacteria, notably *Treponema pallidum*, although in primary syphilis the spirochaete probably enters through minute abrasions which are present even in healthy skin. Primary skin infection such as *impetigo* is due to *Staph. aureus* or *Str. pyogenes*, or both, gaining access to abrasions, usually in children. This may occur in association with ectoparasite infestation, in particular, scabies. Dermatophyte fungi are specialized to grow well in keratinized tissue.

Skin lesions are a feature of some virus infections, such as warts, herpes simplex and molluscum contagiosum. In other virus diseases, including rubella, measles, chickenpox (and, before its eradication, smallpox), a characteristic rash follows the viraemic phase of the illness. *Wound infections* may be accidental or postoperative and many organisms can cause sepsis. Even after surgery many wounds are infected with the endogenous flora of the patient. Swabs, or preferably pus, obtained directly from the wound or abscess, are adequate to find the causative organisms. *Anaerobic* sepsis most commonly occurs following amputations or in contaminated traumatic wounds, particularly if the blood supply has been compromised or the bowel perforated. In classic *gas gangrene*, bubbles of gas may be felt in the wound and surrounding tissues, and the muscle and fascia have a black necrotic appearance. Less florid examples of anaerobes causing extensive cellulitis are more commonly seen in situations where deep wounds are contaminated with endogenous flora.

## GENITAL TRACT INFECTIONS

In the male, acute urethritis is a common condition, usually due to a sexually transmitted microbe such as *N. gonorrhoeae*, *Chlamydia trachomatis* or *Ureaplasma urealyticum*. If untreated these organisms can cause prostatitis or epididymitis, and gonorrhoea may produce unpleasant consequences such as urethral stricture or sterility. Genital ulcers in both sexes may be due to herpes simplex virus, syphilis or chancroid (*H. ducreyi*).

The more complicated female reproductive organs are subjected to many more infections with a greater scope for sequelae. Vaginitis may present as vaginal discharge or irritation and often these symptoms are due to infections that are not always exogenously acquired. *Trichomonas vaginalis* is the most common sexually acquired microbe, although both *N. gonorrhoeae* and chlamydia may also present as discharge. Thrush due to *Candida* species is especially common in pregnancy and in diabetics. It is usually an endogenous condition due to disturbances in the normal commensal flora. Another cause of vaginal discharge, but usually without inflammatory cells and irritation, is associated with an alteration of local pH with proliferation of *Gardnerella vaginalis* and anaerobic spiral bacteria, now termed *Mobiluncus* species. The alkaline conditions and characteristic amines found in *bacterial vaginosis* allow a diagnosis to be easily made on examination of the patient. This condition, which used to be called non-specific vaginitis, is a common condition in sexually active women, although probably not a venereal disease in the usual sense.

The endocervical canal is the site of infection with *N. gonorrhoeae* and *C. trachomatis* in the sexually mature woman. During parturition both organisms may be passed to the baby's eyes to give rise to *ophthalmia neonatorum*. The cervix may also be infected with human papillomavirus (HPV), the cause of genital warts. Some types are associated with a high risk of cervical cancer (see Ch. 45).

Ascending genital infection may present as *acute salpingitis* with fever and pelvic pain. On vaginal examination, there is referred lower abdominal pain on moving the cervix (*cervical excitation*) and tenderness in the iliac fossa on abdominal palpation. Signs and symptoms in cases due to *C. trachomatis* are much less pronounced than those due to gonococci. Some women may develop chronic *pelvic inflammatory disease* (PID) without having suffered a recognizable acute episode. PID, although most often initiated by these two common sexually transmitted pathogens, is usually a polymicrobial infection, in which endogenous commensals, particularly anaerobes, play an important role.

## EYE INFECTIONS

Various microbes may cause acute conjunctivitis. During birth *N.gonorrhoeae* and *C.trachomatis* may be passed to the baby's eyes from the maternal genital tract to give rise to ophthalmia neonatorum. In the newborn, *Staph. aureus* is commonly found in 'sticky eyes', either as a primary cause of conjunctivitis or after infection with another pathogen. In older infants and children, *H. influenzae* and *Str. pneumoniae* are common. Chlamydiae give rise to *trachoma*, the most common cause of blindness in the world, and to a milder form of inclusion blennorrhoea in sexually active individuals.

Primary viral conjunctivitis often occurs in epidemics when certain types of adenovirus are

| Table 65.5 | Causes of choroidoretinitis |
|---|---|
| Viruses | Cytomegalovirus, rubella |
| Bacteria | *Treponema pallidum* |
| Protozoa | *Toxoplasma gondii* |
| Helminths | *Toxocara canis, Onchocerca volvulus* |

implicated. This is usually a mild condition with few sequelae compared with the keratitis due to herpes simplex virus or in shingles when the ophthalmic division of the trigeminal nerve is infected with varicella–zoster virus.

Corneal damage due to fungi as well as herpesviruses is seen in immunosuppressed patients, and keratitis caused by free-living amoebae (*Acanthamoeba* species), though rare, is becoming more common, particularly in wearers of contact lenses.

Penetrating injuries of the eye and ophthalmic surgery may introduce a wide range of bacteria and fungi into the chambers of the eye, which may give rise to *hypopyon* (pus in the eye). This condition requires prompt surgical drainage and instillation of appropriate antibiotics such as gentamicin. *Ps. aeruginosa* and *Proteus* species are among the more common organisms isolated.

Infections of the back of the eye (choroidoretinitis) are seen in many diverse infectious diseases (Table 65.5).

## SYSTEMIC AND GENERAL SYNDROMES

### Pyrexia of unknown origin

PUO may be defined as a significant fever (greater than 38°C) for a few days without an obvious cause, i.e. no apparent infection of an organ or system. In the classic studies of PUO only patients with persistent fever for at least 3 weeks were included. These chronic cases are often due to non-infective causes such as malignancy (especially lymphomata) or autoimmune and connective tissue diseases (such as systemic lupus erythematosus).

In determining an infective aetiology some of the most important questions to be asked of the patient are:

1. Have you been abroad recently?
2. What is your occupation (especially, is animal contact involved)?
3. What immunizations have you had – in particular, have you had BCG?
4. Have you or your family ever had tuberculosis?
5. Are you taking or have you recently had any drugs (especially antibiotics)?

## Character of fever

The individual with suspected PUO should be admitted to hospital so that measurements can be regularly made by skilled staff. Rarely, malingerers may be found out and drug reactions discovered by controlling intake. Rhythmical fevers such as the quartan fever (every 72 h) of *Plasmodium malariae* or undulant fever of *Brucella melitensis* may be rarely found and point to the aetiology. More commonly, fevers are intermittent with rises at the end of the day and falls after rigors or extensive sweating.

The degree of temperature depends also on the host response as well as the pyrogens produced by microbes. Generally, the older the patient the less able they are to mount a pyrexia. Many elderly patients with septicaemia may have normal or subnormal temperatures whereas infants can have fevers of 40°C and febrile convulsions with otherwise mild respiratory viral infections.

## Endocarditis

Infections of the tissue of the heart usually involve damaged valves, either after rheumatic fever or with atheroma. Another important group of patients are those who have had heart surgery, in particular prosthetic valve replacements. In addition, injecting drug users (IUDs) or patients who have had indwelling vascular devices are liable to bacteraemia and, occasionally, endocarditis may follow. The most common causative organisms are listed in Table 65.6.

## Septicaemia

It is not clinically useful to distinguish between *bacteraemia*, organisms isolated from the bloodstream, *septicaemia*, which is a clinical syndrome, and *endotoxaemia*, which is circulating bacterial endotoxin. The spectrum of clinical disease ranges from hypotensive shock and disseminated intravascular coagulation (DIC) with a high mortality, to transient bacteraemia, which may occur in healthy individuals during dental manipulations.

The vascular compartment is sterile and usually intact. Microbes gain entry from breakages of blood vessels adjacent to skin or mucosal surfaces or by phagocytic cells carrying organisms into capillaries or the lymphatic system. Active multiplication within the bloodstream probably only occurs terminally, but in many cases of septicaemia there are high numbers of bacteria recovered from blood cultures, which often only sample 10 mL at a time. This occurs from a heavily contaminated site such as an indwelling

**Table 65.6** Some causes of infective endocarditis (approximate %)

| Organism | Non-operative (%) | IDU or surgery (%) |
|---|---|---|
| Viridans group of streptococci | 70 | 35 |
| Enterococci | 5 | 3 |
| Other streptococci (group G, F) | 10 | <1 |
| *Staphylococcus epidermidis* | 10 | 25 |
| *Staph. aureus* | 5 | 25 |
| Gram-positive rods (diphtheroids) | <1 | 5 |
| *Haemophilus* spp. and other fastidious Gram-negative organisms[a] | <1[b] | <1 |
| Gram-negative bacilli (coliforms, *Pseudomonas* spp.) | 0 | 5 |
| *Coxiella burnetii* (Q fever) | <1[b] | 0 |
| *Chlamydia psittaci* | <1 | 0 |
| Fungi (*Candida* spp.) | <1 | 2 |

IDU, injecting drug user.
[a]*Neisseria, Brucella, Cardiobacterium, Streptobacillus* spp.
[b]These are rough UK figures; in some parts of the Middle East, brucellae and Q fever cause significant numbers of infective endocarditides.

urinary catheter which releases bacteria into veins on movement. Septic shock may be due to Gram-negative lipids (endotoxins) or Gram-positive toxins (e.g. staphylococcal enterotoxin), which are usually proteins. The end result of both is to initiate a cascade of events involving cytokines, especially tumour necrosis factor and interleukin-2, vascular mediators and platelets, which combined lead to DIC and hypotension. This process becomes irreversible and produces failure of all major organs. Patients die from a variety of terminal events which make up the syndrome of *septic shock*. The main microbial causes are listed with approximate frequency in Table 65.7.

Clinical features may occasionally suggest the aetiological agent, e.g. the characteristic purpuric rash of meningococcal disease and the black lesions (*ecthyma gangrenosum*) seen on the skin of compromised patients with pseudomonas septicaemia, but in the majority of bacteraemias the agent can only be determined after blood culture. Sometimes, prior antibiotic therapy may render cultures negative and new methods of antigen detection or gene probes may be useful. Non-specific investigations, such as those shown in Figure 65.1, may offer some help that the cause of the illness is infective. C-reactive protein (CRP), an acute-phase protein which is often greatly elevated in the serum during bacterial infections, may be the most useful of these but, as with peripheral leucocyte counts, there are a significant number of errant results.

## Imported infections

An important group of patients with fever are those who have recently returned from abroad. In whichever country a doctor may practice, travellers with unfamiliar disease will be encountered. Knowledge of medical geography is useful but conditions vary greatly within one country and with time. Up-to-date information is held, often on computer, by communicable disease centres and tropical disease hospitals and schools. The World Health Organization and the

Centers for Disease Control, Atlanta, USA, publish international notification data and maps (see Ch. 70 for websites). Undoubtedly the most important condition to diagnose is malaria due to *Plasmodium falciparum*, which may be rapidly fatal without appropriate treatment in the non-immune subject. The wide distribution of drug resistance in *P. falciparum* has led to difficulties in giving adequate prophylaxis and in treating an acute attack. Other common febrile illnesses which are imported into northern countries are typhoid and paratyphoid. These do not usually

**Table 65.7** Major causes of septicaemia (approximate %)

| Organism | Community acquired (%) | Hospital acquired (%) | Sources and comments |
|---|---|---|---|
| *Escherichia coli* | 35 | 30 | UTI (catheters), biliary tract |
| Other enterobacteria | 5 | 10 | UTI, chest |
| *Pseudomonas* spp. | 5 | 5 | UTI, immunocompromised |
| Other Gram-negative rods | 2 | 5 | Ventilator pneumonia |
| *Neisseria meningitidis* | 3 | 0 | Characteristic skin rash |
| *Staphylococcus aureus* | 30 | 25 | Vascular, postoperative |
| *Staph. epidermidis* | <1 | 20 | Vascular devices |
| *Streptococcus pneumoniae* | 10 | 0 | Pneumonia |
| *Str. pyogenes* | 5 | 2 | Skin, soft tissue |
| Other Gram-positive cocci | 2 | 0 | Skin |
| *Listeria monocytogenes* | <1 | 0 | Bowel, foods |
| *Clostridium* spp. | <1 | 0 | Bowel, gangrenous wounds |
| *Bacteroides* spp. | 3 | 1 | Bowel, pelvis, wounds |
| Mixed infection | 10 | 7 | Bowel, intensive care |

UTI, urinary tract infection.
Data from Dr P. Ispahani, Nottingham Public Health Laboratory, UK.

**Table 65.8** Some important infective conditions imported to temperate regions from the tropics

| Causative organism | Tourists[a] | Expatriates[a] | Immigrants[a] |
|---|---|---|---|
| Viruses | Hepatitis A<br>Influenza | HIV<br>Yellow fever (other arboviruses) | Hepatitis B<br>Haemorrhagic fever |
| Rickettsiae and chlamydiae | Tick typhus | Q fever | Trachoma |
| Bacteria | Legionnaires' disease<br>Toxigenic *Escherichia coli* | Brucellosis<br>Shigellosis | Tuberculosis, enteric fever<br>Cholera |
| Protozoa | Cryptosporidiosis<br>Falciparum malaria<br>Cutaneous leishmaniasis | Giardiasis<br>Malaria (all)<br>Schistosomiasis | Amoebiasis<br>Vivax malaria<br>Kala azar (visceral leishmaniasis) |
| Helminths | – | Tapeworm<br>Filariasis<br>Stronglyloidiasis | Roundworm<br>Hookworm |
| Ectoparasites (ticks, mites and insects) | Ticks | Myiasis jigger flea | Scabies |
| Fungi | – | Dermatophytosis Histoplasmosis | Mycetoma |

[a]These categories are not mutually exclusive.

**Table 65.9** Some common sites of infection in pyrexia of unknown origin

| | |
|---|---|
| Abdomen | Subphrenic abscess |
| | Appendiceal abscess |
| | Ileal tuberculosis |
| | Pelvic abscess |
| Liver and biliary tract | Intrahepatic abscess |
| | Empyema of gallbladder |
| | Ascending cholangitis |
| | Cholecystitis |
| | Viral hepatitis |
| Kidney and urinary tract | Perinephric abscess |
| | Renal tuberculosis |
| | Pyelonephritis (especially children) |
| Bones | Vertebral osteomyelitis |
| | Tuberculosis |
| | Prosthetic infections |
| Cardiovascular | Endocarditis |
| | Graft infections |
| Respiratory | Tuberculosis |
| | Empyema and lung abscess |
| Nervous system | Cryptococcal or tuberculous meningitis |
| | Brain or spinal abscess |

patients which are considered separately, but the separation of diseases and microbes is not exclusive:

1. Short-term travellers or *tourists* who usually visit major cities or special holiday areas, stay in good accommodation and have minimal contact with the indigenous population.
2. Long-term visitors who may be engaged in lengthy overland trips or be working abroad as *expatriates*.
3. *Immigrants* who were brought up abroad and visit or have residence in the host country; also settled immigrants who pay short-term visits to their country of origin.

Individuals who travel abroad vary in their risk behaviour and their exposure to potential pathogens. Generally, advice given by travel operators, tourist offices, embassies and medical sources has greatly improved in the past few years. Companies sending out expatriate workers tend to look after their staff well. Nevertheless, many tourists (up to 50% in some studies) have episodes of travellers' diarrhoea, which in some cases results in admission to hospital. The major groups who are missed in preventative programmes are overland travellers and immigrants returning to their homeland, often with young families who have never been exposed to the infectious risks of their parents' home. Immigrants returning for visits to malarious areas seldom take prophylactic advice, believing themselves to be immune, but protective immunity wanes with prolonged absence.

## Cryptogenic infections

Some of the commonly encountered sites of infection which may give rise to fever, and must be considered in the differential diagnosis of PUO, are listed in Table 65.9.

present with diarrhoea so the possibility of an enteric fever may not be considered. It is also obvious, but sometimes overlooked, that the fever may not be related to the travel history and that the cause is a microbe which could have been caught at home.

Table 65.8 lists some of the more common causes of infectious diseases imported from tropical countries into temperate regions where the diseases are not normally transmitted. There are three groups of

RECOMMENDED READING

Armstrong D, Cohen J, editors: *Infectious Diseases*, Mosby, St Louis, 2011, Elsevier.

Conlon C, Snydman D: *Color Atlas and Text of Infectious Diseases*, Mosby, St Louis, 2000, Elsevier.

Long SS, Pickering LK, Prober CG, editors: *Principles and Practice of Paediatric Infectious Diseases*, Saunders, Philadelphia, 2009, Elsevier.

Mandell GL, Bennett JE, Dolin R: *Principles and Practice of Infectious Diseases*, ed 6, Churchill Livingstone, Philadelphia, 2009, Elsevier.

Warrell DA, Cox TM, Firth JD: *Oxford Textbook of Medicine*, ed 5, Oxford, 2010, Oxford University Press.

# 66 Diagnostic procedures

*R. C. B. Slack*

---

## KEY POINTS

- A central aim in choosing antimicrobial therapy is to match the most appropriate agent to the specific microbial aetiology. In practice, this is constrained by urgency of the situation, the diagnostic information available and policy decisions about antimicrobial use that are made on a local basis consistent with national policies.
- The initial decision on whether or not to give an antimicrobial and on the agent chosen is generally made before microbiological information is available but, where possible, after microbiological samples have been taken.
- In the UK, local and specific guidance is generally available for chemotherapy of common infective syndromes. The strategy reflects the likely causal agents and their local susceptibility patterns, the need to control antimicrobial resistance, and

cost. This guidance is reflected in the local *antibiotic policy.*
- The laboratory will assist in modifying or initiating therapy by determining in vitro susceptibilities and by monitoring antimicrobial drug concentrations in specific circumstances. These analyses may lead to modification of therapy.
- Certain organisms such as streptococci and anaerobes have predictable susceptibilities, whereas others, such as enterobacteria, must be monitored continuously.
- Prophylactic antimicrobials are recommended in highly defined settings and following precise regimens. Ad hoc usage is to be avoided.
- Antimicrobial combinations may be given to increase efficacy, extend the spectrum of cover or prevent the development of resistance during therapy.

---

The role of the laboratory in assisting clinicians in the diagnosis of infection is illustrated in the specimen flow diagram shown in Figure 66.1. The choice of specimen depends on following the principles outlined in Chapter 65. The microbiology laboratory requires enough information on the request card accompanying the specimen to use the optimal methods necessary for identification of potential pathogens in particular infective syndromes. At the most basic level, it is obvious that, when a swab is received in the laboratory, it is necessary to know if it comes from the throat or the vagina! But additional information is also essential: is the patient being investigated for pharyngitis or diphtheria; for vaginal discharge or septic abortion? Furthermore, the specimen must be obtained with care and transported to the laboratory without delay in an appropriate manner. The value of the result is in direct proportion to the attention given to these details, as well as to the skill and efficiency

of the laboratory. For further details of laboratory methods, including specimen containers and culture media used, the reader is encouraged to consult the recommended reading section.

## COLLECTION OF SPECIMENS

Samples for microbiological examination need to be carefully collected, if possible without contamination with commensals or from external sources. Some points to remember with specimens from individual sources are shown in Table 66.1. It is essential to use sterile containers which are leak-proof and able to withstand transportation through the post if necessary. It is more convenient for both the clinician and microbiologist if the laboratory provides request cards, containers and an efficient transport system. There is a need for staff to be aware of safety

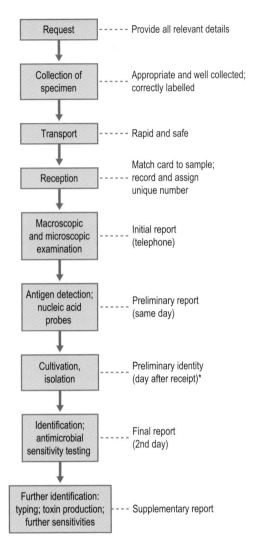

| | |
|---|---|
| Request | - - - - - Provide all relevant details |
| Collection of specimen | - - - - - Appropriate and well collected; correctly labelled |
| Transport | - - - - - Rapid and safe |
| Reception | - - - - - Match card to sample; record and assign unique number |
| Macroscopic and microscopic examination | - - - - - Initial report (telephone) |
| Antigen detection; nucleic acid probes | - - - - - Preliminary report (same day) |
| Cultivation, isolation | - - - - - Preliminary identity (day after receipt)* |
| Identification; antimicrobial sensitivity testing | - - - - - Final report (2nd day) |
| Further identification: typing; toxin production; further sensitivities | - - - - - Supplementary report |

*Viruses, fungi and some bacteria may take longer

**Fig. 66.1** Steps in the isolation and identification of pathogens from an infected patient.

regulations and for all parties to understand who has responsibility for each step of the process and how to minimize handling by untrained people. Special precautions required for 'high-risk' specimens need to be defined by the laboratory and hospital management. Storage of clinical material must be separate from food and drugs, and this may necessitate provision of additional refrigerator space and transport facilities.

### Food, water and environment

The examination of nonclinical specimens is beyond the scope of this book and readers are referred to

appropriate reading. However, an outbreak of gastrointestinal disease inevitably leads to the question of identifying the source and comparing strains isolated. When disease is due to preformed toxins, as with staphylococcal food poisoning, faecal examination is unhelpful, and the diagnosis can only be made by testing the food. Frequently, the offending item has been discarded and the examination of food and water related to specific patients is often unrewarding. Routine sampling of water sources and potentially contaminated food such as poultry at various critical points of production is essential in maintaining good public health. As part of the investigation of an outbreak it may be necessary to collect samples under controlled conditions which can be used as evidence in any prosecution. Laboratories need to be able to receive and process such specimens in an approved way.

## TRANSPORT

Many microbes may perish on transit from the host's body to a laboratory incubator. Some contaminants, especially coliforms, may overgrow the pathogen and so mask its presence. These two constraints make it essential that any material for cultivation of microbes is transported as quickly as possible to the laboratory in a manner expected to protect the viability of any pathogens. Such problems may be minimized by the use of antigen or gene probe detection because of the relative stability of the chemical structures identified on dry swabs.

The ideal situation is to bring the patient to the laboratory for specimen collection or take the laboratory to the clinic. Both approaches are used for special purposes but are obviously inconvenient for many patients and inappropriate and costly for complicated techniques such as virus isolation which need specialized (and safe) facilities.

To overcome any drawbacks due to delay in reaching the microbiology department the following methods may be used:

1. *Transport media.* See Table 66.2.
2. *Boric acid.* The addition of boric acid to urine at a concentration of 1.8% (v/w) will stop bacterial multiplication but lower concentrations are ineffective and higher ones may kill the pathogen.
3. *Dip slides.* These provide a convenient way of inoculating urines at the clinic. They comprise small plastic spoons or strips holding a thin layer of agar which is dipped into the urine and then put in a screw-topped bottle for transport. The agar adsorbs a fixed volume of urine and, after

incubation, colony counts of bacteria give a semiquantitative estimation of numbers.

4. *Refrigeration.* Storage at 4°C before processing will prevent multiplication of most bacteria. However, delicate microbes such as neisseriae may not survive whereas certain organisms, notably listeriae, flourish at low temperatures.

5. *Freezing.* Temperatures of −70°C or below, which can be achieved in liquid nitrogen or special deep freezes, will preserve many microbes, providing

**Table 66.1**  Some important points to remember in the collection of specimens for microbiological examination

| Type of specimen | Comments |
|---|---|
| **Respiratory secretions** | |
| Nasal swab (anterior) | Only for carriage of staphylococci and streptococci |
| Nasopharyngeal swab | For pertussis and meningococci |
| External ear swab | Wide range of microbes, including fungi |
| Myringotomy and sinus samples | As for abscesses – including anaerobes |
| Throat (pharyngeal) swab | Specify if only for streptococci; mention if diphtheria possible; use special transport media for virology |
| Saliva | Used for antibody detection (gingival swab); otherwise discard |
| Laryngeal swab | Specify if for mycobacteria |
| Expectorated sputum | Often poorly collected; specify mycobacteria, legionellae, pneumocystis |
| Transtracheal aspirate, bronchoscopy specimens, lung biopsy | Specify likely diagnosis; ask for specific tests |
| Pleural fluid | Treat as pus; always look for mycobacteria |
| **Gastrointestinal specimens** | |
| Vomitus | Only for virology |
| Gastric washings | For mycobacteria (particularly in children) |
| Gastric biopsy | For *Helicobacter pylori* |
| Duodenal/jejunal aspirates | Protozoa (*Giardia lamblia*, microsporidia, etc.) |
| Liver aspirates | As for pus (anaerobes); consider amoebae |
| Spleen puncture | For *Leishmania* spp. |
| Rectal biopsy | Schistosomiasis |
| Rectal swab | Only for gonococci and chlamydia |
| Colonic biopsy | Histopathological diagnosis of amoebiasis, pseudomembranous colitis (*Clostridium difficile*) |
| Colonic scrapings | Protozoa; amoebic trophozoites (deliver to laboratory immediately) |
| Faeces | Specify possible diagnosis; ask for clostridial toxins, parasite examination if suspected |
| Peri-anal swab | For eggs of threadworm |
| **Urine** | |
| Mid-stream (MSU) | Suitable for most patients |
| Clean catch | Infants and elderly – increased contamination |
| Suprapubic aspirate | Infants and neonates |
| Ureteric/bladder washout | To localize infection |
| Prostatic massage | Collect samples before, during and at end of micturition |
| Terminal urine | Schistosome ova, chlamydia DNA amplification |
| Complete early morning or 24-h urine | Mycobacteria (tubercle) |
| **Central nervous system** | |
| Cerebrospinal fluid by spinal tap | For meningitis collect sample for protein and glucose – test blood sugar simultaneously, specify virology, fungi or syphilis serology |
| Ventricular tap | Specify if through an indwelling shunt or catheter |
| Brain abscess | As for pus (include anaerobes) |
| **Skin and soft tissue** | |
| Skin scraping/nail clipping | Dermatophyte fungi |
| Skin swab | Rarely valuable without pus |
| Skin snips | Onchocerciasis – seek advice |
| Vesicle fluid | Suitable for electron microscopy for viruses |
| Wound swab | Obtain pus if possible; record site |
| Pus, tissues, aspirates | Describe site and any relevant operative details |

**Table 66.1** Continued

| Type of specimen | Comments |
|---|---|
| **Genital** | |
| Urethral swab | Pus for gonococci, scrape for chlamydia |
| Vaginal swab (adult) | Candida, trichomonas, bacterial vaginosis or chlamydia DNA |
| Vaginal swab (prepubertal) | State age; caution required if abuse possible |
| Cervical swab | Separate media for chlamydia |
| Ulcer scrape | Immediate dark-ground microscopy; separate media for virology or chancroid |
| Uterine secretions | Specify puerperium or post-abortion |
| Pelvic aspirates | As for pus |
| Laparoscopy specimens | Include chlamydia specimen |
| **Eye** | |
| Conjunctival swab | Separate virology; scrape for chlamydia |
| Aspirates | As for pus |
| **Blood** | |
| Culture | Strict aseptic technique; take large sample in special media before antibiotics |
| Bone marrow | Valuable for leishmania, mycobacteria, brucella |
| Film | Malaria (thick and thin), filaria, borrelia, trypanosomes |
| Whole blood | Filaria (day or night samples as appropriate) |
| Serum antigen | Rapid diagnosis of many microbial diseases (e.g. hepatitis B) |
| Serum antibody | Retrospective diagnosis of common viral diseases, syphilis and other selected infections; need rising titre or specific IgM |

**Table 66.2** Types of transport medium

| Type of organism | Medium | Comments |
|---|---|---|
| Bacteria | Stuart's semi-solid agar | Contains charcoal to inactivate toxic material |
| Anaerobic bacteria | Various systems, including gassed-out tubes and anaerobic bags | Not widely used, but essential for some strict anaerobes |
| Viruses | Buffered salts solution containing serum | Contains antibiotics to control bacteria and fungi |
| Chlamydiae | Similar to viral transport medium, but without agents that inhibit chlamydiae | Chlamydial antigen media contain detergent to lyse infected cells |
| Protozoa, helminths | Merthiolate–iodine–formalin | Kills active protozoa, but preserves cysts and ova in a form suitable for concentration and microscopy |

they are protected by a stabilizing fluid such as serum or glycerol.

## RECEPTION

The importance of good documentation cannot be overstressed. No matter how well the specimen was taken, transported and processed in the laboratory, the end result depends on communication between people. The clinician making the request must give complete details on the request card and specimen to reduce errors. Staff receiving specimens in the laboratory must match them with the cards and record them into a book or computer. This is usually done by assigning a unique number to each specimen and labelling both the specimen and the request.

When parts of the specimen are separated from the original bottle (e.g. after centrifugation of serum), the laboratory number becomes the only recognizable identification. Transcription errors are far more common than is supposed and are especially important for requests for human immunodeficiency virus (HIV) or syphilis serology, which may have disastrous consequences and medicolegal implications if wrong results are given.

## EXAMINATION

Looking at clinical material with the naked eye or hand-lens should be part of the examination of a patient at the bedside. Sadly, many doctors delegate this to the laboratory staff. Many unnecessary laboratory tests could be avoided if unsuitable specimens were rejected on the ward or in the general practitioner's surgery. These would include: crystal-clear urine from patients with 'cystitis'; well-formed stools from patients with 'diarrhoea'; and mouth washings or saliva from patients with respiratory symptoms.

It was once common practice to carry out certain basic investigations in ward side-rooms, and kits offering 'near-patient testing' are becoming available. However, there are cogent arguments against bedside pathology, including issues of safety, time, competence and quality control.

## Microscopy

Microscopy is an important part of the examination of many specimens. For bacteriology, the Gram and acid-fast (Ziehl–Neelsen or Auramine) stains are usually sufficient, but for the demonstration of fungi or parasites special stains or concentration techniques may be required. 'Wet' mounts, i.e. unstained preparations of fluid material, are widely used in looking at cells in urine, cerebrospinal fluid (CSF), faeces and vaginal secretions. None of these procedures takes more than 5 or 10 min and all are inexpensive in reagent costs and capital equipment. They are therefore ideal rapid methods and new diagnostic techniques have to be judged against microscopy. An initial report, such as 'Gram-negative diplococci and pus cells seen' from meningitic CSF, can be issued within minutes of receiving the specimen and will aid the clinician in confirming the diagnosis and starting appropriate antibiotics.

Similarly, a rapid diagnosis of falciparum malaria can be lifesaving. Indeed, suspected pyogenic meningitis and falciparum malaria are among the few conditions for which it is clearly justifiable to call upon emergency laboratory services outside normal working hours.

Electron microscopy (EM) requires more elaborate preparation than does light microscopy and it is therefore much slower. It was valuable in the diagnosis of certain viral infections, including viral diarrhoea but the availability of antigen (ELISA) and molecular probes has largely replaced EM. The nonspecific nature of electron microscopy gives it an advantage in that any type of viral agent, if present in sufficient numbers, may be recognized.

## Nonculture methods

There are many situations where isolation of microbes in vitro or in tissue culture is impossible or is insufficiently sensitive to make a microbiological diagnosis. Some microbes are so fastidious or slow-growing that useful information cannot be given to clinicians. The isolation of many viruses requires laborious tissue culture methods that are too slow to influence patient management. Microscopy is usually of low sensitivity, e.g. the threshold of detection of acid-fast bacilli in sputum is about $10^5$ microbes per millilitre. Microscopy also has low specificity; for example, Gram staining of faeces would yield millions of Gram-negative rods, but it is not possible to recognize those that are pathogenic by this means.

To overcome these deficiencies probes have been developed which combine a part that reacts with a specific microbial structure and a part that will produce a signal (colour, fluorescence or radioactivity) after the reaction. Many microbes are detectable in this way. Antibodies labelled with fluorescent molecules are widely used in diagnostic virology, e.g. for respiratory secretions to find respiratory syncytial virus. Enzyme-linked antibodies are available as enzyme-linked immunosorbent assay (ELISA) kits for chlamydia detection, and many other *immunoprobes* are commercially produced or under investigation. The explosion in molecular biology has led to the widespread availability of DNA and RNA probes, which have changed from complicated research techniques requiring radioisotopes to relatively simple methods that can be carried out with minimal expertise. Use of amplified nucleic acid tests (e.g. *polymerase chain reaction*, PCR) has greatly increased the sensitivity of probes. Provided a unique sequence of nucleotides is used, the method is highly specific. None the less, as the new technology becomes more commonplace traditional methods will not be discarded. It is more likely that it will complement them.

One of the chief advantages of probes – their specificity – is also one of their major disadvantages. For example, in the investigation of diarrhoea, it would be impossibly laborious to have to use a separate probe for each of the possible microbial causes. Furthermore, use of probes leaves little scope for detection of the unexpected and hampers the discovery of previously unsuspected aetiological agents of disease. The advent of 'chip' technology (*microarrays*) may overcome this deficiency (see Ch. 6).

## Serology

In situations in which microbial isolation is impossible and probes are unavailable, evidence of infection may be obtained by finding a rise in antibody titre or the presence of specific IgM. Serology is still used for diagnosing the causes of 'atypical' pneumonia (mycoplasmal pneumonia, psittacosis, Legionnaires' disease), syphilis, brucellosis and many viral infections, including HIV. It is preferable to take a blood sample early in the illness (the *acute serum*) and another 10–14 days after the onset (the *convalescent serum*); a four-fold or greater rise in antibody titre in the second specimen is diagnostic of acute infection. With some infections, such as HIV and hepatitis B and C, much longer times must elapse.

## Isolation of micro-organisms

The basis of the study of medical microbiology was laid over a century ago by the isolation of microbes in pure culture outside the host animal. The methods used by the fathers of bacteriology have been adapted, simplified and, in some cases, automated for the modern diagnostic laboratory. The principles remain the same: use sterile equipment and media (with cell lines if necessary) and add clinical material. After incubation at 37°C, for a variable time, from a few hours for enterobacteria to weeks for mycobacteria and some viruses and fungi, a visible effect will be produced. This might be colonies growing on agar or a cytopathic effect (CPE) in tissue culture. The skill of microbiology is in identifying the microbes responsible for the effect.

There are limits to the methods that can be used in a routine hospital laboratory to isolate microbes. The choice of media used is dictated by the specimen and by the clinical condition of the patient. For example, in some areas of the world there is little point in looking for *Corynebacterium diphtheriae* in every throat swab, so that the specific media needed are not routinely used. It is therefore incumbent on the doctor to make sure that the laboratory is alerted to look for diphtheria bacilli in any suspicious case. Similarly, clinicians need to know which microbes are routinely sought from particular specimens so that they can make a special request if they suspect the unusual.

'New' causes of illness are often found and new methods of investigating old diseases regularly appear on the market. It is a difficult decision for the laboratory manager to assess at what point a 'new' pathogen becomes sufficiently important to be routinely sought, or to balance the advantages of new (and expensive) technology against cheap and well tried techniques especially in resource poor countries.

## Identification

The full identification of each microbe isolated in a clinical laboratory is both uneconomic and

**Table 66.3** Examples of bacterial identification in medical laboratories

| | Extent of identification | |
|---|---|---|
| Reason for request | Example 1 | Example 2 |
| Test of sterility | Bacteria present | |
| Initial blood culture report | Gram-negative rod | Gram-positive cocci |
| Urine examination | 'Coliforms' | *Staphylococci* |
| Wound swab | *Escherichia coli* | *Staphylococcus aureus* |
| Outbreak epidemiology | *E. coli* O157 | *Staph. aureus* phage type 80/81 |
| Pathogenicity tests | *E. coli* O157 vero toxin-producing | *Staph. aureus* enterotoxin A-positive |

unnecessary. Shortcuts must be made to satisfy the clinical demand of a final report which the doctor can understand and which is available in time to influence management of the patient. In practice, most laboratories use simple and incomplete methods of identification, depending on the level of useful information required. Typing of isolates is for epidemiological or other special reasons, and this is usually done in national reference centres using standardized methods.

Examples of the extent of identification are shown in Table 66.3. This shows that the same organism may not be identified even to the genus level, or it may have extensive genetic investigation depending on the reason for the request. In a cost-conscious climate you get what you pay for and what the service thinks you need!

## Antimicrobial sensitivity testing

One advantage of good bacterial identification is that it helps greatly in choosing antibiotics and in some situations in-vitro tests of susceptibility may be unnecessary. However, the widespread occurrence of bacterial resistance, even in genera such as *Neisseria* and *Haemophilus* in which sensitivity to β-lactam antibiotics was previously assumed, has meant that tests are usually performed on all significant clinical isolates of bacteria. The relevance of information generated in the extremely artificial conditions of the laboratory is discussed in Chapter 67.

As there are technical problems in carrying out sensitivity tests at the same time as the primary culture, the report will be delayed for at least 24 h after isolation of the pathogen. Tests of slow-growing bacteria such as mycobacteria take much longer and tests involving fungi, viruses and protozoa are not ordinarily available. In general, all patients with acute symptoms will receive treatment before the report returns to the doctor so that the result will merely confirm that correct treatment had been chosen. Sometimes, the laboratory report will allow speculative antimicrobial therapy to be modified, e.g. by allowing one or more drugs in a precautionary mixture to be discontinued.

A frequent difficulty facing microbiologists is which, out of a rapidly increasing number of agents, should be tested and, of those tested, which should be reported. Most laboratories test a few representative compounds from among the many penicillins, cephalosporins, aminoglycosides, tetracyclines, quinolones, etc., and restrict those reported to the clinician to two or three agents selected for their appropriateness in the particular infection. In this way, institutional antibiotic policies are reinforced and the impact of the promotional activities of pharmaceutical companies is lessened.

## REPORTS OF RESULTS

Just as it is important to obtain as accurate a result as possible, so it is vital to transfer the information rapidly to the user of the laboratory in a form that is easily intelligible. Laboratory workers need to tailor their reports to suit their customers and to recognize their needs. Trained microbiologists are used to the vagaries of microbial taxonomy and the profusion of antibiotics with similar names, but physicians and surgeons are easily confused by laboratory jargon and changes in nomenclature. On the other hand, clinicians rightly expect laboratory reports to be explicit and helpful. As in so many spheres of health care, a spirit of mutual respect and cooperation is in the best interests of the patients, and this is most likely to happen if microbiologists regularly visit the wards and if clinicians are encouraged to discuss problems with laboratory staff.

In these days of computers and facsimile machines it is attractive to use the latest technology to transfer results, but the personal touch is essential, particularly for important results such as positive blood or CSF cultures. Clinicians dealing with difficult problems enjoy the reassurance that the laboratory has found the cause of a patient's illness and advice on management is generally well received. Seeing the problem for oneself and discussing it with the responsible doctors is the ideal. The telephone is a satisfactory substitute in many cases and is far preferable to a report form printed by a computer and arriving after the crisis is over. It behoves us all to communicate better and faster.

**Box 66.1** List of notifiable diseases in England and Wales

- Acute encephalitis/meningitis
- Acute infectious hepatitis
- Acute poliomyelitis
- Anthrax
- Botulism
- Brucellosis
- Cholera
- Diphtheria
- Dysentery (amoebic or bacillary)
- Enteric fever (paratyphoid/typhoid)
- Food poisoning
- Haemolytic uraemic syndrome
- Infectious bloody diarrhoea
- Invasive Group A streptococcal disease and scarlet fever
- Legionnaires' disease
- Leprosy
- Malaria
- Measles
- Meningococcal septicaemia
- Mumps
- Plague
- Rabies
- Rubella
- SARS
- Smallpox
- Tetanus
- Tuberculosis
- Typhus
- Viral haemorrhagic fever
- Whooping cough
- Yellow fever

Health Protection Regulations 2010.

## NOTIFICATION OF INFECTIOUS DISEASES

In addition to making a clinical diagnosis and treating the individual there is a need with some infectious diseases to determine the source and prevent further spread. In some countries there are public health laws specifying the method of reporting these. The list of *notifiable diseases* in England and Wales is shown in Box 66.1. This reporting system requires a clinical diagnosis, with or without laboratory confirmation, which is notified separately. In England and Wales each health district has a consultant responsible for communicable disease control, who is usually the 'proper officer' for the local government authority. Notifications are sent to the Health Protection Agency (HPA), previously the Communicable Disease Surveillance Centre (CDSC).

There is also an obligation, which in some circumstances may be statutory, for laboratories to report isolates of certain pathogens to central authorities for surveillance purposes. For HIV/AIDS infection the system is voluntary and confidential, yet over 90% of cases are reported in the UK. In an outbreak, or where the pathogen is highly infectious, it is essential for the head of the laboratory to inform both the clinician looking after the patient and local public health staff. In this way a coordinated approach can be made

to prevent further spread of infection. In particular, if there is any indication that the infection may have been acquired by staff working in the laboratory this must be reported to the relevant authority; in the UK that is the Health and Safety Executive.

---

## RECOMMENDED READING

American Society for Microbiology: *Manual of Clinical Microbiology*, ed 10, Washington, DC, 2011, American Society for Microbiology.

Forbes BA, Sahm DF, Weissfeld AS: *Bailey and Scott's Diagnostic Microbiology*, ed 10, St Louis, 2002, Mosby.

Johnson FB: Transport of viral specimens, *Clinical Microbiology Reviews* 3:120–131, 1990.

# 67 Strategy of antimicrobial chemotherapy

*R. C. B. Slack*

## KEY POINTS

- A central aim in choosing antimicrobial therapy is to match the most appropriate agent to the specific microbial aetiology. In practice, this is constrained by urgency of the situation, the diagnostic information available and policy decisions about antimicrobial use that are made on a local basis consistent with national policies.
- The initial decision on whether or not to give an antimicrobial and on the agent chosen is generally made before microbiological information is available but, where possible, after microbiological samples have been taken.
- In the UK, local and specific guidance is generally available for chemotherapy of common infective syndromes. The strategy reflects the likely causal agents and their local susceptibility patterns, the need to control antimicrobial resistance, and cost. This guidance is reflected in the local *antibiotic policy*.
- The laboratory will assist in modifying or initiating therapy by determining in vitro susceptibilities and by monitoring antimicrobial drug concentrations in specific circumstances. These analyses may lead to modification of therapy.
- Certain organisms such as streptococci and anaerobes have predictable susceptibilities, whereas others, such as enterobacteria, must be monitored continuously.
- Prophylactic antimicrobials are recommended in highly defined settings and when following precise regimens. Ad hoc usage is to be avoided.
- Antimicrobial combinations may be given to increase efficacy, extend the spectrum of cover or prevent the development of resistance during therapy.

In the previous chapter the work of the laboratory in assisting doctors in making a definitive microbiological diagnosis was described and summarized in Figure 66.1. Ideally, management of an infection should involve these stages plus choice of an appropriate antimicrobial agent (if necessary) and follow-up tests of cure. Chapter 5 listed the different classes of antimicrobial agents from which the doctor may prescribe. The objectives of an antibiotic strategy are to implement clinical guidelines that cover the treatment of an individual patient and policies based on these will have a maximum public health effect. These include cost-effectiveness and limiting the spread of antibiotic resistance.

## CHOICE OF TREATMENT

Infections are so common in general practice that it is not practical for each patient to be fully investigated and a rational choice of antimicrobial agent made on the results. Because many have a viral aetiology and most respond rapidly to simple symptomatic relief, the choice is not which agent to use but whether to prescribe at all. Many patients who make the effort to see a doctor expect drug treatment. Although the time taken to educate the public and convince the individual is often longer than that needed to write a prescription, it is important that prescribers do not yield to pressure if antibiotics are not indicated. Figure 67.1 shows a flow diagram of choice of antibiotics that is applicable to many common conditions. There are three main points in the diagram:

1. Patients may be categorized on clinical grounds into those with mild, moderate or severe infection and also into those who were previously healthy or have underlying disease that may affect their

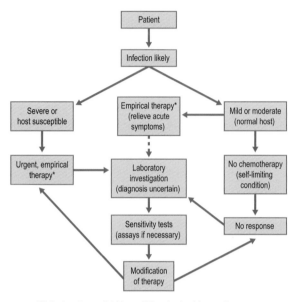

*Choice based on predictable sensitivity or local resistance patterns.
Broken line indicates a course of action that will depend on circumstances

**Fig. 67.1**  General strategy of antimicrobial chemotherapy.

response to therapy; for example, impaired immunity or the presence of a foreign body. In the latter situation it is more important to send specimens to the laboratory and start empirical therapy to cover likely pathogens.

2. The organisms causing many common clinical syndromes have predictable antibiotic sensitivities, allowing a rational choice to be made.

3. The results of laboratory tests may lead to modification or withdrawal of chemotherapy.

Although 'best guess' or empirical therapy is commenced before the results of laboratory tests are available, it is wrong to argue that this approach is incorrect since early administration of an antimicrobial is sometimes life-saving.

## LABORATORY MONITORING

### Susceptibility tests

As well as providing routine tests of sensitivity on individual isolates, the laboratory should provide a general picture of the prevalence of different pathogens occurring in the local population and their pattern of resistance. Different lists should be prepared and regularly circulated to general practitioners, hospital consultants and specialized units. The

methods used and limitations of susceptibility testing are outlined in Chapter 5. Sometimes individual patients will need to be monitored for the efficacy of treatment and to determine if failure has occurred due to acquired resistance or replacement with a more resistant organism. This is especially important in the assessment of new agents in clinical trials.

### Antibiotic assay

Rapid methods are now available to determine the amount of antibiotic in serum and other body fluids during treatment. These assays can be used to monitor the adequacy of dosage or to avoid possible toxic effects of overdosage.

In practice, it is necessary to carry out such assays only in a small minority of patients who are seriously ill with infections such as endocarditis or those receiving potentially toxic agents such as aminoglycosides and vancomycin. Urine samples may be screened for antibacterial activity. This can be of value in determining patient compliance during therapy for tuberculosis.

The interpretation of the results of antibiotic assays may be difficult if the patient is receiving multiple antibiotics. In such cases, the power of the body fluid to inhibit or kill the infecting organism in vitro may be a more useful measurement of adequate dosage; for example, in bacterial endocarditis, the patient's serum should kill the causative organism at a dilution of 1 in 4 or more.

It is important to know the relationship of the sample being assayed to the time of dosage: maximum or *peak* levels are usually measured in serum 0.5–1 h following a dose; minimum or *trough* levels are from a sample taken shortly before the next dose.

Assays should always be carried out in close collaboration with the microbiologist to ensure the correct timing of samples and to avoid errors of interpretation.

### Clinical correlation of laboratory tests

The epithet *sensitive* or *resistant* is a clinical description; in laboratory tests it is usual to select a concentration of the agent which is known to be easily attained in serum, other body fluids or tissue after normal recommended dosage. Organisms susceptible to this, or lower concentrations, are regarded as sensitive; those able to grow are resistant. These terms relate to the *minimum inhibitory concentration* (MIC) of the microbe (see p. 66). The correlation between this interpretation and clinical results is generally good, but not perfect. Discrepancies may be due to a failure to attain adequate concentrations at the site of infection, resulting in clinical failure. However, there are many factors on which the outcome of the host–parasite relationship in infection depends, and it would be surprising if a complete correlation between in-vitro tests and the results of chemotherapy was observed.

## PREDICTABLE SENSITIVITY

Once the identity of an infecting organism is known, the sensitivity pattern is often predictable with a fair degree of accuracy. Not surprisingly, however, the susceptibility of common pathogens may change with time. Thus, predictable sensitivity of micro-organisms, while useful, is a changing concept and will have local variations, so that the advice of local microbiologists should be sought.

### Organisms with predictable sensitivity patterns

*Streptococcus pyogenes* is a good example of an organism that has retained a sensitivity pattern that has changed little in 70 years. Thus, penicillin is always the drug of choice for the treatment of haemolytic streptococcal infections. Other β-lactam antibiotics are also active against *Str. pyogenes*. Erythromycin is an alternative if the patient cannot be given penicillin because of allergy, but an increasing number of strains in some areas show some resistance to this antibiotic in vitro.

Until recently, most strains of *Str. pneumoniae* were highly sensitive to penicillin. An increasing number of penicillin-resistant pneumococci are now found in cases of invasive disease in some institutions, and are posing a major problem worldwide. Fortunately, this is much rarer with strains of *N. meningitidis* which appear to be penicillin-sensitive in most places.

Reproducible patterns of sensitivity to antimicrobial drugs can be shown for many other groups of bacteria and offer a useful guide to the choice of chemotherapy (Table 67.1). However, exceptions to these patterns occur and resistant variants may become prevalent in some localities, particularly under the pressure of intensive antibiotic usage.

In the same way that organisms may exhibit predictable sensitivity to some agents, they may be predictably resistant. Some examples are shown in Table 67.2.

## ORGANISMS OF VARIABLE SENSITIVITY

Many groups of pathogenic bacteria, notably staphylococci and enterobacteria, vary unpredictably in

**Table 67.1** Examples of organisms and antimicrobial agents for which susceptibility is usually predictable

| Organism | Antimicrobial agents normally active |
| --- | --- |
| Streptococci | Penicillin, erythromycin, vancomycin |
| Enterococci | Ampicillin, vancomycin |
| Anaerobic cocci | Penicillin, erythromycin, metronidazole |
| Staphylococci | Flucloxacillin, clindamycin, fusidic acid, gentamicin, vancomycin |
| *Haemophilus influenzae* | Co-amoxiclav, tetracycline, cefotaxime, erythromycin |
| *Escherichia coli* *Proteus mirabilis* | Gentamicin, cefotaxime, co-amoxiclav, ciprofloxacin |
| *Pseudomonas aeruginosa* | Gentamicin, ceftazidime, azlocillin, ciprofloxacin, imipenem |
| *Bacteroides fragilis* | Metronidazole, cefoxitin, co-amoxiclav |
| Rickettsiae Chlamydiae | Tetracyclines, macrolides, rifampicin |
| Mycoplasmas | Tetracyclines, erythromycin |
| *Candida albicans* | Nystatin, amphotericin B, azoles |
| Herpes simplex virus | Aciclovir |

**Table 67.2** Examples of organisms and antimicrobial agents for which resistance is usually predictable

| Organism | Antimicrobial agents *NOT* normally active |
| --- | --- |
| Streptococci Enterococci | Aminoglycosides, nalidixic acid, aztreonam |
| Staphylococci | Most penicillins[a], nalidixic acid, aztreonam |
| *Escherichia coli* | Penicillin, vancomycin, erythromycin, metronidazole |
| *Klebsiella* spp. | Most penicillins, erythromycin, metronidazole |
| *Pseudomonas aeruginosa* | Most penicillins and cephalosporins, erythromycin, metronidazole |
| Anaerobes | Aminoglycosides, aztreonam, nalidixic acid, fluoroquinolones |

[a]Except isoxazolylpenicillins.

their sensitivity to antimicrobial drugs. With these organisms there is a greater need to carry out sensitivity tests on individual isolates.

### Staphylococci

Staphylococci, including coagulase-negative strains, show great variability in susceptibility, and this can severely limit choice of antibiotics. Four main kinds of staphylococci may be encountered:

1. *Penicillin-sensitive strains.* Before the widespread use of penicillin in the 1940s, most *Staphylococcus aureus* isolates were sensitive. Usually these strains are susceptible to other antistaphylococcal agents (macrolides,

aminoglycosides and fusidic acid). Penicillin-sensitive strains now account for about 10% of isolates.

2. *β-Lactamase-producing strains*. Staphylococcal penicillinase confers resistance to all penicillins except methicillin, the isoxazolyl group (cloxacillin, etc.) and nafcillin. These strains usually retain susceptibility to cephalosporins. Most *Staph. aureus* and *Staph. epidermidis* strains found in clinical practice belong to this group.

3. *Methicillin-resistant strains* (MRSA). Methicillin, the first penicillinase-stable penicillin, is used as the test compound to identify these strains in the laboratory. Strains of *Staph. aureus* resistant to methicillin are also resistant to virtually all β-lactam agents. MRSA have epidemiological significance as a group and have been isolated from hospital outbreaks in different countries. Many of these epidemic strains are multiresistant, exhibiting resistance to aminoglycosides, macrolides and other antistaphylococcal agents, including the topical compound, mupirocin, which has been used to eradicate the organism from carriers of MRSA. Vancomycin, teicoplanin or linezolid may be the only agents available for treatment.

4. *Other antibiotic-resistant strains*. Multiple resistance to antistaphylococcal antibiotics may be seen in strains that are methicillin-sensitive. They are found in similar situations to MRSA, namely hospital units with severely debilitated patients and problems with cross-infection. Such resistance patterns are more common in coagulase-negative staphylococci.

## Enterobacteria

*Escherichia coli* includes many strains of variable sensitivity, but among the general population in the UK half of the strains isolated from urinary tract infections are sensitive to ampicillin and amoxicillin, and an even higher proportion are sensitive to cephalosporins, co-amoxiclav (the combination of amoxicillin and clavulanic acid) and trimethoprim.

Variable sensitivity is also a feature of other enterobacteria. There has been an increase in *E. coli* resistant to expanded spectrum β-lactams (ESBLs) in many countries. Where these organisms are also quinolone and trimethoprim resistant, treatment with oral agents is limited. Multiresistant typhoid is a particular problem in many countries where the disease is endemic. If there is doubt about the clinical response, or the sensitivity of the strain, laboratory tests should be carried out.

## Other organisms

Several pathogens which were formerly reliably sensitive to standard agents, including neisseriae, *Haemophilus influenzae*, pneumococci, enterococci, mycobacteria and *Plasmodium falciparum*, are now commonly resistant to first-line therapy. In some cases, options for treatment of infection with these organisms have become severely constrained.

## ANTIBIOTIC POLICIES AND THE CONTROL OF RESISTANCE

The benefits of the use of antibiotics, not only in medicine but also in animal husbandry, must be taken into account in considering the merits of restrictive policies undertaken to control antibiotic resistance.

There is, without doubt, a problem of resistance among many commonly occurring micro-organisms. However, most of the problems of resistance occur among patients within closed communities such as hospitals. This is most marked in areas of intensive care, where large amounts of antibiotics are used in highly susceptible patients with low immunity to infection. In the general community, multiple resistances to antibiotics is presently not a major problem in the UK, but the spread of MRSA out of hospitals into nursing and residential homes may herald a change in this situation.

Accordingly, attention should be directed to those hospital units in which the problem of resistance is significant and which may be the most important source of spread to the general community. As resistance in bacteria has many of the features of an epidemic disease, the application of classic rules and precautions for the prevention of infection may halt this spread.

## Restrictive policies

The use of antibiotics by general practitioners and clinicians is influenced by the prescribing habits of other medical colleagues and by the promotional efforts of the pharmaceutical companies. Thus, an ordered and systematic use of antimicrobial drugs might be of benefit in the general strategy of chemotherapy. Since the use of antibiotics acts as a powerful selective factor in the emergence and spread of resistant micro-organisms, restriction of use should have the opposite effect. The acceptance of this thesis has encouraged restrictive policies involving temporary bans on the use of certain antibiotics. Such policies

**Table 67.3**   Main groups of antibiotics available for clinical use

| Antibacterial agent | Route of administration | Antibacterial spectrum[a] | Some indications for therapy |
|---|---|---|---|
| Phenoxymethylpenicillin | O | + | Streptococcal infections |
| Benzylpenicillin | P | + | Community-acquired pneumonias or meningitis |
| Ampicillin | O, P | + and − | Respiratory, hepatic, biliary infections |
| Amoxicillin | | | |
| Flucloxacillin | O, P | + | Staphylococcal infections |
| Co-amoxiclav | O, P | + and − | Infections due to β-lactamase-producing organisms |
| Imipenem | P | + and − | Serious infections with mixed organisms |
| Cephalosporins | O, P | + and − | Respiratory and urinary infections; staphylococcal infections |
| Aminoglycosides | P | − | Gram-negative coliform infections; endocarditis (with penicillin); pseudomonas infections |
| Macrolides | O, P | + | Streptococcal and staphylococcal infections and those due to legionellae, campylobacters, chlamydiae and coxiellae |
| Tetracyclines | O, P | + and − | Respiratory infections and those due to chlamydiae, mycoplasmas and rickettsiae |
| Chloramphenicol | O, P | + and − | Serious infections due to *Haemophilus influenzae*, salmonellae and rickettsiae |
| Fusidic acid | O, T | + | Staphylococcal infections |
| Glycopeptides | O, P | + | Resistant staphylococcal infections; *Clostridium difficile* enteritis |
| Trimethoprim | O, P | + and − | Urinary and respiratory infections; salmonellosis |
| Co-trimoxazole | | | |
| Imidazoles | O, P | + and − | Anaerobic infections |
| Sulphonamides | O, T | + and − | Intestinal and eye infections |
| Fluoroquinolones | O, P | + and − | Urinary infections; pseudomonal infections; salmonellosis |

O, oral; P, parenteral; T, topical; +, active mainly against Gram-positive bacteria; −, active mainly against Gram-negative bacteria.
[a]See also Table 5.1, p. 55.

---

may also lead to a reduced chance of prescription error and some cost benefits.

## Rotational policies

Periodic changes of antibiotics used in treatment might also help to avoid the emergence of resistant strains by altering the selective pressures and discouraging opportunistic pathogens such as *Pseudomonas* and *Acinetobacter* species. Such a rotational policy might help to retain the therapeutic value of antibiotics over a longer period. The availability of a large range of clinically useful antibacterial substances (Table 67.3) makes this kind of policy more practicable.

## PROPHYLACTIC USE OF ANTIBIOTICS

The unnecessary prophylactic use of antibiotics should be discouraged as this may result in increased selection of resistant variants or superinfection with resistant flora. However, there are several circumstances in which chemoprophylaxis is clearly beneficial.

A widely accepted use of antimicrobial agents for the prevention of infection is in patients who have suffered from rheumatic fever, or are thought otherwise to be at risk of rheumatic carditis to prevent further streptococcal infection. Among other indications for chemoprophylaxis are the use of peri-operative antibiotics in patients undergoing joint replacement to reduce the chance of potentially disastrous infection. Similarly, patients undergoing lower bowel resection receive peri-operative treatment with combinations of agents intended to suppress the lower bowel flora. The clinical and laboratory evidence for the benefit of these kinds of prophylaxis is now well established.

Chemoprophylaxis is also justified in preventing pneumococcal infection in splenectomized patients and pneumocystis pneumonia in people with human immunodeficiency virus (HIV). In healthy individuals who are close contacts of infectious diseases such as meningococcal meningitis, short courses of antibiotics are justified to prevent acquisition of the organism or to eradicate carrier status. Travellers to regions in which malaria is endemic should take antimalarial prophylaxis.

## HOST FACTORS INFLUENCING RESPONSE

In most individuals with normal immune systems an antimicrobial drug assists in a more rapid recovery from infection, but the choice of agent is often not critical providing it has some effect on the causative organisms. In very serious infections or when the patient is at a disadvantage because of impaired or absent immunity, the role of the antibiotic becomes more important and more care should be taken in its selection, dosage and administration.

### Problems of toxicity

The final choice of the most appropriate antimicrobial drug may be influenced by the history and response of the patient. Known hypersensitivity to a drug such as penicillin means that neither this antibiotic nor other penicillins can be safely given and alternatives must be used. Side-effects such as nausea, vomiting, diarrhoea or pruritis may be severe enough to warrant a change in treatment. Some antibiotics have potentially serious side-effects, such as the ototoxicity of the aminoglycosides, and care must be taken to avoid these by laboratory monitoring of drug levels, as such toxicity is usually dose-related. Intercurrent disease may require modification of the dosage of certain antibiotics because of specific organ deficiency, e.g. liver failure or impaired renal function. Ototoxicity of the aminoglycosides must always be borne in mind in patients who have poor renal function.

### Failure to reach the site of infection

The absorption of oral antibiotics varies widely from patient to patient and, if poor, may be a cause of treatment failure. Alternatively, infection may be localized within a large collection of pus or at an anatomical site that is penetrated by antibiotics with difficulty. Obstruction to the flow of body fluids may likewise militate against success; this is important in infections of the urinary tract, biliary system and central nervous system. In some of these cases more radical interference may be indicated to relieve the obstruction.

### Alteration of normal flora

Antibiotic therapy may upset the patient's microflora and result not only in the selection of resistant strains of commensals, such as staphylococci on the skin, or *E. coli* in the intestinal tract, but also colonization with species not normally present. This can lead to antibiotic-induced infection, such as candidosis. Diarrhoea is frequently associated with antibiotic therapy, and reflects disturbance of the normal bowel flora. In a few patients the clinical condition can be severe and proceed to pseudomembranous colitis associated with the toxins of *Clostridium difficile* (see p. 254).

### Intravenous administration

When antibiotics are given intravenously, they should normally be administered directly into the vein and not added to other infusion fluids; otherwise adequate blood levels of the drug may not be attained owing to excretion outpacing administration. There is also the possibility of incompatibility between the antibiotic and the contents of the fluid. In all cases, the manufacturer's instructions and recommendations about the administration of the drug should be closely followed.

## COMBINATIONS OF ANTIBIOTICS

The clinical benefits of the use of combinations of antibacterial agents tend to be exaggerated. The combination of two or more agents has been long accepted in the treatment of tuberculosis, so limiting the selection of mutants resistant to the individual components. The use of β-lactam antibiotics with an aminoglycoside in the treatment of streptococcal endocarditis is also accepted, as the mixture is more bactericidal than the individual components.

A combination of a β-lactam antibiotic with a β-lactamase inhibitor may prevent destruction of the antibiotic. Thus, the enzyme inhibitor clavulanic acid in combination with amoxicillin (co-amoxiclav) restores the activity of the antibiotic against many β-lactamase-producing bacteria.

Potentiation of the antibacterial effect by combinations is referred to as *synergy*; some combinations exhibit a lesser effect than the individual components, and this is called *antagonism*. These interactions are generally displayed in vitro, and it is difficult to establish evidence of advantages or disadvantages in the patient. Thus, the combination of trimethoprim and sulphamethoxazole (co-trimoxazole) can be shown to be synergistic in the test tube, but it has been difficult to demonstrate any clinical benefit, and trimethoprim is now often used on its own to avoid the chance of toxic reactions to sulphonamides.

## ANTIVIRAL THERAPY

An increasing number of agents are being used in the prophylaxis or treatment of viral infections (see Ch. 5).

Aciclovir is the most widely used agent at present, and is prescribed for the treatment of herpes simplex and herpes zoster. This drug can be given orally, but in severely ill patients it is administered intravenously; for example, in treating herpes encephalitis. Aciclovir is also used in the prophylaxis and treatment of varicella, particularly in immunocompromised patients. The related compound ganciclovir is available for the treatment of cytomegalovirus infection, but is associated with considerable toxicity.

Amantadine is active against influenza A virus, but not against influenza B virus. This drug, and the related rimantadine, have been chiefly used for the prophylaxis of influenza. Zanamivir and oseltamivir are active against both A and B viruses and have been used to modify infection and prevent spread of influenza.

Ribavirin (tribavirin) is useful in the treatment of respiratory syncytial virus infections in children, hepatitis B and C (in combination with interferon) and some haemorrhagic fever viruses, such as Lassa fever.

Zidovudine (azidothymidine) is an inhibitor of HIV and was the first drug used in the management of patients with acquired immune deficiency syndrome (AIDS). There are now a number of other antiretroviral agents used in combination (see Ch. 55).

## ANTIFUNGAL THERAPY

Superficial fungal infections are very common. Systematic fungal disease is relatively rare in the UK, except in patients who are immunosuppressed or otherwise compromised. There are few effective antifungal agents that can be used systemically (see Table 5.4, p. 61 and Ch. 61) and some have considerable toxicity.

For many years the chemotherapy of superficial fungal infections depended on preparations of benzoic, salicylic or undecanoic acid. More effective is griseofulvin, given orally, sometimes over long periods, for the treatment of dermatophytoses; the new allylamine, terbinafine, seems to be at least as effective in these conditions. Nystatin and other polyenes are used for the topical treatment of superficial candidosis (thrush). Imidazoles such as clotrimazole are also used in the treatment of vaginal yeast infections.

Amphotericin B is used parenterally for the treatment of systemic candidosis, cryptococccal infections and aspergillosis. Flucytosine is also active against yeasts and has been used in combination with amphotericin B. Amphotericin B is toxic and treatment has to be carefully monitored to obtain the most satisfactory clinical results. Liposomal formulations of the drug appear to be safer and more effective.

The increasing range of antifungal agents used to treat human infections are described in Chapter 61. These are being used more widely in the treatment of systemic fungal disease because of their relative lack of toxicity, although the development of resistance may be a problem. This includes ketoconazole, and triazoles such as itraconazole, fluconazole, voriconazole and posiconazole and the echinocardins (caspofungin and micafungin).

## CHEMOTHERAPY OF SYSTEMIC INFECTIONS

### Serious generalized infection

Patients with serious and often overwhelming generalized infection include those with *bacterial shock syndrome* and others with the symptomatology of acute infection without localizing signs. These syndromes may be related to postoperative infection, to instrumentation, or to the aggravation of a previously mild infection (e.g. extension of a middle ear infection to the brain). Generalized infection may also follow a reduction in the natural resistance of the patient. Such a situation may arise in renal failure, immune deficiency states, blood dyscrasias and neoplastic disease. Specific measures used in the treatment of these diseases may further reduce resistance to infection and the clinical features characteristic of infection may be muted or absent.

Appropriate specimens should be submitted to the laboratory before treatment is begun, in an effort to isolate the causative organisms. However, these patients may require immediate treatment and often there will be little indication of the nature of the infecting organism; more than one species may be involved, especially when the source of the infection is within the abdomen. Empirical chemotherapy must therefore cover Gram-positive cocci, Gram-negative bacilli and anaerobes such as bacteroides. A combination of amoxicillin, an aminoglycoside and metronidazole is suitable. Co-amoxiclav improves the spectrum of amoxicillin and allows omission of the metronidazole. Alternatively, an expanded-spectrum cephalosporin such as cefotaxime can be used. Therapy may be subsequently changed according to the results of laboratory tests. If the patient fails to respond after treatment for 3 days, the use of alternative agents should be considered.

In some patients in intensive care and in the immunocompromised, the possibility of systematic fungal infection or activation of dormant viruses, such as cytomegalovirus, must be considered.

It must always be remembered that bacterial toxins are unaffected by antibacterial therapy. Supportive treatment will include correction of fluid and electrolyte imbalance and appropriate treatment of any co-existing organ failure. In future, immunotherapy such as the use of anti-endotoxins and drugs that alter the cytokine and clotting cascades may find a place in treatment.

## Infective endocarditis

Whenever possible, treatment of endocarditis should be related to the results of sensitivity tests made on the organism isolated from the blood. Formerly, viridans streptococci were the most common isolates and penicillin was the drug of choice. Viridans streptococci are now isolated from only about one-third of patients and the organisms from the remainder are usually relatively resistant to penicillin. Bactericidal therapy with penicillin in combination with an aminoglycoside is usually indicated. It is sometimes helpful to carry out bactericidal tests against the causative organism and it may also be useful to monitor the progress of the patient by assays of the bactericidal activity of the serum against the causative organism.

After operations for the replacement of heart valves it may be difficult to isolate an organism and there may be doubt as to whether or not infection has become superimposed. The risk of withholding treatment, however, is so great that empirical treatment may be indicated, and as staphylococcal infection may occur in such circumstances, it is best to include an antistaphylococcal antibiotic. Injecting drug users are also prone to staphylococcal endocarditis.

For the prevention of bacterial endocarditis in patients at risk following dental extraction, 3 g of amoxicillin, given orally 1 h before surgery, is recommended.

Rare causes of infective endocarditis in which blood cultures are negative include infections with *Coxiella burnetti* or certain chlamydiae. The diagnosis of these conditions depends largely upon serological evidence as it is difficult to isolate the organisms. An aetiological diagnosis is important, as treatment with an appropriate antibiotic, usually tetracycline, may be life-saving.

## Urinary tract infections

### Uncomplicated cystitis

Uncomplicated urinary infections and asymptomatic bacteriuria are common in adolescent and adult women seen in general practice and maternity clinics. Most infections are due to *E. coli*, and most are sensitive to a wide range of drugs. In most cases eradication of the organism is achieved after a short course of therapy with an oral agent such as trimethoprim. The remainder will often respond to a second course of treatment, but if the bacteriuria still persists, fuller urological investigation is required as failure of treatment is more usually related to an abnormality of the urinary system than to resistance of the organism.

### Infections following catheterization

Infection of the urinary tract sometimes occurs after instrumentation such as catheterization or cystoscopy; it is almost unavoidable if indwelling catheters are used. Often the strains causing these infections are derived from the hospital environment, and include resistant strains of Gram-negative bacilli, sometimes in mixed culture. Frequently, the patient is not greatly inconvenienced by such infection, and chemotherapy is not indicated in most areas. If therapy is required, elimination of the organisms can be difficult, particularly if there is residual pathology or a degree of urinary obstruction. Sensitivity tests must be carried out to assist in the choice of therapy. The most useful agents are cephalosporins, trimethoprim and ciprofloxacin; for more serious or refractory cases, in which there is the hazard of systemic spread of the infection, parenteral treatment with an aminoglycoside or an expanded-spectrum cephalosporin must be considered.

### Recurrent infection

In chronic pyelonephritis and recurrent bacteriuria it may be important to control infection by continuous treatment with antibiotics such as trimethoprim. Unfortunately, some patients may become re-infected with resistant species so that alternative drugs must be used. Thus, long-term therapy may require periodic bacteriological reassessment and sensitivity tests on the flora isolated to indicate when changes in therapy are required.

## Respiratory infections

Respiratory tract infections are extremely common, and, although many are primary virus infections, those that are more severe and prolonged usually indicate secondary bacterial invasion. Laboratory diagnosis of these conditions is important since effective treatment depends on use of an antibiotic specifically active against the causative organisms.

## Upper respiratory tract infections

A number of bacteria may be associated with sore throat, pharyngitis and sinusitis, including *Str. pyogenes, Str. pneumoniae, H. influenzae* and Vincent's organisms. The most important infections from the point of view of the development of sequelae are those due to *Str. pyogenes*, for which the treatment of choice is penicillin given for at least 7 days to ensure eradication of the organism. All the other important bacterial pathogens will also respond to this treatment, with the exception of *H. influenzae*, for which treatment with amoxicillin, tetracycline, co-trimoxazole or erythromycin is appropriate.

If for some reason penicillin cannot be prescribed, the antibiotic of choice is erythromycin or co-trimoxazole. Ampicillin and amoxicillin should be avoided if there is any likelihood of glandular fever because these antibiotics tend to cause a rash and prolong the disease. Tetracyclines should be avoided in young children because of the risk of discoloration of developing teeth.

## Lower respiratory tract infections

Lobar pneumonia is most frequently caused by pneumococci and penicillin is the drug of choice; erthyromycin or cefotaxime are good alternatives as are some of the newer fluoroquinolones such as levofloxacin. Infections due to klebsiellae or other organisms will require treatment with antibiotics according to the results of sensitivity tests; cefotaxime or cefuroxime are usually effective if laboratory confirmation is not available. Other coliform bacilli are rarely involved in pulmonary infections although they often colonize the upper respiratory tract; they seldom require specific treatment.

Among atypical pneumonias, mycoplasma infections respond best to a tetracycline or erythromycin; legionella infections respond to macrolides, alone or combined with rifampicin.

Bronchopneumonia is most frequently associated with pneumococci or haemophilus, so that amoxicillin, tetracycline or trimethoprim should be effective. More rarely, bronchopneumonia is caused by *Staph. aureus*, and flucloxacillin, fusidic acid or clindamycin is urgently required for treatment.

Acute exacerbations of chronic bronchitis are almost invariably associated with either *Str. pneumoniae* or *H. influenzae*. Amoxicillin, tetracycline or trimethoprim is usually effective.

In bronchiectasis, lung abscess or cystic fibrosis, antimicrobial treatment should be prescribed according to laboratory culture and sensitivity test results. Combinations of antibiotics may be effective in some of these patients. In pulmonary tuberculosis, combination treatment, usually with rifampicin, isoniazid and pyrazinamide, is mandatory.

## Meningitis

A Gram film and cell count of cerebrospinal fluid (CSF) will usually differentiate viral from bacterial meningitis. If bacteria cannot be seen, initial treatment is with cefotaxime or ceftriaxone. This choice ensures adequate treatment of infections with Gram-negative bacilli (most common in neonates) and of infections with *Neisseria meningitidis, H. influenzae* and *Str. pneumoniae*, which are the most common causes of meningitis in young children. Care must be taken to differentiate *Listeria monocytogenes* infection, as this organism is less sensitive to penicillin and cefotaxime; a combination of amoxicillin and gentamicin is usually used.

When the causative organism is isolated, therapy may be altered to penicillin for meningococcal or pneumococcal infections. *Pseudomonas aeruginosa* meningitis may occasionally occur as a nosocomial infection and should be treated with full doses of gentamicin plus a β-lactam agent such as azlocillin. It is rarely necessary to give intrathecal antibiotics.

Where there is increased CSF pressure, as in spina bifida, shunts are inserted to facilitate the circulation of fluid. These often become contaminated, usually with staphylococci, probably derived from the skin. Antistaphylococcal antibiotics are used to control the growth of the infecting organism in anticipation of replacement of the prosthesis.

## Intestinal infections

Mild bacillary dysentery, salmonella food poisoning and other forms of bacterial diarrhoea do not ordinarily require chemotherapy. Indeed, such therapy may make intestinal carriage more likely and increase the risk of the selection of antibiotic-resistant strains. The most important treatment is correction of fluid balance.

Patients with invasive infection (e.g. typhoid and paratyphoid fever) and those with severe bacillary dysentery or cholera may warrant treatment (see appropriate chapters). Even potentially fatal intestinal infections with *E. coli* O157 fare worse with antimicrobials than fluids alone. This may be due to excess toxin release.

Many intestinal infections are due to viruses, for which there is presently no specific chemotherapy. Cryptosporidiosis is now being diagnosed more frequently, but is usually self-limiting except in the immunocompromised. Infection with other protozoa, such as *Giardia lamblia* or *Entamoeba histolytica*, requires treatment with metronidazole.

Spread of infection from the bowel may give rise to serious infections and associated toxaemia. If subphrenic, retrocolic or pelvic abscesses form, drainage is the most important aspect of treatment, but antibiotics can assist recovery of the patient. Cephalosporins or an aminoglyoside plus ampicillin are useful in empirical treatment, and metronidazole should be added if bacteroides is likely to be present. Acute peritonitis after non-specific inflammation of the bowel, such as appendicitis, is usually effectively treated with amoxicillin (with or without clavulanate) or cefotaxime combined with metronidazole.

## Liver infections

Bacterial infections of the liver and portal pyaemia are best treated with large doses of cefuroxime, cefotaxime, or an antibiotic chosen on the basis of laboratory findings (e.g. ampicillin against enterococci). Liver abscesses occur most frequently by spread via the portal tract of intestinal Gram-negative bacilli, or by retrograde spread in the biliary passages of streptococci (especially *Str. milleri*) and anaerobes from the gallbladder. Ampicillin is selectively concentrated in the bile, and is often useful in treatment of cholecystitis. Amoebic abscess requires prompt and specific treatment with metronidazole, and its possibility should always be kept in mind, particularly in a patient who has been abroad.

Infection caused by the hepatitis viruses B and C has been treated by α-interferon with ribavirin and lamivudine with variable success.

## Bone and joint infections

Most infections of bones and joints are due to *Staph. aureus*. Large doses of flucloxacillin should be given in combination with either fusidic acid or clindamycin unless antibiotic resistant strains are involved which may limit the choice to a glycopeptide or linezolid.

Penicillin in prolonged high dosage is the drug of choice for streptococcal arthritis. Where other organisms, such as *H. influenzae*, neisseriae or Gram-negative rods are involved, specifically directed therapy is required.

## Genital tract infections

Venereal infections such as syphilis and gonorrhoea were traditionally treated with penicillin, but a high proportion of isolates of gonococci are now resistant to this agent, in which case ceftriaxone, co-amoxiclav or ciprofloxacin should be used depending on local patterns.

Non-specific infections of the genital tract are common in women; aerobic and anaerobic bacteria, *Candida* species or *Trichomonas vaginalis*, may be involved. Frequently, an abnormal flora is isolated in the absence of an inflammatory exudate, and it may be difficult to decide on the necessity for chemotherapy. Bacterial vaginosis is such a clinical syndrome associated with *Mobiluncus* spp., which responds to metronidazole or amoxicillin. Vaginal candidiasis is usually treated topically with nystatin or an antifungal imidazole. In trichomoniasis, metronidazole is indicated.

More serious pelvic infection in women is often associated with chlamydiae, and tetracycline or erythromycin is the drug of choice. Azithromycin is a useful single dose agent for uncomplicated genital infection due to chlamydiae. Infection of the fallopian tubes usually involves anaerobic bacteria and metronidazole or co-amoxiclav may be prescribed.

## Surgical wound infections

Most surgical infections are caused by the patient's own organisms, but some arise exogenously, often by cross-infection. In orthopaedic units, most exogenous infections are due to staphylococci, but in gastrointestinal units, Gram-negative bacilli and anaerobes are more common. The situation may change from time to time as a result of ecological movements in the microbial flora within the unit, associated with selective pressures of antibiotic use.

Specimens from infected lesions should always be sent to the laboratory, since the identity of the isolate may have epidemiological significance as well as being of importance in the management of the patient. The microbiologist should always be informed of any therapy as this may affect the interpretation of bacteriological tests.

## Superficial infections

Skin and soft tissue infections are common in general practice. Most are of bacterial origin, although some have a fungal or viral aetiology.

Common lesions such as boils, carbuncles, impetigo and infected wounds are associated with *Staph. aureus* and *Str. pyogenes*. Systemic treatment with appropriate antibiotics may be indicated in some patients, but topical treatment is often effective. The use of antibiotics commonly prescribed for systemic infections should be avoided in favour of antiseptics or topical antibiotics such as mupirocin.

RECOMMENDED READING

Finch RG, Davey PG, Wilcox MH, Irving W: *Antimicrobial Chemotherapy*, ed 6, Oxford, 2011, Oxford University Press.

Finch RG, Greenwood D, Whitley RJ, Norrby SR: *Antibiotic and Chemotherapy*, ed 9, Churchill Livingstone, Edinburgh, 2011, Elsevier.

Grayson ML, editor: *Kucer's The Use of Antibiotics*, ed 6, Butterworth-Heinemann, Oxford, 2010, Elsevier.

Mandell GL, Douglas RG, Bennett JE, editors: *Principles and Practice of Infectious Disease*, ed 7, Churchill Livingstone, Philadelphia, 2010, Elsevier.

### Websites

WHO Essential Drug Monitor: http://www.who.int/medicines/publications/monitor/en/

British Society for Antimicrobial Chemotherapy: http://www.bsac.org.uk/

# 68 Epidemiology and control of community infections

*D. Reid and D. Goldberg*

## KEY POINTS

- The surveillance of infection provides the basis for appropriate investigation and preventive action.
- The infectious process involves three main factors: the micro-organism, the host and the environment.
- Herd immunity indicates the degree to which a community is susceptible to infection.
- Infection is spread in five ways: from person to person, from healthy carriers, from animal sources, from environmental sources and as a result of an organism situated in an area of the body where it is harmless gaining access to a more dangerous site.
- Infection may manifest itself as: a sporadic case, an outbreak, an epidemic or a pandemic.
- Outbreaks have three main patterns of spread: from a single source, from one person to another, or from a single source with subsequent person-to-person spread.
- The epidemiological investigation of an outbreak involves an analysis concerning: the persons involved, the place it occurred and the time those infected became ill.
- Vigilance and high-quality surveillance are necessary in order to have an early warning of emerging infections.

*When you can measure what you are speaking about and express it in numbers, you know something about it; when you cannot express it in numbers, your knowledge is of a meagre and unsatisfactory kind.*

William Thomson, Lord Kelvin
(Popular Lectures and Addresses, 1891)

*Good surveillance does not necessarily mean the making of right decisions but it reduces the chances of wrong ones.*

Alexander Langmuir, 1963

*Once is happenstance, twice is coincidence, the third time it's enemy action.*

Ian Fleming
(Goldfinger, Jonathan Cape, 1959)

Attempts to observe and record diseases in order to devise means of determining their cause and control have a long history. Hippocrates (460–361 BC), 'the father of medical science', and Herodotus (484–425 BC), 'the father of history', both related environmental factors to health. Hippocrates, when writing of the occurrence of diseases, distinguished between the 'steady state', the 'endemic state' and the abrupt change in incidence, the 'epidemic'.

Probably the first public health measures based on case reports of infectious diseases, taken by a European government, occurred in 1348 when the Republic of Venice excluded ships with affected people on board in order to control outbreaks of pneumonic plague (the *black death*). Fifty years later, again in Venice, the concept of *quarantine* was introduced when ships from plague-stricken areas had to stay outside the harbours for 40 days (*quaranta giorni*).

In addition, because of the fear of a plague epidemic, the first of the *Bills of Mortality*, in which causes of death were recorded, was published in London in 1592. In 1662 John Graunt (1620–1674), in his book *Natural and Political Observations Made Upon the Bills of Mortality*, was the first to count the number of persons dying in London from specific illnesses and to advocate the value of obtaining numerical data on a population in order to study the causes of disease (Table 68.1). In 1837 the office of the Registrar General was established to develop the work started by John Graunt; the English physician William Farr (1807–1883) added reports to those of

**Table 68.1** Selection of causes of death in London taken from the Bills of Mortality, 1632

| Causes of death | No. of deaths |
| --- | --- |
| Chrisomes[a] and infancy | 2268 |
| Consumption[b] | 1797 |
| Fever | 1108 |
| Aged | 628 |
| Smallpox | 531 |
| Teeth | 470 |
| Abortive and stillborn | 445 |
| Bloody flux[c], scouring[d] and flux | 348 |
| Dropsy[e] and swelling | 267 |
| Convulsions | 241 |
| Childbed | 171 |
| Measles | 80 |
| Ague[f] | 43 |
| King's evil[g] | 38 |

[a]A child who died during the first month of life or a child who died unbaptized.
[b]Usually pulmonary tuberculosis.
[c]Dysentery
[d]Diarrhoea.
[e]Oedema.
[f]Malaria.
[g]Tuberculosis of the skin.

the Registrar General that dealt with infectious diseases, occupational diseases, accidents or hazardous work conditions.

The importance of keen observation of disease in order to deduce the likely cause has been demonstrated on many occasions. In 1849, 34 years before the identification of *Vibrio cholerae* by Robert Koch (1843–1910), John Snow (1813–1858), a London physician, proved by epidemiological observation that cholera was mainly spread by drinking infected water and not through the air in the form of miasmas, as was commonly thought at the time. Similarly, William Budd (1811–1880), a general practitioner from Devon, showed in 1873 how typhoid was spread, even though it was not until 1885 that the typhoid bacillus was first isolated in the laboratory. More recently, William Pickles (1885–1969), a general practitioner in Wensleydale, Yorkshire, was able to elucidate many of the epidemiological characteristics of hepatitis and other infections well before microbiological advances were to confirm his observations.

From these beginnings the surveillance of infection has assumed national and international proportions. National surveillance is carried out in different countries, for example at the Centers for Disease Control and Prevention (CDC) in Atlanta, USA. In the UK, information on infectious diseases and environmental hazards is collated for each devolved

country by different public health agencies. General Practitioners and other clinicians also undertake regular recording of disease voluntarily. The European Centre for Disease Prevention and Control in Stockholm collects such data for each European country and, on a worldwide basis, the World Health Organization (WHO) provides important liaison and support. This international co-operation is vital as 'germs do not recognize boundaries'.

Probably the most outstanding achievement of international surveillance was the development of a programme for smallpox eradication. The multi-disciplinary approach adopted by the WHO, in which programmes were community based with measurable goals and constant monitoring, resulted in the last endemic case being recorded in October 1977; smallpox was officially declared eradicated in December 1979.

## EPIDEMIOLOGY: DEFINITIONS AND PRINCIPLES

Epidemiology is usually defined as *the study of the nature, distribution, causation, mode of transfer, prevention and control of disease*. It has also been regarded as 'the natural history of disease' or as 'the human face of ecology'. Closely linked with the study of epidemiology is the concept of surveillance, which is probably the most effective infection control technique available. Surveillance is defined as: *the epidemiological study of a disease as a dynamic process involving the ecology of the infectious agent, the host, the reservoirs, the vectors as well as the complex mechanisms concerned in the spread of infection and the extent to which this spread will occur*. There are three main elements of surveillance of infection:

1. the systematic collection of pertinent data
2. the orderly consolidation and evaluation of the data
3. the prompt dissemination of the findings, especially to those who can take appropriate action.

Surveillance provides for the recognition of acute problems requiring immediate local, national or international action, and for further assessment by revealing trends or facilitating forecasts. It also provides a rational basis for planning and implementing efficient control measures and for their evaluation and continuing assessment. Although particularly appropriate to the study of infectious diseases, epidemiological principles are also used to elucidate the causes of non-communicable diseases.

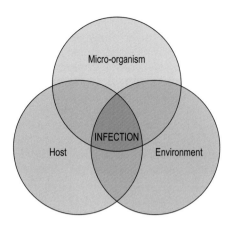

**Fig. 68.1** The three main factors involved in the infectious process.

The infectious process is a dynamic state involving three main factors: the micro-organism, the host and the environment (Fig. 68.1).

## The micro-organism

Since few micro-organisms are harmful to man, the concept of *virulence* (the degree of pathogenicity of an infectious agent indicated by fatality rates and/or its ability to invade and damage the tissues of the host) must be recognized. The degree of virulence depends on *invasiveness* (the capacity of the organism to spread widely through the body) and *toxigenicity* (the toxin-producing property of the organism) (see Ch. 13). A further variable is the *dose* of the organism, as well as virulence. A small number of organisms of high virulence is usually sufficient to cause disease in a susceptible person, whereas if the organism is of low virulence it often fails to cause disease. Another variable is the *portal of entry*. Many organisms have a predilection for a particular tissue or organ. For example, the causal organism of typhoid fever, *Salmonella typhi,* usually causes disease only when it enters the human body through the mouth in food or water (see Ch. 24).

## The host

The reaction of the host to a micro-organism will depend on the ability to resist infection. The individual may not possess sufficient resistance against a particular pathogenic agent to prevent contraction of infection when exposed to the organism. Alternatively, the individual may possess specific protective antibodies or cellular immunity as a result of previous infection or immunization. However, immunity is relative and may be overwhelmed by an excessive dose

of the infectious agent or if the person is infected via an unusual portal of entry; it may also be impaired by immunosuppressive drug therapy, concurrent disease or the ageing process. These properties were particularly evident in the influenza H1N1 pandemic of 2009 when infection was mainly seen in younger persons as those over the age of 60 had acquired immunity from previous exposure.

### Herd immunity

Herd immunity is an important element in the balance between the host population and the micro-organism, and represents the degree to which the community is susceptible or not to an infectious disease as a result of members of the population having acquired active immunity from either previous infection or prophylactic immunization (see p. 731).

Herd immunity can be measured:

1. *Indirectly* from the age distribution and incidence pattern of the disease if it is clinically distinct and reasonably common. This is an insensitive and inadequate method for infections that manifest subclinically.
2. *Directly* from assessments of immunity in defined population groups by antibody surveys (sero-epidemiology) or skin tests; these may show 'immunity gaps' and provide an early warning of susceptibility in the population. Although it may be difficult to interpret the data in absolute terms of immunity and susceptibility, the observations can be standardized to reveal trends and differences between various defined population groups in place and time.

The decision whether to introduce herd immunity artificially by immunization against a particular disease will depend on several epidemiological principles.

• The disease must carry a substantial risk.
• The risk of contracting the disease must be considerable.
• The vaccine must be effective.
• The vaccine must be safe.

The effectiveness and safety of immunization programmes are monitored by observing the expected and actual effects of such programmes on disease transmission patterns in the community by appropriate epidemiological techniques.

### The environment

The environment plays a major role in the causation, spread and control of infection. In the UK, the

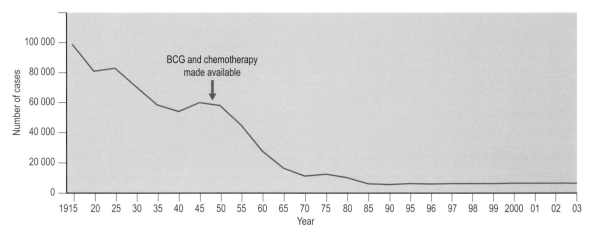

**Fig. 68.2**  Notifications of tuberculosis in U.K., 1915–2008.

disappearance of relapsing fever, plague and cholera, the rarity of indigenous typhoid fever and the relative infrequency of bacillary dysentery are all indications of the improvements that have taken place in environmental conditions.

The decrease in overcrowding and infestation, together with the demand for cleaner water supplies and better sanitation, have been of paramount importance in producing these dramatic advances. This is well illustrated in the case of tuberculosis, which was declining before the availability of chemotherapy and mass Bacillus Calmette–Guérin (BCG) vaccination in countries where socio-economic conditions were improving (Fig. 68.2). Paradoxically, better living conditions may unexpectedly create new problems; for example, poliovirus infection, previously experienced mainly in early childhood, is usually postponed in more favoured communities to older ages when paralysis is a more likely complication unless there is an adequate immunization programme.

In recent years, areas of urban deprivation, particularly in western countries, have been blighted by the culture of illicit drug injection and its associated infections, such as human immunodeficiency virus (HIV) and hepatitis C, acquired through the sharing of injecting equipment. These may also be associated with spore forming bacteria, such as clostridia and anthrax bacilli contracted through soil contamination of drugs.

## THE SPREAD OF INFECTION

Infection spreads in well-defined epidemiological patterns. Knowledge of these will lead to an understanding of the best methods of control, or even eradication, and enables an estimate to be made of the likelihood of this happening.

### Infection spread directly from one person to another

Among this group can be included such highly infectious diseases as chickenpox. Infection is passed directly from a person with the disease to a susceptible contact. Diseases in this category are usually clinically apparent and healthy carriers are not a feature. When it is possible to diminish the number of susceptibles in the target population then eradication becomes feasible, as has happened with smallpox.

### Infection in which healthy carriers are involved

Because apparently healthy individuals may harbour the bacilli responsible for such diseases as typhoid, paratyphoid and diphtheria, often for long periods after having acquired the infection, it is possible for such infections to be transmitted to others and the source remains undetected. For certain infections, such as hepatitis C virus infection, the healthy carrier state may last several decades.

### Infection in which persons harbour the organism before the onset of clinical illness

Organisms such as *Streptococcus pneumoniae* may not cause the person any harm until an event such as a skull fracture allows for the transfer of the bacterium from the middle ear to the cerebrospinal space where it can cause a potentially fatal meningitis.

## Infection derived from animal sources

Diseases derived from animals, such as leptospirosis, Q fever, anthrax, rabies and brucellosis, are known as *zoonoses*. These diseases are spread by direct contact with the animal concerned or indirectly by such means as the ingestion of infected milk and contact with infected bone products, etc.

## Infections derived from environmental sources

The spread of legionellae from cooling towers and air conditioning units to cause legionnaires' disease is an example of illness derived from an infected environment. By dealing appropriately with the infected source by use of biocides in the water, the population can be protected.

## OUTBREAKS OF INFECTION

The crowding together of human beings (or for that matter animals) provides the necessary conditions to allow micro-organisms to multiply and spread. When human beings led nomadic lives there was less opportunity for outbreaks to occur; the main opportunities came when large numbers gathered for a pilgrimage or had other reasons for a meeting. These clusterings facilitated the spread of infection, resulting in outbreaks; the subsequent dispersal of the group enabled the causative organism to be carried elsewhere.

The threat of outbreaks in overcrowded and difficult conditions is particularly well illustrated in military history; on many occasions the germ has been as important in determining the outcome of a campaign as the sword or gun. The typhoid bacillus caused severe effects during both the American Civil War (1861–1865) and the Boer War (1899–1902). The use of typhoid vaccine in the latter years of the First World War meant that the main impact of typhoid in this war subsided after 1916. The pandemic of influenza in 1918–1919, in which about 700 million people were infected with approximately 22 million deaths, was a scourge of military camps and affected many servicemen returning home from the First World War. Several outbreaks of meningococcal meningitis have occurred in pilgrims to Mecca.

## Nomenclature of outbreaks

The term *outbreak* is often confused with other epidemiological terms used to enumerate infection:

1. *Sporadic case*: a person whose illness is not apparently connected with similar illnesses in another person.
2. *Outbreak*: the occurrence of cases of a disease associated in time or location among a group of persons. A *household outbreak* involves two or more persons resident in the same private household and not apparently connected with any other case or outbreak. A *general outbreak* involves two or more persons who are not confined to one private household.
3. *Epidemic*: the large-scale temporary increase in the occurrence of a disease in a community or region that is clearly in excess of normal expectancy.
4. *Pandemic*: the occurrence of a disease that is clearly in excess of normal expectancy and is spread over a whole geographical area, usually crossing national boundaries.

## Types of outbreak

There are three main patterns of outbreak that may be revealed by the construction of graphs of occurrence of cases over time:

1. *The explosive outbreak*. This is characterized by the occurrence of a large proportion of cases in a relatively short period of time (Fig. 68.3); there is a sharp rise and fall in the number of infected persons, because the usual cause of such an event is a common source that infects the people concerned. This type of outbreak is also frequently termed a *common source outbreak* or *a point source outbreak*. This pattern of infection is often discovered when water or food becomes contaminated, although other vehicles of infection can also be responsible for this type of outbreak.
2. *Person-to-person spread*. Outbreaks caused by infections that are spread from person to person

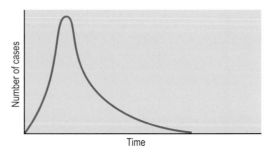

**Fig. 68.3** Epidemic curve apparent when there is an explosive (common or point source) outbreak.

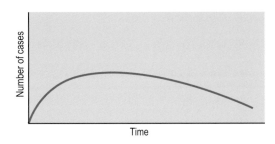

Fig. 68.4 Epidemic curve apparent when there is person-to-person spread of infection.

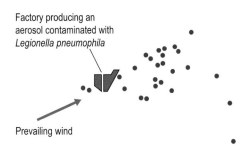

Factory producing an aerosol contaminated with *Legionella pneumophila*

Prevailing wind

Fig. 68.6 Occurrence of legionnaires' disease in persons living downwind from a factory with an evaporative condenser contaminated with *Legionella pneumophila*.

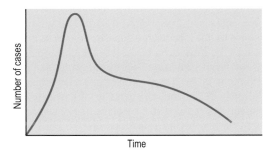

Fig. 68.5 Epidemic curve apparent when there is person-to-person spread subsequent to a common source outbreak.

usually have a more protracted course, taking longer than explosive outbreaks to build up and to subside. An infective agent may be passed from person to person by a variety of routes. Diseases such as dysentery, hepatitis type A and gastroenteritis, which are usually spread by the faecal–oral route, often follow this pattern of spread (Fig. 68.4).

3. *Explosive outbreaks with subsequent person-to-person spread.* This pattern is often apparent when there is contamination of a common water or food source and the initial cases subsequently infect their contacts. Thus, the pattern of the outbreak is a combination of that seen with an explosive outbreak, but followed by a slower decline (Fig. 68.5).

## Analysis of outbreaks

The investigation of an outbreak should be approached in a logical and methodical way. The cause may be elucidated by determining details of the *persons* involved, the *place* where they had been and the *time* when they became ill.

The fundamental pieces of information that should be sought whenever an outbreak occurs are as follows:

1. *WHO gets infected?* What is their age? For example, if a possible food-borne outbreak affects mainly children, could the source be milk or ice-cream?
2. *WHERE were those who became infected?* Where have they recently been? For example, in a hospital outbreak were they all in the same surgical ward? Could a member of the operating staff be a carrier of a pathogen? In a community outbreak of legionnaires' disease were those affected living downwind from a source of infection (Fig. 68.6)?
3. *WHEN did the infection occur?* By knowing the incubation period of the infection and the date of onset of symptoms, it may be possible to trace back to an event that was attended by all those affected.
4. *WHAT was the common factor?* For example, in a food poisoning episode, the ingestion of an article of food by most of those affected but not by those unaffected may be a vital piece of evidence.
5. *HOW did those involved become infected?* For example, abscess formation among recently immunized persons might be due to contaminated vaccine.
6. *WHY did the infection occur?* For example, the reheating of meat may be the cause of a *Clostridium perfringens* food-poisoning outbreak.

## Investigation of outbreaks

In the investigation of outbreaks it is important to have a standardized approach to the various steps involved. Such an approach might have the following as a basis:

1. *Verify the diagnosis.* It is always prudent to confirm that the clinical history is compatible

with the diagnosis. Occasional 'pseudo-epidemics' can occur, sometimes resulting from contamination of specimens.

2. *Establish the existence of an outbreak.* The increased interest of an investigator or a change in the mechanism of reporting can sometimes result in an increase in the number of reports of illness. It is important to check the previous level of investigation of a clinical entity or alteration in laboratory methods.

3. *Establish the extent of an outbreak.* Often the number of cases notified is only a proportion of the total number of those affected. It is necessary to seek out the additional cases or vital information may be lost.

4. *Identify common characteristics or experiences of the affected persons.* An individual history from each confirmed or suspected case is required to detect any common factor among those affected (e.g. eating the same item of food).

5. *Investigate the source and vehicle of infection.* In addition to ascertaining the general characteristics of the material suspected as being the source or vehicle of infection, appropriate laboratory investigation will often have to be done. Good co-operation with laboratory staff is vitally important. Increasingly, putative links between individuals who present with the same infection or infectious disease are confirmed or dispelled through the typing or sequencing of the genes of the organism involved.

6. *Analyse the findings.* The data should be analysed by various epidemiological criteria, especially persons, time and place. Denominators should be obtained to calculate attack rates.

7. *Construct and test a hypothesis.* On the basis of the evidence a hypothesis should be constructed concerning the origin of the outbreak. This may be confirmed by laboratory findings but action to control the outbreak may be needed in advance. The hypothesis may be tested by comparing information from cases with matched controls (case/control study).

## Control of outbreaks

The investigation of an outbreak should be carried out as swiftly as possible so that adequate control measures can be started without delay. Knowledge of the *source of infection*, the *route of transmission* and the *persons at risk* should allow appropriate action to be taken to achieve success.

### Sources of infection

These may be:

- human cases or carriers
- animal cases or carriers
- the environment.

If the initial cases have readily identifiable clinical features (e.g. chickenpox) then control is often easier as it is much more likely that the index case will be located.

On the other hand, it is more difficult to control diseases in which apparently healthy carriers are responsible, as it is necessary to search for an infected person who may be asymptomatic.

It may be important to isolate the case or carrier, and possibly to institute appropriate treatment, until the patient is no longer infectious. The degree of isolation will depend on the type of disease, as not all infections require strict isolation. For example, a patient with a highly infectious disease may require very strict isolation whereas the salmonella excreter will usually need only to cease food-handling activities and observe a high standard of personal hygiene until free from infection. In contrast to 'isolation', the term 'quarantine' applies to restrictions on the healthy contacts of an infectious disease.

If an animal reservoir is responsible, action has to be directed at ensuring that the source of infection is eradicated, withdrawn from consumption or rendered harmless, for example by the pasteurization of milk or the adequate cooking of meat.

When the environment is the source of an outbreak the control measures required will depend on the nature of infection and the mode of spread. In recent years, waterborne spread of legionnaires' disease (e.g. from shower-heads, air-conditioning systems or droplet spread from cooling towers) has become increasingly recognized (Fig. 68.7). Environmental measures, such as the use of biocides, can destroy the causative legionellae at their source and so prevent further cases.

The hospital setting is particularly dangerous as the presence of compromised patients can result in tragic consequences. Moreover, the increasing use of invasive techniques and the appearance of antibiotic-resistant strains of micro-organisms further compound the problem. The early detection of infection by effective surveillance, the emphasis on the cleanest possible environment and awareness among the staff of potential problems are among the measures that need to be stressed to control infection among hospital patients (see Ch. 69).

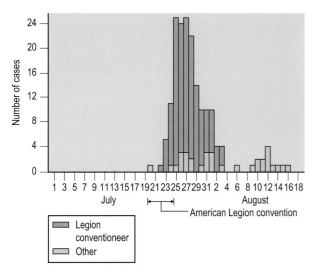

**Fig. 68.7** Legionnaires' disease among those associated with a convention in a hotel in Philadelphia (July–August 1976); an example of an explosive outbreak.

### Route of transmission

Infection may be spread by:

- direct or indirect contact
- air-borne transmission
- food and water-borne transmission
- insect-borne transmission
- percutaneous transmission
- sexual transmission
- transplacental transmission.

There are various ways in which the routes of transmission occurring during an outbreak may be blocked by measures appropriate to the route involved: effective hand washing; disinfection or disposal, if necessary, of the patient's belongings. Strict adherence to high standards of personal hygiene by the contacts of a case are also important measures.

When the disease is air-borne, overcrowding should be avoided and, where appropriate, dormitory or ward beds should be well spaced. In certain instances major isolation measures, such as those adopted to control the outbreak of severe acute respiratory syndrome (SARS) in 2003, need to be implemented. Indeed, the spread of the coronavirus, the air-borne infection responsible for SARS, throughout regions of the Far East (China, Vietnam and Singapore) and North America (Toronto), before it was brought under control, demonstrates how effectively international travel and overcrowding in major cities can facilitate the transmission of serious air-borne infections.

*Food* and *water* should be as free as possible from infection; otherwise their consumption can cause major outbreaks. To prevent *insect-borne transmission*, insect eradication policies and repellents should be considered. HIV is an infection that, commonly, is transmitted through the percutaneous, sexual and transplacental routes; the elimination of infected blood donations by blood donor testing, the provision of sterile needles and syringes for infected drug users, the use of condoms and the treatment of HIV-infected pregnant women with anti-retroviral therapy are measures that prevent the spread of this infection through these routes.

### Persons at risk

Where indicated and feasible, susceptible persons at risk should be protected as soon as possible. Among the measures available, the following may need to be considered:

- immunization
- chemoprophylaxis for close contacts.

Immunity against several infectious diseases can be obtained by either active or passive immunization (see Ch. 70). Examples of rapid effective protection of communities by active immunization are the 'ring vaccination' policy used to protect close contacts of poliomyelitis and so stop more widespread dissemination of poliovirus, and the early (within 72 h of exposure) administration of measles vaccine to close contacts in an institution. Passive immunization, usually by means of human specific immunoglobulin, gives rapid protection to contacts of certain infections, such as hepatitis B, although protection is short lived. Chemoprophylaxis is effective in the protection of close contacts of meningococcal infections and diphtheria.

## MATHEMATICAL MODELS

Mathematical modelling techniques attempt to define, by use of relatively simple estimates and assumptions, the dynamic conditions governing transmission of communicable agents.

Details of the multiplication and growth rates of micro-organisms and the spread of infection under natural or experimental conditions need to be known to simulate spread in defined communities. Measurable factors include:

- the number of infective persons or sources of introduction of infection

- the proportion of susceptible persons in a community at risk
- the duration of immunity
- the introduction of new susceptibles
- the removal rate of infective persons (by isolation, immunity or death)
- the response to vaccines and chemotherapeutic agents.

Mathematical models can be used to predict institutional outbreaks and epidemics.

This approach has been used to attempt to forecast the number of cases of acquired immune deficiency syndrome, variant Creutzfeldt–Jakob disease and bovine spongiform encephalopathy that are likely to occur and the effect of control measures.

## ASSOCIATION AND CAUSATION OF INFECTION

A problem commonly encountered by microbiologists and epidemiologists is the attribution of an infectious disease to a particular micro-organism. How do we determine whether the relationship is one of causation or merely a chance association?

Koch addressed this when he formulated his 'postulates' in 1891. These state that:

1. The organism must always be found in the given disease.
2. The organism must be isolated in pure culture.
3. The organism must reproduce the given disease after inoculation of a pure culture into a susceptible animal.
4. The organism must be recoverable from the animal so inoculated.

For many organisms pathogenic to man it is not possible to fulfil all of Koch's postulates; moreover, they are not applicable to the study of the transmission of infection within a population. For this purpose it is more appropriate to consider the following factors, suggested by the medical statistician Bradford Hill, to establish whether a disease is caused by a particular infectious agent:

1. *Strength*. What is the strength of the association? During the cholera epidemic in London in 1854, John Snow compared the death rates among persons drinking the sewage-polluted drinking water of the Southwark and Vauxhall Company with those receiving the purer water of the Lambeth Company; he discovered that the rate in the former was 14 times greater (Table 68.2). This

| Table 68.2 | Deaths in London during the cholera epidemic of 1854 according to source of water supply | | |
|---|---|---|
| Water source | No. of houses supplied | Deaths |
| Southwark and Vauxhall Company (polluted) | 10 000 | 71 |
| Lambeth Company (non-polluted) | 10 000 | 5 |

strength of association allowed Snow to consider that polluted water was a cause of cholera, although at that time the causative organism itself had not been identified.

2. *Consistency*. Similar observations, made by different people at different times in different places, add confidence to a conclusion that causation is likely.

3. *Specificity*. If the association is limited to a specific group of persons, with a specific type of illness, who have all been subjected to the same specific infection, then a cause-and-effect relationship can be more strongly suspected.

4. *Temporality*. This can be of especial importance when persons in particular occupations become infected (e.g. leptospirosis in sewerworkers). The history of working in a particular environment *before* infection rather than vice versa is particularly relevant.

5. *Biological gradient*. If a dose–response curve is apparent then the evidence for causation is much stronger.

6. *Plausibility*. Is the possibility biologically plausible? The likelihood of veterinary surgeons becoming ill with a zoonotic infection from affected cattle which they have recently been treating seems biologically plausible.

7. *Coherence*. If all the evidence is coherent (e.g. if the same micro-organism is isolated from the index case, the vehicle of transmission and from the victims), this is strong support for causation.

8. *Experiment*. Is the frequency of infection reduced if certain preventive measures are taken? The beneficial effects of the pasteurization of milk to diminish the number of cases of milk-borne salmonellosis is presumptive evidence of a zoonotic relationship.

9. *Analogy*. Has there been similar evidence in the past? The known capacity of the rubella virus to cause congenital abnormalities in the infants of infected mothers makes it easier to accept the possibility of other viruses causing similar problems if maternal infection occurs.

## CONCLUSION

Because of the multifactorial causation of infection it is usually necessary to study the epidemiology of infection in a *multidisciplinary* manner. The microbiologist, the clinician, the epidemiologist, the infection control nurse, the veterinarian, the environmental health officer, and other appropriate personnel, must all be involved; the extent of the involvement will depend on the nature of the infection. Success will depend on the expertise and co-operation of these members of the team.

RECOMMENDED READING

Detels R, Beaglehole R, Lansang MA, Gulliford M: *Oxford Textbook of Public Health*, Oxford, 2009, Oxford University Press.

Donaldson LJ, Scally G: *Essential Public Health*, ed 3, Oxford, 2009, Radcliffe.

Giesecke J: *Modern Infectious Disease Epidemiology*, ed 2, London, 2001, Edward Arnold.

Ekdahl K: *Communicable Disease Control and Health Protection Handbook*, Chichester, 2012, Wiley Blackwell.

Heymann DL, editor: *Control of Communicable Diseases Manual*, ed 19, Washington, DC, 2008, American Public Health Association.

Ksiazek TG, Erdman D, Goldsmith CS et al: A novel coronavirus associated with severe acute respiratory syndrome, *New England Journal of Medicine* 348:1953–1966, 2003.

Mandell G, Douglas RG, Bennet J, editors: *Principles and Practice of Infectious Diseases*, ed 7, Churchill Livingstone, Philadelphia, 2010, Elsevier.

Porta M, Last JM, editors: *A Dictionary of Epidemiology*, Oxford, 2008, Oxford University Press.

### Websites

Centers for Disease Control and Prevention: http://www.cdc.gov/

Cymru NHS Wales: http://www.wales.nhs.uk

European Centre for Disease Prevention and Control: http://www.ecdc.europa.eu/

Health Protection Agency: http://www.hpa.org.uk/

Health Protection Scotland: http://www.hps.scot.nhs.uk/

Public Health Agency Northern Ireland: http://www.publichealth.hscni.net

World Health Organization: http://www.who.int/en/

# 69 Hospital infection

*R. C. B. Slack*

## KEY POINTS

- Hospitals constitute a special environment where the epidemiology of infection is distinct. The chief contributing factors are the accumulation of patients with particular features, the special activities undertaken in hospitals, and the special environment created by the patients and the activities.
- Patients may constitute a special hazard because they are infectious, or they may be unusually susceptible to infection because they have particular conditions or are receiving immunosuppressive treatments.
- Special activities include surgery and extensive use of intravascular devices. Needlestick injuries are a constant hazard.
- The extensive use of antibiotics and disinfectants, and the need to reuse equipment and areas that may become contaminated, contribute to the special environment.
- Certain organisms such as methicillin-resistant *Staphylococcus aureus* (MRSA), *Pseudomonas aeruginosa* and *Clostridium difficile* are important agents of hospital-acquired infection owing to the factors outlined above.
- Careful and detailed attention must be paid to controlling the routes of transmission of infection, through the establishment and maintenance of an *infection control policy.*

The battle between man and microbe is at its most obvious in institutions where vulnerable people are crowded together. Historically, hospitals have a notorious reputation for infection. The hazards of puerperal sepsis and the horrors of septic infection in the pre-Listerian era have been well documented; admission to hospital in the mid-nineteenth century was associated with the fear of gangrene and death.

Since then, surgical and medical techniques have developed dramatically, basic standards of building and hygiene have greatly improved, and the identification and treatment of most infecting micro-organisms have become possible. Despite such changes, infection acquired in hospitals remains a major cause of morbidity and mortality, leading directly or indirectly to an enormous increase in the cost of hospital care and to the emergence of new health hazards for the community. In the past two decades enormous advances in biomedical technology and therapeutics have produced greater numbers of highly susceptible patients requiring treatment in hospitals, and this is aggravated by the occurrence of transferable resistance to antibiotics in pathogenic bacteria and the emergence of new pathogens transmitted by a variety of routes. In spite of these advances in medical care, in many countries pressures on health care facilities and shortages of trained staff make it difficult to practise adequate infection control. There has also been a mistaken view among many health professionals that the advent of the antibiotic era made such precautions unnecessary, and many studies have shown poor compliance with simple hygiene.

## CLASSIFICATION

To measure the extent of hospital and healthcare-associated infection (HAI) and conduct surveillance the following definitions should be considered:

1. Community-acquired infections: either those contracted and developing outside hospitals which require admission of the patient (e.g. pneumococcal pneumonia) or those contracted outside hospital or those which become clinically

apparent within 48 hours of admission or when the patient has been admitted to hospital for other reasons (e.g. chickenpox or zoster).
2. Infections contracted and developing within hospital (e.g. device-associated bacteraemias).
3. Infections contracted in hospital but not becoming clinically apparent until after the patient has been discharged (e.g. many postoperative wound infections).
4. Infections contracted by healthcare staff as a consequence of their work, whether or not this involves direct contact with patients (e.g. hepatitis B).

On average, around 9% of all hospitalized patients will develop an infection as a result of their stay in hospital. Urinary, respiratory and wound infections are the most common.

## FACTORS THAT INFLUENCE INFECTION

Hospital infection, also known as *nosocomial infection*, may be exogenous or endogenous in origin. The exogenous source may be another person in the hospital (*cross-infection*) or a contaminated item of equipment or building service (*environmental infection*). A high proportion of clinically apparent hospital infections are endogenous (*self-infection*), the infecting organism being derived from the patient's own skin, gastrointestinal or upper respiratory flora.

Most infections acquired in hospital are caused by micro-organisms that are commonly present as commensals in the general population. Thus, contact with micro-organisms is seldom the sole or main event predisposing to infection. Various risk factors, alone or in combination, influence the frequency and nature of hospital infection. In comparing rates of HAI it is important to be aware of the frequencies of risk factors such as age, drug treatment or preexisting diseases in the population surveyed as well as the medical or surgical procedures used.

## CONTACT WITH OTHER PATIENTS AND STAFF

In common with any large institution or workplace, the patients and staff of a hospital share many facilities in close or crowded conditions. Outbreaks of diarrhoeal and food-borne disease may be traced to a common source via the hospital water or food supplies. The specific role of hospitals in admitting infected patients or carriers for treatment clearly serves as a potential source of infection for others. Patients with comparable susceptibility to infection tend to be concentrated in the same area, e.g. in neonatal units, burns units or urological wards, where infected and non-infected patients may be cared for by the same staff, thus creating numerous opportunities for the spread of micro-organisms by direct contact. The more susceptible patients usually require the most intensive care with far more daily contacts with staff who act as vectors in the transmission of microbes like insects spreading parasites.

## Inanimate reservoirs of infection

Equipment and materials in use in hospitals often become contaminated with micro-organisms which may subsequently be transferred to susceptible body sites on patients. Gram-positive cocci, derived from skin scales of the hospital population, are found in the air, dust and on surfaces where they may survive along with fungal and bacterial spores of environmental origin. Gram-negative aerobic bacilli are common in moist situations and in fluids, where they often survive for long periods, and may even multiply in the presence of minimal nutrients. An important example of this is legionellae in hospital domestic water supplies. Awareness of the common reservoirs of environmental and contaminating hospital micro-organisms provides the basis for maintaining standards of hygiene (cleaning, disinfection, sterilization) throughout the hospital as well as good engineering and building.

## Role of antibiotic treatment

At least 30% of patients receive antibiotics during their stay in hospital, and this exerts strong selective pressures on the microbial flora, especially of the gastrointestinal tract, leading to the development of antibiotic-associated diarrhoea due to *Clostridium difficile* (see Ch. 22), one of the commonest causes of outbreaks of hospital infection. Sensitive species or strains of micro-organisms which normally maintain a protective function on the skin and other mucosal surfaces tend to be eliminated, whereas those that are more resistant survive and become endemic in the hospital population. This may restrict the range of agents available for treatment and may lead to the transmission of plasmid-mediated antibiotic resistance into strains that show increased virulence, survival and spread within the hospital.

## MICRO-ORGANISMS CAUSING HOSPITAL INFECTION

The most important micro-organisms responsible for hospital infection are listed in Table 69.1.

Outbreaks of *Staphylococcus aureus* infection were often seen in surgical wards and maternity units before the advent of penicillinase-stable penicillins such as methicillin in the early 1960s. Some strains, such as the notorious phage type 80/81, demonstrated particular virulence and colonizing capabilities. Subsequently, epidemic or pandemic strains characterized by resistance to methicillin (MRSA) have been found in many hospitals worldwide, presenting a daunting challenge. Some strains are better able to colonize patients or staff than to produce systemic disease. This illustrates the adaptation and evolutionary changes possible within common hospital bacteria revealed by careful epidemiological typing and observation. The changing patterns may be related to particular events and infection control measures, so that lessons can be learnt for future control and prevention.

With the advent of more elaborate surgery and intensive care, combined with the use of broad-spectrum antibiotics and immunosuppressive drugs, Gram-negative bacteria increased in importance. Many, such as *Pseudomonas aeruginosa*, are *opportunists* capable of causing infection in compromised patients. Such organisms may be found in the patient's own flora, or in damp environmental sites, including patient equipment and medicaments. They may exhibit natural resistance to many antibiotics and antiseptics, and have the ability to colonize traumatized skin such as burns and areas with poor tissue viability such as decubitus ulcers and bed sores.

In recent years, groups of micro-organisms which formerly played no recognized part in hospital infection have emerged. These include the coagulase-negative staphylococci and *Acinetobacter baumanii* present in normal skin flora. Viral or fungal infection, particularly of the immunocompromised patient, has become more important. *Legionella pneumophila*, disseminated from environmental sources such as air conditioning and hot water systems, causes sporadic cases or outbreaks of respiratory infection in hospitals. Awareness of the risks of blood-borne viruses, including hepatitis B and C, human immunodeficiency virus (HIV) and of many agents such as cytomegalovirus, which can be transmitted by organ or cellular transplants, has increased in patients and in staff. The possible risk of iatrogenic spread of the prion causing Creutzfeldt–Jakob disease (see Ch. 60) has persuaded the UK government to take stringent measures on decontamination of surgical instruments and the US blood transfusion service to ban British donors.

**Table 69.1** Commonly occurring micro-organisms in hospital infection

| Type of infection | Micro-organisms responsible |
|---|---|
| Urinary tract infections | *Escherichia coli*<br>*Klebsiella, Serratia, Proteus* spp.<br>*Pseudomonas aeruginosa*<br>*Enterococcus spp.*<br>*Candida albicans* |
| Respiratory infections | *Haemophilus influenzae*<br>*Streptococcus pneumoniae*<br>*Staphylococcus aureus*<br>Enterobacteriaceae<br>Respiratory viruses (influenza, respiratory synctial)<br>Fungi (*Candida* spp., *Aspergilli*) |
| Wounds and skin sepsis | *Staph. aureus*<br>*Str. pyogenes*<br>*Esch. coli*<br>Proteus spp.<br>Anaerobes<br>Enterococcus spp.<br>Coagulase-negative staphylococci |
| Gastro-intestinal infections | *Salmonella* serotypes<br>*Clostridium difficile*<br>Viruses (norovirus, rotavirus) |

## ROUTES OF TRANSMISSION

The hospital offers many opportunities for the exchange of microbes, many of which are harmless and a normal part of the balance between man and his environment. For there to be a significant risk of infection, several factors, including the right susceptible host and the appropriate inoculum of infecting micro-organism, must be linked via an appropriate route of transmission. Understanding of the sources and spread of hospital infection enables efforts to be concentrated in more effective preventive measures.

Common routes of transmission for different micro-organisms are shown in Table 69.2.

**Table 69.2** Hospital infection: sources and spread

| Route | Source | Examples of disease |
|---|---|---|
| 1. Aerial (from persons)<br>Droplets<br>Skin scales | Mouth<br>Nose<br>Skin exudate, infected lesion | Measles, tuberculosis, pneumonia<br>Staphylococcal sepsis<br>Staphylococcal and streptococcal sepsis |
| 2. Aerial (from inanimate sources)<br>Particles | Respiratory equipment<br>Air-conditioning plant | Gram-negative respiratory infection<br>Legionnaires' disease, fungal infections |
| 3. Contact (from persons)<br>Direct spread<br>Indirect via equipment | Respiratory secretions<br>Faeces, urine, skin and wound exudate | Staphylococcal and streptococcal sepsis<br>Enterobacterial and viral diarrhoea, Pseudomonas aeruginosa sepsis |
| 4. Contact (environmental source) | Equipment, food, medicaments, fluids | Enterobacterial sepsis (Klebsiella/Serratia/ Enterobacter spp.)<br>Ps. aeruginosa and other pseudomonads |
| 5. Inoculation | Sharp injury, blood products | Hepatitis B, HIV, malaria |

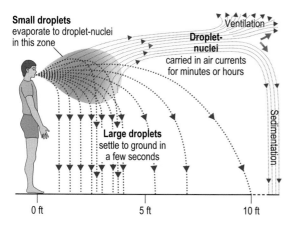

**Fig. 69.1** Spread of respiratory infections by droplets and droplet nuclei.

**Fig. 69.2** Infection of the air with dust particles derived from nasal and oral secretions contaminating hands, handkerchief, clothing and surrounding surfaces: (A) hand soiled with secretions from lips or nose-picking; (B) clothing contaminated by hand; (C) soiled handkerchief; (D) infected dust from handkerchief; (E) dust from clothing (e.g. from near handkerchief pocket); (F) infected dust raised after settling on floor.

## Airborne transmission

Infections may be spread:

- By airborne transmission from the respiratory tract (talking, coughing, sneezing).
- From the skin by natural shedding of skin scales during wound dressing or bed-making.
- By aerosols from equipment such as respiratory apparatus and air-conditioning plants.

Infectious agents may be dispersed as small particles or droplets over long distances (Fig. 69.1). Staphylococci survive well on mucosal secretions, skin scales and dried pus and may be redistributed in the air after initial settlement during periods of increased activity (Fig. 69.2). Gram-negative bacilli do not generally survive desiccation in air, and this route of transmission is therefore limited to conditions of high humidity such as ventilatory equipment, showers or other fine water aerosols.

## Contact spread

The most common routes of transmission for hospital infection are:

- By *direct* contact spread from person to person.
- By *indirect* contact spread via contaminated hands or equipment.

Human secretions as well as contaminated dust particles or fluids may be carried on thermometers, bedpans, bed-linen, cutlery or other shared items. Hands and, to a lesser extent, clothing of hospital staff serve as vectors of Gram-negative and Gram-positive infection. Procedures involving contact with mucosal surfaces, e.g. insertion of a urinary catheter, may introduce micro-organisms from the contaminated hands of the operator or from the patient's own urethral flora into the normally sterile bladder.

## Food-borne spread

Infection may originate in the hospital kitchen, or in special diets, infant feeds, kitchen or commercial supplies. Deteriorating hygiene standards may support the proliferation of flies, cockroaches and other insects or rodents which damage stored products and act as carriers of microbes.

## Blood-borne spread

The accidental transmission of infections such as HIV, hepatitis B or C by needlestick or contaminated 'sharp' injuries has been well documented. In areas of high prevalence of these blood-borne viruses, malaria or syphilis stringent precautions should be taken to minimize transmission between patients and from healthcare workers by strict use of single-use items and screening blood products.

## Self-infection and cross-infection

The interaction between different sources of infection may be illustrated by the example of a patient undergoing lower bowel surgery. *Self-infection* may occur due to transfer into the wound of staphylococci (or occasionally streptococci) carried in the patient's nose and distributed over the skin, or of coliform bacilli and anaerobes released from the bowel during surgery. Alternatively, *cross-infection* may result from staphylococci or coliform bacilli derived from other patients or healthy staff carriers. The organisms may be transferred into the wound *during operation* through the surgeon's punctured gloves or moistened gown, on imperfectly sterilized surgical

instruments and materials, or by airborne theatre dust. *Postoperatively*, organisms may be transferred in the ward from contaminated bed-linen, by airborne ward dust or in consequence of a faulty wound dressing technique.

Of all the possible routes, by far the most likely in this example is self-infection from the patient's own bowel flora and it is therefore against this route that most specific preventive measures in colorectal surgery are directed. Understanding of possible sources of infection and the methods available to block transmission to susceptible sites forms the basis of hospital infection control.

Cross-infection is more often caused by 'hospital' strains selected for characteristics of antimicrobial resistance and virulence. An important example at present is MRSA, which can be easily identified by the microbiology laboratory, which should have a system for alerting the infection control team who need to collect the following basic epidemiological data:

- patient details
- the site and extent of infection
- the dates of admission, operative procedures, first recognition of infection
- specimens and laboratory isolates and typing results
- ward and staff details.

The clustering of cases according to a common surgical team or location in the ward may suggest a common source and may be the first firm indication of an outbreak of hospital infection.

Soon after admission to hospital, individuals commonly become contaminated with the 'hospital flora'. This has been shown with *Staph. aureus* in studies of patients before and during hospital treatment. Those patients who need to stay longer in hospital, e.g. those requiring intensive care or the elderly, are more susceptible to infection and the risks of HAI are greater.

## PREVENTION AND CONTROL

### Infection control policy

The establishment of an effective infection control organization is the responsibility of good management of any hospital. There will normally be two parts:

1. An *infection control committee*, meeting regularly to formulate and update policies for the whole hospital on matters having implications for infection control, and to manage outbreaks of nosocomial infection.

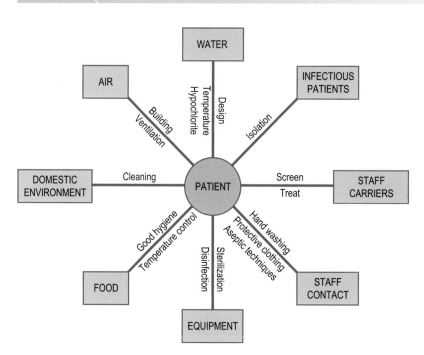

2. An *infection control team* of workers, headed by the *infection control doctor* (usually the microbiologist), to take day-to-day responsibility for this policy.

The functions of this team include surveillance and control of infection and monitoring of hygiene practices, advising the infection control committee on matters of policy relating to the prevention of infection and the education of all staff in the microbiologically safe performance of procedures. The *infection control nurse* is a key member of this team. Close working links between the microbiology laboratory, infection control nurse and the different clinical specialties and support services (including sterile services, laundry, pharmacy and engineering) are important to establish and maintain the infection control policy, and to ensure that it is rationally based and that the recommended procedures are practicable. It is important for all members of the committee to ensure that everyone in the organization makes infection control and hospital hygiene their business. Campaigns should be launched locally raise the profile of proven methods of control such as hand washing. Some of the control measures in which the infection control team should be involved are shown in Figure 69.3.

## Decontamination and sterilization

The provision of sterile instruments, dressings and fluids is of fundamental importance in hospital practice. Items that are reused for procedures in normally sterile sites, such as surgical equipment, must be decontaminated by thorough washing before sterilization by heat. High-vacuum autoclaves have become accepted hospital practice. The development of these sterilizers for processing wrapped goods facilitated the provision of a centralized service of sterile supply to wards, complementing the existing theatre service. The availability of a wide range of prepacked single-use items (syringes, needles, catheters and drainage bags) sterilized commercially by γ-irradiation or ethylene oxide has further improved aseptic procedures and removed the need for reprocessing items that are difficult to clean and therefore impossible to sterilize. The scientific basis of sterilization is mentioned in more detail in Chapter 4.

Most fluids for topical use or intravenous administration are now prepared commercially or in regional units where standards of quality control and efficiency for bulk processes are more readily achieved than in individual hospital pharmacies.

## Aseptic techniques

The provision of sterile equipment will not prevent the spread of infection if there is carelessness in its use. Wherever possible, *no-touch* techniques must be used, coupled with strict personal hygiene on the part of the operator. These routines are rigidly laid down in operating theatre practice and may be modified as required for other procedures such as wound dressing and insertion of intravenous catheters.

## Cleaning and disinfection

The general hospital environment can be kept in good order by attention to basic cleaning, waste disposal and laundry. The use of chemical disinfectants for walls, floors and furniture is necessary only in special instances, such as spillages of body fluids from patients with blood-borne virus infections. Ward equipment such as bed-pan washer/disinfectors and dishwashers should be monitored to ensure reliable performance, and cleaning materials such as mop-heads and cloths should be heat-disinfected and stored dry after use. Pre-cleaning of contaminated instruments and equipment, preferably by means of an automatic washing process with an ultrasonicator, is an essential step before disinfection or sterilization.

## Skin disinfection and antiseptics

The ease of acquisition and transfer of transient hospital contaminants, particularly staphylococci and Gram-negative bacilli on the hands of staff, is an important factor in the spread of hospital infection. Thorough handwashing after any procedure involving nursing care or close contact with the patient is essential. Alcohol-based hand antiseptics or 'rubs' have been introduced in wards where routine handwashing with water and detergent is not practicable. Gloves may be worn for many dirty contact procedures, such as emptying a urinary drainage bag or bedpan, although it should not be forgotten that the gloved hand may also become colonized by transient hospital flora.

Procedures for preoperative disinfection of the patient's skin and for surgical scrubs are mandatory within the operating theatre. Dilute 'in-use' solutions of antiseptics may readily become colonized with Gram-negative bacteria and should be replaced regularly. Ideally, *single-use* preparations should be used. Restriction should be placed on the indiscriminate use of antiseptics and disinfectants by means of a *disinfectant policy* agreed by pharmacists, microbiologists and key users, such as theatre staff.

## Decontamination and disinfectant policy

All hospitals should agree a policy to ensure all clinical staff are familiar with the agents used and procedures involved in decontamination. The policy should consider the following:

- The sources (equipment, skin and environment) for which the choice of process is required.

- The processes and products available for sterilization and disinfection. One objective of the policy is to include a limited range of options and chemicals to be used.
- The category of process required for each item in a simple table: sterilization for surgical instruments, heat disinfection for laundry and crockery, cleaning for floors and furniture.
- The specific products and method to be used for each item and staff responsible.

Effective implementation of the policy requires liaison and training of staff and regular updating as new methods and agents become available. Safety consideration for staff and patients require that a risk assessment is made of procedures and chemicals to minimize hazards and comply with local health and safety regulations. This includes the use of fume cupboards, air scavenging equipment and sealed washer-disinfectors. These requirements take decontamination of equipment out of small clinics into centralized sterile supply departments and increase the use of disposables in medical practice.

## Prophylactic antibiotics

Widespread and haphazard use of antibiotics hastens the emergence of antibiotic-resistant bacteria and increases both the incidence of toxic side-effects and the cost of treatment. However, rational antibiotic prophylaxis plays an important role in infection control. Specific indications include perioperative prophylaxis in gastrointestinal and gynaecological surgery directed predominantly against anaerobic infection and for patients known to have bacteriuria at the time of urological surgery or instrumentation, directed against the urine isolate. An *antibiotic policy* which limits the choice of broad-spectrum agents is important both for prophylaxis and treatment (see Ch. 67).

## Protective clothing

Different activities within the hospital require different degrees of protection to staff and patients. In operating theatres the wearing of sterile gowns, gloves, head gear and face masks minimizes the shedding of micro-organisms. The properties of fabrics available for theatre use have improved, and now include close-weave ventile fabrics that are comfortable to wear and allow evaporation of moisture. 'Total protection' of the operating site may be considered for certain high-risk clean surgery such as hip replacements, during which the surgical team may wear exhaust-ventilated suits and operate under conditions of ultraclean laminar airflow.

For many ward procedures in which there may be soiling, or for simple *barrier nursing* of patients with communicable diseases, plastic aprons and gloves are used. Gloves, face masks and goggles are also indicated for specific procedures when blood contact is likely through splashes or aerosols, such as dental procedures. These should conform to international standards and staff should be trained in their use and disposal.

## Isolation

The isolation policy should list facilities and procedures needed to prevent the spread of specific infections to other patients (*source isolation*) and to protect susceptible or immunocompromised patients (*protective isolation*). Effective isolation demands a highly disciplined approach by all staff to ensure that none of the barriers to transmission (airborne, direct and indirect contact) are breached. Multi-bedded rooms may be used, and even wards converted during hospital outbreaks, but the simplest solution wherever possible is to use single rooms.

'Cubicle' isolation, by which the patient is nursed alone in a room separated by a door and corridor from other patients, confers a substantial measure of protection. Preferably, each isolation room has its own toilet and washing facility. Clean, filtered air is supplied to the room, which should be at negative pressure (*exhaust-ventilated*) to the corridor for source isolation or at positive pressure (*pressure-ventilated*) to the corridor for protective isolation. If, however, there is a small airlock vestibule separating the room from the outer corridor, then exhaust ventilation of the airlock will give effective isolation for either situation. The vestibule or lobby should contain a wash basin and include space for gowning and equipment.

In some critical situations such as bone marrow transplant units, where airborne contamination with environmental fungal spores is a problem, the efficiency of air filtration may be increased and laminar airflow maintained as a barrier around the patient. Stringent isolation in a plastic tent isolator is required only for patients with highly contagious infections and such contingencies usually require transfer to a specialist hospital.

## Hospital building and design

The routine maintenance of the hospital building is important, ensuring that surfaces wherever possible are smooth, impervious and easy to clean. Major rebuilding works on or near the hospital site may generate dust containing fungal and bacterial spores, with implications for specialized units serving immunocompromised patients. Close communications with the works department and hospital administration are necessary to coordinate any protective action. When a new hospital or modification of existing building is planned, the infection control team should be closely involved in discussing the plans. In many countries, guidance on new building design exists to minimize potential hospital-acquired infection. Areas requiring special attention include operating theatres, kitchens, acute wards, laboratories and air-conditioning systems. The risk of Legionnaires' disease is reduced by regular flushing all outlets and installing water supplies that circulate below 20°C for the cold and above 60°C for the hot circuit.

## Equipment

Any object or item of equipment for clinical use should be assessed to determine the appropriate method, frequency and site of decontamination. Wherever possible, heat processes are preferred, although this may be precluded for certain thermolabile items such as fibreoptic endoscopes. Dedicated washer-disinfectors in sealed units are necessary for these items. In many situations, especially in community settings, disposable instruments should be used, although monetary and environmental costs need to be balanced against availability and transport of the item.

## Personnel

An occupational health service should screen staff before employment for serious communicable diseases, such as tuberculosis, and check their immunization status. Hepatitis B vaccine should be given to all health care workers if they have not been fully immunized. Those at special risk performing exposure-prone procedures, such as invasive surgery, should be screened for blood-borne viruses. All healthcare staff (including students and those working in the community) should receive occupational health advice and protection. Staff who have contracted infections such as impetigo or diarrhoea should report and be screened if necessary. Those that sustain needlestick injuries from potentially contaminated sources should have access to advice and post-exposure prophylaxis with antivirals and immunization. There should be an educational programme tailored to the needs of different cadres of staff both on induction and as part of continuing professional development.

## Monitoring

Routine microbiological sampling of the environment is of little benefit, although monitoring of the physical performance of air-conditioning plants and machinery used for disinfection and sterilization is essential. In the event of an outbreak of hospital infection such as Legionnaires' disease, more specific monitoring targeted at the known or likely causative micro-organism should be considered.

Microbiological screening of staff or patients is not undertaken routinely, but it may be needed for specific purposes: to detect carriers of MRSA and hepatitis viruses in those performing some types of surgery or where transmission to patients has occurred.

## Surveillance and the role of the laboratory

The detection and characterization of hospital infection incidents or outbreaks rely on laboratory data that alert the infection control team to unusual clusters of infection, or to the sporadic appearance of organisms that may present a particular infection risk or management problem. This is sometimes referred to as the *'alert organism'* system. Bacterial typing schemes and antibiograms (see Ch. 3) are very important in this regard. In some situations mandatory surveillance of cases of infection with particular pathogens such as MRSA or *C. difficile* may be useful to compare hospitals or units and reduce hospital infection by regular, timely feedback to clinicians and managers. Regular visits to the wards are also important to record data on infected patients from whom no specimens have been received and to respond to problems as they occur. Such visits

also serve to provide opportunities for practical teaching, which is another important element of the infection control team's responsibility. Advances in surgical practice have lead to short stays in hospital so that some postoperative infections are only detected after discharge. Surveillance of surgical site infection should include data collected post-discharge.

## EFFICACY OF INFECTION CONTROL

The evidence base in the literature for acceptable proof of efficacy for infection control measures is limited. These include sterilization, hand-washing, closed-drainage systems for urinary catheters, intravenous catheter care, perioperative antibiotic prophylaxis for contaminated wounds and techniques for the care of equipment used in respiratory therapy. Isolation techniques are assumed to be reasonable as suggested by experience or inference. Measures which are now considered to be ineffective include regular chemical disinfection of floors, walls and sinks, and routine environmental monitoring.

Effective surveillance and action by the infection control team have been shown to reduce infection rates. One important role of the team is to monitor compliance with practices known to be effective and to eliminate the many rituals or less effective practices which may even increase the incidence or cost of cross-infection. As further advances occur in medical care and limited health care resources are spread across hospital and community needs, innovations in infection control will need to be evaluated for efficacy and cost-effectiveness. With this understanding it is possible that hospital infection can be controlled and largely prevented. The dictum of Florence Nightingale, made over a century ago, that 'the very first requirement in a hospital is that it should do the sick no harm', remains the goal.

---

RECOMMENDED READING

Fraise AP, Bradley C, editors: *Ayliffe's Control of Hospital Infection*, ed 5, London, 2009, Hodder Arnold.
Fraise AP, Lambert P, Maillard J-Y, editors: *Russell, Hugo and Ayliffe's Principles and Practice of Disinfection, Preservation and Sterilization*, ed 4, Oxford, 2004, Blackwell.
Wenzel RP, editor: *Prevention and Control of Nosocomial Infection*, ed 4, Baltimore, 2002, Lippincott, Williams and Wilkins.

## Websites

Centers for Disease Control: Healthcare-associated Infections (HAIs). http://www.cdc.gov/hai/

Department of Health (England): Reducing Healthcare Associated Infection. http://hcai.dh.gov.uk/
Health and Safety Executive: http://www.hse.gov.uk/
Hospital Infection Society: http://www.his.org.uk/
Infection Prevention Society (formerly Infection Control Nurses Association): http://www.ips.uk.net/
Medicines and Healthcare Products Regulatory Agency: http://www.mhra.gov.uk/
National Resource for Infection Control (NRIC): http://www.nric.org.uk/
Thames Valley University Evidence Based Guidelines: http://www.wolfson.tvu.ac.uk/research

# 70 Immunization

*R. C. B. Slack*

## KEY POINTS

- Immunization is a major means by which infections may be controlled and, in some cases, eradicated.
- Passive immunization involves the administration of immunoglobulin-containing preparations that provide protection against one or more infections. The immunity is short-lived. Preparations providing protection against tetanus, hepatitis B, rabies, varicella–zoster and vaccinia are available.
- Active immunization produces more enduring immunity. Live-attenuated, killed (inactivated) and subunit (e.g. toxoid or capsular antigen) vaccines are used widely.
- The use of particular vaccines is contraindicated in certain individuals, such as the use of live vaccines in immunocompromised individuals.
- Where immunization prevents transmission, the objective of immunization programmes is to achieve *herd immunity* such that, once a threshold level of immunization has been achieved, no further transmission can take place in that community.
- The standard immunization schedule in the UK provides for active immunization in childhood against diphtheria, tetanus, pertussis, seven serotypes of pneumococci, *Haemophilus influenzae* capsule type B (Hib), *Neisseria meningitidis* capsule type C, polio, and measles, mumps and rubella.
- Additional active immunization may be considered against hepatitis B, varicella, tuberculosis and influenza for specific groups, and travellers are routinely offered additional vaccines specific to the locations visited.

It is appropriate that the last chapter of this book should be devoted to immunization, which is only one of the measures that may be used for the control of infectious diseases (see Ch. 68) yet has dramatically and successfully rid the world of the scourge of smallpox and is well on the way to eradicating poliomyelitis. With rapid advances in understanding host responses to antigens and the means to make and deliver vaccines, the future looks exciting for eradicating other communicable diseases in humans and animals. The cost and efficacy of immunization programmes must be assessed against other forms of defence, (Box. 70.1), such as:

- environmental sanitation
- safe sewage disposal
- a secure water supply
- food hygiene
- clean air and adequate ventilation
- good animal husbandry with effective quarantine arrangements where necessary
- insect vector control
- improved nutrition.

Much of the morbidity and mortality of infection is still not preventable by immunization or presents great difficulties. For example, at present, many of the parasitic, diarrhoeal and respiratory infections that take a heavy toll of life and health among young children in poor and overcrowded communities are not amenable to control by specific vaccines; nor are the common bacterial infections associated with haemolytic streptococci, staphylococci and coliform bacilli.

## RATIONALE OF IMMUNIZATION

The objective is to produce, without harm to the recipient, a degree of resistance sufficient to prevent a clinical attack of the natural infection and to prevent the spread of infection to susceptibles in the community. There is therefore both a personal gain from being immunized and a public health benefit to the population. The degree of resistance conferred may not protect against an overwhelming challenge, but exposure may help to boost immunity.

> **Box 70.1** Approaches to the prevention of infectious disease: An indication of priorities
>
> - Preventive engineering: water, sewage, ventilation, food production and food processing
> - Surveillance and diagnostic awareness
> - Prompt management: recognition, treatment, isolation and contact tracing where necessary
> - Improvement and maintenance of good socio-economic conditions: housing, nutrition, education, medical and social care
> - Increased resistance to infection by appropriate active immunization policies and in some special circumstances by passive immunization

## PASSIVE IMMUNIZATION

*Artificial passive immunization* is used in clinical practice when it is considered necessary to protect a patient at short notice and for a limited period. Antibodies, which may be antitoxic, antibacterial or antiviral, in preparations of human or animal serum are injected to give temporary protection. Human preparations are referred to as *homologous*, and are much less likely to give rise to the adverse reactions occasionally associated with the injection of animal (*heterologous*) sera. An additional advantage of homologous antisera is that, although they do not confer durable protection, their effect may persist for 3–6 months, whereas the protection afforded by a heterologous serum is likely to last for only a few weeks. The use of monoclonal antibodies against specific pathogens, such as respiratory syncytial virus, is likely to widen the scope of passive immunization in future.

Antiserum raised in the horse against diphtheria toxin (*equine diphtheria antitoxin*) is available in some countries for the prophylaxis and treatment of diphtheria. A similar heterologous antiserum is available for emergency use in cases of suspected botulism and to protect those thought to be at risk. Equine tetanus antitoxin is still used in some parts of the world, but it should be abandoned in favour of human tetanus immunoglobulin (see Ch. 22, p. 251). It is most important to give an intended recipient of equine serum a prior test dose to exclude hypersensitive subjects who may have been sensitized by a previous dose of equine serum and may suffer 'serum sickness'.

### Pooled immunoglobulins

Protective levels of antibody to a range of diseases are present in pooled normal human serum. *Human normal immunoglobulin* (HNIG) is available for the short-term prophylaxis of hepatitis A in contacts or travellers who intend to visit countries where hepatitis A is common. However, active immunization is a much better alternative against hepatitis A for frequent travellers to endemic areas. HNIG also protects those with agammaglobulinaemia and has been used in cases of Gram-negative sepsis and *C. difficile* infection.

### Specific immunoglobulins

Preparations of specific immunoglobulins are available for passive immunization against the following:

- tetanus (human tetanus immunoglobulin; HTIG)
- hepatitis B (HBIG)
- rabies (HRIG)
- varicella–zoster (ZIG).

## ACTIVE IMMUNIZATION

### Types of vaccine

#### Toxoids

If the signs and symptoms of a disease can be attributed essentially to the effects of a single toxin, a modified form of the toxin that preserves its antigenicity but has lost its toxicity (a *toxoid*) provides the key to successful active immunization against the disease. This has been spectacularly successful with tetanus and diphtheria.

#### Inactivated vaccines

If the disease is not mediated by a single toxin, it may be possible to stimulate the production of protective antibodies by using the killed (inactivated) organisms. This is done as a routine with vaccines against pertussis (whooping cough), influenza and the inactivated polio (Salk) vaccine.

#### Attenuated live vaccines

In some cases, the inactivation procedure to make a killed vaccine destroys or modifies the protective antigenicity (*immunogenicity*) of the organisms. Hence, another approach is to use suspensions of living organisms that are reduced in their virulence (*attenuated*) but still immunogenic. This strategy has yielded mumps, measles, rubella and varicella vaccines (now combined), the live-virus polio (Sabin) and yellow fever vaccines.

Sometimes, it is possible to use a related organism with shared antigens. Thus, the vaccinia virus vaccine was used to eradicate smallpox, and a bovine tubercle bacillus was modified by Calmette and Guérin to make bacille Calmette–Guérin (BCG), which protects humans against tuberculosis and leprosy (see pp. 220 & 225).

## Special procedures

Some vaccines, such as influenza (virus) vaccine, can be refined by a process that removes unwanted protein and other reactive material but retains the important protective antigens. Some others must be conjugated to proteins to render them immunogenic. Some vaccines, such as hepatitis B vaccine, can be bioengineered. There is much current interest in the possibility of developing *subunit vaccines* consisting of purified fragments of the major immunogenic components of micro-organisms, particularly viruses.

## Immune response

Antibodies against the agents of some bacterial and viral infections may be present in the mother's blood and be passively acquired by the baby (see Part 2 of this book). This gives some protection to the infant at a time when it is poorly equipped to produce specific antibodies, but it may interfere to a varying extent with the infant's capacity to respond to the stimulus of injected or ingested vaccines in the very early months of life. Although the capacity of the infant to produce specific antibody to injected antigens is poorly developed in the first few months of life, this problem can often be resolved by the use of *adjuvants*. Thus, effective responses are produced to powerful antigens such as alum-adsorbed toxoids. Pertussis whole-cell vaccines have an adjuvant effect of their own, so the combination of adsorbed toxoids and whole-cell pertussis vaccine (the triple diphtheria, tetanus and pertussis vaccine; DTP) is an effective immunizing complex that used to be given in the UK at 2, 3 and 4 months of age to cover the period when the lethal potential of pertussis is greatest (see below and Ch. 32). The tissues of the newborn respond effectively to BCG vaccine because the protection here is cell-mediated. The use of a high-potency measles vaccine at 6–9 months of age is likely to be exploited in countries where measles kills or severely injures the very young.

When a good specific antibody response is being sought to a toxoid or a killed antigen, the usual procedure is to give three doses of the antigen at spaced intervals. The first or 'priming' dose evokes a low level of antibody after a latent period of about 2 weeks, but the second dose elicits a much greater (secondary) antibody response, and this is further boosted by the third dose. The efficacy of injected antigen preparations can be enhanced by slow-release agents such as mineral carriers which have adjuvant effects. With most antigens, the response is better if the first two doses are separated by an interval of a month or two. A third dose is generally recommended at some time thereafter, and further booster doses may be given to maintain immunity.

## Duration of immunity

After an effective course of active immunization, a protective amount of antibody may persist in the blood for some years and a subsequent booster injection may maintain protection for a further decade. Much depends upon circumstances that will vary for different vaccines and different groups of people. The duration of active protection cannot be absolutely equated with the presence of demonstrable antibody because factors such as the sensitivity of the test and the actual protective role of the antibody detected have to be taken into consideration.

## Age of commencement of active immunization

This must take account of the immaturity of the antibody-forming system in the very early months (see above) and the infectious challenges that a person may encounter early in life and in later years. The start of any immunization programme must be adjusted to the known epidemiology of the diseases that are prevalent in the country in which it is to be instituted, and it must also be related to any serious infective challenges that may be imported from time to time. Poliomyelitis is a good example of a disease that has been largely eradicated from many communities; however, the disease is quick to strike back if the immunization shield is lowered.

## CONTROLLED STUDIES OF VACCINES

Combined field and laboratory studies aim to provide confidence in the efficacy of vaccines. A field trial can show only whether or not the actual preparation of vaccine used was successful under the circumstances prevailing at the time. Accordingly, trials require very sophisticated design and much care in their execution. In order to satisfy the requirement for reproducibility, the method of preparation of the vaccine must be meticulously described and controlled. Much work continues to define and to refine laboratory tests for the protectiveness of a particular vaccine that might be correlated with its efficacy in field trials. The laboratory test that gives results most closely corresponding to the protective value in the field trials may then be adopted as the test for standardizing future batches of vaccine.

Manufacturers of vaccines for commercial use are required in the UK and in many other countries to satisfy certain standards relating to the purity, safety, potency and stability of their products. In addition, the World Health Organization (WHO) has established internationally agreed requirements. At the national level, a system for continuing surveillance of the efficacy of prophylactic vaccines with continuing notification of any suspected adverse reactions is essential.

## CONTRAINDICATIONS TO THE USE OF VACCINES

In the delivery of an important immunization programme there is a balance between the rights of the individual (and often this is the parent or carer not the person being immunized) and the benefit to the public. It is necessary not to take too legalistic a view of theoretical hazards and thus err on the side of opting out. The risk of opting out of an immunization schedule should be clearly appreciated and shown to be greater than the adverse effects.

There are some useful general principles about contraindications:

- do not give a vaccine to a patient with an acute illness
- do be sure that the postponed immunization is subsequently given
- do not give a live vaccine to a pregnant woman, unless there is a clear balance of risk in favour of vaccination
- avoid giving any vaccine in the first trimester of pregnancy
- do not give live vaccines to patients receiving immunosuppressive drugs or irradiation, or to patients suffering from malignant conditions of the reticulo-endothelial system – delay until after successful therapy when they are in remission.

Experience with human immunodeficiency virus (HIV) antibody-positive patients with or without the signs and symptoms of the acquired immune deficiency syndrome (AIDS) indicates so far that measles, mumps, rubella and polio (live virus) vaccines can be given, but that BCG vaccine should not be given. Inactivated vaccines, e.g. pneumococcal, are not contraindicated and are of great benefit.

## Hazards of immunization

Possible adverse reactions to immunization are:

- mild or moderate pain at the site of injection
- fever and malaise for a day or two after
- anaphylactic reactions are very rare but, as they may be fatal, doctors and nurses should be aware of the possibility and should be prepared for such an emergency by carrying drugs and equipment for resuscitation (a 'shock box') to all immunization sessions.

During the first few years of life when many vaccines are given, children tend to have various health problems that include occasional febrile convulsions and may, sadly, include an unexplained cot death or other tragedy. It is inevitable that some of these events will coincide with the period shortly after a vaccine was given to a child and the possibility of a causal relationship will be entertained. The probability of such a link certainly deserves to be considered, but it is most important to bear in mind that the issue is emotive and that ill-balanced or ill-informed adverse publicity can do irreparable harm to an immunization programme. For example, annual notifications of whooping cough in England and Wales dropped from more than 100 000 in the early 1950s to some tens of thousands in the late 1950s as the vaccine gained ground. By the early 1970s (and after modification of the vaccine to take account of a possible deficiency in its protective cover), whooping cough was largely controlled in the UK, with about 75% of children immunized. In the late 1970s, after some ill-informed adverse publicity, acceptance rates for the vaccine fell steeply to 30% or lower, and the uptake of other vaccines was also affected. Epidemics of whooping cough followed in the UK in 1978 and 1982, with tens of thousands of children affected and a number of deaths. As a result of efforts to restore confidence in pertussis vaccine, uptake figures increased in the 1980s and the disease again began to be brought under control. Preliminary results of tests with new (acellular) pertussis vaccines indicate that these are safe and probably more effective.

Over the past few years there has been considerable publicity about claims that autism and inflammatory bowel disease were associated with MMR vaccine. Although several well-conducted studies have failed to confirm the original study, which first drew attention to this hazard, the media in the UK have supported the hypothesis and cover of the vaccine fell to the point that cases and deaths from measles reemerged. Mathematical models of the dynamics of measles in a population show that if the number of susceptibles in the population exceeds 5% there is a possibility of transmission.

Children who are most vulnerable are likely to be least protected. Pertussis, polio and measles spread most effectively when living conditions are overcrowded and unhygienic. To some extent, these diseases depend upon population density for their spread. Some underprivileged groups in a community are in very real danger when the average rate of vaccine uptake falls, because they often have the lowest cover.

In view of the stringency of the regulations that control the quality and efficacy of vaccines, the probability of error lies more with the vaccinator than with the producer. There is a special obligation to ensure that vaccines are properly stored, reconstituted (if relevant) and correctly administered (Box 70.2). Many preparations rapidly lose their potency if frozen and thawed or exposed to temperature variation. This means it is vital to maintain the 'cold chain' in which the vaccines are held between 2–8°C. The appropriate instructions and local protocols should be followed in detail. *An injectable vaccine must be given with a sterile syringe and needle, a separate sterile syringe and needle must be used for each injection, and the equipment must be disposed of properly.* The dangers of contamination with blood-borne viruses such as HIV and hepatitis B and C have led to the search for alternative methods of delivery by air jets or via mucosal surfaces.

## Site of injection

This will vary with the vaccine to be given. Specific instructions should be followed. In general, and with the exception of BCG, injectable vaccines are given by intramuscular or deep subcutaneous injection. The anterolateral aspect of the thigh or upper arm is the preferred site for infants. Some doctors and nurses use the upper outer quadrant of the buttock, but fat in this area may interfere with the efficacy of the vaccine, especially hepatitis A and B. In future, the technological advances in delivery methods mentioned above will revolutionize the immunization clinics feared by countless school children.

## HERD IMMUNITY

When most people in a community are immune to a particular infection that is spread from person to person, the natural transmission of the infection is effectively inhibited. Thus, if almost all children in a residential school have been immunized against measles, the school is most unlikely to have an outbreak of measles; even the few children who have not been immunized will enjoy a measure of protection afforded by the general herd immunity in that they will not be challenged within the school. This will only apply so long as the school population is largely composed of immune pupils and a nonimmune pupil does not encounter a visitor who is infected with measles. If there is an influx of susceptibles, the level of herd immunity will fall and the general protection will be lost. When the pupils go into other communities at holiday times, the nonimmune individuals are liable to get measles at their first contact with an infective case.

For herd immunity to operate well in a community or a country, vaccine uptake rates must exceed 90%. For some highly transmissible infections, such as measles, uptake rates above 95% are the target. Bear in mind that herd immunity operates only for infections transmitted from person to person. Tetanus is not transmitted in this way; a nonimmune person is fully vulnerable to tetanus even if he or she is surrounded by fully immunized colleagues in a closed community (Fig. 70.1).

## IMMUNIZATION PROGRAMMES

An immunization campaign carried out without provision for its continuation as a routine procedure will not give satisfactory results unless complete eradication of the disease is achieved. Thus, in planning immunization schedules, consideration must be given to ensuring that the general public is receptive and understands the policy. It is essential to secure the trust and cooperation of parents who have to bring their children to the doctor or clinic for a series of inoculations and who will undoubtedly seek reassurance that the benefits are considerable and the risks negligible. Appropriate consent must be obtained for each immunization.

In the planning and execution of a programme, immunological points that merit special attention are:

- the use of combined antigens and the simultaneous administration of killed and live vaccines

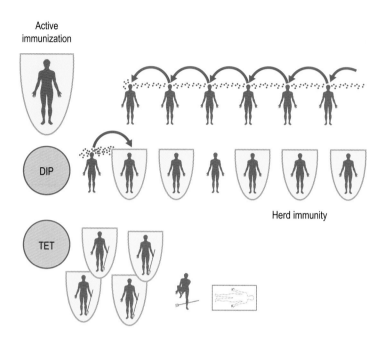

Active immunization

DIP

TET

Herd immunity

**Fig. 70.1** If almost all of the members of a community receive active immunization against a disease that is normally transmitted from person-to-person, the resulting herd immunity confers some advantage even upon an occasional nonimmune member because rapid transmission of the disease through the community is prevented. This is true for diphtheria, but not for tetanus, which is not dependent on person-to-person spread.

- the incorporation of adjuvants in killed vaccines and toxoids
- the age of commencement
- the dosage and spacing of antigens.

## IMMUNIZATION SCHEDULES

The provision of a programme of active immunization to a community should be governed by considerations of need, efficacy, safety and ease of administration. An overriding consideration is the cost and the availability of skilled manpower and the safe delivery and supply of vaccines. Circumstances vary widely in different countries, and priorities vary. The WHO Expanded Programme on Immunization (EPI) has been adopted by most countries of the world as a minimum schedule to protect children in parts of the world where transmission rates are particularly high. Single measles is given at about 9 months rather than the combined MMR given at 12–15 months in industrialized countries. This is a balance between mean age of infection and response to the vaccine. Also, the EPI recommends hepatitis B immunization from birth (see below).

In the UK, it is generally agreed that protection of the susceptible population against diphtheria, whooping cough and tetanus, poliomyelitis, *Haemophilus influenzae* type b (with an inactivated conjugated Hib vaccine), *Neisseria meningitidis* group C (with protein conjugated to group polysaccharide as menC),

common serogroups of *Streptococcus pneumoniae*, and mumps, measles and rubella (with a combined live vaccine) merit priority in the very early years of life. BCG vaccine is offered to some high-risk populations neonatally. In the UK it is now recommended that the DTP Hib and polio vaccine are started early as a single injection given at the same time as menC, at 2 months, with further doses at 3 and 4 months (Table 70.1). This secures earlier protection against pertussis in the months when the disease is most dangerous to the young child.

## NOTES ON SOME VACCINES IN COMMON USE

### Adsorbed tetanus toxoid

The preparation in routine use in the UK is adsorbed onto an aluminium salt; it is more effective and less reactive than simple toxoid. A course of three injections given at intervals of about 4 weeks and boosters prior to, and on leaving, school, i.e. a total of five doses, should protect for life, although studies show that the elderly have low levels of protective antibody. Prevention of tetanus should be considered in relation to the management of wounds (see Ch. 22, p. 251).

### Diphtheria toxoid

The adsorbed preparation used in the UK and incorporated into the triple DTP vaccine contains

**Table 70.1**  Schedule of immunization for children in the UK*

| Age | Vaccine | Notes |
|---|---|---|
| During year 1 | Diphtheria<br>Tetanus<br>Pertussis<br>Polio<br>Hib<br>Pneumococcal (PCV)<br>Meningococcal C (MenC) | DTaP/IPV/Hib 5valent vaccine: start at 2 months; second dose at 3 months and third dose at 4 months intramuscularly<br><br>Give at same time as first and third DTaP/IPV/Hib<br><br>Give at the same times as the second and third DTaP/IPV/Hib injections |
| During year 2 | Measles/ Mumps/ Rubella<br>Hib/MenC<br>PCV | MMR vaccine: give one injection of the combined live vaccine at age 12–13 months<br>Give at same time as MMR |
| At 3–5 years | Diphtheria<br>Tetanus<br>Pertussis<br>Polio<br>MMR | Pre-school boosters |
| Girls 12–13 years | Human papillomavirus | Three doses |
| At 13–18 years | Tetanus<br>Low-dose diphtheria<br>Polio | Booster |

*May 2011.

aluminium phosphate and affords good protection which is boosted at school entry age. This preparation is not used for adults; a dilute adsorbed diphtheria vaccine preparation is used for people who are more than 10 years old and is now incorporated with tetanus toxoid for school leavers as Td. Active immunization of adults against diphtheria is not practised in the UK as a routine, unless there is a potentially high occupational risk of encountering the organism in laboratory or clinical work, or unless a person has been in contact with a case of diphtheria or is travelling to an endemic area and protection is deemed necessary. A course of erythromycin gives further protection to a close contact, and this has replaced the use of diphtheria antitoxin in contacts. The falling level of immunity to diphtheria among adults in communities that regard themselves as having good preventive medical services gives some cause for concern and calls for continuing vigilance.

## Pertussis vaccine

The vaccines in general use are either whole-cell preparations of killed *Bordetella pertussis* or acellular vaccines containing antigenic components of the organism. The protection afforded by the whole-cell vaccines is generally acknowledged to be considerable, but the acellular vaccine seems to be more effective and appears to have fewer adverse reactions so it is now included in the UK schedule. Adverse reactions that may be associated with pertussis vaccine include soreness at the site of injection, irritability and pyrexia. Reactions such as persistent screaming, shock, vomiting and convulsions have been reported, but the association with pertussis vaccine is not invariably clear.

## *Haemophilus influenzae* type b (Hib) vaccine

Invasive encapsulated strains of *H. influenzae*, almost always of serotype b, are associated with meningitis, bacteraemia, epiglottitis and other serious infections particularly affecting young children. The risks of severe morbidity and mortality are highest in children in the age range 3–18 months. Hib conjugate vaccines containing the capsular polysaccharide linked to a protein are immunogenic and reduce pharyngeal carriage of the organism. The Hib vaccines used in the UK are given combined as part of the primary immunization. Children in the age range 1–4 years who have not received Hib vaccine can be protected by a single dose of Hib vaccine. Routine immunization of older children or adults with Hib vaccine is not generally recommended unless they are immunocompromised.

## Meningococcal group C (MenC) vaccine

In 1999, following an increase in fatal cases of invasive meningococcal disease especially due to group C, the UK government was the first in the world to introduce MenC vaccine to the routine programme. Although it is now given as part of primary immunization at 3, 4 and 13 months, when the campaign started it was necessary to protect the whole population up to 18 years of age. The design of the antigen is similar to Hib in that the relatively poorly immunogenic polysaccharide is covalently linked to a protein carrier which produces a prolonged immune response in naïve infants. As with Hib there are few adverse reactions and the introduction universally to children has led to a great reduction in cases of meningitis and carriage in the nasopharynx of group C meningococci.

## Poliomyelitis vaccines

The control of poliomyelitis is one of the great success stories of active immunization, and the worldwide eradication of poliomyelitis is a goal of the WHO which has nearly been achieved. The Salk vaccine came first; this is a killed mixture of the three types of poliovirus (1, 2 and 3). A course of three injections is given at appropriate intervals and in the UK it is combined with the other infant vaccines.

The oral polio vaccine (OPV) was favoured in the UK and many other countries. It is the live-attenuated form developed by Sabin. This is a mixture of the three types, and it is given orally on three occasions, usually at the same time as the infant vaccinations in the early months. As it is a live preparation, the vaccine must be stored and held according to the manufacturer's instructions. OPV colonizes the gut and gives rise to local and humoral antibodies. The faeces contain live virus for some time, and poliomyelitis caused by a vaccine strain is a rare, but recognized, hazard which is why at the end stage of eradication of the disease it is recommended for countries to swap to the injectable form.

## Pneumococcal vaccines

The 23 valent polysaccharide vaccine has been available for over three decades but its place in universal protection of vulnerable patients has not been established. Splenectomized and immunocompromised people should be routinely immunized preferably before surgery or therapy. A conjugate vaccine, produced initially against 7 types of pneumococci is commercially available in many countries and with the inclusion of other common serotypes, has been used either for universal vaccination or to protect infants at highest risk. There is evidence from North America that the universal infant programme has produced a significant decrease in pneumococcal disease in the elderly. There is hope that these vaccines will become more widely available in resource-poor countries where the need is greatest.

## Measles, mumps and rubella (MMR) vaccine

This is a mixture of live-attenuated strains of these three viruses in freeze-dried form; it has to be stored at 2–8°C (not frozen), reconstituted according to the manufacturer's instructions and used promptly. One injection of the mixture is given between 12 and 15 months in the UK schedule, and the second dose in the fifth year, before entry to school.

The measles component may give rise to fever or malaise and sometimes a rash about a week after inoculation. The mumps component may cause some parotid swelling, seen about 3 weeks after inoculation. Very occasional cases of mumps vaccine-associated meningo-encephalitis occur; these generally occur at 3 weeks after use of the Urabe strain. It is usually benign, but there may be confusion with other more serious syndromes in this age group. The rubella component is not usually associated with reactions in this age group, though temporary malaise, mild fever and arthralgia occurring about the ninth day after vaccination have been noted in some older recipients of rubella vaccine.

It is hoped that high vaccine coverage with two doses of MMR vaccine in the UK schedule will eradicate measles, mumps and rubella in this country as it nearly has done in North America. Much depends upon public faith in the immunization programme, which has been undermined by media-led campaigns about the safety of MMR.

All seronegative women of childbearing age and seronegative professional attendants who might come into contact with pregnant women should be offered rubella vaccine after a test for immunity. Although it is not thought to be teratogenic, any woman of childbearing age who is given the vaccine should avoid pregnancy for a month.

## BCG

The attenuated strain of bovine tubercle bacillus known as bacille Calmette–Guérin (BCG) produces cross-immunity to human tuberculosis and has significantly contributed to the control of that disease and to the other important mycobacterial disease, leprosy, in many countries. An intradermal injection of the live-attenuated vaccine is given on the lateral aspect of the arm at the level of the deltoid insertion, but not higher, or on the upper lateral surface of the thigh. Instruction on the reconstitution of the freeze-dried vaccine, the dosage and the detailed technique of giving a truly intradermal injection, should be most carefully observed. With the exception of newborn children, any recipient of BCG vaccination should have been tested for hypersensitivity to tuberculin and found to be negative. Tuberculin tests include the *Mantoux test*, in which diluted tuberculin is injected intradermally, and the *Heaf test*, which is done with a multiple puncture apparatus (see Ch. 18).

## Hepatitis B vaccine

For the protection of groups of people considered to be at special risk of acquiring hepatitis B, a bioengineered vaccine is now in common use. A course of three intramuscular injections is given (not into the buttock) at intervals of 1 and 5 months; thus, it takes 6 months to complete the course, and this is of practical importance. Following needlestick injuries or known contact with the virus it is possible to give an accelerated course although efficacy may not be as good. Protective antibody responses are generally achieved in about 90% of those given the vaccine, with a range of responses from weak to strong, but there is a worrying minority of nonresponders (10–15% in those over 40 years of age). Antibody responses should be checked at least 6 weeks after completion of a course, and it may be prudent to give poor responders or nonresponders a booster dose or a repeat course. Nonresponse rates are particularly worrying among patients on maintenance haemodialysis, for whom a higher dose preparation is available. In the general population, the protection afforded to responders is thought to last for about 5 years, when a booster dose of vaccine may be given. Established policy must await further experience with hepatitis vaccines, which in many countries are being given universally as part of the routine schedule. Great success has been claimed in Asia in reducing prevalence and preventing cancer.

## Other vaccines

Various vaccines are available for the protection of special groups of people or for individuals in special circumstances (Box 70.3). The reader is referred to the appropriate chapters for more detailed consideration of such topics as:

- the prevention of tetanus in wounded patients (Ch. 22)

---

**Box 70.3** Vaccines for active immunization of people at special risk

- Anthrax
- Cholera*
- Hepatitis A*
- Hepatitis B*
- Influenza*
- Japanese B encephalitis*
- Meningococcal infection*
- Plague
- Pneumococcal infection*
- Q fever
- Rabies
- Tick-borne encephalitis
- Typhoid*
- Typhus
- Varicella-zoster*
- Yellow fever

*Some problems (see text).

---

- the indications for pneumococcal vaccine (p. 197)
- the management of rabies (Ch. 58)
- the control of Q fever (Ch. 40)
- the protection of those at special risk from chickenpox or hepatitis B (Chs. 43 & 46)
- the protection of the immunocompromised such as HIV/AIDS patients (Ch. 55)
- the prevention of cervical cancer by human papillomavirus vaccines (Ch. 45)
- the indications for rotavirus vaccine (Ch. 54).

## PROTECTING THE TRAVELLER

An intending traveller to another country should seek advice in advance about the prevailing diseases and the precautions that should be taken. Advice on immunization is unlikely to be of much help if the traveller unwisely runs the risk of drinking raw water or eating uncooked salads and vegetables in a country where sanitation is inadequate and water supplies are insecure.

In advising travellers about exotic diseases, do not forget that diseases now uncommon in countries with developed medical services may still be common in countries that lack such services. Healthcare workers need to include the risk of diphtheria and check immunity to tuberculosis, hepatitis B, measles and poliomyelitis. If the traveller is going to Central Africa or Central America, bear in mind the need for protection against yellow fever or to Mecca for the Hajj to include meningitis vaccine. Other specific vaccines may be indicated such as those against rabies, typhoid and encephalitis. Some of the special vaccines listed in Box 70.3 may also merit inclusion, especially if the traveller's activities when abroad are likely to expose him or her to the relevant diseases. Japanese B encephalitis vaccine may provoke more adverse events than the risk entailed. Travellers to rural areas in the tropics must always put insecticides and anti-malarials on the top of their list of necessities because although there is some progress in the development of an effective malaria vaccine none is available commercially. Practical, simple advice is often of more value than a typhoid or hepatitis immunization.

## UNRESOLVED PROBLEMS

No product is perfect (Box 70.4). Some vaccines are more imperfect than others, and some circumstances pose special problems. The influenza virus has shifts and drifts in its antigenic pattern, so vaccines must be frequently updated. Then decisions have to be made on the patients who merit this special protection. As these include old people and many other patients with chronic medical conditions, the logistics are quite difficult. Most temperate climate countries immunize the elderly and vulnerable before winter and this has been shown in the USA to reduce mortality and hospital admissions.

Cholera vaccines have had a chequered record, with very little evidence of real efficacy for the traveller, who is much better protected by a basic knowledge of hygiene. Results with the use of the oral vaccine are more promising and may protect against ETEC (enterotoxigenic *E. coli*) as well as cholera.

Acute purulent (bacterial) meningitis is a dramatic clinical problem. The MenC vaccine has afforded protection against group C meningitis and group A has been widely used in sub-Saharan Africa, but a group B vaccine is not routinely available at the time of writing and group B strains are more common in many areas.

Several vaccines have been developed against various herpesviruses, including herpes simplex, varicella–zoster and Epstein–Barr viruses. There have been many difficulties, but a live-attenuated varicella vaccine has been developed which is useful for susceptible staff who work in paediatric or maternity wards and is given universally to all infants in some countries.

A vaccine effective against HIV is being urgently sought in the fight against AIDS. There have been many disappointments, and there is now a glimmer of hope. Advances in molecular technology will herald a new generation of immunogens such as DNA vaccines. Delivery of products without using traditional needles and syringes is another target that is getting nearer and will save infections caused by the reuse of unsterile equipment.

## RECOMMENDED READING

Anonymous: Immunological products and vaccines. In: British National Formulary. British Medical Association and Royal Pharmaceutical Society of Great Britain, London (revised at intervals of about 6 months)

Centers for Disease Control and Prevention, Brunette GW, editor: *CDC Health Information for International Travel 2012*, Oxford and New York, 2011, Oxford University Press.

Department of Health, Welsh Office, Scottish Home and Health Department: *Health Information for Overseas Travel*, London, 2001, HMSO.

Department of Health, Welsh Office, Scottish Home and Health Department, DHSS (Northern Ireland): *Immunisation against Infectious Disease*, London, 2006, HMSO.

Kassianos GC: *Immunization: Childhood and Traveller's Health*, ed 4, Oxford, 2001, Blackwell.

Mackett M, Williamson JD: *Human Vaccines and Vaccination*, Oxford, 1995, Bios Scientific Publications.

Plotkin S, Orenstein W, Offit P, editors: *Vaccines*, ed 5, Philadelphia, 2008, WB Saunders.

World Health Organization: *International Travel and Health. Vaccination Requirements and Travel Advice*, Geneva, 2000 WHO.

### Websites

British National Formulary: http://www.bnf.org/

Centers for Disease Control and Prevention. Travelers'Health: http://www.cdc.gov/travel/

Centers for Disease Control and Prevention: Vaccines & Immunizations. http://www.nc.gov/vaccines/

Department of Health (England): Green book. Immunisation against infectious disease. http://www.dh.gov.uk/en/Publichealth/Immunisation/Greenbook/index.htm

Department of Health (England): Immunisation. http://www.dh.gov.uk/en/Publichealth/Immunisation/index.htm

Health Protection Agency: http://www.hpa.org.uk/

Health Protection Scotland: http://www.hps.scot.nhs.uk/

National Travel Health Network and Centre: http://www.nathnac.org/

NHS (Scotland): Fit For Travel. http://www.fitfortravel.nhs.uk/

World Health Organization: Immunization, Vaccines and Biologicals. http://www.who.int/immunization/

World Health Organization: International travel and health. http://www.who.int/ith/

Page numbers followed by "f" indicate figures, "t" indicate tables, and "b" indicate boxes.

Cidal (lethal) antibiotics, 48
Cidofovir, 63, 63t
　polyomavirus treatment, 463
CIE, aspergillosis diagnosis, 635
CIEBOV *see* Côte d'Ivoire ebolavirus
　(CIEBOV)
Ciliostasis, coronavirus infections, 589
CIN (cervical intra-epithelial neoplasia),
　458
Cinoxacin, 60t
Ciprofloxacin, 242
Cirrhosis, chronic hepatitis B infection,
　468
*Citrobacter*, 296–297
　bacteraemia, 297
*Citrobacter koseri*, 297
CJD *see* Creutzfeldt–Jakob disease
　(CJD)
*Cladophialophora carrionii* infection,
　627–628
Class I fusion proteins, virus entry, 84
Class II fusion proteins, virus entry, 84
Classical complement pathway,
　114–115, 115f
Classification (of micro-organisms), 10f,
　24–38, 567
　Adansonian (numerical), 25–26, 26f
　clinical practice, 27–29, 27t
　definition, 24–25
　DNA composition, 26
　DNA homology, 26
　methods, 25–27
　　*see also specific methods*
　ribosomal RNA sequencing, 26–27
　　*see also* Identification (of
　　micro-organisms);
　　Nomenclature
Class switching, antibodies, 103, 125
Clathrin-coated pits, virus entry, 84
Clavams, 58
Clavulanic acid, 58
　structure, 57f
Cleaning, infection control, 724
CLED (cystine–lactose–electrolyte-
　deficient) agar, 318
Clindamycin, 59
　*Clostridium difficile* infection, 254
Clinical correlations, antimicrobial
　drugs, 698–699
Clofazimine, 224
Clonal selection, lymphocytes, 122
*Clonorchis sinensis*, 661, 662t
　eggs, 662f
Closed (batch) broth culture growth, 41
*Clostridium*, 245–255, 363
　biochemistry, 245
　classification, 29
　as commensal, 360t
　morphology, 245
　septicaemia, 687t
　toxins, 245
*Clostridium botulinum*, 253
　infection *see* Botulism
*Clostridium difficile*, 254
　enterotoxins, 165
*Clostridium novyi*, 249–250

*Clostridium perfringens*, 246–249
　α-toxin, 247
　collagenase, 247
　enterotoxins, 165
　hyaluronidase, 247
　infection
　　colitis, 249
　　enteritis necroticans (pigbel), 249
　　food poisoning, 248–249
　　gas gangrene *see* Gas gangrene
　　peritoneal infections, 247
　　septic abortion, 247
　Nagler reaction, 245
*Clostridium septicum*, 249
*Clostridium sporogenes*, 249–250
*Clostridium tetani*, 250–253
　infection *see* Tetanus
　toxins, 250
Clumping factor, *Staphylococcus
　aureus*, 177
CMV *see* Cytomegalovirus (CMV)
COAD (chronic obstructive airway
　disease), 326
Coagulase, *Staphylococcus aureus*, 176
Co-amoxiclav, 701t
Coccidia, 646–647
　*see also individual species*
*Coccidioides*
　infection *see* Coccidioidomycosis
　morphology, 629, 629f
Coccidioidomycosis, 618, 629–630
　disseminated, 629–630
Coccus, morphology, 11, 12f
Cockroaches, 669
Cold foods, astrovirus/calicivirus
　infection, 585
Cold sores, *Herpes simplex virus*
　infection, 423
Coleoptera, 669
Colistin (polymyxin E), 61
　*Pseudomonas aeruginosa* infection,
　301
Coli surface (CS) antigens, *Escherichia
　coli*, 282
Colitis, *Clostridium perfringens*
　infection, 249
Collagenases, 167
　*Clostridium perfringens*, 247
Colonies
　bacteria identification, 30
　bacterial growth, 40, 42
　definition, 10
　morphology, *Enterobacter*, 293
Colonization, bacterial pathogenicity,
　158–160
Colonization factor antigens (CFAs),
　159
　enterotoxigenic *Escherichia coli*, 285t,
　286
　*Escherichia coli*, 282
Colony-forming units (cfu)
　bacterial death, 49
　definition, 41
Colony-stimulating factors
　parasitic infections, 148
　*see also specific types*

Colorado tick fever, 526
*Coltivirus*
　classification, 559
　infections, 525t, 560
　transmission, 560
Columbia agar, *Gardnerella vaginalis*,
　321
Combination antiretroviral therapy
　(cART), 65
　HIV infection treatment, 569, 572
Combination assays, HIV infection,
　572
Combined active-passive immunization,
　tetanus prevention, 253
Commensal micro-organisms
　innate immunity, 113
　*Neisseria*, 256–257
　*Streptococcus*, 193–194
Common cold (coryza), 680
　adenovirus infections, 415
　coronavirus infection, 590–591
　*see also* Rhinovirus infection
Community-acquired infections,
　718–719
Community-acquired methicillin-
　resistant *Staphylococcus
　aureus*, 178–179
Community infections, 708–717
　associations, 716
　historical aspects, 708
　mathematical models, 715–716
　outbreaks, 712–715
　　analysis, 713
　　control, 714–715
　　investigations, 713–714
　　nomenclature, 712
　　types, 712–713
　*Pseudomonas aeruginosa* infection,
　299–300
　spread of, 711–712
　　*see also specific infections*
Compartment for peptide loading,
　antigen-presenting cells, 124
Complement, 114–116
　activation, antibodies, 104–105
　alternative pathway, 115
　anaphylatoxins, 116
　cell lysis, 116
　classical pathway, 114–115, 115f
　defects, 132
　functions, 116
　inflammation, 119t
　lectin pathway, 113
　*Leishmania tropica*, 149
　membrane attack complex, 115–116,
　116f
　parasitic infections, 145, 147
　regulation, 115
　schistosomiasis, 145
　*T spiralis*, 145
　virus infections, 139
Complementary determining region
　(CDR), 103
Complement fixation tests (CFTs)
　adenovirus infections, 417–418
　coccidiomycosis diagnosis, 630